Scott-Brown's Otolaryngology

Sixth edition

Basic Sciences

Scott-Brown's Otolaryngology

Sixth edition

General Editor

Alan G. Kerr FRCS

Consultant Otolaryngologist, Royal Victoria Hospital, Belfast and Belfast City Hospital;
Formerly Professor of Otorhinolaryngology, The Queen's University, Belfast

Other volumes

2 **Adult Audiology** *edited by* Dafydd Stephens

3 **Otology** *edited by* John B. Booth

4 **Rhinology** *edited by* Ian S. Mackay and T. R. Bull

5 **Laryngology and Head and Neck Surgery** *edited by* John Hibbert

6 **Paediatric Otolaryngology** *edited by* David A. Adams and Michael J. Cinnamond

Basic Sciences

Editor

Michael Gleeson MD, FRCS

Professor of Otolaryngology, UMDS, Guy's Hospital; Consultant Otolaryngologist and Skull Base
Surgeon to Guy's, St Thomas' and King's College Hospitals

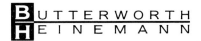

Butterworth-Heinemann
Linacre House, Jordan Hill, Oxford OX2 8DP
A division of Reed Educational and Professional Publishing Ltd

℞ A member of the Reed Elsevier plc group

OXFORD   BOSTON   JOHANNESBURG
MELBOURNE   NEW DELHI   SINGAPORE

First published 1952
Second edition 1965
Third edition 1971
Fourth edition 1979
Fifth edition 1987
Sixth edition 1997

British Library Cataloguing in Publication Data
A catalogue record for this book is
available from the British Library

Library of Congress Cataloguing in Publication Data
A catalogue record for this book is
available from the Library of Congress

ISBN 0 7506 0595 2 (Volume 1)
       0 7506 0596 0 (Volume 2)
       0 7506 0597 9 (Volume 3)
       0 7506 0598 7 (Volume 4)
       0 7506 0599 5 (Volume 5)
       0 7506 0600 2 (Volume 6)
       0 7506 1935 X (set of six volumes)
       0 7506 2368 3 (Butterworth-Heinemann International Edition, set of six volumes)

Printed and bound in Great Britain by Bath Press, Bath

Contents

Colour plates in this volume

Between pages 1/15/14 and 1/15/15

Plate 1/15/I   The arteries of the central skull base. (From Goldenberg, 1984, with permission of the author and publishers, *Laryngoscope*)

Plate 1/15/II   The veins of the central skull base. (From Goldenberg, 1984, with permission of the author and publishers, *Laryngoscope*)

Plate 1/15/III   The nerves of the central skull base. (From Goldenberg, 1984, with permission of the author and publishers, *Laryngoscope*)

Plate 1/15/IV   The structures in the jugular foramen. (From Goldenberg, 1984, with permission of the author and publishers, *Laryngoscope*)

Plate 1/15/V   The deep muscles of the central skull base. (From Goldenberg, 1984, with permission of the author and publishers, *Laryngoscope*)

Plate 1/15/VI   The superficial muscles of the central skull base. (From Goldenberg, 1984, with permission of the author and publishers, *Laryngoscope*)

Contributors to this volume

C. M. Bailey BSc, FRCS
Consultant Otolaryngologist, Royal National
Throat, Nose and Ear Hospital and The Hospitals for
Sick Children, Great Ormond Street, London

Ian Barker LLB
Solicitor, Hempsons, London

P. Beasley FRCS, DLO
Consultant Otolaryngologist, The Royal Devon and
Exeter Hospital, Exeter

J. A. S. Carruth PhD, FRCS
Consultant Otolaryngologist, Southampton
University Hospital, Southampton

Roderick Cawson MD, FRCPath
Emeritus Professor of Oral Medicine and Pathology,
UMDS, Guy's Hospital, London

Stephen J. Challacombe PhD, FDS, FRCPath
Professor of Oral Medicine, UMDS, Guy's Hospital,
London

Henry J. L. Craig MD, FRCA, FFARCSI
Consultant Anaesthetist, Royal Victoria Hospital,
Belfast

Adrian Drake-Lee PhD, FRCS
Consultant ENT Surgeon, The University Hospital,
Birmingham

M. Dyson PhD, MIBiol, CBiol
Reader in Anatomy and Cell Biology, Head of the
Tissue Repair Research Unit, UMDS, Guy's Hospital,
London

Joseph C. Farmer MD
Professor of Otolaryngology, Head and Neck
Surgery, Duke University Medical Center, Durham,
North Carolina, USA

Adrian Fourcin PhD
Professor of Experimental Phonetics, University
College, London

Cameron A. Gillespie MD
Assistant Professor of Otolaryngology, Head and
Neck Surgery, Duke University Medical Center,
Durham, North Carolina, USA

Michael Gleeson MD, FRCS
Professor of Otolaryngology, UMDS, Guy's Hospital;
Consultant Otolaryngologist and Skull Base Surgeon
to Guy's, St Thomas' and King's College Hospitals

J. J. Grote MD
Professor of Otolaryngology, University of Leiden,
The Netherlands

Maurice Hawthorne FRCS
Consultant Otolaryngologist, North Riding
Infirmary, Middlesbrough

Mark Huckvale PhD
Lecturer in Experimental Phonetics, University
College, London

Alan Johnson FRCS
Consultant Otolaryngologist, The University
Hospital, Birmingham

Charles G. Kelly PhD
Senior Lecturer in Immunology, UMDS, Guy's
Hospital, London

Geoffrey A. Land PhD, FAAM, CLD
Director of Clinical Microbiology, Methodist Medical
Center, Dallas, Texas; Professor of Microbiology,
Texas Christian University, Fort Worth, Texas, USA

Gavin Lavery MD, FFARCSI
Consultant in Anaesthesia/Intensive Care Medicine,
Royal Hospitals Trust, Belfast

V. J. Lund MS, FRCS
Professor of Rhinology, Royal National Throat, Nose
and Ear Hospital, London

Linda M. Luxon BSc, FRCP
Professor of Audiological Medicine, The Institute of
Laryngology and Otology and the National Hospital
for Neurology and Neurosurgery, London

Alexander W. McCracken MD,FRCPath, FACP, DCP,
DTM&H
Chairman of the Department of Pathology,
Methodist Medical Center, Dallas, Texas; Professor of
Pathology, University of Texas; Consultant
Pathologist, Baylor University Medical Center,
Dallas, Texas, USA

Julian McGlashan FRCS
Senior Lecturer and Consultant Otolaryngologist,
Queen's Medical Centre, University of Nottingham

Wilson C. Mertens MD
Associate Professor of Medicine, Wayne State
University School of Medicine, Michigan, USA

Brian C. J. Moore MA, PhD
Reader in Auditory Perception, University of
Cambridge

John Philip Patten BSc, FRCP
Consultant Neurologist, King Edward VII Hospital,
Midhurst, West Sussex

Adrian Pearce FFARCS
Consultant Anaesthetist, Guy's Hospital, London

P. D. Phelps MD, FRCS, FFR, FRCR, DMRD
Consultant Radiologist, Royal National Throat, Nose
and Ear Hospital, London

James O. Pickles MA, MSc, PhD, ScD
Head of Hearing Unit, Vision, Touch and Hearing
Research Centre, University of Queensland,
Brisbane, Australia

Neil Pride MD, FRCP
Professor of Respiratory Medicine, Royal
Postgraduate Medical School, Hammersmith
Hospital, London

William J. Primrose FRCSI
Consultant Otolaryngologist, Royal Victoria
Hospital, Belfast

David W. Proops BDS, MB, ChB, FRCS
Consultant Otolaryngologist, The University
Hospital, Birmingham

Lee S. Rayfield BSc, PhD
Assistant Curate in the Parish of Woodford, Wells,
Essex; Formerly Lecturer in Immunology, UMDS,
Guy's Hospital, London

Peter Savundra MA, MSc, MRCP, DCH
Senior Registrar, The National Hospital for
Neurology and Neurosurgery, London

Margaret F. Spittle FRCR, DMRT
Consultant Clinical Oncologist, The Middlesex
Hospital, London

J. Watkinson MS, FRCS, DLO
Consultant Otolaryngologist, Head and Neck
Surgeon, The University Hospital, Birmingham

Neil Weir MB BS, FRCS
Consultant Otolaryngologist, Royal Surrey County
Hospital, Guildford; Honorary Consultant Neuro-
otologist, St George's Hospital, London

Anthony Wright MA, DM, FRCS, TechRMS, LLM
Professor of Otorhinolaryngology and Head of
Department, Institute of Laryngology and Otology,
London

S. R. Young PhD
Senior Research Fellow, Tissue Repair Research
Unit, Division of Anatomy and Cell Biology, UMDS,
Guy's Hospital, London

Introduction

When I started work on this Sixth Edition I did so in the belief that my experience with the Fifth Edition would make it straightforward. I was wrong. The production of the Fifth Edition was hectic and the available time short. The contributors and volume editors were very productive and in under two and a half years we produced what we, and happily most reviewers, considered to be a worthwhile academic work. On this occasion, with a similar team, we allowed ourselves more time and yet have struggled to produce in four years. One is tempted to blame the health service reforms but that would be unfair. They may have contributed but the problems were certainly much wider than these.

The volume editors, already fully committed clinically, have again been outstanding both in their work and in their understanding of the difficulties we have encountered. Once again there was an excellent social spirit among the editors. They have been very tolerant of the innumerable telephone calls and it has always been a pleasure to work with them. The contributors have also been consistently pleasant to deal with, even those who kept us waiting.

There have been technical problems in the production of this work and I want to pay tribute to the patience of all those who suffered under these, not least the publishing staff at Butterworth-Heinemann. One of the solutions to the problems has been the use of a system of pagination that I consider to be ugly and inefficient for the user and I wish to apologize in advance for this. Unfortunately anything else would have resulted in undue delay in the publication date.

Medicine is a conservative profession and many of us dislike change. Some will feel that we have moved forward in that most Latin plurals have been replaced by English, for example we now have polyps rather than polypi. We have also buried acoustic neuromata, with an appropriate headstone, and now talk about vestibular schwannomas. It has taken about two decades for this to become established in otological circles and may take even longer again, to gain everyday usage in the world of general medicine.

I am pleased with what has been produced. Some chapters have altered very little because there have been few advances in those subjects and we have resisted the temptation of change for change's sake. There have been big strides forward in other areas and these have been reflected in the appropriate chapters.

Despite, and because of, the problems in the production of these volumes, the staff at Butterworth-Heinemann have worked hard and have always been pleasant to deal with. I wish to acknowledge the co-operation from Geoff Smaldon, Deena Burgess, Anne Powell, Mary Seager and Chris Jarvis.

It would be impossible to name all those others who have helped, especially my colleagues in Belfast, but I want to pay tribute to the forbearance of my wife Paddy who graciously accepted the long hours that were needed for this work.

As I stated in my introduction to the Fifth Edition, I was very impressed by the goodwill and generosity of spirit among my Otolaryngological colleagues and am pleased that there has been no evidence of any diminution of this during the nine years between the editions. I remain pleased and proud to be a British Otolaryngologist and to have been entrusted with the production of this latest edition of our standard textbook.

Alan G. Kerr

Preface

The practice of Otolaryngology continues to change and expand as the current generation of surgeons break new ground and claim for our specialty aspects of surgery previously reserved for others. Those that we train are now expected to gain experience in subjects as diverse as oncology, immunology, audiological medicine, facial plastics, voice and skull base surgery. It is our expectation that in time they will develop these sub-specialties still further to the benefit of subsequent generations of patients and surgeons. It would be unwise to acquire clinical skills without a prior, thorough, grounding in the basic sciences particularly as they relate to otolaryngology. New technologies dictate that our interpretation of these basic sciences is constantly revised and updated. It is hoped that the information contained in this volume fulfils this need.

It was pleasing that so many of the authors who contributed to the Fifth edition of *Scott-Brown's Otolaryngology* wished to do so again and have made substantial revisions to their chapters. Some, however, have retired and been replaced by new authors, each a recognized authority in their chosen subject. A few of our previous contributors have selected co-authors to help them add new data to their texts. In addition, two completely new chapters have been added which reflect current change in clinical practice. The first, 'Principles and use of nuclear medicine' has been contributed by John Watkinson and provides all necessary information for the clinician or trainee to understand this form of imaging and its application in the diagnosis of numerous conditions and the treatment of thyroid disease in particular. The second, 'Medical negligence in otolaryngology' written by Maurice Hawthorne and Ian Barker, should be compulsory reading for all. Its position at the end of this volume bears no relationship to its importance; better to consider it as preceding all the clinical chapters in subsequent volumes. The end result is that the overall shape of this new edition has changed a little while the content has moved on considerably.

I would like to thank all my contributing authors for their industry and enthusiasm over the last few years while this work has been compiled. Writing chapters is hard enough but, almost without exception, all of those involved have had additional service burdens thrust upon them during this period which must have impacted significantly on their personal timetables. Countless otolaryngologists will be grateful to them for their dedication. My thanks go also to my registrars, Paul Pracy and Rory Walsh, for assisting me in proofreading, detecting my mistakes and correcting them politely.

There are five other very important people to acknowledge. First, my wife, Ann, and our children, Andrew, Clare and Mark for hours of peace and quiet to concentrate and work unhindered. Finally, to Alan Kerr my sincere thanks for giving me the opportunity to edit this work and, in doing so, join a very distinguished group of otolaryngologists who have undertaken this task in the past. There would be no *Scott-Brown* without Alan. His enthusiasm, perseverance, patience and inexhaustible energy are truly legendary and a model for all. Through him and *Scott-Brown*, my education has been furthered and I hope that those who refer to, or read, this text find all the information they require.

Michael Gleeson

Errata

Page 1/1/49

Due to a printing error Figure 1.52 has been wrongly attributed. This illustration should be attributed to Pickles (1988) *An Introduction to the Physiology of Hearing*, 2nd edition, p.236, Academic Press.

Pages 1/7/25 and 1/7/26

The captions for figures 7.6, 7.7 and 7.8 have been incorrectly positioned.
The caption below Figure 7.6 should appear below Figure 7.7; the caption below Figure 7.7 should appear below Figure 7.8; and the caption below Figure 7.8 should appear below Figure 7.6.

Volume index

1

Anatomy and ultrastructure of the human ear

Anthony Wright

Development of the human ear

In accordance with long-standing convention, the adult ear is described here in terms of its three portions, namely the outer, the middle and the inner ears. The inner ear, comprising the bony and membranous labyrinth with its central connections, arises from a set of structures quite distinct from those which give rise to the outer and middle ears. The development of the inner ear, which is the first organ of the special senses to become fully formed in man, is considered first, following a short, general description of the growth of the nervous system.

Prenatal development is divided into a number of separate periods. The first period extends from the time of implantation of the developing blastocyst into the uterine wall until an intraembryonic circulation has started to develop. During this short period of about 21 days, the three layers of ectoderm, mesoderm and endoderm develop to form a flat, elongated plate containing the notochord. This rod-like structure is derived from the ectodermal layer and extends along the length of the embryonic disc from the buccopharyngeal membrane to the cloacal membrane, where ectoderm and endoderm are in direct contact (Figure 1.1). The second brief period of about 35 days, i.e. until the end of the eighth week, is termed the embryonic period. During this time there is rapid growth and cellular differentiation, so that by the fifty-sixth day all the major systems and organs are formed and the embryo has an external shape that is recognizably human. The remaining 7 months of gestation form the fetal period, during which there is rapid growth characterized by changes of shape, and by alterations in the position of one structure to another, rather than by the differentiation of new cell types.

During the embryonic period, the thickened mesoderm on each side of the notochord separates into paired cubical blocks called somites. The first occipital somite lies just behind the head end of the notochord, and no other somites develop further forward from this for the reason that here the mesoderm gives rise to, among other structures, the branchial (or pharyngeal) arches. Forty-one to 43 more pairs of somites develop in a tailward direction during the first 9 days of the embryonic period.

The ectoderm not only assumes the shape of the underlying, developing mass of mesoderm but also thickens in the region of the notochord to form the midline neural plate. On each side of this plate, a longitudinal band of ectoderm, called the neural crest,

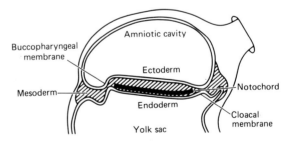

Figure 1.1 Highly diagrammatic representation of a longitudinal section of the developing embryonic disc. The structure never looks like this at any one time since development is progressing at different rates. Nevertheless, mesoderm lies between ectoderm and endoderm except at the buccopharyngeal and cloacal membranes where the two layers are in contact. The notochord, a derivative of the ectodermal layer, lies within the mass of mesoderm. A connecting stalk attaches the developing disc with its amniotic cavity and yolk sac to the uterine wall, and these structures lie within the extra-embryonic coelom at this stage of development

develops. The neural plate subsequently sinks in to form the neural groove, the walls of which eventually close over to produce the neural tube surrounding the neural canal (Figure 1.2). While the neural groove is closing, the neural crest cells sink in from the surface to lie alongside the completed neural tube. At the head end, the neural tube undergoes rapid enlargement and dilatation to form the hindbrain, the midbrain and the forebrain. These last two extend forward past the notochord and buccopharyngeal membrane, which by now has broken down to allow the formation of the buccal cavity.

The neural crest cells, lying alongside the developing brain and spinal cord, develop into a chain of cell clusters which, at the head end of the embryo, form three groups: trigeminal; facial and auditory; and glossopharyngeal and vagal. These clusters contain uni- or bipolar nerve cells and form the cranial sensory nerve ganglia. They link the peripheral sensory receptors with the afferent nuclei in the hindbrain. Motor nerve fibres arise directly from the cell bodies in the three efferent columns in the hindbrain and pass directly to striated muscles or, by way of a synapse, to non-striated muscle and glandular tissue.

The membranous labyrinth

When the embryo has reached the seventh somite stage (about 22 days), a thickening of the ectoderm forms just in front of the first occipital somite on each side of the still open neural groove. This thickening is the otic placode. The mesoderm surrounding this region proliferates and elevates the ectoderm around the placode, which subsequently sinks below the surface to become the otic pit. The ectoderm of the pit undergoes rapid growth, the mouth of the pit narrows and eventually closes, so that by the thirtieth somite (30 days) stage, an enlarging otocyst separated from the surface has been formed and lies anterior and medial to the combined facial and auditory cluster of neural crest cells. The geniculate ganglion migrates from this cluster leaving the auditory (vestibulocochlear) ganglion in close proximity to the otocyst (Figure 1.3).

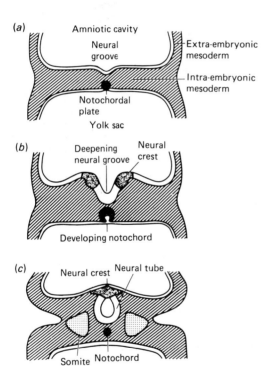

Figure 1.2 Transverse section of the developing embryonic disc at various stages of development. In the early presomite stage (*a*) a midline neural groove is present above the notochordal plate which is fused with the endodermal layer. The neural groove deepens (*b*) and specialized neural crest cells develop on the lips of the groove. The notochord separates from the endodermal layer. By the somite stage (*c*) the neural tube has formed and the neural crest cells are about to migrate to form cell clusters which, at the head end of the embryo, become the cranial sensory nerve ganglia. Cells from the neural crest also form the posterior root ganglion of the spinal cord and the cells of the sympathetic ganglia

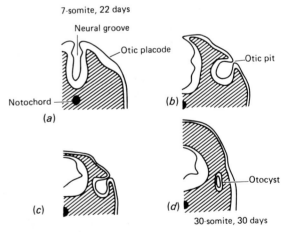

Figure 1.3 Diagram to represent the development of the otocyst from the otic placode which in turn is derived from the ectoderm cranial to the first occipital somite. During the 7 days of its development the neural groove has also become converted into the future brain stem

Within 1 or 2 days, the otocyst has lengthened and an apparent infolding of the wall marks off a medial compartment, the endolymphatic duct, from a more lateral compartment, the utriculosaccular chamber. This period is a time of rapid change, and complex alterations in the shape of different parts of the otocyst take place synchronously. The walls of the chamber grow inwards so that a number of constrictions and folds appear, separating the utricle from the saccule. The major change is an ingrowth of the lateral wall assisted by an enlargement of the initial fold (now called the utricular fold) that together separate the utricular chamber from the endolymphatic duct, and thus form the utricular duct. A lesser change is a separate ingrowth from the medial wall that divides the saccular chamber from the endolymphatic duct and thereby forms the saccular duct (Figure 1.4).

Meanwhile, the endolymphatic system is elongating in a medial direction towards the hindbrain; a proximal dilatation, the endolymphatic sinus, a middle narrow endolymphatic duct and a widened distal endolymphatic sac are formed.

At the same time, other changes are developing in the utricular chamber. At 35 days, three flattened hollow pouches push out approximately at right angles to each other, to form superior, posterior and lateral ridges. At the centre of each curved ridge, the opposing epithelial walls meet, fuse and break down to be replaced by the surrounding mesoderm. In this way, the superior ridge, at about 6 weeks, is transformed into the superior semicircular duct, with the transformation of the other two, the posterior before the lateral, taking place soon afterwards.

While the semicircular ducts are developing, and before the complete formation of the utricular and saccular duct has taken place, the saccule is putting out a single medially directed pouch which is the beginning of the cochlear duct. This grows medially and starts to coil, with the result that at the beginning of fetal life one coil is present, and by 25 weeks the adult form of two-and-one-half coils has been achieved. As the cochlear duct develops, it becomes isolated from the saccule by a constriction called the ductus reuniens.

During this period of complex growth there are other changes within the otocyst. Thickened epithelial areas develop in certain portions of its walls in relationship to the ingrowth of nerve fibres from the bipolar cells of the vestibulocochlear ganglion. The specialized areas of neuroepithelium are the maculae, the cristae and the organ of Corti.

The maculae

The maculae develop from the epithelium that overlies the areas where nerves enter the walls of the saccule and utricle. Two cell types differentiate: the sensory cells, with a single kinocilium and many stereocilia, projecting into the cavity of the otocyst; and the supporting cells. These latter cells appear to be responsible for the formation of the otoconia, although the early stages are not well understood. It seems likely that very small calcium-containing primitive otoconia are produced by the supporting cells and it is these that provide the nucleus for the multilayered deposition of the calcite form of calcium carbonate to produce mature otoconia with their characteristic shape (see section on adult anatomy) (Figure 1.5). The supporting cells also produce a gelatinous matrix that subsequently forms the gelatinous layer of the definitive otoconial membrane. In the very early stages of otoconial formation in man this matrix is not present. However, by 14–16 weeks, the individual parts of the maculae have assumed an adult form with the sensory and supporting cells being overlaid by the mature otoconial membrane (Lim, 1984).

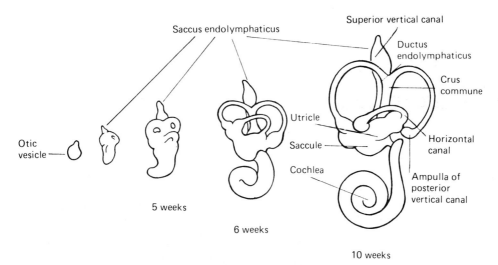

Figure 1.4 Development of the membranous labyrinth from the otocyst. This rapid and complex change occurs over a 6-week period

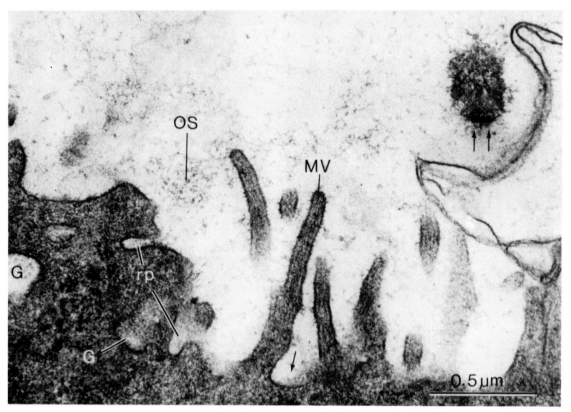

Figure 1.5 A small primitive otoconial crystal with recognizable shape (double arrows) is being formed near the long microvilli (MV) of the supporting cells of 16.5-day mouse embryo. The specific granules that go to form the core of the crystal seem to come from pinocytic vesicles (G) that eventually fuse with the cytoplasmic membrane to release granules (single arrow). Various organic substances (OS) which possibly form the gelatinous layer of the otoconial membrane seem to be secreted by reverse pinocytosis from the supporting cells. (Photograph courtesy of David Lim)

The cristae of the semicircular ducts

At one end of each semicircular duct, a portion of the epithelial lining proliferates and heaps up to form the ridge-like cristae. Differentiation into sensory and supporting cells continues and this takes place on what will eventually become the convex side of the definitive semicircular canal. The membranous duct in this region enlarges to form the ampulla and, subsequently, a fibrogelatinous structure – the cupula – develops within the lumen. It probably originates from the supporting cells and is present in the 24-week-old fetus. Both the cupula and the otoconial membrane (as well as the tectorial membrane) are extremely sensitive to distortion and shrinkage during routine histological preparation; therefore, the shape seen in such preparations does not represent that found in life. Especial care has to be taken to preserve the real shape and form of these structures.

As the ampulla enlarges, the crista grows with it, so that by the time it has reached its adult size, at about 23 weeks, it has become a curved ridge covering the floor and extending part way up the side walls of the ampulla (Figure 1.6).

The organ of Corti

The coils of the cochlear duct are initially circular in cross-section but, with the growth of the surrounding mesoderm, they are converted into a triangular form with a floor and an outer wall at right angles to each other, and a sloping roof completing the triangle. The epithelium lining this duct is originally stratified; however, in the roof, it undergoes regression through columnar, then cuboidal stages changing finally into a simple squamous epithelium that remains as the lining of the future Reissner's membrane. The epithelium of the outer wall develops into the stria vascularis, a three-layered structure which rests on, and is supplied by, a highly vascular strip developed in the surrounding mesoderm. The epithelium of the floor undergoes a series of spectacular changes to form the

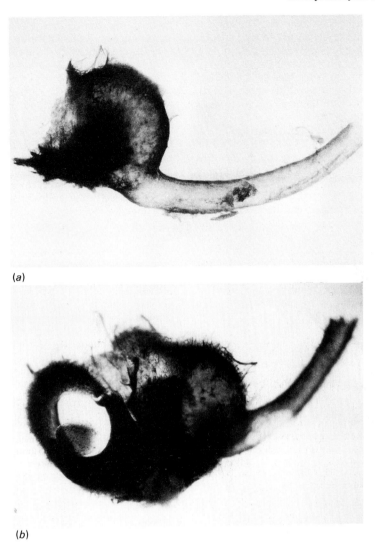

(a)

(b)

Figure 1.6 (a) Light micrograph of part of an osmium-stained semicircular duct and attached ampulla. This specimen comes from a young adult human. Within the ampulla the darkened crista can be seen. (b) View of the ampullae of the lateral and superior semicircular ducts. The crista is now seen more clearly as a saddle-shaped ridge in the open ampulla. Lying in the ampulla is the wedge-shaped cupula. With this method of preparation the cupula has shrunken considerably, but *in vivo* it extends to reach the walls of the ampulla

highly ordered organ of Corti. The structure of this is described in detail in the section on adult anatomy. During development, however, the stratified epithelium, under the influence of nerve terminals arriving from the cochlear ganglion, heaps up to form a ridge-like structure. This starts at about 11 weeks and the process is more rapid in the basal than the apical regions.

The future tectorial membrane, which is an ill-defined gelatinous membrane, develops and extends over the surface of the neuroepithelium. By 16 weeks, the ridge in the basal coil is more pronounced, so

that an inner and outer sulcus are apparent. The inner sulcus is roofed by the tectorial membrane while in the outer sulcus the epithelial cells regress to a flattened low cuboidal form. Within the organ of Corti, sensory and supporting cells are developing. A space – the tunnel of Corti – appears within this mass of cells and separates the inner from the outer sensory cells. A cluster of stereocilia and a more laterally placed single kinocilium develop from the surface of each sensory cell. The kinocilium subsequently degenerates and is not present in man at birth leaving clusters of stereocilia which has resulted in the sensory cells being called hair cells. The supporting cells become highly differentiated. Inner and outer pillar cells, on each side of the tunnel of Corti, give mechanical rigidity to the structure. Deiters' cells surround the base of the outer hair cells and send their processes up to the surface of the organ of Corti, which then expand to form the phalangeal processes that separate the upper surface of the outer hair cells. Hensen's and Claudius' cells form the lateral bulk of the organ of Corti, and it is to these that the tectorial membrane is attached laterally. The cells around the outer hair cells separate, so that definite spaces – the spaces of Nuel – develop and communicate with the tunnel of Corti.

As mentioned earlier, differentiation proceeds in a basal to apical direction, so that at any one time most stages of development can be seen in different parts of the cochlea as the duct is elongating. As the cochlear duct grows and coils, the cochlear ganglion also changes shape, the new form becoming known as the spiral ganglion. By 25 weeks, the organ of Corti and the spiral ganglion are complete and resemble those in the adult.

The bony labyrinth

Mesoderm surrounds the membranous labyrinth, and it is this which undergoes a series of changes that result in the formation of both the bony otic capsule and the perilymphatic spaces of the inner ear. The relatively unspecialized mesoderm of the presomite embryo becomes known as the mesenchyme in subsequent embryonic development as it undergoes differentiation into more specialized tissue. The mesenchyme surrounding the derivatives of the otocyst is initially quite dense and becomes chondrified to form the otic capsule. As the membranous labyrinth increases in size, the adjacent cartilage de-differentiates to form loose periotic tissue. This subsequently regresses to form fluid-filled spaces adjacent to most of the membranous structures. These are the perilymphatic spaces and they arise first in the region destined to become the vestibule. Subsequently, spaces develop around the cochlear duct, the scala tympani preceding the scala vestibuli. While this latter space is developing, other spaces form around the semicircular ducts so that the completed canals are formed. The perilymphatic space does not develop where vestibular and cochlear nerve fibres enter the sensory cell regions, and so these remain in close proximity to the cartilaginous otic capsule. Elsewhere the developing perilymphatic spaces finally become continuous with the result that a tortuous but uninterrupted perilymph-filled space is formed.

The ossification of the remaining cartilaginous otic capsule takes place from up to 14 centres and begins in the fifteenth or sixteenth week. The last centre to begin ossification does so at 21 weeks, an indication that the otic capsule has, by this time, attained its maximum size. Each ossification centre develops as a three-layered structure comprising an inner periosteal layer, a central layer where mixed ossification of cartilage takes place and an outer periosteal layer. In the central layer, the cartilage cells enlarge, the matrix becomes calcified and the cells then shrink, atrophy and disappear leaving lacunae. Vascular invasion of the calcified cartilage proceeds and osteogenic buds enter the lacunae and deposit an osseous lamina on the walls of the space. This is endochondral bone and its formation results in the development of a series of islands of bone enclosed in cartilage. Other osteoblasts derived from the vascular buds lay down endochondral bone on the surface of the remaining cartilage so that, with progressive growth, the vascular spaces are obliterated and the middle layer of the otic capsule will consist of one type of bone (intrachondral) embedded in another (endochondral), with remnants of calcified cartilage. Unlike all other cartilage-derived bones, there is no remodelling, and the fetal architecture is maintained throughout life. The inner periosteal layer ossifies but remains thin, while the outer layer becomes greatly thickened by the laying down of interconnected plates of bone that form a dense hard petrous structure.

The 14 separate ossification centres fuse to form a single bony box (Figure 1.7), without the presence of a single suture line. (For a complete review, see Anson and Donaldson, 1981.) The interior of the bony labyrinth 'communicates' with the outside through seven or eight channels, and the facial nerve passing across and around it in a sulcus eventually becomes enclosed by a bony sheath on the lateral, tympanic aspect (Table 1.1).

The blood supply of the developing otic capsule is derived mainly from the arteries of the tympanic plexus, which are supplied in turn predominantly by the stylomastoid arteries and its branches. The devel-

Table 1.1 Development of communication channels passing through the bony labyrinth

Internal auditory meatus	Persisting channel in cartilage model around VII and VIII nerves
Subarcuate fossa	Persisting vascular channel
Vestibular aqueduct	Fifth and sixth ossification centres fuse around the endolymphatic duct
Cochlear aqueduct	Resorption of precartilage
Fossula ante fenestram	Resorption of precartilage
Fossula post fenestram (inconstant)	Resorption of cartilage
Oval window	Otic capsule becomes footplate of stapes and annular ligament
Round window	Persisting cartilage becomes round window niche and membrane

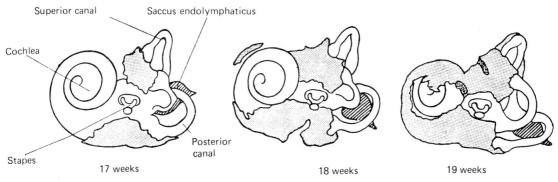

Figure 1.7 Diagram illustrating the progression of ossification of the cartilaginous labyrinth from 14 separate centres, not all of which are shown here. (Derived from Anson and Donaldson, 1981)

oping membranous labyrinth, however, is supplied almost entirely by branches of the internal auditory artery, and this pattern persists throughout life.

The outer and middle ears

The mesenchyme surrounding the primitive pharynx differentiates into paired maxillary and mandibular processes above and below the level of the buccopharyngeal membrane. Shortly after the appearance of these processes, the membrane breaks down and the buccopharyngeal cavity is formed. Behind the level of the membrane, the mesenchyme which surrounds the pharyngeal tube separates on each side into five or six bars running around the pharynx; these are the pharyngeal (branchial) arches. In each arch, a bar of cartilage, together with its associated muscles, differentiates from the mesenchyme. The muscle is supplied by a nerve (one of the special visceral efferents) and the endoderm which covers the arch internally is supplied not only by the nerve of the arch (post-trematic) but also by a branch from the arch behind (pre-trematic). Each arch also has an artery associated with it, at least for a short while during embryonic development. Between successive arches, the endoderm of the pharynx forms pouches which come into contact with the covering ectoderm which has sunk between the arches as the pharyngeal grooves (or clefts). In land-living vertebrates, a thin layer of mesoderm intervenes between the pouch and the cleft which does not break down, so that true gill clefts are never formed.

The first and second arches and their associated structures give rise to the middle and outer ears, Table 1.2 outlines the details of the derivatives of these arches.

The auricle

The development of the auricle begins with the appearance of six hillocks around the first pharyngeal groove between the first and second arches. Three hillocks develop on each side of the groove; but as growth proceeds they tend to become obscured, and of those of the first (mandibular) arch, only that which later forms the tragus can be obviously identified throughout the process (Figure 1.8). It seems that the bulk of the auricle is derived from the mesenchyme of the second (hyoid) arch, which

Table 1.2 Derivatives of the first and second branchial arches

	Cartilage	Post-trematic nerve	Pre-trematic nerve	Artery
First arch derivatives	Meckel's Malleus Incus 'Mandible' Anterior malleolar ligament Sphenomandibular ligament	Mandibular V	Chorda tympani VII	
Second arch derivatives	Reichert's Stapes superstructure Styloid process Lesser cornu of hyoid Stylohyoid ligament	Facial VII	Tympanic branch IX	Stapedial

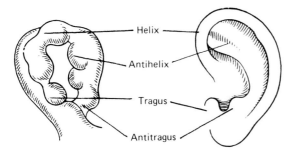

Figure 1.8 Early stages in the development of the auricle. Six cartilaginous hillocks are visible around the first pharyngeal groove. During subsequent development these become the cartilage of the auricle although the bulk of the auricle appears to be derived from the cartilage of the second arch

extends around the top of the groove to form a flattened extension that subsequently becomes the helix (Streeter, 1922). The cartilage of the auricle extends inwards partially to surround the future external meatus. The rudimentary pinna has formed by 60 days and in the fourth month the convolutions have attained their adult form, although further generalized enlargement continues during the remaining months of gestation and also in the postnatal period.

The external canal

The external canal develops from the upper portion of the first pharyngeal groove. It extends inwards as a funnel-shaped tube and the meatus deepens by proliferation of its ectoderm which forms an epithelial plug. The ectoderm at the depths of this plug is in contact with the endoderm of the first pharyngeal pouch for a short while before the mesenchyme intervenes to become the middle fibrous layer of the future tympanic membrane.

The subsequent development of the stratified squamous epithelium of the tympanic membrane and deep external canal is a complex process and so is depicted in diagrammatic form (Figure 1.9). Because the evolution of this part is in three dimensions, both horizontal and vertical diagrams are given for each stage. In brief, a solid anterior bud of epithelial cells is derived from the fundus epithelium, extends vertically to form the drum face, and then opens up as a slit from the primary canal lumen to produce both pars tensa and deep external canal epithelium.

Figure 1.9a represents the primary external canal in the late embryo. Anterior budding of a solid mass of epithelium – the meatal plate – from the primary

canal is the first stage in the development of the tympanic membrane. At this early stage and thereafter, four distinct zones of stratified squamous epithelium may be recognized. Zone 1 is the epithelium at the fundus of the primary external canal. Zone 2 is the medial and zone 3 the lateral epithelium of the meatal plate. Zone 4 is the epithelium of the side walls of the primary external canal which will develop into the adnexal-bearing skin of the cartilaginous external canal. Zone 2 epithelium is always thin and flat. In Figure 1.9a the primary external canal is shown as 'open', i.e. not filled in by superficial epidermal squames. This is the case in the earliest stage of meatal plate development, but not later when it is 'closed' by a solid mass of stratified squamous epithelium until the eighteenth week of development.

The two vertical sections in Figure 1.9a indicate stages in the development of the meatal plate and fundus of the primary external canal. The small complete ring, in the posterior superior region of the developing eardrum, represents the zone 1 epithelium of the fundus of the primary canal from which the meatal plate, here shown as enlarging segments of a circle, emanates. The numbers within the segments denote the zones of stratified squamous epithelium lining the outside of the tympanic membrane and deep external canal precursor in that region. Both zones 2 and 3 are present on the external surface of the developing tympanic membrane. Zone 1 forms a downwardly projecting tongue of epithelium in the course of its early development.

The next stage (Figure 1.9b), which is one of opening up and clearing of the deep canal and meatal plate, commences at 18 weeks' gestation at the same time as cornification of the stratified squamous epithelium of the rest of the skin surface. Zones 2 and 3 are in continuity along the rim of the tympanic membrane (except in the region of the pars flaccida), although now separated by a thin gap elsewhere. The circular extent of the now fully formed drum face is shown in the lower diagram. The solid dark areas in this figure external to the tympanic membrane (and in Figures 1.9c and 1.9d) indicate the anterior and posterior limbs of the bony tympanic ring which have now formed.

The next stage (Figure 1.9c) involves widening of the whole canal, a process which is prominent in later fetal life. During this process, zone 1 is now clearly the covering of the pars flaccida in the en face view. The tongue of its epithelium, running parallel with the handle of the malleus, is prominent. The drum face is covered only by zones 1 and 2, zone 3 now forming most of the deep external canal.

In early childhood (Figure 1.9d), flattening of the external canal epithelium proceeds concomitantly with formation of the mastoid bone, mastoid air cells, and tympanic part of the temporal bone (solid dark

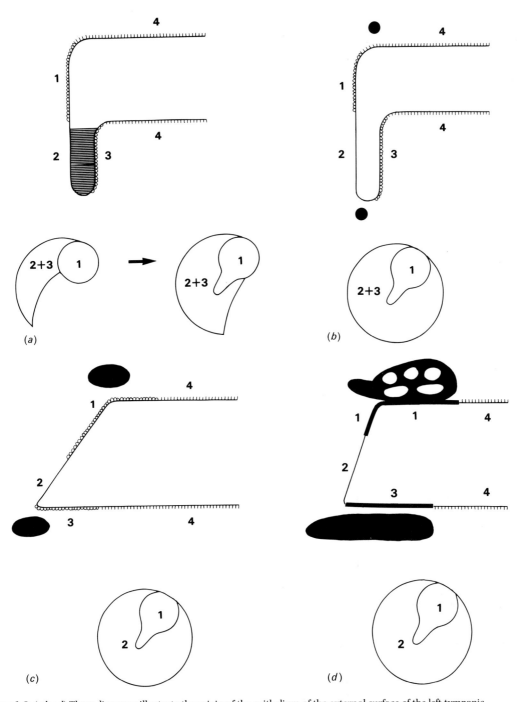

Figure 1.9 (*a,b,c,d*) These diagrams illustrate the origin of the epithelium of the external surface of the left tympanic membrane and deep external canal. They show the meatal plate, the opening up of that plate in the process of clearing the canal and the separation of the medial and lateral epithelia as the deep canal widens. In each of the four illustrations a 'horizontal' section is shown at the top and a corresponding 'vertical' section is shown below. In each horizontal section, posterior is at the top, anterior towards the bottom, medial to the left and lateral to the right; this orientation is approximate. Each vertical section shows the tympanic membrane as it would be seen if it could be viewed along a patent ear canal. The numbers indicate the different epithelial zones that are described in the text which should be consulted for an explanation of the changes. (Courtesy of Professor Leslie Michaels)

areas outside canal) and also widening of the external canal. The stratified squamous epithelium in zones 1 and 3 is still thicker than the flattened epithelium in zone 2, a state of affairs which persists throughout life. In this mature ear, the drum face vertical view shows zone 1 covering the pars flaccida and the tongue of epithelium emanating downward from it, parallel with the handle of the malleus. The pars tensa is covered by zone 2 (see Michaels and Soucek, 1989).

Within the mesenchyme around the external meatus, four small centres of ossification arise in the ninth week. These are destined to fuse and to become the tympanic ring (not an accurate name as it is never a complete ring) and subsequently the tympanic bone. The ring develops a groove on its inner concave face, and this becomes the tympanic sulcus. The bony ring grows in diameter and extends laterally and inferiorly throughout fetal life to occupy the space between the mandibular fossa and the anterior surface of the developing mastoid bone, where it provides a sheath for the developing styloid process. By later fetal life, the tympanic plate is widely open and the definitive bony canal unformed. After birth, anterior and posterior bony prominences, which have developed on the inner aspect of the ring, grow inwards and eventually fuse to form the floor of the canal. As the tips of the processes fuse, a space surrounded by bone is created; this is the foramen of Huschke which is usually obliterated by adolescence. The completed tympanic bone, therefore, makes contact with the mastoid process and part of the squamous bone posteriorly, and with another portion of the squamous and part of the petrous bone anteriorly. The petrotympanic fissure between the more medial aspect of the tympanic bone and the mandibular fossa allows the passage of the chorda tympani nerve, the pre-trematic nerve of the first arch. The tympanic ring is deficient superiorly in the external meatus and this is the tympanic incisura.

The middle ear

The cavity and lining of the middle ear cleft and eustachian tube arise from the expanding first pharyngeal pouch with probably some contribution at the medial end from the second. By the 4-week stage, the distal end lies against the ectoderm of the first pharyngeal groove and expands to form a flattened sac, the precursor of the tympanic cavity. Mesenchyme grows between the ectoderm and the endoderm to form the third layer of the future tympanic membrane. The slit-like space within the sac expands and, as it reaches the developing ossicles and otic capsule, the epithelium lining the sac is draped over the lateral (tympanic) portion of the labyrinth, the bodies of the ossicles, and their developing ligaments and muscular tendons, so that a complex and variable network of mucosal folds is formed. 'Pneumatiza-

tion' of the meso- and hypotympanum is complete at 8 months, while the epitympanum and mastoid antrum have developed by birth. The spaces are not filled with air but with amniotic fluid, and this is replaced shortly after birth. The mastoid antrum, which is an extension of the epitympanum, has started to develop in midfetal life. A few mastoid 'air-cells' are present late in fetal life, but the bulk of their development takes place in infancy and childhood.

The ossicles

The outer lateral ends of the first (Meckel's) and second (Reichert's) arch cartilages lie, respectively, above and below the developing first pharyngeal pouch. Before these arch cartilages are fully defined, condensations in the mesenchyme appear in this region at about 4–5 weeks. As development proceeds, the condensations form cartilage models which, by 6.5 weeks, are well-defined as malleus, incus and stapes. By 5 weeks, the stapes can be recognized as a circular mass at the end of the precursor of Reichert's (second arch) cartilage. Approximately 1.5 weeks later, this becomes annular as it is pierced by the first arch (stapedial) artery, and is now attached to the developing Reichert's cartilage by a membranous bar, the interhyale. At this time, the malleus and incus are developing from cartilage at the end of the precursor of Meckel's (first arch) cartilage. A groove represents the site of the future incudomalleolar joint, and the handle of the malleus and long process of incus are already apparent. By 7.5 weeks, the handle of the malleus lies between the layers of the developing tympanic membrane.

The stapes continues to grow and its ring-like shape is converted into the definitive arch-like stapedial form. It seems likely that the footplate of the stapes is formed primarily from the otic capsule, and that part of the stapedial ring which fuses with the otic capsule during ossification usually regresses. In the adult, therefore, the stapedial arches are derived from second arch cartilage, while the footplate is part of the labyrinthine capsule. Frequently, however, regression of the base of the stapedial ring is incomplete so that a dual origin for the mature footplate is possible. Ossification in the stapedial cartilage starts from a single centre at 4.5 months and is followed by a complex pattern of resorption, with the result that the base, the crura and the adjoining head are eventually hollowed out.

The malleus and incus start ossifying at the 4-month stage and progress is so rapid that, in the 25-week fetus, they are already of adult size and form.

The muscles of the tympanic cavity develop from the first and second arch mesenchyme to become the tensor tympani, which is supplied by a branch of the nerve of the first arch (mandibular), and the stapedius, which is supplied by the nerve of the second arch (facial). The pre-trematic nerve of the first arch is the chorda tympani and, with expansion of the tympanic cavity and resorption of the mesenchyme, its final course is within the layers of the tympanic membrane as it passes from the facial nerve to its destination in the floor of the mouth.

The temporal bone

The temporal bone is derived from four separate morphological elements that fuse with one another. The elements are the tympanic bone, already described previously, the squamous portion, the petromastoid complex, and the styloid process.

The squamous portion of the temporal bone, like the tympanic ring, develops in mesenchyme rather than in a preformed cartilage model. It is ossified from one centre that, as early as 8 weeks, appears close to the root of the zygomatic arch, and extends radially and also into the arch itself. The posteroinferior portion grows down behind the tympanic ring to form the lateral wall of the fetal mastoid antrum.

The petromastoid is morphologically a single element, although it is conveniently described in the adult in two separate units, the petrous and mastoid bones. The development of the cartilaginous otic capsule of embryonic and fetal life has already been described. Rapid progression of ossification completes the formation of the bony labyrinth. However, changes in the outer periosteal layer continue. A cartilaginous flange grows downwards and outwards from the lateral part of the petrosal cartilages, above the tubotympanic cavity, to form the roof of the middle ear and of the lateral bony wall of the eustachian tube. A separate flange grows outwards below the developing middle ear cavity to form the jugular plate. The facial nerve, which lies in a sulcus on the lateral, tympanic, aspect of the otic capsule, is also enclosed by growth from the capsule. Other changes gradually develop in the outer layers of the capsule. The subarcuate fossa, which carried a leash of blood vessels and was as large as the internal meatus, becomes progressively smaller. Anteriorly, the outer periosteal layer enlarges to form the petrous apex.

The styloid process develops from two centres at the cranial end of Reichert's (second arch) cartilage. That part closest to the tympanic bone is the tympanohyal and its ossification centre appears before birth. It fuses with the petromastoid during the first year of life and is surrounded at its root by a portion of the tympanic bone. The ossification centre for the distal part – the stylohyal – does not appear until after birth and fusion with the tympanohyal does not occur, if at all, until after puberty.

The tympanic ring unites with the squamous por-

tion shortly before birth, while the petromastoid fuses during the first year of life, so that tympanosquamous (anterior) and tympanomastoid suture lines are present in the bony external meatus. At birth, the tympanic annulus lies beneath the skull in an almost horizontal plane. By the third month, as a result of the upward and lateral rotation of the petrous bone, caused by rapid enlargement of the forebrain, the annulus appears on the inferolateral aspect of the skull, and it is not until some months later that its accessible oblique position is attained.

The mastoid portion of the petromastoid is at first flat, and the stylomastoid foramen with the facial nerve lies on the lateral surface behind the tympanic bone. With the development of air cells in the mastoid, its lateral portion grows downwards and forwards so that the stylomastoid foramen is carried on to the undersurface of the bone and the facial nerve canal elongates. During the second year of life, the portion of the squamous bone adjoining the petromastoid enlarges and grows downwards to form the mastoid tip. A squamopetrous suture line is usually visible on the outer surface of the mastoid process. Within this process, a variable extension of the antral air cells is found and a septum may be left between deep and superficial air cells. This is Korner's septum and is a remnant of the petrosquamous suture line. As the tympanic bone and the mastoid process develop, the lateral surface of the temporal bone takes up its vertical adult position.

Anatomy of the human ear

For the purpose of anatomical description, the ear is divided into four separate portions. These are the auricle (or pinna), the external auditory canal, the middle ear and its derivatives and, finally, the inner ear.

The auricle

The auricle (or pinna) projects at a greater or lesser angle from the side of the head and has some function in collecting sound (see Chapter 2). The lateral surface of the auricle has several prominences and depressions (Figure 1.10). The curved rim is the helix. At its posterosuperior aspect a small auricular tubercle (Darwin's tubercle) is often present. Anterior to and parallel with the helix is another prominence, the antihelix. Superiorly, this divides into two crura between which is the triangular fossa; the scaphoid fossa lies above the superior of the two crura. In front of the antihelix, and partly encircled by it, is the concha. The anterior superior portion of the concha is usually covered by the descending limb of the anterior superior portion of the helix (the crus of the helix). This region is the cymba conchae. It is the

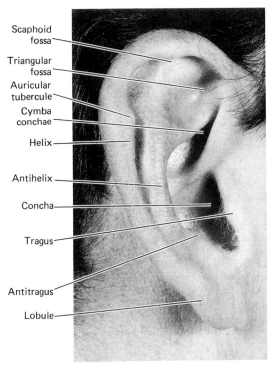

Scaphoid fossa

Triangular fossa

Auricular tubercle

Cymba conchae

Helix

Antihelix

Concha

Tragus

Antitragus

Lobule

Figure 1.10 The author's right auricle, the growth of tragal hairs indicating the passing of youth

direct lateral relation to the suprameatal triangle of the temporal bone. Below the crura of the helix and opposite the concha, across the external auditory meatus, is the tragus, which is a small blunt triangular prominence. This points posteriorly and overlaps the orifice of the external canal. Opposite the tragus, at the inferior limit of the antihelix, is the antitragus. The tragus and antitragus are separated by the intertragic notch. The lobule lies below the antitragus and is soft, being composed of fibrous and adipose tissue. The medial (cranial) surface of the auricle has elevations corresponding to the depressions on the lateral surface, and possesses corresponding names, e.g. the eminentia conchae.

The body of the auricle is composed of a thin plate of cartilage covered with skin, and it is connected to surrounding parts by ligaments and muscles. It is continuous with the cartilage of the external meatus.

The skin of the auricle is thin and closely adherent to the perichondrium on the lateral surface. There is a definite but thin layer of subdermal adipose tissue on the medial (cranial) surface. The skin is covered with fine hairs which have sebaceous glands opening into their root canals. The glands are most numerous in the concha and scaphoid fossa. On the tragus and intertragic notch coarse, thick hairs may develop in the middle-aged and older male.

The cartilaginous skeleton comprises a single piece of elastic fibrocartilage which is absent in the lobule and deficient between the crus of the helix and the tragus, i.e. in the anterior superior portion, where it is replaced by dense fibrous tissue. The cartilage, in the same way as cartilage elsewhere, is dependent on its perichondrium for supply of nutrients and removal of by-products. The cartilage is connected to the temporal bone by two extrinsic ligaments. The anterior ligament runs from the tragus and from a cartilaginous spine on the anterior rim of the crus of the helix to the root of the zygomatic arch. A separate posterior ligament runs from the medial surface of the concha to the lateral surface of the mastoid prominence. Intrinsic ligaments connect various parts of the cartilaginous auricle; that between helix and tragus has already been described and another runs from the antihelix to the posteroinferior portion of the helix.

Extrinsic and intrinsic muscles are, in the same way as ligaments, attached to the perichondrium of the cartilage. The extrinsic muscles are supplied by temporal and posterior auricular branches of the facial nerve and, while being functionally unimportant, they do give rise to the postauricular myogenic response following appropriate auditory stimulation (Gibson, 1978). There are three extrinsic muscles: auricularis anterior, superior and posterior, the last being supplied by the posterior auricular branch of the facial nerve. All three radiate out from the auricle to insert into the epicranial aponeurosis. The intrinsic muscles, six in number, are small, inconsistent and without useful function, other than that of entertaining children in those who possess the ability to alter the shape of the pinna.

Three arterial branches of the external carotid supply the auricle. The posterior auricular provides twigs that supply the medial (cranial) surface and, by extension around the helix, the extremities of the lateral surface. The anterior auricular branches of the superficial temporal artery supply the bulk of the lateral surfaces, and a small auricular branch from the occipital artery assists the posterior auricular in supplying the medial surface.

Many nerves make up the sensory supply of the auricle. Their distribution is variable and the overlap may be extensive. The essential features are described in Table 1.3.

The lymphatic drainage from the posterior surface is to the lymph nodes at the mastoid tip, from the tragus and from the upper part of the anterior surface to the preauricular nodes, and from the rest of the auricle to the upper deep cervical nodes.

The external auditory canal

The external auditory canal extends from the concha of the auricle to the tympanic membrane. The dis-

Table 1.3 Sensory innervation of the auricle

Nerve	Derivation	Region supplied
Greater auricular	Cervical plexus C2,3	Medial surface and posterior portion of lateral surface
Lesser occipital	Cervical plexus C2,3	Superior portion of medial surface
Auricular	Vagus X	Concha and antihelix
		Some supply medial surface (eminetia concha)
Auriculotemporal	Vc mandibular	Tragus, crus of helix and adjacent helix
Facial VII		Probably supplies small region in the root of concha

tance from the bottom of the concha to the tympanic membrane is approximately 2.5 cm, although the length of the anterior canal wall is 1–1.5 cm more because of the length of the tragus, the obliquity of the tympanic membrane and the curvature of the canal wall. The supporting framework of the canal wall is cartilage in the lateral one-third and bone in the medial two-thirds. In adults, the cartilaginous portion runs inwards slightly downwards and forwards. The canal is straightened, therefore, by gently moving the auricle upwards and backwards to counteract the direction of the cartilaginous portion. In the neonate, there is virtually no bony external meatus as the tympanic bone is not yet developed, and the tympanic membrane is more horizontally placed so that the auricle must be gently drawn downwards and backwards for the best view of the tympanic membrane.

In the adult, the lateral cartilaginous portion is about 8 mm long. It is continuous with the auricular cartilage and is deficient superiorly, this space being occupied by the intrinsic ligament between the helix and tragus. The medial border of the meatal cartilage is attached to the rim of the bony canal by fibrous bands.

The bony canal wall, about 1.6 mm long, is narrower than the cartilaginous portion and itself becomes smaller closer to the tympanic membrane. The anterior wall is longer by about 4 mm than the posterior wall because of the obliquity of the tympanic membrane. The medial end of the bony canal is marked by a groove, the tympanic sulcus, which is absent superiorly. Although the tympanic bone makes up the greater part of the canal, and also carries the sulcus, the squamous bone forms the roof. Therefore, there are two suture lines in the canal wall with the tympanosquamous anteriorly and the tympanomastoid posteriorly. Both these suture lines may be more or less developed; they project into the canal and the overlying skin is closely adherent. The tympanomastoid suture is a complex suture line between the anterior wall of the mastoid process, a portion of the squamous bone and the tympanic bone.

Apart from these intrusions into the canal, there are two constrictions: one at the junction of the cartilaginous and bony portions and the other, the isthmus, 5 mm from the tympanic membrane where a prominence of the anterior canal wall reduces the diameter. Deep to the isthmus, the anteroinferior portion of the canal dips forward so that a wedge-shaped anterior recess is formed between the tympanic membrane and the canal.

The skin itself has some properties not found in skin elsewhere. Instead of maturation taking place directly towards the surface there is lateral growth of the epidermis, with the consequence that layers of keratin are shed towards the surface opening of the external meatus (Johnson and Hawke, 1985). This is also true of the epidermal layers of the tympanic membrane, and Alberti (1964) has shown that the rate of migration is about 0.05 mm/day, which approximates the same rate of growth as that of fingernails.

The skin overlying the cartilaginous portion contains hairs and glands. The hairs are narrow and short and project towards the external opening of the meatus. The external surface of individual hairs has a series of overlapping 'scales' which are also directed externally (Figure 1.11).

The glands are of two types, ceruminous and sebaceous. The sebaceous glands are typical of sebaceous glands elsewhere and consist of a single wide duct from which arise a cluster of pear-shaped alveoli. Each alveolus consists of a basement membrane enclosing a mass of epithelial cells. The central cells, which contain fat, break down to form the sebaceous material (sebum), and are in turn replaced by a proliferation of epithelial cells at the edge of the mass. The sebum passes along the ducts which nearly always open into hair follicles (Figure 1.12).

The ceruminous glands lie slightly deeper in the dermis and are simple coiled tubular structures lined with cuboidal secretory cells and surrounded by a myoepithelium. This contains smooth muscle, and its contraction compresses the duct which thus empties its contents into the root canal of the hair follicle from which these cells nearly always originate. The

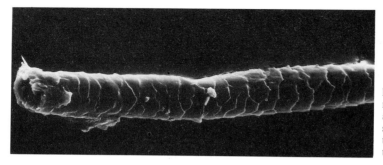

Figure 1.11 Scanning electron micrograph of a single short hair from an adult human external ear canal. A series of overlapping scales is present on the surface of the hair and directed to the external opening of the ear canal

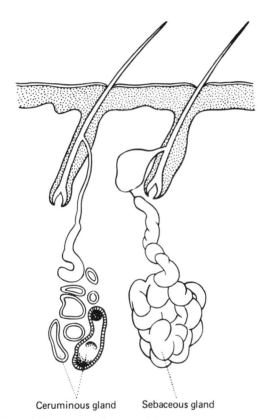

Ceruminous gland   Sebaceous gland

Figure 1.12 Diagram of section of skin of external auditory canal showing ceruminous and sebaceous glands arising from hair follicles. (Courtesy of David Lim)

Wax (cerumen)

The mixture of the products of the sebaceous and ceruminous glands results in the formation of wax, of which there are two distinct forms – dry and wet. Dry wax is yellowish or grey, and is dry and brittle, while wet wax is yellowish brown, and is wet and sticky. The type of wax possessed by an individual is probably monofactorially inherited with the wet phenotype dominant over the recessive dry type. The Japanese, other mongoloid populations and the American Indians tend to carry the recessive gene and, in general, have dry wax, whereas in white and black populations, the wet gene predominates.

Wax contains various amino acids, fatty acids, lysozymes and immunoglobulins and is to some extent bactericidal, being especially potent at killing dividing bacteria (Stone and Fulghum, 1984).

Blood supply and lymphatic drainage

The arterial supply of the external meatus is derived from branches of the external carotid. The auricular branches of the superficial temporal artery supply the roof and anterior portion of the canal. The deep auricular branch of the first part of the maxillary artery arises in the parotid gland behind the temporomandibular joint, pierces the cartilage or bone of the external meatus, and supplies the anterior meatal wall skin and the epithelium of the outer surface of the tympanic membrane. Finally, auricular branches of the posterior auricular artery pierce the cartilage of the auricle and supply the posterior portions of the canal. The veins drain into the external jugular vein, the maxillary veins and the pterygoid plexus.

The lymphatic drainage follows that of the auricle.

The relationships of the external canal are depicted in Figure 1.13.

secretion is initially white and watery, but as it dries and is oxidized, it becomes sticky and semisolid, and thereafter slowly darkens in colour. The ceruminous glands are modified apocrine sweat glands and both react to the same stimuli. Adrenergic drugs, emotion and fever result in an intrinsic release of adrenalin and noradrenalin, and mechanical manipulation, all produce a small increase in secretion.

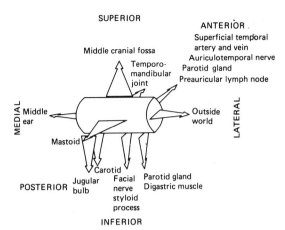

Figure 1.13 Relationships of the right external auditory canal

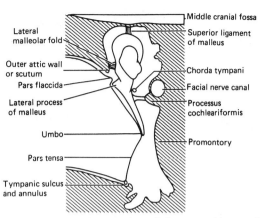

Figure 1.14 Coronal section through the external ear canal and middle ear at the level of the malleus handle

The middle ear cleft

The middle ear cleft consists of the tympanic cavity (tympanum), the eustachian tube and the mastoid air cell system. Included in this section are the extensions of the air cell system into the anterior and posterior petrous apex.

The tympanic cavity

The tympanic cavity is an irregular, air-filled space within the temporal bone and contains the auditory ossicles and their attached muscles. Other structures run along its walls to pass through the cavity. For descriptive purposes, the tympanic cavity may be thought of as a box with four walls, a roof and a floor. The corners are not sharp and, therefore, the precise localization of features lying at the edge of one wall may not be possible with this model.

The lateral wall of the tympanic cavity

The lateral wall of the tympanic cavity is part bony and part membranous. The tympanic membrane forms the central portion of the lateral wall, while above and below there is bone, forming the outer lateral walls of the epitympanum and hypotympanum respectively. The lateral wall of the epitympanum also includes that part of the tympanic membrane lying above the anterior and posterior malleolar folds – the pars flaccida. This lateral epitympanic wall is wedge-shaped in section and its lower bony portion is also called the outer attic wall or scutum (Latin = shield). It is thin and its lateral surface forms the superior portion of the deep part of the external meatus (Figure 1.14).

Three holes are present in the bone of the medial surface of the lateral wall of the tympanic cavity. The opening of the posterior canaliculus for the chorda

tympani nerve is situated in the angle between the junction of the lateral and posterior walls of the tympanic cavity. It is often at the level of the upper end of the handle of the malleus, but a lower situation is very common. The opening leads into a small bony canal which descends through the posterior wall of the tympanic cavity. Near the tympanic opening, the chorda tympani lies anterior and lateral to the facial nerve; it descends obliquely to join the nerve, often at some point within the bone, but occasionally the channel remains separate and the two nerves join outside the skull. A branch of the stylomastoid artery accompanies the chorda tympani into the tympanic cavity.

The petrotympanic (Glaserian) fissure opens anteriorly just above the attachment of the tympanic membrane. It is a slit about 2 mm long which receives the anterior malleolar ligament and transmits the anterior tympanic branch of the maxillary artery to the tympanic cavity. The chorda tympani enters the medial surface of the fissure through a separate anterior canaliculus (canal of Huguier) which is short and is sometimes confluent with the fissure.

The tympanic membrane, forming the lateral wall of the mesotympanum and a small part of the epitympanum, separates the tympanic cavity from the external meatus. It is a thin, nearly oval disc slightly broader above than below, forming an angle of about 55° with the floor of the meatus. Its longest diameter from posterosuperior to anteroinferior is 9–10 mm, while perpendicular to this the shortest diameter is 8–9 mm. Most of the circumference is thickened to form a fibrocartilaginous ring, the tympanic annulus, which sits in a groove in the tympanic bone, the tympanic sulcus. The sulcus does not extend to the roof of the canal which is formed by part of the squamous bone. From the superior limits of the sulcus, the annulus becomes a fibrous band which runs centrally as anterior and posterior malleolar folds to the lateral process of the malleus, the handle of which lies within the tympanic membrane. This leaves a small, rather squat, triangular region of tympanic membrane above the malleolar folds. It does not have a tympanic annulus at its margins, is lax and is called the pars flaccida. The pars tensa forms the rest of the tympanic membrane. It is taut and, when seen from the ear canal, is concave, with the maximum depression at the inferior tip of the malleus handle (the umbo). However, each portion of the membrane, as the latter passes from the annulus to the umbo, is not flat but is gently curved, being slightly convex when seen from the middle ear (Figures 1.14 and 1.15).

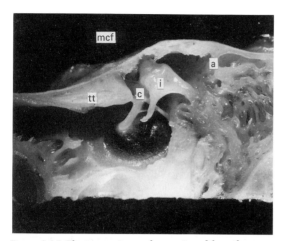

Figure 1.15 The tympanic membrane viewed from the middle ear. The chorda tympani runs superior to the tensor tympani in its passage across the tympanic membrane. The aditus to the mastoid antrum lies posterosuperior to the short process of the incus. a: aditus to mastoid antrum; c: chorda tympani; i: incus; mcf: middle cranial fossa; tt: tensor tympani

The tympanic membrane has three layers: an outer epithelial layer, the epidermis, which is continuous with the skin of the external meatus; a middle, mainly fibrous layer, the lamina propria; and an inner mucosal layer continuous with the lining of the tympanic cavity.

The epidermis is divided into the stratum corneum, the stratum granulosum, the stratum spinosum and stratum basale. In man (Hentzer, 1969), the stratum corneum, which is the outermost layer, consists of between one and six compressed layers of almost acellular structures, without organelles but with recognizable membranes and intercellular junctions (desmosomes). The stratum granulosum contains one to three layers of cells with smooth borders, and interconnecting desmosomes. Keratohyaline granules and lamellar granules are present among occasional tonofilaments, but other cell constituents are lacking. The cells of the stratum spinosum, which are two or three layers deep, have prominent interdigitations

with neighbouring cells to which they are bound by desmosomes. These cells contain bundles of tonofilaments, with mitochondria and ribosomes also present, but have a high nucleus to cytoplasm ratio. The stratum basale, which is the deepest layer, consists of a single layer of cells separated from the lamina propria by a basement membrane. These cells have a polyhedral shape, or are elongated in a line parallel to the basement membrane. Occasionally, prolongations of the deep surface of the cell extend down into the lamina propria. Nerve endings and melanin granules have not been seen in any of the cell layers of the epidermis.

The predominant feature of the lamina propria, in both the pars tensa and the pars flaccida, is the presence of collagen fibrils. In the pars tensa, the fibrils closest to the epithelial layers are usually in direct contact with the basement membrane of the epidermal layer, although in places a thin layer of loose connective tissue intervenes. These lateral fibres are radial in orientation, while the deeper ones are circular, parabolic and transverse. A loose connective tissue layer, containing fibroblasts, macrophages, nerve fibres (mainly unmyelinated) and many capillaries, lies between the deep layers of the lamina propria and the inner mucosal layer. Neither the capillaries nor the nerves appear to penetrate the basement membrane or enter the mucosal layer.

In the pars flaccida, the lamina propria is less marked, but it still contains collagen fibres although they appear to lie in an almost random orientation.

The mucosal epithelium of the pars tensa varies in height from a low simple squamous or cuboidal type to a pseudostratified columnar epithelium. The adjoining cell borders have marked interdigitations with tight junctions between the apices of the cells facing the tympanic cavity. The free surface of the cells, i.e. the surface facing the middle ear, possesses numerous microvilli and, where the epithelium is cuboidal or columnar, cilia with the typical 'nine plus two' internal ultrastructure are found. These true cilia are patchy in their distribution and a continuous sheet, such as that which covers the respiratory mucosa of, say, the eustachian tube, is not found. No goblet cells have been found in this layer, but in cells without cilia, secretory granules are present. The cytoplasm and nuclei of the cells are otherwise unremarkable. The mucosal layer is separated from the lamina propria by a basement membrane. In the pars flaccida, the overall picture is the same except that taller ciliated cells are not found.

Blood supply of the tympanic membrane

The arterial supply of the tympanic membrane is complex and arises from branches supplying both the external auditory meatus and the middle ear. These two sources interconnect through extensive anastomoses, but the vessels are found only in the connective tissue layers of the lamina propria. Within this layer there appears to be a peripheral ring of arteries connected by radial anastomoses, with one or two arteries that run down each side and around the tip of the malleus handle. The arteries involved include the deep auricular branch of the maxillary artery coming from the external auditory meatus; and, from the middle ear, the anterior tympanic branches of the maxillary artery, twigs from the stylomastoid branch of the posterior auricular artery and probably several twigs from the middle meningeal artery.

The venous drainage returns to the external jugular vein, the transverse sinus, dural veins and the venous plexus around the eustachian tube.

Nerve supply of the tympanic membrane

The nerves, in the same way as the blood vessels, run in the lamina propria and arise from the auriculotemporal nerve (Vc) supplying the anterior portion, from the auricular branch of the vagus (X), the posterior portion, and from the tympanic branch of the glossopharyngeal nerve (IX). The variations and overlap are considerable, but both the vascular supply and innervation are relatively sparse in the middle part of the posterior half of the tympanic membrane.

The roof of the tympanic cavity

The tegmen tympani is the bony roof of the tympanic cavity, and separates it from the dura of the middle cranial fossa. It is formed in part by the petrous and part by the squamous bone; and the petrosquamous suture line, unossified in the young, does not close until adult life. Veins from the tympanic cavity running to the superior petrosal sinus pass through this suture line.

The floor of the tympanic cavity

The floor of the tympanic cavity is much narrower than the roof and consists of a thin plate of bone which separates the tympanic cavity from the dome of the jugular bulb. Occasionally, the floor is deficient and the jugular bulb is then covered only by fibrous tissue and a mucous membrane. At the junction of the floor and the medial wall of the cavity there is a small opening that allows the entry of the tympanic branch of the glossopharyngeal nerve into the middle ear from its origin below the base of the skull.

The anterior wall of the tympanic cavity

The anterior wall of the tympanic cavity is rather narrow as the medial and lateral walls converge. The lower portion of the anterior wall is larger than the upper and consists of a thin plate of bone covering the carotid artery as it enters the skull and before it turns anteriorly. This plate is perforated by the super-

ior and inferior caroticotympanic nerves carrying sympathetic fibres to the tympanic plexus, and by one or more tympanic branches of the internal carotid artery. The upper, smaller part of the anterior wall has two parallel tunnels placed one above the other. The lower opening is flared and leads into the bony portion of the eustachian tube which will be described in more detail later on in this chapter. The upper tunnel is separated from the eustachian tube by a thin plate of bone, and contains the tensor tympani muscle which subsequently runs along the medial wall of the tympanic cavity enclosed in a thin bony sheath. This muscle will also be further described in the section on the auditory ossicles.

The medial wall of the tympanic cavity

The medial wall separates the tympanic cavity from the inner ear. Its surface possesses several prominent features and two openings (Figure 1.16). The promontory is a rounded elevation occupying much of the central portion of the medial wall. It usually has small grooves on its surface and these contain the nerves which form the tympanic plexus. Sometimes the grooves, especially the groove containing the tympanic branch of the glossopharyngeal nerve, are covered by bone, with the consequence that small canals are present instead. The promontory covers part of the basal coil of the cochlea and in front merges with the anterior wall of the tympanic cavity.

Behind and above the promontory is the fenestra vestibuli (oval window), a nearly kidney-shaped opening that connects the tympanic cavity with the vestibule, but which in life is closed by the base of the stapes and its surrounding annular ligament. The long axis of the fenestra vestibuli is horizontal, and the slightly concave border is inferior. The size of the fenestra vestibuli naturally varies with the size of the base of the stapes, but on average it is 3.25 mm long and 1.75 mm wide. Above the fenestra vestibuli is the facial nerve and below is the promontory. The fenestra, therefore, lies at the bottom of a depression or fossula that can be of varying width depending on the position of the facial nerve and the prominence of the promontory.

The fenestra cochleae (round window), which is closed by the secondary tympanic membrane (round window membrane), lies below and a little behind the fenestra vestibuli from which it is separated by a posterior extension of the promontory, called the subiculum. Occasionally, a spicule of bone leaves the promontory above the subiculum and runs to the pyramid on the posterior wall of the cavity. This spicule is called the ponticulus. The fenestra cochleae, which faces inferiorly and a little posteriorly, lies completely under cover of the overhanging edge of the promontory in a deep niche and is, therefore, usually out of sight. The niche is most commonly triangular in shape, with anterior, posterosuperior and posteroinferior walls. The latter two meet posteri-

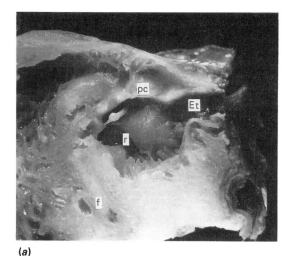

(a)

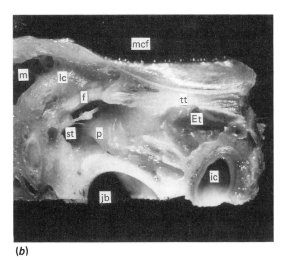

(b)

Figure 1.16 Two separate specimens cut at slightly different levels to show the medial wall of the tympanic cavity and the associated structures. (*a*) Section cut through a block of temporal bone just medial to the inferior part of the annulus; (*b*) section cut deeper, i.e. slightly more medial in a different temporal bone so as to expose the jugular bulb. Et: eustachian tube orifice; f: facial nerve in descending and intratympanic segments; ic: internal carotid; jb: jugular bulb; lc: dome of lateral semicircular canal; m: mastoid antrum; mcf: middle cranial fossa; p: promontory; pc: processus cochleariformis; r: round window niche; st: sinus tympani; tt: tensor tympani. Other structures, i.e. subiculum and ponticulus can be seen clearly but are not labelled to avoid confusion. They are described in the text

orly and lead to the sinus tympani. The average length of the walls of the niche are: anterior – 1.5 mm; superior – 1.3 mm; and posterior – 1.6 mm

(Nomura, 1984). There is great variation in the depth of the niche and, to enable the secondary tympanic membrane to be seen, bone frequently has to be removed from the anterior wall of the niche. Within the niche are mucosal folds or even complete membranes that partly or completely exclude the secondary tympanic membrane from view and may even be mistaken for it during surgery. In the adult, the secondary tympanic membrane lies almost horizontally in the roof of the niche. This membrane is not flat but curves towards the scala tympani of the basal coil of the cochlea, so that it is concave when viewed from the middle ear. It appears to be divided into an anterior and posterior portion by a transverse thickening within the membrane. The shape of the membrane varies, in different temporal bones, from round through oval and kidney-shaped to spatulate, with average longest and shortest diameters of 2.30 mm and 1.87 mm respectively.

The membrane consists of three layers: an outer mucosal, a middle fibrous and an inner mesothelial layer. The mucosal layer is rather like the mucosal layer of the primary tympanic membrane with flattened or cuboidal cells possessing microvilli and, occasionally, clusters of cilia on their surfaces. This layer is separated from the basement membrane by a single layer of loose connective tissue and often contains melanocytes. It is this layer that contains the capillaries and nerves. The rest of the middle layer, which forms the bulk of the membrane, contains fibroblasts and collections of collagen and elastic fibres. The fibres are not, however, ordered in the same way as in the pars tensa and do not form discrete bundles. The inner layer is a continuation of the cell layer lining the scala tympani. There are two or three layers of overlapping, flat mesothelial cells with wide intercellular spaces, but no tight junctions nor any connective tissue layer between this and the middle layer.

The membrane of the fenestra cochleae does not lie at the end of the scala tympani but forms part of its floor. The scala tympani terminates posterior and medial to the membrane. The ampulla of the posterior semicircular canal is the closest vestibular structure to the membrane and its nerve (the singular nerve) runs almost parallel to, and 1 mm away from, the medial attachment of the deep portion of the posterior part of the membrane. The membrane is therefore a surgical landmark for the singular nerve (Gacek, 1983).

The facial nerve canal runs above the promontory and fenestra vestibuli in an anteroposterior direction. It has a smooth rounded lateral surface that is occasionally deficient, and is marked anteriorly by the processus cochleariformis. This is a curved projection of bone, concave anteriorly, which houses the tendon of the tensor tympani muscle as it turns laterally to the handle of the malleus. Behind the fenestra vestibuli, the facial canal starts to turn inferiorly as it begins its descent in the posterior wall of the tympanic cavity.

The region above the level of the facial nerve canal forms the medial wall of the epitympanum. The dome of the lateral semicircular canal extends a little lateral to the facial canal and is the major feature of the posterior portion of the epitympanum. In well-aerated mastoid bones, the labyrinthine bone over the superior semicircular canal may be prominent, running at right angles to the lateral canal and joining it anteriorly at a swelling which houses the ampullae of the two canals. In front and a little below this, above the processus cochleariformis, may be a slight swelling corresponding to the geniculate ganglion, with the bony canal of the greater superficial petrosal nerve running for a short distance anteriorly.

The posterior wall of the tympanic cavity

The posterior wall is wider above than below and has in its upper part the opening (aditus) into the mastoid antrum. This is a large irregular hole that leads back from the posterior epitympanum. Below the aditus is a small depression, the fossa incudis, which houses the short process of the incus and the ligament connecting the two. Below the fossa incudis and

medial to the opening of the chorda tympani nerve is the pyramid, a small hollow conical projection with its apex pointing anteriorly. It contains the stapedius muscle, the tendon of which passes forward to insert into the stapes. The canal within the pyramid curves downwards and backwards to join the descending portion of the facial nerve canal. Between the pyramid and the tympanic annulus is the facial recess (Figure 1.17). This is less marked lower down where the facial nerve canal forms only a slight prominence on the posterior wall. The facial recess is, therefore, bounded medially by the facial nerve and laterally by the tympanic annulus, but running through the wall between the two, with a varying degree of obliquity, is the chorda tympani nerve. This always runs medial to the tympanic membrane, which means that the angle between the facial nerve and the chorda allows access to the middle ear from the mastoid without disruption to the tympanic membrane. This angle can be small or large depending on the site of origin of the chorda from the facial nerve.

Deep to both the pyramid and the facial nerve is a posterior extension of the mesotympanum – the sinus tympani. This extension of air cells into the posterior wall can be extensive, and Anson and Donaldson (1981) reported that, when measured from the tip of

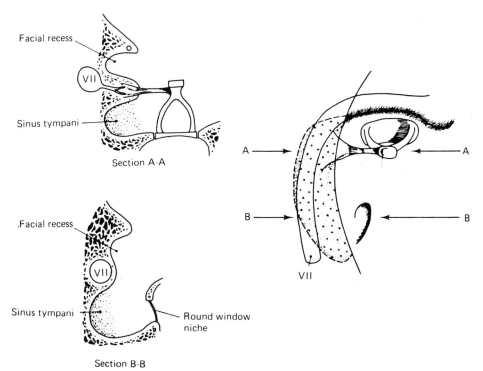

Section A-A

Section B-B

Figure 1.17 The facial recess and sinus tympani at different levels in the middle ear. Section AA is at the level of the pyramid where the facial recess is relatively deep. In section BB, at the level of the round window, the facial recess is quite shallow. The extent of the sinus tympani, deep and posterior to the facial nerve, is variable

the pyramid, the sinus can extend as far as 9 mm into the mastoid bone. The medial wall of the sinus tympani becomes continuous with the posterior portion of the medial wall of the tympanic cavity where it is related to the two fenestrae and the subiculum of the promontory.

The relationships of the middle ear space are shown diagrammatically in Figure 1.18.

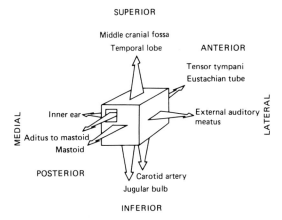

Figure 1.18 The relationships of the right middle ear

The contents of the tympanic cavity

The tympanic cavity contains a chain of three small movable bones – the malleus, incus and stapes – two muscles, the chorda tympani nerve and the tympanic plexus of nerves.

The malleus

The malleus (hammer), the largest of the three ossicles, comprises a head, neck and three processes arising from below the neck. The overall length of the malleus ranges from 7.5 to 9.0 mm (Figure 1.19). The head lies in the epitympanum and has on its posteromedial surface an elongated saddle-shaped, cartilage-covered facet for articulation with the incus. This surface is constricted near its middle and the smaller inferior portion of the joint surface lies nearly at right angles to the superior portion. This projecting lower part is the cog, or spur, of the malleus. Below the neck of the malleus, the bone broadens and gives rise to the following: the anterior process from which a slender anterior ligament arises to insert into the petrotympanic fissure; the lateral process which receives the anterior and posterior malleolar folds from the tympanic annulus; and the handle. The handle runs downwards, medially and slightly backwards between the mucosal and fibrous layers of the tympanic membrane. On the deep, medial surface of the handle, near its upper end, is a small projection into which the tendon of the tensor tympani muscle in-

serts. Additional support for the malleus comes from the superior ligament which runs from the head to the tegmen tympani.

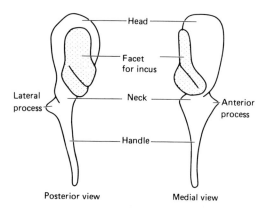

Figure 1.19 The left malleus. The stippling represents the cartilage of the synovial joint that articulates with the incus. Figures 1.20 and 1.21 are on the same scale

The incus

The incus (Figure 1.20) articulates with the malleus and has a body and two processes. The body lies in the epitympanum and has a cartilage-covered facet corresponding to that on the malleus. The short process projects backwards from the body to lie in the fossa incudis to which it is attached by a short ligament. The long process descends into the mesotympanum behind and medial to the handle of the malleus, and at its tip is a small medially directed lenticular process which articulates with the stapes.

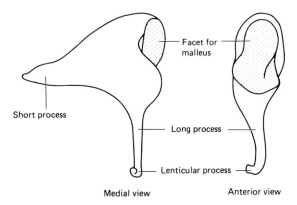

Figure 1.20 Left incus

The stapes

The stapes consists of a head, neck, two crura (limbs) and a base or footplate (Figure 1.21). The head points laterally and has a small cartilage-covered

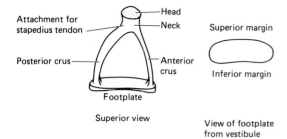

Figure 1.21 Left stapes

depression for articulation with the lenticular process of the incus. The stapedius tendon inserts into the posterior part of neck and upper portion of the posterior crus. The two crura arise from the broader lower part of the neck and the anterior crus is thinner and less curved than the posterior one. Both are hollowed out on their concave surfaces. The two crura join the footplate which usually has a convex superior margin, an almost straight inferior margin and curved anterior and posterior ends. The average dimensions of the footplate are 3 mm long and 1.4 mm wide, and it lies in the fenestra vestibuli where it is attached to the bony margins of the labyrinthine capsule by the annular ligament. The long axis of the footplate is almost horizontal, with the posterior end being slightly lower than the anterior.

The stapedius muscle

The stapedius arises from the walls of the conical cavity within the pyramid and from the downward curved continuation of this canal in front of the descending portion of the facial nerve. A slender tendon emerges from the apex of the pyramid and inserts into the stapes. The muscle is supplied by a small branch of the facial nerve.

The tensor tympani muscle

This is a long slender muscle arising from the walls of the bony canal lying above the eustachian tube. Parts of the muscle also arise from the cartilaginous portion of the eustachian tube and the greater wing of the sphenoid. From its origins, the muscle passes backwards into the tympanic cavity where it lies on the medial wall, a little below the level of the facial nerve. The bony covering of the canal is often deficient in its tympanic segment where the muscle is replaced by a slender tendon. This enters the spoon-shaped processus cochleariformis where it is held down by a transverse tendon as it turns through a right angle to pass laterally and insert into the medial aspect of the upper end of the malleus handle. The

muscle is supplied from the mandibular nerve by way of a branch, from the medial pterygoid nerve, which passes through the otic ganglion without synapse.

The chorda tympani nerve

This branch of the facial nerve enters the tympanic cavity from the posterior canaliculus at the junction of the lateral and posterior walls. It runs across the medial surface of the tympanic membrane between the mucosal and fibrous layers and passes medial to the upper portion of the handle of the malleus above the tendon of tensor tympani to continue forwards and leave by way of the anterior canaliculus, which subsequently joins the petrotympanic fissure.

The tympanic plexus

The tympanic plexus is formed by the tympanic branch of the glossopharyngeal nerve and by caroticotympanic nerves which arise from the sympathetic plexus around the internal carotid artery. The nerves form a plexus on the promontory and provide the following:

1 Branches to the mucous membrane lining the tympanic cavity, eustachian tube and mastoid antrum and air cells
2 A branch joining the greater superficial petrosal nerve
3 The lesser superficial petrosal nerve, which contains all the parasympathetic fibres of IX. This nerve leaves the middle ear through a small canal below the tensor tympani muscle where it receives parasympathetic fibres from VII by way of a branch from the geniculate ganglion. The completed nerve passes through the temporal bone to emerge, lateral to the greater superficial petrosal nerve, on the floor of the middle cranial fossa, outside the dura. It then passes through the foramen ovale with the mandibular nerve and accessory meningeal artery to the otic ganglion. Occasionally, the nerve runs not in the foramen ovale but through a separate small foramen next to the foramen spinosum. Postganglionic fibres from the otic ganglion supply secretomotor fibres to the parotid gland by way of the auriculotemporal nerve.

The mucosa of the tympanic cavity

The middle ear mucosa is to some degree a respiratory mucosa carrying cilia on its surface and being able to secrete mucus (Sade, 1966). The extent of the mucociliary epithelium varies in normal middle ears, being more widespread in the young. However, three distinct mucociliary tracts or pathways can be identified – epitympanic, promontorial and hypotympanic, the latter being the largest. Each of these pathways coalesces at the tympanic orifice of the eustachian tube (Gleeson, Felix and Neivergelt, 1991).

Mucus comes from goblet cells and from mucous glands which are collections of mucus-producing cells linked to the surface by a short duct. In the middle ear, the glands are sometimes absent; however, in most ears they are present and tend to be clustered around the orifice of the eustachian tube, although they are never present in large numbers. Goblet cells eject mucus directly into the middle ear space (Figure 1.22) and are in highest concentration close to the eustachian tube opening (Tos and Bak–Pedersen, 1976). Again, large numbers of goblet cells are rarely seen, but their presence is indicative of the potential ability of the middle ear mucosa to undergo changes typical of respiratory epithelium.

The mucous membrane lines the bony walls of the tympanic cavity, and it extends to cover the ossicles and their supporting ligaments in much the same way as the peritoneum covers the viscera in the abdomen. The mucosal folds also cover the tendons of the two intratympanic muscles and carry the blood supply to and from the contents of the tympanic cavity. These folds separate the middle ear space into compartments. The epitympanic space is only connected to the mesotympanum and is, therefore, ventilated only by way of two small openings between the various mucosal folds – the anterior and posterior isthmus tympani (Figure 1.23). The mucosal folds have been described in detail by Proctor (1964) and are depicted in Figure 1.23.

The blood supply of the tympanic cavity

Arteries supplying the walls and contents of the tympanic cavity arise from both the internal and external carotid system. The overlap between branches is extensive and there is great variability in the supply between individuals. Table 1.4 outlines the general distribution of the arterial supply although the anterior tympanic and stylomastoid arteries are the biggest. Because of the great variability of the blood supply, and the difficulty of interpretation of injected specimens, an 'average' view of the blood supply has been presented. Different authors give different names to what appear to be the same vessels, and attach varying importance to the contribution made by each. However, most believe that a major contribution to the supply of the stapes and incudostapedial joint comes from a plexus of vessels derived from the stylomastoid artery and which surrounds the facial nerve to enter the tympanic cavity by way of the pyramid or directly through its posterior wall. Additional vessels reach the stapes from the meshwork of arterioles on the promontory, and probably derive mainly from the anterior and inferior tympanic arteries.

The eustachian tube (auditory or pharyngotympanic tube)

The eustachian tube is a channel connecting the tympanic cavity with the nasopharynx. In the adult, it is about 36 mm long and runs downwards, forwards and medially from the middle ear. There are two elements to the tube: a lateral bony portion arising from the anterior wall of the tympanic cavity,

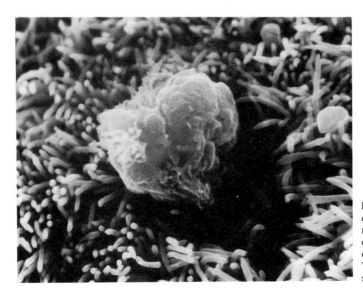

Figure 1.22 High magnification scanning electron micrograph of the surface of the respiratory mucosa from the nasopharyngeal end of the eustachian tube. A small volume of mucus is being secreted from a goblet cell. The cilia of the surrounding cells are clearly seen. Picture width 10 μm

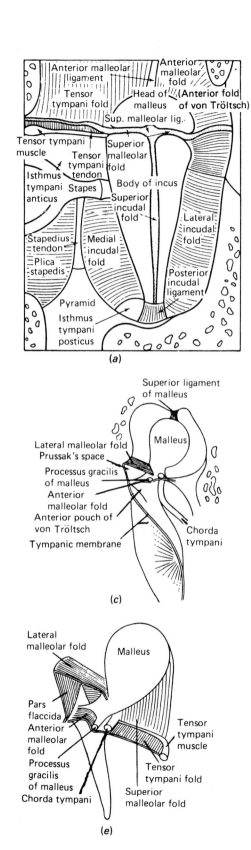

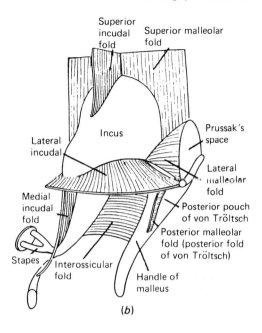

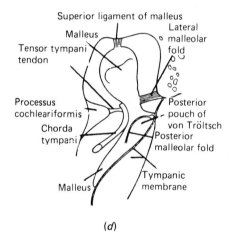

Figure 1.23 The compartments and folds of the middle ear (after Proctor, 1964). (*a*) The attic folds. (*b*) Posterosuperior and lateral view of the right middle ear. (*c*) The anterior pouch of von Tröltsch viewed from an anterior aspect. (*d*) The posterior pouch of von Tröltsch viewed from a posterior aspect. (*e*) Prussak's spaces showing the posterior two-thirds of the space, seen from the front

Table 1.4 Blood supply to the middle ear

Branch	Parent artery	Region supplied
Anterior tympanic	Maxillary artery	Tympanic membrane, malleus and incus, anterior part of tympanic cavity
Stylomastoid	Posterior auricular	Posterior part of tympanic cavity, stapedius muscle
Mastoid	Stylomastoid	Mastoid air cells
Petrosal	Middle meningeal	Roof of mastoid, roof of epitympanum
Superior tympanic	Middle meningeal	Malleus and incus, tensor tympani
Inferior tympanic	Ascending pharyngeal	Mesotympanum
Branch from artery	Artery of pterygoid canal	Meso- and hypotympanum
Tympanic branches	Internal carotid	Meso- and hypotympanum

and a medial fibrocartilaginous part entering the nasopharynx. The tube is lined with respiratory mucosa containing goblet cells and mucous glands and has a carpet of ciliated epithelium (Figure 1.24) on its floor. At its nasopharyngeal end, the mucosa is truly respiratory; but in passing along the tube towards the middle ear, the number of goblet cells and glands decreases, and the ciliary carpet becomes less profuse.

The bony portion is about 12 mm long and is widest at its outer tympanic end. It runs through the squamous and petrous portions of the temporal bone and gradually narrows to the isthmus which is the narrowest part of the whole tube, having a diameter of only 2 mm or less. The roof of the tube is formed by a thin plate of bone, above which is the tensor tympani muscle. The carotid artery, also separated by a plate of bone, lies medial to the tube. In cross-section, the tube is triangular or rectangular with the horizontal diameter being the greater.

The cartilaginous part of the tube is about 24 mm long and has a plate of cartilage forming its back (posteromedial) wall. At the upper border, the cartilage is bent forwards to form a short flange that makes up part of the front (anterolateral) wall. The rest of the front wall comprises fibrous tissue (Figure 1.25). The apex of the cartilage is attached to the isthmus of the bony portion, while the wider medial end lies directly under the mucosa of the nasopharynx and forms the tubal elevation. The cartilage is fixed to the base of the skull in a groove between the petrous part of the temporal bone and the greater wing of the sphenoid. The groove terminates near the root of the medial pterygoid plate. In the nasopharynx, the tube opens 1–1.25 cm behind and a little below the posterior end of the inferior turbinate. The opening is almost triangular in shape and is surrounded above and behind by the tubal elevation. The salpingopharyngeal fold stretches from the lower part of the tubal elevation downwards to the wall of the pharynx. The levator palati, as it enters the soft

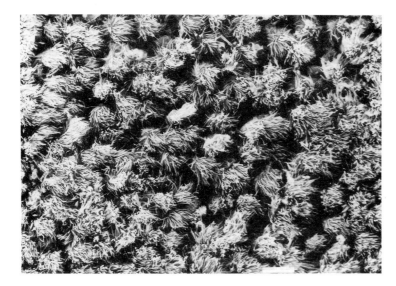

Figure 1.24 Scanning electron micrograph of the surface of respiratory epithelium from nasopharyngeal end of human eustachian tube. A dense carpet of cilia is present on the surface. Marker 10 μm

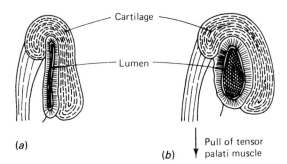

(a)

(b)   Pull of tensor palati muscle

Figure 1.25 Schematic diagram of the cartilaginous portion of the right eustachian tube. (*a*) Tube closed. (*b*) Tube open demonstrating the pull of the tensor palati muscle

palate, results in a small swelling immediately below the opening of the tube. Behind the tubal elevation is the pharyngeal recess or fossa of Rosenmüller. Lymphoid tissue is present around the tubal orifice and in the fossa of Rosenmüller, and may be prominent in childhood.

Muscles attached to the eustachian tube

The tensor palati muscle arises from the bony wall of the scaphoid and from along the whole length of the short cartilaginous flange that forms the upper portion of the front wall of the cartilaginous tube. From these origins, the muscle descends, converges to a short tendon that turns medially around the pterygoid hamulus and then spreads out within the soft palate to meet fibres from the other side in a midline raphe. The tensor palati separates the tube from the otic ganglion, the mandibular nerve and its branches, the chorda tympani nerve and the middle meningeal artery. It is supplied by the mandibular nerve.

The salpingopharyngeus is a slender muscle attached to the inferior part of the cartilage of the tube near its pharyngeal opening, and it descends to blend with palatopharyngeus.

The levator palati contains a few fibres that arise from the lower surface of the cartilaginous tube. This muscle, which also originates from the lower surface of the petrous bone, just in front of the opening for the entrance of the carotid, and from fascia forming the upper part of the carotid sheath, first lies inferior to the tube, then crosses to the medial side and spreads out into the soft palate. Both the salpingopharyngeus and the levator palati are supplied from the pharyngeal plexus.

The mechanism of tubal opening during swallowing and yawning is not well understood. The tensor palati probably plays a major role, assisted by the levator palati and possibly by the salpingopharyngeus which is too slender to have much effect in raising the pharynx and larynx.

The tube is supplied by the ascending pharyngeal and middle meningeal arteries. The veins drain into the pharyngeal plexus and the lymphatics pass to the retropharyngeal nodes. The nerve supply arises from the pharyngeal branch of the sphenopalatine ganglion (Vb) for the ostium, the nervus spinosus (Vc) for the cartilaginous portion and from the tympanic plexus (IX) for the bony part.

The aditus to the mastoid antrum

This is a large irregular opening leading from the posterior epitympanum into the air-filled spaces of the mastoid antrum, often referred to as the aditus ad antrum. On the medial wall is the prominence of the lateral semicircular canal. Below and slightly medial to this is the bony canal of the facial nerve. The short process of the incus is closely related to these two structures, and the average distances between them are: VIIth nerve to semicircular canal – 1.77 mm; VIIth nerve to short process incus – 2.36 mm; and short process incus to semicircular canal – 1.25 mm (Anson and Donaldson, 1981) (Figure 1.26).

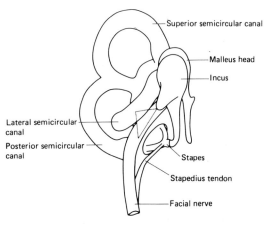

Superior semicircular canal

Malleus head

Incus

Lateral semicircular canal

Posterior semicircular canal

Stapes

Stapedius tendon

Facial nerve

Figure 1.26 Diagram illustrating the relationship between the short process of the incus, the VIIth nerve and the semicircular canal (lateral). The average dimensions are given in the text. This is the right ear with the structures viewed from behind and laterally

The mastoid antrum

The mastoid antrum is an air-filled sinus within the petrous part of the temporal bone. It communicates with the middle ear by way of the aditus and has mastoid air cells arising from its walls. The antrum, but not the air cells, is well developed at birth and by adult life has a volume of about 1 ml, being 14 mm from front to back, 9 mm from top to bottom and 7 mm from side to side. The medial wall of the antrum is related to the posterior semicircular canal and more deeply and inferiorly is the endolymphatic sac and the dura of the posterior cranial fossa. The roof forms part of the floor of the middle cranial fossa and separates the antrum from the temporal lobe of the brain. The posterior wall is formed mainly by the bony covering of the sigmoid sinus. The lateral wall is part of the squamous portion of the temporal bone and increases in thickness during life from about 2 mm at birth to 12–15 mm in the adult. The lateral wall in the adult corresponds to the suprameatal (Macewen's) triangle on the outer surface of the skull. This region can be felt through the cymba conchae of the auricle and is defined by the supramastoid crest – which is the posterior prolongation of the upper border of the root of the zygoma – by a vertical tangent through the posterior margin of the external meatus and, finally, by the posterosuperior margin of the external meatus itself.

The floor of the mastoid antrum is related to the digastric muscle laterally and the sigmoid sinus medially, although in a poorly aerated mastoid bone these structures may be 1 cm away from the inferior antral wall. The anterior wall of the antrum has the aditus in its upper part, while lower down, the facial nerve passes in its descent to the stylomastoid foramen. The relationships of the mastoid antrum are shown in Figure 1.27.

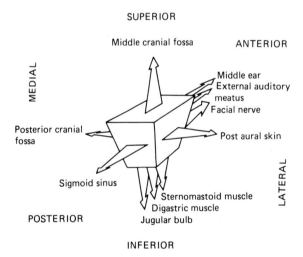

Figure 1.27 Relationships of the right mastoid antrum

The mastoid air cell system

In the majority of the adult population, a more or less extensive system of interconnecting air-filled cavities arises from the walls of the mastoid antrum, and sometimes even from the walls of the epi- and mesotympanum. These air cells can extend throughout the mastoid process and may be separated from the sigmoid sinus and posterior and middle cranial fossae by thin bone, which is occasionally deficient. Cells often extend medially to the descending portion of the facial nerve as the retrofacial cells, down to the digastric muscle as the tip cells, and around the sigmoid sinus as the perisinus cells. They can reach the angle between the sigmoid sinus and the middle fossa dura (the sinodural angle), and may even extend out of the mastoid bone into the root of the zygoma and into the floor of the tympanic cavity underneath the basal turn of the cochlea. Occasionally, the apex of the petrous bone is pneumatized (see following subsection).

These air cells, like the mastoid itself, are lined with a flattened non-ciliated squamous epithelium. Pneumatization can be very extensive, as described previously, when the mastoid process is referred to in terms such as cellular, well-aerated, or by some similar name. Alternatively, the mastoid antrum may be the only air-filled space in the mastoid process when the name acellular or sclerotic is applied. This condition is present in perhaps 20% of adult temporal bones. In between these two forms are the so-called diploeic or mixed types where air cells are present but are interspersed with marrow-containing spaces that have persisted from late fetal life.

The petrous apex

The petrous apex is, surgically, the most inaccessible portion of the temporal bone, and has the shape of a truncated pyramid with a base and three sides making up the medial part of the bone (Figure 1.28). The base of this pyramid is formed, from front to back, by the canal for the tensor tympani and the carotid artery, by the cochlea, the vestibule and the semicircular canals. The superior surface is the floor of the middle cranial fossa extending forwards from the line of the superior semicircular canal (indicated by the arcuate eminence) to the foramen lacerum and the impression for the ganglion of the trigeminal nerve (V). The posterior surface forms the bony wall of the posterior cranial fossa and extends, again from back to front, from the endolymphatic sac and the line of the posterior semicircular canal to the pointed anterior tip of the petrous bone, from which arises the petroclinoid ligament. The junction between the superior and posterior surfaces is marked by the superior petrosal sinus, and the lower limit of the posterior surface is the suture line with the occipital bone. The third face of the pyramid has the jugular bulb and inferior petrosal sinus at its margins and the external opening of the carotid canal in the middle.

Two structures run through the petrous apex – the carotid artery and internal auditory meatus. The latter structure, on entering the posterior surface, divides the petrous apex into anterior and posterior parts. Chole (1985), from whom this description of the petrous apex is derived, reported that about 10%

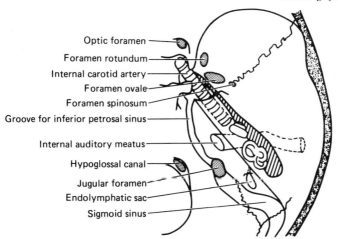

Figure 1.28 Diagram showing the floor of the middle and posterior cranial fossae of the right side of the skull. The eustachian tube, middle ear and mastoid air spaces are represented by the dark cross-hatching while the paths of the internal and external auditory canals are shown by interrupted lines. The text contains the description of the boundaries of the petrous apex

of normal human temporal bones have air cells within the anterior part, while perhaps 30% have a pneumatized posterior segment.

It is also of interest that the carotid artery loses its thick muscular medial layer as it enters the temporal bone from the neck, with the result that the mean thickness of the wall is only 0.15 mm. Sometimes, also, the medial bony wall of the eustachian tube is deficient or extremely thin, so that the carotid is separated from the mucosal lining of the tube by just a thin layer of fibrous connective tissue.

The internal auditory meatus

This is a short canal, nearly 1 cm in length and lined with dura, which passes into the petrous bone in a lateral direction from the cerebellopontine angle. It is closed at its outer lateral end, or fundus, by a plate of bone which is perforated for the passage of nerves

and blood vessels to and from the cranial cavity. The meatus transmits the facial, cochlear and vestibular nerves and the internal auditory artery and vein.

Although various authors, having used different techniques for measurement, report dissimilar dimensions, on average the vertical diameter of the meatus in 90% of normal subjects lies between 2 mm and 8 mm, with an average of about 4.5 mm, and the difference between the two sides in an individual does not exceed 1 mm. The average length of the posterior wall is 8 mm, and the difference between the two sides does not exceed 2 mm (Valvassori and Pierce, 1964; Papangelou, 1972).

The bony plate separating the fundus from the middle and inner ears has a transverse crest on its inner medial surface. This is the crista falciformis and it separates a small upper region from a larger lower area (Figure 1.29). Above the crest and anteriorly is the opening of the facial canal carrying the facial

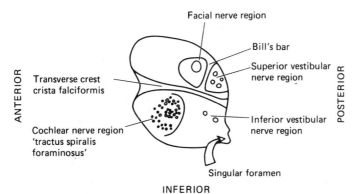

Figure 1.29 The right internal auditory meatus, viewed along its axis and from the posterior cranial fossa

nerve (VII). This is separated, by a small vertical ridge (Bill's bar), from the posterior region which transmits the superior vestibular nerve through several small foramina to the superior and lateral semicircular canals, to the utricle and a part of the saccule. Below the transverse crest, the cochlear nerve lies anteriorly and leaves the meatus through the cochlear area which comprises a spiral of small foramina and a central canal. The inferior vestibular nerve passes through one or two foramina behind the cochlear opening to supply the saccule. Just behind and below the inferior vestibular foramen is the foramen singulare which contains the singular nerve. This runs obliquely through the petrous bone close to the fenestra cochleae (round window) to supply the sensory epithelium in the ampulla of the posterior semicircular canal.

The inner ear

The inner ear, or labyrinth, lies in the temporal bone, and for descriptive purposes it is divided into a bony and a membranous portion. The membranous labyrinth, containing the sensory epithelium of the cochlea and vestibular structures, lies within cavities surrounded by the bony labyrinth.

The bony labyrinth

This is derived from the inner periosteal layer of the otic capsule, and in adult life consists of a thin, but dense, bony shell surrounding the vestibule, the semicircular canals and the cochlea.

The vestibule

The vestibule is the central portion of the bony labyrinth and is a small flattened ovoid chamber lying between the middle ear and the fundus of the internal auditory meatus. It is about 5 mm long, 5 mm high, but only 3 mm deep. On its lateral wall is the opening of the fenestra vestibuli closed in life by the footplate of the stapes and its annular ligament. On the medial wall anteriorly is the spherical recess which houses the macula of the saccule and which is perforated by small holes that carry fibres from the inferior vestibular nerve (Figure 1.30). Behind the spherical recess is a ridge named the vestibular crest. At its lower end, the ridge divides to encompass the cochlear recess which carries cochlear nerve fibres to the very base of the cochlea. Above and behind the crest is an elliptical recess which contains the macula of the utricle. Nerve fibres, destined for the utricle and superior and lateral semicircular canals, perforate the bony wall in an area which corresponds to the superior vestibular nerve region at the fundus of the internal auditory meatus. The opening of the vestibular aqueduct lies below the elliptical recess, and the aqueduct itself passes through the temporal bone to open in the posterior cranial fossa but outside the dura. It carries the endolymphatic duct and several small blood vessels. The posterior wall of the vestibule contains five openings that lead into the semicircular canals. The anterior wall of the vestibule contains an elliptical opening into the scala vestibuli of the cochlea.

The semicircular canals

There are three semicircular canals – superior, posterior and lateral – situated above and behind the vestibule. Each occupies about two-thirds of a circle and the canals are unequal in length, although the lumen of each has a diameter of about 0.8 mm. At one end of each canal is a dilatation called the

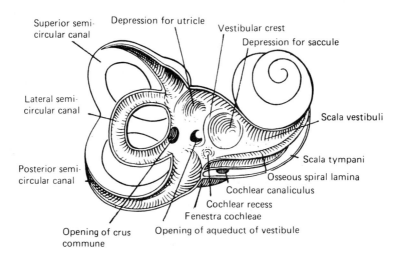

Figure 1.30 Interior of the right bony labyrinth viewed from the lateral aspect

ampulla which contains the vestibular sensory epithelium and opens into the vestibule. For the superior and lateral canals, the ampullae are next to each other at their anterolateral ends, while the ampulla of the posterior canal lies inferiorly near the floor of the vestibule. The non-ampullated ends of the superior and posterior canals meet and join to form the crus commune which enters the vestibule in the middle of its posterior wall. The non-ampullated end of the lateral canal opens into the vestibule just below the crus commune.

In the two ears, the lateral canals lie nearly in the same plane which slopes downwards and backwards at an angle of about 30° to the horizontal when the individual is standing. The other canals are at right angles to this, so that the superior canal of one ear lies nearly parallel with the posterior canal of the other.

The lateral canal bulges the medial wall of the epitympanum, while the apex of the superior canal lies very close to the floor of the middle cranial fossa. The arcuate eminence of this portion of the petrous bone often, but not always, overlies this part of the superior canal.

The cochlea

The bony cochlea lies in front of the vestibule and has an external appearance rather like the shell of a snail (Figure 1.31). It is, however, a coiled tube, with the inside of one coil being separated from the lumen of an adjacent coil by a dense, but thin bony wall. The shell has approximately two-and-one-half turns

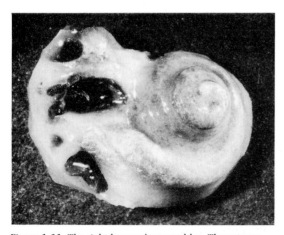

Figure 1.31 The right human bony cochlea. The petrous temporal bone has been drilled down until only a thin bony capsule enclosing the membranous labyrinth remains. The stapes has been removed from the oval window, and the bone overhanging the round window membrane partly removed. In this cochlea there are slightly more than two-and-one-half turns

and its height is about 5 mm, while the greatest distance across the base is about 9 mm. The coils of the cochlea turn about a central cone or modiolus which arises from the cochlear nerve portion of the fundus of the internal auditory meatus, and points laterally and forwards, tapering from a wide base to a narrow apex. The apex of the cochlea, therefore, faces laterally and forwards towards the upper part of the medial wall of the tympanic cavity, while the basal coil forms the bulge of the promontory below this. Arising from the modiolus is a thin shelf of bone that spirals upwards within the lumen of the cochlea as the bony spiral lamina. A membrane – the membranous spiral lamina – extends from the edge of the bony spiral lamina to the outer wall of the cochlea, thereby dividing each coil into the major portions – the scala vestibuli and scala tympani.

Conventional anatomical nomenclature becomes very difficult within the cochlea because of its coiled shape and orientation, so that a separate system has arisen which defines the position of structures relative to the modiolus which is thought of as rising vertically from base to apex (Figure 1.32). Structures close to the modiolus are inner or medial, while other more distant structures are outer or lateral. A coil at the apex is above or apical to a coil at the base, while within one coil a structure on the apical side of the spiral lamina is above one below it. The scala vestibuli, therefore, lies above the scala tympani. This has greatly simplified relating one structure to another, and the terminology will be continued in this chapter.

At the apex, the spiral lamina continues for a short distance as a spur or crescent that is not attached to the modiolus (Figure 1.33). There is, therefore, communication between the perilymph spaces each side of the spiral lamina, and this channel is called the helicotrema.

At the base of the cochlea, the scala vestibuli opens into the vestibule with the fenestra vestibuli and stapes footplate close by on the lateral wall of the vestibule. The scala tympani is a blind-ended tube, but has in its floor the fenestra cochleae (round window) closed by the secondary tympanic membrane (round window membrane). A small opening into the cochlear aqueduct also arises from the basal end of the scala tympani. This aqueduct runs through the petrous bone and into the posterior cranial fossa well below the internal auditory meatus, establishing a communication between the subarachnoid space and the scala tympani.

The modiolus contains many small canals that spread out to enter the bony spiral lamina. The most central canals carry fibres to and from the apical regions, while the outermost canals carry fibres from more basal parts of the cochlea. Close to the origin of the bony spiral lamina, these canals dilate to accommodate the bipolar ganglion cells of the spiral

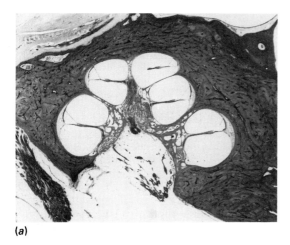

(a)

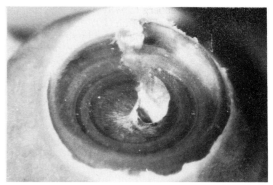

Figure 1.33 The apex of the cochlea. The bone overlying the apex of the cochlea has been removed to show the spiral lamina within. At the apex the spiral lamina continues on for a short distance as a spur or crescent not attached to the modiolus. The scala vestibuli and scala tympani are therefore in communication, and this channel is termed the helicotrema

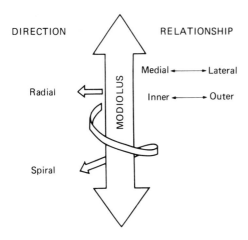

(b)

Figure 1.32 (a) Standard mid-modiolar section of the human cochlea. The spiral lamina is attached to the modiolus and separates the scala tympani below from the scala vestibuli above. The triangular scala media, or cochlear duct lies on the lateral or outer portions of the spiral lamina. (Courtesy of Professor L. Michaels, Institute of Laryngology and Otology.) (b) Diagram representing the nomenclature of the spatial relationships within the cochlea

(cochlear) ganglion, and the confluence of the dilated spaces has given rise to the name of the spiral canal of the modiolus. The name is slightly misleading as only a few unmyelinated efferent nerve fibres run along this apparent canal, with the vast majority of acoustic nerve fibres running across it from the organ of Corti, by way of the spiral ganglion, to form the cochlear nerve in the modiolus.

Perilymph

As well as containing the membranous labyrinth, the bony labyrinth is filled with perilymph. The exact origin of this fluid is not known, although it resembles plasma, interstitial fluid and cerebrospinal fluid in its make-up with major differences being the concentration and type of proteins present.

The membranous labyrinth

The membranous labyrinth is a series of communicating sacs and ducts derived from ectoderm and filled with endolymph. Within the walls of the membranous labyrinth, the epithelium has become specialized to form the sensory receptors of the cochlear and vestibular labyrinth.

The cochlear duct (scala media)

The duct of the cochlea consists of a spirally arranged tube lying on the upper surface of the spiral lamina against the outer wall of the bony canal of the cochlea. The length of the cochlea, as measured by the length of the organ of Corti, varies enormously between individuals and much more than in experimental animals. The average length is around 34 mm (standard deviation about 2 mm) while the range is from 29 to 40 mm, which has interesting implications when the physiology of cochlear function is considered (see Chapter 2). The length measurements are derived from the works of

Retzius (1884), Bredberg (1968), Walby (1985) and Ulehlova, Voldrich and Janisch (1987).

The cochlear duct is triangular in section with a floor formed by the outer part of the bony spiral lamina and all of the membranous spiral lamina; with an outer wall lying against a fibrous thickening of the bony cochlear wall – the spiral ligament; and with a thin sloping roof – Reissner's membrane – that runs from the bony spiral lamina to the upper part of the outer wall. The scala vestibuli lies above the cochlear duct, the scala tympani below (Figure 1.34).

The floor of the cochlear duct

The inner part of the floor is formed by the bony spiral lamina which separates into two ridges one above the other. The upper ridge is the spiral limbus from which the tectorial membrane originates, while the lower ridge gives rise to the membranous spiral lamina and has acoustic nerve fibres running through it to the organ of Corti. The membranous spiral lamina has the flattened epithelium of the scala tympani on its underside, a fibrous middle layer and the organ of Corti on its upper surface. This is separated from the spiral limbus by the inner sulcus, and from the lateral wall by the outer sulcus. The

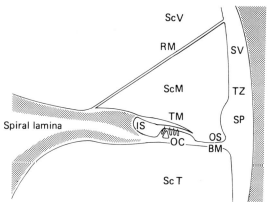

Figure 1.34 Diagram illustrating the structures and relationship of the cochlear duct. ScV: scala vestibuli; ScM: scala media; ScT: scala tympani; RM: Reissner's membrane; TM: tectorial membrane; OC: organ of Corti; BM: basilar membrane; IS: inner sulcus; OS: outer sulcus; SV: stria vascularis; TZ: transitional zone; SP: spiral prominence. ▨ : Bone

organ of Corti is a ridge-like structure containing the auditory sensory cells and a complex arrangement of supporting cells. The sensory cells are arranged in two distinct groups as inner and outer 'hair cells' (Figure 1.35). They are called hair cells because a

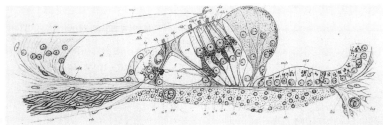

(a)

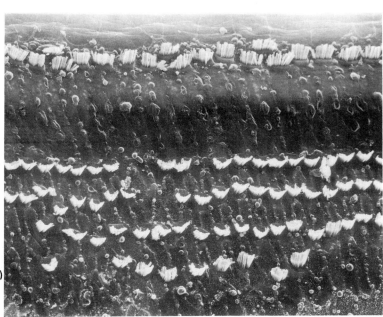

(b)

Figure 1.35 (*a*) Conventional light microscopic section of the human organ of Corti and tectorial membrane (from Retzius, 1884). (*b*) Scanning electron micrograph of a portion of the human organ of Corti. There is a single irregular row of inner hair cells with occasional extra inner hair cells. The outer hair cells lie in several irregular rows with gaps where the hair cells have been replaced by phalangeal scars. The rodent cochlea is by comparison remarkably regular. Picture width 200 μm

cluster of fine filaments, resembling hairs, projects from the upper surface of each sensory cell. There is a single row of inner hair cells, although occasionally extra hair cells may be apparent, and also three, four or five irregular rows of outer hair cells, with frequent gaps where individual hair cells are absent. The distribution of hair cells is markedly different from that seen in rodents (guinea-pigs, rats, etc.) where there is nearly always a highly regular arrangement.

Each hair cell consists of a body, which lies within the organ of Corti, and a thickened upper surface called the cuticular plate, from which projects a cluster of stereocilia or 'hairs'. The stereocilia are not true cilia in that they do not have a central 'nine plus two' core of microtubules, but are more like large microvilli comprising a core of actin molecules packed in a paracrystalline array and covered with a cell membrane (Tilney, Derosier and Mulroy, 1980). The name 'cilia' is, therefore, inappropriate, but its use, like that of the term 'hair cell', has become entrenched in the literature and is unlikely to be replaced by a more convenient and correct term. The inner hair cells are separated from the outer ones by the tunnel of Corti. The bodies of the inner hair cells are flask-shaped, with a small apex and large cell body. The long axis of the cell is inclined towards the tunnel of Corti, and nerve fibres and nerve endings are located around the lower half of the body (Figure 1.36). The stereocilia projecting from the thickened cuticular plate are arranged in two or three rows parallel to the axis of the cochlear duct. The shortest row of stereocilia is innermost, while the longest row is outermost (Figure 1.37). Along the length of the cochlear duct, the height of the longest stereocilia increases linearly with distance from the base, although the variation from base to apex is not great.

The body of the outer hair cell is cylindrical, with the nucleus lying close to the lower pole where afferent and efferent nerve endings are attached. The stereocilia that project from this have a different arrangement from those of the inner hair cells. There are several rows of stereocilia but the configuration varies from a W-shape at the base, through a V-shape in the middle coil, to an almost linear array at the apex. The number of stereocilia also decreases in the passage from base to apex, whereas the length increases, although not in linear fashion (Wright, 1984) (Figure 1.38). Within a single cluster of stereocilia, individual members are linked by short transverse fibrils, and the tips of shorter stereocilia have fine fibrillar extensions running laterally to adjoining longer stereocilia (Furness and Hackney, 1985). These linkages are also found between the stereocilia of both the inner hair cells and vestibular sensory cells (Figure 1.39). The role of these structures in cochlear mechanics is described in Chapter 2.

In the fetus and the newborn there are about 3500 inner hair cells and 13 000 outer hair cells (Bredberg, 1968), although the number of hair cells varies with the length of the cochlea, shorter cochleae having far fewer inner and outer hair cells. The distribution of hair cells, in terms of hair cell density related to place in the cochlea, can be plotted as a cytocochleogram, and it is found that with age there is a generalized reduction in the number of hair cells and an additional loss both at the base and, to a lesser extent, at the apex. These changes are most marked at the outer cells but are also found in the inner hair cell population (see Figure 1.38e). This loss starts at birth and progresses throughout life in a regular and linear fashion, although the rate of loss varies in different parts of the cochlea (Wright *et al.*, 1987).

The hair cells are supported within the organ of Corti by several types of specialized, highly differentiated cells. These are the pillar cells, Deiters' cells and Hensen's cells.

The tectorial membrane arises from the spiral limbus and extends over the organ of Corti to attach close to the Hensen cell region (Kronester–Frei, 1979). The membrane is an acellular gel-like matrix containing fibrillar strands, and is extremely sensitive to distortion and shrinkage during most preparation techniques. The tips of the longest stereocilia of the outer hair cells are attached to, or embedded in, the undersurface of the tectorial membrane and leave an impression on this surface. In adults, however, no impression or attachment of the inner hair cells has ever been noted.

The lateral wall of the cochlear duct

The lateral wall of the cochlear duct has three distinct zones; the stria vascularis above, the spiral prominence below and a transitional zone between the two. The stria vascularis forms the bulk of the lateral wall and consists of three cell layers. The marginal cells face the endolymph and are separated by the intermediate cells from a basal cell layer which is rich in capillaries. The marginal cells have a carpet of microvilli on their endolymphatic surface and tight junctions between neighbouring cells, so that the stria vascularis is effectively isolated from the endolymph. These cells are also rich in mitochondria, have an extensive Golgi apparatus and endoplasmic reticulum, and complex foldings of their basal membranes, which interdigitate with the intermediate and basal cells. The stria is a metabolically active tissue and is thought to play an active role in the maintenance of the ionic composition and electrical potential of the endolymph.

The roof of the cochlear duct (*Reissner's membrane*)

Reissner's membrane is a thin membrane stretching from the bony spiral lamina to the upper part of the

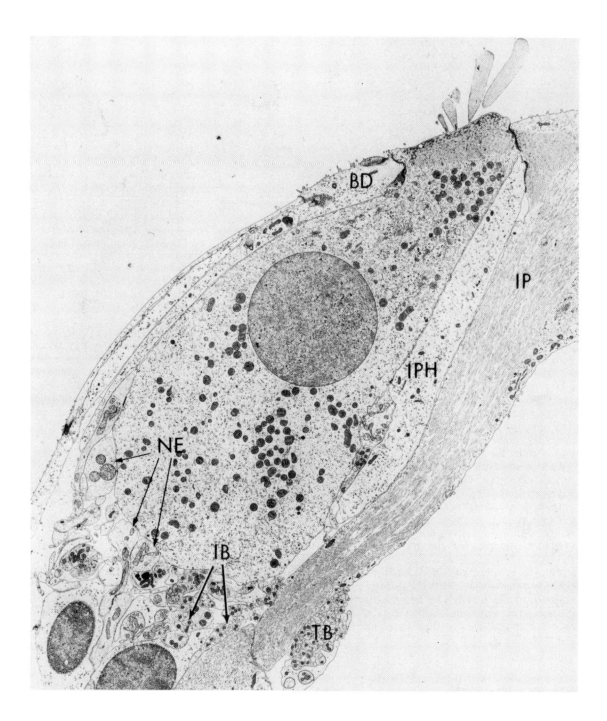

Figure 1.36 Transmission electron micrograph of an ultrathin section of a monkey's inner hair cell. The cell body is flask-shaped with a small apex, a large cell body and a central nucleus. Nerve fibres and nerve endings (NE) are located at the lower half of the cell body. Mitochondria are particularly plentiful in the lower half of the cell cytoplasm. The cell body makes contact with the inner phalangeal cell (IPH) laterally and with the border cell (BD) medially. IP: inner pillar cell; TB: tunnel spiral nerve bundle; IB: inner spiral nerve bundle. Picture width 13.5 μm (courtesy Robert Kimura)

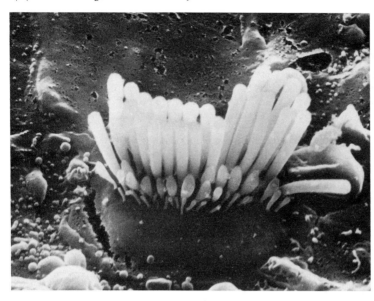

Figure 1.37 Scanning electron micrograph of a human inner hair cell. The stereocilia arise from a smooth circular plate and are arranged in an almost linear array. The short stereocilia are closer to the modiolus. Picture width 8 μm

lateral wall of the cochlear duct. The endolymphatic surface consists of typical squamous epithelial cells with microvilli on their surface and joined together by tight junctions. Two types of epithelial cell have been recognized. The first type are flat and polygonal, their surfaces being covered by short microvilli. Although distributed throughout Reissner's membrane, they are conspicuous by forming a zone two to three cells wide at the limbic margin. The second type of epithelial cell are rounded in surface outline. They are arranged in distinct patterns along Reissner's membrane; bands, strands, whorls or clusters (Felix *et al.*, 1993). A thin basement membrane separates these cells from those of the upper, scala vestibuli, side of the partition. These perilymphatic cells are thicker but have a dense cytoplasm only around the nucleus. Melanocytes are also found in this layer.

All of the cells lining the scala media are joined by tight junctions which effectively separate the endolymph from the outside and help to maintain the unusual ionic content of this fluid (see Chapter 2 for details of the ionic constituents of endolymph).

The vestibular labyrinth

The vestibular labyrinth consists of a complex series of interconnecting membranous ducts and sacs which contain the vestibular sensory epithelium. Unlike the cochlea, the sensory epithelium is found in localized collections in the three ampullae of the semicircular ducts and in the maculae of the saccule and utricle. The saccule lies in the spherical recess near the opening of the scala vestibuli of the cochlea. It is almost globular in shape but is prolonged posteriorly

where it makes contact with the utricle. In the anterior wall there is an oval thickening – the macula. The saccule lies connected anteriorly to the cochlea by a narrow duct, the ductus reuniens. From the posterior part arises the endolymphatic duct. This is joined by the utriculosaccular duct at an acute angle, and continues medially through the vestibular aqueduct to end as a blind pouch, the endolymphatic sac. The junction between the endolymphatic and utriculosaccular ducts has a Y-configuration with the lower limb continuing to the sac.

The utricle is the larger of the two vestibular sacs and is irregularly oblong in shape, occupying the posterosuperior part of the bony vestibule. The lower part of the lateral wall of the pouch contains the comma-shaped macula, the plane of which lies at right angles to that of the macula of the saccule. Apart from the utriculosaccular duct, there are five openings into the utricle which correspond to the utricular ends of the semicircular ducts.

The three semicircular ducts are about 0.2 mm in diameter and resemble the bony canals. Each duct has an ampulla at one end, and within this the sensory cells are collected on a saddle-shaped ridge – the crista – that runs across the lumen.

The vestibular sensory epithelium

The sensory cells of the ampullae and maculae have the same structure and comprise type I and type II cells. Type I cells are flask-shaped with a rounded base and a short neck. The body is surrounded by a large goblet-shaped nerve terminal, or chalice, which often extends to enclose more than one type I cell.

The upper surface of the cell is thickened in the form of a cuticular plate and has a single kinocilium and between 20 and 100 stereocilia projecting from its surface. The kinocilium is slightly thicker than the stereocilia and has the internal structure of a true cilium with a 'nine plus two' arrangement of microtubules and an associated basal body and centriole. The stereocilia have the same internal structure as those of the cochlear sensory cells (Figure 1.40).

Type II cells are cylindrical in shape with the same collection of kino- and stereocilia as the type I cells. The cell body, however, is not surrounded by a nerve chalice but has many button-like nerve terminals associated with it. These button terminals are either granulated and thought to be efferent in origin, or non-granulated and presumed, conversely, to be afferent. The fibres arising from the type I cells are larger in diameter than those of the type II cells, and they are afferent. Efferent fibres to the type I cells appear to terminate on the nerve chalice itself rather than on the cell body (Figure 1.41).

The location of the kinocilium gives the sensory cells polarity and this is related to changes in the neural output when the ciliary bundle is deflected. Deviation in the direction of the kinocilium results in an increase in the resting output of nerve impulses of the afferent neurons, while deflection away from the kinocilium inhibits the resting discharge (Figure 1.42). The sensory cells are arranged in the cristae and maculae, so that there are strict patterns of orientation in the polarity of the cells.

The sensory cells are surrounded by supporting cells. The apical surfaces of the supporting cells are covered with microvilli and it would appear that these cells have a secretory function. Close to the edges of the sensory cell regions of the cristae and maculae, and separated by a transitional zone in much the same way that the stria vascularis is separated from the organ of Corti, is a region occupied by 'dark cells'. These have an irregular surface, and resemble the marginal cells of the stria vascularis. Objects resembling degenerating otoconia are often found on the surface of the dark cells whose function is unclear but may, like the stria vascularis, have some role to play in the maintenance of the composition of the endolymph and, in addition, in the resorption of otoconia.

Recent experimental work using the ototoxic aminoglycoside antibiotics has shown that mammalian vestibular sensory epithelium is capable of regeneration after being damaged by application of the drug (Forge *et al.*, 1993). Such regeneration has been seen in some cold-blooded, non-mammalian groups where there is a continuous production of hair cells and in warm-blooded birds, but the discovery of this process in mammals possibly opens the way to therapeutic intervention. The topic is discussed in depth in Volume 3 Chapter 20.

Structures associated with the vestibular sensory cells

In each ampulla, a gelatinous, wedge-shaped cupula sits astride the crista (Figure 1.43). The cupula, like the tectorial membrane, is extremely sensitive to alterations in its ionic environment and shrinks when standard preparative techniques are employed. In life, the cupula extends to the roof and lateral walls of the ampulla, and is attached firmly to each end of the crista. The rest of the dome of the ampulla also contains a loose fibrillar meshwork but there does appear to be a space between the cupula and the surface of the crista. The 'cilia' of the sensory cells project into this and the longest 'cilia' appear to enter the cupula. It seems most likely that during angular acceleration the cupula remains fixed, and the angle of the junction of the semicircular duct and the ampulla, along with the loose matrix within the dome of the ampulla, serve to direct endolymph into the subcupular space where deflection of the ciliary bundles takes place, with resulting stimulation or inhibition of the neural output of the sensory cells (Dohlman, 1981).

In each macula, a gelatinous material overlies the sensory cells, the ciliary bundles of which appear to project into a honeycomb meshwork in its undersurface. Embedded in the upper surface of the gelatinous layer are the otoconia. These have a characteristic shape with a barrel-shaped body and pointed ends (Figure 1.44). The size of the otoconia is not constant but varies across each macula. Small crystals are found near the central strip, or striola, and near to the margins, while the intervening zone has large, sometimes very large, crystals present in it. The term 'otoconial membrane' is used to describe the combination of the otoconia and the gelatinous membrane.

When the surface of the maculae is examined more closely, small globular bodies can be seen, apparently arising from the supporting cells (Figure 1.44). In experimental animals, these structures have a high calcium content and it has been suggested that the calcium of the otoconia is derived from this source (Harada, 1979). The otoconia are not static structures but appear to have a slow turnover with degenerating otoconia probably being resorbed by the dark cell regions (see Lim, 1984, for review).

The endolymphatic system

The endolymphatic system consists of a duct formed from the endolymphatic duct of the saccule and the utriculosaccular duct from the utricle, and a sac. The sac comprises three distinct portions. The proximal portion or isthmus is the first portion; it is wider than the duct and lies within the bony vestibular aqueduct, as does the intermediate or rugose

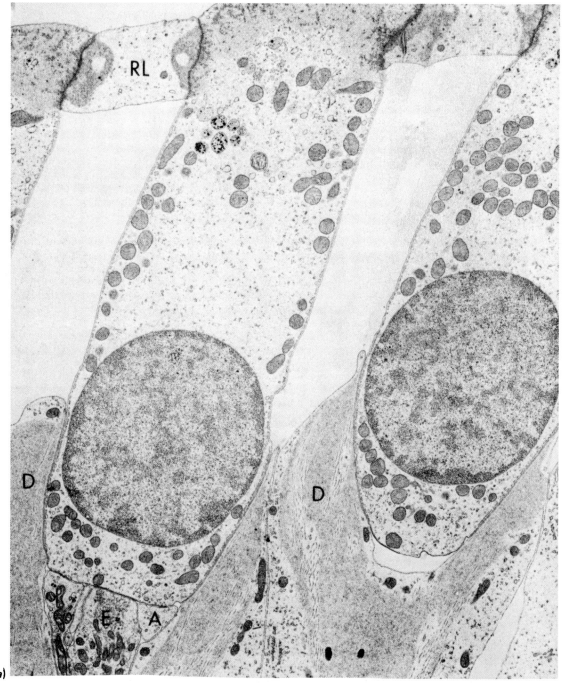

(a)

Figure 1.38 (*a*) Transmission electron micrograph of an ultrathin section of a monkey's outer hair cell. The cell body is cylindrical with the nucleus located in the lower pole. Mitochondria are present throughout the cell body but tend to be localized to the lateral cell membranes where, unlike the inner hair cell, there is a well-developed cisternal system. The apex of the cell is thickened to form the cuticular plate from which the stereocilia arise. The cell is supported at the apex by the phalangeal processes of Deiter's cells which form the reticular lamina (RL). At the base of the outer hair cell, the bodies of Deiter's cells (D) provide support. Afferent (A) and efferent (E) nerve endings synapse at the lower pole. The body of the hair cell is not supported but lies surrounded by perilymph in the spaces of Nuel. Picture width 13 μm (courtesy Robert Kimura). (*b*) Scanning electron micrograph of the outer hair cell region of the human organ of Corti. Three rows of outer cells are shown with a gap in the third row. Picture width 30 μm. (*c*) A single human outer hair cell. The stereocilia are arranged

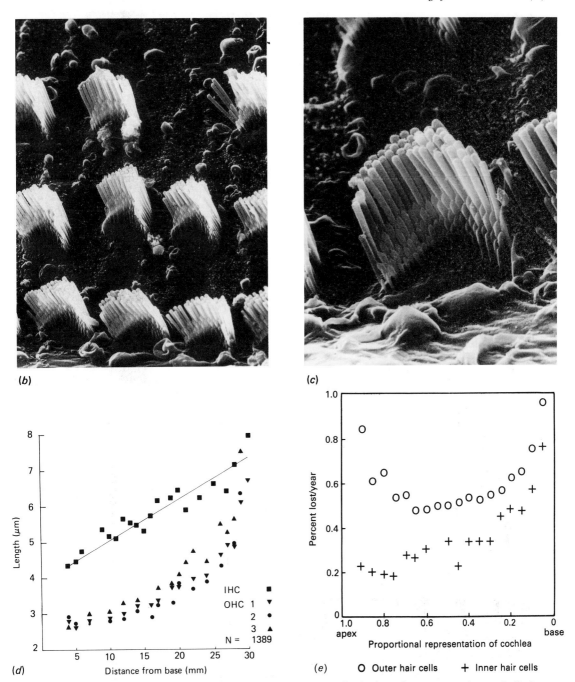

(b)

(c)

(d)

(e) **O** Outer hair cells **+** Inner hair cells

with the shortest ones being closest to the modiolus. Unlike the outer hair cells of rodents there are several rows of tall cilia. Picture width 9 μm. (*d*) Graphic representation of the length of the longest stereocilia of inner and outer hair cells related to position in the cochlea in terms of distance from the base in millimetres. There is a linear increase in the length of the stereocilia of the inner hair cells, but a more complex relationship for the stereocilia of the outer hair cells. (*e*) Graphic representation of the relationship between the percentage of hair cells lost per year and their location within the cochlea. The values for the inner hair cells are represented by crosses, those for the outer hair cells by open circles. The figures have been derived from 53 human cochleae and the wide variation in the length of the cochlear duct between individuals has been compensated for by assuming that each cochlea was of unit length so that distances along the cochlea were presented as a proportion of that length. The base was designated as zero and the apex as one unit. The convention of having the apex to the left and the base to the right allows some comparison with the audiogram

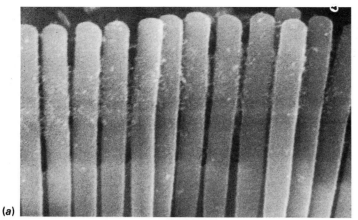

(a)

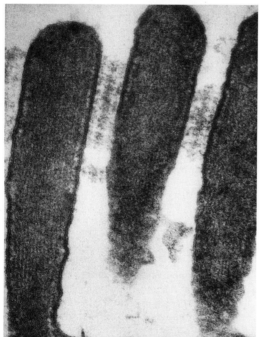

(b)

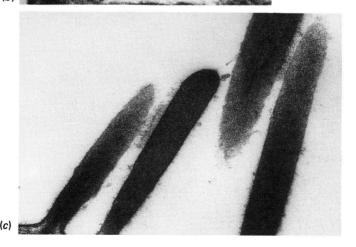

(c)

Figure 1.39 (*a*) Scanning electron micrograph of the inner hair cell stereocilia from a guinea-pig. The fine transverse cross-links can be seen near the tips. Picture width 6.5 μm. (*b*) Transmission electron micrograph of an ultrathin section of guinea-pig stereocilia showing not only the ordered structure of actin molecules that form the core of these structures but also the nature of the cross-links. Picture width 1.5 μm. (*c*) Transmission electron micrograph of the stereocilia showing the very fine apical cross-link which connects the tip of one stereocilium with the body of an adjacent one. (Figures (*a*), (*b*) and (*c*) courtesy of Dr A. Forge, EM Unit, Institute of Laryngology and Otology)

portion. The distal part of the sac is flattened and lies between the dura of the posterior fossa and the petrous bone. This arrangement is quite different from that found in most experimental animals where

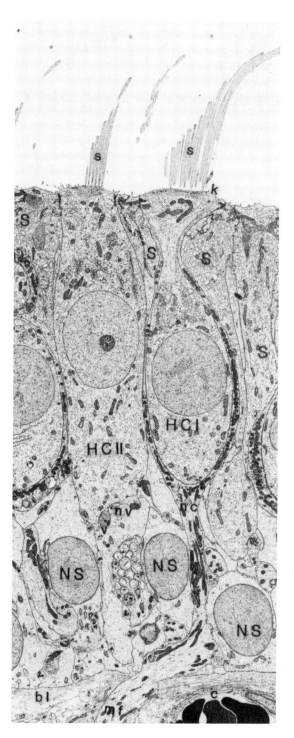

the rugose position, along with the distal position, is extradural.

The proximal part of the sac is lined with low cuboidal epithelium, whereas the intermediate and rugose portion has a columnar epithelium that is extensively folded and, on cross-section, appears to consist of many small channels. The ultrastructural features suggest that the cells have an absorptive or secretory function. The distal part of the sac – that part which is surgically accessible – has a low cuboidal epithelium with no features suggestive of much metabolic activity, and an extremely narrow lumen as the opposing layers of the lining of the sac are frequently in contact (Lundquist *et al.*, 1984).

Innervation of the cochlea

The cochlea is connected with the brain stem by afferent and efferent nerves. The afferent nerves, carrying sensory information to the brain stem, have their cell bodies in the spiral ganglion and their terminal dendrites make contact with the hair cells. The efferent nerves pass directly through the spiral ganglion, their cell bodies being located within the brain stem.

There are major differences in the make-up of the cochlear nerve and spiral ganglion between the frequently studied small mammals and man, and because of the difficulty in obtaining suitable material much remains to be learnt about the anatomy in man. Nevertheless, each cochlear nerve in young, normal individuals contains about 30 000 myelinated nerve fibres. These are virtually all afferent, as the efferent fibres travel initially in the superior vestibular nerve (see below). The afferent fibres pass through the modiolus to the spiral canal where their cell bodies are found. Ninety-five per cent of the spiral ganglion cells are large type I cells, but unlike those found in other species the majority are unmyelinated as the afferent fibre loses its myelin sheath a short distance before entering the cell body. These type I cell bodies, both myelinated and unmyelinated,

Figure 1.40 A portion of the macula of the utricle of the cat showing type I (HCI) and type II (HCII) sensory cells separated by supporting cells. Type I cells are partially surrounded by a nerve chalice (nc) which is the unmyelinated ending of a large myelinated nerve fibre (mf) seen crossing the basal lamina (bl). Vesiculated (v) and non-vesiculated (nv) nerve endings make synaptic contact with the infranuclear portion of type II cells. The nuclei of the supporting cells (NS) are located at the base of the epithelium. Each sensory cell has a single kinocilium (k) and many stereocilia (s) projecting from its free, endolymphatic surface. c: Capillary containing red blood cells. Picture width 26 μm (courtesy Ivan Hunter-Duvar and Raul Hinojosa)

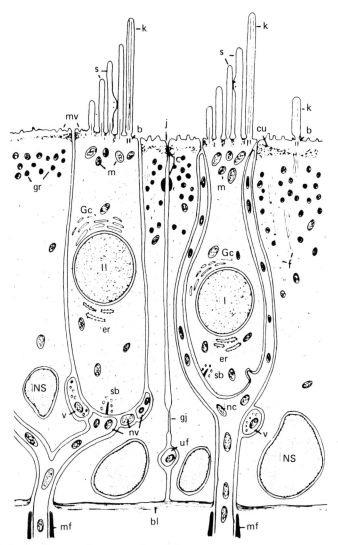

Figure 1.41 Diagram illustrating the general structure of vestibular sensory epithelium. The type I cell (I) is flask-shaped and is almost completely surrounded by a nerve chalice (nc). The type II cell (II) is cylindrical and innervated by vesiculated (v) and non-vesiculated (nv) button-like nerve terminals. b: Basal body; j: junctional complex; cu: cuticular plate; m: mitochondria; Gc: Golgi complex; er: endoplasmic reticulum; sb: synaptic bar; f: tonofilaments; gr: cytoplasmic vesicles in supporting cells; gj: gap junctions between supporting cells; uf: unmyelinated fibres; mf: myelinated fibres; NS: nucleus of supporting cell; bl: basal lamina. (Courtesy Ivan Hunter-Duvar and Raul Hinojosa)

through the modiolus to the spiral canal where their cell bodies are found. Ninety-five per cent of the spiral ganglion cells are large type I cells, but unlike those found in other species the majority are unmyelinated as the afferent fibre loses its myelin sheath a short distance before entering the cell body. These type I cell bodies, both myelinated and unmyelinated, are bipolar and their terminal dendrites subsequently become myelinated for a short distance as they pass through the bony spiral lamina to reach the inner hair cells (Ota and Kimura, 1980). Each inner hair cell has about 10 dendrites synapsing around the lower part of the cell body. The other 5% of spiral ganglion cells are small and may be myelinated or unmyelinated. The cell bodies can be unipolar or bipolar, and by analogy with animal work, it seems likely that the dendrites of these type II cells supply the outer hair cells. The fibres leave the spiral ganglion, run first across the floor of the tunnel of Corti and then descend the cochlea for up to 1 mm within an outer spiral bundle of nerve fibres before being distributed to 10 or more outer hair cells in various rows (Figure 1.45).

The efferent fibres are few in number and arise in

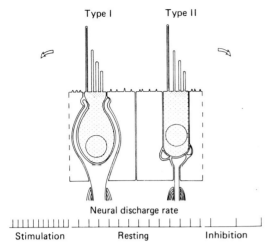

Type I   Type II

Neural discharge rate

| | | | | | | | | | | | | | | | | | | | | | | | | | | | | |
Stimulation   Resting   Inhibition

Figure 1.42 Diagram illustrating neural discharge pattern of vestibular sensory epithelium. As the capillary bundle is deflected towards the kinocilium the resting discharge increases as the cell is stimulated. Inhibition and a decreased firing rate occur when the opposite deflection occurs. The cells therefore have 'polarity'

from the superior cervical ganglion and are independent of the blood supply, whereas others originate in the stellate ganglion and arise from the plexus that surrounds the vertebral, basilar, anterior, inferior, cerebellar and labyrinthine arteries (see Spoendlin, 1984 for review).

The vestibular nerve

The vestibular nerve, like the cochlear nerve, contains afferent and efferent fibres as well as adrenergic sympathetic fibres. Unlike the cochlear nerve, however, there is a large number of efferent fibres and only 19 000 to 20 000 afferent fibres in the young adult. The calibre of the afferent fibres varies considerably between 2 and 15 μm (Spoendlin, 1972) but are, on the whole, larger than their cochlear counterparts. The distribution of the various branches has already been described.

The vestibular ganglion (Scarpa's ganglion) contains the bipolar cell bodies of the afferent neurons as well as the efferent fibres that pass straight through. The ganglion lies at the lateral end of the internal auditory meatus partly covering the vestibular crest and being partially separated into a superior and inferior portion. The human vestibular ganglion is distinct from all other species examined in that the perikaryon is not myelinated, instead it is covered by thin layers of satellite cells. Often the cells are arranged in pairs, closely abutting each other, an arrangement that has led to speculation that incoming information may be modulated by, or transmitted to, adjacent ganglion cells through ephases (Felix *et*

quently supply the inner hair cells, but the majority run out across the tunnel of Corti as tunnel crossing fibres, to branch and terminate as large vesiculated nerve endings on several outer hair cells. The efferent innervation is most dense at the base of the cochlea but gradually diminishes towards the apex.

The other class of fibres entering the cochlea are adrenergic sympathetic fibres, some of which come

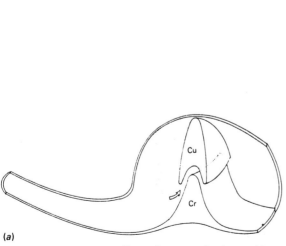

(a)

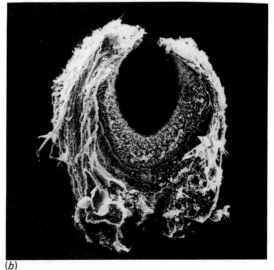

(b)

Figure 1.43 (a) Diagram of bisected semicircular duct and its associated ampulla (see also Figure 1.6). The arrow indicates that, during angular acceleration, the endolymph flows across the surface of the crista, beneath the cupula. Cu: Cupula; Cr: crista. (b) Scanning electron micrograph of the crista from the ampulla of the lateral semicircular canal of a young adult human. The dense carpet of stereocilia is apparent. Marker 100 μm

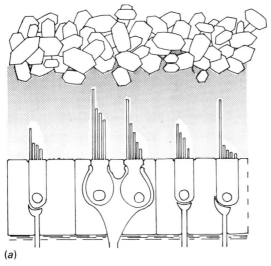

(a)

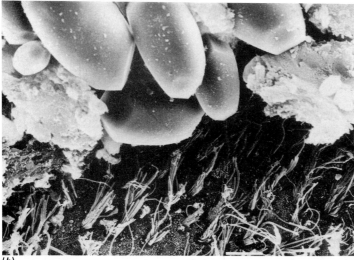

(b)

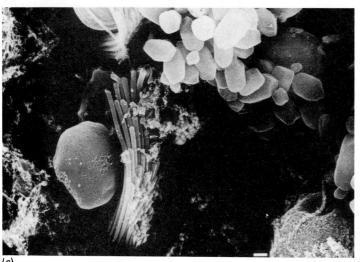

(c)

Figure 1.44 (*a*) Diagrammatic relationship of the sensory cells of the macula to the otoconial membrane. The ciliary bundles are embedded in the honeycomb-like meshwork of the gelatinous layer, which also contains the otoconia. (*b*) The surface of the human saccular macula. Some of the otoconia have been dislodged to reveal the amorphous gelatinous layer and the underlying sensory epithelium with the clusters of cilia. Picture width 100 μm. (*c*) A closer view of a single sensory cell and the otoconia from the striolar region. The wide range in size of the otoconia can be appreciated from this and the preceding micrograph. A fine fibrillar meshwork, the remains of the gelatinous layer, clings to the surface of the cilia and macula. A globular body is seen on the surface of the macula partly obscured by the bundle of stereocilia

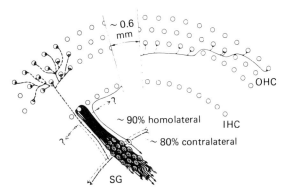

Figure 1.45 Horizontal innervation scheme of the organ of Corti in the cat. Although there are some differences between this animal and man the general pattern is much the same. The afferent nerve fibres are represented by solid lines, the efferent by interrupted lines. The efferent innervation of the outer hair cells (thick interrupted lines) originates (up to 80%) from the contralateral superior olivary complex while the efferents of the inner hair cell system (thin interrupted lines) originate (up to 90%) from the homolateral superior olivary complex. Virtually all of the afferent fibres (thick solid lines) arise from the inner hairs, only a few from the outer hair cells (thin solid lines). (Courtesy of Heinrich Spoendlin)

al., 1987). Proximal to this, the vestibular nerve is a single bundle on its way to the brain stem by way of the cerebellopontine angle.

The course of cochleovestibular bundle

In the internal auditory meatus the vestibular nerve, comprising the superior, inferior and singular nerves, runs medially to merge with the cochlear division. The two major divisions, now one bundle, can be identified more medially by a shallow groove running longitudinally along the bundle. This is a helpful guide to separating the cochlear and vestibular divisions during a vestibular neurectomy, although it is common for some of the outer fibres of the cochlear division to be sacrificed. These fibres carry high-frequency information and their loss may not be clinically significant.

The facial and cochleovestibular nerves rotate about 90° in passing through the internal auditory meatus and cerebellopontine angle so that by the time they reach the brain stem the facial nerve is rostral to the cochleovestibular bundle (i.e. it is further up the brain stem). The two bundles, facial and cochleovestibular, are nearly always separated at the brain stem by the anterior inferior cerebellar artery or a branch of it which is therefore a useful surgical landmark and is protective of the facial nerve. The anterior inferior cerebellar artery supplies the inferior and lateral parts of the under surface of the cerebellum, and has as a branch the labyrinthine artery. Preservation of the anterior inferior cerebellar artery

is therefore extremely important during surgery in this region.

The central connections of the vestibular nuclei are described in more detail in Chapter 4.

The blood supply of the labyrinth

The labyrinth is supplied principally from the labyrinthine artery which is usually a branch of the anterior inferior cerebellar artery, although it may arise directly from the basilar or even the vertebral arteries. The artery passes down the internal auditory meatus to divide into an anterior vestibular and a common cochlear artery, which subsequently divides into the cochlear artery and the vestibulocochlear artery.

The anterior vestibular artery supplies the vestibular nerve, much of the utricle and parts of the semicircular ducts.

The vestibulocochlear artery, on arrival at the modiolus, in the region of the basal turn of the cochlea, divides into its terminal vestibular and cochlear branches, which take opposite directions. The vestibular branch supplies the saccule, the greater part of the semicircular canals, and the basal end of the cochlea; the cochlear branch, running a spiral course around the modiolus, ends by anastomosing with the cochlear artery. The vestibular and cochlear branches both supply capillary areas in the spiral ganglion, the osseous spiral lamina, the limbus, and the spiral ligament.

In the internal auditory canal, the cochlear artery runs a spiral course around the acoustic nerve. In the cochlea, it runs a serpentine course around the modiolus, as the spiral modiolar artery, which is an end artery. Arterioles leave the artery, to run either into the spiral lamina or across the roof of the scala vestibuli (Figure 1.46). Both sets of arteries end in

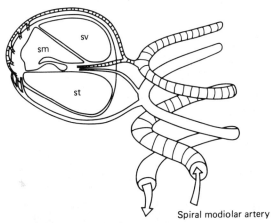

Figure 1.46 Diagram of the vascular supply to the organ of Corti and stria vascularis. sv: Scala vestibuli; sm: scala media; st: scala tympani

capillary networks either in the spiral lamina or the stria vascularis on the lateral wall of the cochlear duct. The capillaries from the lateral wall drain into venules which run under the floor of the scala tympani to empty into modiolar veins which run spirally down the modiolus. The apical regions are drained by way of an anterior spiral vein, while the basal regions drain into the posterior spiral vein. These two branches of the spiral vein join with the anterior and posterior branches of the vestibular vein, in the region of the basal turn, to form the vein of the cochlea, which empties into the jugular bulb.

The vestibular labyrinth is drained from the anterior part by the anterior vestibular vein, which becomes the labyrinthine vein and accompanies the artery of the same name, usually ending in the superior petrosal sinus; and also from the posterior part by the vein of the vestibular aqueduct which passes alongside the endolymphatic duct to the sigmoid sinus.

This description of the vascular supply of the cochlea is based on the work of Axelsson (1968).

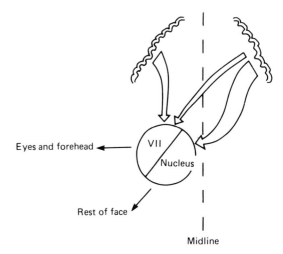

Figure 1.47 Schematic representation of innervation of nerve VII nucleus. The major supply is from the contralateral motor cortex but there is also a contribution from the ipsilateral side which supplies that part of the nucleus involved with innervating the muscles of the forehead and those around the eye

The facial nerve

The VIIth cranial nerve – the facial or intermediofacial – is a mixed nerve containing:
1 Motor fibres to the muscles of facial expression, the buccinator, stapedius, digastric and stylohyoid
2 Taste fibres from the palate and anterior two-thirds of the tongue
3 Secretomotor parasympathetic fibres to the lacrimal and nasal glands, and to the submandibular and sublingual salivary glands
4 Sensory fibres supplying part of the concha of the auricle and sometimes an area of skin behind the ear and part of the mucous membrane in the supratonsillar recess.

The motor fibres have their cell bodies in the facial nucleus in the pons. The nucleus receives pyramidal fibres from the contralateral motor cortex and a smaller number from the same side. The contralateral fibres reach all of the nucleus, while the ipsilateral fibres supply those parts of the motor nucleus involved with innervating the forehead and the muscles around the eyes (Figure 1.47). Other fibres also play on the facial motor nucleus and are involved in reflex movements. They come from the superior colliculus (an optic reflex centre), from the superior olive (acoustic reflex), as well as from sensory V nuclei and the nucleus of the solitary tract. The various inputs are involved in blinking and closing the eyes in response to strong light or touch on the cornea (corneal reflex), contraction and relaxation of the stapedius in response to sound, and sucking movements following the introduction of food into the mouth. Other fibres arrive from higher centres by way of the red nucleus, the mesencephalic reticular formation and probably the globus pallidus, and have been assumed to be involved with emotional facial movement.

The motor fibres leaving the facial nucleus do not pass directly out of the pons but first run medially and dorsally towards the floor of ventricle IV, turn around the nerve VI nucleus and then stream out laterally to leave the pons on the lateral aspect of the brain stem.

The sensory root of the facial nerve enters the brain stem as a separate nerve – the nervus intermedius. It carries the sensory fibres from the conchal skin and the supratonsillar recess, and the taste fibres from palate and tongue. The ganglion associated with these sensory fibres is the geniculate ganglion and the central processes of the unipolar ganglion cells leave the trunk of the facial nerve in the internal auditory meatus, as the nervus intermedius, to enter the brain stem at the lower border of the pons, and pass to the upper part of the nucleus of the solitary tract (tractus solitarius).

Secretomotor parasympathetic fibres also run in the nervus intermedius and have the superior salivatory nucleus as their origin.

At the fundus of the internal auditory meatus, the motor facial nerve which, with the addition of the nervus intermedius, is now complete, enters the facial canal. In this canal, the nerve, surrounded by cerebrospinal fluid, runs between the cochlea anteriorly, the superior semicircular canal posteriorly and with the vestibule beneath it. This labyrinthine segment is the narrowest part of the facial canal with an average diameter of only 0.68 mm at the site of entry of the nerve (Fisch, 1979). As the nerve reaches the medial wall of the epitympanic recess, it turns sharply backwards to make an angle of about 60° with the subsequent tympanic segment. At this turn – the geniculum – lies the geniculate ganglion which is a reddish asymmetric swelling (Figure 1.48).

The tympanic portion of the nerve now begins as it runs posteriorly on the medial wall of the tympanic cavity. The nerve is surrounded by a bony shell and stands out clearly just above the promontory and oval window recess, but below the prominence of the lateral semicircular canal. The anterior end of the tympanic portion is marked by the processus cochleariformis which is a stable landmark rarely eroded by disease. From this level, the nerve slopes downwards and backwards at an angle of about 30° from the horizontal. Above the oval window recess the nerve starts to curve inferiorly, and at the level of the pyramid enters the descending or mastoid portion of its intratemporal course. At this pyramidal turn, the short process of the incus always lies lateral to the nerve. In the descending portion, the nerve lies posterior and deep to both the tympanic annulus and the tympanomastoid suture line in the posterior wall of the external auditory meatus. This descending portion of the nerve lies deep within the mastoid portion of the temporal bone, rarely less than 1.8 cm from the outer surface of the bone in the adult (Figure 1.49).

The nerve emerges from the stylomastoid foramen to enter the neck. The posterior belly of digastric is attached to the digastric groove on the inferior surface of the mastoid process. This groove leads forwards to the stylomastoid foramen and the muscle provides a valuable landmark for the nerve. From the stylomastoid foramen, the nerve turns forward and passes laterally to the base of the styloid process and enters the parotid gland. Within the gland, the nerve separates into two primary divisions – an upper temporofacial and a lower cervicofacial. Each of these

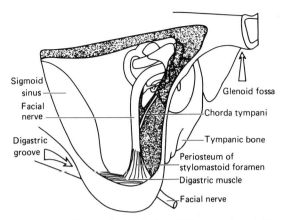

Figure 1.49 The facial nerve in the middle ear and mastoid segment as seen from a cortical mastoidectomy approach combined with a posterior tympanotomy. The stippling indicates the surface of bone that has been drilled during the cortical mastoidectomy

breaks up into several terminal branches which interconnect as the parotid plexus. From this plexus arise the terminal branches of the nerve.

During its course, the facial nerve makes communication with many other nerves, although the precise function of these is often unknown (Table 1.5).

Branches of the facial nerve

From the geniculate ganglion

1 *Greater (superficial) petrosal nerve*. This leaves the geniculate ganglion anteriorly, runs forwards and receives a twig from the tympanic plexus. It enters the middle cranial fossa outside the dura, and runs in a groove in the bone to pass beneath the trigeminal ganglion where it is joined by the deep petrosal nerve from the sympathetic plexus on the internal

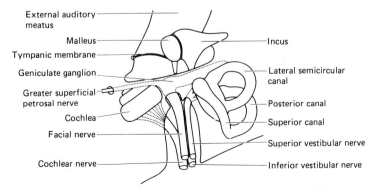

Figure 1.48 Passage of the facial nerve through the right internal auditory meatus and middle ear, as seen from an approach through the middle cranial fossa

Table 1.5 Branches of communication of the facial nerve

Location	Connection
Internal auditory meatus	Vestibulocochlear nerve
Geniculate ganglion	Greater superficial petrosal nerve to pterygopalatine ganglion
	Via lesser petrosal nerve to otic ganglion
	Sympathetic plexus on middle meningeal artery
Facial canal	Auricular branch of vagus
At stylomastoid foramen	IX, X, greater auricular and auriculotemporal nerves
Behind the ear	Lesser occipital nerve
On the face	V nerve
In neck	Transverse cutaneous nerve of neck

carotid artery. The nerve is now called the nerve of the pterygoid canal and it runs through this canal to end in the pterygopalatine ganglion. Taste fibres pass on without interruption in the palatine branches of the ganglion. The secretomotor fibres in the nerve synapse within the ganglion and carry on by way of the zygomatic and lacrimal nerves to the lacrimal gland, and through the nasal and palatine nerves to the nasal and palatine glands.

Branches within the facial canal

1 *Nerve to stapedius.* This arises from the facial nerve as the latter begins its descent, and reaches the muscle through a small canal in the base of the pyramid.
2 *The chorda tympani.* This usually arises above the stylomastoid foramen but can occasionally leave the facial nerve outside the temporal bone and re-enter by way of a separate foramen. Its course in the middle ear has been described already and the nerve leaves the temporal bone by the petrotympanic fissure. It descends, sometimes grooving the medial surface of the spine of the sphenoid, and passes deep to the lateral pterygoid muscle to join the lingual nerve. The parasympathetic secretomotor fibres leave the lingual to enter the submandibular ganglion, which is suspended from the nerve by two fine neural filaments. The secretomotor fibres synapse within the ganglion and continue to supply the submandibular and sublingual salivary glands as well as other minor salivary glands in the floor of the mouth.

The majority of fibres in the chorda tympani are, however, taste fibres and these are derived from the mucous membrane of the presulcal part of the tongue but not from the vallate papillae which lie just in front of the sulcus.

Branches in the neck and face

1 *The postauricular branch* arises close to the stylomastoid foramen and runs up between the external auditory canal and anterior surface of the mastoid. It has connections with other nerves as it continues on to supply the posterior auricular muscle, the intrinsic muscles of the posterior aspect of the pinna and the occipital muscle.
2 *The digastric branch* also arises close to the stylomastoid foramen and supplies the posterior belly of the digastric.
3 *The stylohyoid branch* supplies the stylohyoid muscle and arises near or in conjunction with the digastric branch.

Branches from the parotid plexus

These are highly variable, as is the site of division of the facial nerve into temporofacial and cervicofacial divisions. Nevertheless, five major branches are nearly always found.

1 *Temporal branches* cross the zygomatic arch and supply intrinsic muscles on the lateral surface of the auricle and the anterior and superior auricular muscles. Other branches supply the frontal belly of the occipitofrontalis, the orbicularis oculi and corrugator.
2 *Zygomatic branches* run parallel to the zygomatic arch and also innervate orbicularis oculi. Some of the lower branches may join with the buccal branches to form an infraorbital plexus which innervates the muscles in the middle part of the face.
3 *Buccal branches* pass horizontally forward to the muscles of the middle part of the face. These include the procerus, orbicularis oculi, zygomaticus, levator anguli oris, levator labii superioris, buccinator, orbicularis oris and the small muscles of the nose.
4 *The mandibular branch* runs forward below the angle of the mandible under platysma and then turns upwards and forwards to cross the mandible under cover of depressor anguli oris which it supplies. It continues onwards and supplies the orbicularis oris and other muscles of the lips and chin.
5 *The cervical branch* leaves the lower part of the

parotid gland and runs down the neck under cover of platysma which it supplies.

Blood supply of the facial nerve

The facial nerve is supplied by the anterior inferior cerebellar artery in its intracranial course, by the superficial petrosal branch of the middle meningeal artery, and by the stylomastoid branch of the post-auricular artery in its intratemporal course. Outside the skull, the stylomastoid artery, the posterior auricular or occipital, the superficial temporal and transverse facial artery are all involved.

The veins form a plexus around the nerve, and efferent veins run from this through the nerve sheath to lie on its outer surface. From the intratemporal portion, the venous drainage leaves the canal at the stylomastoid foramen and at the geniculum where it enters the venae comitantes of the stylomastoid and superficial petrosal arteries respectively.

The central auditory system

The brain stem nuclei

The central auditory system consists of a series of ascending or afferent connections (in common with

other sensory pathways) between the cochlea and the auditory cortex.

The ascending pathway consists of fibres running from the cochlea to make connections within the first nucleus of the system, the cochlear nucleus. From this point onwards, connections are made between a series of nuclei, by tracts, some travelling contralaterally and others remaining ipsilateral (Figure 1.50).

From the cochlear nuclei, tracts lead to further brain stem nuclei. Connections are then made in the ipsilateral and contralateral superior olivary complex – thus bilateral representation is present at this point, and from then on. From the superior olivary complex, tracts travel via the lateral lemniscus to the inferior colliculus, and from this to the medial geniculate body. Finally, they leave the brain stem and terminate in the auditory cortex.

The cochlear nuclei

Each afferent auditory nerve fibre runs into the ventral cochlear nucleus where it divides or branches, sending an ascending branch forward or rostrally to the anteroventral cochlear nucleus and one posteriorly and dorsally through the posteroventral cochlear nucleus into the dorsal cochlear nucleus. Each division of the cochlear nuclei, like all other higher auditory nuclei, is tonotopically arranged, and the best or characteristic frequencies of the neurons make a spatially ordered map. Thus the orderly spatial representation of fibres with various characteristic frequencies in the cochlear nerve is preserved in the three divisions of the cochlear nuclei (Figure 1.51).

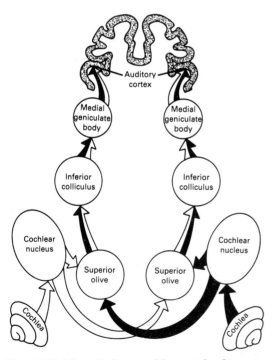

Figure 1.50 Schematic diagram of the central auditory system. The main pathways and nuclei are shown for both cochleae. Bilateral representation of the input from both cochleae is achieved at the superior olive and in all areas above this level

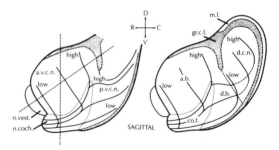

Figure 1.51 Cochlear nuclei cut at two levels in a sagittal plane to show the bifurcation pattern of tonotopic afferent fibres. D; dorsal, C; caudal, V; ventral, R; rostral. Branches that represent high and low frequencies are labelled accordingly: a.b.: ascending cochlear branches; a.v.c.n.: anteroventral cochlear nucleus; co.f.: cochlear nerve fibre; d.b.: descending cochlear branches; d.c.n.: dorsal cochlear nucleus; gr.c.l.: granular cell layer; m.l.: molecular layer; n.coch.: cochlear nerve; n.vest.: vestibular nerve; p.v.c.n.: posteroventral cochlear nucleus; (From Osen 1969)

In the anteroventral cochlear nucleus, the ascending branch of each afferent contacts a spherical cell by means of a particularly large synaptic ending

1/1/48 *Anatomy and ultrastructure of the human ear*

known as an end-bulb of Held. Recordings made from these cells suggest that they have 'primary-like' responses, in other words, their responses are very similar to those recorded in the auditory nerve fibres, being well-preserved by this particularly 'secure' type of synaptic connection.

A number of other cell types are also found in the ventral cochlear nucleus; examples include multipolar cells, globular cells and octopus cells. These cells may be contacted by collaterals from the branches of the afferent fibres and different kinds of physiological responses can be correlated with some of these cell types with varying degrees of certainty.

The dorsal cochlear nucleus is a layered structure, at least in cats and rodents. Interestingly, the dorsal cochlear nucleus is comparatively small in primates and cetaceans (whales). The outermost molecular layer contains few cells but consists mostly of closely packed axons and dendrites of cells from the dorsal cochlear nucleus. The next layer, the granular layer, is identified by a concentration of small granule cells which are local or intrinsic excitatory neurons. Within this layer lie the larger cell bodies of the pyramidal or fusiform cells (the nomenclature used depends on the author). These cells have two groups of dendrites, one orientated towards the surface of the nucleus (the apical dendrites) and one group towards the centre (basal dendrites). The descending branches of at least some of the auditory nerve fibres apparently terminate on the basal dendrites and bodies of these cells. Between the molecular layer and granular layer lie the cell bodies of a group of inhibitory interneurons called the cartwheel cells. When recordings are made from the granule layer of the dorsal cochlear nucleus, complex firing patterns are recorded from the pyramidal cells which suggest that both excitatory and inhibitory inputs are playing on these cells. The details of this circuitry have not yet been determined, but in contrast to the spherical cells of the anteroventral cochlear nucleus, it seems that the pyramidal cells may be extracting features from the auditory stimulus which require a modification of the primary input.

Thus the three divisions of the cochlear nucleus show broadly different response properties, and may have correspondingly different functions. In general, the neurons of the anteroventral cochlear nucleus have properties rather similar to those of auditory nerve fibres and may well function as a simple relay for afferent information. Cells of the dorsal cochlear nucleus, on the other hand, have more complex response properties, and may contribute to complex signal analysis even at this early stage in the auditory pathway. Their output axons bypass the next nucleus in the auditory pathway, the superior olivary complex and end in the nuclei of the lateral lemniscus and the inferior colliculus. The properties of many neurons of the posteroventral cochlear nucleus are intermediate between those of the other two nuclei.

Superior olivary complex

The anteroventral and posteroventral cochlear nuclei project mainly to the superior olivary complex. This superior olivary complex has several component nuclei. The largest, known as the lateral superior olivary nucleus, appears S-shaped in frontal sections. It receives an input from both sides. The ipsilateral input is predominantly excitatory and the contralateral input predominantly inhibitory. The nucleus is therefore responsive to interaural intensity disparities and may use these to code the direction of a sound in space. Another component nucleus, the medial superior olivary nucleus, is responsive to disparities in interaural timing and therefore can be said to code the direction of a sound in space on the basis of timing differences. The spherical cells of the anteroventral cochlear nucleus are known to send axons to both these nuclei.

Inferior colliculus

The next major nucleus of the auditory pathway is the inferior colliculus which receives afferents bilaterally from the superior olivary complex and from the cochlear nuclei, mainly from the contralateral dorsal cochlear nucleus. The inferior colliculus is tonotopically organized (as are the nuclei of the superior olivary complex described above) and seems to play an important part in many auditory reflexes.

Medial geniculate body

The medial geniculate body is the specific thalamic auditory relay. It receives its input from the inferior colliculus and projects to the auditory cortex. It has three divisions, only one of which, the ventral division, is a specifically auditory area. The medial and dorsal divisions receive other kinds of inputs as well, e.g. somatosensory.

The auditory cortex

The auditory cortex is situated on the surface of the brain in cats, but is hidden in the lateral or Sylvian fissure in primates. The core area, which is the primary auditory cortex, receives its input from the ventral division of the medial geniculate body. It is tonotopically organized into isofrequency strips – low frequencies are represented rostrally and high frequencies caudally. (It is interesting to note here that tuning curves recorded from individual cells retain their sharpness at all levels of the auditory pathway.) A discrete columnar organization of frequency is obvious in the auditory cortex, but although cells lying in the same radial direction have similar characteristic frequencies, there do not appear to be any sudden jumps in frequency as an electrode is moved tangentially through the cortex. Binaural dominance, on the other hand, does seem to relate to the existence of discrete columns. Cells of the same binaural dominance (e.g. ipsilateral ear excitatory, contralateral ear inhibitory) lie in the same radial direction in the cortex and are segregated into discrete strips running along the cortical surface at roughly right angles to the isofrequency strips.

The centrifugal pathways

The centrifugal or efferent pathways are parallel to the afferent pathways along the entire length of the system from the cortex down to the hair cells. At many points along the auditory pathway, they run adjacent to, but not actually in, the tracts and nuclei principally associated with the ascending system. The descending pathways are thought to perform some sort of control function but the details are not well known.

The olivocochlear bundle, which was mentioned earlier in connection with the cochlea, may reduce the auditory input when the subject is attending to stimuli in another modality. The olivocochlear bundle also seems to affect auditory discrimination in the presence of noise. The cochlear nucleus receives branches of the olivocochlear bundle and other centrifugal fibres from the superior olivary complex and from higher auditory nuclei including the nuclei of the lateral lemniscus and the inferior colliculus. The centrifugal fibres are both inhibitory and excitatory (Figure 1.52).

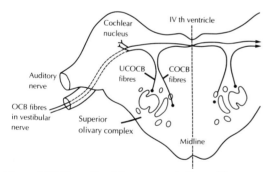

Figure 1.52 The paths of the uncrossed olivocochlear bundle (UCOCB) and the crossed olivocochlear bundle (COCB) are shown on a schematic cross-section of the cat's brain stem. OCB indicates the combined olivocochlear bundle. (From Osen 1969)

(I am indebted to Carol Hackney for this description of the central auditory pathways.)

References

ALBERTI, P. W. (1964) Epithelial migration over tympanic membrane and external canal. *Journal of Laryngology and Otology*, **78**, 808–830

ANSON, B. J. and DONALDSON, J. A. (1981) *Surgical Anatomy of the Temporal Bone*, 3rd edn. Philadelphia: W. B. Saunders

AXELSSON A, (1968) The vascular anatomy of the cochlea in the guinea pig and in man. *Acta Otolaryngologica Suppl*, **243**, 6–134

BREDBERG, G. (1968) Cellular pattern and nerve supply of the human organ of Corti. *Acta Otolaryngologica Suppl*, **236**, 1–135

CHOLE, R. A. (1985) Petrous apicitis: surgical anatomy. *Annals of Otology, Rhinology and Laryngology*, **94**, 251–257

DOHLMAN, G. F. (1981) Critical review of the concept of cupula function. *Acta Otolaryngologica Suppl*, **376**, 1–30

FELIX, H., DE FRAISSINETTE, A., JOHNSSON, L.-G. and GLEESON, M. J. (1993) Morphological features of human Reissner's membrane. *Acta Otolaryngologica*, **113**, 321–325

FELIX, H., HOFFMAN, V., WRIGHT, A. and GLEESON, M. J. (1987) Ultrastructural findings on human Scarpa's ganglion. *Acta Otolaryngologica*, Suppl. 436, 85–92

FISCH, U. (1979) Facial paralysis. In: *Clinical Otolaryngology*, edited by A. G. D. Maran and P. M. Stell. Oxford: Blackwell. pp. 65–84

FORGE, A., LIN, L. I., CORWIN, J. T. and NEVILL, G. (1993) Ultrastructural evidence for hair cell regeneration in the mammalian inner ear. *Science*, **259**, 1616–1619

FURNESS, D. N. and HACKNEY, C. M. (1985) Cross links between stereocilia in the guinea pig cochlea. *Hearing Research*, **18**, 177–188

GACEK, R. R. (1983) Cupulolithiasis and posterior ampullary nerve transection. *Annals of Otology, Rhinology and Laryngology*, Suppl. 112, 25–30

GIBSON, W. P. R. (1978) The myogenic (sonomotor) responses. In: *Essentials of Clinical Electric Response Audiometry*. Edinburgh: Churchill Livingstone. pp. 133–156

GLEESON, M. J., FELIX, H. and NEIVERGELT, J. (1991) Quantitative and qualitative analysis of the human middle ear mucosa. In: *The Eustachian Tube, Basic Aspects*, edited by J. Sade. Amsterdam: Kugler and Ghedini. pp. 125–131

HARADA, Y. (1979) Formation area of statoconia. *Scanning Electron Microscopy*, **III**, 963–966

HENTZER, E. (1969) Ultrastructure of the human tympanic membrane. *Acta Otolaryngologica*, **63**, 376–390

JOHNSON, A. and HAWKE, M. (1985) Cell shape in the migratory epidermis of the external auditory canal. *Journal of Otolaryngology*, **14**, 273–281

KRONESTER-FREI, A. (1979) Localization of the marginal zone of the tectorial membrane *in situ* unfixed and with *in vivo* like ionic milieu. *Archives of Otorhinolaryngology*, **224**, 3–9

LIM, D. J. (1984) The development and structure of otoconia. In: *Ultrastructural Atlas of the Inner Ear*, edited by I. Friedmann and J. Ballantyne. London: Butterworths. pp. 245–249

LUNDQUIST, P. -G. R., ANDERSEN, H., GALEY, F. R. and BAGGERSJO-BACK, D. (1984) Ultrastructural morphology of endolymphatic duct and sac. In: *Ultrastructural Atlas of the Inner Ear*, edited by I. Friedmann and J. Ballantyne. London: Butterworths. pp. 309–325

MICHAELS, L. and SOUCEK, S. (1989) Development of the stratified squamous epithelium of the human tympanic membrane and external canal: the origin of auditory epithelial migration. *American Journal of Anatomy*, **184**, 334–344

NOMURA, Y. (1984) Otological significance of the round window. *Advances in Oto-Rhinolaryngology*, no. 33, edited by C. R. Pfaltz. Basel: Kargel. pp. 1–184

OSEN, K. K. (1969) The intrinsic organization of the cochlear nuclei in the cat. *Acta Otolaryngologica,* **67,** 352–359

OTA, C. Y. and KIMURA, R. S. (1980) Ultrastructural study of the human spiral ganglion. *Acta Otolaryngologica,* **89,** 53–62

PAPANGELOU, L. (1972) Study of the human internal auditory canal. *Laryngoscope,* **82,** 617–624

PROCTOR, B. (1964) The development of the middle ear spaces and their surgical significance. *Journal of Laryngology and Otology,* **78,** 631–649

RETZIUS, G. (1884) *Das Gehororgan der Wilbetiere,* vol. II. Stockholm: Samson and Wallin

SADE, J. (1966) Middle ear mucosa. *Archives of Otolaryngology,* **84,** 137–143

SPOENDLIN, H. (1972) Innervation densities of the cochlea. *Acta Otolaryngologica,* **73,** 233–243

SPOENDLIN, H. (1984) Primary neurons and synapses. In: *Ultrastructural Atlas of the Inner Ear,* edited by I. Friedmann and J. Ballantyne. London: Butterworths. pp. 133–164

STONE, M. and FULGHUM, R. S. (1984) Bactericidal activity of wet cerumen. *Annals of Otology, Rhinology and Laryngology,* **93,** 183–186

STREETER, G. L. (1922) Development of the auricle in the human embryo. *Contributions to Embryology,* **14,** 111–138

TILNEY, L. G., DEROSIER, D. J. and MULROY, M. J. (1980) The organization of actin filaments in the stereocilia of cochlear hair cells. *Journal of Cell Biology,* **86,** 244–258

TOS, M. and BAK-PEDERSEN, K. (1976) Goblet cell population in the normal middle ear and eustachian tube of children and adults. *Annals of Otology,* **85,** (Suppl. 25), 44–50

ULEHLOVA, L., VOLDRICH, L. and JANISCH, R. (1987) Correlative study of sensory cell density and cochlear length in humans. *Hearing Research,* **28,** 147–151

VALVASSORI, G. E. and PIERCE, R. H. (1964) The normal internal auditory canal. *American Journal of Roentgenology,* **92,** 1233–1242

WALBY, A. P. (1985) Scala tympani measurement. *Annals of Otology, Rhinology and Laryngology,* **94,** 393–397

WRIGHT, A. (1984) Dimensions of cochlear stereocilia in man and the guinea pig. *Hearing Research,* **13,** 89–98

WRIGHT, A., DAVIS, A., BREDBERG, G., ULEHLOVA, L. and SPENCER, H. (1987) Hair cell distributions in the normal human cochlea. *Acta Otolaryngologica,* Suppl. 444, 1–48

2

Physiology of hearing

James O. Pickles

Sound and its analysis

An understanding of some of the basic physical properties of sound is a prerequisite for understanding the performance of the auditory system. The transmission of a sound wave from a loudspeaker can be seen in Figure 2.1. The wave shows variations in the pressure of the air, and the velocity and displacement of the molecules. This wave is traversing freely and, in such a case, when the pressure of the wave is at a maximum, the forward velocity of the air molecules is also at a maximum. However, the *displacement* of the molecules lags by one-quarter of a cycle. The displacement is around the mean position; the sound wave does not cause any net flow of air in the direction of motion, and the actual air pressure variations are only a small variation around the mean atmospheric pressure. A sound which is loud enough to be at the pain threshold, 130 dB sound pressure level (SPL), is nevertheless only sufficient to produce pressure variations which are 0.2% of the resting atmospheric pressure. A sound wave as shown in Figure 2.1 has two basic properties: *intensity*, which has the subjective correlate of loudness; and

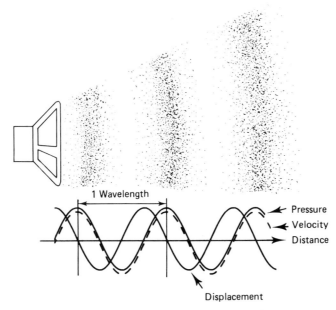

Figure 2.1 The pressure, velocity, and displacement relations in a progressive sound wave

frequency, which has the subjective correlate of pitch.

The pressure and intensity of sound waves

Basic relations

The peak pressure of the sound wave (P) can be related to peak velocity of the air molecules (V) by a constant of proportionality R:

$$P = RV \qquad (1)$$

Here, R is called the impedance, and is a function of the medium in which the sound is travelling. From Figure 2.1, it can be seen that the pressure and velocity of the waveform vary together during the cycle. For such a wave, the same constant of proportionality holds over the whole cycle. This is the case if the wave is travelling freely and progressively in its medium. On the other hand, the situation becomes more complex if there are edges or other boundaries making reflections because, in such cases, the peak of pressure does not necessarily coincide with the peak of velocity. The ratio varies over the cycle and a simple number cannot be used to represent the ratio, and hence the impedance, of the air. Therefore, the impedance is a function not only of the medium alone, but also of its surroundings.

One basic property of the sound wave is that it involves the transfer of energy. The *intensity* is the *power* transmitted by the wave through a unit area. The intensity depends on both the pressure and the velocity, and is an average taken over a whole cycle. If the sound wave is sinusoidal (as in Figure 2.1), then there is a very simple relation between the power, the peak velocity and the peak pressure:

$$\text{Intensity} = \text{Peak pressure} \times \text{peak velocity}/2 \quad (2)$$

The factor of 2 is a function of the shape of the waveform. By using the dependence on R, it can also be expressed as a function only of P or V:

$$\begin{aligned} \text{Intensity} &= \text{Peak pressure}^2/2R \\ &= R \times \text{peak velocity}^2/2 \end{aligned} \quad (2a)$$

This equation reveals the important parameters of the sound wave intensity. If the intensity of the sound wave is constant, the peak velocity and the peak pressure are also constant. The relation does not depend on the frequency of the sound wave. By contrast, the *displacements* produced by a sound wave do vary with frequency if the sound intensity is constant. The displacements vary in inverse proportion to the frequency, so that for a constant intensity, low frequency vibrations produce greater displacements.

The relation in equation (**2**) depends on the exact shape of the waveform. This dependency can be removed by measuring not the *peak* velocities and

pressures but what is known as the root mean square (RMS) values. The RMS value is calculated by taking the value of the pressure or velocity at each moment in the waveform, squaring it, and then taking the average of all the squared values over the waveform. Finally, the square root is taken of the average. The RMS value is useful because the same relation between intensity, pressure and velocity holds over all shapes of waveform:

$$\begin{aligned} \text{Intensity} &= \text{RMS pressure}^2/R \\ &= \text{RMS velocity}^2 \times R \end{aligned} \quad (3)$$

The intensity of sound in air (i.e. in a medium with a constant and known value of R) can be measured by using the RMS pressure to specify the intensity of the wave. Pressure variations are also easily measurable by microphones. Therefore, the term 'sound pressure' is often used interchangeably with the term intensity. Caution is necessary, however, because in a medium of very different impedance, such as water, the intensity for a certain sound pressure will be very different (less in this case).

Decibels

A physicist would measure the RMS pressure in physical units, such as newtons/square metre (N/m² or pascals). Nevertheless, from the point of view of understanding the performance of the auditory system, it is easier to use a scale in which the vast range of sound pressures, from absolute threshold to pain threshold, is described by a convenient range of numbers. A wide range of numbers can be compressed into a smaller range by expressing the numbers as logarithms. The use of this method has other advantages, because the final scale corresponds in certain respects with the way in which sounds are heard. For instance, equal increments in sensation correspond approximately to equal increments in numbers on the logarithmic scale. The scale is constructed by taking the logarithm of the sound intensity. However, the logarithm operation is best performed on quantities without dimensions, e.g. ratios rather than, for instance, intensities. Therefore, the ratio of sound intensity to a reference intensity is used. If logarithms to the base 10 are used, the resulting units are called bels, after Alexander Graham Bell, the inventor of the telephone, since the scale was first used in telephony. The bel turns out to be rather too large to be convenient; therefore, the numbers are multiplied by 10 to obtain units in terms of a smaller unit, one-tenth the size, known as the decibel. The formula for calculating decibels (abbreviated dB) is therefore as follows:

$$\text{Number of dB} = 10\log_{10}\left[\frac{\text{sound intensity}}{\text{reference intensity}}\right] \quad (4)$$

Because it is usual to measure pressures rather than intensities, and because the intensity varies as the *square* of the pressure, decibels can be expressed in terms of pressure ratios, multiplying the logarithm by 20 instead of by 10. Finally, a reference pressure has to be chosen. Any appropriate reference can be used. One scale in common use, the decibel sound pressure level (dB SPL) scale, uses a reference pressure of 2×10^{-5} N/m^2 RMS (20 μPa or 2×10^{-4} dyn/cm^2). At standard temperature and pressure, air impedance is such that this corresponds to a power flow of approximately 10^{-12} W/m^2. In this scale, therefore,

$$\text{Intensity (dB SPL)} = 20 \log_{10} \left[\frac{\text{RMS sound pressure}}{2 \times 10^{-5} \text{ N/m}^2} \right] \quad (5)$$

Any other convenient reference pressure may be used. If the reference pressure is the subject's own absolute threshold at the frequency in question, the measure is known as decibels sensation level. Here, the subject's threshold is by definition 0 dB sensation level. The International Standards Organization (ISO) scale uses as a reference the ISO standard human absolute threshold for the frequency being considered. Scales constructed in these ways are convenient for describing auditory performance. For instance, negative values of decibels sound pressure level (dB SPL; that is pressures below the reference) rarely have to be considered, since the reference is near the lowest absolute threshold. The range of numbers that has to be used is small, since 130 dB SPL is the human being's pain threshold. Similarly, step sizes less than 1 dB rarely have to be taken into consideration, since 1 dB is approximately the minimum intensity step detectable. Moreover, changes in intensity of equal numbers of decibels correspond to approximately equal steps in loudness.

The frequency of sound waves

Frequency, wavelength and velocity

The velocity of sound waves in free air is independent of the frequency, and at sea level has a value of 330 m/s. If the frequency of a wave is *f* cycles/s (or Hz), then *f* waves must pass any point in one second. The length of one wave is therefore 330/*f* metres. As an example, a 1-kHz wave has a wavelength of 0.33 m and, as the equation shows, wavelengths become shorter with increasing sound frequency.

Relation between frequency and sensation

Frequency has the important subjective correlate of pitch. However, in complex sounds, the position is not necessarily clear. It is for instance important to specify what is meant by frequency in a complex sound. Sounds can be analysed mathematically into many separate frequency components, as will be discussed in detail below. This way of decomposing a complex sound is useful in discussing the physics and physiology of the system. While that approach is useful for some purposes, it does not necessarily

mean that the individual frequency components in a complex sound can always be perceived, or that for certain stimuli the perceived pitch is always simply related to the frequency of the individual components in the complex.

The propagation of sound waves

Attenuation by distance

The way that sound waves progress through a medium depends on the nature of the medium, on the irregularities and inhomogeneities it contains, and on the boundaries of the medium. For the simplest source possible conceptually (although impossible to realize in practice), there is a point source of sound, situated in a completely even medium of infinite extent. The sound waves spread out evenly in all directions, so that the wave fronts make a series of expanding spheres centred on the source. In the idealized situation, the wave front will not lose, or indeed gain, energy with time. Because the energy over the total area of the wave front is constant, the energy in each unit area of wave front decreases with distance. The total area increases as the square of the distance, and so the power passing through a unit area, which is the definition of sound intensity, falls as the inverse square of the distance. Thus the sound gets quieter with distance. In many practical situations, however, obstructions will hinder the passage of the sound waves. Even where there is a clear path from the source to the receiver, objects may be present at the side, and often these serve to reflect the sound and prevent it spreading as rapidly as described above. Under these circumstances, the intensity will fall less rapidly than suggested by the square of the distance. A further factor affects the attenuation of sound with distance. When the air is compressed, at the peak of the pressure wave, its temperature rises, and some of the energy of the sound wave is stored as heat. The reverse process takes place, and the energy is passed back into the wave, when the pressure is reduced in the trough of the wave. However, if heat is allowed to flow from the warmer to the cooler regions of the wave, some of the energy in the wave is irredeemably lost. This factor is particularly important for high frequency waves, where the short wavelength allows flow of heat between the peaks and the troughs of the wave.

Transmission between different media

If a medium, of which air is an example, is light and compressible, only small sound pressures will be needed to give a certain velocity of vibration, and hence displacement, of the air molecules. The pressures will be inadequate to give similar velocities of vibration in a denser, less compressible medium – in other words, in a medium with a higher impedance.

If, therefore, a sound wave in air meets a medium of higher impedance, the sound pressures developed on the air side of the boundary will be inadequate to give the same amplitude of vibration of the medium on the other side of the boundary. The result is that much of the sound is reflected, with only a small proportion being transmitted. The pressure at the boundary stays high, but because the reflected wave travels in the reverse direction, it produces movements of the molecules in the reverse direction. Near the boundary, the movements arising from the incident and reflected waves substantially cancel one another, and the net velocity of the air molecules will be small. The resulting ratio of velocity to pressure in the air near the boundary is similar to that in the higher-impedance medium. Near the boundary, therefore, the impedance of the air is raised. This shows that the impedance of a medium is determined by its surroundings as well as by its intrinsic properties. It can be shown mathematically, that if the impedances of the two media are R_1 and R_2 the proportion of the incident power transmitted is $4R_1R_2/(R_1 + R_2)^2$.

This point is important physiologically when transmission of sound from the air into the cochlea is considered. The impedance of the cochlea is much higher than that of air. If the sound waves met the oval window directly, then, as can be calculated from the measured input impedance of the cochlea, only about 1% of the incident energy would enter the cochlea, with the rest being reflected. However, the following will show how the middle ear apparatus, by its action as an impedance transformer, improves this proportion considerably.

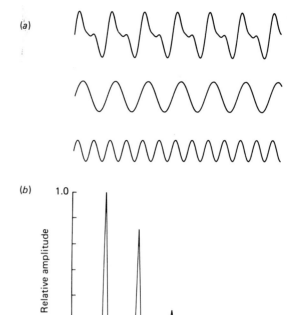

Figure 2.2 (*a*) A portion of a complex waveform. The waveform can be closely approximated by adding together the two waves shown. (*b*) A Fourier analysis of the waveform in part (*a*) shows the two main components, together with smaller ones of higher frequency

Fourier analysis

Figure 2.2 shows a portion of the waveform of a complex sound. The waveform has a regularly repeating pattern with two peaks per cycle. This pattern can be approximated by adding together the two sinusoids shown in the figure, one at 1 kHz, the other at 2 kHz. Such an analysis of a complex sound into its constituent sinusoids is known as Fourier analysis. The small irregularities in the waveform show that other frequency components, vibrating at higher frequencies, are present as well. If all the different sinusoids that have to be added together to give the waveform of Figure 2.2*a* are determined, and the required amplitude of each component is plotted as a function of the frequency of the component, a spectrum of the signal (Figure 2.2*b*) will result. The analysis of signals into spectra, Fourier analysis, is one of the essential tools for those trying to understand the workings of the auditory system.

There are several reasons why it is useful to analyse waveforms into sine waves (sinusoids) rather than into any other waveforms. A primary reason is mathematical, as any realistic waveform can be made out of sums of sinusoids. A second reason is that sinusoidal sound waves behave in a relatively simple way in many complex environments, such as a reflecting environment (e.g. the external auditory meatus), or one that has complex mechanical properties, such as the middle ear. In these cases, it is much easier to describe the way that sinusoidal waves would be affected by the system, and then, knowing how the complex sound can be described as the sum of sinusoids, to use this as a basis of working out how a complex wave would be transformed. A third reason, which is very important in understanding how the ear and the brain analyse sounds, is that the cochlea itself seems to perform a Fourier analysis. Therefore, if a complex sound has been analysed into sinusoids, it is often possible to understand how the auditory system itself would analyse it.

The principles of Fourier analysis can be illustrated most easily by the reverse process of Fourier synthesis, i.e. the process of taking many sinusoids and adding them together to make a complex wave. Figure 2.3 shows how, by adding sinusoids together, a good approximation to a square wave can be made. If this process were continued for more compo-

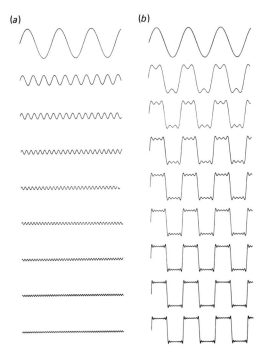

Figure 2.3 A square wave can be approximated by the addition of sinusoids of relative frequencies 1, 3, 5, 7, 9, 11, 13, 15 and 17. The column in (b) shows the effect of successively adding the sinusoids in (a)

at the beginning of the fundamental cycle, each frequency component is moving upwards from its zero-crossing. However, the ear is relatively insensitive to the phase relations between components, so it is not always necessary to specify them.

Non-periodic sounds

Mathematically, a sinusoid repeats for an infinite time, and has a spectrum consisting of a line. The sounds encountered in everyday life do not continue for an infinite time. If the process of Fourier analysis is undertaken on a sound which is ramped on and off (e.g. Figure 2.4c), it will be found that the spectrum now contains not a certain discrete frequency or frequencies but rather a continuous range of frequencies. Moreover, what would be a single line in the spectrum (Figure 2.4a) is spread out into a band (Figure 2.4c). The fewer the number of cycles in the waveform, the wider is the band. In fact, the width of the band, in hertz, is inversely proportional to the time, in seconds, for which the sound is present.

The spectra of many everyday sounds can now be understood. For instance, spoken vowel sounds have a complex repeating waveform, which may continue steadily for half a second or so. In this case, there will be an approximation to a line spectrum, in which the components are harmonics of a fundamental. However, if the sound lasts for 0.5 s, each component

nents, it would be possible to make a waveform indistinguishable from a square wave. Fourier analysis is simply the reverse of this – finding the elementary sinusoids which, when added together, will give the required waveform.

Periodic sounds

The sinusoids in Figure 2.3 have 1, 3, 5, 7, 9 and so on, cycles respectively in the same time interval. Their frequencies are therefore multiples of the lowest, or fundamental, frequency. If the summed wave were repeated indefinitely, without any change of form in each period, then the higher frequencies would have to be *exact* multiples of the fundamental frequency. If the spectra of perfectly periodic sounds (Figure 2.4a and b) are drawn, it will be seen that the components are present only at certain discrete frequencies, as represented by the lines in the spectra, all of which are at exact multiples of the fundamental frequency. Such components at exact multiples of a frequency are called harmonics of the frequency.

In analysing complex sounds, not only do the frequency and amplitude of each frequency component have to be taken into consideration, but also the latter's timing, or phase. In Figure 2.3, each frequency component is in the same phase because,

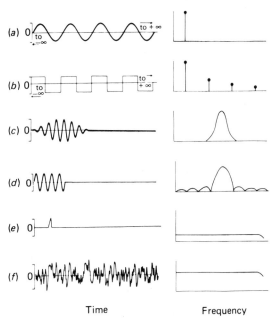

Figure 2.4 Waveforms (left) and their Fourier transforms (right). (a) Sine wave; (b) square wave; (c) and (d) gated sine waves; (e) click; (f) white noise. (From Pickles, 1988)

is spread into a band of closely adjacent frequencies, although in this case the frequency spread will be only about 2 Hz. The shorter the time for which the sound is present, the greater the frequency spread of each component.

A click is a sound which is present for only a short time. In this case, the spectrum has a very wide and uniform spread (see Figure 2.4e). Other transient sounds, which nevertheless give rise to some sort of a pitch sensation, such as the clash of a cymbal, will give rise to a wide frequency spectrum, with some frequency components present at greater intensities than others. Another sound with a wide spectrum is a continuous white noise, or hiss. Here, if the spectrum were averaged for a long period, a spectrum with a wide and uniform spread would be obtained. This differs from a click in the relative phases of the components, which are random in the case of white noise.

Linear systems

One concept which is useful in understanding hearing is that of a linear system. If a system, e.g. the middle ear, is linear it means that it transmits sounds without distortion. In this context, one particular kind of distortion, that of amplitude distortion, is meant. If a system is linear, it means that if the amplitude of the input signal is multiplied by a factor of, say, 10, the amplitude of the output also changes by a factor of 10 times. It also means that when two signals are presented at the same time, the response to both together is the same as the sum of the responses that would be obtained if the signals were presented separately. In other words, linearity means that the presence of one signal does not change the responsiveness of the system to other signals. In the context of Fourier analysis, amplitude linearity has a simple implication. It means that the only frequencies (Fourier components) that are produced by the system are the ones that are put into it.

In some contexts, linearity is used differently: it is used to imply that the gain of a system is independent of frequency. Linearity will not be used in this sense in this chapter. It will be used only, as defined at the beginning of this section, in the sense of amplitude linearity, which is the way that it is used in most of the physiological literature.

The outer ear

In man, the pinna forms a flat cartilaginous flange, with a raised rim and a dip in the centre called the concha. The external ear, which includes the pinna, concha, and external auditory meatus, is considered as having two main influences on the incoming sound. First, it increases the pressure at the tympanic membrane in a frequency-sensitive way, thus empha-sizing certain frequencies in the input. Second, it increases the pressure in a way that depends on the direction of the sound source, and can therefore be used as an aid to sound localization. Although these two actions will be discussed separately, they are two aspects of the same phenomenon.

The gain in sound pressure at the tympanic membrane

In a free field, a portion of the incident sound is reflected off the head. This effect is at its maximum when the source is in the horizontal plane, and 90° to the side, being about 6 dB above 2 kHz, and becoming smaller at lower frequencies. If the sound source is on the opposite side of the head, there will be shadowing around the head, which can reduce the amplitude drastically. On top of this, the pinna–concha system itself can act like an ear trumpet, catching sound over a large area and concentrating it in the smaller area of the external meatus. Thus the total energy available to the tympanic membrane is increased.

A resonance in the external auditory meatus changes the sound pressure at the tympanic membrane in a frequency-selective way. If a tube is one-quarter of a wavelength long, and one end is open while the other is blocked with a hard termination, the pressure will be low at the open end and high at the closed end when the tube is placed in a sound field. This phenomenon is seen in the human external meatus at a frequency of about 3 kHz. Here, the resonance adds 10–12 dB at the tympanic membrane, over the mid-concha position (Shaw, 1974).

Other resonances increase the sound pressure at other frequencies. The most important is a broad resonance, adding about 10 dB around 5 kHz, arising in the concha. The two main resonances are therefore complementary, and increase the sound pressure relatively uniformly over the range from 2 to 7 kHz. The total effect of reflections from the head and pinna, and the various external ear resonances, is to add 15–20 dB to the sound pressure, over the frequency range from 2 to 7 kHz (Figure 2.5) (Stinson and Khanna, 1989).

The meatal quarter-wave resonance as described above can develop only if the meatus is terminated by a boundary with a higher impedance than the air in the canal. This implies that there is a mismatch of impedance between the ear canal and the tympanic membrane, with a loss of efficiency of transfer of energy. Such a mismatch can be measured in man from the standing wave pattern of sound reflected from the eardrum. The point made above is confirmed; although there is variation between the results of different investigators, the impedance of the tympanic membrane in man seems to be three or four times that of the air in the ear canal over a wide

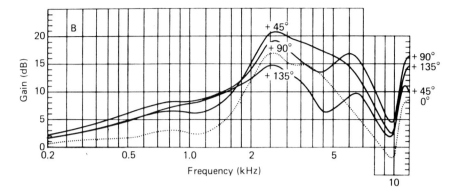

Figure 2.5 The pressure gain of the human external ear, for different frequencies of stimulation and different directions of the sound source. 0° is straight ahead. (From Shaw, 1974)

frequency range above 1 kHz. This leads to some 50% of the energy being reflected back into the meatus (Lawton and Stinson, 1986). A function of the resonances is to reduce the loss of the incident energy around the resonant frequencies. An analysis of the performance of the whole system shows that performance is best in the range of the resonant frequencies (2.5 kHz and above), where performance is between 0 dB and 20 dB of the theoretically perfect value (Rosowski, Carney and Peake, 1990).

Sound localization and the outer ear

The most powerful cues for sound localization are provided by binaural interactions. However, the outer ear provides important cues which are useful in monaural localization and, where binaural hearing is concerned, in enabling us to distinguish in front from behind and up from down (Middlebrooks, Makous and Green, 1989).

Figure 2.5 shows that as a sound source is moved around the head, starting in front and moving round to the side, the main change produced is an attenuation of up to 10 dB in the frequency range from 2 to 7 kHz. This arises from interference between the wave transmitted directly, and the wave scattered off the pinna. Changes in this frequency range could therefore indicate whether the source was in front of the subject or behind. In addition, the dip in the transfer function around 10 kHz gives information as to the elevation of the sound source. As a sound source is raised above the horizontal plane, the low frequency edge of the dip moves to higher frequencies. The dip arises from cancellation between multiple out-of-phase reflections off the back wall of the pinna and concha. While such transformations in the spectrum theoretically contain information about the direction of the source, it would appear that judgement of direction of the source would require either previ-

ous familiarity with the spectrum of the sound, or the possibility of varying the transformation by making searching movements of the head.

At very high frequencies, where the wavelength is short compared with the dimensions of the pinna, it is possible for the pinna to become strongly directional and to produce a high gain on a narrow axis. This is taken advantage of in animals such as cats and bats. For instance, Phillips *et al.* (1982) showed that at 16 kHz the cat pinna could provide 25 dB or more of amplification, but only for sound sources in a narrowly defined direction some 20° or less across. Combined with a mobile pinna, this would permit very accurate monaural localization of high-frequency sound sources.

The middle ear

The middle ear couples sound energy to the cochlea. As well as providing physical protection for the cochlea, the middle ear serves to match the impedance of the air to the much higher impedance of the cochlear fluids. The middle ear apparatus also serves to apply sound preferentially to only one window of the cochlea, thus producing a differential pressure between the windows, required for the movement of the cochlear fluids.

The mode of vibration of the middle ear structures

Calculation of the transformer action requires a detailed knowledge of the way that the middle ear structures move in response to sound. The measurements required are difficult to make, because the movements are complex ones in three dimensions, submicroscopic and depend on the physiological state of the subject. For these reasons, the most reliable information available has come from experimental animals.

Békésy (1941, 1960), after measuring the vibration of the tympanic membrane in human cadavers, suggested that it moved like a stiff plate up to 2 kHz, hinging around an axis of rotation at one edge (Figure 2.6a). He found that the inferior edge of the membrane was flaccid and it was here that the movements were greatest. Khanna and Tonndorf (1972), working with live cats, did not confirm this pattern of movement at any frequency; rather, there were two maxima of vibration, one on either side of the manubrium (Figure 2.6b). Their results suggested that as the tympanic membrane moved to and fro, it buckled in the regions between the manubrium of the malleus and the anterior and posterior edges. The pattern of movement is shown in cross-section in Figure 2.6c. It suggests that the movement of the malleus is somewhat less than the mean movement of the tympanic membrane, and so of the air that drives it. Khanna and Tonndorf (1972) showed that for frequencies below 6 kHz the displacement of the malleus is some 0.5 times the mean displacement of the membrane. At frequencies above 6 kHz the pattern becomes much more complex: the vibration breaks up into many small zones with a reduction in the efficiency of the transfer of vibration to the malleus (Decraemer, Dirckz and Funnell, 1991).

The axis of rotation of the ossicles and the axis of suspension by their ligaments nearly coincide with their centre of rotational inertia. Therefore, the bones are able to vibrate with very little loss through the suspending ligaments (Figure 2.6d). The relatively massive head of the malleus and incus in some species, including man, would therefore appear to aid determination of the appropriate centre of inertia. However, this factor is dominant only at mid frequencies. At low frequencies, where the mass effects are small, the ligaments play an important role in maintaining the position of the ossicles. Békésy (1941, 1960) showed this, by cutting the ligaments. Changing the suspension in this way affected transmission below, but not above, 200 Hz. At high frequencies, above 4 kHz, the axis of rotation changes in a complex way so that there is no simple axis of rotation (Decraemer, Khanna and Funnell, 1991b).

At low frequencies, the coincidence of the centre of inertia of the ossicles with their centre of rotation, will help reduce the perception of bone-conducted sound. Otherwise, the cochlea would be strongly driven by the inertial lag of the ossicles when the skull was vibrated.

The actual mode of movement of the middle ear bones, like the mode of vibration of the tympanic membrane, has been a matter of controversy. It is not known whether the controversy has arisen as a consequence of species differences, or the better methods of measurement which have been used more recently, although of necessity in experimental animals rather than in human beings. For instance, Békésy (1941, 1960), experimenting on human cadavers, suggested that the stapes rocked in the oval window as well as moving in and out. He ascribed this to an asymmetry in the annular ligament, which fits more tightly on its posterior edge. However, Guinan and Peake (1967) found that, in cats, the stapes simply moved in and out like a piston.

The impedance transformer action of the middle ear

Examination of the middle ear as an impedance transformer must begin with a consideration of the impedance of the structure to which it is connected, namely the cochlea.

Following the provisional and tentative conjecture made by Wever and Lawrence (1954), many authors have described the cochlea as having an impedance to sound equal to that of sea water (that is 1.5×10^6 N.s/m^3). While this comparison gains apparent precision by including the main solutes of the perilymph, although in concentrations four times too great, the basis of the comparison, as was indeed emphasized by Wever and Lawrence themselves, is in fact quite wrong. The above impedance is the specific impedance defined for progressive waves in an effectively infinite medium. However, the cochlea is many times smaller than the wavelength of sound in water, and it cannot develop such waves. Instead, the actual impedance of the cochlea is determined by factors such as the mass of the cochlear fluids, the stiffness of the round and oval windows and the other membranes, and by the pattern of motion of the cochlear fluids. Determination of the cochlear impedance is a complex matter, since it appears that the measurement must be made in a living specimen in good physiological condition. For this reason, the only reasonable measurements of cochlear input impedance that are available have been made on experimental animals. Probably the most reliable measurements to date are those of Lynch, Nedzelnitsky and Peake (1982), made on the cat. They showed that over a wide frequency range the input impedance of the cat cochlea had a value of 1.5×10^5 N.s/m^3 (calculated here as a specific impedance), one tenth that expected on Wever and Lawrence's approximation. Earlier authors had obtained much higher values than this, particularly at low frequencies. Lynch, Nedzelnitsky and Peake pointed out that these high values probably arose because the ligaments had dried out to some extent, thus increasing the stiffness of the system. Because air has a specific impedance of 415 N.s/m^3, the formula given above, where the transmission of sound between media of different impedances was considered (see Transmission between different media), would lead to the assumption that only 1% of the incident energy would be conveyed to the

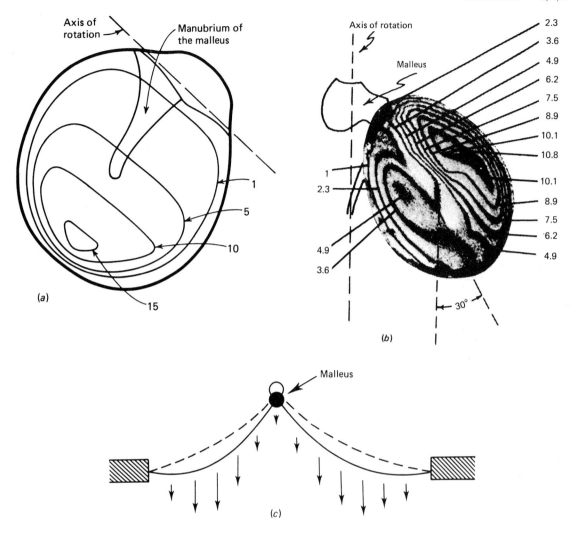

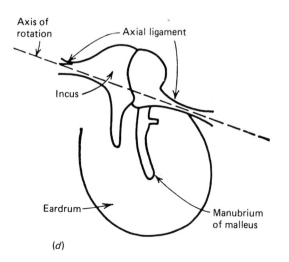

Figure 2.6 The mode of vibration of the human tympanic membrane, according to Békésy. The lines are contours of equal amplitudes of vibration. (From Békésy, 1960; copyright McGraw-Hill, 1960.) (*b*) Vibration contours in the living cat's tympanic membrane, according to Khanna and Tonndorf (1972). The contours are produced by laser interference fringes. The corresponding amplitudes of vibration are shown by the numbers in units of 0.1 μm. (From Khanna and Tonndorf, 1972.) (*c*) The curved membrane principle. (*d*) The axis of rotation of the ossicles. (From Békésy, 1960; copyright McGraw-Hill, 1960)

cochlea in the absence of a middle ear mechanism. This corresponds to an attenuation of the sound by 20 dB.

An efficient impedance transformer will change the low-pressure, high-displacement vibrations of the air into high-pressure, low-displacement vibrations suitable for driving the cochlear fluids. Three components have been identified in the mechanism by which this happens.

1 By far the most important factor depends on the large area of the tympanic membrane in comparison with the area of the footplate of the stapes in the round window. The force collected over the tympanic membrane is expressed over the much smaller stapes foot plate, with a corresponding increase in pressure. The pressure therefore increases in inverse proportion to the ratio of the areas.
2 The ossicles act as a lever, with the malleus being longer than the incus. The displacement at the stapes is therefore decreased, while the force is increased.
3 As described above, the tympanic membrane buckles as it moves to and fro (see Figure 2.6c). The reduction in the movement of the malleus means that the tympanic membrane acts as a mechanical lever, although of rather subtle shape. It therefore again increases the force and decreases the displacement at the stapes.

Measurements of the lever action of the ossicles suggest that the effective length of the manubrium of the malleus, taking into account the complex way that the vibration is connected to it, is some 1.15 times the length of the incus. A value for the impedance transformer ratio can be calculated by multiplying these factors together. In the cat, the area of the tympanic membrane is 0.42 cm^2, and the area of the stapes foot plate is 0.012 cm^2. The pressure is therefore increased 0.42/0.012 = 35 times. The lever ratio increases the force 1.15 times, and decreases the displacement (and therefore velocity) 1.15 times. The

impedance ratio, which is the pressure/velocity ratio, is therefore changed $1.15^2 = 1.32$ times. Finally, the buckling factor decreases the displacement 2.0 times, and increases the force 2.0 times, thus changing the impedance ratio 4.0 times. The overall transformer ratio, expressed as the pressure/velocity ratio is 35 × 1.32 × 4.0 ≃ 185. The middle ear impedance transformer will therefore make the cochlear input impedance of 1.5×10^5 N.s/m^3 appear as $1.5 \times 10^5/185 = 810$ N.s/m^3 at the tympanic membrane. This is nearly twice the specific impedance of air which is 415 N.s/m^3. It agrees with the finding described above that the impedance of the tympanic membrane is rather higher than that of air, although it does not predict the exact value of the impedance which, measurements suggest, is nearer three to four times the specific impedance of the air (Hudde, 1983).

The result of the transformer action of the middle ear (combined with the effect of the outer ear) is that up to 50% of the incident energy is transmitted to the cochlear, as against the 1% expected in the absence of a middle ear transformer (Rosowski, Carney and Peake, 1990).

Transfer as a function of frequency

In order properly to describe the action of the middle ear, it is necessary to consider transmission over the whole audible frequency range, and not only at the mid frequency (1 kHz) for which the calculations above are most nearly valid. Again, this is a measurement that is most easily made in experimental animals. The most direct way to measure the efficiency of transfer is to measure the sound pressure in the scala vestibuli, just behind the oval window, for a certain sound pressure at the tympanic membrane. Nedzelnitsky (1980) showed that in cats transmission reached a peak around 1 kHz; the transmission was less effective at lower and higher frequencies (Figure 2.7). Similar results were obtained with excised

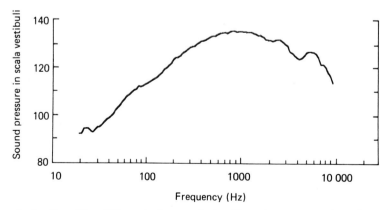

Figure 2.7 The transfer function of the middle ear in the cat, calculated from the pressure in the scala vestibuli, compared with that at the tympanic membrane. Sound pressure level at tympanic membrane = 105 dB. (From Nedzelnitsky, 1980)

human temporal bones by Kringlebotn and Gundersen (1985); they also showed a band pass transfer characteristic, with peak transmission being achieved at around 1 kHz, when their data are used to plot the velocity of the inner ear input as a function of stimulus frequency.

The drop in transmission at low frequencies is probably due to the elastic stiffness of various components of the middle ear. One structure contributing considerable stiffness is the annular ligament that fixes the circumference of the foot plate of the stapes in the oval window. Lynch, Nedzelnitsky and Peake (1982), by comparing the movements produced by pressures applied to the stapes with the effect of pressures applied directly to the cochlear scalae, showed that this ligament contributed stiffness to the system below 500 Hz. Another factor is the air in the middle ear cavity. As the tympanic membrane moves in, the air is compressed, reducing the movement of the tympanic membrane. If the middle ear cavity is vented to the atmosphere, this effect disappears, and low-frequency transmission is improved (Guinan and Peake, 1967).

Stiffness is particularly important at low frequencies because, for constant sound pressure level, the displacement of the air, and so of auditory structures, increases in inverse proportion to frequency. The force on an elastic element is a function of its displacement, and so elasticity has most influence at low frequencies. The inverse relation between frequency and displacement is reflected in the curve shown in Figure 2.7, since at low frequencies transmission to the cochlea declines by almost exactly 20 dB/decade, that is in almost exact inverse proportion to stimulus frequency. The contention that elastic stiffness limits the movement at low frequencies is also supported by the phase data, which at these frequencies show that the tympanic membrane is displaced in phase with the sound pressure. This is the phase relation expected for a stiffness limited system, whereas a 90° phase lag would be expected if the energy were being coupled efficiently into the resistance of the cochlea.

The drop at high frequencies is affected by many factors. One important factor is the pattern of vibration of the tympanic membrane, which, above 6 kHz, breaks up into many independent zones, reducing the coupling to the malleus (Khanna and Tonndorf, 1972). A second factor, giving the dip around 4 kHz in the cat, depends on acoustic resonances within the middle ear cavity, with air resonating between the different compartments within the cavity. The mass of the middle ear system would also appear to have a significant effect at high frequencies. Mass is particularly important in limiting the movements at high frequencies because the forces on a mass are a function of the accelerations involved, which increase with frequency.

The data in Figure 2.7 also allow the calculation of the transformer ratio to be made in a different way, this time directly from the pressure ratio. In the mid-frequency range, the factors leading to transmission losses will be small, and the theoretical calculations detailed above will be most nearly accurate. The calculations lead to the assumption that the area ratio would increase the pressure 35 times, the lever ratio by 1.15 times, and the buckling factor by two. By multiplying these together, a total pressure increase of 80.5 times, corresponding to a 38 dB increase in pressure, is obtained. This is of the same order as, although rather greater than, the 30 dB maximum increase found by Nedzelnitsky (1980). The remaining discrepancy is probably mainly due to transmission losses in the middle ear, including friction in the tympanic membrane, ligaments, and ossicular joints, since they account for some 6 dB of transmission loss at the particular frequency under consideration. Shaw and Stinson (1983) described the different sites of loss in man.

If the total effect of outer and middle ear transmission on the power delivered to the cochlea at different frequencies is calculated, a curve is obtained that closely approximates the air-conduction audiogram for the absolute threshold between 200 Hz and 20 kHz (see for example Rosowski *et al.*, 1986). This suggests that the shape of the human audiogram is determined mainly by factors peripheral to the cochlea, at least until the sharp upper frequency cut-off of hearing is reached.

The role of the middle ear has been described so far as one of transferring sound from the ear canal to the cochlea. However, as in any matched system, transfer in the reverse direction is possible. The importance of this was recognized with the discovery of the cochlear echo (Kemp, 1978), a phenomenon in which sound is generated in the cochlea, either spontaneously or following an external stimulus, and transmitted to the external ear.

Influence of the middle ear muscles

The tensor tympani inserts on the top of the manubrium of the malleus, and contraction pulls the malleus medially and anteriorly, nearly at right angles to the normal direction of vibration. The second muscle, the stapedius muscle, inserts on the posterior aspect of the stapes. Contraction of the muscle, therefore, pulls the stapes posteriorly. Contraction of the tensor tympani can be detected as an inward movement of the tympanic membrane (Møller, 1964). On the other hand, different investigators have reported different effects for contraction of the stapedius muscle. Whereas Møller (1964) reported inward movements of the tympanic membrane in some experiments, and outward movements in others, Pang and Peake (1986) reported that stapedius contraction in cats was effective without *any* detectable movement of the incus, malleus, or tympanic membrane. Contraction of both muscles, however, influences transmission in the same way, by increasing the stiffness of the ossicular chain. The stapedius muscle achieves this by rocking the stapes in the oval window, so increasing the inward tension on the posterior edge of the annular ligament, and the outward tension on the anterior edge.

As pointed out above, when the factors limiting transmission through the middle ear at different frequencies were considered, stiffness has its greatest effects at low frequencies. Pang and Peake (1986) found that the strongest stapedius contractions could reduce transmission by up to 30 dB for frequencies less than 1–2 kHz. At higher frequencies, the effect was limited to 10 dB. However, the fact that any effects at all could be produced above the frequency range in which stiffness can be expected to limit the movement (i.e. above 1–2 kHz), suggests that contraction can do more than increase the stiffness. It may, for instance, change the direction of vibration of the ossicles so that the movement is less effectively coupled to the cochlea. Contraction of the muscles may also serve to damp out unwanted resonances in the middle ear system at these higher frequencies. In support of this, Simmons (1964) showed that, in cats, the middle ear muscles could remove a sharp dip in middle ear transmission which was seen around 4 kHz.

The middle ear muscles contract in response to sound. In man, only the stapedius can be driven acoustically, unless the sound is loud enough to give a startle reflex (Møller, 1974). However, in experimental animals such as cats and rabbits, both the stapedius muscle and tensor tympani contract in response to sound. The reflex arcs for such contractions contain only a few neurons (Borg, 1973). The arc to the stapedius muscle has three to four synapses, ending in the facial nerve, and that to the tensor tympani has four, ending in the trigeminal nerve. The few neurons lead to very fast reaction times; latencies as low as 6–7 ms in the responses to intense tones have been reported in cats and rats, although under the more limited range of experimental conditions possible in man, the limit is nearer 25 ms (Metz, 1951; van der Berge *et al.*, 1990). The latency is a function of the intensity of the stimulus, with longer latencies being found for low intensity stimuli. In man, the reflex threshold, below which no effects are found, has been reported to be some 80 dB above the subject's absolute threshold for stimuli in the frequency range from 250 Hz to 4 kHz (Møller, 1974). Both middle ear muscles can contract in response to stimuli other than external sound, including stimulation of the cornea by a puff of air, touching the skin around the eye or external ear, closing of the eyes, body movements, vocalization and, in some subjects, by voluntary effort (for review see Møller, 1974).

The middle ear muscle reflex has various functions, which include the following. First, the reflex provides protection from noise damage. Although the reflex is too slow to protect the ear from sudden impulsive noise, it does seem to have an effect with longer lasting noises. Zakrisson and Borg (1974) showed that patients with Bell's palsy and paralysis of the stapedius muscle had greater temporary threshold shifts in response to intense frequency noises in the affected than in the unaffected ear. The reflex may, under some circumstances, also be useful with impulsive sounds; Hilding (1961) showed that if a sudden sound such as a gunshot is preceded by a 100 dB tone, the reflex contraction to the tone can provide protection from the gunshot. Second, the reflex may provide selective attenuation of low frequency stimulus components. Such stimuli are particularly effective at masking stimuli in the higher frequency range, and at high intensities they reduce the cues available concerning, for instance, the upper formants of speech sounds. Selective attenuation of the low frequency components by the middle ear muscle reflex could therefore be expected to improve the intelligibility of speech at high intensities. This received experimental support from Borg and Zakrisson (1973), whose patients with Bell's palsy showed deterioration in speech perception at stimulus intensities 25 dB lower than normal subjects. On the other hand, middle ear muscle contraction does not seem to reduce the masking produced by *internally* produced sounds (Irvine *et al.*, 1983), as has sometimes been suggested. Third, the reflex may also have a beneficial effect in reducing the influence of some of the resonances in the middle ear (Simmons, 1964). The reflex has been usefully reviewed by Silman (1984).

Transmission through damaged middle ears

If the middle ear is disordered, transmission can change by way of several mechanisms. The stimulus may be inadequately coupled to the tympanic membrane, the impedance transformer action may be lost, the ability of the ossicles to move may be reduced, and the differential application of sound pressure to the round and oval windows may be affected (Peake, Rosowski and Lynch, 1992).

In the case of a total removal of the middle ear apparatus, the impedance transformer action and the differential application of pressure to the round and oval windows are lost. The loss of transformer action alone would be expected to lead to an increase of some 20 dB in auditory thresholds in the mid-range of frequencies. Békésy (1960) showed in excised human temporal bones that, under such circumstances, the pressures delivered to the round and oval windows were nearly equal. He argued that the scala vestibuli was more yielding than the scala tympani, because its blood vessels could be displaced out of the osseous labyrinth, so allowing equal pressures applied to the two windows to set up differential movements in the scalae of the cochlea. This conjecture received support from the experiments of Tonndorf (1966), who showed that pressure release through structures such as the cochlear aqueduct was possible and could aid the detection of sound. As a second factor, the small compliance of the annular ligament of the stapes, in comparison with the much larger compliance of the round window membrane, will tend to enhance the differential movement. At the present time, it is not known whether the 40–60 dB loss observed clinically can be explained by known mechanisms. In the case of these severe losses, hearing by bone conduction may become significant.

If the middle ear apparatus is lost, but the round window is protected in some way from the incoming sound waves, then a differential pressure can be set up across the round and oval windows. Theoretically, the change in sensitivity is that resulting from the loss of the transformer mechanism alone. If the tympanic membrane is intact and connected directly to the oval window, either by direct contact between the drum head and the stapes or by means of a prosthesis, the major component of the impedance transformer, the area ratio, remains, although the lever action of the ossicles and possibly the buckling action of the tympanic membrane will be lost. As these two latter factors have a comparatively small influence on the impedance transformation, the transformation produced by the middle ear will be only a little affected, and good hearing is theoretically possible.

A hole in the tympanic membrane will reduce the effective area of the membrane in contact with the sound wave. Holes will also reduce the pressure differential across the tympanic membrane and, depending on their position, reduce the mechanical coupling between the remaining intact portions of the membrane and the malleus. The effects of different lesions were studied experimentally in the cat by Payne and Githler (1951). Averaging over all positions in which holes were made, small lesions (10% of the membrane) produced losses of 10–15 dB below 3 kHz, with smaller losses at higher frequencies. It would seem plausible that the pressure differential across the membrane would be maintained more at high frequencies, because the air has less time to flow through the perforation. However, large lesions produced severe losses over the whole range, particularly at the highest frequencies. With these lesions, the sound waves were acting directly on the round and oval windows. The size of the effects was highly dependent upon the site of the lesions. Small and moderate lesions (10–40% of area) had far more severe effects when placed on the posterior and supe-

rior margin of the membrane than when placed on the anterior and inferior margin. Fixation of the stapes will cause decreased transmission of sound to the cochlea through decreased mobility. In severe cases, sound pressure changes arriving directly at the round window should still result in some differential movement of the cochlear fluid, because a release of pressure should be possible through the blood vessels and cochlear aqueduct. In this case, where the sound pressure has its effects directly at the round window, the impedance transformer action of the middle ear will also be lost.

Static pressure changes across the tympanic membrane, whether positive or negative, will increase the tension in the tympanic membrane and so increase its stiffness in response to applied sound. The increased stiffness will attenuate the transmission of sound in the frequency region in which it is stiffness limited, i.e. below about 1 kHz. The lowest stiffness is recorded when the static pressure differential across the membrane is zero and, in the normal case, transmission decreases symmetrically for positive and negative changes in the pressure differential.

Mechanisms of bone conduction

Bone conduction is the normal route for hearing some of the components of one's own voice, is useful with severe conductive loss, and is used as a tool of considerable diagnostic power. The mechanisms of bone conduction have been a matter of controversy over the years and present knowledge of them owes much to the experiments of Tonndorf (1966). Tonndorf (1976) gives a useful review of these and other experiments.

By measuring cochlear microphonics in cats during bone stimulation, Tonndorf was able to measure the different factors leading to effective stimulation by bone conduction. He showed that it was determined by a multiplicity of factors, arising in the inner ear, the middle ear and the external ear.

Inner ear factors

In the most basic experiment, the skull was stimulated with a bone vibrator, and microphonics measured in a cochlea from which the middle ear apparatus had been entirely removed and the cochlear aqueduct blocked. If both the oval and round windows were sealed with rigid cement, bone conduction was substantial, although several decibels worse than in the normal animal. If, however, only the oval window was occluded, the microphonic responses of the cochlea were *better* than normal by some 10 dB over the frequency range below 1 kHz.

The fact that substantial responses to bone conduction remained with the cochlear outlets sealed would suggest that differential flow of cochlear fluids between the windows, or to another opening such as the aqueduct, is not entirely necessary for the detection of bone vibrations. Tonndorf suggested that there was an intrinsic detection of distortional vibrations of the cochlear bone. Differential distortion of the bony walls of the cochlea, and of the walls of the other labyrinthine spaces closely connected to it, would produce a movement of the cochlear fluids. These would be coupled into the cochlear partition since the scala vestibuli is larger than the scala tympani. This is the distortional vibration factor.

Although detection is possible with the windows sealed, the windows will normally have some effect. As sealing the oval window while leaving the round window open actually improved bone conduction, it is apparent that a differential compliance can enhance the detection of bone vibration. Tonndorf suggested that leaving the round window open would release pressure and produce movements in phase with those resulting directly from the distortional vibration. On the other hand, increasing the mobility of the oval window would produce a shunt for the pressure changes, allowing them to bypass the cochlear partition and so reduce the response. This gives an explanation of the Weber test: an increased stiffness of the ossicular chain will reduce the shunting and so increase the detection of bone vibration. The good response with one window sealed was seen, however, only when the vibrations were introduced into the bone. If the cochlea was stimulated by air vibrations led directly into the middle ear, it was necessary to have both windows open to obtain a response.

The experiment also suggested that release of pressure through the cochlear aqueduct, and hence also through the blood vessels, would influence the fluid flow resulting from bone vibration. Sealing the aqueduct reduced the response to vibration. This supports the notion of a 'third window' in the cochlea. Evidence was also presented for its role in the production of movements resulting from the inertia of the cochlear fluids, with a differential flow between the third window and the oval window.

Middle ear factors

The centre of inertia of the middle ear bones does not coincide exactly with their points of attachment. Translational vibrations of the skull will therefore produce a rotational vibration of the bones, which can be coupled to the inner ear. Obviously, this factor will be affected by any pathology in the mobility of the middle ear apparatus. It will also be affected by any natural resonances in the middle ear system. The middle ear acts as a broadly tuned band pass filter with peak transmission around 1 kHz at its natural resonant frequency. If the degree of resonance of the system is reduced by damping the stapes, the main losses will be produced around the natural

resonant frequency. This is the explanation given for the appearance of Carhart's notch with mild stapes fixation, although the notch usually appears at rather higher frequencies, namely 2 kHz.

Outer ear factors

Vibration of the bone is coupled to the walls of the ear canal and so to the air within it. These vibrations escape externally when the ear canal is open. When, however, the ear is occluded, the sound pressure changes in the canal are increased and are transmitted to the inner ear by the normal middle ear route (Békésy, 1941; Tonndorf, 1976). Occlusion therefore increases bone conduction, but only if a significant area of the canal, or other part of the external ear which can radiate, is included behind the occlusion. Because the external radiation of sound is normally best for low frequencies, the change with occlusion is greatest for those frequencies.

The cochlea
The fluid spaces of the cochlea

The principal divisions of the fluid space in the cochlea are the *perilymphatic space*, consisting of the scala vestibuli and the scala tympani, and the *endolymphatic space*, consisting of the scala media. The walls surrounding the endolymphatic space have occluding tight junctions between the cells, obstructing the movement of ions into and out of the endolymph (e.g. Smith, 1978). Figure 2.8 shows the commonly-accepted borders of the endolymphatic space in a cochlear cross-section. Between the scala media and the scala tympani the border is drawn around the top edge of the organ of Corti, along the reticular lamina.

The endolymphatic and perilymphatic spaces extend along the inner ear as shown diagrammatically in Figure 2.9. The perilymphatic space surrounds the membranous labyrinth and opens into the CSF by way of the cochlear aqueduct. The endolymphatic space, as well as continuing throughout the membranous labyrinth, is joined to the endolymphatic sac by means of the endolymphatic duct.

Formation and absorption of the endolymph and perilymph
Endolymph

It is generally agreed that the endolymph of the cochlea is formed by the stria vascularis (for review see Sterkers, Ferrary and Amiel, 1988). The cells here have the morphological and biochemical properties of secreting cells. Under the light microscope, the cells of the stria vascularis can be divided into superficially-located darkly staining cells, called the marginal cells, and more lightly staining basal cells

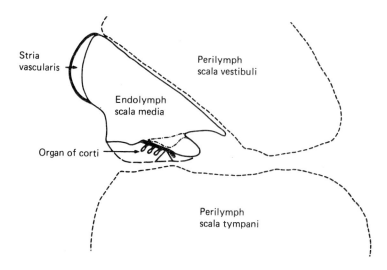

Figure 2.8 The compartments in the cochlea formed by occluding junctions. The thin continuous line surrounds the endolymphatic space, and the dotted line the perilymphatic space. (From Smith, 1978)

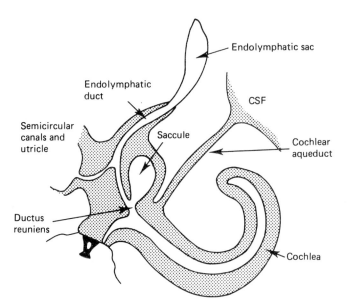

Figure 2.9 Schematic diagram of the perilymphatic space in the cochlea (stippled area) and the endolymphatic space (central clear area, running into the endolymphatic sac)

(e.g. Fawcett, 1986). Under the electron microscope it can be seen that the marginal cells have long infoldings on their basal edge, i.e. on the edge farthest away from the endolymph. The infoldings contain many mitochondria. This is the membrane across which most of the energy-consuming pumping of the stria vascularis takes place. There are also numerous capillaries coursing through the epithelium. The stria vascularis has a high concentration of N^+/K^+-ATPase, adenyl cyclase and carbonic anhydrase, which are enzymes associated with active pumping of ions and transport of fluid into the endolymph. The cells also contain high levels of oxidative enzymes associated with glucose metabolism, as would be needed to provide fuel for a vigorous active transport system (Feldman, 1981; Sterkers, Ferrary and Amiel, 1988). The immediate precursor for endolymph appears to be the perilymph rather than the blood plasma, because radiolabelled ions appear more rapidly in the endolymph after perilymphatic than after intravenous administration (Sterkers *et al.*, 1982).

Endolymph is absorbed in the endolymphatic sac. The cells here have a columnar shape and appear specialized for absorption, containing long microvilli on the luminal surface, and many pinocytotic vesicles and vacuoles. It has also been suggested that free phagocytic cells cross the epithelium to remove cellular debris and foreign material from the endolymph.

Obliteration of the endolymphatic sac and duct in experimental animals causes endolymphatic hydrops, again confirming the view that it is the normal site of absorption of the endolymph (e.g. Kimura, 1967).

Perilymph

The perilymphatic space appears to be continuous between the vestibular and cochlear divisions. In contrast to the position with the endolymph, the site of production of the perilymph is controversial. The perilymph is not a simple ultrafiltrate of plasma, because none of the ions distribute between plasma and perilymph according to a Gibbs-Donnan equilibrium. Several ions and other solutes (e.g. K^+, glucose, amino acids, and proteins) have higher concentrations in the perilymph of the scala vestibuli than in the CSF or the perilymph of the scala tympani. Moreover, when the cochlear aqueduct is blocked, interrupting communication between the CSF and scala tympani, the concentration of solutes in the scala tympani rises towards the levels found in the scala vestibuli, while those in the scala vestibuli do not change. These results suggest that the perilymph of the scala vestibuli originates primarily from the plasma, while the perilymph of the scala tympani originates from both the plasma and CSF (Sterkers, Ferrary and Amiel, 1988). Tracer injections also suggest that the origins of the perilymphs of the scala vestibuli and scala tympani are different, with more rapid equilibration between the plasma and the perilymph of the scala vestibuli than between the plasma and the perilymph of the scala tympani or the CSF.

The composition and electric potentials of the cochlear fluids

Endolymph

Endolymph is unique among the extracellular fluids of the body in that it has a high K^+ content, and a low Na^+ content, resembling intracellular fluid.

The K^+ content of the endolymph can be measured by microsampling or with ion-specific electrodes, although the measurements are tricky because of the small volume of the endolymphatic space. Values obtained by different workers and a variety of techniques are in the range 144–188 mM, isotonic with intracellular K^+ (see Table 2.1). Na^+ concentrations are much more difficult to determine accurately because the Na^+ is present in low concentrations and the samples are susceptible to contamination from the higher levels of Na^+ in the surrounding perilymph. Thus, the earliest measurements of Smith, Lowry and Wu (1954), measured by means of microsampling, showed relatively high values, for example 38 mM. Much lower concentrations have been measured more recently with ion-selective electrodes or by micro-

sampling small (0.1 μl) volumes of fluid (Johnstone and Sellick, 1972; Konishi, Hamrick and Mori, 1984). The latter measurements are generally in the range 0.2–2 mM. These values are also supported by some of the X-ray analyses of crystals of endolymph from the frozen cochlea (Ryan, Wickham and Bone, 1980). Because of the difficulties of making the measurements, the older tables of ionic values should be treated with suspicion as far as the endolymph is concerned. Some of the later measurements are shown in Table 2.1.

Although the endolymph has a high K^+ concentration similar to that found intracellularly, its electric potential, unlike that usually found inside cells, is strongly positive. Values obtained range from + 50 to + 120 mV with respect to the plasma, the higher values being found in the basal turn (Békésy, 1952). The potentials are also higher near the stria vascularis (Tasaki, Davis and Eldredge, 1954).

The positive values suggest that the endocochlear potential is not a simple K^+ diffusion potential, such as is seen inside nerve cells. In other words, the potential is *not* produced by K^+ ions moving passively down their concentration gradient out of the endolymphatic space, taking positive charge with them, as this would leave the endolymph with a negative potential. Instead the positive endocochlear potential is directly dependent on an energy-consuming Na^+, K^+-ATPase in the marginal cells of the stria vascularis (Kuijpers and Bonting, 1969). Inhibition of the ATPase with ouabain reduces the endocochlear potential, and Kuijpers and Bonting suggested that the potential arose from a novel type of electrogenic ATPase, which pumped three K^+ ions into the endolymph for every two Na^+ ions that it pumped out (Kuijpers and Bonting, 1970). However, there has been no evidence for such a unique ATPase. Intracellular recording shows that the marginal cells of the stria vascularis have a high K^+ concentration, a high positive potential, and a low Na^+ concentration, comparable to those of the endolymph (Melichar and Syka, 1987; Offner, Dallos and Cheatham, 1987; Ikeda and Morizono, 1989). While a number of models have been proposed, the different authors all suggest that the basolateral membranes of the marginal cells contain a possibly electrically neutral Na^+, K^+-ATPase, which lowers the Na^+ concentration, and raises the K^+ concentration, inside the marginal cells. The low Na^+ concentration (1.7 mM; Ikeda and Morizono, 1989) would be in equilibrium with plasma at an intracellular potential of + 112 mV; in one attractive version of the models, it is this potential that ultimately underlies the endocochlear potential. Perfusion of the endolymphatic space with low Na^+, in the absence of a vascular circulation, lowers the endocochlear potential immediately, showing that Na^+ is involved in the generation of the potential (Offner, Dallos and Cheatham, 1987). The high positive potential in the marginal cells also drives K^+ into

Table 2.1 Electrolyte concentrations of the endolymph (mequiv./l unless stated otherwise)

Species	Cochlear duct			Utricle			Investigator
	Na^+	K^+	Cl^-	Na^+	K^+	Cl^-	
Guinea-pig	0.6	166					Bosher (1980)
	0.1–2.7			14.3			Sellick and Johnstone (1972)
	1.5*	152.3*	131.0 ± 2.1				Konishi and Hamrick (1978)
	150		117		150	119	Morgenstern, Amano and Orsulakova (1982)
Rat	0.91	154					Bosher and Warren (1968)
	2.9 ± 0.44	156.6 ± 2.1	132.7 ± 1.8				Sterkers et al. (1982)
Cat	1.6	188	206				Peterson et al. (1978)
Human	16.0 ± 5.8[b]	144.2 ± 13.6	114				Rauch and Kostlin (1958)
	16[b]	151[a]					Silverstein (1972)

* mM; [a] patients with Menière's disease; [b] Possibly too high. Modified from Anniko and Wroblewski (1986), Table I

the endolymph, so accounting for the high K^+ concentration in the endolymph.

In experiments in which the Na^+,K^+-ATPase is inactivated, the positive endocochlear potential is replaced by a potential of some -40 mV, which can take several hours to disappear. This negative potential (called $-EP$) is thought to be a conventional diffusion potential, arising because K^+ diffuses across the boundaries of the endolymphatic space (mainly in this case through the organ of Corti), taking positive charge with it, and leaving the endolymph negative. The negative potential remains until the ionic concentrations decay.

Perilymph

Measurement of perilymphatic ionic concentrations does not pose the same problems as that of endolymphatic concentrations, and the results are not controversial. Table 2.2 shows that the results from different investigators are in close agreement. The values are in the range of normal extracellular concentrations, although the K^+ concentrations in the scala vestibuli are somewhat higher than in the scala tympani.

Johnstone and Sellick (1972) reported the electric potential of the scala tympani ($+7$ mV) to be a little more positive than that of the scala vestibuli ($+5$ mV). Voltages are given with respect to blood plasma. The small extra positivity may arise from leakage of K^+ through the organ of Corti, or may reflect small differences in ionic diffusion potentials because of the difference in the K^+ concentrations.

Organ of Corti and subtectorial space

The true border of the perilymphatic space in the organ of Corti is not the basilar membrane, but is likely to be situated more apically in the organ, for instance at the reticular lamina (see Figure 2.8). This is supported by measurements of ionic concentrations in the spaces of the organ of Corti by X-ray microprobe analysis of quick-frozen tissue (Anniko, Lim and Wroblewski, 1984). These measurements show it to have the same ionic composition as perilymph. The basilar membrane is readily permeable to macromolecular tracers, giving them access to the spaces in the organ of Corti. The same is therefore likely to be true for ions which are much smaller. However, Ryan, Wickham and Bone (1980) found that, with their freezing technique, fluid in the spaces of the organ of Corti did not give rise to crystals, suggesting that its protein content was relatively high. Fluid in this space has been named 'cortilymph'.

The fluid in the inner spiral sulcus and in the subtectorial space (between the tectorial membrane and the reticular lamina) has generally been thought to be continuous with the endolymph, and so would have a high positive potential. The chemical and electrical border between the endolymph and the perilymph would then be the reticular lamina, and would include the transducing surfaces of the hair cells. This is supported by direct measurements of the ion concentrations, and by the finding of stimulation-dependent changes in the K^+ concentration of the organ of Corti, confirming that the transducer surfaces of the hair cells are bathed in endolymph (Ryan, Wickham and Bone, 1980; Anniko, Lim and Wroblewski, 1984; Johnstone et al., 1989).

Cochlear mechanics

The mechanical travelling wave in the cochlea forms the basis of the frequency selectivity of the whole organism and, in addition, is the basis of our extreme sensitivity to sounds. A normal travelling wave is therefore fundamental to normal auditory function, and a pathological wave, as probably happens in

Table 2.2 Electrolyte concentrations of the perilymph (mM unless stated otherwise)

Species	Cochlear duct			Utricle			Investigator
	Na^+	K^+	Cl^-	Na^+	K^+	Cl^-	
Guinea-pig			127.8 ± 2.0			128.6 ± 1.9	Konishi and Hamrick (1978)
	154.5	7.3	123.2	124.3	3.5	155.4	Konishi, Salt and Hamrick (1979)
	133.5 ± 2.7	7.4 ± 0.57	120 ± 5.8	138.6 ± 2.6	3.7 ± 0.33	107 ± 4.2	Makimoto, Takedo and Silverstein (1980)
Cat	147 ± 0.94	10.5 ± 0.31	138.5 ± 3.6	157.1 ± 1.1	3.8 ± 0.11	130.0 ± 2.3	Makimoto, Takedo and Silverstein (1980)
Rat	137.5 ± 1.2	4.0 ± 0.15	127.1 ± 0.9	137.0 ± 0.96	3.1 ± 0.15	127.7 ± 0.71	Sterkers *et al.* (1982)
		5.9	119				Bosher and Warren (1968)
Human	129			142*	7*		Silverstein (1972)
				138.0 ± 10.0	10.7 ± 2.6	118.5*	Rauch and Kostlin (1958)

* mequiv/l. Reproduced from Anniko and Wroblewski (1986), Table 2.

most cases of cochlear sensorineural hearing loss, can cause severe deficit.

The cochlear travelling wave was originally described by Békésy (1943, 1960). Working in excised human temporal bones, he opened a stretch of the cochlea, sprinkled reflecting particles on Reissner's membrane, and observed the movement of the membrane stroboscopically in response to applied sound stimuli. Intensities were in the range of 130–140 dB SPL. He showed the now-classic travelling wave (Figure 2.10). He suggested that the pattern was similar to the pattern of movement of the other membrane, the basilar membrane, which carries the organ of Corti. The wave travels along the cochlea, comes to a peak, and dies away rapidly. Figure 2.10 shows the response, as a function of distance, for sinusoidal stimulation of a single frequency. Békésy made plots such as these for a variety of stimulus frequencies, and showed that high frequencies produced a travelling wave peaking near the base of the cochlea, whereas low frequencies produced a wave stretching further up to the apex.

Békésy (1943) also made plots in a different way. He opened the cochlea at single points, and measured the amplitude of vibration at the individual points as he varied the stimulus frequency. If the plots are recalculated for input stimuli of constant sound pressure, the basilar membrane is seen to have a purely low-pass filtering characteristic at each point. That is, the membrane vibrates with a constant amplitude for all low frequencies, until above a certain frequency the response drops abruptly. On the basis of Békésy's results, the capacity of the basilar membrane for frequency filtering is therefore very poor indeed.

It is now known that single neurons of the auditory nerve have very sharp band pass frequency filtering characteristics. That is, the response is large for only a very narrow range of sound frequencies and, if the sound frequency is changed either way, either increased or decreased, the response drops sharply (see below). This led to the suspicion that the sharp tuning might be derived from the mechanics, and that the basilar membrane was much more sharply tuned than Békésy had shown. The most recent measurements, in which great care has been taken by the experimenters, and in which very sensitive methods have been used to make the measurements, have in fact shown that the mechanical response is very sharply tuned. Extensive measurements are now available for the 20 kHz region in the basal turn of the guinea-pig from Johnstone and colleagues (e.g. Sellick, Patuzzi and Johnstone, 1982), and the 7–10 kHz region of the basal turn of the chinchilla from Ruggero and colleagues (e.g. Robles, Ruggero and Rich, 1986). Responses are plotted for one or more individual points on the basilar membrane, and the stimulus frequency is varied. However, instead of plotting the amplitude of response for a fixed input intensity, the converse is shown. That is, the stimulus

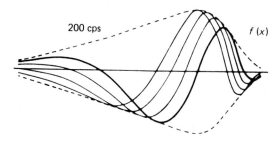

Figure 2.10 The travelling wave in the cochlea, according to Békésy. The base of the cochlea is towards the left, and the apex towards the right. The solid lines show the displacements at four successive instants. The dotted lines show the envelope, which is static. Stimulus frequency: 200 Hz. (From Békésy, 1960; copyright McGraw-Hill, 1960)

intensity necessary to give a certain criterion amount of vibration is plotted for different stimulus frequencies. The resulting curves are called 'tuning curves' or frequency threshold curves (FTCs). A tuning curve for the mechanical response of one point on a basilar membrane of the guinea-pig is shown in Figure 2.11.

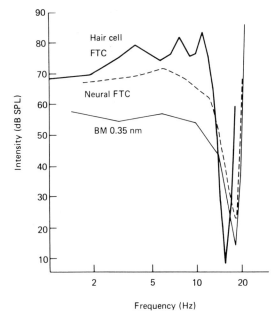

Figure 2.11 axis labels: Intensity (dB SPL) on vertical axis (10–90); Frequency (Hz) on horizontal axis (2, 5, 10, 20). Curves labelled: Hair cell FTC, Neural FTC, BM 0.35 nm.

Figure 2.11 Tuning curve (frequency-threshold curve) for the mechanical vibration of the basilar membrane at 0.35 nm displacement criterion (——). The measurements were made at the 18 kHz place. Also shown is the tuning curve for an auditory nerve fibre (– – –) innervating the same place, and the tuning curve for an inner hair cell (━━) situated a little more apically in the cochlea and so responding best to a lower frequency (14 kHz). (Basilar membrane and neural data from Sellick, Patuzzi and Johnstone, 1982, and hair cell data from Russell and Sellick, 1978. Reproduced from Pickles, 1985)

Two important points can be made from the response shown in Figure 2.11. First, the sharp dip around one frequency, 18 kHz, shows that only very low intensities of sound were necessary to give a response at that frequency. In the experiment illustrated in Figure 2.11, the criterion level of response (0.35 nm) was produced by a sound pressure level at the tympanic membrane of only 12 dB SPL. This is an indication that the mechanical system has a great responsiveness and sensitivity to sound. In fact, if the amplitude of the vibration of the membrane is calculated and compared with the vibration of the stapes at the input to the cochlea, it is found that the travelling wave amplifies the movement by about 40 dB. Second, the intensity necessary to give the criterion response rises sharply on either side of that frequency. The steep

slopes of the function show that the system is very sharply tuned or, in other words, has great frequency selectivity. Sensitivity and frequency selectivity are two important properties of the normally functioning auditory system. The indications are that the sensitivity and frequency selectivity shown by the whole organism are derived from those of the basilar membrane.

Figure 2.11 also shows the tuning curves for the electrical response of a hair cell and an auditory nerve fibre, measured at nearly the same point along the basilar membrane. All three curves have similar, sharply tuned tips. This shows that they have the same degree of tuning.

Why was the sharply tuned response not seen by Békésy? Two reasons have been suggested. First, the cochlea has to be in extremely good physiological condition to show a sharply tuned mechanical response. Any deterioration due to, for instance, anoxia, mixing of the endolymph or perilymph, interference with the blood supply, or bleeding into the scalae, will reduce the response. These factors set very stringent limits where it is necessary to open the cochlear scalae and place measuring instruments on the cochlear partition. In contrast, Békésy performed his measurements on cadavers. Second, it is now known that the response becomes more broadly tuned at high intensities. It should be noted that the measurements of Figure 2.11 are made down to 12 dB SPL. Békésy, because of the relative insensitivity of his measuring instruments, had to use far higher sound pressures, 130–140 dB SPL.

Although the sharpness of tuning shown by Békésy has to be revised, the tonotopicity of the cochlea does not. The modern evidence agrees with Békésy in showing that high frequency tones produce their greatest effects near the base of the cochlea, and low frequency tones at the apex, with a gradation in between for intermediate frequencies.

The fact that the basilar membrane tuning becomes less selective at high stimulus intensities is a reflection of the non-linearity of its response. That is, if the sound pressure is increased 10 times, the amplitude of the movement does not go up 10 times correspondingly, but by rather less. This is shown in the *amplitude functions* of Figure 2.12. If the responses increased in proportion to stimulus pressure, the lines on the graph would all be parallel to the dotted line, which has been drawn for linear growth. However, the lines for stimuli of 18, 19 and 20 kHz (shown by the numbers on the curves) grow with a shallower slope, i.e. non-linearly, for some of their range. If, for instance, the sound pressure at 18 kHz is increased from 30 to 50 dB SPL, the formula for calculation of decibels (see Decibels) will show that the amplitude of the air vibration has gone up 10 times. However, the amplitude of response in the basilar membrane grew from 0.3 to 0.45 mm/s, an increase of only 1.5 times. The non-linearity makes the tuning less selective at high intensities because the responses in the

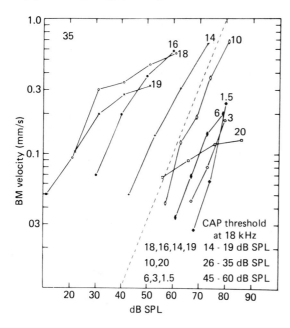

Figure 2.12 Amplitudes of basilar membrane vibration as a function of stimulus intensity, for different frequencies of stimulation (parameter on curves, in kHz). Responses were measured at the 18 kHz point on the basilar membrane. (From Sellick, Patuzzi and Johnstone, 1982, slightly modified)

high intensity stimulation, and is reduced with cochlear pathology. Under these circumstances, the cochlea becomes more broadly tuned and relatively less sensitive. Because of this, Békésy was able to see only the first component in his experiments.

The evidence for this process is still indirect, although all the individual elements of the sequence have been shown. For instance, mathematical models of cochlear mechanics have not been able to imitate the sharp tuning of Figure 2.11 with purely passive mechanical systems. A feedback of mechanical energy has been required in the models, whereupon they have been successful in producing patterns as in Figures 2.11 and 2.12. It is known that the hair cells can move actively in response to stimulation. There is also strong evidence for active mechanical processes in the cochlea, because under some circumstances the cochlea can produce sound, either spontaneously or when triggered by acoustic stimulation (Kemp, 1978). Finally, the changes in tuning and sensitivity, observed with deteriorated cochleae in experimental animals, or psychophysically in human beings with sensorineural hearing loss of cochlear origin, are precisely the changes that would be expected with loss of the active process (see below). Ruggero (1992) and Dallos (1992) reviewed current evidence in favour of the hypothesis. The details of the evidence require consideration of hair cell responses, the influence of the efferent nerve supply, and pathological changes. These will be discussed in the following section, and points of relation to the active mechanical process pointed out.

Transduction by hair cells

The mechanism of signal transduction by hair cells is becoming more clearly understood, as a result of electrophysiological recordings from hair cells, and anatomical observations on the structures that couple the stimulus-induced movements within the hair bundle (e.g. Hudspeth and Corey, 1977; Pickles, Comis and Osborne, 1984; Assad, Shepherd and Corey, 1991). Recent results have been reviewed by Pickles and Corey (1992).

The individual stereocilia on the apical surface of the hair cell are mechanically rigid, and are braced together with cross-links so that they move as a stiff bundle. Therefore, as the bundle is deflected, the different rows of stereocilia could be expected to slide relative to one another (Figure 2.13). There are fine links running upwards from the tips of the shorter stereocilia on the hair cell, which join the adjacent taller stereocilia of the next row (Pickles, Comis and Osborne, 1984). As suggested by Pickles, Comis and Osborne, when the stereocilia are deflected in the direction of the tallest stereocilia, the links are stretched, opening ion channels in the cell membrane. When the stereocilia are deflected in the oppo-

sharply tuned tip of the tuning curve are influenced most by the non-linearity.

It has been questioned why the basilar membrane shows these very sharply tuned and non-linear responses, and why they are so vulnerable. The surprising answer suggested by many lines of evidence is that the basilar membrane contains an *active mechanical amplifier* which uses biological energy to boost the mechanical vibration of the basilar membrane.

It is now believed that as a wave moves up the cochlea, towards its peak, it encounters a region in which the membrane is mechanically active. Triggered by the movement, the membrane starts putting energy into the wave. The amplitude of the movement then grows very sharply, but also dies away sharply because the wave soon reaches a region in which further wave motion for this frequency of stimulation is not possible. The travelling wave can therefore be considered as consisting of two components. There is a broadly tuned, relatively small component, which depends on the purely passive mechanical properties of the basilar membrane and cochlear fluids. In addition, there is a relatively large-amplitude active component, which gives sharp tuning and great frequency selectivity. The second component is produced by an input of biological energy from the cochlea. It is most prominent for low intensities of stimulation. It is less prominent with

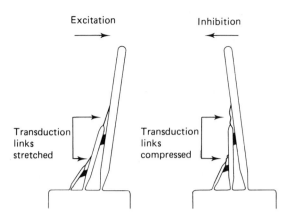

Figure 2.13 The role of tip links between stereocilia in transduction, according to Pickles, Comis and Osborne (1984). Three rows of stereocilia on a hair cell are shown in cross-section. (From Pickles, Comis and Osborne, 1984)

site direction, the tension is taken off the links, and the channels close. This hypothesis is consistent with all the present electrophysiological evidence on transduction in hair cells (Pickles and Corey, 1992). It has received striking recent confirmation from experiments in which the Ca^{2+} is removed from around the hair bundle by perfusion with a calcium-chelating agent; when this is done, the tip links break selectively, and mechanotransduction disappears permanently (Assad, Shepherd and Corey, 1991). There is also considerable evidence that the mechanotransducer channels are in the upper part of the hair bundle. For instance, the spatially-localized application of the channel blocker gentamicin has the greatest effects on mechanotransduction when applied at the tip of the bundle (Jaramillo and Hudspeth, 1991).

The tip links, responsible for coupling the stimulus movements to the transducer channels, are shown for an outer hair cell in Figure 2.14. Inner hair cells have similar links. The actual mechanotransducer channels are likely to be situated at one or both of the points of insertion of the tip links.

The stimulus is coupled to the stereocilia by means of a shear or relative motion between the tectorial membrane and the reticular lamina. As the basilar membrane and organ of Corti are driven upwards and downwards by a sound stimulus, the stereocilia are moved away from and towards the modiolus (Figure 2.15*a* and *b*). Because the tallest stereocilia are situated on the side of the hair cell furthest away from the modiolus, an upwards movement of the basilar membrane is translated into a movement of the stereocilia in the direction of the tallest, as is shown in the left panel of Figure 2.13. This is the direction associated with opening of the ion channels. This is confirmed by recordings of the resistance variations of hair cells, which show that the resistance becomes low when the stereocilia are deflected in the direction of the tallest. The effective direction of shear between the tectorial membrane and the reticular lamina is therefore radial across the cochlear

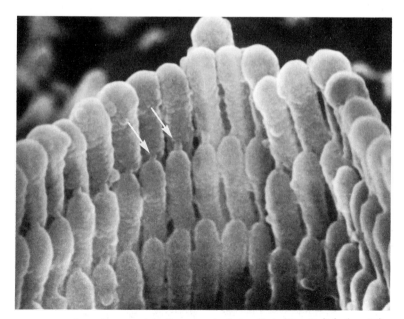

Figure 2.14 Guinea pig: stereocilia at the apex of the V on an outer hair cell, showing tip links (arrows)

duct. It is no surprise that in both inner and outer hair cells the tip links are organized in such a way that they run in a direction most suited for picking up radial shear (Comis, Pickles and Osborne, 1985). In outer hair cells, where the stereocilia are closely packed in a hexagonal array, the rows of stereocilia

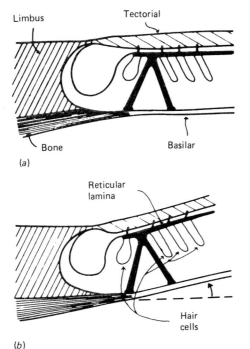

(a)

(b)

need to be set diagonally across the cochlear duct if the tip links are to run radially (see Figure 2.15c). This is apparently the reason for the rows of stereocilia on outer hair cells having a V- or W-shaped arrangement. However, on inner hair cells the packing is looser, and these cells achieve a radial orientation of their tip links while the rows of stereocilia run in a straight line.

When the channels on the stereocilia are open, ions will enter or leave the cell depending on the electrical and chemical gradients across the apical cell surface. It appears that the ion channels are rather large and non-selective, so that, for instance, Na^+, K^+, and Ca^{2+} will enter with nearly the same efficacy (Corey and Hudspeth, 1979). The apical surface of hair cells is faced by endolymph with a high positive potential ($+80$ mV) and a high K^+ concentration. Inside the cell, however, there is a negative intracellular potential, which is -45 mV for inner hair cells and -70 mV for outer hair cells. The potentials combine to give 125 mV (inner hair cells) or 150 mV (outer hair cells) of potential drop across the channel. When the channels are open, K^+ from the endolymph will tend to be driven into the cell by this big potential gradient, thus making the cell become more positive inside (Figure 2.16). When the channels are completely shut, as during the opposite phase of the sound wave, even the resting current is shut off, and the cells will become more negative. Most of the transducer current may be carried by K^+, as this is the predominant ion in the endolymph. K^+ flowing through the mechanotransducer channels and out of

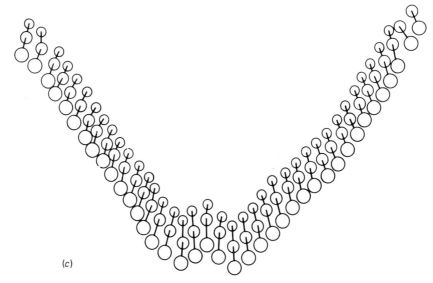

(c)

Figure 2.15 *(a, b)* Coupling of the movement of the basilar membrane to the stereocilia, by means of a shear between the tectorial membrane and the reticular lamina, in a direction radial across the cochlear duct. (From Davis, 1958). *(c)* The direction of tip links on an outer hair cell, showing that they run nearly parallel to the cell's axis of bilateral symmetry, and so nearly radially across the cochlear duct. (From Comis, Pickles and Osborne, 1985)

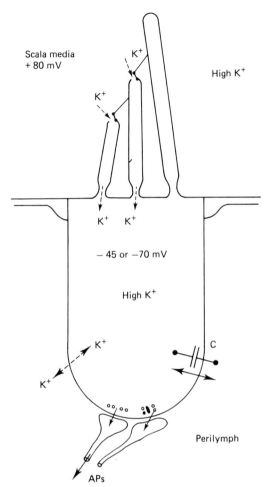

Figure 2.16 Suggested ion flows in a hair cell resulting from transduction. The transducer channels are shown on the ends of the shorter stereocilia, at the lower ends of the tip links, although their exact position is not known. After entering through the transducer channels, K^+ can redistribute itself passively across the basal membrane of the hair cell. The capacitance (C) of the basal cell membranes provides a low-impedance path for high frequency alternating currents. APs = action potentials

the basolateral membranes of the hair cells has been detected as an increase in the K^+ concentration within the space of the organ of Corti during sound stimulation (Johnstone *et al.*, 1989). However, it is possible that some of the transducer current is also carried by other ions, such as Ca^{2+}. It is appropriate for K^+ to be the main carrier of the transducer current. As K^+ is automatically in equilibrium across the basal membrane of the hair cell, any excess K^+ entering the cell through the transducer channel will flow out through the basal membrane without any pumping being necessary. The energy for the whole process comes

from the stria vascularis which, by ion pumping, stores energy in the 'battery' of the endolymph. This is the 'battery' or 'resistance modulation' theory of Davis (1965), as it appears in the light of modern evidence.

Because the stereocilia are driven by a radial shear between the tectorial membrane and the reticular lamina, and because this shear is produced by a vertical movement of the cochlear partition, the hair cells would be expected to have, to a first approximation at least, the same frequency tuning as the mechanical vibration of the basilar membrane. This is supported by the records available so far (see for example Figure 2.11), although it is still open as to whether there are differences of detail, particularly in the low-frequency part of the tuning curve.

The electrical responses of cochlear hair cells

Inner hair cells

The inner hair cells make a large number of synaptic contacts with the afferent fibres of the auditory nerve. In fact, some 95% of all afferent auditory nerve fibres make contact with the inner hair cells, and each inner hair cell has terminals from about 20 afferent fibres (Spoendlin, 1972). It must, therefore, be assumed that the role of inner hair cells is to detect the movement of the basilar membrane and transmit it to the auditory nerve.

If the electrical potential of an inner hair cell is measured during a low-frequency acoustic stimulus, approximately sinusoidal oscillations of the membrane potential are obtained, as the transducer channels open and close (Figure 2.17*a*, top traces). If such records are used to plot the instantaneous value of the input sound pressure against the intracellular voltage, the curves are obtained as in Figure 2.17*b*. This record was obtained from an inner hair cell of the guinea-pig cochlea, driven by an acoustic stimulus. The values along the horizontal axis of Figure 2.17*b* are therefore plotted as sound pressure at the input, rather than as a direct deflection of the stereocilia. Where it is possible to manipulate the stereocilia directly, as in explants of the neonatal mouse cochlea where the tectorial membrane has not developed, similar curves are obtained as a function of direct stereociliar displacement (Kros, Rüsch and Richardson, 1992).

The function in Figure 2.17*b* is asymmetrical in two ways. First, the resting or zero point of the function shows that at rest only about 20% of the channels are open. Second, maximum channel opening is achieved much more gradually and for much more extreme deflections than is the case with channel closing. These asymmetries mean that, in response to sinusoidal stimulation, a distorted response will be obtained in the hair cell. The predominant

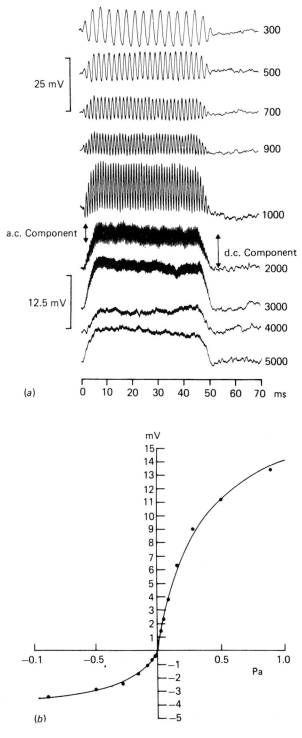

(a)

(b)

Figure 2.17   (*a*) Intracellular voltage changes on an inner hair cell of the guinea-pig cochlea, for different frequencies of stimulation (number on left of traces, Hz). (From Palmer and Russell, 1986). (*b*) Relation between instantaneous sound pressure (horizontal axis) and intracellular voltage change (vertical axis) for an inner hair cell. (From Russell and Sellick, 1983)

distortion is that the positive excursions will be greater than the negative excursions and, as shown by some of the traces in Figure 2.17a, the whole record appears to shift upwards. Therefore, the responses of inner hair cells can be divided, to a first approximation, into an oscillating AC response, occurring at the stimulus frequency, and a DC depolarization.

The importance of these asymmetries is seen when the stimulus frequency is increased above about 1 kHz. Above this frequency, the electrical circuit properties of the hair cell walls begin to affect the response. The basal walls of the hair cell begin to act as a capacitor, and as the frequency is raised, more and more of the transducer current will flow out through the capacitance of the basal walls of the hair cells (see Figure 2.16). It therefore tends to short-circuit the AC component of the transducer current and, consequently, the a.c. (alternating coupled) voltage response in the cell drops (Russell and Sellick, 1983). This is why in Figure 2.17a, the AC changes become relatively smaller as the stimulus frequency is raised. However, the DC component is not affected by this process and remains large even at high frequencies of stimulation (see Figure 2.17a). The different roles of the AC and DC components of the response will be seen when the activity of auditory nerve fibres is discussed.

Consideration of inner hair cell responses is not complete without including the mode of coupling of the movement to the stereocilia. The tips of the inner hair cell stereocilia are not embedded in the tectorial membrane as are the tips of outer hair cell stereocilia. Rather, they are thought to fit loosely into a groove in Hensen's stripe. The stereocilia would therefore appear to be driven by viscous drag of the endolymph. Viscous forces increase with the velocity of the movements, and recordings show that inner hair cells respond to the velocity, rather than just the displacement, of the basilar membrane (Russell and Sellick, 1983).

Outer hair cells

The great majority of the afferent auditory nerve fibres make their synaptic contact with inner rather than outer hair cells. Only a few make contact with outer hair cells. It does not, therefore, appear that outer hair cells form an essential step in transferring information about the basilar membrane vibration to the central nervous system. Rather, the outer hair cells are probably involved in generating the active mechanical amplification of basilar membrane vibration, which gives rise to the relatively large amplitude and sharply tuned mechanical travelling wave. They also generate the cochlear microphonic, and this may be an essential step in the mechanical amplification.

Outer hair cells are relatively difficult to record from in the mammalian cochlea: possibly, the way that the cell body is suspended by its two ends in the spaces between the Deiters' cells means that it is difficult for microelectrodes to penetrate cleanly. In addition, the position of the outer hair cells, partway across the cochlear duct, means that acoustic stimulation is more likely to throw out the microelectrode. Where outer hair cells have been recorded from *in vitro*, they show responses to direct manipulation of their stereocilia in the same way as do inner hair cells (Figure 2.17) (Kros, Rüsch and Richardson, 1992). However, the position *in vivo* is more controversial. Outer hair cells in the apical turns of the cochlea (recorded in the chinchilla, in the 1 kHz frequency region) show responses similar to the isolated outer hair cells. The input–output function (Figure 2.17b) is asymmetric, with the point for zero input near the foot of the function (Dallos, 1985). Outer hair cells in the basal turns of the cochlea (recorded in the guinea pig, in the 20 kHz region), show entirely symmetrical input–output functions, with the resting point in the centre of the function. It is possible that the difference in response depends on a standing bias applied to the stereocilia by the tectorial membrane in the basal turn of the intact cochlea, and this is absent in the apical turns and *in vitro*. Whatever is the cause, the result is that outer hair cells in the basal turns of the cochlea produce only AC responses, and not DC responses at moderate levels of stimulation (for further explanation, see section on inner hair cells above). This means that outer hair cells in the basal turn must be having their effects via their AC responses. At the moment, it is a puzzle how basal turn outer hair cells carry out their function, because at high frequencies the capacitance of the basal walls of the outer hair cells offer a low impedance to AC currents, meaning that outer hair cells produce negligible intracellular a.c. voltage responses, as well as negligible DC responses (Santos-Sacchi, 1992).

The motile response of outer hair cells, thought to be part of the mechanism by which the outer hair cells amplify the travelling wave to increase the cochlea's sensitivity and frequency selectivity (see cochlear mechanics, above), is currently thought to consist of a length change in the outer hair cell body (e.g. Brownell *et al.*, 1985; Santos-Sacchi, 1992). The length changes have been recorded as a.c. movements at up to 15 kHz in isolated fragments of the organ of Corti (Reuter *et al.*, 1992). The motile mechanism appears to reside in the membrane, because if all else in the cell is disrupted but the membrane remains intact, the motile response remains (Holley and Ashmore, 1988). The most recent idea is that the outer hair cell membrane is tightly packed with geometrically and electrically anisotropic protein particles (Kalinec *et al.*, 1992). A voltage across the membrane will reorientate the particles, changing the surface area of the cell membrane. A system of filaments just underlying the membrane constrains the areal change, forcing the cell to keep to the same diameter, so that the cell increases in length instead (Holley, Kalinec and Kachar, 1992). It is not, however, known how a length change in the outer hair cell body feeds back to amplify the vibration of the basilar membrane in return.

The gross electrical responses of the cochlea

If an electrode is placed within one of the cochlear scalae, or on the walls of the cochlea, or indeed anywhere in the vicinity of the cochlea, electric potentials can be recorded in response to acoustic stimuli. They can be divided into three components. First, there is the cochlear microphonic, which is an AC response that follows the waveform of the stimulus (Figure 2.18). Superimposed on that, a DC shift in the baseline of the microphonic is often seen. This is the summating potential. At the beginning of the stimulus, and sometimes at the end, a series of deflections in the negative direction can be seen, making the neural potentials. The first phase is called the N_1 potential and the second smaller phase, which is not always visible, the N_2 potential.

The cochlear microphonic is derived almost entirely from the outer hair cells, for if the cells are destroyed by the ototoxic antibiotic kanamycin, the response will drop drastically (Dallos, 1973). Electrode penetration through the organ of Corti shows the microphonic to be generated at the reticular lamina, which is the interface across which the transducing surface of the hair cell is situated (Tasaki, Davis and Eldredge, 1954). It is likely that the microphonic represents the massed effects of the transducer currents flowing through outer hair cells. Intracochlearly, the microphonic may be essential for the mechanical amplification of the travelling wave.

The summating potential can appear as either a positive or a negative shift, depending on the stimulus

conditions. Unlike the cochlear microphonic, it can take some time to reach maximum amplitude after the onset of a stimulus. Evidence concerning the origin of the summating potential is still incomplete, but it is most likely generated as a distortion component of the outer hair cell response, with perhaps a small contribution from inner hair cells. At present there is insufficient information available about the responses of outer hair cells.

The neural potentials arise from the massed action potentials in the auditory nerve which are produced at the onset of a stimulus. They depend on the sum of a large number of synchronous action potentials, with the N_1 potential arising from the fibres firing the first time in response to the stimulus, and N_2 from the fibres firing a second time. The summed effect is thought to be realized as the action potentials emerge from the internal auditory meatus (Teas, Eldredge and Davis, 1962). With tone pips at low intensities, the N_1 potential will be dominated by fibres with characteristic, or most sensitive, frequencies near the stimulus (see below). However, at higher intensities, fibres of a wider range of characteristic frequencies will be activated. The delays involved in the travelling wave will affect the synchrony. Because the wave travels most rapidly in the base of the cochlea, fibres nearer the base come to dominate the response, and this also means that the latency of the response is reduced as the intensity is raised (Ozdamar and Dallos, 1976).

The responses of auditory nerve fibres
The activation of nerve fibres: phase locking and frequency selectivity

Neurotransmitter is released in the synapses at the base of inner hair cells, and this gives rise to action potentials in the auditory nerve fibres. Single auditory stimuli are always excitatory, never inhibitory. Transmitter is released as a result of depolarization of the inner hair cells. For low-frequency stimuli, the transmitter will be released in packets concentrated during the depolarizing phases of the hair cell response (e.g in the upward phases of the top five traces of Figure 2.17a). Because these take place in synchrony with the sound stimulus, transmitter release and action potential generation is also in synchrony with the individual cycles of the stimulus. This is known as *phase-locking*; an example from an experimental record is shown in Figure 2.19. Phase-locking is seen only at low frequencies, however, where the cyclic changes in inner hair cell intracellular potential are large. As explained earlier (see The electrical responses of cochlear hair cells), the AC component of the intracellular response becomes smaller above about 1 kHz. The degree to which action potentials are phase locked, therefore, declines above this frequency. By 3–5 kHz, the a.c. responses in the inner hair cells are so small that phase-locking of action

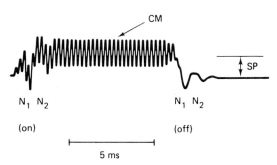

Figure 2.18 Diagram of the gross electrical responses to a tone burst, including the N_1 and N_2 neural potentials, the cochlear microphonic (CM) and the summating potential (SP). (From Pickles, 1988)

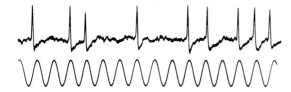

Figure 2.19 Phase-locked action potentials (upper trace), evoked by a 0.3 kHz tone (lower trace). In this record, the action potentials always occur just before the peak of the sound waveform. (From Evans, 1975)

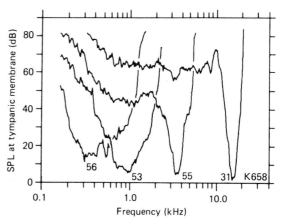

Figure 2.20 Tuning curves of four auditory nerve fibres. (From Kiang, 1980)

potentials is negligible. Only the DC component of the intracellular change can play a part in the generation of action potentials, and then the action potentials are evoked equally in all phases of the sound stimulus (Palmer and Russell, 1986).

Phase-locking represents one way in which information about the sound stimulus is transmitted up the auditory nerve. For stimulus frequencies below some 5 kHz, therefore, the timing of the action potentials in the nerve is able to signal details of the temporal properties of the sound waveform. This is known as the *temporal coding* of stimuli.

A second important way that auditory nerve fibres code information is by means of their frequency selectivity. It should be recalled that inner hair cells detect the movement of the basilar membrane at one point along the cochlear duct, and that the mechanical response of the membrane is very sharply tuned (see Figure 2.11). Auditory nerve fibres, therefore, share the tuning characteristics of single points on the membrane and of the inner hair cells. If recordings are made from fibres at different points on the cochlear duct, the sharply-tuned responses will be centred on different frequencies (Figure 2.20). Figure 2.20 shows tuning curves (frequency-threshold curves) in which the sound pressure level to give a certain criterion increase in firing has been measured automatically by computer for different frequencies of stimulation. Each fibre has a frequency of stimulation for which it is most sensitive, that is for which the sound pressure level was lowest for the criterion response. This is known as the best, or characteristic, frequency. As expected from the tonotopic organization of the mechanical travelling wave in the cochlea, fibres innervating the base have the highest best frequencies, and those innervating the apex the lowest.

Coding based on frequency selectivity is called place coding, for the reason that the fibres responding best to different frequencies arise from different places in the cochlea. It would therefore be possible to determine the frequency of a stimulus by telling which fibres were activated. It should be noted that the temporal code and the place code are not mutually exclusive. A low frequency stimulus will be frequency filtered, according to the place principle, before the fibre is

stimulated. When stimulated, the pattern of firings will carry information about the frequency filtered waveform of the stimulus. The relative extent to which these two principles are actually used by the nervous system under different circumstances is at the moment a matter of debate. Pickles (1986) reviewed and analysed stimulus coding in auditory nerve fibres.

Figure 2.20 also shows that the auditory nerve fibres have their lowest thresholds at around 0 dB SPL. It is indeed a general finding that the most sensitive fibres have their lowest thresholds in an intensity range close to the behavioural absolute threshold. In fact, some 75% of fibres have their best thresholds within a 15-dB range of this (Liberman and Kiang, 1978). These low threshold fibres have particularly high rates of spontaneous activity (that is random firing seen in the absence of any stimulation). It is likely that the low thresholds arise because the fibres have very sensitive synapses on the hair cells. A second minor population of fibres have much higher thresholds, in some cases 70 dB or more above the behavioural threshold. These fibres have particularly low rates of spontaneous activity (Liberman and Kiang, 1978).

The frequency selectivity of auditory nerve fibres can be characterized in a variety of ways. One way is to measure the bandwidth of the tuning curve at a set distance above the tip; bandwidths are often measured 10 dB above the tip. In that case, the bandwidth of cat auditory nerve fibres, in the range in which they are most frequency selective (around 10 kHz) is one-eighth of their characteristic frequency (e.g. Evans, 1975). If the inverse of this is taken, and the 10-dB bandwidth divided by the characteristic frequency is measured, a number that increases with sharpness of tuning is obtained. This is called 'Q_{10dB}', by analogy with the Q value of electrical filters. In the cat, it averages about 8 at 10 kHz.

Intensity responses of auditory nerve fibres

As the stimulus intensity is increased, the amplitude of basilar membrane vibration grows (see Figure 2.12). The activation of inner hair cells grows similarly and, as shown in Figure 2.21, so also does the firing rate of auditory nerve fibres. The functions for the different stages have many points of similarity. The slopes of the rate intensity functions, like the basilar membrane functions, are steeper for stimuli below the characteristic frequency than for those above it. Moreover, stimuli below the characteristic frequency can drive a fibre to greater firing rates than can stimuli above the characteristic frequency. It should also be noted that for stimuli at the characteristic frequency of the fibre, the maximum, or saturated rate has been reached by about 30 dB SPL. Therefore, it would seem that the intensity of an acoustic stimulus can be coded in the firing rates of the auditory nerve fibres at least up to this intensity. A minority of fibres, with high thresholds, do not reach their maximum firing rates until much higher intensities (e.g. above 100 dB SPL), and these fibres would therefore be capable of coding stimulus intensity in the middle and upper part of the intensity range (e.g. Yates, Winter and Robertson, 1990).

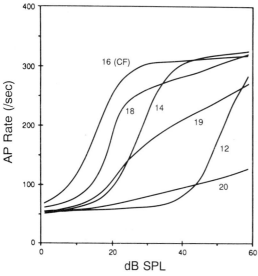

Figure 2.21 Firing rate plotted as a function of stimulus intensity for a guinea-pig auditory nerve fibre (characteristic frequency = 16 kHz), for different frequencies of stimulation, shown by numbers on each curve. (From Yates, Winter and Robertson, 1990, Fig. 2)

Non-linear interactions in the cochlea and auditory nerve

Although single auditory stimuli are always excitatory, one stimulus can change the responsiveness of auditory nerve fibres to other stimuli. This derives from the non-linear mechanical response of the basilar membrane vibration, where the application of one stimulus can reduce the response to a second stimulus (Ruggero, Robles and Rich, 1992). The reduction of activity is called two-tone suppression, because it is seen only during the interaction of two or more stimuli. It can, therefore, be distinguished from inhibition mediated by inhibitory synapses because spontaneous activity cannot be inhibited. The actual mechanisms of two-tone suppression are a matter of debate. The generally favoured mechanism is that the suppressor drives the outer hair cells to the upper limits of their amplitude range of sensitivity (see Figure 2.17b). This reduces the extent to which the hair cells can increase their response to a second superimposed stimulus, and so contribute to the active mechanical amplification of the travelling wave to the second stimulus (Johnstone, Patuzzi and Yates, 1986). Two-tone suppression may well be important functionally. In the firing of the auditory nerve fibre array, it aids in keeping separate the representation of the different elements of a complex stimulus.

Basilar membrane vibration and auditory nerve responses in pathological cochleae

As studied physiologically, it is apparent that most types of cochlear sensorineural hearing loss are related to loss of the sharply tuned portion of the mechanical travelling wave. This has been seen directly in the travelling wave, in the responses of hair cells, and in the responses of auditory nerve fibres. The loss probably happens because outer hair cells are among the most vulnerable elements in the organ of Corti, leading to the loss of their contribution to the active mechanical component of the travelling wave. Moreover, it is likely that small deteriorations in the outer hair cell travelling wave system are immediately noticeable. In the more severe cases, loss of inner hair cells and auditory nerve fibre responses will also reduce the detection of sounds. Here, it is possible that the great redundancy arising from the large number of auditory nerve fibres affords some protection from the effects of small losses.

The changes in the mechanical travelling wave resulting from the effects of cochlear damage are shown in Figure 2.22a. In this instance, as the experiment progressed, the tuning curve changed shape from a sharply-tuned, low-threshold curve, to a higher-threshold and broadly-tuned curve. This prob-

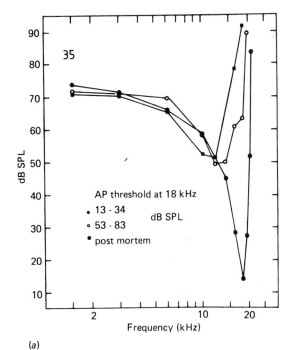

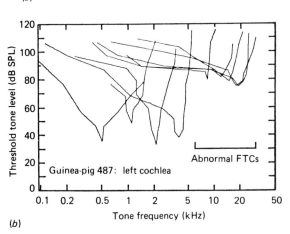

Figure 2.22 (a) Basilar membrane tuning measured when the cochlea was in good condition (●), poor condition (○), or after death (■). (From Sellick, Patuzzi and Johnstone, 1982). (b) Auditory nerve fibre tuning curves in a guinea-pig treated with kanamycin. Fibres at the high-frequency end of the cochlea had high thresholds and broad tuning ('abnormal FTCs'). (From Evans and Harrison, 1976)

ably happened as a result of trauma from the acoustic stimuli used in making the measurements. After death, the curve had a still higher threshold and still broader tuning (Figure 2.22a). Here there would be complete loss of the active component of cochlear mechanics, and a resulting loss of the active mechanical amplification of the travelling wave. There would

then be a return to a broadly-tuned wave similar to the one shown originally in cadavers by Békésy (1943, 1960).

Similar changes can be seen in the tuning curves of auditory nerve fibres in guinea-pigs that have been treated with kanamycin, an aminoglycoside antibiotic which preferentially destroys outer hair cells. Figure 2.22b shows that auditory nerve fibres recorded from the region of cochlear damage had high thresholds and broad tuning, comparable to the pathological basilar membrane responses of Figure 2.22a. Corresponding changes can be seen experimentally with a variety of challenges, including anoxia, the infusion of ototoxic agents, and ageing (e.g. Schmeidt, Mills and Adams, 1990; Martin et al., 1993).

The changes initially produce a rise in the best thresholds of auditory nerve fibres, and then, with larger losses, a deterioration in the fibres' frequency resolving power. This is shown as an increase in the widths of the tuning curves. Such changes have an obvious correlate with the changes observed in man in many cases of sensorineural loss of cochlear origin, with an increase in absolute threshold and a loss of frequency resolution, apparent as a deterioration in the ability to understand complex sounds such as speech. Recruitment is commonly seen with sensorineural hearing loss, and this too has its correlates in the activity of auditory nerve fibres. First, when the low-threshold tip of the tuning curve is lost, the rate-intensity functions steepen. It should be noted that, as in Figure 2.21, in a normal fibre the intensity function is relatively shallow for frequencies of stimulation at and above the fibre best frequency. This is a result of the active amplification of the cochlear travelling wave, which produces a shallow growth in the basilar membrane intensity functions at and above best frequency (see Figure 2.12). When the active component of the travelling wave is lost, the shallow growth disappears and the rate-intensity functions come to have a similar, steep, slope at all frequencies (Harrison, 1981). A second reason relates to the spread of activity along the array of nerve fibres. If the tuning curves are much broader than normal – say by a factor of 10 times – then for a certain level above fibre threshold, 10 times as many fibres will be activated as in the normal case. Increases in stimulus level will then produce changes in 10 times as many fibres as in the normal case, and loudness will grow correspondingly more quickly.

A different pattern of changes is seen with experimental endolymphatic hydrops. Harrison and Prijs (1984) showed that, in guinea-pigs with long-term experimental hydrops, low-frequency nerve fibres were affected most, with increases in their best thresholds, and a deterioration in sharpness of tuning. This can be contrasted with the pattern usually seen with cochlear damage, where the high frequency fibres seem most vulnerable. A specific effect on low frequency fibres can be expected if the *stiffness* of the cochlear partition has been increased by the hydrops, because this is the characteristic pattern of change with increases in stiffness in a mechanical system.

The centrifugal innervation of the cochlea

The cochlea receives a centrifugal, or efferent, nerve supply, arising in the superior olivary complex of the brain stem; it is called the olivocochlear bundle. One component of the bundle (the medial olivocochlear system), which arises from the medial borders of the superior olivary complex and projects mainly contra-laterally, innervates the outer hair cells directly. A smaller number of fibres, making the lateral olivocochlear system, arise laterally in the superior olivary complex, mainly on the ipsilateral side, and innervate the afferent dendrites below the inner hair cells (Guinan, Warr and Norris, 1983).

The functional importance of the olivocochlear bundle has long been a mystery. Speculations built on recent evidence suggest that, by affecting the state of the outer hair cells, the olivocochlear bundle can modify the active mechanical amplification of the travelling wave in the cochlea. Although effects on the basilar membrane vibration have not yet been measured directly, activation of the fibres can modify the extent to which the cochlea returns energy to the ear canal (see next section), suggesting an influence on the mechanics (Mountain, 1980). The changes that it can produce in inner hair cell and auditory nerve fibre tuning curves also suggest that it has its effect via an influence on mechanical tuning (Wieder-hold, 1970; Brown, Nuttall and Masta, 1983), while acetylcholine, the major neurotransmitter of the olivo-cochlear bundle, affects the gain of the active motile response in isolated outer hair cells (Sziklai and Dallos, 1993). Rajan and Johnstone (1983) showed that stimulation of the bundle could protect the ear against moderate levels of noise damage, which is understandable if the olivocochlear bundle reduced the magnitude of the travelling wave. There is also the suggestion that it may be involved in selective attention, although this result is controversial (Puel, Bonfils and Pujol, 1988).

Cochlear echoes

One of the most intriguing discoveries has been that the cochlea can emit sounds. It appears that the vibrations arise from the hair cells themselves, or at least that the hair cells are an essential component of the process producing the sounds. It also seems likely that the production of sound by the cochlea is a by-product of the active mechanical amplification of the travelling wave. Cochlear echoes also open the possi-

bility of a new objective tool for diagnosing cochlear abnormalities.

Cochlear echoes were discovered by Kemp (1978), who sealed a small microphone and speaker into the ear canals of human subjects. In response to a click applied to the speaker, there was a peak of pressure in the canal. However, there was also a later, and much smaller, peak. Amplification of the traces showed that the second peak was a complex wave, with a form different for each subject (Figure 2.23). If the wave had predominantly high frequency compo-nents, they appeared soon after the stimulus, and if it had predominantly low frequency components, they appeared later. It is suggested that, as the travelling wave progressed up the cochlea, it might meet imped-ance discontinuities, perhaps formed by irregularities in the active system feeding energy back into the travelling wave. The discontinuities would reflect a reverse pressure wave, which would emerge through the middle ear and be recorded in the canal. This model would account for the relation between the predominant frequency in the response, and the time delay after the stimulus.

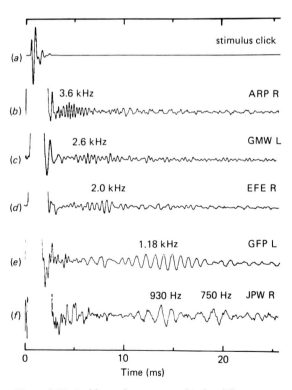

Figure 2.23 Cochlear echoes measured in five different subjects. (*a*) Sound pressure in canal produced by a click. (*b–f*) Sound pressures in canal, shown with a much magnified vertical scale. The input click has clipped (first 3 ms), but the waveform of the echo is visible (3–22 ms). The predominant frequency in each echo is marked on the trace. (From Wilson, 1980)

It can be shown that an active mechanical amplifier is involved in the echo, because for very low intensity stimuli more energy can be returned to the ear canal than was originally introduced (Kemp, 1978). In other cases, where the subject was hearing a tonal tinnitus, the tinnitus could be detected as a sound pressure fluctuation in the canal (Kemp, 1979). However, it is recognized that this is probably not the clinically important form of tinnitus, which is likely to arise by means of a different mechanism, perhaps centrally. Echoes can be detected in both entirely healthy cochleae and those showing small losses, while strong spontaneous emissions seem to be associated with localized hair cell pathology in the presence of normal hair cells (e.g. Clark *et al.*, 1984). The presence of emissions or echoes can therefore be used as an objective indication of the state of the cochlea, with an echo at normal levels indicating a threshold within 30 dB of normal (for review see Probst, Lonsbury-Martin and Martin, 1991). The method has been developed into an automated testing system of objective audiometry, which has the advantage that it is rapid, does not require sedation of infants, and does not require high levels of screening against ambient sounds (Bray and Kemp, 1987).

References

ANNIKO, M. and WROBLEWSKI, R. (1986) Ionic environment of cochlear hair cells. *Hearing Research*, **22**, 279–293

ANNIKO, M., LIM, D. and WROBLEWSKI, R. (1984) Elemental composition of individual cells and tissues in the cochlea. *Acta Otolaryngologica*, **98**, 439–453

ASSAD, J. A., SHEPHERD, G. M. G. and COREY, D. P. (1991) Tip-link integrity and mechanical transduction in vertebrate hair cells. *Neuron*, **7**, 985–994

BÉKÉSY, G. VON (1941) Uber die Messung der Schwingungsamplitude der Gehorknochelchen mittels einer kapazitiven Sonde. *Akustische Zeitschrift*, **6**, 1–16

BÉKÉSY, G. VON (1943) Uber die Resonanzkurve und die Abklingzeit der verschiedenen Stellen der Schneckentrennwand. *Akustische Zeitschrift*, **8**, 66–76

BÉKÉSY, G. VON (1952) Resting potentials inside the cochlear partition of the guinea pig. *Nature*, **169**, 241–242

BÉKÉSY, G. VON (1960) *Experiments in Hearing*, edited by E. G. Wever. New York: McGraw Hill

BORG, E. (1973) On the neuronal organization of the acoustic middle ear reflex. A physiological and anatomical study. *Brain Research*, **49**, 101–123

BORG, E. and ZAKRISSON, J. E. (1973) Stapedius reflex and speech features. *Journal of the Acoustical Society of America*, **54**, 525–527

BOSHER, S. K. (1980) The effects of inhibition of the strial Na$^+$-K$^+$-activated ATPase by perilymphatic ouabain in the guinea pig. *Acta Otolaryngologica*, **90**, 219–229

BOSHER, S. K. and WARREN, R. L. (1968) Observations on the electrochemistry of the cochlear endolymph of the rat: a quantitative study of its electrical potential and ionic composition as determined by means of flame spectrophotometry. *Proceedings of the Royal Society, Series B*, **171**, 227–247

BRAY, P. and KEMP, D. T. (1987) An advanced cochlear echo technique suitable for infant screening. *British Journal of Audiology*, **21**, 191–204

BROWN, M. C., NUTTALL, A. L. and MASTA, R. I. (1983) Intracellular recordings from cochlear inner hair cells: effects of stimulation of the crossed olivocochlear efferents. *Science*, **222**, 69–72

BROWNELL, W. E., BADER, C. R., BERTRAND, D. and RIBAUPIERRE, Y. DE (1985) Evoked mechanical responses of isolated cochlear outer hair cells. *Science*, **227**, 194–196

CLARK, W. W., KIM, D. O., ZUREK, P. M. and BOHNE, B. A. (1984) Spontaneous otoacoustic emissions in chinchilla ear canals: correlation with histopathology and suppression by external tones. *Hearing Research*, **16**, 299–314

COMIS, S. D., PICKLES, J. O. and OSBORNE, M. P. (1985) Osmium tetroxide postfixation in relation to the cross linkage and spatial organization of stereo cilia in the guinea-pig cochlea. *Journal of Neurocytology*, **14**, 113–130

COREY, D. P. and HUDSPETH, A. J. (1979) Ionic basis of the receptor potential in a vertebrate hair cell. *Nature*, **281**, 675–677

DALLOS, P. (1973) Cochlear potentials and cochlear mechanics. In: *Basic Mechanisms in Hearing*, edited by A. R. Møller. New York: Academic Press. pp. 335–372

DALLOS, P. (1985) Response characteristics of mammalian cochlear hair cells. *Journal of Neuroscience*, **5**, 1591–1608

DALLOS, P. (1992). The active cochlea. *Journal of Neuroscience*, **12**, 4575–4585

DAVIS, H. (1958) Transmission and transduction in the cochlea. *Laryngoscope*, **68**, 359–382

DAVIS, H. (1965) A model for transducer action in the cochlea. *Cold Spring Harbor Symposia on Quantitative Biology*, **30**, 181–189

DECRAEMER, W. F., DIRCKX, J. J. J. and FUNNELL, W. R. J. (1991) Shape and derived geometrical parameters of the adult, human tympanic membrane measured with a phase-shift moiré interferometer. *Hearing Research*, **51**, 107–122

DECRAEMER, W. F., KHANNA, S. M. and FUNNELL, W. R. J. (1991) Malleus vibration mode changes with frequency. *Hearing Research*, **54**, 305–318

EVANS, E. F. (1975) Cochlear nerve and cochlear nucleus. In: *Handbook of Sensory Physiology Vol 5/2*, edited by W. D. Keidel and W. D. Neff. Berlin: Springer. pp. 1–108

EVANS, E. F. and HARRISON, R. V. (1976) Correlation between cochlear outer hair cell damage and deterioration of cochlear nerve tuning properties in the guinea pig. *Journal of Physiology*, **256**, 43–44P

FAWCETT, D. W. (1986) *A Textbook of Histology*. Philadelphia: W. B. Saunders

FELDMAN, A. M. (1981) Cochlear biochemistry. In *Pharmacology of Hearing*, edited by R. D. Brown and E. A. Daigneault. New York: Wiley. pp. 52–80

GUINAN, J. J. and PEAKE, W. T. (1967) Middle-ear characteristics of anesthetized cats. *Journal of the Acoustical Society of America*, **41**, 1237–1261

GUINAN, J. J., WARR, W. B. and NORRIS, B. E. (1983) Differential olivocochlear projections from lateral versus medial zones of the superior olivary complex. *Journal of Comparative Neurology*, **221**, 358–370

HARRISON, R. V. (1981) Rate-versus-intensity functions and related AP responses in normal and pathological guinea pig and human cochleas. *Journal of the Acoustical Society of America*, **70**, 1036–1044

HARRISON, R. V. and PRIJS, V. F. (1984) Single cochlear fibre responses in guinea pigs with long-term endolymphatic hydrops. *Hearing Research*, **14**, 79–84

HILDING, D. A. (1961) The protective value of the stapedius reflex: an experimental study. *Transactions of the American Academy for Ophthalmology and Otolaryngology*, **65**, 297–307

HOLLEY, M. C. and ASHMORE, J. F. (1988) On the mechanism of a high-frequency force generator in outer hair cells isolated from the guinea pig cochlea. *Proceedings of the Royal Society of London B*, **232**, 413–429

HOLLEY, M. C., KALINEC, F. and KACHAR, B. (1992) Structure of the cortical cytoskeleton in mammalian outer hair cells. *Journal of Cell Science*, **102**, 569–580

HUDDE, H. (1983) Measurement of the eardrum impedance of human ears. *Journal of the Acoustical Society of America*, **73**, 242–247

HUDSPETH, A. J. and COREY, D. P. (1977). Sensitivity, polarity, and conductance change in the response of vertebrate hair cells to controlled mechanical stimuli. *Proceedings of the National Academy of Sciences of the USA*, **74**, 2407–2411

IKEDA, K., and MORIZONO, T. (1989) Electrochemical profiles for monovalent ions in the stria vascularis: cellular model of ion transport mechanisms. *Hearing Research*, **39**, 279–286

IRVINE, D. R. F., CLAREY, J. C., MORTON, R. E. and NEWMAN R. G. (1983) Masking by internally generated noise and protection by middle ear muscle activity. *Hearing Research*, **10**, 371–374

JARAMILLO, F. and HUDSPETH, A. J. (1991) Localization of the hair cell's transduction channels at the hair bundle's top by iontophoretic application of a channel blocker. *Neuron*, **7**, 409–420

JOHNSTONE, B. M. and SELLICK, P. M. (1972) The peripheral auditory apparatus. *Quarterly Reviews of Biophysics*, **5**, 1–57

JOHNSTONE, B. M., PATUZZI, R. and YATES, G. K. (1986) Basilar membrane measurements and the travelling wave. *Hearing Research*, **22**, 147–153

JOHNSTONE, B. M., PATUZZI, R., SYKA, J. and SYKOVA, E. (1989) Stimulus-related potassium changes in the organ of Corti of the guinea pig. *Journal of Physiology*, **408**, 77–92

KALINEC, F., HOLLEY, M. C., IWASA, K. H., LIM, D. J. and KACHAR, B. (1992) A membrane-based force generation mechanism in auditory sensory cells. *Proceedings of the National Academy of Sciences of the USA*, **89**, 8671–8675

KEMP, D. T. (1978) Stimulated acoustic emissions from within the human auditory system. *Journal of the Acoustical Society of America*, **64**, 1386–1391

KEMP, D. T. (1979) Evidence for mechanical nonlinearity and frequency selective wave amplification in the cochlea. *Archives of Oto-Rhino-Laryngology*, **224**, 37–45

KHANNA, S. M. and TONNDORF, J. (1972) Tympanic membrane vibration in cats studied by time-averaged holography. *Journal of the Acoustical Society of America*, **51**, 1904–1920

KIANG, N.-Y.-S. (1980) Processing of speech by the auditory nervous system. *Journal of the Acoustical Society of America*, **68**, 830–835

KIMURA, R. S. (1967) Experimental blockage of the endolymphatic duct and sac and its effect on the inner ear of the guinea pig. *Annals of Otology, Rhinology and Laryngology*, **76**, 664–687

KONISHI, T. and HAMRICK, P. E. (1978) Ion transport in the cochlea of guinea pig. II. Chloride transport. *Acta Otolaryngologica*, **86**, 176–184

KONISHI, T., HAMRICK, P. E. and MORI, H. (1984) Water permeability of the endolymph-perilymph barrier in the guinea pig cochlea. *Hearing Research*, **15**, 51–58

KONISHI, T., SALT, A. N. and HAMRICK, P. E. (1979) Effects of exposure to noise on ion movement in guinea pig cochlea. *Hearing Research*, **1**, 325–342

KRINGLEBOTN, M. and GUNDERSEN, T. (1985) Frequency characteristics of the middle ear. *Journal of the Acoustical Society of America*, **77**, 159–164

KROS, C. J., RÜSCH, A. and RICHARDSON, G. P. (1992) Mechano-electrical transducer currents in hair cells of the cultured neonatal mouse cochlea. *Proceedings of the Royal Society B*, **249**, 185–193

KUIJPERS, W. and BONTING, S. L. (1969) Studies on the (Na^+-K^+)-activated ATPase. XXIV. Localization and properties of ATPase in the inner ear of the guinea pig. *Biochimica et Biophysica Acta*, **173**, 477–485

KUIJPERS, W. and BONTING, S. L. (1970) The cochlear potentials. I. The effect of ouabain on the cochlear potentials of the guinea pig. *Pflügers Archiv European Journal of Physiology*, **320**, 348–358

LAWTON, B. W. and STINSON, M. R. (1986) Standing wave patterns in the human ear canal used for estimation of acoustic energy reflectance at the ear drum. *Journal of the Acoustical Society of America*, **79**, 1003–1009

LIBERMAN, M. C. and KIANG, N.-Y.-S. (1978) Acoustic trauma in cats. *Acta Otolaryngologica Supplementum*, **358**, 1–63

LYNCH, T. J., NEDZELNITSKY, V. and PEAKE, W. T. (1982) Input impedance of the cochlea in cat. *Journal of the Acoustical Society of America*, **72**, 108–130

MAKIMOTO, K., TAKEDA, T. and SILVERSTEIN, H. (1980) Species differences in inner ear fluids. *Archives of Oto-Rhino-Laryngology*, **228**, 187–194

MARTIN, W. H., SCHWEGLER, J. W., SCHEIBELHOFFER, J. and RONIS, M. L. (1993) Salicylate-induced changes in cat auditory nerve activity. *Laryngoscope*, **103**, 600–604

MELICHAR, I. and SYKA, J. (1987) Electrophysiological measurements of the stria vascularis potentials in vivo. *Hearing Research*, **25**, 35–43

METZ, O. (1951) Studies on the contraction of the tympanic muscles as indicated by changes in the impedance of the ear. *Acta Otolaryngologica*, **39**, 397–405

MIDDLEBROOKS, J. C., MAKOUS, J. C. and GREEN, D. M. (1989) Directional sensitivity of sound-pressure levels in the human ear canal. *Journal of the Acoustical Society of America*, **86**, 89–108

MØLLER, A. R. (1964) Effect of tympanic muscle activity on movement of the eardrum, acoustic impedance, and cochlear microphonics. *Acta Otolaryngologica*, **58**, 525–534

MØLLER, A. R. (1974) The acoustic middle ear muscle reflex. In: *Handbook of Sensory Physiology Vol. 5/1*, edited by W. D. Keidel and W. D. Neff. Berlin: Springer. pp. 519–548

MORGENSTERN, C., AMANO, H. and ORSULAKOVA, A. (1982) Ion transport in the endolymphatic space. *American Journal of Otolaryngology*, **3**, 323–327

MOUNTAIN, D. C. (1980) Changes in endolymphatic potential and crossed olivocochlear bundle stimulation alter cochlear mechanics. *Science*, **210**, 71–72

NEDZELNITSKY, V. (1980) Sound pressures in the basal turn of the cat cochlea. *Journal of the Acoustical Society of America*, **68**, 1676–1689

OFFNER, D. L., DALLOS, P. and CHEATHAM, M. A. (1987) Positive endocochlear potential: mechanism of production by marginal cells of the stria vascularis. *Hearing Research*, **29**, 117–124

ÖZDAMAR, Ö. and DALLOS, P. (1976) Input-output functions of cochlear whole-nerve action potentials: interpretation in terms of one population of neurons. *Journal of the Acoustical Society of America*, **59**, 143–147

PALMER, A. R. and RUSSELL, I. J. (1986) Phase-locking in the cochlear nerve of the guinea-pig and its relation to the receptor potential of inner hair-cells. *Hearing Research*, **24**, 1–15

PANG, X. D. and PEAKE, W. T. (1986) How do contractions of the stapedius muscle alter the acoustic properties of the ear? In: *Peripheral Auditory Mechanisms*, edited by J. B. Allen, J. L. Hall, A. Hubbard, S. T. Neely and A. Tubis. Berlin: Springer. pp. 36–43

PAYNE, M. C. and GITHLER, F. J. (1951) Effects of perforations of the tympanic membrane on cochlear potentials. *Archives of Otolaryngology*, **54**, 666–674

PEAKE, W. T., ROSOWSKI, J. J. and LYNCH, T. J. (1992) Middle-ear transmission: acoustic versus ossicular coupling in cat and human. *Hearing Research*, **57**, 245–268

PETERSON, S. K., FRISHKOPF, L. S., LECHENE, C., OMAN, D. M. and WEISS, T. F. (1978) Element composition of inner ear lymph in cats, lizards and skates determined by electron probe microanalysis of liquid samples. *Journal of Comparative Physiology*, **126**, 1–14

PHILLIPS, D. P., CALFORD, M. B., PETTIGREW, J. D., AITKIN, L. M. and SEMPLE, M. N. (1982) Directionality of sound pressure transformation at the cat's pinna. *Hearing Research*, **8**, 13–28

PICKLES, J. O. (1985) Hearing and listening. In: *Scientific Basis of Clinical Neurology*, edited by M. Swash and C. Kennard. Edinburgh: Churchill Livingstone. pp. 188–200

PICKLES, J. O. (1986) The neurophysiological basis of frequency selectivity. In: *Frequency Selectivity in Hearing*, edited by B. C. J. Moore. London: Academic Press. pp. 51–121

PICKLES, J. O. (1988) *An Introduction to the Physiology of Hearing*, 2nd edn. London: Academic Press

PICKLES, J. O. and COREY, D. P. (1992) Mechanoelectrical transduction by hair cells. *Trends in Neurosciences*, **15**, 254–259

PICKLES, J. O., COMIS, S. D. and OSBORNE, M. P. (1984) Cross-links between stereocilia in the guinea pig organ of Corti, and their possible relation to sensory transduction. *Hearing Research*, **15**, 103–112

PROBST, R., LONSBURY-MARTIN, B. L. and MARTIN, G. K. (1991) A review of otoacoustic emissions. *Journal of the Acoustical Society of America*, **89**, 2027–2067

PUEL, J. L., BONFILS, P. and PUJOL, R. (1988) Selective attention modifies the active micromechanical properties of the cochlea. *Brain Research*, **447**, 380–383

RAJAN, R. and JOHNSTONE, B. M. (1983) Crossed cochlear influences on monaural temporary threshold shifts. *Hearing Research*, **9**, 279–294

RAUCH, S. and KOSTLIN, A. (1958) Aspects chimiques de l'endolymphe et de la perilymphe. *Practica Oto-RhinoLaryngologica*, **20**, 287–291

REUTER, G., GITTER, A. H., THURM, U. and ZENNER, H-P. (1992) High frequency radial movements of the reticular lamina induced by outer hair cell motility. *Hearing Research*, **60**, 236–246

ROBLES, L., RUGGERO, M. A. and RICH, N. C. (1986) Basilar membrane mechanics at the base of the chinchilla cochlea. I. Input-output functions, tuning curves, and response

phases. *Journal of the Acoustical Society of America*, **80**, 1364–1374

ROSOWSKI, J. J., CARNEY, L. H., LYNCH, T. J. and PEAKE, W. T. (1986) The effectiveness of external and middle ears in coupling acoustic power into the cochlea. In: *Peripheral Auditory Mechanisms*, edited by J. B. Allen, J. L. Hall, A. Hubbard, S. T. Neely and A. Tubis. Berlin: Springer. pp. 3–12

ROSOWSKI, J. J., CARNEY, L. H. and PEAKE, W. T. (1990) The radiation impedance of the external ear of the cat: measurements and applications. *Journal of the Acoustical Society of America*, **84**, 1695–1708

RUGGERO, M. A. (1992) Responses to sound of the basilar membrane of the mammalian cochlea. *Current Opinion in Neurobiology*, **2**, 449–456

RUGGERO, M. A., ROBLES, L. and RICH, N. C. (1992) Two-tone suppression in the basilar membrane of the cochlea: mechanical basis of auditory-nerve rate suppression. *Journal of Neurophysiology*, **68**, 1087–1099

RUSSELL, I. J. and SELLICK, P. M. (1978) Intracellular studies of hair cells in the mammalian cochlea. *Journal of Physiology*, **284**, 261–290

RUSSELL, I. J. and SELLICK, P. M. (1983) Low-frequency characteristics of intracellularly recorded receptor potentials in guinea-pig cochlear hair cells. *Journal of Physiology*, **338**, 179–206

RYAN, A. F., WICKHAM, M. G. and BONE, R. C. (1980) Studies of ion distribution in the inner ear: scanning electron microscopy and x-ray microanalysis of freeze-dried cochlear specimens. *Hearing Research*, **2**, 1–20

SANTOS-SACCHI, J. (1992) On the frequency limit and phase of outer hair cell motility: effects of the membrane filter. *Journal of Neuroscience*, **12**, 1906–1916

SCHMEIDT, R. A., MILLS, J. H. and ADAMS, J. C. (1990) Tuning and suppression in auditory nerve fibers of aged gerbils raised in quiet or noise. *Hearing Research*, **45**, 221–236

SELLICK, P. M. and JOHNSTONE, B. M. (1972) Changes in cochlear endolymph Na$^+$ concentration measured with Na$^+$ specific micro electrodes. *Pflügers Archiv European Journal of Pathology*, **336**, 11–20

SELLICK, P. M., PATUZZI, R. and JOHNSTONE, B. M. (1982) Measurement of basilar membrane motion in the guinea pig using the Mössbauer technique. *Journal of the Acoustical Society of America*, **72**, 131–141

SHAW, E. A. G. (1974) The external ear. In: *Handbook of Sensory Physiology Vol. 5/1*, edited by W. D. Keidel and W. D. Neff. Berlin: Springer. pp. 455–490

SHAW, E. A. C. and STINSON, M. R. (1983) The human external and middle ear: models and concepts. In: *Mechanics of Hearing*, edited by E. de Boer and M. A. Viergever. The Hague: Martinus Nijhoff. pp. 3–18

SILMAN, S. (1984) *The Acoustic Reflex*. Orlando: Academic Press

SILVERSTEIN, H. (1972) A rapid protein test for inner ear fluid analysis. *Transactions of the American Academy for Ophthalmology and Otolaryngology*, **76**, 1030–1031

SIMMONS, F. B. (1964) Perceptual theories of middle ear muscle function. *Annals of Otology, Rhinology and Laryngology*, **73**, 724–740

SMITH, C. A. (1978) Structure of the cochlear duct. In: *Evoked Electrical Activity in the Auditory Nervous System*, edited by R. F. Naunton and C. Fernandez. New York: Academic Press. pp. 3–19

SMITH, C. A., LOWRY, O. H. and WU, M. L. (1954) The

electrolytes of the labyrinthine fluids. *Laryngoscope*, **64**, 141–153

SPOENDLIN, H. (1972) Innervation densities of the cochlea. *Acta Otolaryngologica*, **73**, 235–248

STERKERS, O., SAUMON, G., TRAN BA HUY, P. and AMIEL, C. (1982) Evidence for a perilymphatic origin of the endolymph. Application to the pathophysiology of Menieres disease. *American Journal of Otolaryngology*, **3**, 367–375

STERKERS, O., FERRARY, E. and AMIEL, C. (1988) Production of inner ear fluids. *Physiological Reviews*, **68**, 1083–1128

STINSON, M. R. and KHANNA, S. M. (1989) Sound propagation in the ear canal and coupling to the eardrum, with measurements on model systems. *Journal of the Acoustical Society of America*, **85**, 2481–2491

SZIKLAI, I. and DALLOS, P. (1993) Acetylcholine controls the gain of the voltage-to-movement converter in isolated outer hair cells. *Acta Otolaryngologica*, **113**, 326–329

TASAKI, I., DAVIS, H. and ELDREDGE, D. H. (1954) Exploration of cochlear potentials in guinea pig with a microelectrode. *Journal of the Acoustical Society of America*, **26**, 765–773

TEAS, D. C., ELDREDGE, D. H. and DAVIS, H. (1962). Cochlear responses to acoustic transients: an interpretation of whole-nerve action potentials. *Journal of the Acoustical Society of America*, **34**, 1438–1459

TONNDORF, J. (1966) Bone conduction: studies in experimental animals. *Acta Otolaryngologica Supplementum*, **213**, 1–132

TONNDORF, J. (1976) Bone conduction. In: *Handbook of Sensory Physiology Vol. 5/3*, edited by W. D. Keidel and W. D. Neff. Berlin: Springer. pp. 37–84

VAN DEN BERGE, H., KINGMA, H., KLUGE, C. and MARRES, E. H. M. A. (1990) Electrophysiological aspects of the middle ear muscle reflex in the rat: latency, rise time and effect on sound transmission. *Hearing Research*, **48**, 209–220

WEVER, E. G. and LAWRENCE, M. (1954) *Physiological Acoustics*. Princeton: Princeton University Press

WIEDERHOLD, M. L. (1970) Variations in the effects of electric stimulation of the crossed olivocochlear bundle on cat single auditory nerve fiber responses to tone bursts. *Journal of the Acoustical Society of America*, **48**, 966–977

WILSON, J. P. (1980) Evidence for a cochlear origin for acoustic re-emissions, threshold fine structure and tonal tinnitus. *Hearing Research*, **2**, 233–252

YATES, G. K., WINTER, I. M. and ROBERTSON, D. (1990) Basilar membrane nonlinearity determines auditory nerve rate-intensity functions and cochlear dynamic range. *Hearing Research*, **45**, 203–220

ZAKRISSON, J. E. and BORG, E. (1974) Stapedius reflex and auditory fatigue. *Audiology*, **13**, 231–235

3

The perception of sound

Brian C. J. Moore

The ear as a frequency analyser

Unlike the sinusoidal tones which are often used in the assessment of hearing, sounds encountered in everyday life are generally complex, containing a number of different sinusoidal frequency components. It is a central characteristic of the auditory system that it acts as a limited-resolution Fourier analyser; complex sounds are broken down into their sinusoidal frequency components. The initial basis of this frequency analysis almost certainly depends upon the tuning which is observed in the cochlea (see Chapter 2 for details). Indeed, it is possible that the tuning observed in the cochlea is sufficient to account for the analysing capacity of the entire auditory system (Moore, 1986; Pickles, 1986). It is largely as a consequence of this frequency analysis that we are able to hear one sound in the presence of another sound with a different frequency. This ability is known as frequency selectivity or frequency resolution.

The frequency analysis which takes place in the ear has consequences for many aspects of auditory perception, including: the audibility of individual components in complex tones; the masking of one sound by another; musical consonance and dissonance; the perception of timbre (sound quality); and the perception of pitch.

Measurement of the frequency analysing capacity of the ear

Audibility of partials in complex sounds

A sinusoid is usually perceived as a single tone with a 'pure' sound. The pitch of the tone is related to its frequency, and the loudness mainly to its intensity. If two sinusoids are presented simultaneously, the percept depends upon their frequency separation. If the two components are widely spaced in frequency, say 100 Hz and 10 000 Hz, two separate tones are perceived; thus the ear behaves as a frequency analyser, splitting the complex sound into its component sinusoids. If, on the other hand, the components are closely spaced in frequency, say 1000 and 1030 Hz, then a single sound is perceived corresponding to the mixture of the two. In this case the ear's frequency resolution is insufficient to separate the components. Thus the limits of the ability to 'hear out' the components in a complex sound reflect the analysing capacity of the auditory system.

A continuum of effects is observed as the frequency separation between two sinusoids is slowly increased from a very small value. When the two sinusoids are separated by a few hertz they sound like a single tone fluctuating in loudness. The fluctuations, known as 'beats', have a physical basis, since the two sinusoids move alternately in and out of phase, producing first reinforcement and then cancellation. The number of beats per second is equal to the frequency separation between the two sinusoids, so that as their frequency separation increases the beats are perceived to be more rapid. For separations exceeding 20 Hz, the amplitude fluctuations are no longer perceived as such, but rather a harsh unpleasant sound is heard, with a quality sometimes called 'roughness'. As the separation increases still further the roughness at first increases, and then decreases, and finally two separate tones are heard, each of which has a 'smooth' quality.

The minimum frequency separation at which the two tones can be heard separately varies depending on their mean frequency. At 500 Hz it is about 35 Hz, while at 5000 Hz it is about 700 Hz (Plomp,

1964a). This gives a first indication of the characteristics of the ear's filtering mechanism; its resolution is not constant as a function of centre frequency, but decreases with increasing centre frequency.

When a complex tone containing many components is presented, some of the individual frequency components or partials may be heard out. Normally we do not listen in this way. For example, the complex tones produced by musical instruments or the human voice are usually heard as having a single pitch (see below). However, it is possible to hear out individual partials provided attention is directed in an appropriate way, for example, by presenting a comparison sinusoid whose frequency coincides with that of one of the partials.

For multi-tone complexes, it is generally slightly more difficult to hear the individual components than when only two are present. Particularly for frequencies below 1000 Hz, the frequency separation between adjacent components required to hear out the components is greater than that required for a two-tone complex (Plomp, 1964a). Figure 3.1, taken from Plomp (1976), summarizes results from Plomp (1964a), Plomp and Mimpen (1968) and Soderquist (1970). It shows the frequency separation between adjacent partials required for a given partial to be heard out from a complex tone with either two equal-amplitude components (solid circles) or many equal-amplitude components (open symbols and crosses). In the latter case, for a centre frequency of 500 Hz the necessary separation is about 80 Hz, increasing to about 800 Hz at 5000 Hz.

The difference between the results for two tone complexes and multi-tone complexes has been explained in terms of the use of information contained in the detailed timing of the firing patterns of neurons in the auditory nerve ('phase locking'; see Moore, 1989, and Chapter 2). When a two-tone complex is used, neurons with characteristic frequencies (CFs) below the frequency of the lower partial phase lock primarily to that partial. Similarly, neurons with characteristic frequencies above the frequency of the upper partial phase lock primarily to that partial. These patterns of phase locking might be used to extract the pitches of the individual partials (Moore, 1989; see also the discussion of pitch perception later in this chapter). When a partial is contained within a multi-tone complex, the patterns of phase locking in neurons with characteristic frequencies both above and below the frequency of the partial are disrupted by the adjacent partials. Thus the partials have to be separated by a greater amount before the partial can be heard out. Consistent with this view, Moore and Ohgushi (1993) showed that the highest and lowest sinusoidal components in a multi-component complex were easier to hear out than the 'inner' components. Notice that, in Figure 3.1, the results for the two-tone complex and the multi-tone complexes converge at about 5000 Hz. This is the highest frequency

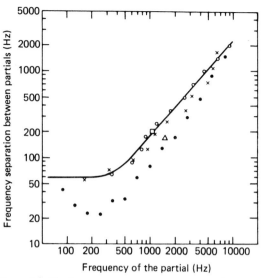

Figure 3.1 The frequency separation between adjacent partials required for a given partial to be 'heard out' from a complex tone with either two equal-amplitude components (solid circles) or many equal-amplitude components (open symbols and crosses), plotted as a function of the frequency of the partial. The open square and triangle show the results of Soderquist (1970) for inharmonic tone complexes for non-musicians and musicians respectively. (From Plomp, 1976, *Aspects of Tone Sensation*, Academic Press, by courtesy of the author and publisher)

for which phase locking has been observed in the auditory nerve of mammals (see Chapter 2).

Soderquist (1970) compared the ability to hear out partials for two groups of four subjects, musicians and non-musicians. The results, shown in Figure 3.1 (triangle – musicians, square – non-musicians), indicate that the frequency separation of the partials required to 'hear out' a given partial in a complex tone is, on average, smaller for musicians than for non-musicians. Fine and Moore (1993) showed that this was not due to greater frequency selectivity in musicians. Thus we must conclude that factors other than frequency selectivity enter into this task.

Periodic complex tones, such as those produced by many musical instruments or the human voice (when the vocal cords are vibrating; see Chapter 14), consist of a fundamental component, whose frequency equals the repetition rate of the sound, and a series of harmonics, whose frequencies are integer multiples of the fundamental frequency. Hence, the harmonics are equally spaced on a linear frequency scale. The results shown in Figure 3.1 indicate that, for a harmonic complex, the lower harmonics are more easily heard out or resolved than the higher harmonics. In fact, for a complex tone with equal-amplitude harmonics, only about the first five to eight harmonics are resolvable. This is an important factor in modern theories of pitch perception for complex tones.

Masking, critical bands and auditory filters

Weak sounds are sometimes rendered inaudible by other sounds, a process known as 'masking'. The amount of masking is defined as the number of decibels by which the threshold for the signal is raised above the absolute threshold (see below for a definition of absolute threshold). One conception of auditory masking, which has had both theoretical and practical success, assumes that the auditory system contains a bank of bandpass filters, with continuously overlapping passbands (Fletcher, 1940). In the simple case of a sinusoidal signal presented in a background noise, it is assumed that the observer 'listens' to the filter whose output has the highest signal-to-masker ratio. The signal is detected if that ratio exceeds a certain value. In most practical situations the filter involved has a centre frequency close to that of the signal.

A good deal of work has been directed towards determining the characteristics of the 'auditory filters'. Fletcher (1940) was one of the first people to apply the auditory-filter concept to the masking of sinusoidal tones by broad-band noise. He assumed that to predict threshold it would be reasonable to approximate the auditory filter as a simple rectangle, with a flat top and vertical edges. Thus all frequency components falling within the flat top or passband would be passed equally, whereas components outside the passband would be rejected. He called the width of this passband the critical bandwidth (CB). If the masker is a white noise, with a flat spectrum (equal amount of power per unit bandwidth), then the amount of noise passing through the auditory filter is the product of the power per unit bandwidth (No) and the critical bandwidth. Thus, if the power of the signal at threshold is P, then

$$P = K(CB)No \qquad (1)$$

where K is a constant of proportionality related to the efficiency of the detector mechanism following the auditory filter. Rearranging this formula,

$$CB = P/(K\,No) \qquad (2)$$

Fletcher pointed out that if K were independent of frequency, it would be possible to determine how the value of the critical bandwidth varies with frequency by measuring the threshold for detecting a sinusoidal signal as a function of frequency in a noise with a flat spectrum. However, recent measurements have suggested that K is not independent of frequency (Patterson and Moore, 1986; Peters and Moore, 1992). Thus the measurement of tone thresholds in white noise does not give a reliable way of estimating

the value of the critical bandwidth. The ratio P/No is often called the critical ratio. The term critical bandwidth is reserved for more direct measures of the auditory filter bandwidth, such as those described below.

Although the approximation of the auditory filter as a simple rectangle works quite well for signals in broad-band noise, it does not work well for maskers which contain only a narrow range of frequencies. An example, taken from the results of Egan and Hake (1950), is given in Figure 3.2. The masker in this case was a narrow band of noise with a centre frequency of 410 Hz, and a bandwidth of 90 Hz. The masker was set at a number of different overall levels, as indicated in the Figure, and for each level the threshold of a sinusoidal signal was determined as a function of signal frequency. The masked audiograms obtained in this way have rounded tops and sloping edges, which clearly indicates that the auditory filter is not a simple rectangle. Notice that at higher masker levels the slope of the masked audiogram tends to decrease on the high-frequency side. This means that at high sound levels low frequencies become relatively more effective at masking high frequencies. This phenomenon is called the 'upward spread of masking'. The masked audiograms obtained using sinusoidal maskers are basically similar to those shown in Figure 3.2, but the results are complicated by the occurrence of beats when the signal and masker are close in frequency. Sometimes the listener may not detect the signal as such, but may detect the beats. The result is a local minimum in the masked audiogram when the signal frequency is close to that of the masker. This problem is avoided with narrow-band noise maskers, since such maskers have inherent random amplitude fluctuations which preclude the use of beats as a cue.

Although masked audiograms of the type described

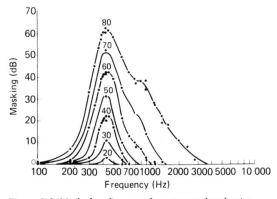

Figure 3.2 Masked audiograms for a narrow band noise masker centred at 410 Hz. Each curve shows the elevation in threshold of the sinusoidal signal as a function of frequency for a particular level of the masking noise. (From Moore, 1989. Original data from Egan and Hake, 1950)

above can give a rough idea of the shape of the auditory filter, they cannot be used to give a direct estimate of this shape. In principle, there is a different auditory filter for each centre frequency, and the shape and bandwidth may change with centre frequency. As the signal frequency changes, the auditory filter used to detect it also changes. One method of solving this problem is analogous to that used by neurophysiologists in determining a neural tuning curve (see Chapter 2). The resulting curves are often called psychophysical tuning curves (PTCs). The signal used is a sinusoid which is presented at a very low level, say 10 dB above the absolute threshold. It is assumed that this will excite only a small number of nerve fibres with characteristic frequencies close to that of the signal. Thus, to a first approximation, only one auditory filter is involved in detecting the signal. The masker is either a sinusoid or a narrow band of noise.

To determine a psychophysical tuning curve the signal is fixed in frequency and level, and the level of the masker required to mask the signal is determined, for various centre frequencies of the masker. If it is assumed that the signal will be masked when the masker produces a fixed amount of activity in the neurons which would otherwise respond to the signal, then the curve mapped out in this way is analogous to the neural tuning curve (Zwicker, 1974). Some examples are given in Figure 3.3. Returning to the concept of the auditory filter, the psychophysical tuning curve can be thought of as representing the masker level required to produce a fixed output from the filter centred at the signal frequency. Normally a filter characteristic is determined by plotting the output as a function of frequency for an input fixed in level. However, if the filter is linear the two methods are equivalent. Thus the filter shape can be obtained simply by turning the tuning curve upside-down.

The shapes of psychophysical tuning curves determined in humans are quite similar to neural tuning curves determined in the auditory nerve of mammals, and this encourages the belief that the basic frequency selectivity of the auditory system is established at the level of the auditory nerve. However, it is important to remember that the assumptions made in interpreting the psychophysical tuning curve may not be quite correct. For example, the detection of the signal inevitably involves activity over an array of neurons, with a range of characteristic frequencies. It is likely that as the frequency of the masker changes, there is a change in the characteristic frequency of the neurons which are most effective in indicating the presence of the signal. An alternative way of expressing this idea is to say that the centre frequency of the filter used to detect the signal may change as the frequency of the masker is altered. When the signal is detected through a filter which is not centred at the signal frequency, this is called 'off-frequency listening'.

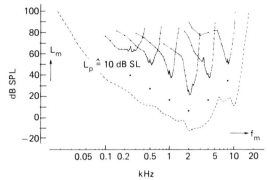

Figure 3.3 Psychophysical tuning curves (PTCs) determined in simultaneous masking using sinusoidal signals 10 dB above absolute threshold (called 10 dB SL). For each curve the solid diamond below it indicates the frequency and level of the signal. The masker was a sinusoid which had a fixed starting phase relationship to the 50-ms signal. The masker level required for threshold is plotted as a function of masker frequency. Since the signal was brief, beats were not audible, but fluctuations in the waveform resulting from the interference of the signal and masker are probably responsible for the slight irregularities around the tips of the PTCs. The dashed line shows the absolute threshold for the signal. (From Vogten, 1974, in *Facts and Models in Hearing*, edited by E. Zwicker and E. Terhardt, Springer-Verlag, by courtesy of the author)

Patterson (1976) has described a method of determining auditory filter shape which effectively prevents off-frequency listening. The method is illustrated in Figure 3.4. The signal is fixed in frequency, and the masker is a noise with a bandstop or notch centred at the signal frequency. The deviation of each edge of the notch from the signal frequency is denoted by Δf. The threshold of the signal is determined as a function of notch width. Usually the

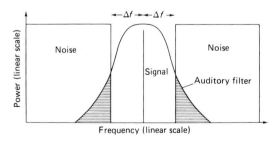

Figure 3.4 Schematic illustration of the method used by Patterson (1976) to determine auditory filter shape. The threshold of the sinusoidal signal is measured as a function of the width of a spectral notch in the noise masker. The amount of noise passing through the auditory filter centred at the signal frequency is proportional to the shaded areas. (From Moore, 1989, by courtesy of the publisher)

notch is symmetrically placed around the signal frequency and the analysis assumes that the auditory
filter is symmetric on a linear frequency scale. This
assumption appears not unreasonable, at least for
the top part of the filter and at moderate sound levels
(Patterson and Nimmo-Smith, 1980). For a signal
symmetrically placed in a notched noise, the highest
signal-to-masker ratio at the output of the auditory
filter is achieved with a filter centred at the signal
frequency, as shown in Figure 3.4. Shifting the filter,
say, upwards reduces the amount of noise passing
through the filter from the lower band, but this is
more than offset by the increase in noise from the
upper band. Hence, it seems reasonable to assume
that for this task the subject only uses the filter
centred at the signal frequency.

As the width of the spectral notch is increased, less
and less noise passes through the auditory filter;
thus, the threshold of the signal drops. The amount
of noise passing through the auditory filter is proportional to the area under the filter in the frequency
range covered by the noise. This is shown as the
shaded areas in Figure 3.4. Given the assumption
that threshold corresponds to a constant signal-to-
masker ratio at the output of the auditory filter, the
change in threshold with notch width indicates how
the area under the filter varies with Δf. The area
under a function between certain limits is obtained
by integrating the value of the function over those
limits. Hence by differentiating the function relating
threshold to Δf, the shape of the filter is obtained. In
other words, the attenuation of the filter at given
deviation, Δf, from the centre frequency is proportional to the slope of the function relating signal
threshold to notch width at that value of Δf.

A typical set of results for such an experiment is
shown in the left-hand panel of Figure 3.5, for three
different signal frequencies. The notch width is plotted
as a proportion of centre frequency, fc, so that the
general form of the results is similar for all three
frequencies; in the range $0.05 < f/fc < 0.3$ the data
form a roughly straight line on these logarithmic-
power versus linear-frequency coordinates, but the
curves tend to flatten at very narrow and very wide
notch widths. Patterson and Nimmo-Smith (1980)
pointed out that this form of threshold function implies that the auditory filter shape is like a pair of
back-to-back exponential functions, but with a
rounded rather than a sharp top, and with shallow
skirts beyond $\Delta f/fc = 0.4$. They called this form of
filter shape a rounded exponential. Although the
auditory filter shapes can be estimated from the slopes
of the functions in the left panel of Figure 3.5, a
better method is to assume a general form for the
auditory filter – a rounded exponential – with a small
number of free parameters. The assumed filter can
then be used to predict the threshold data, and the
parameters varied to find the values giving the smallest mean-squared deviation between the obtained

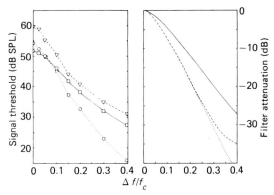

Figure 3.5 The left-hand panel shows the threshold of a
sinusoidal signal plotted as a function of the relative width
of a spectral notch in a noise masker ($\Delta f/fc$). The notch was
always centred at the signal frequency which was either
0.4 ($\square$), 1.0 ($\bigcirc$) or 6.5 ($\triangledown$) kHz. The right-hand panel
shows the shapes of the auditory filters derived from the
data on the left: 0.4 (—), 1.0 ($\cdots$), 6.5 (– – –). (From
Shailer and Moore, 1983, by courtesy of the publisher)

and predicted thresholds. This procedure gives relatively robust estimates of auditory filter shape when
the data are subject to errors, as is inevitably the case
in psychophysical experiments.

Patterson *et al.* (1982) suggested that a good approximation to the auditory filter shape was given by
the expression:

$$W(g) = (1 - r)(1 + pg) \exp(-pg) + r \qquad (3)$$

where g is the normalized frequency deviation from
the centre of the filter; $g = (f-fc)/fc$. The parameter
p determines the sharpness of the passband of the
auditory filter, and the parameter r approximates the
shallower tail of the auditory filter. Details of how to
use this expression to derive filter shapes from
notched-noise data are given in Patterson *et al.*
(1982) and Patterson and Moore (1986). The filter
shapes in the right-hand panel of Figure 3.5 were
derived in this way. Only half of each filter is shown
since the filters are assumed to be symmetric on a
linear frequency scale. For the values of r which are
typically found, the equivalent rectangular bandwidth (ERB) of the auditory filter is equal to $4fc/p$.
(The equivalent rectangular bandwidth is a measure
of the 'effective' bandwidth of a filter. It is the bandwidth of an ideal rectangular filter which has the
same peak transmission as the filter being studied,
and which passes the same power of white noise. For
the auditory filter, the equivalent rectangular bandwidth is about 10% greater than the 3-dB bandwidth.) The equivalent rectangular bandwidth of the
auditory filter may be considered as a measure of the
critical bandwidth.

Auditory filter shapes derived using notched-noise
maskers have equivalent rectangular bandwidths

which increase with increasing centre frequency. However, when expressed as a proportion of centre frequency the bandwidth tends to be narrowest at middle to high frequencies. Over the range 100 to 10 000 Hz, and at moderate sound levels, the equivalent rectangular bandwidth is well approximated by:

$$ERB = 24.7(4.37F + 1) \qquad (4)$$

where F is frequency in kHz (Glasberg and Moore, 1990). This expression is shown in Figure 3.6, together with estimates of the equivalent rectangular bandwidth from several different experiments. The Figure also shows the 'traditional' critical bandwidth function, as suggested by Zwicker and Terhardt (1980). Notice that the traditional critical bandwidth function flattens off below 500 Hz, whereas the estimates of auditory filter bandwidth continue to decrease. When the 'traditional' values were estimated, the data were sparse for frequencies below 500 Hz, and some of the older measures did show a continuing decrease below 500 Hz (Greenwood, 1961). Recent data support the idea that the critical bandwidth continues to decrease with decreasing frequency below 500 Hz (Sek and Moore, 1994).

The results described so far apply at moderate

sound levels (noise spectrum levels up to 40 dB). There is now considerable evidence that the shape of the auditory filter changes somewhat with level, and that at high levels it can be markedly asymmetric. The asymmetry of the auditory filter can be investigated by using notched noise with the notch placed both symmetrically and asymmetrically about the signal frequency. The auditory filter shape can be derived on the assumption that the subject always uses the filter giving the highest signal-to-masker ratio (Patterson and Nimmo-Smith, 1980; Glasberg and Moore, 1990). The results of such experiments indicate that the low-frequency side of the auditory filter becomes shallower with increasing level, whereas the high-frequency side may become slightly steeper (Patterson and Nimmo-Smith, 1980; Lutfi and Patterson, 1984; Moore and Glasberg, 1987; Glasberg and Moore, 1990, 1994). Thus the filter becomes increasingly asymmetric at high levels, and its equivalent rectangular bandwidth tends to increase. Figure 3.7 shows auditory filter shapes as a function of level for a centre frequency of 1 kHz. The shapes were obtained by combining the data from a number of experiments, interpolating where necessary. The decrease in slope of the low-frequency side

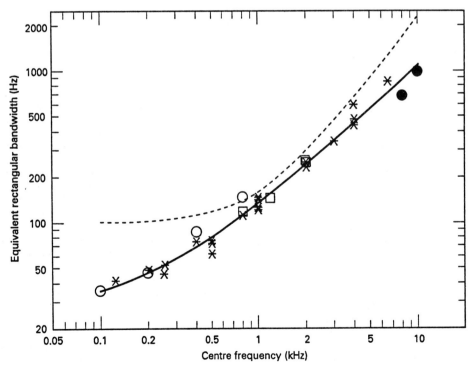

Figure 3.6 Estimates of the auditory filter bandwidth (ERB) from a variety of experiments, plotted as a function of centre frequency. The solid line gives a good fit to the data; ERB = 24.7 (4.37F + 1). The dashed line shows the traditional critical bandwidth function; CB = 25 + 75 (1 + 1.4F²)⁰·⁶ᵃ. ○ Moore, Peters and Glasberg 1990; ● Shailer *et al.*, 1990; □ Dubno and Dirks, 1989; * Moore and Glasberg 1983

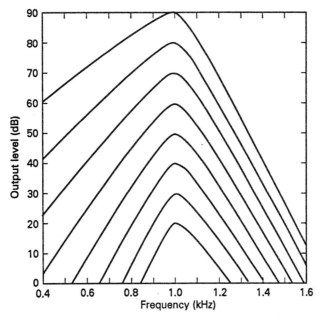

Figure 3.7 Auditory filter shapes for various input sound levels (20–90 dB sound pressure level) for a centre frequency of 1 kHz. With increasing sound level the upper branch of the filter becomes slightly steeper and the lower branch becomes considerably less steep

of the auditory filter with increasing level corresponds to the classical 'upward spread of masking'; at high levels, maskers well below the signal in frequency can have a pronounced masking effect (see Figure 3.2).

The excitation pattern

Measures of the auditory filter shape all use a fixed signal frequency, and attempt to characterize frequency selectivity at that frequency. An alternative approach is to characterize the distribution of excitation across frequencies (or places within the cochlea) for a given masker: this distribution has been referred to as the excitation pattern of the masker. In terms of the filter bank analogy, the excitation pattern can be considered as the output of the auditory filters as a function of filter centre frequency (Moore and Glasberg, 1983). Many workers have attempted to derive the excitation pattern of a masker by measuring signal threshold as a function of signal frequency, on the assumption that the signal threshold is directly proportional to the masker excitation at the signal frequency/place (e.g. Zwicker and Feldtkeller, 1967). Thus the masked audiograms shown in Figure 3.2 might be considered as giving a crude measure of the excitation pattern of the masker at each masker level. However, off-frequency listening and the detection of beats can markedly influence the form of the results.

It is instructive to consider in more detail the relationship between filter shapes and excitation patterns. This is easiest to explain using a simplified equation for the auditory filter shape:

$$W(g) = (1 + pg) \exp(-pg) \qquad (5)$$

This simplified equation gives a good description of the main passband of the auditory filter. The equivalent rectangular bandwidth of the auditory filter is assumed to vary with centre frequency according to equation 4. The value of p at a given centre frequency can be derived from equation 4 by recalling that ERB = $4fc/p$. It is then a simple matter to calculate the filter output as a function of filter centre frequency for any given input stimulus. Figure 3.8 illustrates this graphically for a 1-kHz sinusoid.

At the top are shown auditory filter shapes at several centre frequencies, with the form given by equation 5. Notice that the filters are assumed symmetric on the linear frequency scale, and that the filter bandwidths increase with centre frequency in accord with equation 4. For the filter with the lowest centre frequency shown, the relative output of the filter in response to the 1-kHz tone is about -40 dB, indicated by the point a. In the lower half of the figure this gives rise to point a on the excitation pattern; the point has an ordinate of -40 dB, and it is positioned on the abscissa at a frequency corresponding to the centre of the lowest filter illustrated. The relative outputs of the other filters shown are indicated, in

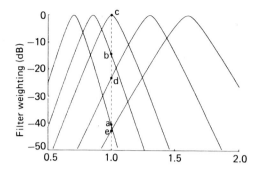

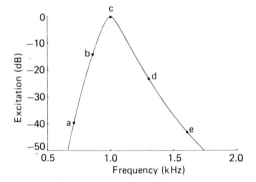

Figure 3.8 The top panel shows auditory filter shapes at several centre frequencies. The dotted line shows a 1-kHz sinusoidal tone which is applied to the filters. The bottom panel shows the output of the auditory filters as a function of filter centre frequency. This is the excitation pattern of the 1-kHz tone. (From Moore and Glasberg, 1983, by courtesy of the publisher)

order of increasing centre frequency, by the points *b* to *e*. These each give corresponding points on the excitation pattern. The entire excitation pattern was derived by calculating the filter output for filter centre frequencies spaced at 10-Hz intervals. Note that the derived excitation pattern is asymmetric; it has the same general form as the masked audiogram for a narrow-band noise masker (see Figure 3.2). This illustrates that the asymmetry seen in masked audiograms is not incompatible with the idea that the auditory filter is roughly symmetric at moderate sound levels.

Non-simultaneous masking and suppression

It is now widely accepted that the normal peripheral auditory system is characterized by significant non-linearity. One manifestation of this non-linearity is suppression, which may be crudely characterized as follows: strong excitation at one characteristic frequency/place will suppress weaker excitation at adjacent characteristic frequencies/places. This re-

sults in the phenomenon of two-tone suppression (Sachs and Kiang, 1968; see Chapter 2). More generally, it produces an enhancement in the sharpness of the excitation pattern produced by the initial filtering process; differences in level between peaks and dips in the excitation pattern are increased by suppression, giving a greater 'contrast' in the pattern. Suppressive interactions between the different frequency components in a complex sound only develop when those components are presented simultaneously. The suppression produced by adding an extra component to a sound begins almost instantaneously, and also ceases very rapidly when the component is removed.

Suppression does not seem to produce measurable effects in simultaneous masking. Houtgast (1972, 1974) has suggested that this is because suppression at a particular characteristic frequency or place does not change the signal-to-masker ratio at that place. The threshold in simultaneous masking appears to depend primarily on that ratio, and so suppression has no effect on threshold. Houtgast presented evidence that non-simultaneous techniques, where the signal is presented out-of-time with the masker, could be used to demonstrate the effects of suppression. The signal can be viewed as a kind of 'probe' for estimating the excitation evoked by the masker in the frequency region of the signal. The signal itself is not suppressed by the masker, since it is not presented simultaneously with the masker. However, if suppression alters the excitation evoked by the masker in the frequency region of the signal, then this is revealed as a change in the threshold of the signal.

One method which has been widely used to study suppression is forward masking. The signal is presented just after the end of the masker. If the effective level of the masker is altered by suppression, that should lead to a change in the amount of masking produced by that masker.

An example of results obtained with this technique is given in Figure 3.9, taken from Shannon (1976). The time pattern of the masker and signal is shown at the top. The masker always contained a 1-kHz tone at a level of 40 dB sound pressure level. The amount of masking produced by the 1-kHz tone is taken as a reference, and is called 0 dB in the five panels to the left of the Figure. The effect of adding a second sinusoidal component to the masker is shown in the five panels by the points plotted as open circles. The frequency, f_v, of this extra component varied from 0.3 to 3.5 kHz, and its level, L_v, varied from 30 dB sound pressure level (bottom panel) to 70 dB sound pressure level (top panel). When f_v was very close to 1 kHz, the second component increased the amount of forward masking, as would be expected. However, when f_v was just above 1 kHz, the second component reduced the amount of forward masking, an effect called 'unmasking'. This effect has been attributed to suppression. It is assumed that the second component suppresses the response to the 1-

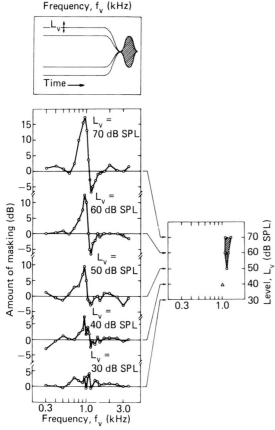

Figure 3.9 Results of an experiment demonstrating 'unmasking' in forward masking. The unmasking has been interpreted in terms of suppression. See text for details. (From Shannon, 1976, *Journal of the Acoustical Society of America*, **59**, 1460–1470, by courtesy of the author and publisher)

and broadband maskers (such as notched noise). The results which will be presented later in this chapter (in the section on Frequency selectivity in impaired hearing) were obtained using stimuli like this.

Absolute thresholds and the perception of loudness

Absolute thresholds

The absolute threshold for a sound is the minimum detectable level of the sound in the absence of any other sounds. The physical method of specifying the sound level is important, and two methods are in common use. In the first method the sound pressure is measured either at some point close to the entrance to the ear canal, or at some point inside the ear canal, preferably close to the eardrum. This gives what is called the minimum audible pressure (MAP), and it is most commonly obtained using sounds delivered by an earphone. In the second method the sound is delivered by a loudspeaker. The sound level at the position of the centre of the listener's head is established after removing the listener from the sound field. This gives what is known as the minimum audible field (MAF). The two methods give slightly different results since the head, pinna and meatus do have an effect on the sound field. However the general form of the results is similar.

The lowest curve in Figure 3.10 shows the average minimum audible field for healthy adult listeners. It should be noted that 'normal' listeners may have thresholds up to 20 dB above or below the average. Thresholds tend to increase with age, particularly at

kHz component when f_v is just above 1 kHz, which reduces the amount of forward masking produced by that component. The suppression increases as L_v is increased. The panel on the right shows values of f_v and L_v for which more than 3 dB of unmasking was observed. The shaded area bounded by these values resembles the upper of the two-tone suppression areas observed neurophysiologically (see Chapter 2).

Forward masking is not without problems in interpretation. It has been suggested that the unmasking produced by adding an extra component to a masker may be partly the result of changes in the cues available to the subjects, rather than being a result of the physiological process of suppression. Many demonstrations of unmasking seem to be confounded in this way (Moore, 1980; Moore and O'Loughlin, 1986). Moore and O'Loughlin have suggested that this problem can be minimized by using sinusoidal signals

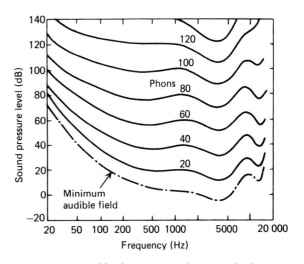

Figure 3.10 Equal-loudness contours for various loudness levels, as indicated on each curve. The dashed-dotted curve shows the absolute threshold (minimum audible field). (Original data from Robinson and Dadson, 1956)

high frequencies (4 kHz and above). The range of frequencies where sensitivity is greatest, 500–5000 Hz, is also the range most important for understanding speech.

Equal-loudness contours

In describing the perception of sound it is useful to have some kind of scale which allows one to compare the loudness of different sounds. A first step towards this is to construct equal-loudness contours for sinusoids of different frequencies. The standard tone, for example, might have a frequency of 1 kHz, and a level of 40 dB sound pressure level, and the listener is asked to adjust the level of a second tone (say, 2 kHz) so that it sounds equally loud. If this is repeated for many different frequencies of the second tone, then the sound level required, plotted as a function of frequency, maps out an equal-loudness contour. Different contours are obtained by using different levels of the 1-kHz standard tone, as shown in Figure 3.10.

When the standard tone is at 1 kHz, its loudness level is defined as being equal to its sound pressure level. Thus the loudness level of any sound is the level (in dB sound pressure level) of the 1-kHz tone to which it sounds equal in loudness. The unit of loudness level is the phon, and each equal-loudness contour in Figure 3.10 is labelled with its phon value. Note that the contours resemble the absolute threshold curve at low levels, but tend to become flatter at high levels. This finding has been taken into account in the design of sound-level meters, which weight the power at different frequencies according to the shapes of equal-loudness contours. At low sound levels, low-frequency components contribute little to the total loudness of complex sounds, and so an 'A' weighting is used, which reduces the contribution of low frequencies to the overall meter reading. At high levels, where the equal-loudness contours are flatter, a more nearly flat weighting characteristic, the 'C' weighting, is used.

It is important to realize two limitations of readings obtained using sound level meters. The first is that readings in phons do not directly indicate the loudness of sounds, even for simple sinusoids. It is not true that a sound with a loudness level of 80 phons is twice as loud as one with a loudness level of 40 phons. The phon scale can only be used to indicate the order in which the loudness of sounds should be ranked. The second limitation is that the loudness of complex sounds, containing many frequency components, depends on how the energy is distributed over frequency (see the section on The role of frequency selectivity in determining loudness), and this is not taken into account in simple sound level meters. In spite of these limitations (and others not mentioned here), sound level meters have been widely used in the measurement of industrial and community noise.

Loudness scaling

Scaling methods have been used as a means of deriving the relationship between the physical intensity of sounds and their subjective loudness. There are many variations of the methods but they usually involve getting the listener to make a 'direct' estimate of the magnitude of the loudness sensation. In one method, called magnitude estimation, the listener is presented with a series of sounds, with various intensities, and is asked to give a number according to how loud each one sounds. In another method, called magnitude production, the listener is asked to adjust the intensity of a sound so that it bears some specified relationship to a reference sound (e.g. twice as loud or one-quarter as loud). On the basis of results obtained with these methods, Stevens (1957) and others have suggested that loudness, L, is a power function of physical intensity, I:

$$L = kI^{0.3} \qquad (6)$$

where k is a constant depending on the subject and the units used. In other words, the loudness of a given sound is proportional to its intensity raised to the power 0.3. Roughly, this means that a two-fold change in loudness is produced by a 10 dB change in level.

Stevens proposed the sone as the unit of loudness. One sone is defined arbitrarily as the loudness of a 1-kHz tone at 40 dB sound pressure level. Thus a 1-kHz tone at 50 dB sound pressure level will have a loudness of 2 sones and a 1-kHz tone at 60 dB will have a loudness of 4 sones. The sone scale has been employed in models which allow the calculation of the loudness of complex sounds, and it has become quite widely used, being incorporated in a number of standard procedures for calculating loudness (Stevens, 1972). However, the interpretation of the scale, and the methods of deriving it, have been the subject of criticism. The results of loudness scaling experiments can show great variability between listeners, and it is known that the exact way in which the experiments are conducted can have a large effect; biases of various kinds can be significant. Warren (1970) attempted to eliminate known biases and found that half-loudness corresponds to a 6 dB reduction in level, rather than the 10 dB suggested by Stevens.

Many researchers are unhappy with the whole concept of asking listeners to judge the magnitude of a sensation. What we do in everyday life is to judge the characteristics of sound sources, so that our estimate of loudness is affected by the apparent distance of the sound source, the context in which it is heard, the nature of the sound, and so on. In other words we are attempting to make some estimate of the properties of the source itself, and introspection as to the nature of the sensation evoked may be an unnatural and difficult process.

The role of frequency selectivity in determining loudness

It has been known for many years that if the total intensity of a complex sound is fixed, its loudness depends on the frequency range over which the sound extends. The basic mechanism underlying this seems to be the same critical band or auditory filter as is revealed in masking experiments (see above). Consider as an example a noise whose total intensity is held constant while the bandwidth is varied. The loudness of the noise can be estimated indirectly by asking the listener to adjust the intensity of a second sound, with a fixed bandwidth, so that it sounds equally loud. The two sounds are presented successively. When the bandwidth of the noise is less than a certain value the loudness is roughly independent of bandwidth. However, as the bandwidth is increased beyond a certain point, the loudness starts to increase. This is illustrated in Figure 3.11, for several different overall levels of the noise. The bandwidth at which loudness starts to increase is known as the critical bandwidth for loudness summation. Its value is approximately the same as the equivalent rectangular bandwidth of the auditory filter.

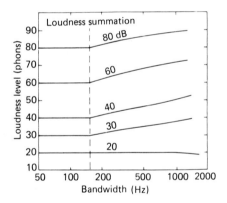

Figure 3.11 The loudness level in phons of a band of noise centred at 1 kHz, measured as a function of the width of the band. For each of the curves the overall level was held constant, and is indicated in the figure. The dashed line shows that the bandwidth at which loudness begins to increase is the same at all levels tested (except that no increase occurs at the lowest level). (Adapted from Feldtkeller and Zwicker, 1956, *Das Ohr als Nachrichtenempfänger*, S. Hirzel, by courtesy of the author and publisher)

The increase in loudness with increasing bandwidth can be understood if we assume that when the bandwidth of a sound is greater than one ERB, the loudness in adjacent, but non-overlapping, bands is summed to give the total loudness. Consider the

effect of taking a band of noise whose width equals one ERB, and doubling the bandwidth, keeping the total intensity constant. The noise will now cover two one-ERB-wide bands, but the intensity in each band will be half that in the original band. According to Steven's power law, $L = kI^{0.3}$, halving intensity is equivalent to a reduction in loudness to 0.81 of the original value. The total loudness in the two bands will be $2 \times 0.81 = 1.62$ times the original value. Thus increasing bandwidth beyond the critical band results in an increase in loudness. At low sound levels the power law appears to break down, and loudness changes in proportion with sound intensity. Thus the change in loudness with bandwidth is reduced or absent, as may be seen in the lowest curve of Figure 3.11.

The perception of pitch
The pitch of pure tones

Pitch is defined as that attribute of auditory sensation in terms of which sounds may be ordered on a musical scale, i.e. that attribute in which variations constitute melody. For sinusoidal stimuli (pure tones) the pitch is closely related to the frequency; the higher the frequency the higher the pitch. One of the classic debates in hearing theory is concerned with the mechanisms underlying the perception of pitch. One theory, called the place theory, suggests that pitch is related to the distribution of activity across nerve fibres. A tone with a given frequency produces maximum activity in nerve fibres with characteristic frequencies close to that frequency, and the 'position' of this maximum is assumed to determine pitch. Shifts in frequency are detected as changes in the amount of activity at the place where the activity changes most. Usually such changes are maximal in neurons with characteristic frequencies below the stimulating frequencies; these characteristic frequencies correspond to the low-frequency side of the excitation pattern, where the slope is steep, and small changes in frequency produce large changes in activity.

The alternative theory, called the temporal theory, suggests that pitch is determined by the time-pattern of neural spikes. For frequencies up to about 5 kHz, neural spikes are phase-locked to the stimulus, so that the time-intervals between successive spikes carry information about the stimulus frequency (see Chapter 2).

One major fact which these theories have to account for is our remarkably fine acuity in detecting frequency changes. This ability is called frequency discrimination, and is not to be confused with frequency selectivity or frequency resolution. For two tones of 500 ms duration presented successively, a difference of about 3 Hz (or less in trained subjects) can be detected at a centre frequency of 1 kHz. It has been suggested that tuning curves (or auditory filters) are not sufficiently sharp to account for this fine acuity in terms of the place theory (see Moore and Glasberg, 1986b, for a detailed discussion of this). A further difficulty for the place theory comes from a consideration of the way frequency discrimination changes with centre frequency. Figure 3.12 shows that discrimination worsens abruptly above 4–5 kHz (Moore, 1973). This is difficult to explain in terms of place theory, since neither neural measures of frequency selectivity (such as tuning curves) nor psychophysical measures of frequency selectivity (such as psychophysical tuning curves or auditory filter shapes) show any corresponding change.

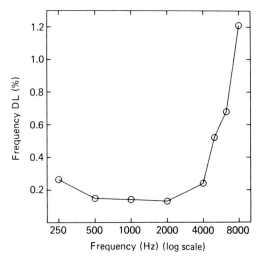

Figure 3.12 The smallest detectable change in frequency (called the frequency DL), expressed as a percentage of frequency, and plotted as a function of frequency. The stimuli were 200-ms sinusoidal tones. Note the worsening in performance above 4–5 kHz. (Data from Moore, 1973)

These facts can be accommodated by the temporal theory. Changes in frequency discrimination with centre frequency (and with tone duration) can be predicted from the information available in inter-spike intervals (Goldstein and Srulovicz, 1977). The worsening performance at 4–5 kHz corresponds well with the frequency at which the temporal information ceases to be available (see Chapter 2). Studies of the perception of musical intervals also indicate a change in mechanism around 4–5 kHz. Below this, a sequence of pure tones with appropriate frequencies conveys a clear sense of melody. Above this, the sense of musical interval and of melody is lost, although the changes in frequency may still be heard.

The evidence, then, supports the idea that, for pure tones, pitch perception and discrimination are determined primarily by temporal information for frequen-

cies below 4–5 kHz, and by place information for frequencies above this. The important frequencies for the perception of music and speech lie in the frequency range where temporal information is available.

The pitch perception of complex tones

In general, any sound which is periodic may have a pitch, provided the repetition rate lies in the range 20–20 000 Hz. The pitch is related to the repetition rate, in the same way that it is related to frequency for pure tones. When a pitch value is assigned to a complex tone this is generally understood to be the frequency of a sinusoid which has the same pitch. Before introducing theories of pitch perception for complex tones, it is useful to consider those physical properties of a complex sound that are important in determining its pitch.

Periodic sounds can be analysed into a series of sinusoids consisting of a fundamental component and a series of harmonics. For example, a brief impulse repeating 200 times per second has a fundamental component of 200 Hz, and harmonics at 400, 600, 800 . . . Hz. The pitch of such a sound is close to that of a 200-Hz sinusoid. What physical characteristics are essential for producing this pitch? The obvious answer, the presence of the fundamental component at 200 Hz, is not correct. The fundamental can be removed, or masked by low-frequency noise, and the pitch remains the same. This is called 'the phenomenon of the missing fundamental'. The pitch remains the same even if the sound is filtered so as to contain only a few harmonics, say 1200, 1400, 1600 and 1800 Hz. The low pitch evoked by a group of harmonics (with a missing fundamental) has been given various names, including residue pitch, virtual pitch and low pitch.

Another possibility, that pitch is determined by the spacing between harmonics, is also incorrect. This can be shown by shifting all of the components upwards in frequency by an equal amount, say to 1219, 1419, 1619 Hz. The spacing between components remains the same, but the pitch is heard to go up slightly (Schouten, Ritsma and Cardozo, 1962).

Consider now the possibility that the pitch is related to some aspect of the time structure of the stimulus. Any sound entering the ear has to pass through the ear's filtering mechanism, so that the effective stimulus for each neuron resembles a bandpass filtered version of the original waveform. A simulation of how the waveforms might look at the outputs of the auditory filters for a typical periodic sound is shown in Figure 3.13. The sound in this case was the vowel /i/ as in *weed*.

The auditory filter bandwidth increases with centre frequency, but the spacing between harmonics is constant. The lower harmonics of the sound are

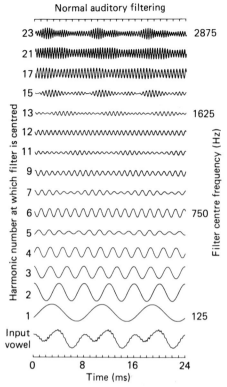

Figure 3.13 The waveforms at the outputs of simulated auditory filters in response to a complex periodic tone, the vowel /i/. See text for details. (From Rosen and Fourcin, 1986, in *Frequency Selectivity in Hearing*, edited by B. C. J. Moore, Academic Press, by courtesy of the author and publisher)

patterns of neural discharge, is probably also important (Moore, Glasberg and Shailer, 1984). In the second stage some form of pattern recognizer determines a fundamental frequency whose harmonics match those of the stimulus as closely as possible (Goldstein, 1973). The perceived pitch corresponds to the frequency of this internally determined fundamental. In one model of this type the pitch is determined by a mechanism which generates subharmonics of components which are present in the stimulus (Terhardt, 1974). These subharmonics coincide at certain frequencies. The frequency with the greatest number of coincidences corresponds to the perceived pitch of the sound. Consider the example shown in Table 3.1. It may be seen that the greatest number of coincidences in the subharmonics is at 200 Hz, which corresponds to the perceived pitch.

Table 3.1 An example illustrating Terhardt's model for the perception of the pitch of complex tones

	Frequency of component (Hz)		
	800	*1000*	*1200*
Frequencies of subharmonics	400	500	600
	266.7	333.3	400
	200	250	300
	160	**200**	240
	133.3	166.7	**200**

The complex tone in this case contains just three sinusoidal frequency components, 800, 1000 and 1200 Hz. A series of subharmonics of each component is generated. These subharmonics coincide at certain frequencies, the greatest number of coincidences occurring at 200 Hz. This corresponds to the perceived pitch.

effectively resolved. Each produces activity in a different auditory filter, and the outputs of those filters are sinusoidal waveforms corresponding to the individual harmonics. The higher harmonics, on the other hand, are not completely resolved and interfere with one another. The waveform resulting from the interference of a group of harmonics has a repetition rate the same as that of the waveform as a whole (shown at the bottom of the figure). Thus the repetition period of the waveforms at the outputs of auditory filters responding to higher harmonics could be the basis for pitch. However, this explanation is not entirely satisfactory. If a complex sound is filtered so as to contain only high unresolved harmonics (say above the 10th), a pitch is still heard, but it is weak and ambiguous compared to that heard when lower harmonics are present (Moore and Rosen, 1979). Apparently the lower, resolvable, harmonics are more important in determining pitch.

Most modern theories of pitch perception assume a two-stage process. In the first stage the lower harmonics are analysed. This analysis depends on the ear's filtering mechanism, but the time structure of the output from each filter, as represented in the temporal

This model can explain the slight pitch shifts which take place when the frequencies of all components are shifted upwards by an equal amount. In this case the subharmonics do not coincide perfectly, since the complex is no longer harmonic, but the frequency at which several subharmonics almost coincide matches the perceived pitch quite well.

In summary, modern theories assume that the pitch perception of complex tones is a kind of pattern-recognition process based on a preliminary analysis of the components present in the sound. The initial analysis may depend on both 'place' and 'temporal' information. When only high harmonics are present, a pitch can still be heard but it is weaker. Presumably in this case the harmonics cannot be resolved and the pitch is based purely on timing information. For a more comprehensive review of recent data and theories on pitch perception the reader is referred to Moore and Glasberg (1986b), Moore (1993) and Houtsma (1995).

The perception of timbre

Timbre may be defined as the characteristic quality of sound that distinguishes one voice or musical instrument from another. Unlike pitch and loudness, which are one-dimensional, timbre is multidimensional; there is no single scale along which the timbres of various sounds can be compared. Timbre, as defined above, depends on several different physical properties of sound, including:

1 Whether the sound is periodic, having a tonal quality for repetition rates from about 20 to 20 000 Hz, or irregular and having a noise-like quality.
2 Whether the sound is continuous or interrupted. For sounds which have short durations the exact way in which the sound is turned on and off can play an important role. For example, in the case of sounds produced by stringed instruments, a rapid onset (a fast rise time) is usually perceived as a struck or plucked string, whereas a gradual onset is heard as a bowed string.
3 The distribution of energy over frequency (i.e. the spectrum), and changes in the spectrum with time. This is the correlate of timbre which has been studied most widely.

For steady-state periodic sounds it is possible to use the more restricted definition of timbre given by the American Standards Association: 'that attribute of auditory sensation in terms of which a listener can judge that two steady-state complex tones having the same loudness and pitch, are dissimilar'. Timbre defined in this way depends primarily on the energy spectrum of the sound (Plomp, 1976). For example, sounds containing predominantly high frequencies have a 'sharp' timbre, whereas those containing mainly low frequencies sound 'dull' or 'mellow'. This is another example of the action of the ear as a frequency analyser. The components in a complex sound are partially separated by the auditory filters, and the distribution of the excitation at the output of the filters, as a function of filter centre frequency (i.e. the excitation pattern), determines timbre.

The temporal resolution of the ear

The auditory system is particularly well adapted to detecting changes in sounds as a function of time. The limits of this ability reflect the temporal resolution of the ear. A particularly straightforward method of assessing temporal resolution is to measure the threshold for detecting a temporal gap in a sound. Many gap-detection experiments have used wideband noise as a stimulus, since introducing a temporal gap in such a noise does not change the spectrum of the noise. The results generally agree quite well, the threshold value being 2–3 ms (Plomp, 1964b; Penner, 1977). More recently, gap thresholds have been measured for band-limited noises, to determine how gap threshold varies with centre frequency and bandwidth. Unfortunately, when a noise band is abruptly switched off and on, to produce the gap, a change in spectrum takes place. Energy is spread or 'splattered' to frequencies outside the nominal bandwidth of the noise. In order to prevent the detection of this 'spectral splatter', the noise bands have been presented with complementary band-reject noise, to mask off-frequency energy (Fitzgibbons and Wightman, 1982; Shailer and Moore, 1983). Some recent results from Eddins, Hall and Grose (1992) are plotted in Figure 3.14. The stimuli were noise bands whose bandwidth was varied while keeping the upper cutoff frequency (UCF) fixed at one of three values.

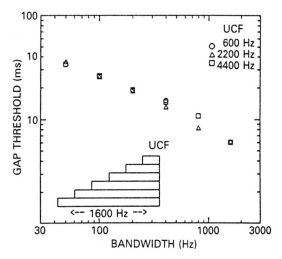

Figure 3.14 Thresholds for the detection of a gap in a band of noise, plotted as a function of noise bandwidth with the upper cut off frequency (UCF) as parameter. The inset shows schematically that the UCF was held constant as the bandwidth was varied. UCF: ○ 600 Hz; △ 2200 Hz; □ 4400 Hz. (Data from Eddins *et al.*, 1992)

The gap threshold increases markedly as the noise bandwidth is made smaller. This can be explained in terms of the inherent random fluctuations in the noise. As the bandwidth decreases, these fluctuations become slower and more confusable with the gap to be detected (Glasberg and Moore, 1992). For a given bandwidth, there is hardly any effect of varying the upper cut off frequency of the noise.

At low sound levels, gap detection improves somewhat with increasing sound level. However, above a certain level (about 25–30 dB spectrum level for bandlimited noise signals) performance changes only slightly with increasing level (Shailer and Moore, 1983).

A more general characterization of temporal resolution can be obtained by measuring the threshold for detecting changes in the amplitude of a sound as a function of the rapidity of the changes. In the simplest case, white noise is sinusoidally amplitude modulated, and the threshold for detecting the modulation is determined as a function of modulation rate. The function relating threshold to modulation rate is known as a temporal modulation transfer function (TMTF) (Viemeister, 1979). An example of the results is shown in Figure 3.15; (data are from Bacon and Viemeister, 1985). The thresholds are expressed as 20 log$m$, where m is the modulation index.

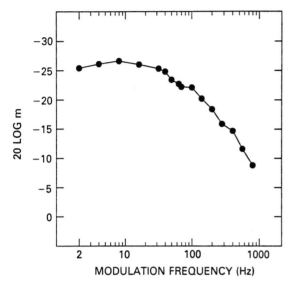

Figure 3.15 A temporal modulation transfer function. The threshold modulation depth is plotted as a function of modulation frequency. Thresholds are expressed as 20 log(m) where m is the modulation index. (Data from Bacon and Viemeister, 1985)

For low modulation rates, performance is limited by the amplitude resolution of the ear, rather than by temporal resolution. Thus, the threshold is independent of modulation rate for rates up to about 16 Hz. As the rate increases beyond 16 Hz, temporal resolution starts to have an effect; performance worsens, and for rates above about 1000 Hz the modulation is hard to detect at all. The shapes of temporal modulation transfer functions do not vary much with overall sound level, but the ability to detect the modulation does worsen at low sound levels.

The localization of sounds

Binaural cues

It has long been recognized that slight differences in the sounds reaching the two ears can be used as cues in sound localization. The two major cues are differences in the time of arrival at the two ears and differences in intensity at the two ears. For example, a sound coming from the left arrives first at the left

ear and is more intense in the left ear. For steady sinusoidal stimulation, a difference in time of arrival is equivalent to a phase difference between the sounds at the two ears. However, phase differences are not usable over the whole audible frequency range. Experiments using sounds delivered by headphones have shown that a phase difference at the two ears can be detected and used to judge location only at frequencies below about 1500 Hz. This is reasonable because the listener must be able to determine which cycle of the sound in one ear corresponds to a given cycle in the other ear. At high frequencies, the wavelength of sound is small compared to the dimensions of the head, so the listener cannot determine which cycle in the left ear corresponds to a given cycle in the right; there may be many cycles of phase difference. Thus phase differences become ambiguous and unusable at high frequencies. On the other hand, at low frequencies our accuracy at detecting changes in relative time at the two ears is remarkably good; changes of 10–20 μs can be detected, which is equivalent to a movement of the sound source of 1–2% laterally.

Intensity differences between the two ears are primarily useful at high frequencies. This is because low frequencies bend or diffract around the head, so that there is little difference in intensity at the two ears whatever the location of the sound source. At high frequencies the head casts more of a 'shadow', and above 2–3 kHz the intensity differences are sufficient to provide useful cues. For complex sounds, containing a range of frequencies, the difference in spectral patterning at the two ears may also be important.

The idea that sound localization is based on interaural time differences at low-frequencies and interaural intensity differences at high frequencies has been called the 'duplex theory' of sound localization, and it dates back to Lord Rayleigh (1907). However, it has been realized in recent years that it is not quite correct (for a review see Hafter, 1984). Complex sounds, containing only high frequencies (above 1500 Hz), can be localized on the basis of interaural time delays, provided that they have an appropriate temporal structure. For example, a single click can be localized in this way no matter what its frequency content. Periodic sounds containing only high-frequency harmonics can also be localized on the basis of interaural time differences, provided that the envelope repetition rate (usually equal to the fundamental frequency) is below about 600 Hz (Neutzel and Hafter, 1981). Since most of the sounds we encounter in everyday life are complex, and have repetition rates below 600 Hz, interaural time differences are used for localization in most listening situations.

The role of the pinna

Although binaural cues are traditionally considered as the most important in sound localization, it is clear that they are not sufficient to account for all of our abilities. For example, a simple difference in time or intensity will not indicate whether a sound is coming from in front or behind, or above or below, but such judgements can clearly be made. Further, under some conditions localization with one ear can be as accurate as with two. In recent years it has been shown that the pinnae play an important role in sound localization (Batteau, 1967). They do so because the spectra of sounds entering the ear are modified by the pinnae in a way which depends upon the direction of the sound source. This direction-dependent filtering provides cues for sound source location. The pinnae are important not just in providing cues about the direction of sound sources, but also in enabling us to judge whether a sound comes from within the head or from the outside world. A sound is only judged as coming from outside if the spectral transformations characteristic of the pinnae are imposed on the sound. Thus sounds heard through headphones are normally judged as being inside the head; the pinnae do not have their normal effect on the sound when headphones are worn. Judgements of the position of a sound within the head are referred to as lateralization. However, sounds delivered by headphones can be made to appear to come from outside the head if the signals delivered to the headphones are synthetically processed (filtered) so as to mimic the normal action of the pinnae. Such processing can also create the impression of a sound coming from any desired direction in space.

The pinnae alter the sound spectrum primarily at high frequencies. Only when the wavelength of the sound is comparable with the dimensions of the pinnae is the spectrum significantly affected. This is mostly above about 6 kHz. Thus, people with high-frequency hearing losses are generally unable to make use of the directional information provided by the pinnae. Hearing aid users also suffer in this respect, since, even if the microphone is appropriately placed within the pinna, the response of most aids is limited to frequencies below 6 kHz.

The precedence effect

In everyday conditions the sound from a given source reaches the ears by many different paths. Some of it arrives via a direct path, but a great deal may only reach the ears after reflections from one or more surfaces. However, listeners are not normally aware of these reflections or echoes, and they do not appear to impair the ability to localize sound sources. The reason for this seems to lie in a phenomenon known as the precedence effect (Wallach, Newman and Rosenzwieg, 1949). When several sounds reach the ears in close succession (i.e. the direct sound and its echoes) the sounds are perceptually fused into a single sound, and the location of the total sound is primarily determined by the location of the first (direct) sound. Thus the echoes have little influence on the perception of direction. Furthermore, there is little direct awareness of the echoes, although they may influence the timbre and loudness of the sound.

The precedence effect only happens for sounds of a discontinuous or transient character, such as speech or music, and it can break down if the echoes are sufficiently intense compared to the direct sound. However, in normal conditions the precedence effect plays an important role in the localization and identification of sounds in reverberant conditions.

Perception of sound by the hearing impaired

Conductive hearing losses can be considered mainly as attenuating the sound reaching the inner ear. They do not have any marked effect on the ability to analyse or discriminate sound. Sensorineural losses, on the other hand, are commonly accompanied by reduced discrimination and/or distortion in the way sound is perceived. This section describes some of the changes in auditory perception associated with cochlear hearing losses.

Frequency selectivity in impaired hearing

There is now considerable evidence that in listeners with hearing impairments of cochlear origin there is a loss of frequency selectivity. This has been demonstrated using most of the masking techniques discussed earlier. In general, greater threshold elevations tend to be associated with broader auditory filters. However, the following cautions should be observed:

1 There can be considerable variability among patients, even when the elevation in absolute threshold is similar. Although the bandwidth of the auditory filter is correlated with the threshold elevation (Pick, Evans and Wilson, 1977; Glasberg and Moore, 1986), some patients have broad filters and almost normal thresholds, while some have elevated thresholds but almost normal filters.

2 The auditory filter becomes broader at high sound levels even in normal listeners (see Figure 3.7). Since measurements with patients usually have to be made at high sound levels, part of the broadening may be attributed to a normal level effect.

Figure 3.16 shows a comparison of auditory filter shapes obtained separately from each ear of five patients with unilateral cochlear hearing losses. The upper panels show filter shapes for the normal ears

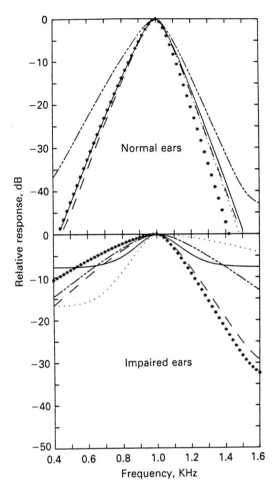

Figure 3.16 Auditory filter shapes for the normal ears (top) and the impaired ears (bottom) of five subjects with unilateral cochlear impairments. The centre frequency was 1 kHz. (Data from Glasberg and Moore, 1986)

and the lower panels show filter shapes for the impaired ears, which had threshold elevations at the test frequency (1 kHz) ranging from about 40 to 60 dB. Losses were relatively flat as a function of frequency. A notched-noise masker was used, as described earlier, and the same noise spectrum level (50 dB) was used for testing all ears, so the results are not subject to the difficulty discussed in (2) above.

It is clear that the auditory filters are considerably broader in the impaired ears. The most obvious feature is that the lower skirts of the filters are consistently and considerably less sharp in the impaired ears. This implies that these subjects are unusually susceptible to the upward spread of masking from low frequencies. This appears to be a common feature in cases of cochlear impairment, even in patients

with relatively flat losses as a function of frequency. It may partially account for the fact that hearing aids are often most effective when their gain is greater at high frequencies than at low. A rising frequency-gain characteristic can help to alleviate the effects of the upward spread of masking.

There is also evidence that the suppression mechanism may be damaged, or even completely inoperative, in cases of cochlear impairment. The auditory filter shape measured in non-simultaneous masking is typically sharper than that measured in simultaneous masking, a difference which is commonly attributed to suppression (Houtgast, 1974, 1977; Moore and Glasberg, 1981; Glasberg, Moore and Nimmo-Smith, 1984). In patients with cochlear impairments the differences are reduced or may even be zero (Festen and Plomp, 1983). However, in cases of moderate impairment (40–50 dB losses), the auditory filter shape measured with a notched-noise masker may still be slightly sharper in forward masking than in simultaneous masking. An example is given in Figure 3.17, which compares auditory filter shapes derived from simultaneous and forward masking for the normal ear and for the impaired ear of a patient with a unilateral cochlear loss (data from Moore and Glasberg, 1986a).

In the example shown the signal level was fixed and the noise spectrum level was varied to determine threshold, as described in Moore and Glasberg (1981). The notched noise was always symmetrically placed around the signal frequency, and so it was not possible to determine the asymmetry of the auditory filter. Hence only half of each filter shape is shown in the lower panel. For each ear, the noise level required for threshold was similar in simultaneous and forward masking for a notch width of zero. Thus the results are not confounded by differences in overall noise level between simultaneous and forward masking. The difference between the filter shapes for simultaneous and forward masking is smaller for the impaired ear than for the normal ear, but a difference nevertheless exists, indicating that suppression may be operating weakly in the impaired ear.

Consequences of impaired frequency selectivity

It is useful to consider briefly the perceptual consequences of a reduction in frequency selectivity. The first major consequence is a greater susceptibility to masking by interfering sounds. In everyday situations, the frequency content (the spectrum) of attended sounds usually differs from that of other sounds which may be present in the environment. At the outputs of auditory filters tuned to the desired frequencies, the signal is passed but much of the background noise is attenuated. When the auditory filters are broader than normal, the rejection of background noise is much less effective. Thus background

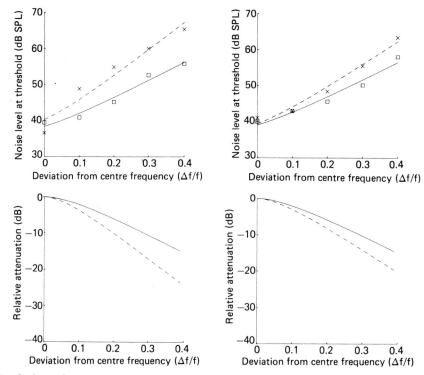

Figure 3.17 Results for a subject with a unilateral cochlear impairment. The top panels show the level of a notched-noise masker needed to mask a 1.5-kHz signal as a function of the width of the notch in the noise (expressed as the deviation of each edge of the notch from the signal frequency divided by the signal frequency). — and □ denote simultaneous masking and – – – – and × denote forward masking. Results for the normal ear are shown on the left, and for the impaired ear on the right. The auditory filter shapes derived from the data are shown in the lower panels. The fact that the filters are sharper in forward masking has been interpreted as resulting from suppression. The results suggest that suppression is still operating in the impaired ear, but more weakly than normal. (From Moore and Glasberg, 1986a, by courtesy of the publisher)

noise severely disrupts the detection and discrimination of sounds, including speech. Indeed, difficulty in understanding speech in noise is one of the commonest complaints among people with hearing impairments of cochlear origin. It has been shown that the intelligibility of speech in noise is related to frequency selectivity, worsening as frequency selectivity decreases (Dreschler and Plomp, 1980; Patterson *et al.*, 1982; Festen and Plomp, 1983; Glasberg and Moore, 1989). Also, smearing the spectra of sounds so as to simulate reduced frequency selectivity has the effect of reducing the intelligibility of speech in noise (ter Keurs, Festen and Plomp, 1992; Baer and Moore, 1993, 1994).

A related difficulty arises in the perceptual analysis of complex sounds such as speech or music. The timbre of a musical note or a vowel sound depends strongly on the spectrum of the sound, and correspondingly on the shape of the excitation pattern evoked by the sound. When the ear's frequency selectivity is impaired, the excitation pattern of a sound becomes 'blurred'; the peaks and dips are less well

represented. The situation may be made even worse if the suppression mechanism, which normally enhances the contrast between peaks and dips in the excitation pattern, is damaged. Thus it is more difficult for the impaired listener to tell the difference between different vowel sounds, or to distinguish musical instruments (for a review see Rosen and Fourcin, 1986).

Loudness perception and recruitment in impaired ears

Damage to the inner ear, such as that produced by noise exposure, often results in an abnormality of loudness perception known as loudness recruitment. Although the absolute threshold may be elevated, the rate of growth of loudness with intensity is more rapid than normal, so that at high intensities the sound appears as loud in the impaired ear as it would in a normal ear. The effect is most easily demonstrated when only one ear is affected, since then loudness matches can be made between the two ears, but it can be detected in other ways. The presence of recruitment can limit the usefulness of conventional hearing aids, since if the gain of the aid is set so as to make sounds of low intensity clearly audible, sounds of high intensity are uncomfortably loud. Hearing aids incorporating 'compression', especially multi-band compression, can be useful in alleviating this effect (Laurence, Moore and Glasberg, 1983; Moore *et al.*, 1992).

It has been suggested (Evans, 1975) that recruitment may be a consequence of the impaired frequency selectivity which is commonly associated with it. If tuning curves (or auditory filters) are broader than normal, then as the intensity of a tone is increased above threshold the activity will spread across the nerve fibre array (or to adjacent auditory filters) more rapidly than it would in the normal ear. This rapid spread of activity could be the reason for the rapid growth of loudness with intensity.

Moore *et al.* (1985) tested this idea by measuring how the rate of growth of loudness of a tone in recruiting ears was affected by presenting that tone in a band-stop or notched noise. They argued that this noise should mask the excitation pattern of the tone at characteristic frequencies far removed from the tone frequency. Thus, if Evans' suggestion were correct, the noise should reduce the rate of growth of loudness of the tone. They found that the noise had little effect on the loudness of the tone, and concluded that recruitment is probably not mediated by an abnormally rapid spread of excitation across the nerve fibre array. It seems likely that recruitment is caused by loss of the active mechanism in the cochlea (see Chapter 2). This mechanism boosts the response to weak sounds in a normal ear, but it has little effect on the response to intense sounds. Hence, when the active mechanism is damaged, the response to weak sounds is reduced (so that they become inaudible), but the response to intense sounds is almost normal.

Pitch perception in impaired hearing

The data on this topic show considerable variability across subjects. Most people with cochlear hearing losses show impaired frequency discrimination, but a few have almost normal discrimination. This applies to both pure and complex tones (Moore and Peters, 1992). The pattern-recognition theories of pitch perception predict an impairment in pitch perception and discrimination of complex tones whenever frequency resolution is impaired, since the perception of pitch is assumed to depend upon the ability to resolve the lower harmonics. However, it may be the case that quite good discrimination is possible on the basis of temporal information alone. Only when temporal processing is also disrupted, will performance become

very poor. Thus some subjects can show very broad psychophysical tuning curves, and almost normal pitch discrimination for complex tones. (For a review of this topic see Rosen and Fourcin, 1986.)

Temporal resolution in impaired hearing

There is some controversy as to whether temporal resolution is affected by cochlear hearing loss; some measures appear to show reduced temporal resolution, while others do not. Several factors can affect measures of temporal resolution in impaired subjects and not all of these are directly connected with temporal processing itself.

One important factor influencing the results is the degree to which the stimuli contain random fluctuations in amplitude. For stimuli that have marked slow fluctuations, such as narrow bands of noise, subjects with cochlear impairment often perform more poorly than normal in tasks such as gap detection (Fitzgibbons and Wightman, 1982; Florentine and Buus, 1984; Buus and Florentine, 1985; Glasberg, Moore and Bacon, 1987). However, gap detection is not usually worse than normal when the stimuli are sinusoids, which do not have inherent amplitude fluctuations (Moore and Glasberg, 1988; Moore *et al.*, 1989). Glasberg, Moore and Bacon (1987) and Moore and Glasberg (1988) suggested that the poor gap detection for narrowband noise stimuli might be a consequence of loudness recruitment. For a person with recruitment, the inherent fluctuations in a narrowband noise would result in larger-than-normal loudness fluctuations from moment to moment, so that inherent dips in the noise might be more confusable with the gap to be detected.

To assess this idea, Glasberg and Moore (1992) simulated the effects of loudness recruitment by processing the envelopes of narrow bands of noise so as to magnify the envelope fluctuations. The ability to detect gaps in the bands of noise was adversely affected by the magnified envelope fluctuations. Conversely, when the envelope fluctuations were compressed, gap detection was improved; this was the case for both normally-hearing and hearing-impaired subjects. These results support the idea that the poorer gap detection found in hearing-impaired subjects is a consequence of their loudness recruitment.

A second important factor influencing measures of temporal resolution is the sound level used. Many measures of temporal resolution show that performance in normally hearing subjects worsens at low sensation levels. It is not generally possible to test hearing-impaired subjects at high sensation levels, because of their loudness recruitment. Thus, on some measures of temporal resolution, such as the detection of gaps in bands of noise or the rate of recovery from forward masking, hearing-impaired subjects appear markedly worse than normal subjects when tested at the same sound pressure levels, but only slightly worse at equal sensation levels, (Fitzgibbons and Wightman, 1982; Tyler *et al.*, 1982; Glasberg, Moore and Bacon, 1987). On some measures, such as the detection of temporal gaps in sinusoids, hearing-impaired subjects can actually perform a little better than normally hearing subjects when tested at equal sensation levels (Moore and Glasberg, 1988; Moore *et al.*, 1989).

A final important consideration is the bandwidth available to the listeners. For example, several studies measuring temporal modulation transfer functions for broadband noise showed that impaired listeners were generally less sensitive to high rates of modulation than normal listeners (Formby, 1982; Lamore, Verweij and Brocaar, 1984; Bacon and Viemeister, 1985). However, this may have been largely a consequence of the fact that high frequencies were inaudible to the impaired listeners (Bacon and Viemeister, 1985); most of the subjects used had greater hearing losses at high frequencies than at low.

Bacon and Gleitman (1992) measured temporal modulation transfer functions for broadband noise using subjects with relatively flat hearing losses. They found that at equal (high) sound pressure levels performance was similar for hearing-impaired and normally hearing subjects. At equal (low) sensation levels, the hearing-impaired subjects tended to perform better than the normally hearing subjects. Moore, Shailer and Schooneveldt (1992) controlled for the effects of listening bandwidth by measuring temporal modulation transfer functions for an octave-wide noise band centred at 2 kHz, using subjects with unilateral and bilateral cochlear hearing loss. Over the frequency range covered by the noise, the subjects had reasonably constant thresholds as a function of frequency, both in their normal and their impaired ears. This ensured that there were no differences between subjects or ears in terms of the range of audible frequencies in the noise. To ensure that subjects were not making use of information from frequencies outside the nominal passband of the noise, the modulated carrier was presented in an unmodulated broadband noise background. They found that performance was similar for the normal and impaired ears, both at equal sound pressure levels, and equal sensation levels, although there was a slight trend for the impaired ears to perform better at equal sensation levels.

In summary, for stimuli with inherent slow amplitude fluctuations (such as narrow bands of noise) temporal resolution is poorer for impaired ears than for normal ears, since the inherent fluctuations are effectively magnified by recruitment in the impaired ears and this adversely affects performance. However, for deterministic stimuli (such as sinusoids) or for broadband noise stimuli, temporal resolution may be as good as or better than in normal ears, when the comparison is made at equal sensation levels. In practice, hearing-impaired subjects often show poor performance on measures of temporal resolution because the stimuli are at low sensation levels and/or because the audible bandwidth of the stimuli is restricted.

General summary and conclusions

A central theme of this chapter has been the frequency-analysing capacity of the auditory system. This capacity plays a role in the ability perceptually to separate simultaneously presented sounds, to detect signals in masking noise, to identify the timbre of speech and musical sounds, and to perceive the pitch of complex tones. The basic properties of these abilities can be understood by conceiving of the peripheral auditory system as containing a bank of bandpass filters, whose centre frequencies cover the whole audible range. The bandwidths of the filters at different centre frequencies are characterized by the value of the auditory filter bandwidth (ERB) or critical bandwidth (CB). The value of the auditory filter bandwidth increases in rough proportion with centre frequency above about 1 kHz (see Figure 3.6).

The basic frequency-analysing mechanisms seem to be well established at the level of the auditory nerve. Information about stimulus frequency, intensity, and spectrum may be carried both in the distribution of activity across nerve fibres and in the temporal patterns of neural firing. Temporal patterns may be particularly important in the perception of pitch.

Damage to the inner ear results in an impairment in the frequency-analysing mechanisms. This has been shown both neurophysiologically, in single fibres in the auditory nerve, and psychophysically, using masking techniques. Thus the ability to detect and discriminate signals in noise, to identify the timbre of sounds, and to perceive the pitch of complex sounds, may all be impaired. Temporal resolution may also be reduced in cases of cochlear hearing loss. This occurs mainly for stimuli with slowly fluctuating envelopes, or stimuli at low sensation levels. In addition changes in the loudness of sounds with changes in stimulus intensity and bandwidth may be abnormal. These disabilities are not corrected with a conventional hearing aid.

References

BACON, S. P. and GLEITMAN, R. M. (1992) Modulation detection in subjects with relatively flat hearing losses. *Journal of Speech and Hearing Research*, **35**, 642–653

BACON, S. P. and VIEMEISTER, N. F. (1985) Temporal modulation transfer functions in normal-hearing and hearing-impaired subjects. *Audiology*, **24**, 117–134

BAER, T. and MOORE, B. C. J. (1993) Effects of spectral smearing on the intelligibility of sentences in the presence of noise. *Journal of the Acoustical Society of America*, **94**, 1229–1241

BAER, T. and MOORE, B. C. J. (1994) Effects of spectral smearing on the intelligibility of sentences in the presence of interfering speech. *Journal of the Acoustical Society of America*, (in press)

BATTEAU, D. W. (1967) The role of the pinna in human localization. *Proceedings of the Royal Society B*, **168**, 158–180

BUUS, S. and FLORENTINE, M. (1985) Gap detection in normal and impaired listeners: the effect of level and frequency. In: *Time Resolution in Auditory Systems*, edited by A. Michelsen. New York: Springer-Verlag. pp. 159–179

DRESCHLER, W. A. and PLOMP, R. (1980) Relations between psychophysical data and speech perception for hearing-impaired subjects. I. *Journal of the Acoustical Society of America*, **68**, 1608–1615

DUBNO, J. R. and DIRKS, D. D. (1989) Auditory filter characteristics and consonant recognition for hearing-impaired listeners. *Journal of the Acoustical Society of America*, **85**, 1666–1675

EDDINS, D. A., HALL, J. W. and GROSE, J. H. (1992) Detection of temporal gaps as a function of frequency region and absolute noise bandwidth. *Journal of the Acoustical Society of America*, **91**, 1069–1077

EGAN, J. P. and HAKE, H. W. (1950) On the masking pattern of a simple auditory stimulus. *Journal of the Acoustical Society of America*, **22**, 622–630

EVANS, E. F. (1975) The sharpening of frequency selectivity in the normal and abnormal cochlea. *Audiology*, **14**, 419–442

FELDTKELLER, R. and ZWICKER, E. (1956) *Das Ohr als Nachrichtenempfänger*. Stuttgart: S. Hirzel

FESTEN, J. M. and PLOMP, R. (1983) Relations between auditory functions in impaired hearing. *Journal of the Acoustical Society of America*, **73**, 652–662

FINE, P. A. and MOORE, B. C. J. (1993) Frequency analysis and musical ability. *Music Perception*, **11**, 39–53

FITZGIBBONS, P. J. and WIGHTMAN, F. L. (1982) Gap detection in normal and hearing-impaired listeners. *Journal of the Acoustical Society of America*, **72**, 761–765

FLETCHER, H. (1940) Auditory patterns. *Reviews of Modern Physics*, **12**, 47–65

FLORENTINE, M. and BUUS, S. (1984) Temporal gap detection in sensorineural and simulated hearing impairment. *Journal of Speech and Hearing Research*, **27**, 449–455

FORMBY, C. (1982) Differential sensitivity to tonal frequency and to the rate of amplitude modulation of broad-band noise by hearing-impaired listeners. *Ph. D. Thesis*, Washington University, St Louis

GLASBERG, B. R. and MOORE, B. C. J. (1986) Auditory filter shapes in subjects with unilateral and bilateral cochlear impairments. *Journal of the Acoustical Society of America*, **79**, 1020–1033

GLASBERG, B. R. and MOORE, B. C. J. (1989) Psychoacoustic abilities of subjects with unilateral and bilateral cochlear impairments and their relationship to the ability to understand speech. *Scandinavian Audiology Supplement*, **32**, 1–25

GLASBERG, B. R. and MOORE, B. C. J. (1990) Derivation of auditory filter shapes from notched-noise data. *Hearing Research*, **47**, 103–138

GLASBERG, B. R. and MOORE, B. C. J. (1992) Effects of envelope fluctuations on gap detection. *Hearing Research*, **64**, 81–92

GLASBERG, B. R. and MOORE, B. C. J. (1994) Growth-of-masking functions for several types of maskers. *Journal of the Acoustical Society of America*, (in press)

GLASBERG, B. R., MOORE, B. C. J. and BACON, S. P. (1987) Gap detection and masking in hearing-impaired and normal-hearing subjects. *Journal of the Acoustical Society of America*, **81**, 1546–1556

GLASBERG, B. R., MOORE, B. C. J. and NIMMO-SMITH, I. (1984) Comparison of auditory filter shapes derived with three different maskers. *Journal of the Acoustical Society of America*, **75**, 536–544

GOLDSTEIN, J. L. (1973) An optimum processor theory for the central formation of the pitch of complex tones. *Journal of the Acoustical Society of America*, **54**, 1496–1516

GOLDSTEIN, J. L. and SRULOVICZ, P. (1977) Auditory-nerve spike intervals as an adequate basis for aural frequency measurement. In: *Psychophysics and Physiology of Hearing*, edited by E. F. Evans and J. P. Wilson. London: Academic Press. pp. 337–346

GREENWOOD, D. D. (1961) Critical bandwidth and the frequency coordinates of the basilar membrane. *Journal of the Acoustical Society of America*, **33**, 1344–1356

HAFTER, E. R. (1984) Spatial hearing and the duplex theory: How viable? In: *Dynamic Aspects of Neocortical Function*, edited by G. M. Edelman, W. E. Gall and W. M. Cowan. New York: Wiley. pp. 425–448

HOUTGAST, T. (1972) Psychophysical evidence for lateral inhibition in hearing. *Journal of the Acoustical Society of America*, **51**, 1885–1894

HOUTGAST, T. (1974) Lateral suppression in hearing. *Ph. D. Thesis*, Free University of Amsterdam

HOUTGAST, T. (1977) Auditory-filter characteristics derived from direct-masking data and pulsation-threshold data with a rippled-noise masker. *Journal of the Acoustical Society of America*, **62**, 409–415

HOUTSMA, A. J. M. (1995) Pitch perception. In: *Handbook of Perception and Cognition, Volume 6. Hearing*, edited by B. C. J. Moore. Orlando, Florida: Academic Press. pp. 267–295

LAMORE, P. J. J., VERWEIJ, C. and BROCAAR, M. P. (1984) Reliability of auditory function tests in severely hearing-impaired and deaf subjects. *Audiology*, **23**, 453–466

LAURENCE, R. F., MOORE, B. C. J. and GLASBERG, B. R. (1983) A comparison of behind-the-ear high-fidelity linear aids and two-channel compression hearing aids in the laboratory and in everyday life. *British Journal of Audiology*, **17**, 31–48

LUTFI, R. A. and PATTERSON, R. D. (1984) On the growth of masking asymmetry with stimulus intensity. *Journal of the Acoustical Society of America*, **76**, 739–745

MOORE, B. C. J. (1973) Frequency difference limens for short-duration tones. *Journal of the Acoustical Society of America*, **54**, 610–619

MOORE, B. C. J. (1980) Detection cues in forward masking. In: *Psychophysical, Physiological and Behavioural Studies in Hearing*, edited by G. van den Brink and F. A. Bilson. Delft: Delft University Press. pp. 222–229

MOORE, B. C. J. (1986) Parallels between frequency selectivity measured psychophysically and in cochlear mechanics. *Scandinavian Audiology Supplement*, **25**, 139–152

MOORE, B. C. J. (1989) *An Introduction to the Psychology of Hearing*, 3rd edn. London: Academic Press

MOORE, B. C. J. (1993) Frequency analysis and pitch perception. In: *Human Psychophysics*, edited by W. A. Yost, A. N. Popper and R. R. Fay. New York: Springer-Verlag. pp. 56–115

MOORE, B. C. J. and GLASBERG, B. R. (1981) Auditory filter shapes derived in simultaneous and forward masking. *Journal of the Acoustical Society of America*, **70**, 1003–1014

MOORE, B. C. J. and GLASBERG, B. R. (1983) Suggested formulae for calculating auditory-filter bandwidths and excitation patterns. *Journal of the Acoustical Society of America*, **74**, 750–753

MOORE, B. C. J. and GLASBERG, B. R. (1986a) Comparisons of frequency selectivity in simultaneous and forward masking for subjects with unilateral cochlear impairments. *Journal of the Acoustical Society of America*, **80**, 93–107

MOORE, B. C. J. and GLASBERG, B. R. (1986b) The role of frequency selectivity in the perception of loudness, pitch and time. In: *Frequency Selectivity in Hearing*, edited by B. C. J. Moore. London: Academic Press. pp. 251–308

MOORE, B. C. J. and GLASBERG, B. R. (1987) Formulae describing frequency selectivity as a function of frequency and level and their use in calculating excitation patterns. *Hearing Research*, **28**, 209–225

MOORE, B. C. J. and GLASBERG, B. R. (1988) Gap detection with sinusoids and noise in normal, impaired and electrically stimulated ears. *Journal of the Acoustical Society of America*, **83**, 1093–1101

MOORE, B. C. J. and O'LOUGHLIN, B. J. (1986) The use of nonsimultaneous masking to measure frequency selectivity and suppression. In: *Frequency Selectivity in Hearing*, edited by B. C. J. Moore. London: Academic Press. pp. 179–250

MOORE, B. C. J. and OHGUSHI, K. (1993) Audibility of partials in inharmonic complex tones. *Journal of the Acoustical Society of America*, **93**, 452–461

MOORE, B. C. J. and PETERS, R. W. (1992) Pitch discrimination and phase sensitivity in young and elderly subjects and its relationship to frequency selectivity. *Journal of the Acoustical Society of America*, **91**, 2881–2893

MOORE, B. C. J. and ROSEN, S. M. (1979) Tune recognition with reduced pitch and interval information. *Quarterly Journal of Experimental Psychology*, **31**, 229–240

MOORE, B. C. J., GLASBERG, B. R. and SHAILER, M. J. (1984) Frequency and intensity difference limens for harmonics within complex tones. *Journal of the Acoustical Society of America*, **75**, 550–561

MOORE, B. C. J., PETERS, R. W. and GLASBERG, B. R. (1990) Auditory filter shapes at low center frequencies. *Journal of the Acoustical Society of America*, **88**, 132–140

MOORE, B. C. J., SHAILER, M. J. and SCHOONEVELDT, G. P. (1992) Temporal modulation transfer functions for band-limited noise in subjects with cochlear hearing loss. *British Journal of Audiology*, **26**, 229–237

MOORE, B. C. J., GLASBERG, B. R., DONALDSON, E., MCPHERSON, T. and PLACK, C. J. (1989) Detection of temporal gaps in sinusoids by normally hearing and hearing-impaired subjects. *Journal of the Acoustical Society of America*, **85**, 1266–1275

MOORE, B. C. J., GLASBERG, B. R., HESS, R. F. and BIRCHALL, J. P. (1985) Effects of flanking noise bands on the rate of growth of loudness of tones in normal and recruiting ears. *Journal of the Acoustical Society of America*, **77**, 1505–1515

MOORE, B. C. J., JOHNSON, J. S., CLARK, T. M. and PLUVINAGE, V. (1992) Evaluation of a dual-channel full dynamic range compression system for people with sensorineural hearing loss. *Ear and Hearing*, **13**, 349–370

NEUTZEL, J. M. and HAFTER, E. R. (1981) Lateralization of complex waveforms: spectral effects. *Journal of the Acoustical Society of America*, **69**, 1112–1118

PATTERSON, R. D. (1976) Auditory filter shapes derived with noise stimuli. *Journal of the Acoustical Society of America*, **59**, 640–654

PATTERSON, R. D. and MOORE, B. C. J. (1986) Auditory filters and excitation patterns as representations of frequency resolution. In: *Frequency Selectivity in Hearing*, edited by B. C. J. Moore. London: Academic Press. pp. 123–177

PATTERSON, R. D. and NIMMO-SMITH, I. (1980) Off-frequency listening and auditory filter asymmetry. *Journal of the Acoustical Society of America*, **67**, 229–245

PATTERSON, R. D., NIMMO-SMITH, I., WEBER, D. L. and MILROY, R. (1982) The deterioration of hearing with age: frequency selectivity, the critical ratio, the audiogram, and speech threshold. *Journal of the Acoustical Society of America*, **72**, 1788–1803

PENNER, M. J. (1977) Detection of temporal gaps in noise as a measure of the decay of auditory sensation. *Journal of the Acoustical Society of America*, **61**, 552–557

PETERS, R. W. and MOORE, B. C. J. (1992) Auditory filter shapes at low center frequencies in young and elderly hearing-impaired subjects. *Journal of the Acoustical Society of America*, **91**, 256–266

PICK, G., EVANS, E. F. and WILSON, J. P. (1977) Frequency resolution in patients with hearing loss of cochlear origin. In: *Psychophysics and Physiology of Hearing*, edited by E. F. Evans and J. P. Wilson. London: Academic Press. pp. 273–281

PICKLES, J. O. (1986) The neurophysiological basis of frequency selectivity. In: *Frequency Selectivity in Hearing*, edited by B. C. J. Moore. London: Academic Press. pp. 51–121

PLOMP, R. (1964a) The ear as a frequency analyzer. *Journal of the Acoustical Society of America*, **36**, 1628–1636

PLOMP, R. (1964b) The rate of decay of auditory sensation. *Journal of the Acoustical Society of America*, **36**, 277–282

PLOMP, R. (1976) *Aspects of Tone Sensation*. London: Academic Press

PLOMP, R. and MIMPEN, A. M. (1968) The ear as a frequency analyzer II. *Journal of the Acoustical Society of America*, **43**, 764–767

RAYLEIGH, LORD (1907) On our perception of sound direction. *Philosophical Magazine*, **13**, 214–232

ROBINSON, D. W. and DADSON, R. S. (1956) A re-determination of the equal-loudness relations for pure tones. *British Journal of Applied Physics*, **7**, 166–181

ROSEN, S. and FOURCIN, A. (1986) Frequency selectivity and the perception of speech. In: *Frequency Selectivity in Hearing*, edited by B. C. J. Moore. London: Academic Press. pp. 373–487

SACHS, M. B. and KIANG, N. Y. S. (1968) Two-tone inhibition in auditory nerve fibers. *Journal of the Acoustical Society of America*, **43**, 1120–1128

SCHOUTEN, J. F., RITSMA, R. J. and CARDOZO, B. L. (1962) Pitch of the residue. *Journal of the Acoustical Society of America*, **34**, 1418–1424

SEK, A. and MOORE, B. C. J. (1994) The critical modulation frequency and its relationship to auditory filtering at low frequencies. *Journal of the Acoustical Society of America*, (in press)

SHAILER, M. J. and MOORE, B. C. J. (1983) Gap detection as a function of frequency, bandwidth and level. *Journal of the Acoustical Society of America*, **74**, 467–473

SHAILER, M. J., MOORE, B. C. J., GLASBERG, B. R., WATSON, N. and HARRIS, S. (1990) Auditory filter shapes at 8 and 10 kHz. *Journal of the Acoustical Society of America*, **88**, 141–148

SHANNON, R. V. (1976) Two-tone unmasking and suppression in a forward masking situation. *Journal of the Acoustical Society of America*, **59**, 1460–1470

SODERQUIST, D. R. (1970) Frequency analysis and the critical band. *Psychonomic Science*, **21**, 117–119

STEVENS, S. S. (1957) On the psychophysical law. *Psychological Review*, **64**, 153–181

STEVENS, S. S. (1972) Perceived level of noise by Mark VII and decibels (E). *Journal of the Acoustical Society of America*, **51**, 575–601

TER KEURS, M., FESTEN, J. M. and PLOMP, R. (1992) Effect of spectral envelope smearing on speech reception. *Journal of the Acoustical Society of America*, **91**, 2872–2880

TERHARDT, E. (1974) Pitch, consonance, and harmony. *Journal of the Acoustical Society of America*, **55**, 1061–1069

TYLER, R. S., SUMMERFIELD, A. Q., WOOD, E. J. and FERNANDES, M. A. (1982) Psychoacoustic and phonetic temporal processing in normal and hearing-impaired listeners. *Journal of the Acoustical Society of America*, **72**, 740–752

VIEMEISTER, N. F. (1979) Temporal modulation transfer functions based on modulation thresholds. *Journal of the Acoustical Society of America*, **66**, 1364–1380

VOGTEN, L. L. M. (1974) Pure-tone masking: a new result from a new method. In: *Facts and Models in Hearing*, edited by E. Zwicker and E. Terhardt. Berlin: Springer-Verlag. pp. 142–155

WALLACH, H., NEWMAN, E. B. and ROSENZWIEG, M. R. (1949) The precedence effect in sound localization. *American Journal of Psychology*, **62**, 315–336

WARREN, R. M. (1970) Elimination of biases in loudness judgements for tones. *Journal of the Acoustical Society of America*, **48**, 1397–1413

ZWICKER, E. (1974) On the psychophysical equivalent of tuning curves. In: *Facts and Models in Hearing*, edited by E. Zwicker and E. Terhardt. Berlin: Springer-Verlag. pp. 132–140

ZWICKER, E. and FELDTKELLER, R. (1967) *Das Ohr als Nachrichtenempfänger*. Stuttgart: Hirzel-Verlag

ZWICKER, E. and TERHARDT, E. (1980) Analytical expressions for critical band rate and critical bandwidth as a function of frequency. *Journal of the Acoustical Society of America*, **68**, 1523–1525

4

The physiology of equilibrium and its application to the dizzy patient

Peter Savundra and Linda M. Luxon

In humans, a highly sophisticated mechanism for maintaining gaze and balance has developed, which is dependent upon visual, vestibular, proprioceptive and superficial sensory information (Figure 4.1). The information is integrated in the central nervous system and is modulated by activity arising in the reticular formation, the extrapyramidal system, the cerebellum and the cerebral cortex. A lesion at any of these sites may produce symptoms associated with a loss of balance, a failure of gaze fixation or an abnormality of perception.

Symptoms may be reported variously by patients as a specific illusion of movement or loss of balance to a much more vague complaint of dizziness, disequilibrium, faintness, giddiness, sensations of swimminess or floating, unexpected falls and anxiety or difficulty thinking in certain environments. The term *vertigo* is usually defined as an illusion of movement (Ludman, 1979) or the disagreeable sensation of instability or disordered orientation in space (Agate, 1963). Cawthorne (1952) defined vertigo as an hallucination of movement, highlighting the reality of the perception of some sufferers, while Ludman's use of the word illusion suggests the understanding by some sufferers that they and their environment are not actually moving. The lay term *dizziness* can be used to cover the less specific synonyms noted above. Other patients have an illusion of horizontal or vertical oscillation of the visual world, sometimes exacerbated by head movements. This is termed *oscillopsia* (Bender, 1965).

Until the advent of magnetic resonance imaging, no part of the human vestibular system could be adequately visualized *in vivo* and the understanding of the physiology of the human system was based on the analysis of reflexes and responses. However, con-

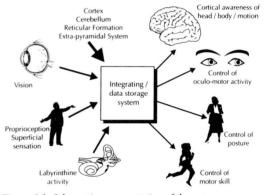

Figure 4.1 Schematic representation of the sensory integration in a balance perception model

siderable progress has been made with the study of vertebrate and invertebrate vestibular systems, where imaging and invasive *in vivo* and *in vitro* analyses are possible.

The vestibular system was present as the statocyst, the most primitive gravity receptor, over 600 million years ago. It is still to be found in the higher members of the phylum Coelenterata. With the evolution of the taxa, the balance receptor organ became increasingly complex, attaining a more sophisticated form in the modern fish some 100 million years ago (Gray, 1955).

Throughout the invertebrate and vertebrate kingdoms, the balance receptor organs have evolved in parallel and there remain considerable similarities. While it is unwise to extrapolate from one species to another, let alone between mammals and invertebrates, information has been gathered and hypotheses proposed, which have enabled human experiments to be formulated. As a result, the understanding of the physiology of human equilibrium has been advanced by the detailed study of the balance receptors of other animals.

As a first step, it is useful to define the role of the vestibular system.

Functions of the vestibular system

The functions of the vestibular system are:

1 The detection of body motion (linear and angular acceleration), as monitored by head motion
2 The detection of the head in space relative to the gravitational vector (tilt).

This information is integrated with other inputs to contribute to:

1 The maintenance of the fovea on the object of visual fixation
2 The maintenance of balance
3 The activity of the autonomic nervous system
4 The level of arousal and mood.

The perception of normal and abnormal balance

Normal

Patients without vestibular function do not experience a turning sensation when rotated in the absence of visual and tactile cues (Guedry, 1974). The sensation of movement is not lost following spinal transection, blindness or oculomotor paralysis. On the other hand, lesions of the non-dominant parietal cortex can produce the illusion of movement (Critchley, 1953; Barlow, 1970) and electrical stimulation of the superior sylvian gyrus and the inferior intraparietal sulcus produces a sensation of rotation or bodily movement (Penfield, 1957).

The subjective awareness of motion is subserved by vestibulocortical projections (Bottini *et al.*, 1994). These were first identified electrophysiologically by Watzl and Mountcastle (1949), who recorded monophasic potentials in the suprasylvian gyrus, following electrical stimulation of the contralateral vestibular nerve. Studies in the cat and the squirrel monkey have demonstrated projections from the vestibular nuclei to the thalamus, and thence to the sensorimotor cortex (Liedgren *et al.*, 1976; Liedgren and Rubin, 1976). Functionally, therefore, the vestibulothalamocortical projections allow some integration of labyrinthine and somatic proprioceptive signals, and thus facilitate conscious awareness of body orientation.

The perception of the magnitude of acceleration does not correlate with physiological variables. This was demonstrated by Van Egmond, Groen and Jongkees (1948), who examined the threshold and dura-

tion of subjective sensation with the threshold and duration of induced nystagmus. With their technique, termed cupulometry, subjects were rotated, at constant velocities, ranging up to 60°/s and then suddenly stopped to record the durations of 'after-turning sensation' and post-rotation nystagmus. The average nystagmus and sensation cupulogram for 15 subjects is shown in Figure 4.2.

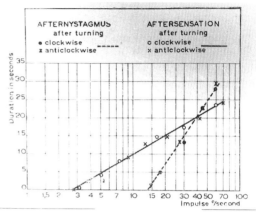

Figure 4.2 Graph of the average nystagmus and sensation cupulograms (from Van Egmond, A. A. J., Groen J. J. and Jongkees L. B. W. The turning test with small regulable stimuli. *Journal of Laryngology and Otology*, **62**, 63–69. 1948 by permission of the Editor)

It is clear that the average slope of the sensation cupulogram differs from that of the nystagmus cupulogram, although both are derived from a single cupular deflection from a given stimulus. This apparent discrepancy is almost certainly the result of the central nervous system altering the stimulus-response relationship (Guedry, 1974). It may be proposed therefore that the central pathways which subserve subjective sensation and nystagmus are different, although they are both dependent upon the same input.

The perception of acceleration is dependent upon the magnitude of the acceleration (Mach, 1875). Below a minimum threshold, a subject does not perceive acceleration and for the perception of rotation the threshold of constant *angular acceleration* is 0.1–0.4°/s² (Clark, 1967), although, the perception of rotation increases with prolonged constant acceleration.

The threshold for the perception of movement with horizontal *linear acceleration* ranges from 5 to 15 cm/s² (Guedry, 1974) and varies with the amplitude of the stimulus. At lower amplitudes, the subject perceives motion without direction, but as the amplitude increases, directionality becomes apparent. At higher amplitudes, there is the additional perception of tilt. The explanation of this is given in Figure 4.3. F_g is the acceleration due to gravity. The force generating the swing has an acceleration F_t. The resulting force

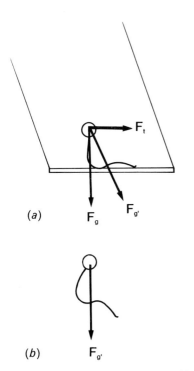

(a)

(b)

Figure 4.3 Diagram to illustrate (*a*) distribution of forces; (*b*) subjective sensation in linear acceleration on a parallel swing. F_g: acceleration due to gravity; F_t: swing acceleration; $F_{g'}$: resultant force which is perceived as the true earth vertical

is $F_{g'}$, which is then perceived as the true earth vertical.

Static tilt experiments (Clark, 1970; Graybiel, 1974), in which subjects are strapped to a tilt platform, in total darkness, and are asked either to estimate the deviation of the head from the earth's vertical or to adjust a luminous line on a dark field to a vertical position, have shown that, up to 40°, normal subjects can perceive as little as 2–4° of tilt.

Abnormal

Sensory inputs are normally combined to provide an accurate model of the physical world, but symptoms arise when there is an unusual combination of sensory inputs triggered by exposure to visual stimuli, such as rapidly changing images on a television screen, striped material or fast-moving traffic and crowds. This is termed *visual vertigo*. Such symptoms can be experienced in the absence of demonstrable vestibular disease and Roberts (1967) has suggested a hypothesis to explain this phenomenon. From birth, the information required for balance is integrated and stored in data centres within different sites in the brain. New information is constantly compared with these data and under normal circumstances 'immediate recognition' of sensory patterns enables vestibular activity to take place at a subconscious level, but new data patterns which are not immediately recognized will precipitate the perception of vestibular activity.

The false perception of motion of self and/or external objects may be provoked by visual, vestibular or neurological disease or by the presentation of unphysiological stimuli, or by the removal or distortion of the stimulus. A common manifestation is the feeling of imbalance caused by the wearing of new spectacles or bifocal lenses. Vertigo can be triggered in supermarkets by lines of shelves under featureless, shadowless fluorescent lighting. The loss of the sense of turning in normal subjects flying in cloud is well-known (Benson, 1978). In the motorist's vestibular disorientation syndrome (Page and Gresty, 1985) patients with vestibular disease develop an illusion of turning and make inappropriate postural or steering adjustments when travelling at speed, particularly in the dark or on open, featureless roads. Symptoms of imbalance can arise if the driver suddenly loses expected environmental cues, as when overtaking high-sided vehicles.

The resulting misleading sense of movement and disorientation may be associated with somatic symptoms, such as nausea and sweating and feelings of panic, anxiety and inadequacy (Brandt and Daroff, 1980a). Similar symptoms have been described in space phobia (Marks, 1981) and the importance of defining and differentiating a vestibular or visual disturbance is crucial in order to institute appropriate treatment.

Vestibular anatomy

To understand the physiology of the vestibular apparatus, an appreciation of the anatomy and ultrastructure of the peripheral vestibular system and its central pathways is required.

Otic capsule

The peripheral vestibular system is an integral part of the labyrinth, which lies in the otic capsule in the petrous portion of the temporal bone. The otic capsule is composed of three chambers: the cochlea anteriorly and the peripheral vestibular system in the vestibule and the posterior vestibular chamber. Three bony semicircular canals open into the posterior vestibular chamber by means of five round apertures. The two vertical canals (the superior and posterior canals) join posteriorly to form a single crus commune.

Membranous labyrinth

The membranous labyrinth (Figure 4.4) is surrounded by perilymph and is suspended by fine connective tissue strands from the bony labyrinth. It consists of an anterior chamber, the cochlear duct, which subserves hearing, and which connects, by way of the round saccule, with the posterior vestibular apparatus. The peripheral vestibular apparatus consists of the saccule, utricle and semicircular canals.

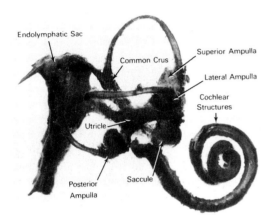

Figure 4.4 Membranous labyrinth (Dissected by K. Watanuki. From Schuknecht, H. F. *Pathology of the Ear*, 2nd edn. Philadelphia: Lea & Fabiger. 1993)

The membranous labyrinth contains endolymph. This is produced by the secretory cells of the stria vascularis of the cochlea and the dark cells of the vestibular labyrinth (Kimura, 1969).

The membranous labyrinth contains five areas of sensory epithelium, the vestibular receptor organs: two maculae of the otolith organs (utricle and saccule) and three cristae ampullares of the semicircular canals. The sensory epithelium, which is comprised of both sensory and supporting cells, rests on connective tissue, which is firmly adherent to the bony labyrinth. The supporting cells secrete the mucopolysaccharide gel of the cupula and the otoconial membrane.

Saccule

The saccule lies in a recess near the opening of the scala vestibuli of the cochlea and is almost globular in shape. It is connected anteriorly by the ductus reuniens to the cochlea and posteriorly via the utriculosaccular duct to the endolymphatic duct. On its anterior, vertical wall is the elliptical saccular macula – a thickened area of sensory epithelium (Figure 4.5).

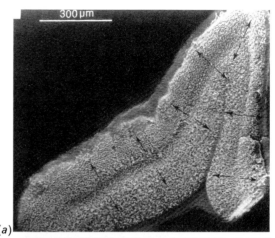

(*a*)

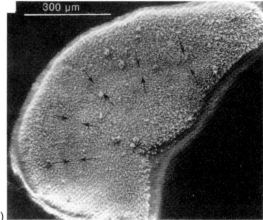

(*b*)

Figure 4.5 Scanning electron microscopic view of the chinchilla (*a*) saccule, (*b*) utricle (arrows indicate the direction of stereociliary polarization). (From Lim, D. J. In: Paparella, M. M., Shumrick D. A., Gluckman, J. L. and Meyershoff, W. L. *Otolaryngology*, vol. 1. *Basic Sciences and Related Disciplines*, 3rd edn, 1991. Philadelphia: W. B. Saunders Co)

Utricle

The utricle is larger than the saccule and lies posterosuperiorly to it. It is irregularly oblong in shape and is connected anteriorly via the utriculosaccular duct to the endolymphatic duct. The three semicircular canals open into it by five openings, the posterior and superior semicircular canals sharing one opening at the crus commune. On the floor of the utricle, tilted anteriorly and rostrally upwards by about 30°, lies the sensory epithelium of the comma-shaped macula (see Figure 4.5).

Semicircular canals

The three semicircular canals are small ring-like structures, each forming two-thirds of a circle with a diameter of about 6.5 mm, and a luminal cross-sectional diameter of 0.4 mm. One end of each canal is dilated to form the ampulla, which contains a saddle-shaped ridge, the crista ampullaris, on which lies the sensory epithelium.

Sensory epithelium

The sensory epithelium is localized to the maculae of the utricle and saccule and the cristae ampullares of the semicircular canals. The sensory cells (see below)

are surrounded by supporting cells, and therefore do not come into direct contact with the bony base of the cristae. The apical surfaces of the supporting cells are covered with microvilli.

Close to the periphery of the sensory epithelium of the utricular macula and the cristae are the dark cell regions. These cells resemble those of the stria vascularis and are thought to secrete vestibular endolymph and contribute to its electrical potential (see below).

Macula (Figure 4.6)

Each macula is a small area of sensory epithelium. The ciliary bundles of the sensory cells (see below)

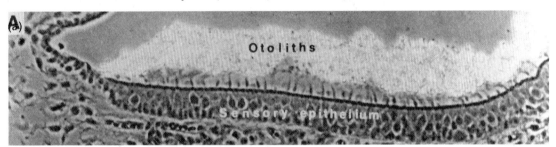

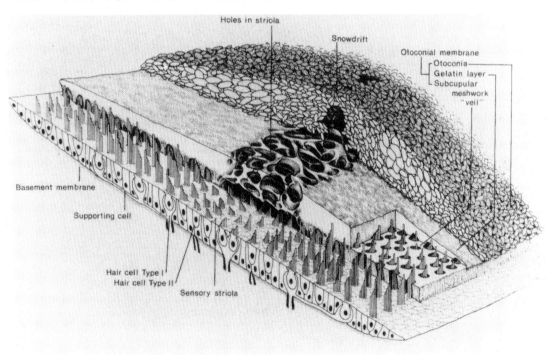

(b)

Figure 4.6 (*a*) Light microscopy of utricular otoconial membrane (From Lim, D. J. and Lane, W. C. *American Academy of Otolaryngology*, 1969, **73**, 866). (*b*) Artist's conception of the cross-section of the saccule showing the substructures of the otoconial membrane with its striolar holes and the snowflake zone of otoconia. (Drawing by Nancy Sally. From Paparella, M. M., Shumrick, D. A., Gluckman, J. L. and Meyershoff, W. L. *Otolaryngology*, vol. 1. *Basic Sciences and Related Disciplines*, 3rd edn, 1991. Philadelphia: W. B. Saunders Co)

project into the overlying statoconial membrane, which consists of an otoconial layer, a gelatinous area and a subcupula meshwork (Lim, 1979). The otoconial layer is comprised of calcareous material: the gelatinous layer, a mucopolysaccharide gel, and the subcupula layer, a honeycomb of ciliary bundles (Lindeman, 1969; Lim, 1979).

The otoconia are of variable size, but are distributed in a characteristic pattern. In the saccule, the largest otoconia are found close to the central strip (the striola) of the saccule, whereas in the utricle, it is the smallest which lie near the striola, with the largest nearer the periphery of the macula.

The sensory cells are also organized with the kinocilia orientated away from the striola in the saccular macula, but towards the striola in the utricular macula. This orientation is of considerable importance in understanding the physiology of the saccule and utricle (see below).

The otoconia appear to have a slow turnover. They appear to be produced by the supporting cells of the sensory epithelium (Harada, 1979), and to be resorbed by the dark cell regions (Lim, 1984).

The specific gravity of the otoconial membrane is approximately 2.7. Therefore, even at rest, it exerts a force on the sensory epithelium.

Crista

The crista ampullaris consist of a crest of sensory epithelium supported on a mound of connective tissue, lying at right angles to the longitudinal axis of the canal (Figure 4.7). The crista is surmounted by

a bulbous, wedge-shaped, gelatinous mass, the cupula. The cilia of the sensory cells project into the cupula. The exact anatomy of the cupula *in vivo* is uncertain as preparation is associated with its shrinkage and the effect of this on its structure is unknown. *In vivo*, it may form a water-tight seal (Figure 4.8) or there might be a small subcupular space (Dohlman, 1981).

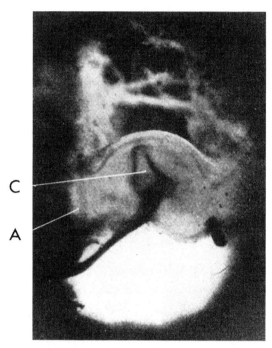

Figure 4.8 Deflection of the cupula in the ampulla of pike's horizontal semicircular canal. A = ampulla, C = cupula. (From Steinhausen 1931)

The specific gravity of the cupula is the same as that of endolymph, though, because of its different composition it may have different solubility coefficients for different solutes, e.g. ethanol. This could lead to differences in specific gravity under different conditions (Brandt, 1991). At rest, under normal conditions, the cupula does not exert a force on the sensory epithelium.

Vestibular receptor cells

There are a total of 23 000 hair cells in the three human cristae (Rosenhall, 1972a) and between 45 000 and 60 000 in the two maculae (Rosenhall, 1972b). The hair cells are surrounded by supporting cells, which are attached to the basement membrane, in which is found the neural and vascular tissue.

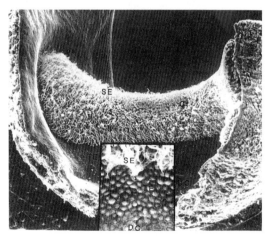

Figure 4.7 Saddle-shaped crista (Cr) of a chinchilla. The cupula has been removed. Higher magnification shows transition from sensory epithelium (SE) to transitional epithelium (TE) to dark cell zone (DC). PS = planum semilunatum. (From Hunter–Duvar, I. and Hinojosa, R. *Ultrastructural Atlas of the Inner Ear.* edited by I. Friedmann and J. Ballantyne. London: Butterworths. 1984)

The vestibular hair cells can be classified into two types: type I and type II. Type I cells are flask-shaped, while type II cells are cylindrical (Figure 4.9), although it is likely that the classification of the vestibular hair cells is more complicated than this. The type I cells are distinguished by being goblet shaped with a basal nucleus, and an afferent neuronal calyx on which the efferent fibres synapse. The type II cells are cylindrical, with a basal nucleus and bouton-type afferent and efferent basolateral synapses. A higher proportion of the type I cells lies near the crests of the cristae, while the type II cells are more equally distributed on the slopes.

The sensory cells are neuroepithelial hair cells, each bearing 50–100 thin stereocilia and a single thick and long kinocilium on the apical surface. The stereocilia, which are non-motile and rigid, are not true cilia, but consist of actin filaments (Flock and Cheung, 1977), in a paracrystalline array, with other cytoskeletal proteins. Micromanipulation demonstrates that they bend at their point of insertion to the cuticular plate and that they fracture if pushed too far (Flock, 1977; Flock, Flock and Murray, 1977). The stereocilia vary in height, but are graded with reference to the kinocilium, the tallest, about 100μm, being closest to the kinocilium. They are longest on the hair cells at the periphery of the cristae and shortest on the maculae, especially near the striolae.

The kinocilium projects from the cell cytoplasm, through a segment of the cell lacking a cuticular plate. Early studies had demonstrated that the vertebrate kinocilium has the complete structure of a motile cilium (Flock and Duvall, 1965; Hamilton,

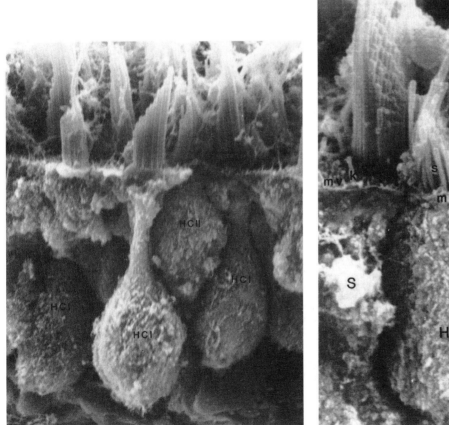
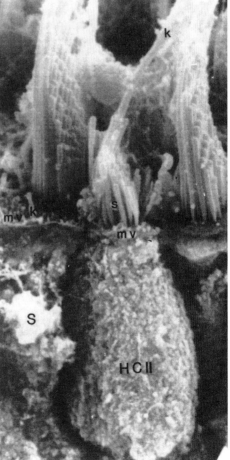

Figure 4.9 Freeze fractures through the chinchilla saccular macula showing type I (HCI) and type II (HCII) vestibular hair cells, supporting cells (S), kinocilia (k), microvilli (mv). (From Hunter–Duvar, I. and Hinojosa, R. *Ultrastructural Atlas of the Inner Ear*, edited by I. Friedmann and J. Ballantyne. London: Butterworths. 1984)

1969; Hunter–Duvar and Hinojosa, 1984) with a basal body, which closely resembles the centriole and the '9 + 2' arrangement of microtubule doublets of true cilia. However, the inner dynein arms are selectively lacking and a central pair of microtubules is not present in the distal portion of the kinocilium (Kikuchi *et al.*, 1989), which would suggest that the vestibular kinocilia may not be motile, or are only weakly motile.

However, the kinocilia are capable of flagella-like movements (Flock, Flock and Murray, 1977; Ross *et al.*, 1987; Rusch and Thurm, 1990), though it is not clear whether these movements take place *in vivo*, or are manifestations of *in vitro* thermal motion or enzymatic deterioration (Wooley and Brammal, 1987). Kinociliary beating can be induced by pressure on the tips and the frequency is in the order of a few Hertz, although, if active, the generator of motility has not been elucidated. In addition, the kinocilia deflect in response to high negative depolarization.

Glycocalyx and extracellular filaments connect the kinocilium with their neighbouring stereocilia (Ernstson and Smith, 1986; Takumida *et al.*, 1990). It has been postulated that one role of this extracellular network is to maintain the spatial organization of the entire kinocilium-stereociliary bundle (Jeffries *et al.*, 1986; Takumida, 1989) which allows mechanical stimuli to be transmitted to the stereocilia via the kinocilium (Hillman and Lewis, 1971; Ross *et al.*, 1987). However, detachment of the kinocilium does not significantly effect the movement of the stereocilia (Hudspeth and Jacobs, 1979).

In cochlear hair cells, some of the extracellular filaments are highly organized. These filaments are called tip links. Each tip link has a fine central filament about 6 nm diameter (Pickles *et al.*, 1988). At its point of insertion to the cell wall of the taller stereocilium, there is an area of increased density between the external membrane and the actin core. Below its lower attachment to the conical extension at the tip of the shorter stereocilium, there is a dense cap over the ends of the actin filaments. The tip links join every stereocilium to its neighbours and are arranged in the direction of the kinocilium. According to the Pickles' 'tip link' model, the tip links play an important role in mechanical-electrical transduction (Pickles, Comis and Osborne, 1984). This model has not been confirmed and its relevance to vestibular hair cells is uncertain. However, Takumida *et al.* (1990) have described in the human vestibule, the presence of interconnections between the tips of the shorter stereocilia to the shafts of their neighbouring taller stereocilia. Each stereocilium tip has one tip link. The tip links, are composed of single thin fibres about 16–26 nm diameter and about 90 nm in length and are orientated in the direction of, but not attached to the kinocilium. There are also numerous horizontal interconnections between stereocilia and between the kinocilium and neighbouring stereocilia. These interconnections may serve to maintain the distance between neighbouring stereocilia.

It has been suggested that the tip links may be intimately related to the mechano-electrical transduction function of the stereocilia, but this is currently a topic of intensive research. In favour of this model are the observations that extracellular current flows appear greatest around the tips of the shorter stereocilia (Hudspeth, 1982), that voltage-sensitive ion channels are present at or near the tips of the stereocilia (Hudspeth, 1985), that each stereocilium appears to possess only one transducer channel and that the greatest effects are produced by deflection of the cilia towards the kinocilium (Flock, 1965) (Figure 4.10).

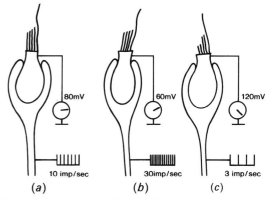

Figure 4.10 Diagram to illustrate the change in firing rate of vestibular nerve: (*a*) when the vestibular hair cell is resting; (*b*) when the vestibular hair cell is depolarized by sterociliary deflection towards the kinocilium; (*c*) when the vestibular hair cell is hyperpolarized by stereociliary deflection away from the kinocilium

The role of the kinocilium has not been elucidated. It is not present in the mammalian cochlea, but whether it has a functional role in the vestibule is not known.

Innervation

The two types of hair cell (see Figure 4.9) differ considerably as regards innervation. The basal portion of the cells synapse with afferent and efferent nerve fibres. Each type I cell is surrounded by a calyx formed by a single afferent nerve with which it makes 10–20 synapses (Hamilton, 1968). Type II cells have multiple bouton-type afferent nerve terminals. In the cristae, some central type II cells have calyceal endings and there is a greater afferent innervation from the type II cells nearer the crest than the slopes. In the crest area, each afferent may have multiple ribbon-type bouton synapses, while in the periphery each afferent may have only one synapse with a type II cell (Lindeman, 1969; Watanuki and Meyer zum Gottesberge, 1971; Baird *et al.*, 1988; Fernandez, Baird and Goldberg, 1988; Goldberg, Lysakowski and Fernandez, 1990).

Type II hair cells have two to six efferent synapses which are sited on the basolateral wall of the cells. The efferent innervation from the type I cells is sparse and does not synapse directly with the hair cells but with the afferent calyx.

The innervation pattern of the two types of hair cell also differs. There are three types of afferent terminal: type I fibres, which form calyx units; type II fibres which form bouton units and dimorphic fibres which innervate both types of receptors. Each type I fibre innervates several neighbouring type I hair cells. Each type II hair cell receives synapses from several different afferent fibres, with each afferent fibre supplying several type II hair cells. Thus, type I hair cells display a convergent afferent innervation pattern, while type II hair cells display a divergent and convergent pattern.

The axon diameters are greatest for the calyceal afferent fibres (up to 20 μm) and least for the type II fibres.

In the cristae, calyx units are confined to the central zone at the crest of the cristae, while bouton units lie in the periphery and dimorphic units predominate between these two areas.

A fine unmyelinated plexus is found at the base of the sensory epithelium. From the plexus arise myelinated fibres (primary vestibular neurons) which pass to large bipolar cells with cell bodies in Scarpa's ganglion in the internal auditory meatus. Scarpa's ganglion may be divided into a superior portion, which innervates the cristae of the superior vertical and lateral semicircular canals, the utricular macula and a small anterosuperior portion of the saccular macula, and an inferior portion, which innervates the major part of the saccular macula and the posterior vertical canal (Gacek, 1968) (Figure 4.11).

The superior portion of the ganglion gives rise to large fibres, which occupy a central portion within the ampullary nerves and terminate as the calyces of the type I hair cells on the crest of the cristae. The inferior portion gives rise to smaller fibres, which end in boutons on the type II hair cells and are more numerous on the slopes of the cristae (Sando, Black and Hemenway, 1972; O'Leary *et al.*, 1974).

The central processes of the primary vestibular neurons form an ascending branch, which synapses superiorly with the vestibular nuclei or cerebellum, and a descending branch, which synapses on the more inferior vestibular nuclei.

The efferent supply to the vestibular sensory epithelium arises bilaterally from the area of the VIth nerve nucleus and adjacent to the lateral and medial vestibular nuclei (Gacek and Lyon, 1974). The fibres emerge

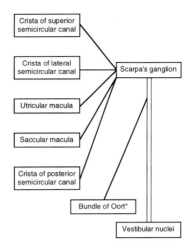

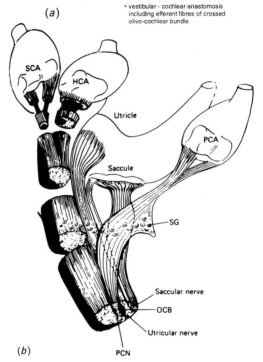

Figure 4.11 (*a*) and (*b*) Schematic diagram of vestibular nerve. (From Gacek, R. R. *Advances in Oto-Rhino-laryngology*, vol 28, Series edited by C. P. Pfaltz, *Vestibular Neurotology*, edited by P. Molina–Negro and R. A. Bertrand. Basel: S. Karger, 1982). SG = Scarpa's ganglion; OCB = olivocochlear bundle ; PCA = posterior crista ampullaris; SCA = superior crista ampullaris ; HCA = horizontal crista ampullaris; PCN = posterior canal nerve

from the brain stem in the olivocochlear bundle, which travels with the afferent fibres of the vestibular nerve. The cochlear efferents leave the vestibular nerve as the bundle of Oort.

Vestibular physiology
Neurotransmitters

The nature and effect of neurotransmitters within the vestibular apparatus are poorly defined but several transmitters have been identified. Glutamate and glutamate-mimetic agents increase spontaneous and stimulus-evoked activity in frog (Valli *et al.*, 1985) and cat (Dechesne, Raymond and Sans, 1984) vestibular neurons, while gamma-aminobutyric acid (GABA) is also a likely afferent neurotransmitter, in that its synthesizing enzyme L-glutamate decarboxylase has been identified exclusively in the hair cell cytoplasm and its degradation enzyme GABA-transaminase has been identified in the nerve calyces, nerve fibres and hair cells, suggesting that it terminates transmitter action (Lopez and Meza, 1988). GABA increases the spontaneous activity of single units in the cat saccular macula, while GABA-receptor blockade, with picrotoxin, inhibits spontaneous and evoked activity in the skate semicircular canal (Flock and Lam, 1974). Monoamine oxidase-depleting agents have also been shown to affect the presynaptic bar structure of frog vestibular hair cells (Osborne and Thornhill, 1972).

Acetylcholine is a likely efferent transmitter as acetylcholinesterase is present in the efferent fibres in the human cochlea (Uchizono, Nomura and Kosaka, 1967) and is lost after vestibular nerve section (Gacek, 1968). Moreover, choline acetyltransferase activity decreases after vestibular nerve section (Lopez and Meza, 1988). Enkephalin, calcitonin gene-related peptide (Tanaka *et al.*, 1989) and substance P (Usami, Hozawa and Ylikoski, 1991) have also been localized to efferent terminals and neural somas (Highstein, 1991), although their role is undefined.

Labyrinthine fluids

There are two distinctly separate fluids in the labyrinth: perilymph and endolymph, which do not mix. Vestibular endolymph is contained within the membranous labyrinth, while the cochlear endolymph compartment is contained by the boundaries of the reticular lamina.

Endolymphatic system

The endolymphatic system consists of the endolymphatic sac, which leads via the endolymphatic duct in the bony vestibular aqueduct, to the utriculosaccular duct.

The endolymphatic duct consists of three portions, of which the proximal part, the isthmus, and the intermediate rugose part, lie within the vestibular aqueduct. The distal part is flattened and lies between the dura of the posterior fossa and the petrous bone.

The isthmus and intracranial parts are lined by low cuboidal epithelium. The rugose part is lined with extensively folded columnar epithelium with numerous small channels, consistent with an active absorptive role and there appears to be active pinocytic activity in this area (Lundquist *et al.*, 1984).

Endolymph

Endolymph is produced at several sites (Tasaki and Spyropoulos, 1959; Sellick, Johnstone and Johnstone, 1972) and circulates through the endolymphatic system of the membranous labyrinth, although endolymph potentials and composition are not uniform (O'Connor *et al.*, 1982; Amano, Orsulakova and Morgenstern, 1983; Morgenstern, Amano and Orsulakova, 1982).

Endolymph is unique among extracellular fluids in having a high potassium (around 145 mmol/l) and low sodium concentration (around 5 mmol/l) (Smith, Lowry and Wu, 1954; Johnstone and Sellick, 1972). Perilymph resembles the composition of extracellular fluid (potassium 10 mmol/l, sodium 140 mmol/l), but both endolymph (around 1.25 g/l) and perilymph (around 2–4 g/l) have a high protein concentration (Anniko and Wroblewski, 1986). CSF protein is 0.2–0.5 g/l.

The cochlear endolymphatic potential is uniquely high at $+80$ mV to $+120$ mV (Bekesy, 1952; Peake, Sohmer and Weiss, 1969; Ono and Tachibana, 1990). In vestibular endolymph, the potential is much lower. Kusakari *et al.* (1986) recorded a saccular endolymphatic potential of $+5 \pm 3.5$ mV. Sellick, Johnstone and Johnstone (1972) recorded a utricular endolymphatic potential of $+1.8 \pm 4.4$ mV. Guinea-pig ampullary endolymphatic potential is $+3.3 \pm 1.2$ mV (Ono and Tachibana, 1990). Vestibular endolymphatic potential is partly independent of cochlear endolymphatic potential (Ono and Tachibana, 1990).

The investigation of the source of endolymph has primarily been directed on the cochlear stria vascularis, in which the marginal cells have the highest positive potential (Melichar and Syka, 1987). Moreover, the stria is the only structure which retains its positive potential after mixing perilymph and endolymph with the destruction of Reissner's membrane. In the stria vascularis, the activity of Na^+/K^+-ATPase is about 12 times higher than in any other area of the cochlea (Kuijpers and Bonting, 1970) and there is also a high concentration of carbonic anhydrase and adenyl cyclase (Drescher and Kerr, 1985). These findings suggest that the stria vascularis is the source of cochlear endolymph and the endolymphatic potential. The channels between the cochlea and vestibule suggest that endolymph can flow between the spaces.

However, there is other evidence that vestibular endolymph is produced in the dark cells of the vestibular labyrinth (Kimura, 1969; Salt and Konishi, 1986). The fine structure of the dark cells of the cristae and utricular macula are similar to those of the marginal cells of the cochlear stria vascularis in that they are particle rich, containing large numbers of vesicles, vacuoles and mitochondria (Jahnke, Meyer zum Gottesberge and Neuman, 1991) and they have an enormously increased surface area due to folded cell processes. These folded membranes have high ATPase (Nakai and Hilding, 1968) and carbonic anhydrase activity (Watanabe and Ogawa, 1984). It has been demonstrated that the utricle (Sellick, Johnstone and Johnstone, 1972) and cristae ampullares (Dohlman, 1965; Tsujikawa *et al.*, 1991) produce endolymph and generate an endolymphatic potential independent of other sources.

Vestibular endolymph flows via the utricle to the endolymphatic duct, which leads to the endolymphatic sac, where endolymph is reabsorbed (Guild, 1927; Kimura and Schuknecht, 1965; Lundquist, 1965; Schuknecht, Northrop and Igarashi, 1968; Kimura, 1976; Lundquist, 1976; Friberg, Bagger–Sjoback and Rask–Andersen, 1985; Wackym, Friberg, and Bagger–Sjoback, 1986, 1987). Cochlear endolymph flows out of the scala media of the cochlea via the ductus reuniens to the saccule and then to the endolymphatic duct (Andersen, 1948).

The underlying mechanisms for the absorption of endolymph through the epithelial lining of the surrounding blood vessels and the mechanisms of regulating endolymph volume and composition are not known, but on the basis of the data collected various hypotheses have been advanced.

Following adrenalectomy, there are changes in rat ampullary dark cell ultrastructure, suggesting that the homeostasis of vestibular endolymph may be partly regulated by adrenocorticosteroids (ten Cate, Patterson and Rarey, 1990).

It is likely that the transport of ions and fluid from the endolymphatic sac is an active process and there is evidence of an active transcellular ion exchange with passive bulk transepithelial flow of water. There are dilated lateral intercellular spaces, leaky tight junctions and membrane bound Na^+/K^+-ATPase (Wackym, Glasscock and Linthicum, 1988) as found in other fluid-transporting epithelia. The rate of fluid transport correlates with the size of the lateral intercellular spaces (Friberg, Wackym and Bagger-Sjoback, 1986), which dilate with high flows and collapse when transport is arrested. A high sodium diet causes an increase in size of the lateral intercellular spaces, a low sodium diet a decrease. The inhibition of membrane bound Na^+/K^+-ATPase with a food factor, found in tea, coffee and red wine (Harlan and Mann, 1982), prevented the dilation in the lateral intercellular spaces following a high sodium diet and, in fact, caused a constriction (Wackym *et al.*, 1990).

Other membrane bound Na^+/K^+-ATPase inhibitors, such as ouabain, ethacrynic acid and amiloride have a similar effect (Takumida and Bagger-Sjoback, 1989).

Perilymph

Perilymph has a similar ionic composition to extracellular fluid and cerebrospinal fluid (Anniko and Wroblewski, 1986). Its potential is about $+5\,mV$ to $+7\,mV$ (Johnstone and Sellick, 1972). The origin of perilymph is uncertain. The perilymphatic space communicates with the subdural space via the cochlear aqueduct and the perineural spaces at the distal end of the internal auditory meatus and perilymph may be produced from cerebrospinal fluid. It may also be a product of ultrafiltration through the perilymphatic capillaries (Feldman, 1981).

The cochlear aqueduct extends from an opening near the round window of the scala tympani to the subarachnoid space near the ganglion of the glossopharyngeal nerve and may contain a net of fibrous tissue in the same plane as the arachnoid (Perlman and Lindsay, 1939; Holden and Schuknecht, 1968). The patency of the cochlear aqueduct is variable (Wlodyka, 1978), but age is associated with closure.

Blocking the cochlear aqueduct does not affect labyrinthine morphology or function (Kimura, Schuknecht and Ota, 1974; Suh and Cody, 1974). However, when the cochlear aqueduct is patent, CSF pressure is close to perilymph pressure (Kerth and Allen, 1963; Carlborg, 1981). The compression of the jugular veins, which raises intracranial pressure, can produce changes in middle ear impedance (Klockhoff, Anggard and Anggard, 1966) and it has been suggested that this is due to a change in load on the stapes footplate allowing a non-invasive method of estimating CSF pressure (Marchbanks *et al.*, 1987). An increase in CSF pressure can cause displacement of the resting position of stapes laterally, so allowing a greater freedom of movement medially with inward-going tympanic membrane displacement, while a decrease in CSF pressure will displace the resting stapes medially, so reducing its inward displacement with inward-going tympanic membrane displacement.

Orientation

The vestibular system transduces into neural activity forces due to angular acceleration in each of the three planes of motion: yaw (horizontal about a vertical axis), pitch (flexion and extension about a vertical axis) and roll (lateral head tilt about a horizontal axis) and linear acceleration in all dimensions (Figure 4.12).

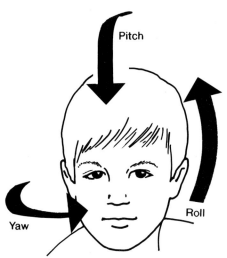

Figure 4.12 The three planes of head motion

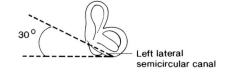

Left lateral semicircular canal

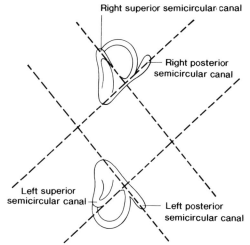

Figure 4.13 Orientation of semicircular canals

The anatomical organization of the components of the vestibular system contributes to the analysis of these stimuli (Spoendlin, 1964). The labyrinths are sited on the horizontal axis of the cranium. The lateral semicircular canals slope downwards and backwards at an angle of approximately 30° to the horizontal. The two vertical canals are approximately orthogonal to each other. The superior vertical canal is anterior and is directed posteromedially to anterolaterally over the roof of the utricle. The posterior vertical canal is posterior and is directed downwards and laterally behind the utricle. The ipsilateral posterior and contralateral superior canals are approximately in the same plane (Figure 4.13), although precise measurements indicate that the canals are not in perfect geometric alignment (Takagi, Sando and Takahashi, 1989).

The sensory epithelium is also spatially arranged. The cristae lie at right angles to the longitudinal axis of the canals and are therefore in the optimal plane for stimulation following displacement of the cupula or endolymph (see Figure 4.7). Both maculae lie along the contours of the labyrinth: the utricular maculae approximately in the horizontal plane and the saccular maculae, on the medial wall, in approximately the vertical plane (Figure 4.14). The contours of the saccule and utricle further enhance the complexity of the orientation of their sensory epithelium.

The hair cells are also spatially orientated: as hair cells are depolarized by displacement of the stereocilia towards the kinocilium and hyperpolarized by displacement away (see above), their orientation is important (see Figure 4.10).

In the maculae, the hair cells are orientated with reference to the S-shaped striolae (see Figure 4.14). In the saccular macula, the kinocilia are orientated

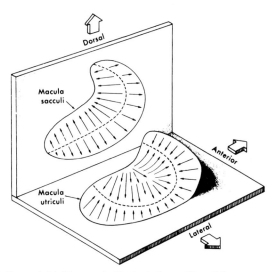

Figure 4.14 Diagram to illustrate the position of the utricular and saccular maculae. The arrows indicate the direction of stereociliary deflection that excites the hair cells in that region of the otolith organ. (From Barber, H. O. and Stockwell, C. W. *Manual of Electronystagmography*, 2nd edn. 1980. St Louis: C. V. Mosby)

away from the striola, while in the utricular macula, the kinocilia are orientated towards the striola.

Therefore, subtle differences in the displacement of the otoconial membrane will produce different patterns of responses from the hair cells. However, the orientation of the utricular macula is likely to make it more sensitive to horizontal (side to side), linear acceleration, while that of the saccular macula is likely to make it more sensitive to vertical (head-toe), linear acceleration.

In the cristae, the kinocilia are uniformly arranged in each canal. In the lateral canals, the kinocilia are orientated towards the utricles. In the vertical canals, they are directed away from the utricles. The different polarization will cause the hair cells in the lateral canals to be stimulated by utriculopetal (ampullopetal) endolymph flow and those in the vertical canals to be stimulated by utriculofugal (ampullofugal) flow (Figure 4.15).

The orientation of the hair cells of the lateral semicircular canals makes them most sensitive to yaw movements. The vertical canals are more sensitive to pitch and roll, with the posterior semicircular canal most responsive to pitch with the head in the yaw position (i.e. with the jaw approximated to the shoulder).

It has been postulated (Benson and Barnes, 1973) that the signals from the hair cells are integrated spatially, so that information is provided with respect to both fore-and-aft and lateral acceleration of the head. This hypothesis is supported by the eye movements resulting from the electrical stimulation of the otoliths

Orientation of the stereocilia in the vestibular hair cells of the crista of the lateral semicircular canal

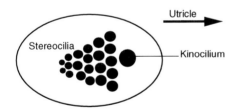

Orientation of the stereocilia in the vestibular hair cells of the crista of the vertical semicircular canal

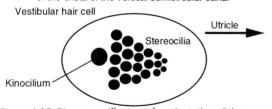

Figure 4.15 Diagram to illustrate the orientation of the hair cells in the lateral semicircular canals which are depolarized by utriculopetal displacement of the cupula and that of the vertical canals depolarized by utriculofugal displacement

(Fluur and Mellstrom, 1971). The combined polarization vectors of neurons over both maculae cover all positions of the head in three-dimensional space.

Otoliths

The structure of the utricle and saccule, in particular the organization of the sensory epithelium on the macula around the striola and the specific gravity of the otoconial membrane, suggest that their function is to transduce gravitational changes. As a linear acceleration leads to a change of the gravitational vector, it is likely that the otolith organs transduce information on linear acceleration and velocity. Similarly, the otolith organs transduce information on head tilt as this leads to a change in the acceleration due to gravity. Tilt and linear acceleration cause deflection of the stereocilia and thus alter the resting rate of afferent neuronal activity (Fernandez and Goldberg, 1976).

Semicircular canals

Rotation of the cranium will not immediately be accompanied by flow of endolymph (due to the inertia of the fluid) and this leads to deflection of the stereocilia and in turn a change in afferent neuronal activity.

The functional role of the semicircular canals was proposed by Flourens in 1842 after he demonstrated characteristic head movements in pigeons following the opening of the semicircular canals. Ewald (1892) attached a cannula to the semicircular canals of pigeons and applied positive and negative pressures to cause ampullofugal and ampullopetal endolymph flow. He made three important observations, known as Ewald's laws:

1 Head and eye movements always take place in the plane of the canal being stimulated and in the direction of endolymph flow
2 In the horizontal canal, ampullopetal endolymph flow causes a greater response than ampullofugal flow
3 In the vertical canals, ampullofugal endolymph flow causes a greater response than ampullopetal flow.

These observations can be explained on the basis of the orientation of the stereocilia and the structures on which the hair cells are aligned as described above.

The exact function of the cupula is not universally accepted, and this, in part, reflects the uncertainty of the exact characteristics of the cupula *in vivo*. During fixation the cupula shrinks and this has led to the hypothesis that the cupula does not completely occlude the ampulla and therefore it does not act as 'a water-tight swing door seal'. According to this hypothesis, the cupula remains fixed, but the dimensions of the structures direct endolymph into a subcupular space where deflection of the ciliary bundles occurs (Dohlman, 1981).

Although the exact way in which the cupula moves in mammals is unknown, the more widely accepted hypothesis is based on Steinhausen's pendulum model (1931). Using Indian ink to visualize the flow of endolymph in the semicircular canals of fish, he demonstrated that the cupula acted as a seal and moved with the endolymph.

According to Newton's third law, if an angular acceleration is applied to the cranium, the displacement of the cupula-endolymph system is resisted by three forces: an *inertial force*, which is a function of the moment of inertia of the system (M) and its acceleration (A), an *elastic force*, which is a function of the moment of elasticity (S) and magnitude of the angular displacement of the system (D), and a *viscous force*, which is a function of the moment of endolymph viscosity (R) and the velocity of displacement (V). If the angular acceleration of the cranium is $\mathring{A}$, the displacement of the cupula-endolymph system can be described by the following equation:

$$MA(t) + RV(t) + SD(t) = M\mathring{A}(t) \qquad 1$$

For small movements, the inertial and elastic forces are negligible. Therefore, the force applied to the cupula-endolymph system is opposed mostly by the force due to viscosity. Therefore,

$$RV(t) \approx M\mathring{A}(t) \qquad 2$$

Integrating equation 2,

$$D(t) \approx MV_h(t)/R$$

where V_h is the velocity of head motion. Therefore, for small movements, the angular displacement of the cupula is proportional to the velocity of cranial movements.

At the beginning of cranial acceleration, the cupula-endolymph does not move immediately. After a lag period, the cupula-endolymph system is displaced. After a few seconds of constant cranial acceleration, the applied and restraining forces balance and the cupula-endolymph system moves with the walls of the labyrinth. However, the cupula has been displaced. At this stage, the inertial force and viscous forces are zero and therefore, equation 1 reduces to,

$$SD(t) = M\mathring{A}(t) \qquad 3$$

Integrating equation 3,

$$D(t) = M\mathring{A}(t)/S.$$

Therefore, the final angular displacement of the cupula is proportional to the magnitude of the constant cranial acceleration.

The displacement of the cupula follows an exponential time course. In support of the pendular model is the fact that the time course of the return of the cupula to the resting position, after the stimulus is terminated, follows the same exponential pattern as that following initial deviation.

The effect of acceleration

The fixation of the sensory epithelium to connective tissue, which is firmly bound to the cranium, means that movement of the cranium will cause movement of the sensory epithelium with no phase or amplitude change. On the other hand, the endolymph, cupula and otoconial membrane are not directly attached to the cranium and therefore phase and amplitude differences do develop. As a result, the cilia, which are bound to the sensory epithelium, but embedded in the cupula or otoconial membrane are deflected.

The maximal stimulus is a force parallel to the surface of the sensory epithelium, which bisects the bundle of the stereocilia and passes through the kinocilium (Bekesy, 1966), while a force perpendicular to the epithelial surface is ineffective in stimulating the hair cells (Fernandez and Goldberg, 1976).

The deflection of the stereocilia causes current flow (Lowenstein and Wersall, 1959; Hudspeth and Corey, 1977; Russell, Richardson and Cody, 1986) with deflection of the stereocilia towards the kinocilium causing cell membrane depolarization, and deflection away from the kinocilium causing hyperpolarization, with the permeability changes taking place on the apical surface of the hair cells. Current pulses cause small intracellular voltage changes when the stereocilia are deflected towards the kinocilium and large voltages changes when the stereocilia are deflected away (Hudspeth and Corey, 1977). Therefore, the depolarization of the cell is associated with a decrease of membrane resistance, suggesting that ionic channels open during depolarization. Using patch-clamp electrodes Ohmori (1985) recorded step-changes in transcellular current when the stereocilia were deflected. This is consistent with the hypothesis that individual or groups of ionic channels are opening (Holton and Hudspeth, 1986).

The greatest potential changes are recorded just over the tapering part at the tips of the stereociliary bundle (Hudspeth, 1982), suggesting that this is the site of ionic flow. Na^+ and K^+ ions and to a lesser extent Ca^{++} ions may carry transducer current (Corey and Hudspeth, 1979). In chick vestibular cells, Ca^{++} and other divalent ions are more effective than Na^+ and K^+, while in the frog sacculus, K^+ appear to carry receptor current (Zucca, Valli and Casella, 1985). This suggests that the membranes are charge-selective. The ionic channel diameter is of the order of 0.7 nm (Hudspeth, 1985) and the channels are Ca-dependent, with the cessation of transduction with a Ca^{++} concentration below 10 μmol/l (Corey and Hudspeth, 1979).

There is a delay of 40 μs at 22°C between transducer current and stereociliary deflection. The time-constants are lower for larger stimulus steps. The latency is temperature dependent decreasing by a factor of 2.5 for every 10°C increase. Corey and Hudspeth (1983) suggested that these data support a direct mechanical effect rather than a biochemical reaction, secondary messenger or enzyme-mediated response. The mechanism of channel opening is not known, but hypotheses include a two-state kinetic model, where the channels oscillate between open and closed states and a three-state kinetic model, where there are two closed states and one open state (Corey and Hudspeth, 1983). However, Pickles, Comis and Osborne (1984) suggested that the deflection of the stereocilia causes the tip links to pull open or close the channels. Pickles *et al.* suggested that in the cochlea, the tip links may be displaced by 0.4Å. While this is subatomic, greater deflections may take place *in vivo* in the vestibular stereocilia, but the Pickles model has yet to be proven. It is supported by documentation of the existence of the tip links, their orientation, points of insertion and the site of the presumed ionic channels.

The depolarization of the hair cells causes neural excitation and excision of the kinocilium does not alter the response to stereociliary deflection (Hudspeth and Jacobs, 1979). Therefore, the deflection of the stereocilia causes the hair cells to act as transducers converting mechanical energy into ionic flow and neural action potentials.

The primary vestibular afferents

In 1932, Hoagland demonstrated the resting neural activity generated in lateral line organs. In squirrel monkeys, the average resting discharge rate of saccular and macular units is approximately 65 spikes per second, while a higher rate of 70–90 spikes per second is recorded from the cristae. Studies of both the cristae (Fernandez and Goldberg, 1971) and the otolith organs (Fernandez and Goldberg, 1976) have demonstrated that some neurons have a regular spontaneous firing rate, while others have an irregular rate. Calyx units discharge irregularly, while bouton units discharge regularly. The response dynamics are closely related to the positioning of the afferents on the sensory epithelium (Goldberg, Lysakowski and Fernandez, 1990) with the more central dimorphic units discharging irregularly, and the more peripheral units discharging regularly. The significance of this has not yet been defined.

The semicircular canal afferents differ in response to head rotation. Calyx units are low-gain units, while type II and dimorphic units are high gain units (Baird *et al.*, 1988). The recording of action potentials within the primary afferent fibres innervating the cupula has provided a direct method of measuring cupula-endolymph dynamics and has enabled the effect of both static (Lowenstein and Roberts, 1950; Vidal *et al.*, 1971; Fernandez, Goldberg and Abend, 1972; Loe, Tomko and Werner, 1973) and dynamic stimuli (Lowenstein and Saunders, 1975; Fernandez and Goldberg, 1976) to be defined. The magnitude of cupular deflection is precisely reflected by changes in neural firing rate which would therefore be proportional to the velocity of cranial movement. A bidirectional response, with a slightly higher gain in the excitatory response has been documented from all vestibular sensory receptors. One explanation for this asymmetry, which serves to clarify Ewald's law is that the firing of the neurons cannot be reduced below zero.

Vestibular efferents

On the basis of an increase in the spontaneous discharge rate of horizontal semicircular canal nerve in the frog following perilymph perfusion with *d*-tubocurarine, Caston and Rousell (1984) suggested that the activity of the vestibular system was under tonic inhibition of the efferent system. The electrical stimulation of efferents in the monkey and fish increases afferent resting discharge and reduces afferent gain to adequate stimulation. The effect is greatest on high-gain velocity-dependent afferents (Highstein *et al.*, 1987), that is, the type II hair cell afferents.

Central vestibular connections

Vestibular nuclei

The majority of afferent fibres from the hair cells terminate in the vestibular nuclei, which lie on the floor of the IVth ventricle, bounded medially by the pontine reticular formation, laterally by the restiform body, rostrally by the brachium conjunctivum and ventrally by the nucleus and spinal tract of the trigeminal nerve. Some primary vestibular neurons pass directly to the cerebellum, in particular the flocculonodular lobe and the vermis. No primary vestibular afferents cross the midline.

In the vestibular nuclei, four major groups of cell bodies (the second order vestibular neurons) may be identified. There is also a number of smaller groups of cells which are closely related to the major nuclei. Some nuclei receive only primary vestibular afferents, but, with the exception of the neurons of the interstitial nucleus, the majority receive afferents from the cerebellum, reticular formation, spinal cord and contralateral vestibular nuclei. The vestibular nuclei also receive a pathway from the visual system (Waespe and Henn, 1977). The largest afferent supply to the vestibular nuclei arises in the cerebellum (Brodal, 1974).

The exact afferent connections to, and efferent projections from, the vestibular nuclei have not been totally identified, but the following generalizations may be made about the four major groupings of vestibular nuclei (Figures 4.16 and 4.17):

Superior vestibular nucleus of Bechterew

The afferent input is from the cristae of the semicircular canals and cerebellum. The efferent output runs in the median longitudinal bundle to innervate the motor nuclei of the extrinsic eye muscles. This nucleus is therefore particularly important in the control of the semicircular canal-ocular reflexes.

Lateral vestibular nucleus of Dieter

The afferent input is primarily from the cerebellum and utricular macula (with a few spinal and commissural afferent fibres). The efferents are primarily involved in vestibulospinal activity by way of the vestibulospinal pathways and reticulospinal pathways and inferior part of the median longitudinal bundle.

The superior and lateral vestibular nuclei project to the thalamus in an anterior projection which runs lateral to the red nucleus and dorsal to the subthalamic nucleus to the ventral posterolateral nucleus of the thalamus. A smaller projection runs in the lateral lemniscus to end near the medial geniculate.

Medial vestibular nucleus of Schwalbe

The afferent input is primarily from the cristae and cerebellum with a few fibres from the reticular formation and utricular macula. The efferent output projects in the median longitudinal bundle to both the oculomotor nuclei and the cervical cord. It is of importance in coordinating eye, head and neck movements. Other efferents from this nucleus run to the vestibulocerebellum, the reticular formation and the contralateral vestibular nuclei.

Descending vestibular nucleus

The afferent input is from the utricular and saccular maculae (with a small supply from the cristae and cerebellum). The efferent output is mainly to the cerebellum and reticular formation. In addition, numerous commissural fibres supply the contralateral ascending medial and lateral vestibular nuclei.

The efferent activity of the vestibular nuclei reflects the integrated and modulated activity from a number of different afferent inputs. The vestibular nuclei connect with the oculomotor nuclei, the spinal cord, the cerebellum, the autonomic nervous system, the thalamus, and the contralateral vestibular nuclei. Commissural connections also pass through the cerebellum (Furuya, Kawano and Shimazu, 1976).

Before neuronal impulses arriving in the vestibular nuclei are transmitted further, they pass at least one synapse and thus may be modified by impulses entering the nuclei from other sources. Therefore, it is likely that, at the level of the vestibular nuclei, labyrinthine information is integrated with information from other somatosensory systems. About 75% of the neurons of the vestibular nuclei are activated by vestibular nerve stimulation and about half are monosynaptically activated (Shimazu and Precht, 1965).

The activity of neurons within the vestibular nuclei during vestibular stimulation has been investigated for canal-dependent units (Shimazu and Precht, 1965; Fuchs and Kimm, 1975; Schneider and Anderson, 1976) and for otolith-dependent units (Peterson, 1970). Electrophysiological studies have identified two groups of secondary vestibular neurons – type I and type II (Shimazu and Precht, 1966). Type I neurons are excited, type II inhibited by ipsilateral rotation of the head. Type I neurons are monosynaptically innervated and type II multisynaptically acti-

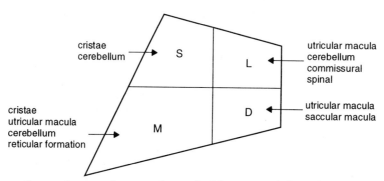

Figure 4.16 Diagram to illustrate the main afferent supply to each of the main vestibular nuclei (S = superior, M = medial, L = lateral, D = descending)

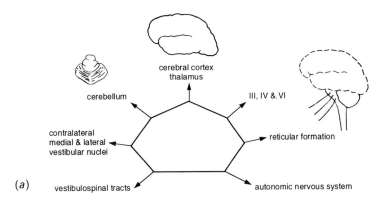

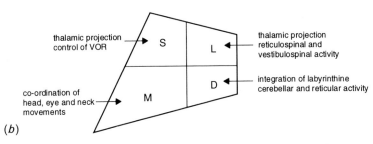

Figure 4.17 Diagrams to illustrate (*a*) the main efferent pathways of the vestibular nuclei; (*b*) the primary functions of the vestibular nuclei (S = superior, M = medial, L = lateral; D = descending)

vated. Type I connections tend to be ipsilateral and excitatory, whereas type II neurons are activated by contralateral type I neurons or by neurons in the reticular substance.

The result of head rotation is to stimulate the ipsilateral labyrinth and inhibit the contralateral labyrinth. The effect is further enhanced by the neuronal pattern of excitation and inhibition. The ipsilateral labyrinth stimulates the ipsilateral type I neurons which, in turn, excite contralateral type II neurons, which inhibit the contralateral type I neurons (Figure 4.18). Further inhibition of the contralateral type I neurons is effected by another inhibitory pathway from the reticular substance (Shimazu and Precht, 1966).

Physiologically the existence of commissural inhibitory connections from one lateral canal to another enhances the sensitivity of the vestibular system (Markham, Yagi and Curthoys, 1977) and may explain the concept of central velocity storage. Such connections are of clinical importance in compensation following a unilateral vestibular disturbance and can also explain certain forms of nystagmus, e.g. periodic alternating nystagmus.

Ascending vestibular projections (Figure 4.19)

Following electrical stimulation of the vestibular nerve, monophasic potentials can be recorded in the contralateral suprasylvian gyrus just anterior to the auditory area (Watzl and Mountcastle, 1949). Studies in the cat and the squirrel monkey have demonstrated projections from the vestibular nuclei to the thalamus, and thence to the sensorimotor cortex (Liedgren *et al.*, 1976; Liedgren and Rubin, 1976). The thalamocortical projections end at the central sulcus near the motor cortex and at the lower end of the inferior parietal sulcus near the post-central gyrus (Fredrickson, Kornhuber and Schwarz, 1974). These thalamic and cortical areas also receive proprioceptive and visual projections.

Electrical stimulation of the superior sylvian gyrus and the region around the inferior parietal sulcus produces a sensation of body displacement (Penfield, 1957). Positron emission tomography displays increased regional perfusion of the temporoparietal junction, anterior cingulate gyrus and primary sensory cortex after contralateral cold vestibular stimulation (Bottini *et al.*, 1994).

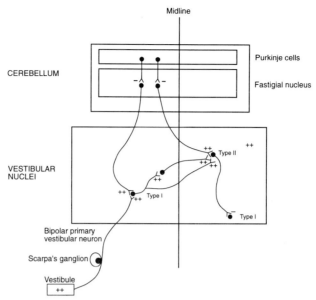

Figure 4.18 Diagram to illustrate the interrelation of type I and type II secondary vestibular neurons. An increase of labyrinthine activity increases ipsilateral type I neuron activity. The type I neuron excites the contralateral inhibitory type II neuron with a subsequent reduction of contralateral type I neuron activity

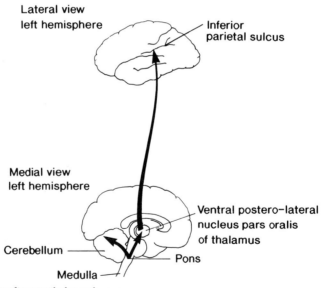

Figure 4.19 Diagram of ascending vestibular pathways

Vestibular responses

There are three types of response following peripheral vestibular stimulation: the vestibulo-ocular reflexes, the vestibulospinal reflexes and the vestibulocollic reflexes.

Vestibulo-ocular reflexes

Vestibulo-ocular reflexes include the semicircular canal-ocular reflexes and the otolith-ocular reflexes. The vestibulo-ocular reflexes provide a simple example of a reflex arc, comprising the vestibular receptor, primary, secondary and tertiary neurons and the effector organ, the oculomotor muscles (Szentagothai, 1950).

Semicircular canal-ocular reflexes

This is the dominant of the vestibulo-ocular reflexes (Bronstein and Gresty, 1991) and the measurement of the lateral semicircular canal-ocular reflexes, by examination of the oculomotor responses to precise vestibular stimuli, is of immense clinical value.

The connections between the individual semicircular canals and the extraocular muscles have been precisely defined by animal experiments, involving stimulation and ablation of individual semicircular canals (Lorente de No, 1933; Fluur, 1959; Cohen, Suzuki and Bender, 1964) (Figure 4.20). The planes of the semicircular canals are not aligned with those of the extraocular muscles and further integration is required to effect this spatial transformation.

Under physiological circumstances, an angular acceleration produces an exact mirror image of events which take place simultaneously in opposite labyrinths. Each utriculopetal stimulus in one labyrinth is matched by an equal, but opposite, utriculofugal displacement in the functionally paired canal of the other ear. In this push-pull arrangement, the lateral canals form one pair, while the posterior canal, because of its anatomical disposition, is parallel to, and therefore paired with, the opposite superior canal. The difference in input to the vestibular nuclei from the left and right labyrinths is the basis of the vestibular response and mediates all labyrinthine reflexes.

With regard to angular acceleration to the right in the plane of the horizontal canals (Figure 4.21), endolymph displacement takes place in the direction opposite to that of rotation, that is leftwards. Accordingly, utriculopetal deviation of the cupula of the right horizontal canal happens with utriculofugal movement of the cupula of the left horizontal canal. This results in an increase in the firing rate of the right ampullary nerve with a decrease in neural activity in the left ampullary nerve. Thus the afferent information coming from the right ampullary nerve exerts an excitatory influence on the agonist muscles and an inhibitory influence on the antagonist muscles, while the response from the left ampullary nerve reduces the excitatory influence on the antagonist muscles and disinhibits the agonist muscles. This results in contraction of the left lateral rectus and the right medial rectus muscles, with relaxation of the

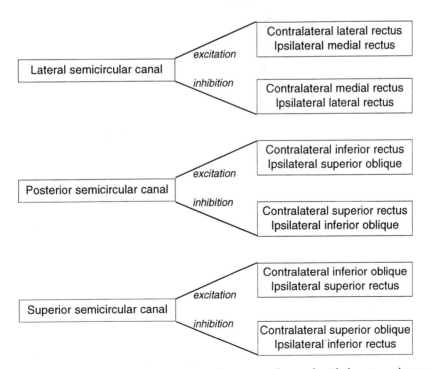

Figure 4.20 Diagram to illustrate the functional connections of the semicircular canals with the extraocular muscles

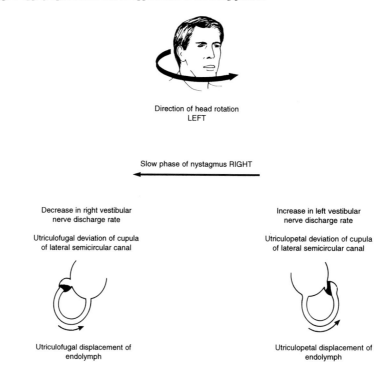

Direction of head rotation
LEFT

Slow phase of nystagmus RIGHT

Decrease in right vestibular
nerve discharge rate

Increase in left vestibular
nerve discharge rate

Utriculofugal deviation of cupula
of lateral semicircular canal

Utriculopetal deviation of cupula
of lateral semicircular canal

Utriculofugal displacement of
endolymph

Utriculopetal displacement of
endolymph

Figure 4.21 Diagram to illustrate the effect of head rotation on the cupulae of the lateral semicircular canals and the compensatory eye movement

left medial rectus and the right lateral rectus muscles, producing deviation of the eyes to the left (Figure 4.22).

Otolith-ocular reflexes

Stimulation of the utricular nerve induces eye movements (Suzuki, Tokumasu and Cohen, 1969), but the otolith control of extraocular muscles has proved more difficult to delineate than semicircular canal relationships. The sensory receptors of the otolith organs are orientated towards many different planes. Hence, any physiological stimulus results in a complex firing pattern of excitation and inhibition of many different units, which cannot be reproduced experimentally. Nevertheless, rotational and torsional compensatory eye movements, produced by static head tilt, are well documented. In humans, counter-torsional movements are produced by lateral tilt (ocular counter rolling), while vertical rotation results in forward/backward tilt (Miller, 1962).

Otolith-ocular reflexes display responses at frequencies between 0.5 to 1 Hz with a gain of $17°/s/g$ where gain is calculated by convention as angular eye velocity in degrees per second evoked per unit of gravitational acceleration (Barnes, 1979; Buizza *et*

al., 1980; Hain, 1986). However, the latency of the response is less than 50 ms (Bronstein and Gresty, 1988). It is therefore extremely valuable in maintaining the eyes on target as the visually-guided slow phase eye movement has a latency of around 125 ms (Robinson, 1965).

Canal and otolith interaction

If a subject is rotated with the head at the centre, the semicircular canals will signal angular acceleration. If the head is placed eccentrically, the otolith organs will signal additionally linear head acceleration (Gresty, Bronstein and Barratt, 1987; Takeda *et al.*, 1990; Viire *et al.*, 1986). The direction of linear movement in this case will complement the direction of angular rotation and the effect will be summated.

In paediatric practice, a clinical test used to assess vestibular function is to swing the child at arm's length, facing the physician. In this case the direction of linear acceleration (e.g. to the left) will conflict with the direction of angular rotation (the child's head will rotate to the right). When canal and otolith signals conflict, Bronstein and Gresty (1991) demonstrated that the canal reflex predominates.

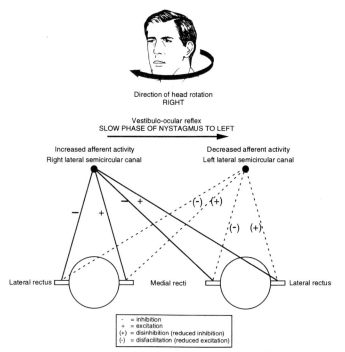

Figure 4.22 Diagram to illustrate the reciprocal arrangements of the canal-ocular reflex

The sensitivity of the otolith-ocular reflex is given by the mean eye velocity in response to the average acceleration and is of the order of $20°/s/g$ (Barnes, 1980). The sensitivity is enhanced by co-directional canal signals (Gresty and Bronstein, 1986) and visual cues (Buizza *et al.*, 1980; Bronstein and Gresty, 1988; Baloh *et al.*, 1988a) with the ocular responses inversely proportional to viewing distance (Schwartz, Busettini and Miles, 1989).

Central velocity storage

The time constant of the vestibulo-ocular reflex is greater than that predicted by cupulo-endolymph mechanics. This is explained by the concept of central velocity-storage – the continuation of activity in the vestibular nuclei after the cessation of the primary afferent signal (Raphan, Matsuo and Cohen, 1979).

The mechanism of central velocity storage is thought to be related to the presence of positive feedback circuits. Type I secondary neurons provide axon collaterals to chains of interneurons on the ipsilateral brainstem and cerebellum (Lorente de No, 1933). Inhibitory interneurons can convert the inhibitory commissural pathways to provide a positive feedback loop to the secondary vestibular neurons (Shimazu and Precht, 1966).

Evidence for the existence of central velocity-storage is offered by the results of unilateral labyrinthectomy, where immediately after ablation, the duration of post-rotation nystagmus is markedly reduced, to be followed by a gradual increase over a period of weeks (Wolfe and Kos, 1977; Jenkins, 1985; Fetter and Zee, 1988).

Vestibulospinal reflexes

The labyrinth influences posture and orientation through neck, axial and limb motoneurons. However, the influence of vestibular activity on postural muscles is more difficult to define and less clearly understood than the labyrinthine control of eye movements (Anderson, Soechting and Terzuolo, 1979). This can be explained partly by the fact that the vestibular system is only one of many afferent inputs to a complex multisensory orientation control system, and partly by the fact that vestibular activity produces postural change only after it has been processed and monitored in the light of other learned responses. Furthermore, vestibular activity affects neck muscles in a different manner to that of the rest of the somatic musculature. Jones and Milsum (1965) have proposed that as changes in vestibular activity are used directly to detect movement, error or deviation in neck position, that the vestibular-neck orientation system be considered a closed loop negative feedback control system, in contrast to the vestibular-limb/torso and the vestibular-oculomotor systems where afferent fibres appear to exert little or no direct effect on the response and have no direct representation within the vestibular nuclei. Thus these are essentially open loop systems.

Alterations in vestibular function can profoundly affect posture (Magnus, 1924). Ewald (1892) demonstrated such changes in posture by rotating animals on a turntable; when rotation ceased, the animal showed a tendency to fall in the direction of the slow phase of eye movement and head deviation. This tendency was counteracted by a reflex increase in extensor tone in the antigravity muscles of the limb on the side towards which the animal was falling, with a simultaneous reduction of extensor tone in the contralateral limbs. The animal, therefore, maintained its balance. These reflexes are mediated by a push-pull mechanism between the extensor and flexor muscles (Figure 4.23).

Roberts (1978) has divided the reflexes which control posture into three categories: *positional reflexes*, which are 'static postural adjustments adopted when the animals reference platform is displaced from its normal earth reference'; *reflex effects of acceleration* on the neck, body and limbs; and *righting reflexes*, which are considered to be specific combinations of vestibular, neck and limb reflex mechanisms. In man, the responses tend to be overridden or dominated by a higher cerebral function such as vision, but the effect of tonic labyrinthine reflexes is observed when the brain stem is disconnected from higher neural centres as happens, for example, with high brain stem tumours.

The vestibular apparatus exerts an influence on the control of posture by way of the myotatic reflex (the deep tendon reflex), which is the elementary unit for the control of tone in the trunk and extremity skeletal muscles. Impulses are transmitted to alpha- and gamma-motoneurons of the spinal cord and body posture is maintained through the maculo-spinal reflex arc (Johanson, 1964). This reflex is under the influence not only of the vestibular system but also of the multiple supraspinal centres, including the basal ganglia, the cerebellum and the reticular formation. The vestibular influence may be demonstrated in animals by the ipsilateral reduction of muscular tone, following unilateral destruction of the labyrinth or the lateral vestibular nucleus (Fulton, Liddell and Rioch, 1930).

Vestibular information influences spinal anterior horn cell activity by means of three major efferent pathways:

1 The lateral vestibulospinal tract
2 The medial vestibulospinal tract
3 The reticulospinal tract.

The first two arise directly from neurons in the vestibular nuclei, while the reticulospinal tract arises from those neurons in the reticular formation that are influenced by vestibular activity as well as by other sensory inputs. In these three neural pathways, cerebellar activity is integrated with the activity of the vestibular apparatus and the reticular formation, in order to maintain equilibrium and coordinate locomotion (Pompeiano, 1974).

The *lateral vestibulospinal tract* originates primarily from neurons in the lateral vestibular nucleus and there is a clear topographic organization. The anterior/superior region of the nucleus supplies the cervical cord, while the posterior/inferior region innervates the lumbosacral cord. Intermediate neurons supply the thoracic cord. Along the entire length of

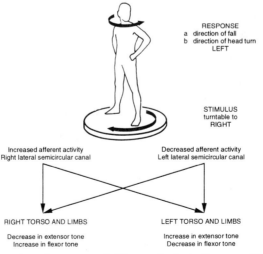

Figure 4.23 Diagram to illustrate the reciprocal arrangement of the canal-spinal reflexes – omitting the influence of cortical, extrapyramidal, cerebellar and reticular pathways

the tract, which runs ipsilaterally in the spinal cord, these fibres terminate on the anterior horn cells directly, or indirectly, by way of interneurons. The lateral vestibulospinal tract fibres synapse with alpha- or gamma-motoneurons, as well as with interneurons in segmental reflex pathways. Direct disynaptic excitatory pathways exist to axial motoneurons, but limb pathways are polysynaptic.

The *medial vestibulospinal tract* originates from neurons of the medial vestibular nucleus, and the fibres descend in the median longitudinal bundle. They synapse terminally with interneurons in the cervical cord, and do not appear to form direct connections with the cervical anterior horn cells. It is smaller than the lateral vestibulospinal tract or the reticulospinal tract, but it is particularly important in cervicovestibulo-ocular reflexes.

The *reticulospinal tract* originates from neurons in the bulbar reticular formation, with both crossed and uncrossed fibres traversing the length of the spinal cord in the grey matter. While inhibitory and facilitatory stimuli are transmitted by this tract to the motoneurons throughout the spinal cord, relatively little is known about the exact neural pathways.

Vestibulocollic reflexes

The role of these reflexes in man is uncertain (Outerbridge and Jones, 1971), however, patients lacking vestibular function have impaired head stabilization in response to unpredictable oscillations (Guitton *et al.*, 1986; Bronstein, 1988). In animals, unilateral labyrinthine lesions can provoke an asymmetric head posture (Magnus, 1924). Peripheral vestibular lesions (Halmagyi, Gresty and Gibson, 1979) may be associated with an asymmetric head posture in man, e.g. in spasmodic torticollis (Bronstein and Rudge, 1986).

Bronstein (1988) reported that following wholebody movements normal subjects and those with vestibular hypofunction responded differently. Normal subjects appeared to respond to acceleration, with a response in advance of trunk movements (i.e. in advance of the velocity dimension) while those with vestibular failure displayed a significant time lag of response and a reduction of gain.

Gaze fixation

An important role of the vestibular system is the maintenance of the fovea on a fixation point during changes of head and body position. The interaction between visual, vestibular and cervical information enables a more precise eye movement to be achieved and thus better ocular stability than would be possible if only one system alone were functioning. The vestibulo-ocular and cervico-ocular reflexes fixate the fovea upon its target with compensatory eye movements which rotate the eyes in the opposite direction to the head movement. These reflexes are modulated by the action of central vestibular structures and depend on the integrity of the pathways mediating eye movements. A disturbance of this function can cause vertigo and oscillopsia. To appreciate the role of the peripheral vestibular apparatus in maintaining gaze fixation and the role that the examination of eye movements has in determining whether sites of pathology reside in the peripheral or central vestibular apparatus, some understanding of the physiology of eye movements is required.

The stability of gaze is a complex phenomenon and the relationship between the head and an object in the environment may change in a number of ways: either the head or the object may remain stationary while the other moves, or both may move simultaneously. The visual, vestibular and proprioceptive systems can work in conjunction to maintain the fovea on newly appearing visual targets, but when vestibular and visual signals conflict, e.g. when the head and a visual target are moving at the same velocity, the vestibulo-ocular reflex is suppressed and gaze is maintained on the moving target, thus the visual system predominates (Melville Jones, 1964; Dichgans *et al.*, 1973). The vestibulo-ocular reflex overrides the cervico-ocular reflex (Takemori and Suzuki, 1971).

It is at the level of the vestibular nuclei that vestibular information is modulated and oculomotor activity generated (Miles, 1974) in conjunction with central vestibular structures. The vestibulocerebellum (flocculonodular lobe) is important in mediating visuovestibular interaction (Ito, 1975; Robinson, 1976). Electrophysiological studies have shown that the Purkinje cells of the flocculonodular lobes receive afferent visual and vestibular information, which is 'compared' and efferent information is related back to the vestibular nuclei (Baker, Precht and Llimas, 1973).

Many areas of the cerebral cortex are involved in eye movement control, including the frontal, occipital and occipitoparietal lobes. In area 8 of each frontal lobe lies the 'frontal eye field', stimulation of which causes contralateral conjugate deviation of the eyes and pathology of which causes ipsilateral conjugate deviation (Penfield and Jasper, 1954) with the inhibition of ipsilateral pursuit eye movements. Areas 18 and 19 of the occipitoparietal lobes are involved with slow pursuit eye movements.

The frontal eye fields project to the internal capsule adjacent to the globus pallidus, through the genu into the thalamus, zona inserta and fields of Forel into the upper brain stem. A smaller projection deviates in Dejerine's bundle through the pes penunculi and substantia nigra, while other projections cross in the corpus callosum to follow a similar pathway on the other side. The fibres pass to the paramedian pontine reticular formation. Fibres from the occipital pathways pass along the medial side of the optic radiation, through the posterior part of the internal capsule and the pulvinar into the mesencephalon, with some fibres passing to the opposite side (Brucher, 1964). There are also connections between the frontal and occipital eye fields.

Discrete lesions in the region of the nucleus of the posterior commissure abolish upgaze (Pasik, Pasik and Bender, 1969). Bilateral lesions in the rubral area of the rostral interstitial nucleus of the medial longitudinal bundle and the fields of Forel inhibit downgaze. Bilateral stimulation of this area causes downgaze (Kompfe *et al.*, 1979). Unilateral lesions in the region of the fields of Forel cause a temporary loss of contralateral horizontal conjugate gaze.

While the response to stimulation of the peripheral vestibular apparatus or cervical proprioceptors is a compensatory eye movement, there are many other causes of eye movement: both voluntary and involuntary. Among the involuntary eye movements are nystagmus, saccadic intrusions, ocular flutter, opsoclonus, ocular spasms, ocular myoclonus and ocular bobbing. Voluntary eye movements are saccades. The volitional or involuntary following of a visual target is effected by a pursuit eye movement or optokinetic nystagmus.

Nystagmus

Nystagmus is a combination of alternating slow phase and fast saccadic eye movements in opposite directions (Figure 4.24). For clinical purposes, the direction of nystagmus is defined by the fast phase. It is graded by its presence in different directions of resting eye position. If it is only observed with the eyes deviated in the same direction as the fast phase, it is described as *first degree*; if it is seen in the primary position, it is *second degree* and if it seen with the eyes deviated contralaterally to the fast phase, it is *third degree*.

Nystagmus may be physiological or pathological. Pathological nystagmus may be congenital or acquired. Physiological nystagmus can be generated by

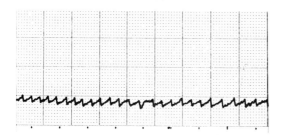

Figure 4.24 Electronystagmogram of nystagmus (fast phase to left)

extremes of eye deviation, e.g. more than 30° laterally from the primary position, or be induced by rotation, caloric and visual stimulation (see below). It can be modified by the degree of mental alertness (Collins, 1974a), by optic fixation (Hood, 1968), by other sensory stimuli, e.g. auditory, tactile or cervical information (Baloh and Honrubia, 1979), by age (Tibbling, 1969), and by drugs (Nozue, Mizuno and Kaga, 1973).

There are three visually controlled oculomotor systems which are of clinical importance in terms of their relationships with the vestibulo-ocular reflexes: the saccadic system, the smooth pursuit system and the optokinetic system.

The saccadic system

A saccade is a fast eye movement around 350–600°/s, increasing with increased amplitude of eye movement (Robinson, 1964) (Figure 4.25). They can be voluntary or involuntary. *Voluntary saccades* are used to move the eyes between targets in the shortest possible time. The rapid eye movements of the fast phase of nystagmus and the REM phase of sleep are *involuntary saccades*. Thus saccades can be generated as part of a reflex, volitionally towards a target or in the absence of a visual target, as for example towards a remembered target. A volitional saccade in the direction opposite to the visual target is termed an *antisaccade*.

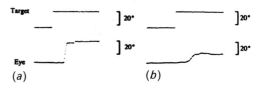

Figure 4.25 Electronystagmogram of saccadic eye movements, (a) normal; (b) slow

The purpose of the involuntary saccadic system is to maintain the target on the fovea. The direction of the saccade is such as to move the orbit rapidly towards targets already moving towards the fovea. That is the saccade resets the fovea on a target. In a rotation to the right, the new target is coming from the right, so the saccade is to the right. If a subject is within an optokinetic drum rotating from the subject's left to right, the new target is coming from the left, so the saccade is to the left. During a saccade there is no useful visual perception (Gresty, Trinder and Leech, 1976).

Normal subjects are accurate up to a target jump of 20°. Above this, a small additional corrective saccade is required, but overshoots are rare. The normal saccadic reaction time between a random target jump and the saccade is 200 ms. For predicted saccades, the reaction time is less and the saccade may anticipate the target jump.

While a saccade may be visually triggered, it can also be of vestibular (Melville Jones, 1964; Barnes, 1979) or cervical origin (Bronstein and Hood, 1986), when the fast phase of nystagmus shifts the eyes in the direction of the ongoing head movement, before there is a slow phase compensatory drift. This is termed the *anticompensatory* function of the vestibulo-ocular reflex – the *compensatory* function being the slow phase eye movement in the opposite direction.

The saccade is generated by groups of 'burst' neurons in the paramedian pontine reticular formation and pretectal region. The burst neurons in the paramedian pontine reticular formation fire in short bursts just before the onset of involuntary horizontal fast saccades or voluntary saccades. The burst neurons in the pretectal region generate vertical saccades (Hoyt and Daroff, 1971). The pretectal areas for downward saccades are distinct from those for upward saccades. The eye position is maintained by 'tonic' cells which continue to fire after the saccade is complete (Cohen and Henn, 1972). The superior colliculus contains cells which exhibit burst activity before saccades (Wurtz and Goldberg, 1972; Wurtz and Mohler, 1976).

The ability to make saccades may depend on the integrity of projections between the frontal eye fields, caudate nucleus, substantia nigra reticulata and the deep and intermediate layers of the superior colliculus. Different pathways are involved under different behavioural conditions (Zee, 1984; Bronstein and Kennard, 1987). Predictive saccades (where the targets are separately delivered at regular time intervals) (Bronstein and Kennard, 1987), acoustically triggered saccades (Zahn, Abel and Dell'Osso, 1978; Zambarbieri *et al.*, 1982) and saccades in the dark without visual targets (Becker and Fuchs, 1969) tend to be slow and hypometric, while randomly elicited visually triggered saccades are accurate, showing the significance of visual input. The superior colliculus receives visual input directly and indirectly via the parietal lobe (Schiller, True and Conway, 1980; Bruce and Goldberg, 1985). The ablation of the superior colliculus leads to a loss of saccades elicited by stimulation of visual pathways (Schiller, 1977; Pierrott–Deseilligny *et al.*, 1991). This supports the role of the superior colliculus in visually elicited saccades. Electrical stimulation of the frontal eye field causes a saccadic deviation (Robinson and Fuchs, 1969), though single unit recordings reveal that the units fire after, rather than before saccadic eye movements (Bizzi and Schiller, 1970). Vision and the occipital cortex are not required for these saccadic eye movements and they can be generated after bilateral occipital lobectomy (Pasik and Pasik, 1964). Lesions of the frontal eye fields do not lead to as profound a loss

of saccadic accuracy as after collicular lesions (Schiller, 1977).

Also projecting to the superior colliculus is a population of GABA-ergic cells from the substantia nigra. These cells have a high baseline firing rate which falls 200 ms before a remembered saccade to the contralateral visual field (Hikosaka and Wurtz, 1983). These cells receive a GABA-ergic input from the corpus striatum (Vincent, Hattori and McGeer, 1978). The injection of the GABA-agonist, muscimol into the superior colliculus produced slow hypometric saccades with long latencies, suggesting that the substantia nigra reticulata projection is inhibitory (Hikosaka and Wurtz, 1985a,b).

The paramedian pontine reticular formation is connected to the ipsilateral abducens nerve nucleus and by the median longitudinal bundle to the contralateral oculomotor nucleus of medial rectus. The pretectal neurons are also connected to the oculomotor nuclei. Both sets of neurons are connected to the vestibular nuclei.

Ocular stabilizing systems

The visual system itself acts to stabilize the fovea on visual targets during head and environmental change using smooth pursuit eye movements and optokinetic nystagmus.

The smooth pursuit system

In humans, the smooth pursuit system is responsible for maintaining gaze on a moving target, so that the target is stabilized on the fovea (Dodge, 1903) (Figure 4.26). It compares and then matches target and eye velocities. In the absence of a target, pursuit eye movements cannot take place and the attempt to move the eye, even slowly, results in a saccade, though subjects can pursue *apparent* target motion in the absence of a target moving across the retina (Steinbach, 1976). While one stimulus, therefore, is the presence of a target moving across the retina, other factors appear to drive the system, including perhaps retinal position, retinal velocity error and perceived target motion (Pola and Wyatt, 1980).

The degree of match between eye and target movement is given by the gain:

$$\text{Gain} = \text{eye velocity/target velocity.}$$

If the target is tracked across a patterned background moving in the opposite direction, there is an opposite optokinetic stimulus. Despite this, pursuit remains smooth, but there is a fall in gain.

In normal subjects, the gain of the pursuit system approaches unity at peak velocities of 30°/s or sinusoidal rotation at 0.1 Hz (Baloh *et al.*, 1988b). Above a peak velocity of 60°/s or sinusoidal rotation at 1 Hz, the gain falls off rapidly and catch-up saccades are required (Meyer, Lasker and Robinson, 1985). In

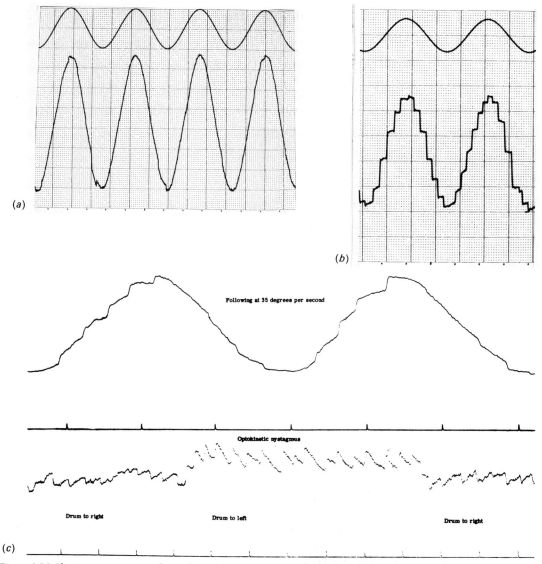

Figure 4.26 Electronystagmogram of smooth pursuit eye movements. (*a*) Normal; (*b*) grossly abnormal pursuit; (*c*) impaired smooth pursuit to the right with associated impairment of slow component of left beating optokinetic nystagmus

man, the gain during sinusoidal oscillation at these levels in the dark (to stimulate the vestibulo-ocular reflex alone) is only 0.4, while, at 1–4 Hz and velocities greater than 100°/s, the gain is near unity (Barnes, 1979). Therefore, the smooth pursuit and the vestibulo-ocular reflex systems are complementary in stabilizing the retinal image with the pursuit system efficient at low target velocities and the vestibulo-ocular system efficient at high input velocities.

The smooth pursuit system is of particular clinical importance as it is considered to be intimately related with the mechanisms by which the vestibulo-ocular reflex is suppressed by optic fixation and this is of the utmost importance in differentiating peripheral from central vestibular pathology.

Lesions of the fovea, lateral geniculate body, calcarine cortex (Yee *et al.*, 1982), parieto-occipital cortex (Lynch and McClaren, 1983), parietotemporal region, dorsolateral pontine nucleus and the cerebellar flocculus result in an impairment of smooth pursuit eye movements (May, Keller and Suzuki, 1988; Zee *et al.*, 1981).

The smooth pursuit system has its origin in the sensory cells of the fovea. The afferent limb passes in the optic nerve to the ipsilateral and contralateral lateral geniculate bodies and calcarine cortex. Unilateral afferent limb lesions spare smooth pursuit eye movements. The efferent pathways originating in Brodmann areas 19 and 39 descend near the posterior limb of the internal capsule through the reticular formation to the cerebellum, predominantly to the contralateral flocculus (Morrow and Sharpe, 1990).

Optokinetic nystagmus

Optokinetic nystagmus (Figure 4.27) is a reflex oscillation of the eyes, induced by movement of large areas in the visual field. The most common example of this phenomenon can be observed in the jerking eye movements of a train passenger as he views a landscape whose features traverse the field of vision with the motion of the train. In everyday life, the optokinetic response rarely acts independently, but interacts with the vestibulo-ocular reflex during the execution of spontaneous head movements, and with the smooth pursuit system during the visual following of a moving target, e.g. a bird in flight. In these situations, the optokinetic stimulation results from the apparent displacement of the surroundings, which is

attributable to eye movements induced by the primary response.

Ter Braak (1936) identified two types of optokinetic nystagmus: the first was 'active' and was elicited by attempting to follow a series of small moving targets; the second was 'passive' and was elicited by the movement of the entire surroundings. The first causes a 'look' nystagmus, the second a 'stare' nystagmus which differ in characteristics (Nelson and Stark, 1962; Hood, 1967; Honrubia *et al.*, 1968). In humans, the 'look' system is predominant except when there is neurological or foveal pathology.

The 'look' response has a time constant of a fraction of a second and consists of large amplitude eye movements with slow component velocities almost linearly related to target velocity up to 60°/s. In the 'look' optokinetic nystagmus, the mean position of the eyes deviates in the direction of the slow component. Nasotemporal and temporonasal stimulation gives symmetrical responses.

In afoveate animals, the 'stare' response has a slow build-up with a time constant of several seconds and consists of lower amplitude, higher frequency movements linearly related to target velocity up to 30°/s. There is a different response between nasotemporal and temporonasal stimulation, with the latter being better (Hobbelen and Collewijn, 1971). This is the optokinetic nystagmus response seen in patients with

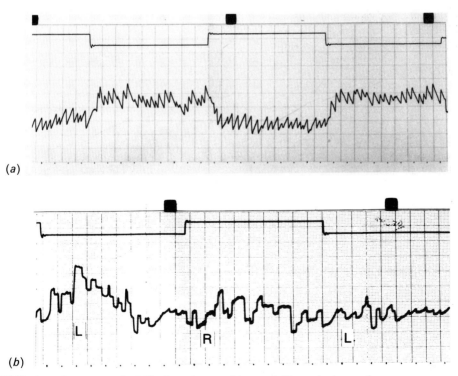

Figure 4.27 Electronystagmogram of optokinetic nystagmus, (*a*) normal; (*b*) grossly abnormal

macular field losses (Baloh, Yee and Honrubia, 1980) and cerebellar disease (Yee *et al.*, 1982). In the 'stare' optokinetic nystagmus, in afoveate animals and man, the eyes deviate in the direction of the fast component, which is not corrective but directs the eye towards the new oncoming target and is more affected by the position of the eye than the velocity of the slow component (Lau, Honrubia and Baloh, 1978).

The slow component velocity has a high variability of greater than 40% and can be reduced by inattention (Dichgans, Nauck and Wolpert, 1973), fatigue, sedatives, and metabolic disease (Baloh, Yee and Honrubia, 1982). Age (Yee *et al.*, 1982) can also cause symmetrical slowing of the slow component.

The 'look' and 'stare' optokinetic nystagmus are mediated by different pathways. The 'look' response involves the fovea and calcarine cortex (Zee *et al.*, 1982) and may share the same pathways as the smooth pursuit system, but a further pathway is necessary to inhibit inappropriate optokinetic nystagmus responses (Holmes, 1938). Also, some patients can display abnormal pursuit eye movements with normal optokinetic nystagmus, e.g. in extrapyramidal disease, while others can display abnormal optokinetic nystagmus with abnormal pursuit, suggesting some separation of pathways, at a cortical level (Lynch and McClaren, 1983).

The 'stare' response involves the peripheral retina and crosses the optic chiasm. Via the accessory optic tract, the afferent pathway reaches the contralateral midbrain nuclei and inferior olive and the ipsilateral flocculus (Maekawa and Simpson, 1973). From the midbrain a further pathway reaches the ipsilateral paramedian pontine reticular formation before crossing to the contralateral vestibular nuclei, thus bypassing the flocculus (Baloh, Yee and Honrubia, 1982; Honrubia *et al.*, 1982; Yee *et al.*, 1982).

Proprioception and cervico-ocular reflex

Proprioception has a role in balance. If the cervical apophyseal joints are infiltrated with local anaesthetic, the subject can feel vertiginous and will tend to fall towards the side of the injection (de Jong *et al.*, 1977), but there appears to be little loss of balance following major joint replacements (Grigg, Finerman and Riley, 1973). Unilateral electrical stimulation of the neck (Wapner, Werner and Chandler, 1951) or trunk tilt with the head fixed (Fischer, 1927) can cause deviation of the subjective vertical.

Cervical proprioception is a function of the deep short muscles of the neck, which are rich in muscle spindles (Voss, 1958; Cooper and Daniel, 1963; Richmond and Bakker, 1982). Proprioception is also mediated by the Pacini receptors and Golgi tendon organs of periarticular tissue. Skin receptors may also contribute position sensing information (McCloskey, 1978).

The role of cervical proprioception in maintaining ocular stability is uncertain (Bizzi, Kalil and Tagliasco, 1971). Horizontal contralateral nystagmus has been reported with cervical anaesthesia (Barré, 1926; Schubert, 1950; de Jong *et al.*, 1977). Cutaneous and limb proprioception also have an uncertain role, but nystagmus can be evoked in stationary subjects seated in darkness inside a rotating cylinder by placing their hands on the inner wall (Brandt, Buchele and Arnold, 1977).

Cervical proprioception mediates two reflexes: the cervico-ocular reflex and tonic postural neck reflexes. In man, tonic postural neck reflexes can only be elicited in the newborn (Gesell, 1938) in the form of the asymmetric tonic neck reflex or with gross brain stem lesions (De Kleyn and Stenvers, 1941).

The difficulties of studying the cervico-ocular reflex in humans is the problem of inadvertent vestibular stimulation with the overriding response of the vestibulo-ocular reflex and the low gain (Takemori and Suzuki, 1971) of the system (a body torsion of 50–60° with respect to the head results in a compensatory eye deviation of only 4–5°).

The cervico-ocular reflex is mediated by the medial and descending vestibular nuclei. Cervical proprioceptive and vestibular inputs are modulated in the vestibular nuclei (Hikosaka and Maeda, 1973), while other cervical inputs to the rostral areas of the cerebellar vermis (Berthoz and Llinas, 1974) allow further scope for interaction.

The potent effect of the cervico-ocular reflex on the vestibulo-ocular reflex has been clearly demonstrated in rabbits (Baloh and Honrubia, 1979) in contradiction to the situation in humans. Following the loss of vestibular function, the cervico-ocular reflex is enhanced with shortening of latencies, enhancement of slow phase velocities, increased gain and absence of stimulation after nystagmus (Dichgans *et al.*, 1973; Bles, de Jong and Rasmussens, 1984; Bronstein and Hood, 1986), indicating the precedence of the vestibulo-ocular reflex.

The gain of the cervico-ocular reflex is greater if the head is oscillated around the stationary trunk than if the trunk is oscillated around the stationary head (Bronstein and Hood, 1987), suggesting the additional effect of retinal inputs.

Clinical relevance of vestibular physiology
The assessment of the giddy patient

This review of the physiology of balance and gaze fixation stresses the interrelationships of the many different systems required. The clinical correlate of this fact is that the assessment of any disorder of equilibrium must be based on a multidisciplinary approach. A full and comprehensive history is essential, together with a complete general medical examination, with particular attention to the eyes, the ears, the central nervous system and the locomotor system. Although the exclusion of otological pathology is essential in any balance disorder, many conditions will elude diagnosis if balance is equated purely with a disorder of vestibular function. Drachman and Hart (1972) have emphasized the importance of multisensory deficits, particularly in the elderly, and have postulated a syndrome, producing dizziness, when two or more of the following conditions are present: visual impairment (not correctable), neuropathy, vestibular deficits, cervical spondylosis and orthopaedic disorders which interfere with ambulation. It is also important to assess cardiac and vascular function. An appreciation and understanding of the concept that disequilibrium may be consequent upon multiple mechanisms is essential if appropriate investigation and interpretation of data are to be achieved.

Having established the need for a general medical approach to the problem of unsteadiness, it is essential to identify the presence or absence of a vestibular component. Clinically, vestibulo-ocular and vestibulo-spinal reflex functions must be assessed.

History

While the clinical examination and the results of neuro-otological investigations will suggest the site of pathology, the history is of considerable value in diagnosing the likely aetiology of the symptoms and it is essential that a careful history facilitates differentiation of vestibular pathology from symptoms suggesting related cardiovascular or neurological disease. Any association with auditory symptoms should be established. Precipitating factors such as head or eye movements, visual stimuli or spontaneous onset should be clarified. The duration of the illness, each bout of symptoms and individual episodes, together with information about clustering may also be helpful. A detailed description of the first attack and any coincident history may be of immense value.

Stance and gait

Vestibulospinal function is assessed crudely by examination of stance and gait, but these tests are non-specific and insensitive in respect of vestibular function in comparison with the assessment of vestibulo-ocular function as they are dependent upon a variety of sensory and musculoskeletal functions other than vestibular function.

Stance

Postural sway is increased pathologically in vestibular, neurological, musculoskeletal and orthopaedic conditions. While the vestibulo-ocular reflex is the established method for objective vestibular assessment, an overall assessment of balance, including strategies is important in defining those factors which may lead to falls and unsteadiness (see below).

The position of the head should be noted. A head tilt may be compensatory for an ocular paresis, e.g. a roll away from a IVth nerve lesion, or be the result of a skew deviation, resulting from otolith or central pathology. The head may turn towards the side of a VIth nerve lesion or a visual field defect.

The Romberg test (Romberg, 1846) is often used clinically to assess the vestibulo-spinal reflexes, but it must be emphasized that this is an inaccurate concept for it assesses the many factors required to achieve 'balance', including posterior column function, and proprioception. The subject stands feet together, hands by the side, with the eyes open and then closed. The patient with vestibular or proprioceptive loss sways more or leans towards the pathological side more with the eyes closed than open. Patients with cerebellar lesions also tend to fall towards the pathological side, but with little enhancement with eye closure.

Gait

Gait testing may be of particular value in providing information about the many systems which give rise to imbalance. Loss of proprioception, as seen in tabes dorsalis, and to a lesser extent in sensory neuropathy, results in a characteristic high-stepping, foot-slapping gait. A hemiplegic gait, with extension and rotation of the hip, extension of the knee and plantar flexion, causing dragging of the leg, with flexion of the affected arm is instantly recognizable, as is the festinant, marche à petit pas of the parkinsonian patient, who walks with the neck and sometimes torso flexed, with little arm swing on the affected side and pill-rolling digits, and the wide-based, shuffling gait of the patient with the Pierre–Marie syndrome of multiple brain stem lacuna infarcts. Midline cerebellar dysfunction tends to give rise to a broad-based, ataxic gait, while unilateral, cerebellar hemisphere pathology, like unilateral peripheral vestibular pathology, causes a tendency to veer to the affected side with the ipsilateral leg abducted. The stiff painful gait of arthritis, or myopathy of the limb girdle muscles, resulting in rotation of the pelvis from side to side with every step, may be noted. A hysterical gait is recognized by the bizarre features, which do not conform to any specific organic disease pattern, but it is extremely important to exclude the bizarre posturing and gait mannerisms seen with extrapyramidal disorders, drug-induced dystonia and dyskinesia and gait apraxia.

A disturbance of the integrating ability of the central nervous system may also give rise to unsteadiness as, for example, in Parkinson's disease or in vascular disease associated with a stroke.

Although vestibular, visual and proprioceptive activity are all vital for the maintenance of perfect balance, spatial orientation can be controlled by any two of these mechanisms (Jongkees, 1953). However, man is unable to maintain his balance satisfactorily by using only one of the three systems. This physiological principal is admirably demonstrated on gait testing of a patient with bilateral vestibular failure. With eyes open and normal proprioception, it may be difficult to observe any gait disturbance, but if the patient is asked to walk in the dark, a marked difficulty and hesitancy of gait will be observed. If the patient is then deprived of all proprioception by being made to walk on a soft rubber mattress, with eyes closed or blindfolded, he will immediately fall to the ground as all three of the main sensory modalities required for balance are removed.

The formal analysis of gait disturbances can be of crucial value in rehabilitation.

Eye movements

A detailed examination of eye movements and nystagmus provides a wealth of information in the siting of both peripheral and central vestibular disorders. An informed and experienced assessment at the bedside will provide diagnostic information, but quantitative data may allow a more accurate interpretation by using precise visual targets and recording the resultant eye movement. Recording techniques include electronystagmography, photoelectric or video recording and scleral coil recording in a magnetic field (Collewijn, van der Mark and Jansen, 1975). Most widely available is electronystagmography, which though less sensitive than direct visual observation and scleral coil techniques is relatively simple to use and offers hard copy data. Electronystagmography also allows eye movements to be documented in the absence of optic fixation in total darkness. Eye closure is not an alternative to darkness as the responses are unreliable (Tjernstrom, 1973). Bell's phenomenon (elevation of the eyes behind the closed lids) and other eye movements intervene with the inhibition of nystagmus and the alteration of arousal can cause changes in eye movements.

It must be emphasized that the results of the examination of eye movements can be used to interpret vestibulo-ocular function only after a detailed assessment of visual acuities, visual fields, and eye movements with the identification of strabismus, gaze paresis, dysconjugate gaze and latent nystagmus.

The choroidoretinal potential

The choroidoretinal potential is the potential difference between the cornea and retina, created by the retinal pigmentary epithelium. The orbit therefore acts like a dipole and its movement will lead to a change of potential recordable with surface electrodes at stationary points on either side of the orbit. This potential forms the basis of eye movement recording by electronystagmography. The signal is enhanced by the careful application of electrodes to well pre-

pared skin and the use of chlorided silver electrodes (to avoid polarization) and electrode gel. The choroidoretinal potential increases with darkness and the subject should be dark-adapted for 10 minutes before recording is commenced. The potential change can be DC amplified and recorded. The use of differential amplification with a third electrode on the forehead, will allow the elimination of unwanted signals such as the ECG, EEG and myogenic activity and further enhance the detection of the ocular movement.

Ocular paresis and gaze palsy

Ocular paresis and gaze palsy describe a poverty of eye movements. Binocular lateral gaze is termed *version*. The bilateral adduction of the eyes is termed *vergence*. The ocular paresis or gaze palsy may be unilateral or bilateral. Eye movements are dysconjugate when the two eyes move independently.

It is important to determine whether the lesion is an ocular paresis, which implies a lesion at the level of, or peripheral to, the oculomotor nuclei or a gaze paresis, which implies a more rostral lesion. An ocular paresis may be due to a retro-orbital space-occupying lesion or due to involvement of the extra-ocular muscles (e.g. in thyroid eye disease or mitochondrial cytopathy). Myasthenia gravis causes a fluctuating unpredictable variable ocular palsy. Lesions of the IIIrd, IVth and VIth cranial nerves or their nuclei cause a paresis in the direction of pull of the muscles they innervate. A lesion of the IIIrd cranial nerve causes the eye to be 'down and out'. There may be an associated ptosis and dilated pupil if the lesion involves the circumferential fibres of the IIIrd cranial nerve (e.g. due to compression from a space-occupying lesion). A lesion of the IVth cranial nerve causes the eye to be slightly elevated. This increases on adduction and the head may roll away from the side of the lesion to reduce diplopia. A lesion of the VIth cranial nerve causes a loss of abduction and may cause the head to be rotated towards the side of the lesion to reduce diplopia.

A gaze palsy may be nuclear or supranuclear with reference to the oculomotor nuclei within the brain stem. A supranuclear gaze palsy is identified by the finding of an improved range of eye movements in response to rotational and caloric stimulation of the vestibulo-ocular reflex, while in a nuclear palsy or an ocular palsy, the eye movements remain limited.

The site of a discrete lesion may be confirmed by magnetic resonance imaging (Bronstein *et al.*, 1990).

Nystagmus

Nystagmus is an invaluable sign in siting vestibular and neurological disease (Rudge, 1983). If maximal diagnostic information is to be obtained, one must document alterations in the nystagmic response produced by: *change of eye position* (30° right and left from midposition of gaze); *presence and absence of optic fixation;* and *various head positions.*

Eye deviation greater than 30° to right and left may result in *physiological end-point nystagmus* in normal subjects.

Experimental lesions at different levels of the vestibulo-ocular pathways in animals have allowed documentation of the resultant nystagmus. Bilateral labyrinthine destruction does not cause nystagmus, as there is no asymmetry of vestibular information. Peripheral vestibular lesions of labyrinthine or VIIIth nerve origin result in spontaneous vestibular nystagmus towards the side opposite to the lesion. Pathology at the level of the vestibular nuclei may produce spontaneous nystagmus either ipsilaterally or contralaterally, depending on the location and extent of the lesion and the imbalance produced between inhibitory and excitatory secondary vestibular neurons (Uemura and Cohen, 1973). Lesions of the vestibulo-ocular pathways in the brain stem may affect either the slow vestibular component of the nystagmus (e.g. gaze paretic nystagmus), the fast saccadic component (as discussed previously) or both phases of nystagmus.

Vestibular nystagmus

Physiological nystagmus can be generated by the vestibular system. If a small rotational head movement is made, a slow compensatory eye movement is generated in the direction opposite to rotation. If a larger stimulus is applied, such that the compensatory eye movement cannot be contained within the confines of the orbit, the slow vestibular-induced eye deviation is interrupted by a fast eye movement in the opposite direction. The slow phase is generated by the vestibular nuclei and the fast phase is an involuntary saccadic eye movement, generated by neurons in the ipsilateral parapontine reticular formation (Raphan and Cohen, 1978). Subjects experiencing repeated angular accelerations, e.g. ice-skaters and dancers, display habituation, that is a reduction or loss of nystagmus with rotation (Collins, 1974b).

Pathological vestibular nystagmus is present in the absence of acceleration and is termed *spontaneous vestibular nystagmus.* It results from an imbalance of the afferent vestibular system. *Alexander's law* states that spontaneous vestibular nystagmus is maximal if the position of the gaze is in the direction of the fast phase, and least if in the opposite direction.

Spontaneous vestibular nystagmus may result from labyrinthine, vestibular nerve, vestibular nuclei or cerebellar lesions. With labyrinthine and vestibular nerve lesions, nystagmus is usually in the direction contralateral to the lesion because of reduced function, but in the presence of an irritative lesion, as for example in the acute phase of Menière's syndrome, the nystagmus may be directed towards the affected

ear. Lesions of the vestibular nuclei may produce nystagmus in either direction, depending on the relative involvement of excitatory and inhibitory pathways, while cerebellar lesions tend to produce nystagmus ipsilateral to the lesion.

If the lesion is small or compensation has taken place, nystagmus may only be elicited with the removal of optic fixation, *spontaneous nystagmus in the absence of optic fixation.* This is an important criterion to allow identification of nystagmus due to peripheral pathology, i.e. that the nystagmus usually displays an increase of amplitude with a reduction of slow phase velocity with the removal of optic fixation (Dix and Hallpike, 1966; Korres, 1978). The nystagmus may be detected in the dark by electronystagmography or by direct observation with either an infrared viewer or Frenzel's glasses.

Gaze paretic nystagmus

Horizontal nystagmus of vestibular origin should be differentiated from *gaze paretic nystagmus,* although this differentiation may be difficult on clinical visual inspection alone. Characteristically, there is an exponential drift away from the intended position of gaze, followed by a corrective saccadic movement. Thus, the nystagmus is always observed in the direction of gaze and, as the angle of gaze increases, so the amplitude of nystagmus increases. Furthermore, in the absence of optic fixation, although the amplitude of gaze paretic nystagmus increases, the frequency and slow component velocity decrease. The underlying abnormality is a failure of gaze maintenance. *Symmetrical* gaze paretic nystagmus is commonly observed in association with deranged pursuit following the ingestion of psychotropic drugs and alcohol. *Asymmetrical* horizontal gaze paretic nystagmus always indicates a structural lesion, e.g. involving the oculomotor nuclei, oculomotor nerves or muscles, ocular myasthenia or a retro-orbital space-occupying lesion. In the case of the cerebellar or cerebellopontine angle disease, the nystagmus is of larger amplitude towards the side of the lesion (Brun's nystagmus).

Head shaking nystagmus

Nystagmus which appears after rapid horizontal head shaking is termed head shaking nystagmus and is attributed to a lesion in the vestibular system (Kamei *et al.,* 1964; Hain, Fetter and Zee, 1987). The test involves shaking the head back and forth ± 30° at a frequency of > 1.5 Hz (peak velocity > 280°/s) for 10–20 seconds and then suddenly stopping. Spontaneous nystagmus is abnormal and indicates an asymmetry in the vestibular system.

The response follows the physiological directional asymmetry in vestibular responses described in Ewald's second law (1892), that is the differential effects of ampullofugal versus ampullopetal endolymph flow, i.e. excitatory inputs versus inhibitory inputs. Normally in head shaking the directional asymmetries balance, but with a unilateral peripheral lesion, there is an asymmetry which is revealed by the nystagmus with the slow phase of nystagmus in the direction of the pathological side.

The direction of the nystagmus is not always that predicted by Ewald's second law (Takahashi *et al.*, 1990). It has been suggested that head shaking nystagmus is a function of the directional preponderance of peripheral vestibular asymmetry and also of the amount of velocity storage (Hain, Fetter and Zee, 1987). For the nystagmus to appear after the head shaking has stopped, the directional asymmetry must have been stored. Some storage would be the result of cupula-endolymph mechanics, but the importance of central velocity-storage is reflected by the loss of head shaking nystagmus in the acute phase after unilateral labyrinthectomy (Fetter *et al.*, 1990). Furthermore, if there is a direction specific asymmetry in the central velocity-storage mechanism, the direction of head shaking nystagmus may not be as predicted according to Ewald's law (Demer, 1985).

Vertical head shaking can also be performed and even normal subjects can display transient vertical head shaking nystagmus.

Downbeat nystagmus

Downbeat nystagmus usually implies central nervous system disease (Fisher *et al.*, 1983; Bogousslavsky, Regli and Hunberbuhler, 1980). It is commonly associated with an intra-axial lesion at the craniocervical junction (Cogan and Burrows, 1954; Cogan, 1968) and is well recognized in association with the Arnold–Chiari malformation and cerebellar disease. Downbeat nystagmus can also be drug-induced by anticonvulsants (Alpert, 1978; Wheeler, Ramsey and Weiss, 1982) and lithium (Halmagyi *et al.*, 1983). It can be congenital. The patient complains of oscillopsia particularly on downgaze. Clues to the site of lesion may be given by a history of swallowing difficulties or choking when laying down and in such patients MRI scanning is indicated. Recognition of a malformation may enable surgical correction.

Downbeat nystagmus is not affected by optic fixation, but the amplitude and slow component velocity are increased by lateral gaze, head extension and head movements in the pitch plane. Downbeat nystagmus may be present only on down and lateral gaze, but it does not always follow Alexander's law and may indeed be maximal only on upgaze. It can be enhanced by convergence. Downbeat nystagmus is associated with impaired smooth pursuit and optokinetic nystagmus.

Downbeat nystagmus may arise from asymmetric vertical canal reflexes (Gresty *et al.*, 1986) due to a lesion which interrupts tonic excitatory activity to

the inferior recti between the vestibular nuclei or to a bilateral lesion of the flocculus which leads to disinhibited excitation of the superior recti (Zee *et al.*, 1981).

Upbeat nystagmus

Upbeat nystagmus is seen with intra-axial lesions of the brain stem in the tegmentum of the pontomesencephalic or the pontomedullary junction (Fisher *et al.*, 1983). It may be congenital (Shibasaki, Yamashita and Motomura, 1978).

It is not affected by lateral gaze. Convergence may enhance or suppress it or reverse it to downbeat (Cox *et al.*, 1981). It may suppress with loss of optic fixation.

Patients experience oscillopsia due to slip of the retinal image and fore-aft imbalance.

The upward vestibulo-ocular reflex is mediated by excitation of the anterior semicircular canals of the superior vestibular nuclei and the contralateral oculomotor nucleus via the brachium conjunctivum (Ito, Nisimaru and Yamamoto, 1976). Therefore the loss of this pathway would lead to a loss of tonic upgaze with a slow drift down and upbeat nystagmus.

Rebound nystagmus

Rebound nystagmus is characteristic of cerebellar dysfunction. It manifests itself as gaze evoked nystagmus, which disappears, or reverses, as the direction of gaze is held and, on recentring, a burst of nystagmus is initiated in the direction of the return saccade (Hood, Kayan and Leech, 1973; Baloh, Konrad and Honrubia, 1975).

Dysconjugate nystagmus

Dysconjugate nystagmus is commonly a correlate of central nervous system disease. Ataxic nystagmus, associated with an internuclear ophthalmoplegia, is the most well-recognized variety. It is the result of a lesion in the median longitudinal bundle (Cogan, Kubik and Smith, 1950) and most commonly develops in multiple sclerosis. *Monocular nystagmus*, by definition, is dysconjugate, and has been reported in a number of ophthalmological and neurological conditions (Nathanson, Bergman and Berker, 1955; Donin, 1967). *See-saw nystagmus* is rare but is associated with lesions near the optic chiasm (Arnott and Miller, 1970; Williams *et al.*, 1982).

Congenital nystagmus

Congenital nystagmus is presumed to be present from infancy, but it may not be noticed until school age or adulthood and sometimes it is only documented at an occupational medical or after the patient has presented with neurological or ophthalmological symptoms. It is, therefore, important to avoid incorrect diagnoses, such as multiple sclerosis or cerebellar degeneration with a resulting iatrogenic handicap through loss of employment.

Nystagmus would be detected in infancy if it were present in the primary position, but congenital nystagmus may be present only on eccentric gaze and there may be a wide neutral zone or null position in which nystagmus is absent. The point of reversal of the direction of congenital nystagmus and the neutral zone may be eccentric. If oscillopsia is a symptom subjects may involuntarily turn their head or develop a compensatory head tremor (Gresty and Halmagyi, 1979) to facilitate fixation by maintaining the eye position in the neutral zone. Pendular nystagmus may be accompanied by head nodding (Cogan, 1956).

Congenital nystagmus consists of very high frequency, up to 6 Hz, oscillations of the eyes. It can be associated with sensory pathology, e.g. ocular albinism or it can be seen in its absence, *motor-defect nystagmus* (Cogan, 1967). Usually the direction is horizontal, but it may be torsional or vertical. The waveforms can consist of pendular and jerk nystagmus. Congenital nystagmus can be characterized by an exponentially increasing or decreasing slow phase or by unidirectional or bidirectional jerks and each subject may display several waveforms, e.g. a pendular nystagmus may convert to a jerk nystagmus with gaze in the direction of the fast phase.

Congenital nystagmus is usually conjugate, though it can be monocular (Walshe and Hoyt, 1969) and it is important with monocular oscillations that retro-orbital lesions and ocular myokymia are excluded. Latent congenital nystagmus is elicited by covering one eye, allowing monocular fixation. The resulting nystagmus beats towards the fixating eye. Latent congenital nystagmus is often associated with concomitant squint and alternating hyperphoria (Dell'-Osso, 1985).

The vestibulo-ocular reflexes elicited by oscillatory stimuli have appropriate phase reversals with a normal gain, but those elicited by unidirectional step rotational stimuli appear to be of short duration and are abnormal in waveform (Gresty *et al.*, 1985). Gresty *et al.* (1985) advanced two possible, not necessarily mutually exclusive, explanations. One is that the induced responses are masked by the congenital spontaneous nystagmus. The other is that because the unidirectional stimulus is predictable, that the time constant is shortened due to the adaptation that might develop in subjects accustomed to a slip of the retinal image.

Attempts to suppress the vestibulo-ocular reflex by optic fixation cause a modulation of the vestibulo-ocular reflex but nystagmus is still observed and subjects with congenital nystagmus report some failure to stabilize the visual target suggesting that the vestibular response has not been fully suppressed (Gresty *et al.*, 1985). On the other hand, the nystag-

mus recorded may be the congenital nystagmus breaking through and often its characteristic waveforms can be recognized. Rotation influences the direction of the congenital nystagmus, e.g. an acceleration to the right brings out the nystagmus that is seen on right gaze with a contralateral shift of the neutral zone. Therefore, the resulting nystagmus is in the same direction as the induced response and as a result electronystagmography is likely to give a misleading impression of the degree of vestibulo-ocular reflex suppression impairment and it becomes a difficult diagnostic problem to assess the degree of impairment of the vestibulo-ocular reflex and its suppression, if any, in congenital nystagmus (see Figure 4.37).

Congenital nystagmus usually attenuates with convergence (Walshe and Hoyt, 1969), with eye closure and in sleep (Daroff, Troof and Dell'Osso, 1978), but this is not due to a loss of fixation (Shibasaki, Yamashita and Motomura, 1978; Yee *et al.*, 1981). Though darkness attenuates nystagmus in some subjects, many demonstrate a persistence (Yee *et al.*, 1981).

Subjects with congenital nystagmus display saccadic (Yee *et al.*, 1976), optokinetic (Yee, Baloh and Honrubia, 1980; Halmagyi, Gresty and Leech, 1980) and smooth pursuit (Gresty, Page and Barratt, 1984) abnormalities.

The saccadic abnormalities are mild and involve their initiation and accuracy, though not their velocity (Yee *et al.*, 1976). Whether the ENG abnormalities are only due to superimposition of the spontaneous nystagmus is uncertain.

Pursuit eye movements are impaired in congenital nystagmus (Gresty, Page and Barratt, 1984). The envelope of the eye movement accurately matches the target trajectory but the spontaneous nystagmus waveform is superimposed causing the ENG to suggest gross impairment (see Figure 4.26). In subjects with a neutral zone, pursuit eye movements shift the neutral zone contralaterally. This can cause the slow component to move in a direction opposite to the target, 'reversed pursuit'. This sign is strongly suggestive of congenital nystagmus, although it can be recorded in centripetal nystagmus and periodic alternating nystagmus.

A characteristic abnormality of optokinetic nystagmus, the 'reversed optokinetic nystagmus' can assist the diagnosis of congenital nystagmus (Halmagyi, Gresty and Leech, 1980). Normally the fast phase of the nystagmus induced by the optokinetic drum is in the opposite direction to the movement of the stimulus (Barany, 1921), but in congenital nystagmus the optokinetic nystagmus may be reversed with the fast phase in the same direction as the movement of the stimulus. This sign is not pathognomonic of congenital nystagmus and a similar ENG can be recorded when there is second and third degree spontaneous nystagmus and no optokinetic nystagmus (Gresty, Page and Barratt, 1984).

The pathophysiology of congenital nystagmus is uncertain. Nystagmus waveforms and the modification of nystagmus by the predominant position of gaze, convergence, eyelid closure, darkness, vestibulo-ocular reflex, vestibulo-ocular reflex suppression, pursuit and optokinetic nystagmus are similar in subjects with and without sensory defects suggesting that the primary defect driving congenital nystagmus is not visual. Subjects with congenital nystagmus have a full range of eye movements, normal saccadic velocities and normal vestibular function excluding pathology in these areas.

A clue to the site of pathology may lie in the pathophysiology of the reversal of optokinetic nystagmus. The stimulus may produce a shift of the neutral zone, but this would imply that the neutral zone is a function not only of eye position but also of eye movement or slip of the retinal image. There is evidence to support the hypothesis that eye movement influences the development of the visual cortex. Numerous neurophysiological studies have demonstrated that neurons in the mammalian visual cortex respond specifically to precise visual patterns (Hubel and Wiesel, 1977). Different cortical cells can be particularly sensitive to different colours, patterns and spatial orientations. This differentiation of the cortical visual neurons takes place in the first few months of postnatal life and it can be manipulated not only by visual input but also by eye movement (Maffei and Bisti, 1976). Buisseret, Gary-Bobo and Imbert (1978), using an extraocular muscle relaxant, demonstrated that area 17 striatal cortical cell differentiation was dependent on ocular mobility even with visual stimulation and sectioning the proprioceptive afferents from the extraocular muscles following the ophthalmic branch of the trigeminal nerve before Gasser's ganglia demonstrated that this stimulus for visual cortical differentiation was dependent on the proprioceptive input (Trotter, Gary-Bobo and Buisseret, 1979).

The afoveate rabbit with an almost complete panoramic visual field fixates with an optokinetic negative feedback control system operating on the input of the movement of the retinal image (Collewijn, 1972). Therefore, if the sign of the signal anywhere in the system were reversed, the system would fail and nystagmus occur. This has been induced in normal rabbits by artificially reversing the optokinetic reflexes in an experiment involving the use of an open-loop positive feed-back system using a mobile covered eye to control the mobile visual scene of an immobile seeing eye (Collewijn and van den Mark, 1972). Albino rabbits display this reversed optokinetic nystagmus when an optokinetic nystagmus stimulus is limited to the anterior visual field, that is to the temporal retina (Collewijn, Winterson and Dubois, 1978). This suggests the hypothesis that congenital nystagmus may be the result of an abnormal decussation of temporal retinal fibres, where a large proportion of

optic nerve fibres originating in the temporal retina, which normally do not decussate, terminate contralaterally. This abnormality has been found in the retinogeniculo-striatal pathways and in the projections to the pretectum and superior colliculus in the albinos of many species, where nystagmus is a feature (e.g. Guillery, Okoro and Witkorp, 1975; Lane, Kaas and Allman, 1974).

Periodic alternating nystagmus

Periodic alternating nystagmus changes direction with a change of head or eye position. Patients complain of oscillopsia. The cycle length varies from 1 to 6 minutes with null periods of 2–20 seconds. The precise site of the lesion is unknown, but both the cerebellum (Baloh, Honrubia and Konrad, 1976; Rudge and Leech, 1976; Furman, Wall and Pang, 1990) and the caudal brain stem (Keane, 1974) have been implicated. There is an abnormality of central vestibular function: the horizontal semicircular canal-ocular reflex during sinusoidal rotation displays an abnormal gain and phase with a variable rate of decay of the post-rotatory responses, canal-otolith interaction is abnormal and the otolith-ocular response displays an enlarged modulation component (Furman, Wall and Pang, 1990), suggesting that there is an abnormality of central velocity storage.

Positional and positioning nystagmus

Nystagmus can be elicited in critical head postures in certain pathological states. *Positional nystagmus* is present if the nystagmus develops while the head is stationary in the critical position and is the result of the gravity vector, while *positioning nystagmus* is present if the nystagmus begins while the head is still moving and is due to linear and angular acceleration forces.

Barany (1921) described two types of positional nystagmus. The first of these was studied further by Dix and Hallpike (1952a), who designated the disorder positional nystagmus of benign paroxysmal type, now termed benign paroxysmal positional nystagmus. The patient experiences vertigo when laying in a critical position, typically with the head to one side after a brief latency of 2–20 seconds. Patients who complain that their vertigo is aggravated by head movements must be examined for positional nystagmus and vertigo. The Hallpike manoeuvre (Dix and Hallpike, 1952a) is a valuable clinical test in such patients and is the only means of diagnosing or excluding benign paroxysmal positional vertigo. The manoeuvre consists of moving the sitting patient rapidly into the laying position with the head held 45° to the right or left (i.e. angled in such a way that during the manoeuvre the posterior semicircular canal of the undermost ear moves through the vertical plane) until the head is hanging over the edge of the couch, relaxed in the physician's hands with little support from the patient's nuchal musculature (Figure 4.28).

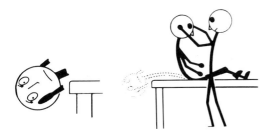

Figure 4.28 Diagram to illustrate the Hallpike manoeuvre

In patients with benign paroxysmal positional vertigo, with the pathological ear undermost, the Hallpike manoeuvre produces a cluster of classical signs. There is a latent period of 2–20 seconds, followed by the development of rotational nystagmus, with the fast phase towards the ground (geotropic) and accompanied by vertigo. The vertigo and nystagmus *adapt* (i.e. resolve) after a short period (up to 50 seconds). On sitting up, the vertigo returns, often with reversal of the nystagmus, before both resolve. On retesting, the vertigo and nystagmus *fatigue* (i.e. disappear or reduce) upon repetition. These characteristics are crucial to the diagnosis. While the aetiology of this type of positional nystagmus is often uncertain, the lesion is usually within the labyrinth.

Although the Hallpike manoeuvre is of immense importance in diagnosing benign paroxysmal positional vertigo, it is crucial to remember that the classical picture can rarely be the result of retrocochlear and central pathology (Harrison and Ozsahinoglu, 1972), e.g. in the cerebellum (Fernandez, Alzate and Lindsay, 1959) or around the floor of the IVth ventricle (Hallpike, 1967). Atypical nystagmus, persisting nystagmus, nystagmus without vertigo, any variability of the direction of nystagmus, the absence of a latent period before the onset of nystagmus and the absence of fatiguability suggest central pathology. In essence, if some of the diagnostic characteristics of benign paroxysmal positional vertigo are met but others are absent, central pathology must be suspected.

It is of no clinical value to perform the Hallpike manoeuvre in the absence of optic fixation as positional nystagmus under these conditions will develop in as many as 30% of cases and the significance is uncertain (Stahle and Terrins, 1965).

Positional vertigo and nystagmus can also be caused by debris in the lateral semicircular canals (McClure, 1985; Baloh, Jacobson and Honrubia, 1993).

Optokinetic nystagmus

The physiology and pathways subserving optokinetic nystagmus have been outlined above. Disorders affect-

ing saccadic eye movements, or smooth eye movement, may result in derangements of optokinetic nystagmus. Neurological disease involving either the brain stem, cerebellum or IIIrd and VIth cranial nerves may result in derangement of the fast saccadic components. Supranuclear lesions cause a tonic deviation of the eyes in the direction of the slow phase of the optokinetic nystagmus with a loss of the contralateral saccade. The slow component may be reduced by ipsilateral lesions of the visual pathways or the efferent motor pathways. Lesions at every level from the brain stem, basal ganglia, cerebellum and cortex have been shown to cause derangement of the slow component velocity of the optokinetic response. In contrast, peripheral vestibular abnormalities of the labyrinth or VIIIth nerve rarely give rise to optokinetic derangements (Abel and Barber, 1981; Yee *et al.*, 1982). Optokinetic nystagmus is, therefore, of great clinical value in distinguishing peripheral from central vestibular disorders.

A qualitative assessment of the optokinetic response may be undertaken at the bedside, or in the outpatient department, by using either a hand-held rotating striped Barany drum or a mechanically driven drum. For quantitative, diagnostic purposes, more precise and reproducible stimulus parameters are obtained by seating a patient inside a large, striped, rotating drum and stimulating the entire visual field. Alternatively, a moving field of parallel bars, projected on to a surface covering approximately 60° of visual angle, may be used.

The optokinetic response may be of value in determining whether nystagmus is congenital. In congenital nystagmus, the optokinetic nystagmus may be 'reversed' (Halmagyi, Gresty and Leech, 1980), but such a reversal can also be found in miner's nystagmus and multiple sclerosis (Hood and Leech, 1974).

Saccadic eye movements

Saccadic eye movements can be assessed by asking the patient to look back and forth between two targets in front of him sited approximately 30° to the right and left of the midline. Increasing the distance between the targets (beyond 30°) increases the chance of detecting a hypometric saccade, while reducing the distance between targets increases the chance of detecting a hypermetric saccade (Zee *et al.*, 1976). Care should be taken to ensure that the visual fields are normal as the commonest cause of unilateral hypometric saccades is an homonymous hemianopia.

Three variables are examined: saccade reaction time (latency), velocity, and accuracy.

Abnormalities may be due to CNS pathology, ocular myasthenia or extraocular muscle pathology (Henriksson *et al.*, 1981). Peripheral vestibular lesions do not cause abnormal saccades.

Unilateral lesions of the parapontine reticular formation cause loss of all types of rapid ipsilateral movement and the eyes move to the contralateral visual field. Pretectal lesions cause a loss of vertical saccades.

With a parapontine reticular formation lesion, during contralateral optokinetic nystagmus or ipsilateral rotation, the eyes display a tonic contralateral deviation with a loss of the fast phase of the nystagmic response. With ipsilateral optokinetic nystagmus or contralateral rotation, there is a normal ipsilateral slow phase response and a normal contralateral saccade (Dix, Harrison and Lewis, 1971).

Internuclear ophthalmoplegia

An internuclear ophthalmoplegia may present as ataxic nystagmus, where adducting saccades towards the side of the lesion are slower than abducting saccades. Subtle early lesions can be revealed by ENG with slowing of the adducting saccade on the side of the lesion, with a normal velocity but hypermetric abducting saccade (Figure 4.29). With more extensive brain stem pathology affecting the ipsilateral parapontine reticular formation and both median longitudinal bundles (Pierrott–Deseilligny *et al.*, 1981), the 'one and a half syndrome' can result with a failure of conjugate gaze in one direction and an internuclear ophthalmoparesis in the other (Fisher, 1967). An explanation for the signs seen in internuclear ophthalmoplegia was offered by Pola and Robinson (1976). The horizontal saccade is generated by a pulse-step in neural activity, part of which excites medial rectus motoneurons on the fibres of the median longitudinal bundle. The median longitudinal

bundle is thought to carry excitatory fibres to the ipsilateral medial rectus and inhibitory fibres to the contralateral medial rectus. Therefore, the interruption of the median longitudinal bundle will reduce excitation to the ipsilateral medial rectus and inhibition to the contralateral medial rectus. Therefore the eye ipsilateral to the median longitudinal bundle lesion will adduct slowly and inadequately, while the contralateral eye will overshoot and there will be a derangement of conjugate contralateral gaze. The effect of this would be a corrective saccade of the contralateral eye, hence *ataxic nystagmus*.

The pathways subserving vertical and horizontal saccades are independent, such that vertical saccades are unimpaired by lesions of the paramedian pontine reticular formation, but impaired by lesions of the mesencephalic reticular formation (Buettner, Buettner–Ennever and Henn, 1977). The relationship between the mesencephalic reticular formation and the paramedian pontine reticular formation is not entirely clear, but vertical saccades can be abolished by stimulation of units in the paramedian pontine reticular formation (Keller, 1974), perhaps due to formations running lateral to the median longitudinal bundle.

In *cerebellar pathology*, the accuracy of the saccades (ocular dysmetria) is impaired with undershooting (hypometria) and/or overshooting (hypermetria) ipsilateral to the lesion (Zee *et al.*, 1976), followed by compensatory saccades. Hypermetria rarely happens in normal subjects and its presence is therefore strongly suggestive of CNS pathology. It is more common in cerebellar lesions than hypometria, while in intrinsic brain stem lesions, due to vertebrobasilar

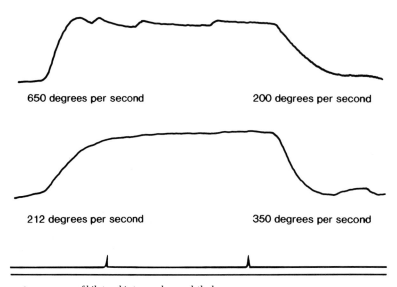

650 degrees per second   200 degrees per second

212 degrees per second   350 degrees per second

Figure 4.29 Electronystagmogram of bilateral internuclear ophthalmopareses

ischaemia, multiple sclerosis, or infiltrating tumours, hypometria is more likely (Goebel *et al.*, 1971).

In *supranuclear degeneration*, multiple system atrophy (Steele-Richardson-Olazewski syndrome, Shy-Drager syndrome, progressive supranuclear palsy) and Huntington's chorea, saccade reaction time is prolonged. In these conditions, hypometria is common. In supranuclear lesions, vertical eye movements are usually affected before horizontal, initially with downgaze often more involved than upgaze (Dix, Harrison and Lewis, 1971) and saccades more affected than pursuit. The velocity of the saccades is usually reduced before the amplitude (Pasik, Pasik and Bender, 1969; Kompfe *et al.*, 1979). The pathological process involves the burst neurons associated with saccades (Newman *et al.*, 1970). The reciprocal innervation of the lateral and medial recti is preserved, but there is a failure of this in the inferior rectus muscle on attempted upgaze (Pinhas *et al.*, 1978).

With *frontal pathology*, there may be hypometria or loss of horizontal saccades contralateral to the side of the lesion (Baloh, Honrubia and Sills, 1977), while vertical saccades are not affected. However, frontal lesions affect voluntary anti-saccades. Normal subjects can direct a saccade in the opposite direction to an illuminated fixation target in the periphery. Subjects with frontal lesions tend to make an involuntary saccade to the target before the antisaccade.

In *ocular myasthenia*, the saccades may be normal at the start of testing, but with repeated testing, a deficiency of acetylcholine may develop and the saccades will slow. Intravenous edrophonium may reverse this deterioration. Fatigue, alcohol and benzodiazepines will also cause slowing but saccadic movements are less impaired than smooth pursuit (Ajodhia and Dix, 1975).

Saccades are not impaired as a result of pure peripheral vestibular dysfunction.

It is important to distinguish ocular myasthenia (with the effect of intravenous edrophonium) from an internuclear ophthalmoparesis (by measuring the different velocities and amplitudes of abducting and adducting saccades) from ocular palsies and gaze palsies (by their classical presentations) from supranuclear gaze palsies (by the increase in eye movements on stimulation of the vestibulo-ocular reflex by head movements, rotation and caloric stimulation).

Pursuit eye movements

The smooth pursuit system can be examined clinically by moving a target (e.g. a finger) slowly back and forth in front of the patient's eyes.

In *chronic peripheral vestibular disorders*, pursuit is normal. In *acute peripheral vestibular disorders*, contralateral pursuit may be impaired (due to superimposed nystagmus). In acoustic neuroma, pursuit movements are usually not impaired until the brain stem is involved. In *pretectal and basal ganglia lesions*, vertical pursuit is usually impaired. There is ipsilateral derangement of pursuit in *cerebellar, pontine and parieto-occipital lesions* (Schalen, Henriksson and Pyykko, 1982).

Pursuit eye movements are *symmetrically* affected by age, psychotropic medication, alcohol, anticonvulsants, and vestibular and CNS sedatives (Ajodhia and Dix, 1975) and this does not necessarily imply pathology.

Vestibular tests

The role of vestibular tests

A careful history and general, neurological and neuro-otological clinical examination, particularly of eye movements will contribute greatly towards the making of the final diagnosis and as a result the value of vestibular tests in clinical medicine has been questioned. In positional and positioning nystagmus, the clinical examination and, where indicated imaging studies, rather than vestibular tests yield the diagnosis. However, in the majority of patients with vestibular pathology, an accurate diagnosis can be made only after the considered application of vestibular tests and usually imaging studies do not contribute to the diagnosis.

A variety of eye movement recording techniques is available. These can be used to examine eye movements in the absence of optic fixation and offer the advantage of supplying hard copy for the measurements of slow and fast phase velocities, frequency, amplitude and response durations and the analysis of disordered eye movements. This is important for the detection of subtle dysconjugacy, e.g. in early internuclear ophthalmoplegia, and the detection of borderline saccadic slowing. Eye movement recording is also valuable in detecting optokinetic nystagmus asymmetries and the failure to suppress the vestibulo-ocular reflex with optic fixation.

Electronystagmography is the most widely available technique, but it should be appreciated that it is less sensitive than fundoscopy in detecting nystagmus and that it is of limited value if the response is torsional or oblique. Here scleral coil and computer supported video-recording are more valuable.

Frenzel's glasses, though helpful in the absence of a dark room, do not adequately eliminate optic fixation and the illumination of the eyes required by the observer can cause artefactual eye movements. Infra-red examination is an alternative, but these techniques should not be seen as a substitute for eye movement recording as no hard data for measurement or comparison purposes can be obtained.

The physiological aspects of the most well established tests are briefly considered.

Caloric tests

The caloric test is the most widely available vestibular test and is the cornerstone of vestibular diagnosis, particularly as it allows each labyrinth to be tested separately. However, in the presence of active external ear or middle ear disease, standard water caloric testing is contraindicated and consideration has to be given to the use of air caloric testing. Care has to be taken to ensure that access to the tympanum is unobstructed and after warm irrigation, the presence of a tympanic flush should be sought. Some patients, e.g. those with cerebellar dysfunction or those with a failure of central mechanisms of compensation, demonstrate a hyperactive response and a shortened irrigation may be required to enable completion of the test.

In the normal situation, a steady stream of electrical activity arises in each vestibular end organ and tends to drive the eyes towards the opposite side, by way of the vestibulo-ocular reflex. For practical purposes, the vestibular system may be considered in two halves, the activity of each being balanced in an equal and opposite manner, such that the eyes are maintained in a central position. The basis of the caloric test lies in the development of an asymmetry of information in the two halves of the vestibular system, as a result of the application of a thermal gradient across the horizontal canal of each labyrinth in turn. The patient lies in the supine position, with the head titled 30° upwards, so that the horizontal semicircular canal is brought into the vertical plane, the position of maximal sensitivity to a thermal gradient (Figure 4.30). The thermal stimulus is standardized for each of the four irrigations, that is

7°C below and above body temperature in the right and left ears. The induced nystagmus may be measured by using a number of parameters (duration, slow component velocity, frequency and/ or amplitude) and reflects the integrity of the vestibulo-ocular reflex derived from each labyrinth independently.

Hot irrigations cause a slow deviation of the eyes away from the irrigated ear, with fast saccadic phases directed towards the irrigated ear, while precisely the converse situation appertains for cold irrigations (Figure 4.31). The nystagmic response from the onset of irrigation to the end of observable nystagmus is documented, in both the presence and absence of optic fixation.

The caloric test, as described, was established on a quantitative basis in 1942 by Fitzgerald and Hallpike, and remains the best method of assessing the integrity of each labyrinth and its central nervous system connections. The results of the test are well documented in a large range of vestibular and neurological conditions. The localizing value in siding and siting vestibular pathology is high, and the value of the test in revealing an organic basis to symptoms of vestibular derangement remains unchallenged.

Mechanism

The conventional explanation for the caloric response is that thermal currents are created, with hot irrigations causing an ampullopetal and cold irrigations an ampullofugal flow of endolymph, leading to stimulation of the cupula. This convection theory proposed

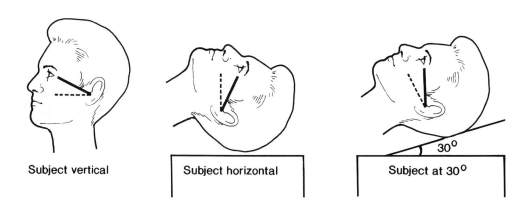

Subject vertical   Subject horizontal   Subject at 30°

Figure 4.30 Diagram to illustrate the vertical disposition of the horizontal semicircular canal as a result of elevation of the head by 30° from the supine position

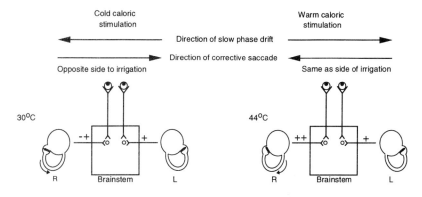

Figure 4.31 Diagram to illustrate the direction of nystagmus produced by cold and warm caloric irrigation of the right external auditory canal. L = Left, R = Right

by Barany (1922) was questioned after the observation of caloric nystagmus under microgravity conditions and in space, where convection currents cannot explain the findings (Baumgarten, Benson and Berthoz, 1984; Scherer *et al.*, 1986). It had also been noted that the duration of nystagmus (McNally *et al.*, 1947) and the maximum slow-phase velocities (Coats and Smith, 1967) were greater in the face-up than face down positions (Figure 4.32). Coats and Smith (1967) suggested that one component of caloric nystagmus was a direct thermal stimulation of the vestibular sensory epithelium and the ampullary nerve endings. Their explanation was that warming would increase neural discharge and would produce nystagmus towards the irrigated ear, regardless of body position. This would add to the convection effect in the face-up position, but would subtract from the convection effect in the face-down position. Further support for this hypothesis came from the re-interpretation of the Coats and Smith data by Hood (1989).

Pathological findings

Pathology may give rise to two distinct patterns of response: '*canal paresis*' and '*directional preponderance*'. These may appear separately, or in combination. They are calculated by the following formulae, into which are entered either the durations of nystagmus from the start of irrigation or the peak or mean slow component velocities:

Canal paresis %

$$= \frac{(L30° + L44°) - (R30° + R44°)}{(L30° + L44° + R30° + R44°)} \times 100$$

Directional preponderance %

$$= \frac{(L30° + R44°) - (R30° + L44°)}{(L30° + L44° + R30° + R44°)} \times 100$$

(Jongkees, Maas and Philipzoon, 1962).

The data can be pictorially represented (Figure 4.33).

The canal paresis is characterized by a reduced response to both hot and cold stimuli applied to one ear, and is a manifestation of depression of function of one labyrinth, the ipsilateral VIIIth nerve (Dix and Hallpike, 1952a), the vestibular nerve at its root entry zone (Uemura and Cohen, 1973) or the vestibular nuclei within the brain stem (Francis *et al.*, 1992). The directional preponderance gives rise to greater nystagmus in one direction, and is a sign of imbalance between the two halves of the vestibular system. This may result from lesions of the labyrinth, the vestibular nerve, the vestibular nuclei, the cerebellum and/or the corticofugal fibres deep in the temporal lobe. A derangement of any of these centres may result in an imbalance between the vestibular inputs, and hence a tendency for the eyes to drift either to the right or to the left. A vestibular stimulus will, therefore produce a nystagmus, which is more exaggerated when the slow component is in the direction of the tendency of eye drift. With more pronounced degrees of tonic imbalance, spontaneous nystagmus will appear.

An understanding of the pathophysiological mechanisms of canal paresis and directional preponderance makes it clear that bithermal testing of both ears is necessary. If both ears are irrigated at one temperature only, it is impossible to be certain whether one is dealing with a canal paresis, a directional

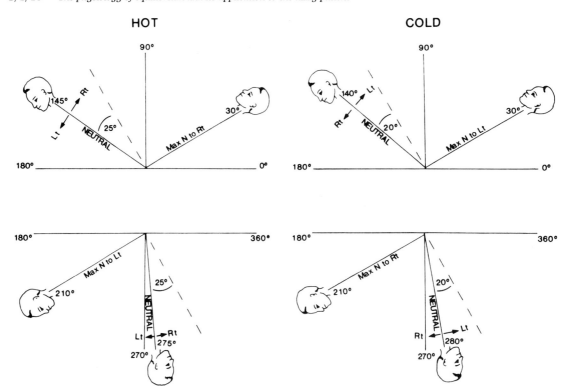

Figure 4.32 Experimental (——) and theoretical (– – – –) neutral head angles and the angles of maximum reactivity. The arrows indicate the direction of nystagmus. The discrepancy between the experimental and theoretical angles is due to the direct thermal-induced neural component. (From Hood J.D. Evidence of direct thermal action upon the vestibular receptors in the caloric test. *Acta Otolaryngologica*, **107**, 161–165, 1989)

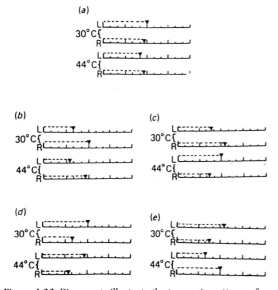

Figure 4.33 Diagram to illustrate the two main patterns of abnormal response observed upon caloric testing. (a) Normal; (b) left canal paresis; (c) directional preponderance to the left; (d) right canal paresis; (e) directional preponderance to the right. L = Left ear; R = Right ear

preponderance, a combined pattern or a normal response (Figure 4.34).

Demanez and Ledoux (1970) demonstrated that a caloric-induced nystagmus is much enhanced by eye closure in normal subjects and in cases of peripheral vestibular lesions, but appreciably less so, or even inhibited, in the case of a central vestibular disturbance. Takemori and Cohen (1974) demonstrated that the suppression of nystagmus by optic fixation is lost after extirpation of the flocculus. This phenomenon is readily explicable on the basis of vestibulo-ocular reflex suppression in the presence of a visual stimulus, and provided that the central nervous system and cerebellar pathways subserving this mechanism are intact, there will be excellent suppression of caloric-induced nystagmus, but if the central pathways are deranged, there will be little suppression. In the caloric test, this phenomenon has been documented by calculation of a '*fixation index*', which compares the magnitude of the response in the absence and presence of optic fixation (Hood and Korres, 1979), e.g. the ratio of the duration of the response with optic fixation to that in the absence of optic fixation.

It must be emphasized that, in the literature, there are many different methods of conducting the caloric test and the foregoing discussion merely underlines

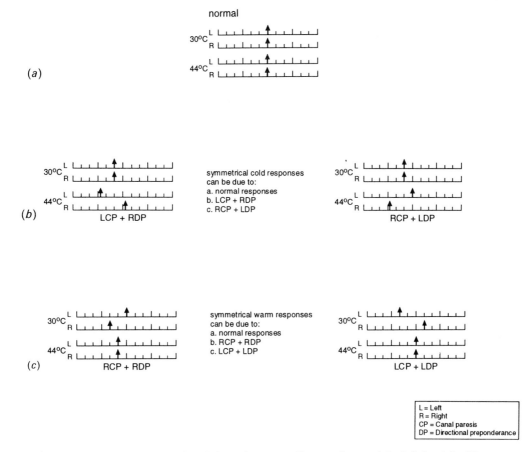

Figure 4.34 Diagram to illustrate the need to perform bithermal irrigation (durational criteria). L = Left, R = right, CP = canal paresis, DP = directional preponderance. Combined abnormalities may give normal responses with cold *or* warm irrigations alone

the relevant physiology and pathophysiological mechanisms of importance in this procedure.

Rotation testing

Rotation about the vertical axis (Figure 4.35) provides another method of modulating the resting activity in the vestibular system. The patient is seated in a chair that rotates about its vertical axis, and the patient's head is tilted 30° downward so that the angular rotation takes place in the plane of the horizontal semicircular canals.

Figure 4.36 illustrates the effect of sinusoidal acceleration. The imbalance generated in the vestibular system by such a stimulus is 'sensed' by the central

nervous system connections, and a compensatory slow eye deviation in the opposite direction to that of rotation is initiated. With increasing rotational stimulus, the slow phase is interrupted by a rapid corrective saccadic eye movement, giving rise to induced nystagmus.

Rotation testing is of particular value in certain situations. If the caloric test reveals no observable response, high frequency oscillation or high intensity acceleration may provide evidence of residual vestibular function. Vestibular thresholds may be identified by applying minimal angular accelerations. Rotation testing may allow the possibility of detecting unilateral *vestibular recruitment*, defined as an abnormally large growth of response with increasing stimulus

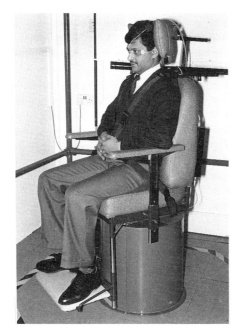

Figure 4.35 Rotation chair (note position of subject's head)

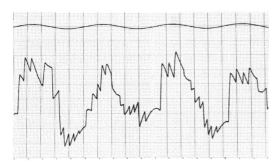

Figure 4.36 Electronystagmogram of vestibulo-ocular reflex stimulated by sinusoidal rotation

intensity. If recruitment is present, the directional preponderance would be greatest at the threshold of the affected ear and the asymmetry would lessen as the damaged end-organ displays recruitment (Mendel, 1971; Matsuhira *et al.*, 1991). However, recruitment is not always detected in damaged end-organs (Furman *et al.*, 1990). *Decruitment*, defined as an abnormally reduced growth or diminution of response with increasing stimulus intensity may be a feature of central vestibular pathology (Torok, 1976). Rotation testing also permits the investigation of visual-vestibular interactions (Baloh *et al.*, 1982) and the failure to suppress the vestibulo-ocular reflex with fixation provides evidence of central cerebellovestibular dysfunction (Figure 4.37).

Limitations of caloric and rotation tests

It should be emphasized that neither rotation nor caloric testing can distinguish between pathology of the vestibule and vestibular nerve. Moreover, neither test enables assessment of all the vestibular receptors.

In monaural irrigation, only the ipsilateral horizontal canal, its ampullary nerve and its central connections are tested, while in binaural irrigation, the vertical canals, their ampullary nerves and central connections are tested (in the presence of normal function of each lateral canal). Caloric testing cannot be used to elicit responses from the utricle and saccule. Rotation tests examine both horizontal canals, their nerve supply and their central connections. Rotation tests can also be used to test otolith function, by placing the head forward of the axis of rotation, so that there will be a tangential linear stimulation of the otoliths during rotation (Gresty, Bronstein and Barratt, 1987). However, the value of this in clinical practice remains uncertain (Barratt, Bronstein and Gresty, 1987).

A disadvantage of rotation testing is that both labyrinths are tested simultaneously. Thus, a unilateral dysfunction may be difficult to identify, although an asymmetrical response to rotatory stimuli may be observed because of the difference in excitation and inhibition between ampullopetal and ampullofugal stimulation of the labyrinth. This asymmetry is most pronounced after high intensity stimuli, but is consistent only in identifying complete unilateral, peripheral, vestibular paralysis (Honrubia *et al.*, 1980).

It should be stressed that the presence of pathology in the vertical canals and the otoliths cannot be elicited routinely by vestibular tests, and may be suspected only by a careful history and clinical examination.

Galvanic testing

Galvanic stimulation of the vestibular system can cause vertigo and activate the vestibulo-ocular reflex. This has been used to differentiate between labyrinthine and retrolabyrinthine pathology (Pfaltz, 1969) as the response depends on the integrity of Scarpa's ganglion and the central vestibular connections (Huizinga, 1931; Dohlman, 1938). The thresholds are raised in vestibular neuronitis and in long standing Ménière's disease (Dix and Hallpike, 1952b).

Galvanic stimulation is carried out by placing saline pads to the tragus, external ear canal, or over the mastoid with a further electrode attached to the sternum. Stimulation can be bilateral or unilateral and the cathode is excitatory. At a threshold of 1–2 mA, in the dark, in healthy volunteers, the body sways away from the cathode and nystagmus is produced with the fast phase towards the cathode. Cessation of stimulation produces a reversed response, though this can be uncomfortable if sudden.

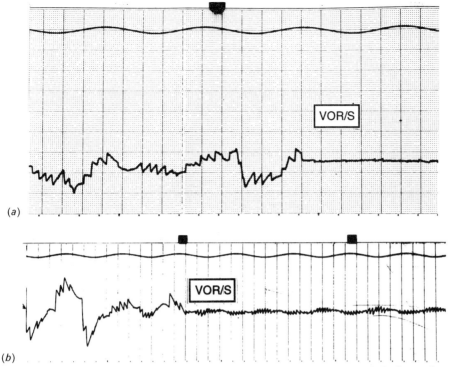

Figure 4.37 Electronystagmogram of sinusoidal vestibulo-ocular reflex suppression. (*a*) Normal; (*b*) abnormal

Pfaltz (1969) described similar thresholds in most of his subjects with Menière's disease, but absent responses with ipsilateral acoustic neuroma. With body sway platforms, the normal threshold for detection of a response is 0.25–1 mA (Baron, 1978).

The early difficulty with galvanic testing lay in the discomfort experienced when the thresholds for nystagmus were raised to 7–10 mA. Moreover, electronystagmography may be complicated due to electrical artefacts, but the markedly lower currents required for posturographic sway measurements have overcome these shortcomings (Kapteyn and De Wit, 1972; Watanabe *et al.*, 1983).

Posturography

Posturography, using a static platform, allows a quantitative assessment of the Romberg test (Jansen, Larsen and Oleson, 1982; Trieson *et al.*, 1982), while dynamic posturography allows other study paradigms to be tested, such as the effect of moving versus stationary visual fields and platforms (Black and Nashner, 1984) giving more physiological and pathophysiological information. Posturography has confirmed the following observations (Nashner, 1973; Barigant, Merlet and Orfait, 1972):

1 The centre of gravity of the erect whole body mass plumbs to a point on the ground a few centimetres in front of the transverse ankle axis from a point in the centre pelvis immediately below the level of the umbilicus

2 Normal standing does not imply a completely static posture – the body is in continuous motion even when attempting to remain still

3 Postural sway activity along the anteroposterior (x) axis is generally much more prominent than along the transverse body (y) axis because of the greater x-axis instability of the ankle joint.

Nashner's experiments with posturography (1973) confirmed that postural control is regulated by local regulation from spinal reflexes commanded by information from muscle spindle and tendon stretch receptors and extraspinal feedback from the visual and vestibular systems.

Frequency analysis of oscillations on a moving platform showed that 1.5–2.5 Hz oscillations were increased by eye closure, while slower oscillations (0.5–1 Hz) were decreased. The faster oscillation could be attenuated with the feet apart or splinting the ankles, suggesting the involvement of the ankle joint. On the other hand slow oscillations were increased with the feet apart. Begbie (1967) suggested that these slower oscillations were the result of re-flexes generated by the vestibular system.

Established posturographic patterns are not yet sufficiently well defined to be diagnostic for vestibular pathology in part because different investigators use different measures: sway area (Sheldon, 1963), sway frequency (Seliktar *et al.*, 1978), total sway path (Diener *et al.*, 1984; Taguchi and Tada, 1988), sway velocity (Taguchi and Tada, 1988), power spectral density (Diener *et al.*, 1984) and mean squared displacement (Black, 1982) and in part because different equipment has different sensitivities. Therefore there are difficulties with standardization. While intra-subject reproducibility has been reported as good (Thyssen *et al.*, 1982), there may be a significant learning effect (Holliday and Fermie, 1979).

Posturography has been used to quantify sway in cerebellar disease. Lesions of the spinocerebellar afferents cause an omnidirectional sway with preserved visual stabilization, while subjects with cerebellar hemisphere lesions have results within normal limits. Patients with vestibulocerebellar lesions display an omnidirectional low frequency sway which stabilizes poorly with vision. In anterior lobe atrophy a 3 Hz tremor is superimposed on low frequency anteroposterior sway oscillations (Dichgans *et al.*, 1976; Diener *et al.*, 1984). In patients with bilateral vestibular hypofunction, there is an increase in anteroposterior sway at 0.4 Hz (Tokita, Maeda and Miyata, 1981). In proprioceptive disorders due either to posterior column involvement or sensory neuropathy sway can be increased with eye closure. It had been claimed that vestibular abnormalities could be detected earlier than with other vestibular tests (Kapteyn and de Wit, 1972) but more recent work has not supported this claim. Voorhees (1989) obtained abnormal posturography scores in only 45% of patients with peripheral vestibular disease and 72% of patients with central vestibular disease. However, by adding head extension and a more complex calculation involving sway energy, Jackson, Epstein and Boyete (1991) increased the sensitivity to 68%. Nonetheless, at the present time, posturography is not a diagnostic tool.

Posturography may have a role in monitoring the course of vestibular compensation (Norre and Forrez, 1986; Shepard *et al.*, 1993).

Vestibular evoked responses

The recording of vestibular evoked responses is a research technique. It is not possible to record near-field vestibular neuronal responses non-invasively, therefore evoked responses have been considered. The criteria necessary to record evoked responses dictate that the response must have resolved before the next stimulus is delivered, and that sufficient stimulus-response data are collected to obtain a sufficiently high signal-to-noise ratio for a response to be recognized. The major difficulty of recording vestibular evoked responses is the long time constant of the mechanics of the vestibular system.

Other problems have complicated the interpretation of the early results (e.g. Greiner *et al.*, 1967; Salami *et al.*, 1975). In particular, the stimulus has to be refined to be specific to the vestibular endorgans and not involve cervical proprioceptive, visual or somatosensory receptors and the response itself can be contaminated by corneoretinal potentials. Hood and Kayan (1985) attempted to resolve the difficulties and determined an evoked response in subjects with vestibular function and none in subjects with absent vestibular function.

The limitations of vestibular tests

A major disadvantage of all types of vestibular test is that the normative data are not standardized and universal, such that normative data have to be collected for each set of equipment before it can be used for clinical diagnosis. The equipment for rotation tests, posturography and evoked responses is expensive. Space and completely darkened rooms are required. The rotating chair and the targets require great precision in being set up. Trained personnel are required. Despite these reservations, the use of posturography and rotation testing have become widespread (Honrubia *et al.*, 1980; Rubin, 1981). The main advantages are the access to hard copy data which allows detailed analysis of results from a variety of test paradigms for documentation purposes and research purposes and enables monitoring of treatment and rehabilitation.

Clinical vestibular syndromes

Unilateral peripheral vestibular lesions

An acute unilateral lesion of a labyrinth causes a typical picture (Magnus, 1924) with the animal developing nystagmus with the fast component directed away from the side of the lesion, the head is rotated to keep the affected ear lowermost, the trunk curling with the concavity on the contralateral side and the contralateral limbs extending.

After a unilateral peripheral vestibular lesion, there is a reduction in activity in the ipsilateral type I vestibular neurons in response to linear and angular acceleration. This leads to a reduction in the excitation of contralateral inhibitory type II neurons and therefore an increase in the activity of the contralateral type I neurons. A positive feedback circuit is set up with a resultant severe imbalance in spontaneous neuronal activity. The resulting data-set of vestibular, visual and proprioceptive inputs does not match the patterns integrated and stored since birth (Roberts, 1967) and so vertigo results with a sensation of rotation or imbalance to the side opposite to the lesion and an objective postural deviation to the side of the lesion by activation of intact vestibulospinal reflexes. There is also an imbalance in the vestibulo-ocular reflex, which causes the eyes to drift towards the side of the lesion with the fast phase in the opposite direction. There is no visual perception during a saccade, but in the slow phase, external objects seem to move in the opposite direction and thus aggravate the vertigo. The patient may automatically lie on the side of the lesion, so that the volitional angle of gaze is in the direction of the saccade, reducing the slow phase drift. If there is second or third degree nystagmus, there may be blurring of vision. After a few days, the ipsilateral type I neurons regain some spontaneous activity and respond to the stimulation of the intact contralateral labyrinth (Yagi and Markham, 1984).

The mechanisms for recovery are uncertain. The return of activity to the type I neurons causes excitation of the contralateral type II neurons and some inhibition of the contralateral type I neurons, so that a degree of compensation returns.

Benign paroxysmal positional vertigo

Benign paroxysmal positional vertigo was described by Barany (1921). In this condition, the patients give a history of positional vertigo – vertigo typically triggered by particular head movements. Although the Hallpike manoeuvre is essential for diagnosis of the clinical syndrome, it is not diagnostic of aetiology. In patients with benign paroxysmal positional vertigo, with the pathological ear undermost, the Hallpike manoeuvre produces a cluster of classical signs. There is a latent period of 2–20 seconds, followed by the development of rotational nystagmus, with the fast phase towards the ground (geotropic) and accompanied by vertigo. The vertigo and nystagmus adapt, but on sitting up, the nystagmus may reverse and is again accompanied by vertigo. Both the symptoms and signs fatigue on retesting.

Benign paroxysmal positional vertigo is unlikely to be the result of a single lesion. Various mechanisms have been postulated, and until recently the most widely accepted hypothesis was the *cupulolithiasis model* according to which degenerated dense material from the utricular macula becomes attached to the cupula of the posterior semicircular canal leading to the ampullofugal stimulation of the posterior semicircular canal when it is undermost (Schuknecht and Ruby, 1973). In support of this model is the specificity of the direction of stimulation required to produce the clinical picture, with the head inclined in the angle which would maximally stimulate the ampulla of the posterior semicircular canal (see Figure 4.28) and the effect of denervation of the posterior semicircular canal ampulla by section of its nerve (Gacek, 1978). While these observations would support the role of the posterior semicircular canal, the 'heavy cupula' concept has been called into question by the results of experiments where a heavy cupula is created by alcohol or deuterium ingestion, when the resulting nystagmus in a particular head position is sustained for long periods of time, rather than the classic picture in benign paroxysmal positional vertigo of transient nystagmus (Money, Johnson and Carlett 1970; Money and Myles, 1974). An alternative and increasingly popular hypothesis is that of the *canalithiasis model*, which suggests that the dense debris is localized in the long arm of the posterior semicircular canal (Hall, Ruby and McClure, 1979; Epley, 1980; Parnes and McClure, 1991). Other hypotheses include that of a single calcified mass (Vyslonzil, 1963) and non-homogeneous layering of endolymph (McClure, 1985).

Horiozontal semicircular canal variants of benign positional vertigo have been described (McClure, 1985; Pagnini, Nute and Vannucchi, 1989; Baloh, Jacobson and Honrubia, 1993). The patient experiences vertigo and exhibits intense geotropic horizontal nystagmus lasting approximately 60 seconds, not fatiguing on retesting when the head is turned (yaw) to the pathological side, reversing with less intense vertigo and nystagmus with a contralateral yaw.

Otolith dysfunction

A feature of vestibular dysfunction is that patients can present with symptoms which may appear bizarre and this is particularly true where the otolith organs are involved. As these organs mediate gravitational acceleration, dysfunction can lead to a false feeling of falling, or lateropulsion (being pushed to the side), or of the ground appearing to rise or fall, or of difficulty finding the visual vertical (aligning objects to the vertical) (Halmagyi, Gresty and Gibson, 1979). They may experience oscillopsia or vertigo when straining, coughing or sneezing (Healy, Strong and Sampogna, 1974). Their heads may tilt in response to loud sounds (Dieterich, Brandt and Fries, 1989) or they may have more obviously organic-sounding symptoms such as postural imbalance or oscillopsia or display ataxia (Brandt and Daroff, 1980a) or positional vertigo (Schuknecht and Ruby, 1973).

The effect of otolith dysfunction is to cause the eyes and head to skew in the vertical and oblique directions (the *ocular tilt reaction*), so patients may complain of diplopia and have a head tilt, for example, destruction of the left labyrinth may cause leftward head roll, leftward ocular counter-rolling with clockwise cyclorotation and the right eye to be higher than the left – a right-over-left skew deviation, i.e. hypotropia of the undermost eye, with deviation of the subjective visual vertical to the left (Halmagyi, Gresty and Gibson, 1979). The ocular tilt reaction can also be a manifestation of central pathology (see below).

Central vertigo

Pathology of the central structures integrating and relaying balance information and gaze fixation can cause vertigo, oscillopsia and imbalance. The clinical picture may be accompanied by symptoms and signs referable to adjacent neural structures.

Lesions of the *vestibular nuclei* cause vertigo and the patient falls or veers towards the side of the lesion. The involvement of central otolith pathways causes difficulty judging the visual vertical (Brandt and Daroff, 1980a). Nystagmus is often directed contralaterally, but may be ipsilateral, bilateral, vertical, torsional or dysconjugate (unequal in the two eyes). The loss of optic fixation causes a reduction in frequency with an increase in amplitude of nystagmus, while eye closure abolishes it, distinguishing it from a peripheral lesion (Korres, 1978). Caloric testing may reveal a canal paresis if the lesion involves the *vestibular nerve root entry zone* (Uemura and Cohen, 1973) or the *vestibular nuclei* (Francis *et al.*, 1992).

Lesions of the *brain stem* and *midbrain* cause vertigo. Nystagmus is usually bilateral and abolished or attenuated by the loss of optic fixation. Lesions of the low brain stem cause severe vertigo accompanied by vomiting and nystagmus, which is directed contralaterally to the lesion. Caloric testing rarely reveals a canal paresis, but there may be a contralateral directional preponderance. There may be downbeat nystagmus and pursuit eye movements downwards may be deranged. Lesions of the tegmentum of the ponto-medullary and pontomesencephalic junctions cause upbeat vertical nystagmus and there may also be an internuclear ophthalmoplegia or a gaze paresis (Troost *et al.*, 1980). Lesions of the posterior commissure cause rapid bilateral saccades without a normal saccadic interval of more than 200 ms (Zee and Robinson, 1979). Lesions around the IIIrd ventricle cause see-saw nystagmus, where one eye rises and intorts, while the other extorts and falls in reciprocal fashion (Daroff, 1965).

Mesencephalic lesions can cause a supranuclear gaze palsy, in which there is a loss of volitional gaze, with vertical movements lost before horizontal ones, but intact eye movements with vestibular stimulation.

Lesions involving the *cerebellum* may occasionally cause vertigo, which is usually most marked on positional testing. In primates, including man, cerebellar lesions have been shown to cause profound abnormalities of eye movements with an inability to maintain ipsilateral eccentric gaze and a loss of smooth pursuit eye movements and optokinetic nystagmus towards the pathological side (Westheimer and Blair, 1973, 1974). If the cerebellar lesion is unilateral, ipsilateral pursuit is impaired and there may be ipsilateral gaze evoked nystagmus. Caloric testing yields an ipsilateral directional preponderance (see below). Highly localized lesions of the flocculus produce vestibular abnormalities of spontaneous and positional nystagmus. Unilateral loss of the flocculus causes an ipsilateral loss of suppression of nystagmus by optic fixation (Takemori and Cohen, 1974), due to a loss of inhibition from cerebellar Purkinje cells (Lisberger and Fuchs, 1977). This leads to a failure of suppression of vestibulo-ocular reflex by optic fixation and a failure to enhance nystagmus with the loss of optic fixation in bithermal caloric testing (see below). Lesions of the flocculus also cause a reduction in slow phase velocity of optokinetic nystagmus (from about 100°/s to 40°/s). Lesions of the cerebellar hemispheres and paraflocculus do not have these effects. In man, cerebellar lesions cause dysmetric, often hypermetric saccades, but saccadic velocities and latencies are normal (Zee *et al.*, 1976).

Irritative lesions of the *cerebral cortex* can cause vertigo. Currie *et al.* (1971) reported that 16% of patients with temporal lobe epilepsy had vertigo as the aura or the entire ictal event. Lesions of the angular gyrus cause an ipsilateral directional preponderance on caloric and optokinetic testing. The caloric asymmetry is present only with fixation and the directional preponderance reverses in the dark (Carmichael *et al.*, 1961).

Ocular tilt reaction

The ocular tilt reaction consists of a coordinated lateral head tilt (roll) and dysconjugate or conjugate skew deviation with cyclorotation of both eyes towards the head tilt (clockwise with head tilt to the left; anti-clockwise with head tilt to the right) and hypotropia of the undermost eye.

It can be seen in lesions involving the otoliths (Halmagyi, Gresty and Gibson, 1979), the lateral medulla, e.g. in Wallenberg's syndrome (Brandt and Dieterich, 1987) and the rostral midbrain tegmentum of the upper brain stem (Brandt, Dieterich and Fries, 1988; Halmagyi *et al.*, 1990).

Patients with tonic ocular tilt reaction do not experience a perceptual tilt in the abnormal head position, but may if the head tilt is passively corrected. If the ocular tilt reaction is paroxysmal the patient may experience rotatory oblique oscillopsia.

Oscillopsia

The vestibulo-ocular reflex stabilizes the eyes during head movements. Therefore vestibular failure causes the eyes to lose fixation during head movements with a loss of dynamic visual acuity (visual acuity with head movement) and blurring of vision on walking. Frequently, the world appears to bob or move around in this condition. When eliciting a history of 'blurred vision' associated with movement, it is important to consider oscillopsia as a possible cause.

Oscillopsia can also be due to central lesions preventing gaze maintenance. Pretectal lesions may be associated with an alternating hypertropia developing spontaneously or on lateral gaze to each side. In this condition, the eye movements are slower and of larger amplitude than in see-saw nystagmus, which consists of alternating skew deviation and cyclodeviation with intorsion of the rising eye and extorsion of the falling eye. See-saw nystagmus is seen in lesions of the diencephalic–mesencephalic junction (Daroff, 1965). Oscillopsia is also sustained with paroxysmal ocular tilt reaction and vertical nystagmus.

Pressure vertigo

Changes in ambient pressure can cause transient disturbances of balance and vertigo even in the absence of aural pathology. This has been recorded in airmen (van Wulfften Palthe, 1922; Jones, 1957; Lundgren and Malm, 1966) and divers (Lundgren, 1973). The symptoms are more likely to develop where there are problems opening the eustachian tubes (Merica, 1942; Ingelstedt, Ivarsson and Tjernstrom, 1974). In some subjects vertigo can be precipitated by sneezing and coughing (Goodhill, 1981) and during the Valsalva manoeuvre.

There have been reports of an association between vertigo and otitis media in children (Busis, 1993) and the resolution of vertigo (Grace and Pfleiderer, 1990; Golz et al., 1991) and positional and spontaneous nystagmus (Golz et al., 1991) following middle ear ventilation. In acute otitis media there may be serous or toxic labyrinthitis (Gates, 1980; Blayney and Colman, 1984). Possibly, in other cases, there may be an asymmetry of pressures delivered to the round and oval windows of each ear with a resulting differential stimulation of the vestibular end-organs causing alternobaric vertigo. Vertigo was precipitated in healthy volunteers when exposed to pressure changes of 8.8 kPa in 25 s. The onset of vertigo and nystagmus occurred when the relative overpressure was > 5.9 kPa provided there was a definite asymmetry of middle ear pressures with different eustachian tube opening pressures (Ingelstedt, Ivarsson and Tjernstrom, 1974).

Some subjects report vertigo when exposed to loud sounds, *Tullio's phenomenon*, and sounds of sufficiently high intensity will induce nystagmus even in normal subjects (Dickson and Chadwick, 1951). Tullio (1929) reported on the effect of sound in normal animals, in rabbits eliciting slow movements in one direction of the head and torso, eyes, pinna, and front and rear legs. The effect is independent of a functioning cochlea, but requires a functioning vestibule (Kwee, 1976). Tullio's phenomenon is seen at < 110 dB in congenital deafness (Kwee, 1976) and in Menière's disease and has been reported in labyrinthitis and acoustic neuroma (Stephens and Ballam, 1974), chronic middle ear disease, particularly with cholesteatoma and perilymphatic fistula (Benjamins, 1938; Pyykko et al., 1992). The pathophysiology

may be multifactorial. The phenomenon can present when there is more than one mobile window on the vestibular side of the vestibular membrane. In subjects with endolymphatic hydrops the cause may be the ballooning of the membranous labyrinth with the saccule coming into contact with the stapes footplate (Kacker and Hinchcliffe, 1970; Nadol, 1974, 1977). It has been reported following the traumatic dislocation of the stapedovestibular joint (Kacker and Hinchcliffe, 1970). Kwee (1976) reported the Tullio's phenomenon in the Mondini–Alexander dysplasia where the enlarged saccule makes contact with the footplate (Altmann, 1950).

In some patients vertigo and nystagmus can be precipitated by transiently increasing or decreasing pressure in the external ear canal. The vertigo can consist of a sensation of rotation, movement or falling, or the patient may see the room tilt or experience oscillopsia. A Politzer bag and an olive tip or a Siegle's otoscope may be sufficient to carry out the test, although it is important to avoid performing an unintentional cold air caloric test. The response may be enhanced in the absence of optic fixation (with Frenzel glasses or in the dark with DC ENG chart recording) and with the affected ear uppermost (Uemura et al., 1977). The pressure test can elicit two signs: the fistula sign and Hennebert's sign (1911), suggesting different underlying pathophysiological mechanisms (Perlman and Leek, 1952).

The fistula sign can be elicited by either positive or negative pressure, although positive pressure usually produces a greater response and results in nystagmus lasting several seconds. The response may appear after a latency of 2–3 seconds, the amplitude may increase during the first few seconds and the response may persist for a few seconds after the removal of the stimulus (Nadol, 1977). Historically the fistula sign was associated with labyrinthine fistula (Lucae, 1881; Dohlman, 1953) and it may be seen in the presence of chronic suppurative otitis media with cholesteatoma as a manifestation of erosion of the bony labyrinth over the lateral semicircular canal. If a labyrinthine fistula were present, a positive pressure would be expected to lead to the ampullopetal deflection of the cupula with the resultant nystagmus towards the stimulated ear, with a negative pressure eliciting the opposite response. However, the opposite can happen (Dohlman, 1953) and, in some instances, both positive and negative pressure can cause nystagmus in the same direction.

Hennebert's sign is more usually present on negative pressure, which causes brief vertigo with two to four beats of eye movement lasting no more than 2 seconds. If it is also present with positive pressure, nystagmus in opposite directions may be elicited by alternating from positive to negative pressure. Horizontal or rotational nystagmus can be observed. A positive Hennebert's sign can be elicited in the absence of a perforation in the tympanic membrane in congenital syphilis (Hennebert, 1911; Asherson,

1931). In congenital syphilis, the pathological mechanisms suggested include gummatous osteitic erosion involving the periosteum, periosteal bone, endochondral bone and endosteum particularly around the semicircular canals (Fraser and Muir, 1917; Karmody and Schuknecht, 1966), loosening of the stapedial annular ligament (Mayer and Fraser, 1936) with abnormal stapes mobility (Perlman and Leek, 1952) and pathological adhesions, vestibulofibrosis, between the membranous labyrinth and the stapes footplate (Nadol, 1974). Nadol (1974) postulated that this is also the mechanism for Hennebert's sign in endolymphatic hydrops. Hennebert's sign has been reported to be present in many cases of perilymph fistula (Kohut, Haenel and Waldorf, 1979; Singleton, 1986), but not in pneumolabyrinth with perilymph fistula where, at exploratory tympanotomy, air bubbles were seen emerging through the ruptured round window (Yanagihara and Nishioka, 1987).

Epley (1981) described two patients with vertigo aggravated by eructation, hiccup or sneeze who exhibited a positive Hennebert's sign. In both cases the symptoms improved after tensor tympani transection, the suggested mechanism being that tensor tympani contraction moves the stapes medially by pulling the manubrium of the malleus anteromedially. However, the first patient also had shortened his Shea Teflon cup prosthesis over an oval window graft and the second underwent an endolymphatic sac decompression, which complicate the interpretation of the results of tensor tympani transection.

Cervical vertigo

The characteristic symptoms following the injection of local anaesthetic to the deep cervical area is a sensation of numbness and floating (de Jong *et al.*, 1977). The low sensitivity of the cervico-ocular reflex and its subordinate role to the vestibulo-ocular reflex suggest that vertigo is unlikely to be the result of cervical kinaesthetic involvement alone. There are also hypotheses that head movements can cause vertigo due to osteophytic compression of the vertebrobasilar arteries (Sheehan, Bauer and Meyer, 1960) or irritation of the cervical sympathetic plexus (Barre, 1926). If the compression of the vertebrobasilar arteries is to cause vertigo, significant pathology would also have to be present in the internal carotid arteries and circle of Willis and such extensive ischaemia is likely to lead to simultaneous neurological and cochlear symptoms. The clinical picture should include significant cervical pathology causing pain and cervical root symptoms and signs. Long tract signs due to spinal cord compression may also be expected. However, Rosengart *et al.* (1993) reported a case of lightheadedness, tinnitus and downbeat nystagmus precipitated by head yaw towards the dominant vestibular artery due to compression by osteophytes with reversal with the head in the primary position.

Falls in the elderly

Falls are common in the elderly (Luxon, 1991). Community studies indicate that over one-third of the population over the age of 65 years and nearly one-half of those over the age of 80 years had suffered one or more falls in the previous year (Campbell *et al.*, 1981; Perry, 1982). Dizziness in the elderly is also common, and was reported by 47% of men and 61% of women over the age of 70 years (Droller and Pemberton, 1953). However, the falls may be abrupt without warning and present as drop attacks. Table 4.1 lists causes of dizziness and falls in the elderly. While it is mandatory to assess the elderly fallers for visual and proprioceptive loss, cardiovascular factors (particularly aortic stenosis and dysrhythmias), musculoskeletal disorders, foot deformities (Gibson *et al.*, 1987) and vestibular dysfunction are common (Belal and Glorig, 1986; McClure, 1986; Norre, Forrez and Beckers, 1987).

There are age-dependent changes in the vestibular end-organs (Johnsson and Hawkins, 1972; Rosenhall and Rubin, 1975) and vestibular nerve (Bergstrom, 1973). However, the effects of these on vestibular function is unclear. A decline in vestibular function above 60 years of age was reported (Mulch and Petermann, 1979) but subsequent work has led to the validity of the results being questioned (Wall, Black and Hunt, 1984).

Age-dependent central vestibular changes may also develop with a loss of vestibular neurons in the vestibular nuclei and a loss of neurons in other areas of the brain stem (Meier–Ruge, Gigax and Wierspergen, 1980), in the Purkinje cells of the cerebellum (Hall, Miller and Corsellis, 1975) and in the temporoparietal cortex (Meier–Ruge, Gigax and Wierspergen, 1980).

There are age-dependent changes in reaction time (Overstall, 1978), the effects of which would be compounded by musculoskeletal factors. Mental tasks can reduce further postural stability in the elderly (Stelmach, Zelaznik and Loire, 1990).

Posturography confirms the degradation of postural stability with age (Sheldon, 1963; Corso, 1975; Black *et al.*, 1977) and demonstrates that a loss of vestibular function tends to cause a greater loss of postural stability in the elderly than the young (Norre, Forrez and Beckers, 1987), confirming that the effect of vestibular dysfunction is compounded by age-dependent changes in visual perception (Bender, 1975), proprioception (Arnold and Harriman, 1977; Wyke, 1979; Pyykko, Jantti and Aalto, 1988) and changes in cervical compensatory mechanisms due to damaged mechanoreceptors in the cervical apophyseal joints (Wyke, 1979). Drachman and Hart (1972) identified multisensory dizziness as the third major cause of unsteadiness in the elderly.

Table 4.1 Causes of dizziness and falls

Otological	Idiopathic	Peripheral vestibular lesions
		Menière's disease
		Benign paroxysmal positional vertigo
		Acoustic neuroma
		Cholesteatoma
		Otosclerosis
		Glomus tumour
		Temporal bone lesions
	Trauma	Labyrinthine contusion
	Infective	Chronic middle ear disease
		Viral labyrinthitis
		Syphilis
		Tuberculosis
		Ramsay Hunt syndrome
Neurological	Ischaemic, haemorrhagic and mitotic	Cerebellopontine angle lesions
		Pontine and medullary lesions
		Cerebellar lesions
		Internal capsule and thalamic lesions
		Cerebral hemisphere lesions
	Idiopathic	Epilepsy
		Parkinsonism
		Steele-Richardson syndrome
		Shy-Drager syndrome
		Demyelination, e.g. multiple sclerosis
		Hydrocephalus
		Spinocerebellar degeneration
		Sensorineuropathy
	Infective	Meningitis, neurosyphilis, borellia
	Trauma	Subdural and extradural haematomas
		Whiplash injury
Visual		Ocular pathology
		Retro-orbital lesions
		Diplopia
Vascular diseases	Cerebrovascular	Vertebrobasilar insufficiency
		Subclavian steal syndrome
		Wallenberg's syndrome
		Vasculitides
	Cardiovascular	Postural hypotension
		Syncope
		Carotid sinus syndrome
		Cardiac dysrhythmia
		Mechanical cardiac dysfunction
Haematological		Anaemia
		Hyperviscosity syndromes, haemoglobinopathies
Skeletal		Foramen magnum abnormalities
		Cervical abnormalities
		Osteoarthritis
		Arthritides
		Paget's disease
Iatrogenic	Pharmacological complications	Hypotension, hypoglycaemia, central vestibular dysfunction, confusion, dyskinesia, dystonia
	Appliances	Inappropriate walking aids
		Inappropriate cervical collars
		Inappropriate lenses
	Surgery	
Psychogenic		
Mitotic	Secondary extension	Nasopharynx
		External ear
	Metastases	
Toxin		Ethanol, carbon monoxide
Endocrine		Hypothyroidism
		Hypoglycaemia

Motion sickness

Consideration of the clinical applications of vestibular physiology must include the entity of motion sickness, which is a normal physiological response to certain types of real or apparent motion. Motion sickness is characterized by nausea, vomiting, pallor and cold sweating, and may be sustained during sea, air, car, space and camel travel. However, it is also commonly encountered in children on swings or at fun fairs, in space and aircraft simulators.

For many years, motion sickness has been ascribed to vestibular 'overstimulation', but this hypothesis is difficult to substantiate as certain observations cannot be explained on this basis. Strong, unfamiliar stimuli, such as the repeated stops of a rotating chair, do not tend to induce motion sickness, whereas combinations of linear and angular accelerations, such as voluntary or involuntary head movements during simultaneous rotation about the vertical axis, are highly provocative (Guedry, 1970). In addition, it is well established that the purely visual stimuli may also produce a 'motion sickness' syndrome (Dichgans and Brandt, 1973). Subjects with a strong history of motion sickness may display a hyperactive vestibulo-ocular reflex, or altered hip sway strategy or positional nystagmus (Hamid, 1991). The currently accepted explanation of motion sickness is based on a suspected mismatch between sensory information arising from the eyes, the labyrinth or other receptors stimulated by motion forces, or between these signals of actual sensory input and those of the expected sensory input, as determined by the central nervous system in the light of previous experience (Reason, 1970, 1978).

The pathways subserving the neurophysiological mechanisms which result in motion sickness are poorly established. It is well recognized that the vestibular apparatus and vestibular projections in the cerebellum are essential for the development of motion sickness. Convergence of vestibular, visual and somatosensory afferents can be identified at the level of the vestibular nuclei (Wilson and Melville-Jones, 1979), and it is at this level, therefore, that matching of actual and expected motion cues may take place. Although supratentorial structures are involved in motion sickness, they are not essential, as the condition has been documented in both the decorticate dog and man (Reason and Brandt, 1975). It therefore seems likely that the vestibulocerebellum and the vestibular nuclei are prerequisites for the development of motion sickness. Although some people are sensitive to the development of motion sickness, others are highly resistant (Jongkees, 1974) and the reasons influencing susceptibility are not understood.

Medical management of vestibular disorders

Vestibular compensation and rehabilitation

Following a unilateral vestibular insult the patient experiences vertigo, but usually, the symptoms are relatively short-lived. Electrophysiological studies indicate that following labyrinthectomy, there is a loss of activity in the unilateral secondary vestibular neurons of the vestibular nuclei, but then there is a return of activity to the deafferented vestibular neurons (Precht, Shimazu and Markham, 1966). In animal studies, if a second labyrinthectomy is performed after compensation, the animal again develops signs of acute vestibular loss with nystagmus directed towards the previously operated ear, as if the first labyrinthectomy had not taken place (Bechterew's compensatory nystagmus 1883). Compensation again takes place, usually faster than after the first labyrinthectomy. This would suggest that the deafferented vestibular neurons recover spontaneous activity.

The recovery of the vestibulo-ocular and vestibulo-spinal reflexes are similar if the lesion is in the peripheral vestibular system, but differ considerably if the lesion is in the central vestibular system (Petrone, de Benedittis and de Candia, 1991). Compensation is also more rapid after labyrinthectomy than vestibular neurectomy, suggesting that the vestibular nerve contributes in some way to recovery (Cass and Goshgarin, 1991).

The vestibular system is also extremely adaptable. Prisms can cause the visual perception of moving targets to be reversed and yet normal subjects can learn to compensate and function well. This compensation extends as far as a reversal of the vestibulo-ocular reflex following rotation in the dark (Gonshor and Melville Jones, 1976).

A bilateral loss of vestibular function will cause oscillopsia. Some recovery of function may be due to the cervico-ocular reflex (Dichgans *et al.*, 1973; Bles, de Jong and Rasmussens, 1984; Bronstein and Hood, 1987), though it is also likely that the slip of the retinal image may be compensated for by central visual mechanisms as occurs in congenital nystagmus (Buchelle, Brandt and Degner, 1983) and oculomotor palsies (Wist, Brandt and Krafczyk, 1983). This hypothesis is supported by the reduced optokinetic response seen in patients with long-standing vestibular failure (Zee, Yee and Robinson, 1976).

In some patients recovery does not happen. The persisting symptoms are usually not the acute symptoms of severe rotational vertigo, but are less dramatic, sometimes mild and continuous, with short-lived exacerbations usually triggered by clear-cut stimuli, such as changes of head position or exposure to visual stimuli, e.g. ironing striped materials, patterned floors and walls, escalators and walking between supermarket shelves. The vertigo is often not rotational, but consists of floating or rocking sensations. These symptoms can cause severe social handicap, including a loss of earning capacity and may result in psychological disorders (Eagger *et al.*, 1992). The reasons why some patients do not compensate is uncertain. Rudge and Chambers (1982) suggested that cerebellar damage, impairment of proprioception and visual impairment will contribute to the persistence of vestibular symptoms.

Vestibular habituation training has been applied in the management of vertigo due to peripheral vestibular dysfunction for over 50 years (Cawthorne, 1944; Cooksey, 1945). Other techniques include the Brandt-Daroff exercises (1980b), the Semont manoeuvre (Semont, Freyss and Vitte, 1988) and the Epley manoeuvre (1992).

Animal studies have offered some insight into the mechanism of vestibular rehabilitation training. Exercise appears to expedite, while physical confinement appears to impair rehabilitation. Lacour, Roll and Appaix (1976) demonstrated that restraining a baboon in a plaster cast inhibited compensation, while Igarashi *et al.* (1981) demonstrated that 2.5 hours daily exercise improved gait deviation in unilateral labyrinthectomized squirrel monkeys. Similarly, visual experience expedites, while deprivation impairs, rehabilitation. Courjon *et al.* (1977) demonstrated that exposure to light caused a more rapid loss of spontaneous nystagmus than captivity in the dark and Fetter, Zee and Proctor (1988) showed that occipital lobectomy prior to labyrinthectomy caused impaired compensation and then only for low speeds of rotation (30–60°/s). A loss of proprioception, due for example to cervical transection delays compensation (Schaefer and Meyer, 1973). Vestibular sedatives also delay compensation (Lacom and Xerri, 1984).

The mechanisms of compensation are unknown, but several hypotheses have been advanced and in particular compensation may be an example of *CNS plasticity* (Dieringer and Precht, 1977). There is considerable evidence for the involvement of the cerebellum in the modulation of the vestibular system in relation to visual input (Ito, 1972). The cerebellum receives not only vestibular information from first and second order vestibular neurons, but also visual information via climbing fibres from the dorsal cap of the inferior olive which pass to the Purkinje cells of the cerebellar flocculus. The ablation of the dorsal cap of the inferior olive compromises the plasticity of the vestibular system (Haddad, Demer and Robinson, 1980). While cerebellectomy, spinal cord section and oblique and vertical midline midbrain section do not reduce the recovery of spontaneous activity in the vestibular nuclei, the cerebellum and the commissural fibres act to reduce the activity of contralateral vestibular nuclei. Therefore, the compensatory process may involve these pathways (McCabe, Ryu and

Sekitani, 1972; Schaefer and Meyer, 1973). Vestibular compensation has been explained on the basis of *reactive synaptogenesis* with the development of new synapses and axonal sprouts. While this has been demonstrated in the frog (Dieringer, Kunzle and Precht, 1984), it has not been demonstrated in mammals. Following denervation, supersensitivity to neurotransmitters can develop but, to date, *denervation supersensitivity* has not been demonstrated in the vestibular nuclei to GABA, acetylcholine (Calza *et al.*, 1989) or glutamate. Compensation may be the result of increased neurotransmitter release into the deafferented nuclei from the remaining inputs (Errington, Lynch and Bliss, 1987). It has also been demonstrated that vestibular nuclei neurons can generate resting activity *in vitro* and in isolated slices, suggesting that there may be intrinsic membrane properties which could explain the recovery of function (Darlington, Smith and Hubbard, 1989). Jones and Nelson (1992) demonstrated a return of function to the ipsilateral vestibular nerve after streptomycin-induced vestibular hair cell loss and suggested that this may be evidence of a return of hair cell function.

In benign paroxysmal positional vertigo, the repositioning of debris from around the cupula (Brandt and Daroff, 1980b; Semont, Freyss and Vitte, 1988) or the cupula (Epley, 1992; Herdman *et al.*, 1993) of the posterior semicircular canal can be curative, indicating that recovery is due to mechanical changes in the labyrinth. In other conditions, physiological or psychological adaptation and the control of hyperventilation (Theunissen, Huygen and Folgering, 1986) have a role as demonstrated in several studies on active vestibular rehabilitation therapy (Dix, 1979; Norre, 1987; Norre and Beckers, 1988; Shepard *et al.*, 1993). Vestibular rehabilitation therapy is also required to expedite recovery after posterior ampullary neurectomy and posterior canal occlusion for benign paroxysmal positional vertigo (Parnes, 1994).

References

ABEL, S. and BARBER, H. O. (1981) Measurement of optokinetic nystagmus for otoneurological diagnosis. *Annals of Otology, Rhinology and Laryngology*, **90**, 1–12

AGATE, J. (1963) *The Practice of Geriatrics*. London: Heinemann. p. 91

AJODHIA, J. M. and DIX, M. R. (1975) Ototoxic effects of drugs. *Minerva Otorhinolaringologica*, **25**, 117–131

ALPERT, J. N. (1978) Downbeat nystagmus due to anticonvulsant toxicity. *Annals of Neurology*, **4**, 471–473

ALTMANN, F. (1950) Histologic picture of inherited nerve deafness in man and animals. *Archives of Otolaryngology*, **51**, 852–890

AMANO, H., ORSULAKOVA, A. and MORGENSTERN, C. (1983) Intracellular and extracellular ion content of the endolymphatic sac. *Archives of Otorhinolaryngology*, **237**, 273–277

ANDERSEN, H. C. (1948) Passage of trypan blue into the

endolymphatic system of the labyrinth. *Acta Otolaryngologica*, **36**, 273–283

ANDERSON, J. H., SOECHTING, J. F. and TERZUOLO, C. A. (1979) Role of vestibular inputs in the organization of motor output to the forelimb extensors. *Progress in Brain Research*, **50**, 582–596

ANNIKO, M. and WROBLEWSKI, R. (1986) Ionic environment of cochlear hair cells. *Hearing Research*, **22**, 279–293

ARNOLD, N. and HARRIMAN, D. G. (1977) The incidence of abnormality in control human peripheral nerves, studied by single axon dissection. *Journal of Laryngology and Otology*, **33**, 55–61

ARNOTT, F. J. and MILLER, S. J. H. (1970) Seesaw nystagmus. *Transactions of the Ophthalmological Society of the UK*, **84**, 251–257

ASHERSON, N. (1931) The ear in congenital syphilis: some clinical observations. *Journal of Laryngology*, **46**, 326–331

BAIRD, R. A., DESMADRYL, G., FERNANDEZ, C. and GOLDBERG, J. M. (1988) The vestibular nerve of the chinchilla. II Relation between afferent response properties and peripheral innervation patterns in the semicircular canals. *Journal of Neurophysiology*, **60**, 182–203

BAKER, R. G., PRECHT, W. and LLIMAS, R. (1973) Cerebellar modullatory action on the vestibulo-cochlear pathway in the cat. *Experimental Brain Research*, **15**, 364–385

BALOH, R. W. and HONRUBIA, V. (1979) *Clinical Neurophysiology of the Vestibular System*. Philadelphia: F. A. Davis Company

BALOH, R. W., HONRUBIA, V. and KONRAD, H. R. (1976) Periodic alternating nystagmus. *Brain*, **99**, 11–26

BALOH, R. W., HONRUBIA, V. and SILLS, A. (1977) Eye tracking and optokinetic nystagmus: results of quantitative testing in patients with well-defined nervous system lesions. *Annals of Otology, Rhinology and Laryngology*, **86**, 108–114

BALOH, R. W., JACOBSON, K. and HONRUBIA, V. (1993) Horizontal semicircular canal variant of benign positioning vertigo. *Neurology*, **43**, 2542–2549

BALOH, R. W., KONRAD, H. R. and HONRUBIA, V. (1975) Vestibulo-ocular function in patients with cerebellar atrophy. *Neurology*, **25**, 160–168

BALOH, R. W., YEE, R. D. and HONRUBIA, V. (1980) Optokinetic asymmetry in patients with maldeveloped foveas. *Brain Research*, **186**, 211–216

BALOH, R. W., YEE, R. D. and HONRUBIA, V. (1982) Clinical abnormalities of optokinetic nystagmus. In: *Functional Basis of Ocular Motility Disorders*, edited G. Lennerstrand, D. S. Lee and E. L. Keller. Oxford: Pergamon. pp. 311–320

BALOH, R. W., BEYKIRCH, K., HONRUBIA, V. and YEE, R. D. (1988a) Eye movements induced by linear acceleration on a parallel swing. *Journal of Neurophysiology*, **60**, 2000–2014

BALOH, R. W., YEE, R. D., HONRUBIA, V. and JACOBSON, K. (1988b) A comparison of the dynamics of horizontal and vertical smooth pursuit in normal human subjects. *Aviation Space and Environmental Medicine*, **59**, 121–124

BALOH, R. W., YEE, R. D., JENKINS, H. A. and HONRUBIA, V. (1982) Quantitative assessment of visual-vestibular interaction using sinusoidal rotatory stimuli. In: *Nystagmus and Vertigo: Clinical Approaches to the Patient with Dizziness*, edited by V. Honrubia and M. A. B. Brazier. New York: Academic Press. pp. 231–239

BARANY, R. VON (1921) Diagnose von Krankheitser-scheinungen im Bereiche des Otolithenapparates. *Acta Otolaryngologica*, **2**, 434–437

BARANY, R. VON (1922) Zur Klinik und Theorie des Eisenbahn-nystagmus. *Acta Otolaryngologica*, **3**, 260–265

BARIGANT, P., MERLET, P. and ORFAIT, J. (1972) New design of ELA statokinestiometer. *Agressologie*, **13C**, 69–74

BARLOW, J. S. (1970) Vestibular and non-dominant parietal lobe disorders. (Two aspects of spatial disorientation in man). *Diseases of the Nervous System*, **31**, 667–673

BARNES, G. R. (1979) Vestibulo-ocular function during coordinated head and eye movements to acquire visual targets. *Journal of Physiology*, **287**, 127–147

BARNES, G. R. (1980) Vestibular mechanisms. *Clinical Physics and Physiological Measurement*, **1**, 3–40

BARON, J. B. (1978) Statokinesimetrie. *Les Feuillets du Practicien*, **2**, 23–31

BARRATT, H., BRONSTEIN, A. M. and GRESTY, M. A. (1987) Testing the vestibular-ocular reflexes: abnormalities of the otolith contribution in patients with neuro-otological disease. *Journal of Neurology, Neurosurgery and Psychiatry*, **50**, 1029–1035

BARRÉ, J. A. (1926) Sur un syndrome sympathique cervical posterieur et sa cause frequente: l'arthrite cervicale. *Revue de Neurologie*, **45**, 1246–1253

BAUMGARTEN, R. VON, BENSON, A. and BERTHOZ, A. (1984) Effects of rectilinear acceleration and optokinetic and caloric stimulations in space. *Science*, **225**, 208–212

BECHTEREW, W. (1883) Ergebnisse der Durchschneidung des N. acusticus, nebst Erorterung der Bedeutung der semicircularen Canale fur das Korpergleichgewicht. *Pflugers Archiv für die Gesamte Physiologie des Menschen und der Tiere*, **30**, 312

BECKER W. and FUCHS, A. F. (1969) Further properties of the human saccadic system: eye movements and correction saccades with and without visual fixation points. *Vision Research*, **9**, 1247–1258

BEGBIE, G. H. (1967) Some problems of postural sway. In: *Myotatic Kinesthetic and Vestibular Mechanisms*, edited by A. V. S. de Reuck and J. Knight. Boston: Little Brown & Co. pp. 80–92

BEKESY, G. (1952) DC resting potentials inside the cochlear partition. *Journal of the Acoustic Society of America*, **24**, 72–76

BEKESY, G. (1966) Pressure and shearing forces as stimuli of labyrinthine epithelium. *Archives of Otolaryngology*, **84**, 122–130

BELAL, A. and GLORIG, A. (1986) Disequilibrium of aging (presbyastasis). *Journal of Laryngology and Otology*, **100**, 1037–1041

BENDER, M. B. (1965) Oscillopsia. *Archives of Neurology*, **13**, 204–213

BENDER, M. (1975) The incidence and type of perceptual deficiencies in the aged. In: *Neurological and Sensory Disorders in the Elderly*, edited by W. S. Fields. New York: Stratton Intercontinental. pp. 15–31

BENJAMINS, C. E. (1938) Les reactions acoustiques de Tullio chez l'homme. *Acta Otolaryngologica*, **26**, 249–257

BENSON, A. J. (1978) Spatial disorientation. In: *Aviation Medicine, Vol. 1. Physiology and Human Factors*, edited by G. Drenin and J. Emsting. London: Tri-Med Books. pp. 405–467

BENSON, A. J. and BARNES, G. R. (1973) Responses to rotating linear acceleration vectors considered in relation to a model of the otolith organs. *Fifth NASA Symposium on the Role of the Vestibular Organs in the Exploration of Space*, Pensacola, Florida. SP-314, Washington DC: NASA. pp. 221–236

BERGSTROM, B. (1973) Morphology of the vestibular nerve. *Acta Otolaryngologica*, **76**, 331–338

BERTHOZ, A. and LLINAS, R. (1974) Afferent neck projections to the cat cerebellar cortex. *Experimental Brain Research*, **20**, 285–401

BIZZI, E. and SCHILLER, P. H. (1970) Single unit activity in the frontal eye fields of unanaesthetised monkeys during eye and head movements. *Experimental Brain Research*, **10**, 151–158

BIZZI, E., KALIL, R. E. and TAGLIASCO, V. (1971) Eye-head coordination in monkeys: evidence for centrally-patterned organisation. *Science*, **173**, 452–454

BLACK, F. O. (1982) Vestibular function assessment in patients with Meniere's disease: the vestibulo-spinal system. *Laryngoscope*, **92**, 1419–1435

BLACK, F. O. and NASHNER, L. M. (1984) Vestibulospinal control differs in patients with reduced versus distorted vestibular function. *Acta Otolaryngologica Supplementum*, **404**, 110–114

BLACK, F. O., O'LEARY, D. P., WALL, C. and FURMAN, J. (1977) The vestibulo-spinal stability test: normal limits. *Transactions of the American Academy of Ophthalmology and Otolaryngology*, **84**, 549–560

BLAYNEY, A. W. and COLMAN, B. H. (1984) Dizziness in childhood. *Clinical Otolaryngology*, **9**, 77–85

BLES, W., DE JONG, J. M. B. and RASMUSSENS, J. J. (1984) Postural and oculomotor signs in labyrinthine defective subjects. *Acta Otolaryngologica*, Suppl. 406, 101–104

BOGOUSSLAVSKY, J., REGLI, F. and HUNBERBUHLER, J. P. (1980) Downbeat nystagmus. *Neuro-ophthalmology*, **1**, 137–143

BOTTINI, G., STERZI, R., PAULESU, E., VALLAR, G., CAPPA, S. F., ERMINIO, F. *et al.* (1994) Identification of the central vestibular projections in man: a positron emission tomography activation study. *Experimental Brain Research*, 99, 164–169

BRANDT, T. (1991) Man in motion. Historical and clinical aspects of vestibular function. A review. *Brain*, **114**, 2159–2174

BRANDT, T. and DAROFF, R. B. (1980a) The multisensory physiological and pathological vertigo syndromes. *Annals of Neurology*, **7**, 195–203

BRANDT, T. and DAROFF, R. B. (1980b) Physical therapy for benign paroxysmal positional vertigo. *Archives of Otolaryngology*, **106**, 484–485

BRANDT, T. and DIETERICH, M. (1987) Pathological eye-head coordination in roll: tonic ocular tilt reaction in mesencephalic and medullary lesions. *Brain*, **110**, 649–666

BRANDT, T., BUCHELE, W. and ARNOLD, F. (1977) Arthrokinetic nystagmus and ego-motion sensation. *Experimental Brain Research*, **30**, 331–338

BRANDT, T., DIETERICH, M. and FRIES, W. (1988) Otolithic Tullio phenomenon typically presents as paroxysmal ocular tilt reaction. *Advances in Oto-Rhino-Laryngology*, **42**, 153–156

BRODAL, A. (1974) The anatomy of the vestibular nuclei and their connections. In: *Handbook of Sensory Physiology: The Vestibular System*, edited by H. H. Kornhuber, Vol. VI, Part 1. New York: Springer-Verlag. pp. 239–352

BRONSTEIN, A. M. (1988) Evidence for a vestibular input contributing to dynamic head stabilization in man. *Acta Otolaryngologica*, **105**, 1–6

BRONSTEIN, A. M. and GRESTY, M. A. (1988) Short latency eye movement responses to transient linear head acceleration: a specific function of otolith-ocular reflex. *Experimental Brain Research*, **71**, 406–410

BRONSTEIN, A. M. and GRESTY, M. A. (1991) Compensatory eye movements in the presence of conflicting canal and otolith signals. *Experimental Brain Research*, **85**, 697–700

BRONSTEIN, A. M. and HOOD, J. D. (1986) The cervico-ocular reflex in normal subjects and patients with absent vestibular function. *Brain Research*, **373**, 399–408

BRONSTEIN, A. M. and HOOD, J. D. (1987) Oscillopsia of peripheral vestibular origin: central and cervical compensatory mechanisms. *Acta Otolaryngologica*, **104**, 307–314

BRONSTEIN, A. M. and KENNARD, C. (1987) Predictive eye saccades are different from visually triggered saccades. *Vision Research*, **27**, 517–520

BRONSTEIN, A. M. and RUDGE, P. (1986) Vestibular involvement in spasmodic torticollis. *Journal of Neurology, Neurosurgery and Psychiatry*, **49**, 290–295

BRONSTEIN, A. M., RUDGE, P., GRESTY, M. A., DU BOULAY, G. and MORRIS, J. (1990) Abnormalities of horizontal gaze. Clinical, oculographic and magnetic resonance imaging findings. II. Gaze palsy and internuclear ophthalmoplegia. *Journal of Neurology, Neurosurgery and Psychiatry*, **53**, 200–207

BRUCE, C. J. and GOLDBERG, M. E. (1985) Primate frontal eye fields. I. Single neurones discharging before saccades. *Journal of Neurophysiology*, **53**, 603–635

BRUCHER, J. M. (1964) *L'aire oculogyre frontal du singe.* Brussels: Arscia

BUCHELLE, W., BRANDT, T. and DEGNER, D. (1983) Ataxia and oscillopsia in downbeat-nystagmus vertigo syndrome. *Advances in Otorhinolaryngology*, **30**, 291–297

BUETTNER, U., BUETTNER–ENNEVER, J. A. and HENN, V. (1977) Vertical eye movements related to unit activity in the rostral mesencephalic reticular formation of the alert monkey. *Brain Research*, **130**, 234–252

BUISSERET, P., GARY-BOBO, E. and IMBERT, M. (1978) Ocular motility may be involved in recovery of orientational properties of visual cortical neurons in dark-reared kittens. *Nature*, **272**, 816–817

BUIZZA, A., LEGER, A., DROULEZ, J., BERTHOZ, A. and SCHMID, R. (1980) Influence of otolithic stimulation by linear acceleration on optokinetic nystagmus and visual motor perception. *Experimental Brain Research*, **39**, 165–176

BUSIS, S. N. (1993) Vertigo. In: *Pediatric Otolaryngology*, edited by C. D. Bluestone and S. E. Stool. Philadelphia: W. B. Saunders Co. pp. 261–270

CALZA, L., GIARDINO, L., ZANNI, M., GALETTI, R., PARCHI, P. and GALETTI, G. (1989) Involvement of cholinergic and GABA-ergic systems in vestibular compensation. In: *Vestibular compensation: Facts, Theories, and Clinical Perspectives*, edited by M. Lacour, M. Toupet, P. Denise and Y. Christen. Paris: Elsevier. pp. 189–199

CAMPBELL, A. J., REINKEN, J., ALLAN, B. C. and MARTINEZ, G.S. (1981) Falls in old age: a study of frequency and related clinical factors. *Age and Ageing*, **10**, 264–270

CARLBORG, B. (1981) On physiological and experimental variation of the perilymphatic pressure in the cat. *Acta Otolaryngologica*, **91**, 19–28

CARMICHAEL, E. A., DIX, M. R., HALLPIKE, C. S. and HOOD, J. D. (1961) Some further observations upon the effect of unilateral cerebral lesions on caloric and rotational nystagmus. *Brain*, **102**, 527–558

CASS, S. P. and GOSHGARIAN, H. G. (1991) Vestibular compensation after labyrinthectomy and vestibular neurectomy in cats. *Otolaryngology – Head and Neck Surgery*, **104**, 14–19

CASTON, J. and ROUSELL, H. (1984) Curare and the efferent vestibular system. An electrophysiological study in the frog. *Acta Otolaryngologica*, **97**, 19–26

CAWTHORNE, T. (1944) The physiological basis for head exercises. *Journal of the Chartered Society of Physiotherapists*, **30**, 106–107

CAWTHORNE, T. E. (1952) Vertigo. *British Medical Journal*, **2**, 931–933

CLARK, B. (1967) Thresholds for the perception of angular acceleration in man. *Aerospace Medicine*, **38**, 443–450

CLARK, B. (1970) The vestibular system. *Annual Review of Psychology*, **21**, 273–306

COATS, A. C. and SMITH, Y. (1967) Body position and the intensity of caloric nystagmus. *Acta Otolaryngologica*, **63**, 515–532

COGAN, D. G. (1956) *Neurology of the Ocular Muscles*. Springfield: C. C. Thomas

COGAN, D. G. (1967) Congenital nystagmus. *Canadian Journal of Ophthalmology*, **2**, 4–10

COGAN, D. G. (1968) Downbeat nystagmus. *Archives of Ophthalmology*, **80**, 757–768

COGAN, D. G. and BURROWS, L. J. (1954) Platybasia and the Arnold–Chiari malformation. *Archives of Ophthalmology*, **52**, 13–29

COGAN, D. G., KUBIK, C. S. and SMITH, W. L. (1950) Unilateral internuclear ophthalmoplegia: report on 8 clinical cases with post-mortem study. *Archives of Ophthalmology*, **44**, 783–796

COHEN, B. and HENN, V. (1972) Unit activity of the pontine reticular formation associated with eye movements. *Brain Research*, **46**, 403–410

COHEN, B., SUZUKI, J. I. and BENDER, M. B. (1964) Eye movements from semicircular canal nerve stimulation in the cat. *Annals of Otology, Rhinology and Laryngology*, **73**, 153–169

COLLEWIJN, H. (1972) An analogue model of the rabbit's optokinetic system. *Brain Research*, **36**, 71–88

COLLEWIJN, H. and VAN DEN MARK, F. (1972) Ocular stability in variable visual feedback conditions in the rabbit. *Brain Research*, **36**, 47–57

COLLEWIJN, H., VAN DER MARK, F., and JANSEN, T. C. (1975) Precise recording of human eye movements. *Vision Research*, **15**, 447–450

COLLEWIJN, H., WINTERSON, B. and DUBOIS M. F. W. (1978) Optokinetic eye movements in albino rabbits: inversion in the anterior visual field. *Science*, **199**, 1351–1353

COLLINS, W. E. (1974a) Arousal and vestibular habituation. In: *Handbook of Sensory Physiology: The Vestibular System*, edited by H. H. Kornhuber. Vol. VI. New York: Springer–Verlag. pp. 361–368

COLLINS, W. E. (1974b) Habituation of vestibular responses with and without visual stimulation. In: *Handbook of Sensory Physiology: The Vestibular System*, edited by H. H. Kornhuber. Vol. VI. New York: Springer–Verlag. pp. 369–388

COOKSEY, F. S. (1945) Rehabilitation of vestibular injuries. *Proceedings of the Royal Society of Medicine*, **39**, 273–278

COOPER, S. and DANIEL, P. M. (1963) Muscle spindles in man: their morphology in the lumbricals and the deep muscles of the neck. *Brain*, **86**, 563–586

COREY, D. P. and HUDSPETH, A. J. (1979) Ionic basis of the receptor potential in a vertebrate hair cell. *Nature*, **281**, 675–677

COREY, D. P. and HUDSPETH, A. J. (1983) Kinetics of the receptor current in bullfrog saccular hair cells. *Journal of Neuroscience* **3**, 962–976

CORSO, J. F. (1975) Sensory processes in man during maturity and senescence. In: *Neurobiology of Ageing: An Interdisciplinary Life-span Approach*, edited by J. M. Ordy and K. R. Brizzee. New York: Plenum Press. pp. 119–145

COURJON, J. H., JEANNEROD, M., OSSUZIO, I. and SCHMID, R. (1977) The role of vision in compensation of vestibuloocular reflex after hemilabyrinthectomy in the cat. *Experimental Brain Research*, **28**, 235–248

COX, T. A., CORBETT, J. J., THOMPSON, H. S. and LENNARSON, L. (1981) Upbeat nystagmus changing to downbeat nystagmus with convergence. *Neurology*, **31**, 891–892

CRITCHLEY, M. (1953) *The Parietal Lobes*. London: Arnold

CURRIE, S., HEATHFIELD, K. W. G., HENSON, R. A. and SCOTT, D. F. (1971) Clinical course and prognosis of temporal lobe epilepsy. *Brain*, **94**, 173–190

DARLINGTON, C. L., SMITH, P. F. and HUBBARD, J. I. (1989) Neuronal activity in the guinea pig medial vestibular nucleus in vitro following chronic unilateral labyrinthectomy. *Neuroscience Letters*, **105**, 143–148

DAROFF, R. B. (1965) See-saw nystagmus. *Neurology*, **15**, 874–877

DAROFF, R. B., TROOF, B. T. and DELL'OSSO, L. F. (1978) Nystagmus and related ocular oscillations. In: *Neuro-Ophthalmology*, edited by J. S. Glaser. Hagarstown: Harper and Row. pp. 219–243

DECHESNE, C., RAYMOND, J. and SANS, A. (1984) Action of glutamate in the cat labyrinth. *Annals of Otology, Rhinology and Laryngology*, **93**, 163–165

DE JONG, P. I. V. M., DE JONG, J. M. V. B., COHEN, B. and JONGKEES, L. B. W. (1977) Ataxia and nystagmus induced by injection of local anaesthetic in the neck. *Annals of Neurology*, **1**, 240–246

DE KLEYN, A. and STENVERS, H. W. (1941) Tonic neck reflexes on the eye muscles in man. *Proceedings of the Koninklijke Nederlandse Akademie van Wetenschappen*, **44**, 385–396

DELL'OSSO, L. F. (1985) Congenital, latent and manifest latent nystagmus – similarities, differences and relations to strabismus. *Japanese Journal of Ophthalmology*, **29**, 351–368

DEMANEZ, J. P. and LEDOUX, A. (1970) Automatic fixation mechanisms and vestibular stimulation. *Advances in Oto-Rhino-Laryngology*, **17**, 90–98

DEMER, J. L. (1985) Hypothetical mechanisms of head-shaking nystagmus (HSN) in man: asymmetrical velocity storage. *Society of Neuroscience Abstracts*, **11**, 1038

DICHGANS, J. and BRANDT, T. (1973) Optokinetic motion sickness and pseudo-Coriolis effects induced by moving stimuli. *Acta Otolaryngologica*, **76**, 339–348

DICHGANS, J., NAUCK, B. and WOLPERT, E. (1973) The influence of attention, vigilance and stimulus area on optokinetic and vestibular nystagmus and voluntary saccades. In: *The Oculomotor System and Brain Functions*, edited by V. Zikmund. London: Butterworths. pp. 273–294

DICHGANS, J., MAURITZ, K. H., ALLUM, J. H. J. and BRANDT, T. (1976) Postural sway in normals and atactic patients: stabilising and destabilising effects of vision. *Agressologie*, **17**, 15–24

DICHGANS, J. E., BIZZI, E., MORASSO, P. and TAGLIASCO, V. (1973) Mechanisms underlying recovery of eye-head coordination following bilateral labyrinthectomy in monkeys. *Experimental Brain Research*, **18**, 548–562

DICKSON, E. D. D. and CHADWICK, D. L. (1951) Observations

on the disturbances of equilibrium and other symptoms induced by jet engine noise. *Journal of Laryngology and Otology,* **65**, 154–165

DIENER, H. C., DICHGANS, J., BACHER, M. and GOMPF, B. (1984) Quantification of postural sway in normals and patients with cerebellar diseases. *Electroencephalography and Clinical Neurophysiology,* **57**, 134–142

DIERINGER, N. and PRECHT, W. (1977) Modification of synaptic output following unilateral labyrinthectomy. *Nature,* **269**, 431–433

DIERINGER, N., KUNZLE, H. and PRECHT, W. (1984) Increased projections of dorsal root fibres to vestibular nuclei after hemilabyrinthectomy in the frog. *Experimental Brain Research,* **55**, 574–578

DIETERICH, M., BRANDT, T. and FRIES, W. (1989) Otolith function in man: results from a case of otolith Tullio phenomenon. *Brain,* **112**, 1377–1392

DIX, M. R. (1979) The rationale and technique of head exercises in the treatment of vertigo. *Acta Oto-Rhino-Laryngologica Belgica,* **33**, 370–384

DIX, M. R. and HALLPIKE, C. S. (1952a) The pathology, symptomatology, and diagnosis in certain disorders of the vestibular system. *Proceedings of the Royal Society of Medicine,* **45**, 341–354

DIX, M. R. and HALLPIKE, C. S. (1952b) The pathology, symptomatology, and diagnosis of certain common disorders of the vestibular system. *Annals of Otology, Rhinology and Laryngology,* **61**, 987–1016

DIX, M. R. and HALLPIKE, C. S. (1966) Observations on the clinical features and neurological mechanisms of spontaneous nystagmus resulting from unilateral neurofibromata. *Acta Otolaryngologica,* **61**, 1–22

DIX, M. R., HARRISON, M. J. G. and LEWIS, P. D. (1971) Progressive supranuclear palsy (the Steele Richardson–Olszewski syndrome): a report of 9 cases with particular reference to the mechanism of the oculomotor disorder. *Journal of Neurological Sciences,* **13**, 237–256

DODGE, R. (1903) Five types of eye movements in the horizontal meridian plane of the field of regard. *American Journal of Physiology,* **8**, 307–329

DOHLMAN, G. (1938) On the mechanism of transmission into nystagmus on stimulation of the semicircular canals. *Acta Otolaryngologica,* **26**, 425–442

DOHLMAN, G. (1953) The mechanism of the fistula test. *Acta Otolaryngologica,* Suppl. **109**, 22–26

DOHLMAN, G. (1965) The mechanism of secretion and absorption of endolymph in the vestibular apparatus. *Acta Otolaryngologica,* **59**, 275–288

DOHLMAN, G. (1981) Critical review of the concept of cupula function. *Acta Otolaryngologica,* Suppl. 376, 1–30

DONIN, J. F. (1967) Acquired monocular nystagmus in children. *Canadian Journal of Ophthalmology,* **2**, 212–215

DRACHMAN, D. A. and HART, C. (1972) An approach to the dizzy patient. *Neurology,* **22**, 323–334

DRESCHER, D. G. and KERR, T. P. (1985) Na$^+$, K$^+$ – activated adenosine triphosphatase and carbonic anhydrase: inner ear enzymes of ion transport. In: *Auditory Biochemistry,* edited by D. G. Drescher. Springfield: Charles C. Thomas. pp. 436–472

DROLLER, H. and PEMBERTON, J. (1953) Vertigo in a random sample of elderly people living in their homes. *Journal of Laryngology and Otology,* **67**, 689–695

EAGGER, S., LUXON, L. M., DAVIES, R. A., COELHO, A. and RON, M. A. (1992) Psychiatric morbidity in patients with peripheral vestibular disorders: a clinical and neuro-otological

study. *Journal of Neurology, Neurosurgery and Psychiatry,* **55**, 383–387

EGMOND, A. A. J. VAN, GROEN, J. J. and JONGKEES, L. B. W. (1948) The turning test with small regulable stimuli. *Journal of Laryngology and Otology,* **62**, 63–69

EPLEY, J. M. (1980) New dimensions of benign paroxysmal positional vertigo. *Otolaryngology – Head and Neck Surgery,* **88**, 599–605

EPLEY, J. M. (1981) Reflexogenic vertigo treated by tensor tympani transection. *Otolaryngology – Head and Neck Surgery,* **89**, 849–853

EPLEY, J. M. (1992) The canalith repositioning procedure: for treatment of benign paroxysmal positioning vertigo. *Otolaryngology – Head and Neck Surgery,* **107**, 399–404

ERNSTSON, S. and SMITH, C. A. (1986) Stereo-kinociliar bonds in mammalian vestibular organs. *Acta Otolaryngologica,* **101**, 395–402

ERRINGTON, M. L., LYNCH, M. A. and BLISS, T. V. P. (1987) Long-term potentiation in the dentate nucleus: induction and increased glutamate release are blocked by D(-) aminophosphonovalerate. *Neuroscience,* **20**, 279–284

EWALD, J. R. (1892) *Physiologische Untersuchungen uber das Endorgan des Nervus Octavus.* Bergmann: Wiesbaden

FELDMAN, A. M. (1981) Cochlear fluids: physiology, biochemistry and pharmacology. In: *Pharmacology of Hearing,* edited by R. D. Brown and E. A. Daigneault. New York: Wiley. pp. 81–97

FERNANDEZ, C. and GOLDBERG, J. M. (1971) Physiology of peripheral neurons innervating semicircular canals of squirrel monkey. II. Response to sinusoidal stimulation and dynamics of peripheral vestibular system. *Journal of Neurophysiology,* **34**, 661–675

FERNANDEZ, C. and GOLDBERG, J. M. (1976) Physiology of peripheral neurons innervating otolith organs of the squirrel monkey. *Journal of Neurophysiology,* **39**, 970–1008

FERNANDEZ, C., BAIRD, R. A. and GOLDBERG, J. M. (1988) The vestibular nerve of the chinchilla. I. Peripheral innervation patterns in the horizontal and superior semicircular canals. *Journal of Neurophysiology,* **60**, 167–181

FERNANDEZ, C., GOLDBERG, J. M. and ABEND, W. K. (1972) Response to static tilts of peripheral neurons innervating otolith organs of the squirrel monkey. *Journal of Neurophysiology,* **35**, 978–997

FERNANDEZ, C. A. R., ALZATE, R. and LINDSAY, J. R. (1959) Experimental observations on positional nystagmus in the cat. *Annals of Otology, Rhinology and Laryngology,* **68**, 816–829

FETTER, M. and ZEE, D. S. (1988) Recovery from unilateral labyrinthectomy in Rhesus monkey. *Journal of Neurophysiology,* **59**, 370–393

FETTER, M., ZEE, D. S., KOENIG, E. A. and DICHGANS, J. (1990) Head-shaking nystagmus during vestibular compensation in humans and Rhesus monkeys. *Acta Otolaryngologica,* **110**, 175–181

FETTER, M., ZEE, D. S. and PROCTOR, L. R. (1988) Effect of lack of vision and occipital lobectomy upon recovery from unilateral labyrinthectomy in rhesus monkey. *Journal of Neurophysiology,* **59**, 394–407

FISHER, A., GRESTY, M. A., CHAMBERS, B. and RUDGE, P. (1983) Primary position upbeating nystagmus. *Brain,* **106**, 949–964

FISHER, C. M. (1967) Some neuro-ophthalmological observations. *Journal of Neurology Neurosurgery and Psychiatry,* **30**, 383–392

FISCHER, M. H. (1927) Messende Untersuchungen uber die

Gegenrollung der Augen und die Localisation der scheinbaren Vertikalen bei seitlicher Neigung. *Albrecht von Graefes Archiv für klinische und experimentelle Ophthalmologie.* **118**, 633–680

FITZGERALD, G. and HALLPIKE, C. S. (1942) Studies in human vestibular function: 1. Observations on the directional preponderance ('Nystagmusbereitschaft') of caloric nystagmus resulting from cerebral lesions. *Brain*, **65**, 115–137

FLOCK, A. (1965) Transducing mechanisms in the lateral line canal organ receptors. *Cold Spring Harbor Symposium on Quantitative Biology*, **30**, 133–145

FLOCK, A. (1977) Physiological properties of sensory hairs in the ear. In: *Psychophysics and Physiology of Hearing*, edited by E. F. Evans and J. P. Wilson. London: Academic Press. pp. 15–25

FLOCK, A. and CHEUNG, H. C. (1977) Actin filaments in sensory hairs of inner ear receptor cells. *Journal of Cell Biology*, **75**, 339–343

FLOCK, A. and DUVALL, A. J. (1965) The ultrastructure of the kinocilium of the sensory cells in the inner ear and lateral line organs. *Journal of Cell Biology*, **25**, 1–7

FLOCK, A. and LAM, D. (1974) Neurotransmitter synthesis in inner ear and lateral line sense organs. *Nature*, **249**, 142–144

FLOCK, A., FLOCK B. and MURRAY, E. (1977) Studies on the sensory hairs of receptor cells in the inner ear. *Acta Otolaryngologica*, **83**, 85–91

FLOURENS, P. (1842) *Recherches Experimentales sur les Proprietes et les Fonctions du Systeme Nerveux dans Les Animaux Vertebres.* Paris: Crevot

FLUUR, E. (1959) Influences of the semicircular canal ducts on extra-ocular muscles. *Acta Otolaryngologica Supplementum*, **149**, 5–46

FLUUR, E. and MELLSTROM, A. (1971) The otolith organs and their influence on oculomotor movements. *Experimental Neurology*, **30**, 139–147

FRANCIS, D. A., BRONSTEIN, A. M., RUDGE, P. and DU BOULAY E. P. G. H. (1992) The site of brain stem lesions causing semcircular canal paresis. An MRI study. *Journal of Neurology, Neurosurgery and Psychiatry*, **55**, 446–449

FRASER, J. S. and MUIR, R. (1917) The pathology of congenital syphilitic disease of the ear. *Journal of Laryngology and Otology*, **32**, 8–30

FREDRICKSON, J. M., KORNHUBER, H. H. and SCHWARZ, J. M. (1974) Cortical projections of the vestibular nerve. In: *Handbook of Sensory Physiology. The Vestibular System* Vol VI, edited by H. H. Kornhuber. New York: Springer-Verlag. pp. 565–582

FRIBERG, U., BAGGER–SJOBACK, D. and RASK–ANDERSEN, H. (1985) The lateral intercellular spaces in the endolymphatic sac. A pathway for fluid transport? *Acta Otolaryngologica*, Suppl. 426, 1–17

FRIBERG, U., WACKYM, P. A. and BAGGER–SJOBACK, D. (1986) Effect of labyrinthectomy on the endolymphatic sac. A histological, ultrastructural and computer aided morphometric investigation in the mouse. *Acta Otolaryngologica*, **101**, 172–182

FUCHS, A. F. and KIMM, J. (1975) Unit activity in vestibular nucleus of the alert monkey during horizontal angular acceleration and eye movement. *Journal of Neurophysiology*, **38**, 1140–1161

FULTON, J. F., LIDDELL, E. G. T. and RIOCH, D. M. (1930) The influence of unilateral destruction of the vestibular nuclei upon posture and the knee jerk. *Brain*, **53**, 327–343

FURMAN, J., WALL, C. and PANG, D. L. (1990) Vestibular function in periodic alternating nystagmus. *Brain*, **113**, 1425–1439

FURMAN, J., DURRANT, J., HYRE, R. and KAMERER, D. (1990) Vestibular recruitment in Meniere's disease. *Annals of Otology, Rhinology and Laryngology*, **99**, 805–809

FURUYA, N., KAWANO, K. and SHIMAZU, M. (1976) Transcerebellar inhibitory interaction between bilateral vestibular nuclei and its modulation by cerebello-cortical activity. *Experimental Brain Research*, **25**, 447–463

GACEK, R. R. (1968) The innervation of the vestibular labyrinth. *Annals of Otology, Rhinology and Laryngology*, **77**, 676–686

GACEK, R. (1978) Further observations of posterior ampullary nerve transection for positional vertigo. *Annals of Otology, Rhinology and Laryngology*, **87**, 300–305

GACEK, R. R. and LYON, M. (1974) Localisation of vestibular efferent neurones in the kitten with horseradish peroxidase. *Acta Otolaryngologica*, **77**, 92–101

GATES, G. A. (1980) Vertigo in children. *Ear, Nose and Throat Journal*, **59**, 358–365

GESELL, A. (1938) The tonic neck reflex in human infant. *Journal of Paediatrics*, **13**, 455–464

GIBSON, M. J., ANDRES, R. O., ISAACS, B., RADEBURGH, T. and WORM–PETERSEN, J. (1987) The prevention of falls in later life. *Danish Medical Bulletin*, **34**, (suppl. 4), 1–24

GOEBEL, H. H., KOMATSUZAKI, A., BENDER, M. B. and COHEN, B. (1971) Lesions of the pontine tegmentum and conjugate gaze paralysis. *Archives of Neurology*, **24**, 431–440

GOLDBERG, J. M., LYSAKOWSKI, A. and FERNANDEZ, C. (1990) Morphophysiological and ultrastructural studies in the mammalian cristae ampullares. *Hearing Research*, **49**, 89–102

GOLZ, A., WESTERMAN, S. T., GILBERT, L. M., JOACHIMS, H.Z. and NETZER, A. (1991) Effect of middle ear effusion on the vestibular labyrinth. *Journal of Laryngology and Otology*, **105**, 987–989

GONSHOR, A. and MELVILLE JONES, G. (1976) Extreme vestibulo-ocular adaptation induced by prolonged optical reversal of vision. *Journal of Physiology*, **256**, 381–414

GOODHILL, V. (1981) Ben H. Senturia lecture. Leaking labyrinth lesions, deafness, tinnitus and dizziness. *Annals of Otology, Rhinology and Laryngology*, **90**, 99–106

GRACE, A. R. H. and PFLEIDERER, A. G. (1990) Disequilibrium and otitis media with effusion: what is the association? *Journal of Laryngology and Otology*, **104**, 682–684

GRAY, O. (1955) A brief survey of the phylogenesis of the labyrinth. *Journal of Laryngology and Otology*, **69**, 151–179

GRAYBIEL, A. (1974) Measurement of otolith function in man. In: *Handbook of Sensory Physiology: The Vestibular System*, edited by H. H. Kornhuber, Vol. VI, Part 2. New York: Springer–verlag. pp. 233–266

GREINER, G. F., COLLARD, M., CONRAUX, C., PICART, P. and ROHMER, F. (1967) Recherche des potentials evoques d'origine vestibulaire chez l'homme. *Acta Otolaryngologica*, **63**, 320–329

GRESTY, M. A. and BRONSTEIN, A. M. (1986) Otolith stimulation evokes compensatory reflex eye movements of high velocity when linear motion of the head is combined with concurrent angular motion. *Neuroscience Letters*, **65**, 149–154

GRESTY, M. A. and HALMAGYI, G. M. (1979) Abnormal head movements. *Journal of Neurology, Neurosurgery and Psychiatry*, **42**, 705–714

GRESTY, M. A., BRONSTEIN, A. M. and BARRATT, H. (1987) Eye

movement responses to combined linear and angular head movement. *Experimental Brain Research*, **65**, 377–384

GRESTY, M. A., PAGE, N. G. R. and BARRATT, H. J. (1984) The differential diagnosis of congenital nystagmus. *Journal of Neurology, Neurosurgery and Psychiatry*, **47**, 936–942

GRESTY, M. A., TRINDER, E. and LEECH, J. (1976) Perception of everyday visual environments during saccadic eye movements. *Aviation Space and Environmental Medicine*, **47**, 991–992

GRESTY, M. A., BARRATT, H. J., PAGE, N. G. R. and ELL, J. J. (1985) Assessment of vestibulo-ocular reflexes in congenital nystagmus. *Annals of Neurology*, **17**, 129–136

GRESTY, M. A., BARRATT, H., RUDGE, P. and PAGE, N. (1986) Analysis of downbeat nystagmus. Otolithic versus semicircular canal influences. *Archives of Neurology*, **43**, 52–55

GRIGG, P., FINERMAN, G. A. and RILEY, L. H. (1973) Joint-position sense after total hip replacement. *Journal of Bone and Joint Surgery*, **55**, 1016–1025

GUEDRY, F. E. (1970) Conflicting sensory cues as a factor in motion sickness. In: *Fourth Symposium on the Role of the Vestibular Organs in Space Exploration*. Report SP-187. Washington, DC: NASA. pp. 45–52

GUEDRY, F. E. (1974) Psychophysics of vestibular sensation. In: *Handbook of Sensory Physiology: The Vestibular System*, edited by H. H. Kornhuber, Vol. VI, Part 2. New York: Springer–Verlag. pp. 3–154

GUILD, S. R. (1927) The circulation of endolymph. *American Journal of Anatomy*, **39**, 57–81

GUILLERY, R. W., OKORO, A. N. and WITKORP, C. J. (1975) Abnormal visual pathways in the brain of a human albino. *Brain Research*, **96**, 373–377

GUITTON, D., KEARNEY, R. E., WERELEY, N. and PETERSON, B. W. (1986) Visual, vestibular and voluntary contributions to human head stabilization. *Experimental Brain Research*, **64**, 59–69

HADDAD, G. M., DEMER, J. L. and ROBINSON, D. A. S. (1980) The effect of lesions of the dorsal cap of the inferior olive on the vestibulo-ocular and optokinetic systems of the cat. *Brain Research*, **185**, 265–275

HAIN, T. C. (1986) A model of the nystagmus induced by off vertical axis rotation. *Biological Cybernetics*, **54**, 337–350

HAIN, T. C., FETTER, M. and ZEE, D. S. (1987) Head-shaking nystagmus in patients with unilateral peripheral vestibular lesions. *American Journal of Otolaryngology*, **8**, 36–47

HALL, T. C., MILLER, A. K. H. and CORSELLIS, J. A. N. (1975) Variations in the human Purkinje cell population according to age and sex. *Neuropathology and Applied Neurobiology*, **1**, 267–292

HALL, S. F., RUBY, R. R. F. and MCCLURE, J. A. (1979) The mechanics of benign paroxysmal vertigo. *Journal of Otolaryngology*, **8**, 151–158

HALLPIKE, C. S. (1967) Some types of ocular nystagmus and their neurological mechanisms. *Proccedings of the Royal Society of Medicine*, **60**, 1–12

HALMAGYI, G. M., GRESTY, M. A. and GIBSON, W. P. R. (1979) Ocular tilt reaction with peripheral vestibular lesion. *Annals of Neurology*, **6**, 80–83

HALMAGYI, G. M., GRESTY, M. A. and LEECH, J. (1980) Reversed optokinetic nystagmus, mechanism and clinical significance. *Annals of Neurology*, **7**, 429–435

HALMAGYI, G. M., RUDGE, P., GRESTY, M. A. and SANDERS, M. D. (1983) Downbeating nystagmus, a review of 62 cases. *Archives of Neurology*, **40**, 777–784

HALMAGYI, G. M., BRANDT, T., DIETERICH, M., CURTHOYS, I. S., STARK, R. J. and HOYT, W. F. (1990) Ocular tilt reaction with unilateral mesodiencephalic lesion. *Neurology*, **40**, 1503–1509

HAMID, M. A. (1991) Vestibular and postural findings in the motion sickness syndrome. *Otolaryngology – Head and Neck Surgery*, **104**, 135–136

HAMILTON, D. W. (1968) The calyceal synapse of type I vestibular hair cells. *Journal of Ultrastructural Research*, **23**, 98–114

HAMILTON, D. W. (1969) The cilium on mammalian vestibular hair cells. *Anatomical Record*, **164**, 253–258

HARADA, V. (1979) Formation area of statoconia. *Scanning Electron Microscope*, **3**, 963–966

HARLAN, D. M. and MANN, G. V. (1982) A factor in food which impairs Na^+, K^+-ATPase in vitro. *American Journal of Clinical Nutrition*, **35**, 250–257

HARISSON, M. S. and OZSAHINOGLU, C. (1972) Positional vertigo: aetiology and clinical significance. *Brain*, **95**, 369–372

HEALY, G. B., STRONG M. S. and SAMPOGNA, D. (1974) Ataxia, vertigo, and hearing loss. A result of rupture of the inner ear window. *Archives of Otolaryngology*, **100**, 130–135

HENNEBERT, C. (1911) A new syndrome in hereditary syphilis of the labyrinth. *Presse Medicale Belge Bruxelles*, **63**, 467–470

HENRIKSSON, N. G., HINDFELT, B., PYYKKO, I. and SCHALEN, L. (1981) Rapid eye movements reflecting neurological disorders. *Clinical Otolaryngology*, **6**, 111–119

HERDMAN, S. J., TUSA, R. J., ZEE, D. S., PROCTOR, L. R. and MATTOX, D. E. (1993) Single treatment approaches to benign paroxysmal positional vertigo. *Archives of Otolaryngology – Head and Neck Surgery*, **119**, 450–454

HIGHSTEIN, S. M. (1991) The central nervous system efferent control of the organs of balance and equilibrium. *Neuroscience Research*, **12**, 13–30

HIGHSTEIN, S. M. GOLDBERG, J. M. MOSCHOVAKIS, A. K. and FERNANDEZ, C. (1987) Inputs from regularly and irregularly discharging vestibular nerve afferents to secondary neurons in the vestibular nuclei of the squirrel monkey. II. Correlation with output pathways of secondary neurons. *Journal of Neurophysiology*, **58**, 719–738

HIKOSAKA, O. and MAEDA, M. (1973) Cervical afferents on abducens motoneurons and their interactions with vestibulo-ocular reflex. *Experimental Brain Research*, **18**, 512–530

HIKOSAKA, O. and WURTZ, R. H. (1983) Visual and oculomotor functions of monkey substantia nigra pars reticulata. Memory-contigent visual and saccade responses. *Journal of Neurophysiology*, **49**, 1268–1283

HIKOSAKA, O. and WURTZ, R. H. (1985a) Modification of saccadic eye movements by GABA related substances I. Effect of muscimol and bicuculline in monkey superior colliculus. *Journal of Neurophysiology*, **53**, 266–291

HIKOSAKA, O. and WURTZ, R. H. (1985b) Modification of saccadic eye movements by GABA related substances II. Effects of muscimol in monkey substantia nigra pars reticulata. *Journal of Neurophysiology*, **53**, 292–308

HILLMAN, D. E. and LEWIS, E. R. (1971) Morphological basis for a mechanical linkage in otolith receptor transduction in the frog. *Science*, **174**, 416–419

HOAGLAND, H. (1932) Impulses from sensory nerves of catfish. *Proceedings of the National Academy of Sciences of the USA*, **18**, 701–705

HOBBELEN, J. F. and COLLEWIJN, H. (1971) Effect of cerebrocortical and collicular ablations upon the optokinetic reactions in the rabbit. *Documenta Ophthalmologica*, **30**, 227–236

HOLDEN, H. and SCHUKNECHT, H. (1968) Distribution pattern of blood in the inner ear following spontaneous subarachnoid hemorrhage. *Journal of Laryngology*, **82**, 321–329

HOLLIDAY, P. J. and FERMIE, G. R. (1979) Changes in measurement of postural sway resulting from repeated testing. *Aggressologie*, **20**, 225–228

HOLMES, G. (1938) The cerebral integration of ocular movements. *British Medical Journal*, **2**, 107–112

HOLTON, T. and HUDSPETH, A. J. (1986) The transduction channel of hair cells from the bull-frog characterised by noise analysis. *Journal of Physiology*, **375**, 195–227

HONRUBIA, V., BALOH, R. W., YEE, R. D. and JENKINS, H. A. (1980) Identification of the location of vestibular lesions on the basis of vestibulo-ocular reflex measurements. *American Journal of Otolaryngology*, **1**, 291–301

HONRUBIA, V., DOWNEY, W. L., MITCHELL, D. P. and WARD, P. H. (1968) Experimental studies on optokinetic nystagmus. II. Normal humans. *Acta Otolaryngologica*, **65**, 441–448

HONRUBIA, V., KOEHN, W. W., JENKINS, H. A. and FENTON, W. H. (1982) Effect of bilateral ablation of the vestibular cerebellum on visuo-vestibular interaction. *Experimental Neurology*, **75**, 616–626

HOOD, J. D. (1967) Observations upon the neurological mechanism of optokinetic nystagmus with special reference to the contribution of peripheral vision. *Acta Otolaryngologica*, **63**, 208–215

HOOD, J. D. (1968) Electronystagmography. *Journal of Laryngology and Otology*, **82**, 167–183

HOOD, J. D. (1989) Evidence of direct thermal action upon the vestibular receptors in the caloric test. *Acta Otolaryngologica*, **107**, 161–165

HOOD, J. D. and KAYAN, A. (1985) Observations upon the evoked responses to natural vestibular stimulation. *Electroencephalography and Clinical Neurophysiology*, **62**, 266–276

HOOD, J. D. and KORRES, S. (1979) Vestibular suppression in peripheral and central vestibular disorders of the brain. *Brain*, **102**, 785–804

HOOD, J. D. and LEECH, J. (1974) The significance of peripheral vision in the perception of movement. *Acta Otolaryngologica*, **77**, 72–79

HOOD, J. D., KAYAN, A. and LEECH, J. (1973) Rebound nystagmus. *Brain*, **96**, 507–526

HOYT, W. F. and DAROFF, F. R. B. (1971) Supranuclear disorders of ocular control in man. In: *The Control of Eye Movements*, edited by P. Bach-Y-Rita, C. C. Collins and J. E. Hyde. New York: Academic Press. pp. 175–263

HUBEL, D. H. and WIESEL, T. N. (1977) Ferrier lecture: functional architecture of macaque visual cortex. *Proceedings of the Royal Society of London B*, **198**, 1–59

HUDSPETH, A. J. (1982) Extracellular current flow and the site of transduction by vertebrate hair cells. *Journal of Neuroscience*, **2**, 1–10

HUDSPETH, A. J. (1985) The cellular basis of hearing: the biophysics of hair cells. *Science*, **230**, 745–752

HUDSPETH, A. J. and COREY, D. P. (1977) Sensitivity, polarity, and conductance change in the response of vertebrate hair cells to controlled mechanical stimuli. *Proceedings of the National Academy of Sciences USA*, **74**, 2407–2411

HUDSPETH, A. J. and JACOBS, R. (1979) Stereocilia mediate transduction in vertebrate hair cells. *Proceedings of the National Academy of Sciences USA*, **76**, 1506–1509

HUIZINGA, E. (1931) De la reaction galvanique de l'appareil vestibulaire. *Acta Otolaryngologica*, **15**, 451–468

HUNTER-DUVAR, I. M. and HINOJOSA, R. (1984) Vestibule: sensory epithelia. In: *Ultrastructural Atlas of the Inner Ear*, edited by I. Friedmann and J. Ballantyne. London: Butterworths. pp. 211–244

IGARASHI, M., LEVY, J. K., O-UCHI, T. and RESCHKE, M F. (1981) Further study of physical exercise and locomotor balance compensation after unilateral labyrinthectomy in squirrel monkeys. *Acta Otolaryngologica*, **92**, 101–105

INGELSTEDT, S., IVARSSON, A. and TJERNSTROM, O. (1974) Vertigo due to relative overpressure in the middle ear. *Acta Otolaryngologica*, **78**, 1–14

ITO, M. (1972) Neural design of the cerebellar motor control system. *Brain Research*, **40**, 81–84

ITO, M. (1975) The vestibulo-cerebellar relationships: vestibulo-ocular reflex arc and flocculus. In: *The Vestibular System*, edited by R. F. Naunton. New York: Academic Press. pp. 129–146

ITO, M., NISIMARU, N. and YAMAMOTO, M. (1976) Pathways for the vestibulo-ocular reflex excitation arising from semicircular canals of rabbits. *Experimental Brain Research*, **24**, 257–271

JACKSON, R. T., EPSTEIN, C. M. and BOYETE, J. E. (1991) Enhancement of posturography testing with head tilt and energy measurements. *American Journal of Otology*, **12**, 420–425

JAHNKE K., MEYER ZUM GOTTESBERGE, A. and NEUMAN, T. (1991) Freeze-fracture studies on vestibular secretory cells and melanocytes. *Journal of Otorhinolaryngology and its Related Specialities*, **53**, 279–286

JANSEN, C., LARSEN, R. E. and OLESON, M. B. (1982) Quantitative Romberg's test. *Acta Neurologica Scandinavica*, **66**, 93–99

JEFFRIES, D. J., PICKLES, J. O., OSBORNE, M. P., RHYS-EVANS, P. H. and COMIS, S. D. (1986) Crosslinks between stereocilia in hair cells of the human and guinea pig vestibular labyrinth. *Journal of Laryngology and Otology*, **100**, 1367–1374

JENKINS, H. A. (1985) Long-term adaptive changes of the vestibulo-ocular reflex in patients following acoustic neuroma surgery. *Laryngoscope*, **95**, 1224–1234

JOHANSON, W. H. (1964) The importance of the otoliths in disorientation. *Aerospace Medicine*, **35**, 874–877

JOHNSSON, L. G. and HAWKINS, J. E. (1972) Sensory neural degeneration with ageing as seen in microdissection of the human inner ear. *Annals of Otology, Rhinology and Laryngology*, **81**, 179–193

JOHNSTONE, B. M. and SELLICK, P. M. (1972) The peripheral auditory apparatus. *Quarterly Reviews of Biophysics*, **5**, 1–57

JONES, G. M. (1957) A study of current problems associated with disorientation in man-controlled flight. *Flying Personnel Research Committee Report*, no 1006. London: Air Ministry

JONES, G. M. and MILSUM, J. H. (1965) Spatial and dynamic aspects of visual fixation. *IEEE Transactions on Biomedical Engineering*, **12**, 54–62

JONES, T. A. and NELSON, R. C. (1992) Recovery of vestibular function following hair cell destruction by streptomycin. *Hearing Research*, **62**, 181–186

JONGKEES, L. B. W. (1953) Uber die Untersuchungsmethoden des Gleichgewichtsorgans. *Fortschritte der Hals-Nasen-Ohrenheilk*, **1**, 1–147

JONGKEES, L. B. W. (1974) Motion sickness. II. Some sensory

aspects. In: *Handbook of Sensory Physiology*, edited by H. H. Kornhuber, Vol. VI, Part 2. New York: Springer–Verlag. pp. 405–411

JONGKEES, L. B. W., MAAS, J. P. M. and PHILIPZOON, A. J. (1962) Clinical nystagmography. *Practica Otolaryngologica*, **24**, 65–93

KACKER, S. K. and HINCHCLIFFE, R. (1970) Unusual Tullio phenomenon. *Journal of Laryngology and Otology*, **84**, 155–166

KAMEI, T., KIMURA, K., KANEKO, H. and NORO, K. (1964) Revaluation of the head-shaking test as a method of nystagmus provocation. Part 1. Its nystagmus eliciting effect. *Japanese Journal of Otolaryngology*, **67**, 1530–1534

KAPTEYN, T. S. and DE WIT, G. (1972) Posturography as an auxiliary in vestibular investigations. *Acta Otolaryngologica*, **73**, 104–111

KARMODY, C. S. and SCHUKNECHT, H. F. (1966) Deafness in congenital syphilis. *Archives of Otolaryngology*, **83**, 18–27

KEANE, J. R. (1974) Periodic alternating nystagmus with downbeating nystagmus: a clinical anatomical case study of multiple sclerosis. *Archives of Neurology*, **30**, 399–402

KELLER, E. L. (1974) Participation of median pontine reticular formation in eye movement generation in monkey. *Journal of Neurophysiology*, **37**, 316–332

KERTH J. D. and ALLEN, G. W. (1963) Comparison of the perilymphatic and cerebrospinal fluid pressures. *Archives of Otolaryngology*, **77**, 581–594

KIKUCHI, T., TAKASAKA, T., TONOSAKI, A. and WATANABE, H. (1989) Fine structure of guinea pig vestibular kinocilium. *Acta Otolaryngologica*, **108**, 26–30

KIMURA, R. S. (1969) Distribution, structure and function of dark cells in the vestibular labyrinth. *Annals of Otology, Rhinology and Laryngology*, **78**, 542–561

KIMURA, R. S. (1976) Experimental pathogenesis of hydrops. *Archives of Otorhinolaryngology*, **212**, 263–275

KIMURA, R. S. and SCHUKNECHT, H. F. (1965) Membranous hydrops in the inner ear of the guinea pig after obliteration of the endolymphatic sac. *Practica Otorhinolaryngologica*, **27**, 343–354

KIMURA, R. S., SCHUKNECHT, H. and OTA, C. (1974) Blockage of the cochlear aqueduct. *Acta Otolaryngologica*, **77**, 1–12

KLOCKHOFF, I., ANGGARD, G. and ANGGARD, L. (1966) Recording of cranio-labyrinthine pressure transmission in man by acoustic impedance method. *Acta Otolaryngologica*, **61**, 361–370

KOHUT, R. I., HAENEL, J. L. and WALDORF, R. A. (1979) Minute perilymph fistulas: vertigo and Hennebert's sign without hearing loss. *Annals of Otology, Rhinology and Laryngology*, **88**, 153–159

KOMPFE, D., PASIK, T., PASIK, P. and BENDER, M. B. (1979) Downward gaze in monkeys: stimulation and lesion studies. *Brain*, **102**, 527–558

KORRES, S. (1978) Electronystagmographic criteria in neuro-otological diagnosis. 2: Central nervous system lesions. *Journal of Neurology, Neurosurgery and Psychiatry*, **41**, 254–264

KUIJPERS, W. and BONTING, S. L. (1970) The cochlear potentials. II. The nature of the cochlear endolymphatic resting potential. *Pflugers Archive European Journal of Physiology*, **320**, 359–372

KUSAKARI, J., KOBAYASHI, T., ARAKAWA, E., ROKUGO, M., OHYAMA, K. and INAMURA, N. (1986) Saccular and cochlear endolymphatic potentials in experimentally induced endolymphatic hydrops of guinea pigs. *Acta Otolaryngologica*, **101**, 27–33

KWEE, H. L. (1976) The occurrence of the Tullio phenomenon in congenitally deaf children. *Journal of Laryngology and Otology*, **90**, 501–507

LACOM, M. and XERRI, C. (1984) Vestibular compensation: new perspectives. In: *Lesion-induced Neuronal Plasticity in Sensorimotor Systems*, edited by H. Flohr and W. Precht. Berlin: Springer–Verlag. pp. 240–253

LACOUR, M., ROLL, J. P. and APPAIX, M. (1976) Modifications and development of spinal reflexes in the adult baboon (*Papio papio*) following unilateral vestibular neurotomy. *Brain Research*, **113**, 255–269

LANE, R. H., KAAS, J. H. and ALLMAN J. M. (1974) Visuotropic organization of the superior colliculus in normal and Siamese cats. *Brain Research*, **70**, 413–430

LAU, C. G. Y., HONRUBIA, V. and BALOH, R. W. (1978). The pattern of eye movement trajectories during physiological nystagmus in humans. In: *Vestibular Mechanisms in Health and Disease*, edited by J. D. Hood. London: Academic Press. pp. 37–44

LIEDGREN, S. R. C. and RUBIN, A. M. (1976) Vestibulo-thalamic projections studied with antidromic technique in the cat. *Acta Otolaryngologica*, **82**, 379–387

LIEDGREN, S. R. C., MILNE, A. C., RUBIN, A. M., SCHWARZ, D. W. F. and TOMLINSON, R. D. (1976) Representation of vestibular afferents in somatosensory thalamic nuclei of squirrel monkey (*Saimiri sciureus*). *Journal of Neurophysiology*, **39**, 601–612

LIM, D. J. (1979) Fine morphology of the otoconial membrane and its relationship to the sensory epithelium. *Scanning Electron Microscopy*, **3**, 929–938

LIM, D. J. (1984) The development and structure of otoconia. In: *Ultrastructural Atlas of the Inner Ear*, edited by I. Friedman and J. Ballantyne. London: Butterworths. pp. 245–269

LINDEMAN, H. H. (1969) Studies on the morphology of the sensory regions of the vestibular apparatus. *Advances in Anatomy, Embryology and Cell Biology*, **42**, 1–113

LISBERGER, G. G. and FUCHS, A. F. (1977) Role of primate flocculus in smooth pursuit eye movements and rapid behavioural modification of the vestibulo-ocular reflex. In *Control of Gaze by Brainstem Neurons*, edited by R. Baker and A. Berthoz. Amsterdam: Elsevier/North Holland. pp. 381–389

LOE, P. R., TOMKO, D. L. and WERNER, G. (1973) The neural signal of angular head position in the primary afferent vestibular nerve axons. *Journal of Physiology*, **230**, 29–50

LOPEZ, I. and MEZA, G. (1988) Neurochemical evidence for afferent GABAergic and efferent cholinergic neurotransmission in the frog vestibule. *Neuroscience*, **25**, 13–18

LORENTE DE NO, R. (1933) Anatomy of the eighth nerve. 1. The central projection of the nerve endings of the internal ear. *Laryngoscope*, **43**, 1–38

LOWENSTEIN, O. and ROBERTS, T. D. M. (1950) The equilibrium function of the otolith organs of the Thornback Ray *Raja Clavata. Journal of Physiology*, **11**, 392–415

LOWENSTEIN, O. and SAUNDERS, R. D. (1975) Otolith controlled responses from the first-order neurones of the labyrinth of the bullfrog (*Rana catesbeina*) to changes in linear acceleration. *Proceedings of the Royal Society of London, Series B*, **191**, 475–505

LOWENSTEIN, O. and WERSALL, J. (1959) A functional interpretation of the electron-microscopic structure of sensory hairs in the cristae of the elasmobranch *Raja clavata* in terms of directional sensitivity. *Nature*, **184**, 1807–1808

LUCAE, A. (1881) Uber optischer Schwindel bei Druckerho-hung im Ohr. *Archiv für Ohrenheilkunde*, 17, 237–245

LUDMAN, H. (1979) Vestibular function. In: *Diseases of the Ear*, 4th edn, edited by S. R. Mawson and H. Ludman. London: Edward Arnold. p. 195

LUNDGREN, G. E. C. (1973) On alternobaric vertigo epidemiological aspects. *Forsvarsmedicin*, 9, 406–409

LUNDGREN, G. E. C. and MALM, L. U. (1966) Alternobaric vertigo among pilots. *Aerospace Medicine*, 37, 178–180

LUNDQUIST, P. G. (1965) The endolymphatic duct and sac in the guinea pig. An electron microscopic and experimental investigation. *Acta Otolaryngologica*, Suppl. 201, 1–108

LUNDQUIST, P. G. (1976) Aspects on endolymphatic morphology and function. *Archives of Otorhinolaryngology*, 212, 231–240

LUNDQUIST, P. G., ANDERSEN, H., GALEY, F. R. and BAGGERSJO-BACK, D. (1984) Ultrastructural morphology of endolymphatic duct and sac. In: *Ultrastructural Atlas of the Inner Ear*, edited by I. Friedmann and J. Ballantyne. London: Butterworths. pp. 245–269

LUXON, L. M. (1991) Disturbances of balance in the elderly. *British Journal of Hospital Medicine*, 45, 22–26

LYNCH, J. C. and MCCLAREN J. W. (1983) Optokinetic nystagmus deficits following parieto-occipital cortex lesions in monkeys. *Experimental Brain Research*, 49, 125–130

MCCABE, B. F., RYU, J. H. and SEKITANI, T. (1972) Further experiments on vestibular compensation. *Laryngoscope*, 82, 381–397

MCCLOSKEY, D. J. (1978) Kinesthetic sensibility. *Physiological Reviews*, 58, 763–820

MCCLURE, J. A. (1985) Horizontal canal BPV. *Journal of Otolaryngology* 14, 30–35

MCCLURE, J. A. (1986) Vertigo and imbalance in the elderly. *Journal of Otolaryngology*, 15, 248–252

MACH, E. (1875) *Grundlinien der Lehre von den Bewegungsempfindungen*. Leipzig: Engelman. Amsterdam: Bonset. (translation) 1967

MCNALLY, W. J., STUART, E. A., JAMIESON, J. S. and GAULTON, G. (1947) Some experiments with caloric stimulation of the human labyrinth to study the relative values of ampullopetal and ampullo-fugal endolymphatic flow (Ewald's laws). *Transactions of the American Academy of Ophthalmology and Otolaryngology*, 52, 513–541

MAEKAWA, K. and SIMPSON, J. I. (1973) Climbing fiber responses evoked in vestibulo-cerebellum of rabbit from visual system. *Journal of Neurophysiology*, 36, 649–666

MAFFEI, L. and BISTI, S. (1976) Binocular interaction in strabismic kittens deprived of vision. *Science*, 191, 579–580

MAGNUS, R. (1924) *Korperstellung*. Berlin: Springer

MARCHBANKS, R. J., REID, A., MARTIN, A. M., BRIGHTWELL, A. P. and BATEMAN, D. (1987) The effect of raised intracranial pressure on intracochlear fluid pressure: three case studies. *British Journal of Audiology*, 21, 127–130

MARKHAM, C. H., YAGI, T. and CURTHOYS, I. S. (1977) The contribution of the contra-lateral labyrinth to second order vestibular neuronal activity in the cat. *Brain Research*, 138, 99–109

MARKS, I. M. (1981) Space 'phobia': a pseudo-agoraphobic syndrome. *Journal of Neurology, Neurosurgery and Psychiatry*, 44, 387–391

MATSUHIRA, T., YAMASHITA, K., YASUDA, M. and OHKUBO, J. (1991) Detection of the unilateral vestibular recruitment phenomenon using the rotation test. *Acta Otolaryngologica*, Suppl. 481, 486–489

MAY, J. G., KELLER, E. L. and SUZUKI, D. A. (1988) Smooth-pursuit eye movement deficits with chemical lesions in the dorsolateral pontine nucleus of the monkey. *Journal of Neurophysiology*, 59, 952–977

MAYER, O. and FRASER, J. S. (1936) Pathological changes in the ear in late congenital syphilis. *Journal of Laryngology and Otology*, 51, 683–714

MEIER-RUGE, W., GIGAX, P. and WIERSPERGEN, N. (1980) A synoptic view of pathophysiology and experimental pharmacology in gerontological brain research. In: *Psychopharmacology of Ageing*, edited by C. Eisdorfer and W. E. Fann. New York: Spectrum. pp. 65–97

MELICHAR, I. and SYKA, J. (1987) Electrophysiological measurements of the stria vascularis potentials in vivo. *Hearing Research*, 25, 35–43

MELVILLE JONES, G. (1964) Predominance of anti-compensatory oculomotor response during rapid head rotation. *Aerospace Medicine*, 35, 965–968

MENDEL, L. (1971) Vestibular recruitment in Meniere's disease. *Acta Otolaryngologica*, 72, 155–164

MERICA, F. W. (1942) Vertigo due to obstruction of the Eustachian tubes. *Journal of the American Medical Association*, 118, 1282–1284

MEYER, C. H., LASKER, A. G. and ROBINSON, D. A. (1985) The upper limit of human smooth pursuit velocity. *Vision Research*, 25, 561–563

MILES, F. A. (1974) Single unit firing patterns in the vestibular nuclei related to voluntary eye movements and passive body rotation in the conscious monkey. *Brain Research*, 71, 215–224

MILLER, E. F. (1962) Counterrolling of the human eye produced by head tilt with respect to gravity. *Acta Otolaryngologica*, 54, 479–501

MONEY, K. E. and MYLES, W. S. (1974) Heavy water nystagmus and effects of alcohol. *Nature*, 247, 404–405

MONEY, K. E., JOHNSON, W. H. and CARLETT, B. A. (1970) Role of semicircular canals in positional alcohol nystagmus. *American Journal of Physiology*, 208, 1065–1070

MORGENSTERN, C., AMANO, H. and ORSULAKOVA, A. (1982) Ion transport in the endolymphatic space of guinea pigs. *American Journal Otolaryngology*, 3, 323–327

MORROW, M. J. and SHARPE, J. A. (1990) Cerebral hemispheric localization of smooth pursuit asymmetry. *Neurology*, 40, 284–292

MULCH, G. and PETERMANN, W. (1979) Influence of age on results of vestibular function tests: review of literature and presentation of caloric test results. *Annals of Otology, Rhinology and Laryngology*, 88, suppl. 56, 1–17

NADOL, J. B. (1974) Positive 'fistula sign' with an intact tympanic membrane. *Archives of Otolaryngology*, 100, 273–278

NADOL, J. B. JR (1977) Positive Hennebert's sign in Meniere's disease. *Archives of Otolaryngology*, 103, 524–530

NAKAI, Y. and HILDING, D. (1968) Vestibular endolymph-producing epithelium. *Acta Otolaryngologica*, 66, 120–128

NASHNER, L. M. (1973) Vestibular and reflex control in normal standing. In: *Control of Posture and Locomotion*, edited by R. B. Stein and K. G. Pearson. New York: Plenum Press. pp. 291–308

NATHANSON, M., BERGMAN, T. S. and BERKER, M. B. (1955) Monocular nystagmus. *American Journal of Ophthalmology*, 40, 685–692

NELSON, G. P. and STARK, L. (1962) Optokinetic nystagmus in man. *Quarterly Progress Report, Research Laboratory of Electronics*, 66, 366–369

NEWMAN, N., GAY, A. J., STROUD, M. H. and BROOKS, J. (1970) Defective rapid eye movements in progressive supranuclear palsy. *Brain*, **93**, 775–784

NORRE, M. E. (1987) Rationale of rehabilitation treatment for vertigo. *American Journal of Otolaryngology*, **8**, 31–35

NORRE, M. E. and BECKERS, A. M. (1988) Vestibular rehabituation training. *Archives of Otolaryngology – Head and Neck Surgery*, **114**, 883–886

NORRE, M. E. and FORREZ, G. (1986) Vestibulospinal function in otoneurology. *Journal for Oto-Rhino-Laryngology and its Related Specialities*, **48**, 37–44

NORRE, M. E., FORREZ, G. and BECKERS, A. (1987) Vestibular dysfunction causing instability in aged patients. *Acta Otolaryngologica*, **104**, 50–55

NOZUE, N., MIZUNO, M. and KAGA, K. (1973) Neuro-otological findings in diphenylhydantoin intoxications. *Annals of Otology, Rhinology and Laryngology*, **82**, 389–394

O'CONNOR, A., LUXON, L. M., SHORTMAN, R. C., THOMPSON, E. J. and MORRISON, A. W. (1982) Electrophoretic separation and identification of perilymph proteins in cases of acoustic neuroma. *Acta Otolaryngologica*, **93**, 195–200

OHMORI, H. (1985) Mechano-electrical transduction currents in isolated vestibular hair cells of the chick. *Journal of Physiology*, **359**, 189–217

O'LEARY, D. P., DENNIS, P., DUNN, R. F. and HONRUBIA, V. (1974) Functional and anatomical correlation of afferent responses from the isolated semicircular canal. *Nature*, **251**, 225–227

ONO, T. and TACHIBANA, M. (1990) Origin of the endolymphatic DC potential in the cochlea and ampulla of the guinea pig. *European Archives of Otorhinolaryngology*, **248**, 99–101

OSBORNE, M. P. and THORNHILL, R. (1972) The effect of monoamine depleting drugs upon synaptic bars in the inner ear of the bullfrog (*Rana catesbiana*). *Zeitschrift für Zellforschung Mikroscopische Anatomie*, **127**, 347–355

OUTERBRIDGE, J. S. and JONES, G. M. (1971) Reflex vestibular control of head movement in man. *Aerospace Medicine*, **42**, 935–940

OVERSTALL, P. W. (1978) Falls in the elderly – epidemiology, aetiology, and management. In: *Recent Advances in Geriatric Medicine*, edited by B. Isaacs. London: Churchill Livingstone. pp. 61–72

PAGE, N. G. R. and GRESTY, M. A. (1985) Motorist's vestibular disorientation syndrome. *Journal of Neurology, Neurosurgery and Psychology*, **48**, 729–735

PAGNINI, P., NUTE, D. and VANNUCCHI, P. (1989) Benign paroxysmal vertigo of the horizontal canal. *Journal for Otorhinolaryngology and its Related Specialities*, **51**, 161–170

PARNES, L. S. (1994) Treatment of benign paroxysmal positional vertigo. *Advances in Otolaryngology*, **8**, 321–339

PARNES, L. S. and MCCLURE, J. A. (1991) Free-floating endolymph particles: a new operative finding during posterior canal occlusion. *Laryngoscope*, **101**, 988–992

PASIK, P. and PASIK, T. (1964) Oculomotor functions in monkeys with lesions of the cerebrum and superior colliculus. In: *The Oculomotor System*, edited by M. B. Bender. New York: Harper Row. pp. 40–80

PASIK, T., PASIK, P. and BENDER, M. B. (1969) The pretectal syndrome in monkeys. *Brain*, **92**, 871–884

PEAKE, W. T., SOHMER, H. S. and WEISS, T. F. (1969) Microelectrode recordings of intracochlear potentials. *Quarterly Progress Report, M.I.T. Research Laboratory of Electronics*, **94**, 293–304

PENFIELD, W. (1957) Vestibular-sensation and the cerebral cortex. *Annals of Otology, Rhinology and Laryngology*, **66**, 691–698

PENFIELD, W. and JASPER, H. (1954) *Epilepsy and Functional Anatomy of Human Brain*. London: Churchill

PERLMAN, H. B. and LEEK, J. H. (1952) Late congenital syphilis of the ear. *Laryngoscope*, **62**, 1175–1196

PERLMAN, H. and LINDSAY, J. (1939) Relation of the internal ear spaces to the meninges. *Archives of Otolaryngology*, **29**, 12–23

PERRY, B. C. (1982) Falls among the aged living in a high rise apartment. *Journal of Family Practice*, **14**, 1069–1073

PETERSON, B. W. (1970) Distribution of neural responses to tilting within vestibular nuclei of the cat. *Journal of Neurophysiology*, **33**, 750–767

PETRONE, D., DE BENEDITTIS, G. and DE CANDIA, N. (1991) Experimental research on vestibular compensation using posturography. *Bollettino – Societa Italiana Biologia Sperimentale*, **67**, 731–737

PFALTZ, C. R. (1969) The diagnostic importance of galvanic tests in neuro-otology. *Practica Oto-Rhino-Laryngologica*, **31**, 193–203

PICKLES, J. O., COMIS, S. D. and OSBORNE, M. P. (1984) Crosslinks between stereocilia in the guinea pig organ of Corti, and their possible relation to sensory transduction. *Hearing Research*, **15**, 103–112

PICKLES, J. O., BRIX, J., GLEICH, O., KOPPL, C., MANLEY, G. A. and OSBORNE, M. P. (1988) The fine structure and organisation of tip links on hair cell stereovilli. In: *Basic Issues in Hearing*, edited by H. Duifhuis, J. W. Horst and H. P. Wit. London: Academic Press. pp. 56–63

PIERROTT-DESEILLIGNY, C., CHAIN, F., SERARA, M., GRAY, F. and L'HERMITTE, F. (1981) The 'One and a half' syndrome: electro-oculographic analyses of five cases with deductions about physiological mechanisms of lateral gaze. *Brain*, **104**, 665–700

PIERROTT-DESEILLIGNY, C., ROSA, A., MASMOUDI, K., RIVAUD, S. and GAYMARD, B. (1991) Saccade deficits after a unilateral lesion affecting the superior colliculus. *Journal of Neurology, Neurosurgery and Psychiatry*, **54**, 1106–1109

PINHAS, I., PINHAS, A., GOLDHAMMER, Y. and BRAHAM, J. (1978) Progressive supranuclear palsy: EMG examination of eye muscles. *Acta Neurologica Scandinavica*, **58**, 304–308

POLA, J. and ROBINSON, D. A. (1976) An explanation of eye movements seen in internuclear ophthalmoparesis. *Archives of Neurology*, **33**, 447–452

POLA, J. and WYATT, H. J. (1980) Target position and velocity: the stimuli for smooth pursuit eye movements. *Vision Research*, **20**, 523–534

POMPEIANO, O. (1974) Cerebello-vestibular interrelations. In: *Handbook of Sensory Physiology: The Vestibular System*, edited by H. H. Kornhuber, Vol. VI, Part 1. New York: Springer–Verlag. pp. 417–476

PRECHT, W., SHIMAZU, H. and MARKHAM, C. H. (1966) A mechanism of central compensation of vestibular function following hemilabyrinthectomy. *Journal of Neurophysiology*, **29**, 996–1010

PYYKKO, I., JANTTI, P. and AALTO, H. (1988) Postural control in the oldest olds. *Advances in Oto-Rhino-Laryngology*, **41**, 146–151

PYYKKO, I., ISHIZAKI, H., AALTO, H. and STARCK, J. (1992) Relevance of the Tullio phenomenon in assessing perilymphatic leak in vertiginous patients. *American Journal of Otology*, **13**, 339–342

RAPHAN, T. and COHEN, B. (1978) Brainstem mechanisms for rapid and slow eye movements. *Annual Review of Physiology*, **40**, 527–552

RAPHAN, T., MATSUO, V. and COHEN, B. (1979) Velocity storage in the vestibulo-ocular reflex arc (VOR). *Experimental Brain Research*, **35**, 229–248

REASON, J. T. (1970) Motion sickness: a special case of sensory rearrangement. *Advances in Science*, **26**, 386–393

REASON, J. T. (1978) Motion sickness adaptation: a neural mismatch model. *Journal of the Royal Society of Medicine*, **71**, 819–829

REASON, J. T. and BRANDT, J. J. (1975) *Motion Sickness*. London: Academic Press

RICHMOND, F. J. R. and BAKKER, D. A. (1982) Anatomical organization and sensory receptor content of soft tissues surrounding upper cervical vertebrae in the cat. *Journal of Neurophysiology*, **48**, 49–61

ROBERTS, T. D. M. (1967) *Neurophysiology of Postural Mechanisms*. New York: Plenum Press

ROBERTS, T. D. M. (1978) *Neurophysiology of Postural Mechanisms*, 2nd edn. London: Butterworths

ROBINSON, D. A. (1964) The mechanics of human saccadic eye movement. *Journal of Physiology*, **174**, 245–264

ROBINSON, D. A. (1965) The mechanics of human smooth pursuit. *Journal of Physiology*, **180**, 569–591

ROBINSON, D. A. (1976) Adaptive gain control of vestibulo-ocular reflex by the cerebellum. *Journal of Neurophysiology*, **39**, 954–969

ROBINSON, D. A. and FUCHS, A. F. (1969) Eye movements evoked by stimulation of frontal eye fields. *Journal of Neurophysiology*, **32**, 637–648

ROMBERG, M. H. (1846) *Lehrbuch der Nerven Krankheiten des Menschen*. Berlin: A. Duncker

ROSENGART, A., HEDGES, T. R., TEAL, P. A., DEWITT, L. D., WU, J. K., WOLPERT, S. *et al.* (1993) Intermittent downbeat nyastagmus due to vertebral artery compression. *Neurology*, **43**, 216–218

ROSENHALL, U. (1972a) Vestibular macular mapping in man. *Annals of Otology, Rhinology and Laryngology*, **81**, 339–351

ROSENHALL, U. (1972b) Mapping of the cristae ampullares in man. *Annals of Otology, Rhinology and Laryngology*, **81**, 882–889

ROSENHALL, U. and RUBIN, W. (1975) Degenerative changes in the human vestibular sensory epithelium. *Acta Otolaryngologica*, **79**, 67–85

ROSS, M. D., KOMOROWSKI, T. E., ROGERS, C. M., POTE, K. G. and DONOVAN, K. M. (1987) Macular suprastructure, stereociliary bonding, and kinociliary/stereociliary coupling in rat utricular macula. *Acta Otolaryngologica*, **104**, 56–65

RUBIN, W. (1981) Sinusoidal harmonic acceleration test in clinical practice. *Annals of Otology, Rhinology and Laryngology*, **90** (suppl. 86), 18–25

RUDGE, P. (1983) *Clinical Neuro-otology*. Edinburgh: Churchill Livingstone

RUDGE, P. and CHAMBERS, B. R. (1982) Physiological basis for enduring vestibular symptoms. *Journal of Neurology, Neurosurgery and Psychiatry*, **45**, 126–130

RUDGE, P. and LEECH, J. (1976) Analysis of a case of periodic alternating nystagmus. *Journal of Neurology, Neurosurgery and Psychiatry*, **39**, 314–319

RUSCH, A. and THURM, U. (1990) Spontaneous and electrically induced movements of ampullary kinocilia and stereovilli. *Hearing Research*, **48**, 247–264

RUSSELL, I. J., RICHARDSON, G. P. and CODY, A. R. (1986)

Mechanosensitivity of mammalian auditory hair cells in vitro. *Nature*, **321**, 517–519

SALAMI, J., POTVIN, A., JONES, K. and LANDRETH, J. (1975) Cortical evoked responses to labyrinthine stimulation in man. *Psychophysiology*, **2**, 55–61

SALT, A. N. and KONISHI, T. (1986) The cochlear fluids: perilymph and endolymph. In: *Neurobiology of Hearing: The Cochlea*, edited by R. A. Altschuler, D. W. Hoffman and R. P. Bobbin. New York: Raven Press. pp. 109–122

SANDO, I., BLACK, F. O. and HEMENWAY, W. G. (1972) Spatial distribution of vestibular nerve in internal auditory canal. *Annals of Otology, Rhinology and Laryngology*, **81**, 305–314

SCHAEFER, K. P. and MEYER, D. L. (1973) Compensatory mechanisms following labyrinthine lesions in the guinea pig. A simple model of learning. In: *Memory and Transfer of Information*, edited by H. P. Zippel. New York: Plenum. pp. 203–232

SCHALEN, L., HENRIKSSON, N. G. and PYYKKO, I. (1982) Quantification of tracking eye movements in patients with neurological disorders. *Acta Otolaryngologica*, **93**, 387–395

SCHERER, H., BRANDT, U., CLARKE, A. H., MERBOLD, U. and PARKE, R. (1986) European vestibular experiments on the Spacelab-I mission 3. Caloric nystagmus in microgravity. *Experimental Brain Research*, **64**, 255–263

SCHILLER, P. H. (1977) The effect of superior colliculus ablation on saccades elicited by cortical stimulation. *Brain Research*, **122**, 154–156

SCHILLER, P. H., TRUE, S. D. and CONWAY, J. L. (1980) Deficits in eye movements following frontal eye-field and superior colliculus ablations. *Journal of Neurophysiology*, **44**, 1175–1194

SCHNEIDER, L. W. and ANDERSON, D. J. (1976) Transfer characteristics of first and second order lateral canal and vestibular neurons in gerbil. *Brain Research*, **112**, 61–76

SCHUBERT, K. (1950) Schwindel und Sympathikus. *Archiv für Ohren-Nasen und Kehlkopfheilkunde versinigt mit Zeitschrift fur Hals-Nasen und Ohrenheilkunde*, **156**, 489–499

SCHUKNECHT, H. F. and RUBY, R. R. (1973) Cupulolithiasis. *Advances in Otorhinolaryngology*, **20**, 434–443

SCHUKNECHT, H. F., NORTHROP, C. and IGARASHI, M. (1968) Cochlear pathology after destruction of the endolymphatic sac in the cat. *Acta Otolaryngologica*, **65**, 479–487

SCHWARTZ, U., BUSETTINI, C. and MILES, F. A. (1989) Ocular responses to linear motion are inversely proportional to viewing distance. *Science*, **245**, 1349–1396

SELIKTAR, R., SUSAK, Z., NAJENSON, T. and SOLZI, P. (1978) Dynamic features of standing and their correlation with neurological disorders. *Scandinavian Journal of Rehabilitation Medicine*, **10**, 59–64

SELLICK, P. M., JOHNSTONE, J. R. and JOHNSTONE, B. M. (1972) The electrophysiology of the utricle. *Pflugers Archiv European Journal of Physiology*, **336**, 21–27

SEMONT, A., FREYSS, G. and VITTE, E. (1988) Curing the BPPV with a liberatory manoeuver. *Advances in Otorhinolaryngology*, **42**, 290–293

SHEEHAN, S., BAUER, R. B. and MEYER, J. S. (1960) Vertebral artery compression in cervical spondylosis. *Neurology*, **10**, 968–986

SHELDON, J. H. (1963) The effect of age on the control of body sway. *Gerontology Clinics*, **5**, 129–138

SHEPARD, N. T., TELIAN, S. A., SMITH-WHEELOCK, M. and ANIL, R. (1993) Vestibular and balance rehabilitation therapy. *Annals of Otology, Rhinology and Laryngology*, **102**, 198–205

SHIBASAKI, H., YAMASHITA, Y. and MOTOMURA, S. (1978)

Suppression of congenital nystagmus. *Journal of Neurology, Neurosurgery and Psychiatry*, **41**, 1078–1083

SHIMAZU, M. and PRECHT, W. (1965) Tonic and kinetic responses of cats vestibular neurons to horizontal angular accelerations. *Journal of Neurophysiology*, **28**, 989–1013

SHIMAZU, M. and PRECHT, W. (1966) Inhibition of central vestibular neurons from the contralateral labyrinth and its mediating pathway. *Journal of Neurophysiology*, **29**, 467–492

SINGLETON, G. T. (1986) Diagnosis and treatment of perilymph fistulas without hearing loss. *Otolaryngology – Head and Neck Surgery*, **94**, 426–429

SMITH, C. A., LOWRY, O. H. and WU, M. L. (1954) The electrolytes of the labyrinthine fluids. *Laryngoscope*, **64**, 141–153

SPOENDLIN, H. (1964) Uber die Polarisation der Vestibularen Rezeptoren. *Pratica Otorhinolaryngologica*, **26**, 418–432

STAHLE, J. T. and TERRINS, J. (1965) Paroxysmal positional nystagmus. *Annals of Otology, Rhinology and Laryngology*, **74**, 69–83

STEINBACH, M. J. (1976) Pursuing the perceptual rather than the retinal stimulus. *Vision Research*, **16**, 1371–1376

STEINHAUSEN, W. (1931) Uber den Nachweis der Bewegung der Cupula in der intaken Bogengangsampulle des Labyrinthes bei der naturlichen und calorishen Reizung. *Pflugers Archiv für die Gesamte Physiologie des Menschen und der Tiere*, **228**, 322–328

STELMACH, G. E., ZELAZNIK, N. H. and LOIRE, D. (1990) The influence of aging and attentional demands on recovery from postural instability. *Aging*, **2**, 155–161

STEPHENS, S. D. G. and BALLAM, H. M. (1974) The sono-ocular test. *Journal of Laryngology and Otology*, **88**, 1049–1059

SUH, K. W. and CODY, D. T. R. (1974) Obliteration of vestibular and cochlear aqueduct. *Laryngoscope*, **84**, 1352–1368

SUZUKI, J. I., TOKUMASU, K. and COHEN, B. (1969) Eye movements from single utricular nerve stimulation in the cat. *Acta Otolaryngologica*, **68**, 350–362

SZENTAGOTHAI, J. (1950) The elementary vestibulo-ocular reflex arc. *Journal of Neurophysiology*, **13**, 395–407

TAGUCHI, K. and TADA, C. (1988) Change of body sway with growth of children in posture and gait. Development, adaptation and modulation. Excerpta Medica, *Amsterdam International Congress Series*, **812**, 59–66

TAKAGI, A., SANDO, I. and TAKAHASHI, H. (1989) Computer-aided three-dimensional reconstruction and measurement of semicircular canals and their cristae in man. *Acta Otolaryngologica*, **107**, 362–365

TAKAHASHI, S., FETTER, M., KOENIG, E. and DICHGANS, J. (1990) The clinical significance of head-shaking nystagmus in the dizzy patient. *Acta Otolaryngologica*, **109**, 8–14

TAKEDA, N., IGARASHI, M., KOIZUKA, I., CHAE, S. and MATSUNAGA, T. (1990) Recovery of the otolith-ocular reflex after unilateral deafferentation of the otolith organs in squirrel monkeys. *Acta Otolaryngologica*, **110**, 25–30

TAKEMORI, S. and COHEN, B. (1974) Visual suppression of vestibular nystagmus in Rhesus monkeys. *Brain Research*, **72**, 203–212

TAKEMORI, S. and SUZUKI, J. I. (1971) Eye deviations from neck torsion in humans. *Annals of Otology, Rhinology and Laryngology*, **80**, 439–444

TAKUMIDA, M. (1989) Glycocalyx and ciliary interconnections of the vestibular end organs: an investigation by high resolution scanning electron microscope. *Journal for Oto-Rhino-Laryngology and its Related Specialities*, **51**, 137–143

TAKUMIDA, M. and BAGGER-SJOBACK, D. (1989) Effects of amilo-

ride on the endolymphatic sac. *Journal of Laryngology and Otology*, **103**, 466–470

TAKUMIDA, M., SUZUKI, M., HARADA, Y. and BAGGER-SJOBACK (1990) Glycocalyx and ciliary interconnections of the human vestibular end organs: an investigation by scanning electron microscope. *Journal for Oto-Rhino-Laryngology and its Related Specialities*, **52**, 137–142

TAKUMIDA, M., TAKEDA, N., SENBA, E., TOHYAMA, M., KUBO, T. and MATSUNAGA, T. (1984) Localisation, origin and fine structure of calcitonin gene related peptide containing fibres in vestibular end organs of the rat. *Brain Research*, **504**, 31–35

TANAKA, M., TAKEDA, N., SENDA, E., TOHYAMA, M., KUBO, T. and MATSUNGA, T. (1989) Localisation, origin and fine structure of calcitonin gene-related peptide containing fibres in vestibular end organs of the rat. *Brain Research*, **504**, 31–35

TASAKI, I. and SPYROPOULOS, C. S. (1959) Stria vascularis as a source of endolymphatic potential. *Journal of Neurophysiology*, **22**, 149–155

TEN CATE, W. F., PATTERSON, K. and RAREY, K. E. (1990) Ultrastructure of ampullar dark cells in the absence of circulating adrenocorticosteroid hormones. *Acta Otolaryngologica*, **110**, 234–240

TER BRAAK, J. W. G. (1936) Untersuchungen ueber optokinetischen Nystagmus. *Archives Neerl de Physiologie*, **21**, 309–376

THEUNISSEN, E. J. M., HUYGEN, P. L. M. and FOLGERING, H. T. (1986) Vestibular hyperreactivity and hyperventilation. *Clinical Otolaryngology*, **11**, 161–169

THYSSEN, H. H., BRYNSKOV, J., JANSEN, E. C. and MUNSTER-SWENDSEN, J. (1982) Normal ranges and reproducibility for the quantitative Romberg's test. *Acta Neurologica Scandinavica*, **66**, 100–104

TIBBLING, L. (1969) The rotatory nystagmus response in children. *Acta Otolaryngologica*, **68**, 459–467

TJERNSTROM, O. (1973) Nystagmus inhibition as an effect of eye closure. *Acta Otolaryngologica*, **75**, 408–418

TOKITA, T., MAEDA, M. and MIYATA, H. (1981) The role of the labyrinth in standing posture control. *Acta Otolaryngologica*, **91**, 521–527

TOROK, N. (1976) Vestibular decruitment in central nervous system disease. *Annals of Otology, Rhinology and Laryngology*, **85**, 131–135

TRIESON, H. H., BRINSCOMBE, J., JANSEN, E. and SWENSON, J. M. (1982) Normal ranges in the reproducibility for the quantitative Romberg's test. *Acta Neurologica*, **66**, 100–104

TROOST, B. T., MARTINEZ, J., ABEL, L. A. and HEROS, R. C. (1980) Upbeat nystagmus and internuclear ophthalmoplegia with brainstem glioma. *Archives of Neurology*, **37**, 453–456

TROTTER, Y., GARY-BOBO, E. and BUISSERET, P. (1979) Restoration of orientation specificity of the visual cells in kittens after section of the ophthalmic branches of the Vth nerve. *Neuroscience Letters*, **53**, 296

TSUJIKAWA, S., NINOYU, O., AMANO, H., YAMASHITA, T. and KUMAZAWA, T. (1991) Positive and negative DC potentials in the vestibular system of pigeons. *Journal for Oto-Rhino-Laryngology and its Related Specialties*, **53**, 6–9

TULLIO, P. (1929) *Das Ohr und die Enstenhung der Sprahe und Schrift*. Berlin–Vienna: Schwartzenberg

UCHIZONO, K., NOMURA, Y. and KOSAKA, K. (1967) Localization of acetylcholinesterase activity in the efferent fiber of the human cochlea. *Journal of the Physiology Society of Japan*, **29**, 241–242

UEMURA, T. and COHEN, B. (1973) Effects of vestibular nuclei lesions on vestibulo-ocular reflexes and posture in monkeys. *Acta Otolaryngologica Supplementum*, **315**, 1–71

UEMURA, T., SUZUKI, J., HOZAWA, J. and HIGHSTEIN, S. M. (1977) *Neuro-otological Examination with Special Reference to Equilibrium Function Tests.* Baltimore: University Park Press

USAMI, S., HOZAWA, J. and YLIKOSKI, J. (1991) Co-existence of substance P and calcitonin gene related peptide like immunoreactivity in rat vestibular end organs. *Acta Otolaryngologica*, Suppl. 481, 168–169

VALLI, P., ZUCCA, G., PRIGIONI, I., BOTTA, L., CASELLA, C. and GUTH, P. S. (1985) The effect of glutamate on the frog vestibular canal. *Brain Research*, **330**, 1–9

VAN WULFFTEN PALTHE, P. M. (1922) Function of the deeper sensibility and of the vestibular organs in flying. *Acta Otolaryngologica*, **4**, 415–448

VIDAL, J., JEANNEROD, M., LIFSCHITZ, W., LEVITAN, H., ROSENBURG, J. and SEGUNDO, J. P. (1971) Static and dynamic properties of gravity-sensitive receptors in the cat vestibular system. *Kybernetik*, **9**, 205–215

VIIRE, E., TWEED, D., MILNER, K. and VILLIS, T. (1986) A re-examination of the gain of the VOR. *Journal of Neurophysiology*, **56**, 439–450

VINCENT, S. R., HATTORI, T. and MCGEER, E. G. (1978) The nigrotectal projection: a biochemical and ultrastructural characterisation. *Brain Research*, **151**, 159–164

VOORHEES, R. L. (1989) The role of dynamic posturography in neuro-otologic diagnosis. *Laryngoscope*, **99**, 995–1001

VOSS, H. (1958) Zahl and Anordnung der Muskelspindeln in den unteren Zungenbeinmuskeln, dem M. sternocleidomastoideus und den Bauch-und tiefen Nackenmuskeln. *Anatomischer Anzeiger*, **105**, 265–275

VYSLONZIL, E. (1963) Uber eine umschriebene anasmmlung von Otokien in hinteren hautigen Bogengange. *Monatsschrift für Ohrenheilkunde*, **97**, 63

WACKYM, P. A., FRIBERG, U. and BAGGER-SJOBACK, D. (1986) Human endolymphatic duct: possible mechanisms of endolymph outflow. *Annals of Otology, Rhinology and Laryngology*, **95**, 409–414

WACKYM, P. A., FRIBERG, U. and BAGGER-SJOBACK, D. (1987) Human endolymphatic sac: possible mechanisms of pressure regulation. *Journal of Laryngology and Otology*, **101**, 768–779

WACKYM, P. A., GLASSCOCK, M. E. and LINTHICUM, F. H. (1988) Immunohistochemical localisation of the Na$^+$, K$^+$-ATPase in the human endolymphatic sac. *Archives of Otorhinolaryngology*, **245**, 221–223

WACKYM, P. A., CACALIS, R. F., FRIBERG, U., RASK-ANDERSEN, H. and LINTHICUM, F. H. (1990) Size variations in the lateral intercellular spaces on the endolymphatic sac induced by dietary factors. *Laryngoscope*, **100**, 217–222

WAESPE, W. and HENN, V. (1977) Neuronal activity in the vestibular nuclei of the alert monkey during vestibular and optokinetic stimulation. *Experimental Brain Research*, **27**, 523–538

WALL, C., BLACK, F. O. and HUNT, A. E. (1984) Effects of age, sex, and stimulus parameters upon vestibulo-ocular responses to sinusoidal rotation. *Acta Otolaryngologica*, **98**, 270–278

WALSHE, F. B. and HOYT, W. H. (1969) *Clinical Neuro-ophthalmology*, vol. 1. Baltimore: Williams and Wilkins

WAPNER, S., WERNER, H. and CHANDLER, K. A. (1951) Experiments on sensory-tonic field theory of perception. *Journal of Experimental Psychology*, **42**, 341–345

WATANABE, K. and OGAWA, A. (1984) Carbonic anhydrase activity in the stria vascularis and dark cells in vestibular labyrinth. *Annals of Otology, Rhinology and Laryngology*, **93**, 262–266

WATANABE, K., OHI, H., SAWA, M., OHASHI, N., KOBAYASHI, H. and MIZOKOSHI, K. (1983) Clinical findings of galvanic body sway test in cases of vestibular disorders. In: *Vestibular and Visual Control on Posture and Locomotor Equilibrium*, edited by M. Igarish and F. O. Black. Basel: Karger. pp. 322–330

WATANUKI, K. and MEYER ZUM GOTTESBERGE, A. (1971) Light microscopic observations of the sensory epithelium of the crista ampullaris in the guinea pig. *Annals of Otology, Rhinology and Laryngology*, **80**, 450–454

WATZL, E. and MOUNTCASTLE, V. (1949) Projection of vestibular nerve to cerebral cortex of the cat. *American Journal of Physiology*, **159**, 594

WESTHEIMER, G. and BLAIR, S. M. (1973) Oculo-motor defects in cerebellectomised monkeys. *Investigative Ophthalmology*, **12**, 618–621

WESTHEIMER, G. and BLAIR, S. M. (1974) Functional organisation of the oculo-motor system revealed by cerebellectomy. *Experimental Brain Research*, **21**, 463–472

WHEELER, S. D., RAMSEY, R. E. and WEISS, J. (1982) Drug-induced downbeat nystagmus. *Annals of Neurology*, **12**, 227–228

WILLIAMS, I. M., DICKINSON, P., RAMSAY, R. J. and THOMAS, L. (1982) Seesaw nystagmus. *Australian Journal of Ophthalmology*, **10**, 19–25

WILSON, V. J. and MELVILLE-JONES, G. (1979) *Mammalian Vestibular Physiology.* New York: Plenum Press

WIST, E. R., BRANDT, T. and KRAFCZYK, S. (1983) Oscillopsia and retinal slip. *Brain*, **106**, 153–168

WLODYKA, J. (1978) Studies of cochlear aqueduct patency. *Annals of Otology, Rhinology and Laryngology*, **87**, 22–28

WOLFE, D. M. and KOS, C. M. (1977) Nystagmic responses of the Rhesus monkey to rotational stimulation following unilateral labyrinthectomy: final report. *Transactions of the American Academy of Ophthalmology and Otolaryngology*, **84**, 38–45

WOOLEY, D. M. and BRAMMAL, A. (1987) Direction of sliding velocities within trypsinised sperm axonemes of *Gallus domesticus*. *Journal of Cell Science*, **88**, 361–371

WURTZ, R. H. and GOLDBERG, M. E. (1972) Activity of superior colliculus in behaving monkey. III. Cells discharging before eye movements. *Journal of Neurophysiology*, **35**, 575–586

WURTZ, R. H. and MOHLER, C. W. (1976) Organization of monkey superior colliculus: enhanced visual response of superficial layer cells. *Journal of Neurophysiology*, **39**, 745–765

WYKE, B. (1979) Cervical articular contributions to posture and gait and their relation to senile disequilibrium. *Age and Ageing*, **8**, 251–258

YAGI, T. and MARKHAM C. H. (1984) Neural correlates of compensation after hemilabyrinthectomy. *Experimental Neurology*, **84**, 98–108

YANAGIHARA, N. and NISHIOKA, I. (1987) Pneumolabyrinth in perilymphatic fistula: report of three cases. *American Journal of Otology*, **8**, 313–318

YEE, R. D., BALOH, R. W. and HONRUBIA, V. (1980) A study of congenital nystagmus: optokinetic nystagmus. *British Journal of Ophthalmology*, **64**, 926–932

YEE, R. D., BALOH, R. W., HONRUBIA, V. and JENKINS, H. A. (1982) Pathophysiology of optokinetic nystagmus. In: *Nystagmus and Vertigo. Clinical Approaches to the Patient with Dizziness*, edited by V. Honrubia and M. Brazier. New York: Academic Press. pp. 251–296

YEE, R. D., BALOH, R. W., HONRUBIA, V. and KIM, Y. S. (1981) A study of congenital nystagmus: vestibular nystagmus. *Journal of Otolaryngology*, 10, 89–98

YEE, R. D., WONG, E. K., BALOH, R. W. and HONRUBIA, V. (1976) A study of congenital nystagmus: waveforms. *Neurology*, 26, 326–333

ZAHN, J. R., ABEL, L. A. and DELL'OSSO, L. F. (1978) Audio-ocular response characteristics. *Sensory Processes*, 2, 32–37

ZAMBARBIERI, D., SCHMID, R., MAGNEES, G. and PRABLANC, C. (1982) Saccadic responses evoked by presentation of visual and auditory targets. *Experimental Brain Research*, 47, 417–427

ZEE, D. S. (1984) Ocular motor control: the cerebral control of saccadic eye movements. In: *Neuro-ophthalmology 1984*, edited by S. Lessell and J. T. W. van Dalen. Amsterdam: Elsevier. pp. 141–156

ZEE, D. S. and ROBINSON, D. A. (1979) A hypothetical explanation of saccadic oscillation. *Annals of Neurology*, 5, 405–414

ZEE, D. S., YEE, R. D. and ROBINSON, D. A. (1976) Optokinetic responses in labyrinthine-defective human beings. *Brain Research*, 113, 423–428

ZEE, D. S., YAMAZAKI, A., BUTLER, P. H. and GUCER, G. (1981) Effects of ablation of flocculus and paraflocculus on eye movements in primate. *Journal of Neurophysiology*, 46, 878–899

ZEE, D. S., YEE, R. D., COGAN, D. G., ROBINSON, D. A. and ENGLE, W. K. (1976) Oculomotor abnormalities in hereditary cerebellar ataxia. *Brain*, 99, 207–234

ZEE, D. S., BUTLER, P. H., OPTICAN, L. M., TUSA, R. J. and GUCER, G. (1982) Effects of bilateral occipital lobectomies on eye movements in monkeys: preliminary observations. In: *Physiological and Pathological Aspects of Eye Movements*, edited by A. Roucoux and M. Crommelinck. Documenta Ophthalmologica Proceedings Series 34. Amsterdam: Junk. pp. 225–232

ZUCCA, G., VALLI, P. and CASELLA, C. (1985) Receptor current in ciliate cells of the frog sacculus. *Bollettino – Societa Italiana Biologia Sperimentale*, 61, 411–417

5

Anatomy of the nose and paranasal sinuses

V. J. Lund

Development of nose and paranasal sinuses

The external nose and nasal cavity

The nose develops from a number of mesenchymal processes around the primitive mouth (Hamilton and Mossman, 1972; Moore, 1982) (Figure 5.1). The nasal cavity is first recognizable in the 5.6 mm (crown–rump distance) embryo in the fourth intra-uterine week as the *olfactory* or *nasal placode*, a thickening of the ectoderm above the stomatodaeum (Streeter, 1945). This placode sinks to form the *olfactory pit* lying between the proliferating mesoderm of the medial and lateral nasal folds of the frontonasal process. This deepens to form the *nasal sac* by the fifth week (Figure 5.2).

In the 12.5 mm embryo, the maxillary process of the first branchial arch grows anteriorly and medially to fuse anteriorly with the medial nasal folds and the frontonasal process which closes the nasal pits off to form widely separated primitive, nasal cavities (Figure 5.3). The primitive nasal cavity and mouth are separated initially by a bucconasal membrane. This gradually thins as the nasal sacs extend posteriorly and eventually breaks down at the 14–15 mm stage to form the primitive choanae. These are more anteriorly placed than the definitive posterior choana due to continuous posterior growth of the palate (Warbrick, 1960). The floor anterior to the choana forms from mesenchymal extensions of the medial nasal folds to produce the premaxilla and ultimately the upper lip and medial crus of the lower lateral cartilages.

The maxillary process also grows ventrally from the dorsal end of the mandibular process (first visceral arch) to join the lateral nasal fold around the naso-

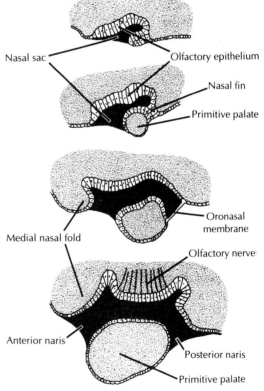

Figure 5.1 The development of the nasal sac, nasal cavity and primitive palate (after Hamilton and Mossman, 1972)

maxillary groove. Ectoderm in this region eventually canalizes to form the nasolacrimal duct. The lateral nasal folds also form the nasal bones, upper lateral

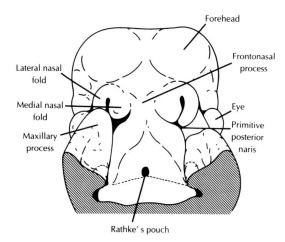

Figure 5.2 The roof of the stomatodaeum of a 12 mm human embryo illustrating the development of the primitive palate and posterior nares by approximation of the maxillary processes to the lateral and medial nasal folds. The previous site of attachment of the buccopharyngeal membrane is represented by a dotted line and part of the left maxillary process has been removed (after Hamilton and Mossman, 1972)

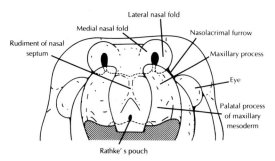

Figure 5.3 The roof of the stomatodaeum of a 12.5 mm embryo (after Hamilton and Mossman, 1972)

cartilages and lateral crus of the lower lateral cartilages.

The palate and nasal septum

The primitive palate begins to form anteriorly with fusion of the maxillary and frontonasal processes by the 13.5 mm embryo stage. A midline ridge develops from the posterior edge of the frontonasal process in the roof of the oral cavity and extends posteriorly to the opening of Rathke's pouch (Figure 5.4). This becomes the nasal septum which is continuous anteriorly with the partition between the primitive nasal

cavities. As the nasal cavities enlarge, the palatal processes, derived from the lateral maxillary mesoderm, grow medially towards each other and the septum. Initially they lie lateral to the tongue, but as this moves ventrally with further growth the palatal processes swing medially and fuse horizontally (Figures 5.5 and 5.6). The fusion begins along the posterior margin of the primitive palate and is complete except for a midline dehiscence at the future site of the incisive canal. Fusion continues between the palatal processes and the septum from anterior to posterior, separating the nasal and oral cavities and most posteriorly the nasopharynx and oral cavity as the palatal processes complete the soft palate and uvula.

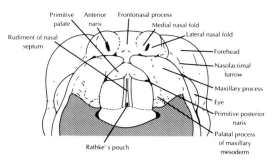

Figure 5.4 The roof of the stomatodaeum of a 13.5 mm human embryo (after Hamilton and Mossman, 1972)

On either side of the anterior septum, in relation to the paraseptal Jacobson's cartilage, an invagination of ectoderm forms the vomeronasal organ, which largely disappears in man, leaving only a blind tubular pouch, 2–6 mm long (Johnson, Josephson and Hawke, 1985). Longitudinal strips of cartilage 7–15 mm in length may be identified in the embryo, lying adjacent to the vomeronasal organ on either side of the septal cartilage. These may occasionally remain as discrete entities in the adult but more usually involute, leaving only a small cartilaginous bulge. The primitive septum is initially made entirely of cartilage. The superior part ossifies to form the perpendicular plate of the ethmoid (from crista galli downwards (Zuckerkandl, 1893; Schultz-Coulon and Eckermeyer, 1976) and the vomer in the posteroinferior portion, leaving an anteroinferior quadrilateral cartilaginous plate. Two ossification centres appear for the vomer at the eighth fetal week on either side of the cartilage, uniting to form a deep bony groove in which the cartilage sits. As growth continues part of the cartilage absorbs as the two bony lamellae fuse. By puberty, the lamellae are almost completely united with everted alae and an anterior groove as indications of the vomer's

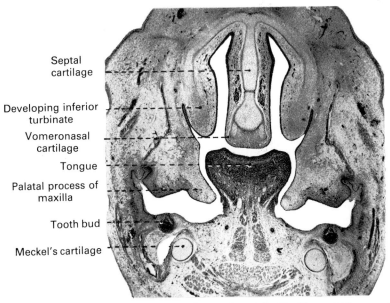

Septal cartilage

Developing inferior turbinate

Vomeronasal cartilage

Tongue

Palatal process of maxilla

Tooth bud

Meckel's cartilage

Figure 5.5 Section through the developing palate of a 20 mm human fetus (after Hamilton and Mossman, 1972)

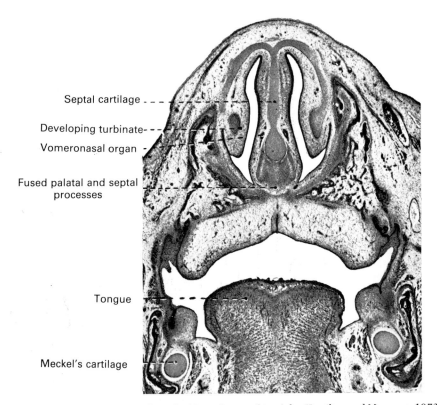

Septal cartilage

Developing turbinate

Vomeronasal organ

Fused palatal and septal processes

Tongue

Meckel's cartilage

Figure 5.6 Section through the developing palate of a 48 mm human fetus (after Hamilton and Mossman, 1972)

bilaminar origin. The nasal bones arise during the tenth and eleventh week.

The paranasal bones and sinuses

The maxilla

The maxilla arises during the sixth and seventh weeks from five ossification centres. In the fourth fetal month these fuse to form the alveolar, palatine, zygomatic and frontal processes and the floor of the orbit. A further centre appears in the medial floor of the pyriform aperture, forming the premaxilla in which the upper incisor teeth develop. The premaxilla forms the anterior nasal spine and fuses with the vomeronasal cartilages laterally and septal cartilage superiorly.

The ethmoid bone

The ethmoid bone ossifies in the cartilaginous nasal capsule from three centres; one for each labyrinth and one for the perpendicular plate. The centres for the labyrinth are present from the fourth or fifth intrauterine month, so they are partially ossified at birth. The perpendicular plate and crista galli develop from one centre during the first year after birth and fuse with the labyrinths at the beginning of the second year. Both this centre and that for the labyrinth contribute to the cribriform plate.

The frontal bone

The frontal bone ossifies in membrane from two centres, one in each superciliary ridge appearing in the eighth intrauterine week. At birth the bone is composed of two halves separated by a frontal or metopic suture, which begin to fuse from the second year. This is usually complete by the eighth year, though may persist in some races such as the Japanese (Warwick and Williams, 1973).

The sphenoid bone

The sphenoid is divided into two parts; a presphenoidal portion anterior to the tuberculum sellae continuous with the lesser wings made up of six separate ossification centres, and the postsphenoidal part composed of the sella turcica and dorsum sellae associated with the greater wings and pterygoid processes derived from eight centres. The pre- and post-sphenoidal parts of the body fuse around the eighth intrauterine month. At birth the bone consists of three pieces, a central portion consisting of the body and lesser wings and two lateral parts, each consisting of the greater wing and pterygoid process which begin to fuse at one year after birth.

The turbinate bones

A series of elevations appear on the lateral wall of the nose from the sixth fetal week which will ultimately form the turbinates. The most inferior or maxilloturbinal forms the inferior turbinate. The middle, superior and supreme turbinates result from reduction of the complex ethmoturbinal system found in lower mammals. Similarly the primitive nasoturbinal is represented by the agger nasi region and uncinate process of the ethmoid.

The maxillary sinus

The maxillary sinus is the first sinus to appear (7–10 weeks) as a shallow groove expanding from the primitive ethmoidal infundibulum into the mass of the maxilla (Figure 5.7). Absorption and expansion results in a small cavity at birth which measures 7 × 4 × 4 mm (Ritter, 1973), and is encroached upon by the orbit and dentition. It continues to grow during childhood at an estimated annual rate of 2 mm vertically and 3 mm anteroposteriorly (Proetz, 1953) and in particular with development of the middle third of the face as the dentition erupts. Thus the floor of the maxillary sinus ultimately comes to lie at a lower level than the floor of the nasal cavity, with mucociliary clearance to the middle meatus consequent upon this development. The sinus may become relatively enlarged in old age as a result of resorption of the alveolus secondary to loss of teeth.

The ethmoid sinus

The ethmoid cells may be detected as furrows in the lateral wall from the fourth intrauterine month (see Figure 5.7) and a few cells are present at birth. The sphenoid sinus is recognizable at around the third

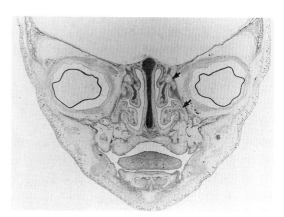

Figure 5.7 Coronal section through the head of a 150 mm human fetus showing early cavitation of maxillary sinus and ethmoids (arrowed)

intrauterine month as an evagination from the spheno-ethmoidal recess and again a small cavity is found at birth ($2 \times 2 \times 1.5$ mm) which reaches full size in adolescence and may expand further in old age. Pneumatization is said to progress at a rate of 0.25 mm each year from the age of 4 years but this is not constant (Hinck and Hopkins, 1965).

The frontal sinus

The frontal sinus is the most variable in size and shape and may be regarded embryologically as an anterior ethmoidal cell. Although a small frontal recess is recognizable from the third intrauterine month, upward expansion does not take place until after birth. Consequently a frontal sinus cavity is not apparent at post mortem until the end of the first year. The configuration of the sinus and the frontal recess is subject to considerable variation. Diverticula, septation and accessory drainage channels are not uncommon. The frontal recess, although frequently a narrow hour-glass segment, may have a longer, more tortuous path encroached upon by adjacent anterior ethmoidal cells. These variations are a direct consequence of the sinus' embryological development as it is the last to complete its growth, in early adulthood.

Anomalies

Fusion of the processes takes place from anterior to posterior. Partial or complete failure of fusion results in abnormalities which range from a bifid uvula to clefts of varying severity. Failure of fusion between a maxillary process and the corresponding premaxilla causes a *cleft lip*. Failure of the maxillary and lateral processes to fuse produces a *facial cleft* with an open nasolacrimal furrow. Non-fusion between the palatine processes and nasal septum results in a *cleft palate*. In its most severe form there is a completely deficient palate and bilateral clefts in the upper lip on either side of the philtrum. Clefts of the lip and palate are seen in just under 0.1% of neonates. Interestingly, more clefts develop on the left than the right (Koelliker, 1882). Occasionally, median clefts are encountered which can produce anomalies ranging from a widened columella and nasal tip to complete dehiscence of the nasal bridge and a bifid nose. Failure of the oronasal membrane to rupture results in *choanal atresia*, which may be either membranous or bony and may lie at a variable distance from the nasopharynx because of changes in the position of the posterior choana during development.

Rarely the olfactory placode fails to develop, with complete or partial absence of the nose. This is usually associated with bilateral choanal atresia and hypoplastic maxillae. Unilateral choanal atresia is much more common. Unilateral maldevelopment of the olfactory placode produces a *proboscis lateralis* where the mesenchyme grows out in a complete ring resembling a trunk and the maxilla and eye are often affected. Median facial anomalies result from abnormal first and second arch development and are generally fatal.

Premature ossification of the sphenoid or fusion of the pre- and post-sphenoidal portions may produce an abnormal depression of the nasal bridge (often seen in achondroplasia) and anomalous fusion of the presphenoid results in *hyperteleorism*.

Cysts arise from epithelial entrapment in the lines of fusion between the various processes. *Nasolabial cysts* develop in the furrow between the maxillary and median nasal elevation and *globulomaxillary cysts* at the junction of the primitive palate and palatine processes, in the alveolar process between lateral incisor and canine teeth. The *dermoid cyst* is a relatively common congenital abnormality. It is a median nasal lesion found on the glabella, dorsum or tip of the nose between the alar cartilages or on the columella. It may be superficial or communicate with a deeper component through a tract between the nasal bones which may extend intracranially through the cribriform plate. Two theories have been proposed for its formation; the cranial theory postulates that as dura mater recedes, it pulls nasal ectoderm forming a sinus. Pinching off of the sinus leads to cyst formation. Alternatively, ectoderm may become trapped between the two medial nasal folds.

Comparative anatomy (Figures 5.8–5.11)

There is a basic pattern to the mammalian nasal cavity which can be recognized in man and offers important teleological information (Negus, 1958; Moore, 1981). In all mammals the nasal fossa is divided into two by a midline septum and its functions are respiratory (moistening, cleaning, and warming inspired air) and olfactory. This is evident in the macroscopic and microscopic configuration of the nose. The lateral nasal wall bears three sets of turbinals; ethmoturbinals, nasoturbinals and maxilloturbinals. The ethmoturbinals are arranged in two rows, the ectoturbinals laterally and endoturbinals medially. They increase surface area for greater olfactory acuity. Ethmoturbinals are particularly well developed in macrosmatic animals and can be very numerous. The olfactory area is augmented by the ethmoturbinals by a factor of five in sheep, 2.5 in the dog and 1.34 in man (Dieulafe, 1906).

The anthropoid and human nose are remarkably similar demonstrating the increasing importance of vision over olfaction (Cave and Wheeler Haines, 1939; Napier and Napier, 1967; Osman Hill, 1970;

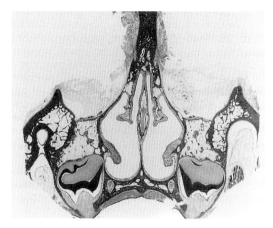

Figure 5.8 Coronal section through midfacial block from *Mandrillus sphinx* (mandrill) showing absence of maxillary sinuses

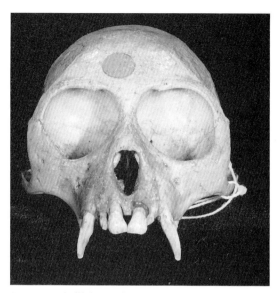

Figure 5.10 Skull of *Miopithecus talapoin* (dwarf gueron). The maxilla is encroached upon by the orbit and dentition. It therefore does not have a functional maxillary sinus

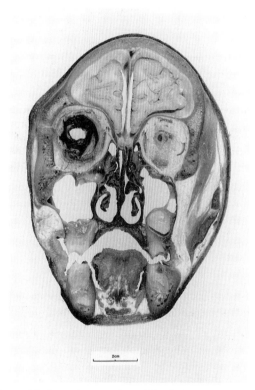

Figure 5.9 Coronal section through head of *Pan troglodytes* (chimpanzee) showing well-developed maxillary sinus and reduced turbinal structure

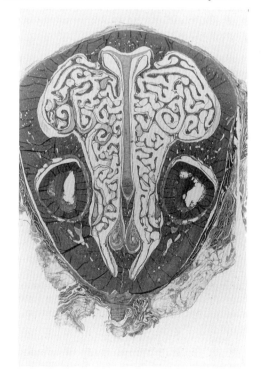

Figure 5.11 Coronal section through nasal cavity of *Castor canadensis* (Canadian beaver) showing extensive ethmoturbinal system

Cave, 1973). There is a reduction in anteroposterior length, resulting in a high-roofed cavity between two large orbits which face forwards. The ectoturbinals disappear during fetal development and the endotur-binals are reduced to three; middle, superior and supreme. The nasoturbinal is represented by the un-cinate process and agger nasi of the ethmoid and the maxilloturbinal is equivalent to the inferior turbinate.

A secondary olfactory organ, the vomeronasal or Jacobson's organ, is found lying either side of the anterior nasal septum usually protected by small cartilages. This organ has an important influence on feeding and oestrus in many mammals, though there is considerable variation in its morphology (Harrison, 1987).

The paranasal sinuses are a characteristic feature of terrestrial, placental, mammals and are absent in monotremes, marsupials and cetacea. The distribution and configuration of the sinuses is varied and despite much consideration and some interesting suggestions (Rhys Evans, 1992), a convincing explanation of their origin and function has not been forthcoming. The maxillary sinus ranges from an extensive cavity, meeting in the midline of the hard palate, e.g. chimpanzee (Bourne, 1972) and pneumatizing the nasal, frontal, lacrimal, palatine and nasoturbinal bones, e.g. bears, horses and elephants, to a shallow lateral recess, e.g. the baboon. The size of the maxillary sinus increases with the size of the skull and orbit in monkeys and higher primates though not with body size (Lund, 1988a). However, the maxillary sinus is not a constant feature and there does not appear to be any specific factor which correlates with its presence or absence among the anthropoids. In the great apes, the maxillary sinus and nasal configuration of the gorilla and chimpanzee resemble that of man with the natural ostium opening into the middle meatus.

Most mammals have additional pneumatized chambers communicating with the olfactory region and opening between the ethmoturbinals into which the olfactory epithelium may extend. These may correspond to ethmoid, frontal or sphenoid sinuses but there is considerable interspecies and intraspecies variation. The big ungulates, elephants and carnivores have considerable frontal pneumatization. In the majority of monkeys, the gibbon and orang there is little frontal development. Humans and the African apes can be distinguished by the presence of an ethmoid complex in addition to a true frontal and sphenoid sinus, though the ethmoid is most highly developed in humans. Examination of these patterns of mammalian sinus pneumatization does not clarify the purpose of the paranasal sinuses.

Anatomy of the nose and paranasal sinuses

External nose and vestibule

A considerable literature is available devoted to descriptions of the external appearances of the nose as it pertains to cosmetic surgery (Figure 5.12).

Vestibule and skin

The vestibule is the dilated passageway leading from the external nares into the nasal fossae, demarcated by the limen nasi, at the superior margin of the lower lateral cartilage. It is lined by skin bearing coarse hairs or vibrissae (though without erector

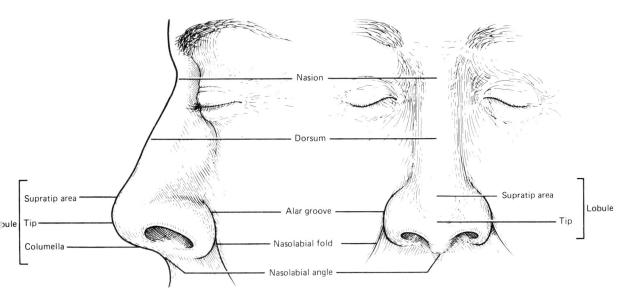

Figure 5.12 External nose showing surface anatomy

muscles), sebaceous glands and sweat glands. With increasing age the overall area of the vestibule enlarges at the expense of the respiratory region of the nasal cavity.

The thickness of the skin and soft tissues of the nasal bridge vary. Over the dorsum and sides of the nose it is thin and loosely adherent. It becomes thicker and more adherent over the tip and alar cartilages where it contains numerous large sebaceous glands. The elasticity and mobility of the skin over the nose also varies dependent upon the quality and anchorage of the collagen fibres running between the skin and underlying layers.

Muscles of the external nose (Figures 5.13 and 5.14)

The nose has a number of muscles which, in man,

have assumed an almost vestigial importance. As muscles of facial expression, they are all supplied by branches of the facial nerve. The *depressor nasi septi muscle* attaches between the alveolus and the medial crus of the lower lateral cartilage. Its function is to depress the septum and tip, expanding the external nares during forced inspiration. The *nasalis muscle* is composed of an alar and a transverse part. The transverse fibres run from the pyriform aperture onto the dorsum of the nose into a thin aponeurosis attached to the transverse muscle fibres of the opposite side. Its action is to contract the nasal aperture. The alar component arises beneath the nasomaxillary suture and runs inferiorly, laterally and anteriorly, attaching by a short thin tendon to the skin of the nasal ala. Contraction produces shortening and dilatation of the nostril.

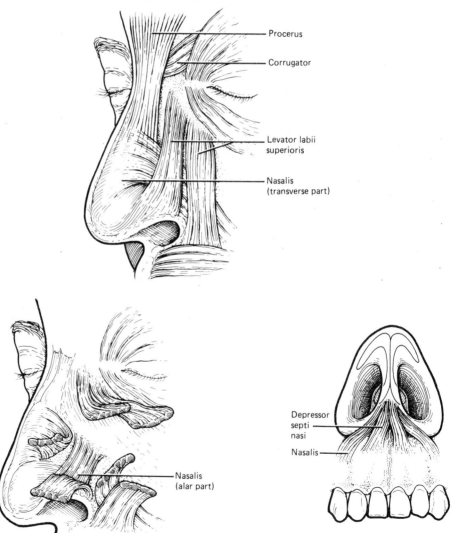

Figure 5.13 External musculature of the nose

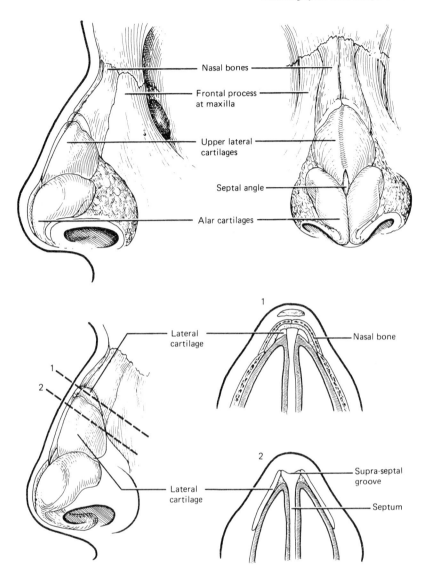

Figure 5.14 Bony and cartilaginous anatomy of the nose

A continuation of frontalis forms the *procerus muscle*. It shortens the nose when contracted but also produces facial movement of the area between the eyebrows hence its alternative name, *depressor glabelli* (Virchow, 1912). The development of this muscle and the associated fat pad is responsible for the shape of the root of the nose. *Levator labii superioris alaequae nasi* arises from the frontal process of the maxilla and blends with the perichondrium of the lateral crus of the lower lateral cartilage. It pulls this superiorly, dilating the nostril and in addition elevates the upper lip, hence its name. Electromyography shows that the nasal dilators are respiratory muscles as their action correlates with ventilatory resistance (Sasaki and Mann, 1976).

The supporting framework of the external nose is composed of a bony skeleton provided by the nasal bones, frontal processes of the maxillae and nasal part of the frontal bone and a cartilaginous framework consisting of septum, upper and lower lateral cartilages and a variable number of minor accessory alar cartilages.

Nasal bones (Figure 5.15)

The nasal bones unite with each other in the midline, with the frontal bone superiorly at the nasofrontal suture and laterally with the frontal process of the maxilla at the nasomaxillary suture. They are supported by the nasal spine of the frontal bone and by

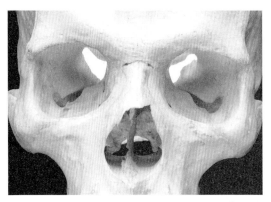

Figure 5.15 Human skull (anterior aspect) showing bones surrounding the pyriform aperture

the perpendicular plate of the ethmoid, both of which groove the bones. The nasal bone is wedge-shaped, usually convex and smooth on its outer surface and concave and roughened internally. The bones are grooved by adjacent neurovascular bundles, producing radiolucencies which may be difficult to interpret on X-rays. There is considerable ethnic and individual variation in the shape and size of the nasal bones (Lang, 1989a).

Pyriform aperture (see Figure 5.15)

The pyriform aperture is bounded below and laterally by the maxilla and above by the nasal bones. The anterior nasal spine lies in the middle of the inferior border. It can be up to 15 mm in length (Lang and Sakals, 1982) and is related superiorly to the antero-inferior free end of the septal cartilage.

Cartilages of the external nose and columella

The nasal cartilages are composed of hyaline cartilage which may be ossified. They prevent collapse of the vestibule on inspiration. The upper cartilages are triangular flat expansions lying inferior to the nasal bones and are overlapped by them, by the adjacent frontal processes of the maxillae and by the lower lateral cartilages in 72% of cases (Lang, 1989b), to all of which they are attached by fibrous tissue. The groove between the upper and lower lateral cartilages is known as the limen nasi, which is the site of intercartilaginous incisions. The medial aspect of the upper lateral cartilages are continuous with the nasal septal cartilage which is bifid in this area.

The lower lateral or alar cartilages form the lower third of the nose. They are each composed of a medial and lateral crus which meet at the dome of the tip, though the highest point can be on the lateral crus. The medial crura are loosely attached to each other in the midline and contribute to the columella, anterior to the quadrilateral cartilage. The lower margin of the lateral crus does not follow the margin of the nostril but ascends away from the margin laterally. Between one and four (average 2.3) minor sesamoid cartilages are found between the upper and lower lateral cartilages.

The part of the septum running between the tip of the nose and philtrum is called the *columella*. It bounds the anterior nares medially and is thicker posteriorly because of the contribution made by the medial crura of the lower lateral cartilages.

Blood supply

Branches of the facial artery supply the alar region while the dorsum and lateral walls of the external nose are supplied by the dorsal branch of the ophthalmic artery and the infraorbital branch of the maxillary. There are significant anastomoses between these vessels on each side and between the right and left sides (Lang, 1989c).

The venous networks do not parallel the arterial supply but correspond to territories termed arterio-venous units (Lang, 1989d). The frontomedian area drains to the facial vein and the orbitopalpebral area to the ophthalmic vein with interconnections to the anterior ethmoidal system and thence cavernous sinus which can be of clinical significance. The facial vein arises by the confluence of the supratrochlear and supraorbital veins at the inner canthus where it is termed the angular vein in its superior portion. Usually a transverse venous anastomosis exists between the right and left supratrochlear veins.

Nerve supply

The skin of the external nose receives its sensory supply from the two upper divisions of the trigeminal nerve; ophthalmic and maxillary. The ophthalmic has an infratrochlear branch supplying the lateral surface of the root of the nose and an external nasal branch supplying the skin over the root and dorsum as far as the tip of the nose. The infraorbital branch of the maxillary nerve gives external and internal nasal branches which supply the nasal alae and skin of the nasal vestibule respectively, inferior palpebral and superior labial branches which form the *pes anserinus minor* with superior buccal branches of the facial nerve, and the anterior superior alveolar branch with its supply to the anterior lateral wall.

Lymphatic drainage

This drains from the external nose with the anterior face to the submandibular and submental nodes, with buccal nodes adjacent to the facial vein some-times intervening. There may also be bilateral drain-age and flow to the parotid region is possible.

Nasal cavity

The nasal cavity extends from the external nares or nostrils to the posterior choanae, where it becomes continuous with the nasopharynx and is narrower anteriorly than posteriorly. Vertically it extends from the palate to the cribriform plate, being broader at its base than superiorly where it narrows to the olfactory cleft. The nasal cavity is divided in two by a septum. The configuration and dimensions show considerable ethnic variation. Each half has a floor, a roof, a lateral wall and a medial (septal) wall. The *floor* is concave from side to side, anteroposteriorly flat and almost horizontal. Its anterior three-quarters are com-posed of the palatine process of the maxilla, its poster-ior one-quarter by the horizontal process of the pala-tine bone. About 12 mm behind the anterior end of the floor is a slight depression in the mucous membrane overlying the incisive canals. This con-tains the terminal branches of the nasopalatine nerve, the greater palatine artery and a short mucosal canal (Stenson's organ). Occasionally incisor and canine teeth can protude into the floor of the nasal cavity.

The *roof* is narrow from side to side, except posteri-orly and may be divided into frontonasal, ethmoidal and sphenoidal parts, related to the respective bones.

As both the frontonasal and sphenoidal parts of the roof slope downwards, the highest part of the nasal cavity relates to the cribriform plate of the ethmoid which is horizontal. This area is covered by olfactory epithelium which spreads down a little distance onto the upper lateral and medial walls of the nasal cavity. The rest of the nasal cavity (with the exception of the nasal vestibule) is lined by respiratory mucous mem-brane which is intimately adherent to the underlying periosteum and perichondrium and is continuous with that of the paranasal sinuses, nasolacrimal duct and nasopharynx.

Nasal septum

Bones and cartilages (Figure 5.16)

The nasal septum is composed of a small anterior membranous portion, cartilage and several bones: the perpendicular plate of the ethmoid, the vomer and two bony crests of the maxilla and palatine. The cartilaginous portion is composed of a quadrilateral cartilage with a contribution from the lower and upper lateral alar cartilages forming the anterior nasal septum. The quadrilateral cartilage is 3–4 mm thick in its centre but increases to 4–8 mm anteroinfer-iorly, an area which has been termed the *footplate*. The upper margin of the cartilage also expands where it is connected to the upper lateral cartilages, forming the anterior septal angle, just cranial to the domes of

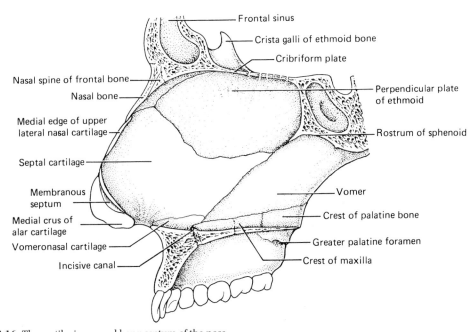

Figure 5.16 The cartilaginous and bony septum of the nose

the lower lateral cartilages. It is bound firmly by collagenous fibres to the nasal bones, and to the perpendicular plate of the ethmoid and vomer and, where it sits inferiorly in the nasal crest of the palatine process of the maxilla, the fascial attachment effects a pseudoarthrosis. It abuts the maxillary spine at the inferior septal angle. Anteriorly it is attached by a thin membranous septum to the medial crura of the lower lateral cartilages.

The perpendicular plate forms the superior and anterior bony septum, is continuous above with the cribriform plate and crista galli and abuts a variable amount of the nasal bones (Lang, 1989e). The vomer forms the posterior and inferior nasal septum and articulates by its two alae with the rostrum of the sphenoid, thereby creating the vomerovaginal canals which transmit the pharyngeal branches of the maxillary artery. Occasionally the sphenoid sinus may pneumatize the vomer. The inferior border of the vomer articulates with the nasal crest formed by the maxillae and palatine bones. The anterior border articulates with the perpendicular plate above and the quadrilateral cartilage inferiorly. The posterior edge of the vomer forms the posterior free edge of the septum.

The nasal septum, and in particular the quadrilateral cartilage is of crucial importance in the development of the middle third of the face. This has been the subject of considerable experimental and longitudinal clinical studies (Scott, 1953, 1956, 1957, 1958, 1959, 1963; Sarnat and Wexler, 1966; Pirsig, 1977; Verwoerd, Urbanus and Nijdam, 1979; Loosen, Verwoerd-Verhoef and Verwoerd, 1988). The surface area of the septum measures between 30 and 35 cm^2 in adults (Gherardi, 1939).

Deflections may develop at any of the septal articulations and spurs may also be found where the quadrilateral cartilage sends small processes between the ethmoid and vomer. Thiele (1855) found septal deviations in 22% of a normal population and these deviations were more often to the left than the right (Zuckerkandl, 1893; Lang, 1989f). As such deflections are far commoner in men than women, they are most likely to be acquired due to trauma than be congenital and this has been substantiated by work on identical twins in relations to deformities of the anterior septum (Grymer and Melsen, 1989).

Histology

The mucoperichondrium and mucoperiosteum of the septum is separate from that overlying the maxillary crest, reflecting its embryological development. The mucous membrane is predominantly respiratory with a small area of olfactory epithelium superiorly adjacent to the cribriform plate. Respiratory epithelium is composed of ciliated and non-ciliated pseudostratified columnar cells, basal pluripotential stem cells and goblet cells. The columnar cells are 25 μm in height

and 7 μm wide, tapering to 2–4 μm at the basement membrane. Each cell bears 300–400 microvilli, irrespective of the presence of cilia. These are finger-like cytoplasmic extensions, 2 μm in length and 0.1 μm diameter. Their function is to increase surface area and thus prevent drying. Where cilia are present, there are 50–100 per cell though the number varies with their position in the nose and age. The cilia are composed of the classical axonema of nine peripheral doublet and two central single microtubules (Figure 5.17). Each peripheral pair (A and B) connects to the next doublet and to the central microtubule with hexin links. The A microtubule bears an outer and inner dynein arm, composed of ATPase which can attach to the B microtubule, leading to axonemal displacement and cilial beating (Figure 5.18).

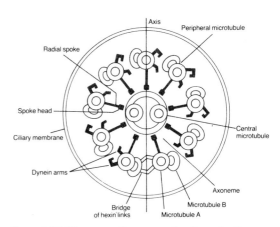

Figure 5.17 Diagrammatic cross-section through cilium near the base, showing the ultrastructure of the axonema and demonstrating the classical 9 + 2 pattern of microtubules

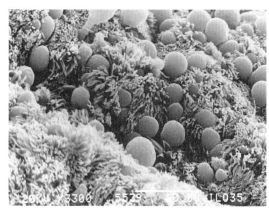

Figure 5.18 Scanning electron micrograph of respiratory epithelium showing ciliated cells with globules of mucus (magnification × 3300)

Seromucinous glands are found in the submucosa and are more important in mucus production in the nasal cavity than the goblet cells which are more numerous in the sinuses. On the septum the number of goblet cells increases from anterior to posterior and from superior to inferior (Tos and Morgensen, 1979). By contrast the glands decrease from anterior to posterior and from superior to inferior and decrease with age. The neonatal septum is 450 mm² with 17–18 glands/mm², compared with the adult septum of 1700 mm² and 8.5 glands/mm².

The olfactory epithelium spreads down from the cribriform plate onto the upper septum. It is composed of receptor cells, supporting cells with microvilli and basal stem cells conferring on olfactory epithelium the capacity for regeneration. Each receptor cell has approximately 17 cilia, but these differ from their respiratory counterparts in their radial arrangement, greater length and poorly developed ultrastructure. Dynein arms are not present preventing linking between the microtubules and conventional beating. The sensory endings have a characteristic knob-like vesicular structure from which olfactory fibres join the axonal bundle (Figure 5.19). There is a sharp transition zone between the olfactory and respiratory epithelium though the relative area of each varies with age and reflects the decrease in olfactory acuity. Secretion for the olfactory epithelium is provided by Bowman's glands.

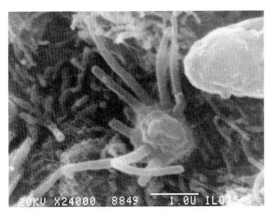

Figure 5.19 Scanning electron micrograph of olfactory epithelium showing a sensory bulb (magnification × 24 000)

Blood supply

The external and internal carotid arteries are responsible for the rich blood supply to the nose. The sphenopalatine artery (branch of the maxillary artery and thus external carotid artery) supplies the posteroinferior septum. The greater palatine artery (also a branch of the maxillary) supplies the anteroinferior portion entering the nasal cavity via the incisive canal. The superior labial branch of the facial artery contributes

anteriorly, in particular to *Kiesselbach's plexus*, which is composed of unusually long capillary loops and is situated in *Little's area* on the anterior septum – a common source of epistaxis. The internal carotid artery supplies the septum superiorly via the anterior and posterior ethmoidal arteries and also contributes to Kiesselbach's plexus (Figure 5.20).

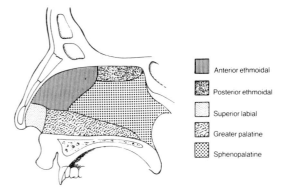

Anterior ethmoidal

Posterior ethmoidal

Superior labial

Greater palatine

Sphenopalatine

Figure 5.20 Blood supply to the nasal septum. (From Maran and Lund, 1990 by courtesy of the publisher Georg Thieme Verlag)

There is a sinusoid system in the nasal submucosa under autonomic control which has been well described in relation to the turbinates but is also present on the septum adjacent to the inferior turbinate and on the most anterior septum (Figure 5.21). This

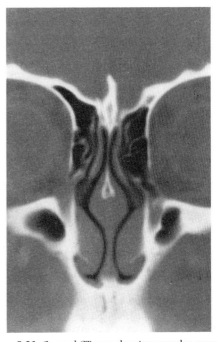

Figure 5.21 Coronal CT scan showing vascular expansion of anterior nasal septum

anterior septal tubercle or intumescence was first described by Morgagni (Zuckerkandl, 1893) and may be related to control of airflow into the olfactory cleft. A similar structure is seen on the posterior septum in two-thirds of individuals.

The cavernous venous system drains via the spheno-palatine vessels into the pterygoid plexus posteriorly and into the facial veins anteriorly. Superiorly the ethmoidal veins communicate with the superior ophthalmic system and there may be direct intracranial connections through the foramen caecum into the superior sagittal sinus.

Nerve supply (Figure 5.22)

The maxillary division of the trigeminal nerve provides the sensory supply to the majority of the nasal septum. The nasopalatine nerve supplies the bulk of the bony septum, entering the nasal cavity via the sphenopalatine foramen, passing medially across the roof to the upper septum and running down and forwards to the incisive canal to reach the hard palate. The anterosuperior part of the septum is supplied by the anterior ethmoidal branch of the nasociliary nerve and a smaller anteroinferior portion receives a branch from the anterior superior alveolar nerve. The posteroinferior septum also receives a small supply from the nerve to the pterygoid canal and a posterior inferior nasal branch of the anterior palatine nerve.

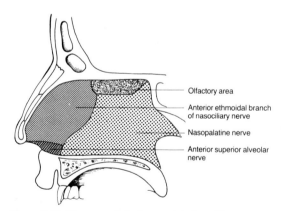

Figure 5.22 Nerve supply to the nasal septum. (From Maran and Lund, 1990 by courtesy of the publisher Georg Thieme Verlag)

The sensory nerves are accompanied by postganglionic sympathetic fibres to blood vessels and postganglionic parasympathetic secretomotor fibres pass to glands with the branches from the pterygopalatine ganglion.

The olfactory epithelium covers the inferior surface of the cribriform plate spreading down to cover a variable area on the upper septum and adjacent lateral wall, over the medial surface of the superior concha. With increasing age the area is encroached upon by respiratory epithelium and in the adult covers an area of approximately 2–5 cm^2. The surface area is considerably increased by the cilia on the receptor cells. Nerve fibres arising from the olfactory receptors are slim (0.2 μm in diameter) and non-myelinated. They join up into approximately 20 bundles which traverse the cribriform plate to reach the olfactory bulbs. Each bundle carries a tubular sheath of dura and pia-arachnoid, which may be sheared in head injuries, destroying olfaction and potentially producing cerebrospinal fluid leakage.

The fibres synapse in the glomeruli of the olfactory bulbs which in turn connect with the olfactory tract and with other cells (mitral and tufted) within the bulb which contribute to feedback loops from higher cortical centres. The olfactory tract passes on the inferior surface of the frontal lobe to the olfactory trigone from which diverging bundles, the medial and lateral olfactory striae, pass around the anterior perforating substance to connect with the hypothalamus, amygdala and hippocampus. These complex linkages subserve the interactions of smell, taste, feeding and reproductive behaviour, representing one of the most primitive areas of the brain.

Lymphatic drainage

The anterior septum drains with the external nose to the submandibular nodes while drainage is to the retropharyngeal and anterior deep cervical nodes posteriorly.

The lateral nasal wall (Figure 5.23)

Inferior meatus (Stammberger and Kennedy, 1995)

The inferior meatus is that part of the lateral wall of the nose lateral to the inferior turbinate. It is the

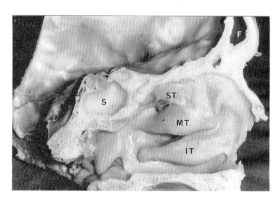

Figure 5.23 Sagittal section through the nasal cavity showing structures of lateral nasal wall (IT: inferior turbinate, MT: middle turbinate, ST: superior turbinate, F: frontal sinus, S: sphenoid sinus)

largest meatus, extending almost the entire length of the nasal cavity. The meatus is highest at the junction of the anterior and middle third. In adults this ranges from 1.6 to 2.3 cm (mean 1.9 cm) at 1.6 cm along the bony lateral wall (Lund, 1988b). The nasolacrimal duct opens into the inferior meatus usually just anterior to its highest point. There is no true valve, the opening being covered by small folds of mucosa. It can be identified in life by gentle massage of the lacrimal sac at the medial canthus.

Inferior turbinate (Figure 5.24)

This structure is composed of a separate bone, the inferior concha which has an irregular surface, perforated and grooved by vascular channels to which the mucoperiosteum is firmly attached. The bone has a maxillary process which articulates with the inferior margin of the maxillary hiatus. It also articulates with the ethmoid, palatine and lacrimal bones, completing the medial wall of the nasolacrimal duct. The inferior concha has its own ossification centre which appears around the fifth intrauterine month.

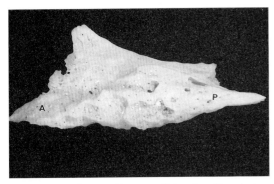

Figure 5.24 Inferior turbinate, medial surface (A: anterior, P: posterior). (From Maran and Lund, 1990 by courtesy of the publisher Georg Thieme Verlag)

The turbinate possesses an impressive submucosal cavernous plexus with large sinusoids under autonomic control which provides the major contribution to nasal resistance. The turbinate is covered by respiratory epithelium, with a high number of goblet cells (approximately 8/mm^2) which decrease in density towards the posterior end (Tos and Morgensen, 1979).

Middle meatus

The middle meatus is that portion of the lateral nasal wall lying lateral to the middle turbinate. It receives drainage from the frontal, maxillary and anterior ethmoidal sinuses. Considerable confusion has arisen with regard to terminology in this area, as many terms originally defined in the last century by the German and French have been used interchangeably.

In the past when radical sinus surgery was predominantly used for most pathology this was of less significance. The advent of endoscopic surgery has led to an increased interest in the detailed anatomy of the region and a need for consensus in terminology.

The configuration of the structures of the middle meatus are complex and variable, but can more readily be understood when the embryological development of the area is considered. If the topographical anatomy is considered in the sagittal plane, a number of structures are apparent, covered by the middle turbinate (Figures 5.25 and 5.26). In a disarticulated skull, the maxillary bone has a large opening in its medial wall, the *maxillary hiatus*. In the articulated skull this is filled in by adjacent bones:

inferior: the maxillary process of the inferior turbinate bone
posterior: the perpendicular plate of the palatine bone
anterosuperior: a small portion of the lacrimal bone
superior: the uncinate process and bulla of the ethmoid.

A portion of the maxillary hiatus is nevertheless left open by these osseous attachments, which in life is filled by the mucous membrane of the middle meatus, the mucous membrane of the maxillary sinus and the intervening connective tissue – the membranous portion of the lateral wall. This membranous area can be defined as lying anterior or posterior to the uncinate process, constituting the anterior and posterior fontanelles respectively. It is in the fontanelles that accessory ostia are found, their formation probably arising as a consequence of infection and consequently, they have been compared to perforations in the tympanic membrane. It is difficult to ascertain a 'natural' incidence for accessory ostia but is probably of the order of 4–5% in the general adult population, increasing to 25% in patients with chronic rhinosinusitis. Accessory ostia are found most frequently in the posterior fontanelle which is generally larger than its anterior counterpart.

The uncinate process (Figure 5.27)

This thin crescent of bone curves posteriorly, parallel with the curve of the anterior face of the ethmoidal bulla. In addition to its anterior attachment to the maxillary hiatus, it attaches superiorly in a variety of ways. It may curve laterally to reach the lamina papyracea, it may attach superiorly to the skull base or occasionally it may fuse with the insertion of the middle turbinate. In the two latter situations there is confluence of drainage from the frontal and maxillary sinuses with the ethmoidal infundibulum leading into the frontal recess, with obvious potential pathological consequences. When the uncinate process inserts on the lamina papyracea, the ethmoidal infundibulum

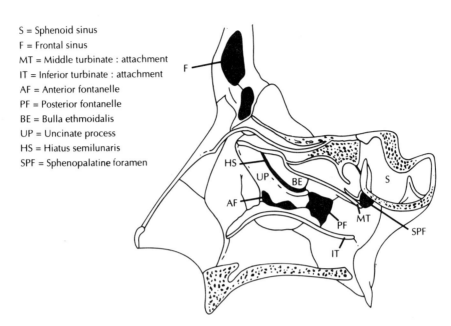

S = Sphenoid sinus
F = Frontal sinus
MT = Middle turbinate : attachment
IT = Inferior turbinate : attachment
AF = Anterior fontanelle
PF = Posterior fontanelle
BE = Bulla ethmoidalis
UP = Uncinate process
HS = Hiatus semilunaris
SPF = Sphenopalatine foramen

Figure 5.25 Bony structures of lateral nasal wall (after Stammberger, 1991)

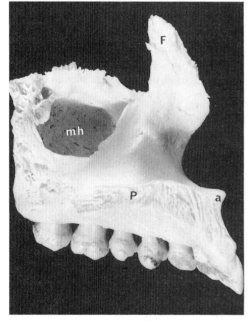

Figure 5.26 Maxillary bone, medial view. (mh: maxillary hiatus, F: frontal process, a: anterior nasal spine, P: palatine process). (From Maran and Lund, 1990 by courtesy of the publisher Georg Thieme Verlag)

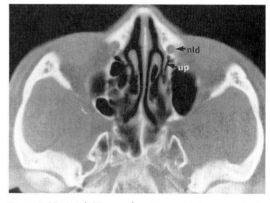

Figure 5.27 Axial CT scan showing uncinate process (up) and nasolacrimal duct (nld)

leads superiorly into a blind pouch, the *terminal recess* (recessus terminalis). Exceptionally, the uncinate process is pneumatized.

The agger nasi

This area has caused considerable confusion but constitutes with the uncinate process, the remnants of the nasoturbinal in lower mammals and is the most anterior part of the ethmoid. It is represented by a small crest or mound on the lateral wall just anterior to the attachment of the middle turbinate. It is occasionally pneumatized, though the incidence in the normal population is probably less than 5%. Pneumatization of the agger nasi region may encroach upon the nasolacrimal duct.

Hiatus semilunaris

The hiatus semilunaris is a two-dimensional space lying between the posterior edge of the uncinate process and the anterior surface of the ethmoidal bulla. The ethmoidal infundibulum is reached from the middle meatus by passing through the hiatus semilunaris.

Ethmoidal infundibulum (Figure 5.28)

The ethmoidal infundibulum is a three-dimensional funnel connecting the natural ostium of the maxillary sinus to the middle meatus via the hiatus semilunaris. It is defined:

medial: uncinate process and hiatus semilunaris
lateral: lamina papyracea
anterior: an acute-angled blind recess where the uncinate process meets the lamina papyracea
posterior: anterior face of the ethmoidal bulla
superior: this will vary according to the attachment of the uncinate process.

Anteriorly the uncinate process may be separated by only 1–2 mm from the lamina papyracea for some distance before they join.

The natural ostium of the maxillary sinus lies in the floor of the ethmoidal infundibulum, usually at the junction of its middle and posterior third and so is not readily visualized until the uncinate process has been removed.

The frontal recess

The frontal recess is found in the most anterosuperior portion of the middle meatus. The term 'fronto-nasal duct' has been generally abandoned as no true duct exists either histologically or topographically in most people. The natural ostium of the frontal sinus is somewhat variable in its configuration but most frequently it presents as an hour-glass narrowing opening directly into the recess. Rarely, a longer narrowed region is found. In 10% of patients, multiple ostia are found (Lund, 1987), though these openings should not be confused with a more laterally placed suprabullar (superior anterior ethmoidal) cell running into the orbital roof.

The frontal recess may be defined:

medial: middle turbinate
lateral: lamina papyracea
superior: skull base
inferior: dependent upon the attachment of the uncinate process.

The ethmoidal bulla (see Figure 5.27)

This is one of the most constant features in the middle meatus containing the largest anterior ethmoidal cell but it may be poorly aerated or completely unpneumatized in 8% of patients (Stammberger, 1991) hence its alternative nomenclature of torus lateralis (lateral bulge) (Zuckerkandl, 1893; Grunwald, 1925). The anterior face forms the posterior margin of the hiatus semilunaris and ethmoidal infundibulum. Posteriorly the bulla may fuse with the basal lamella of the middle turbinate and superiorly it may reach the roof of the ethmoids forming the posterior wall of the frontal recess. Sometimes a cleft is encountered between the posterior wall of the bulla and the basal lamella of the middle turbinate, the *lateral sinus* or *recessus supraethmoidalis*. If the bulla does not reach the skull base, the lateral recess will connect above the bulla with the frontal recess anteriorly. It may be defined:

medial: middle turbinate
lateral: lamina papyracea
superior: roof of ethmoid
inferior and anterior: roof and posterior wall of the ethmoidal bulla
posterior: basal lamella of the middle turbinate.

Anatomical variations (Figures 5.29–5.32; Table 5.1)

There is a considerable range of anatomical variation in this area which has been implicated in the aetiology of sinus infection (Zinreich, Kennedy and Gayler,

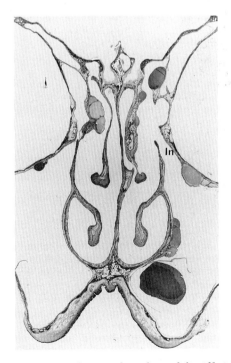

Figure 5.28 Coronal section through an adult midfacial block, in the region of infundibulum (In)

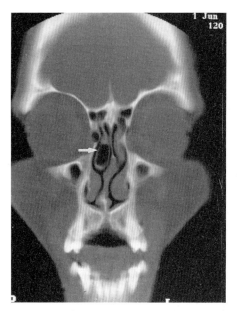

Figure 5.29 Coronal CT scan showing concha bullosa (arrow)

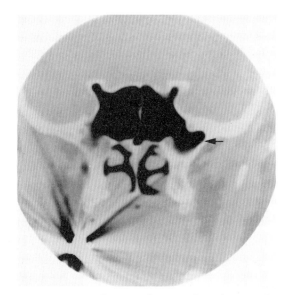

Figure 5.31 Coronal CT scan showing sphenoid sinus with extensive lateral pneumatization (arrow)

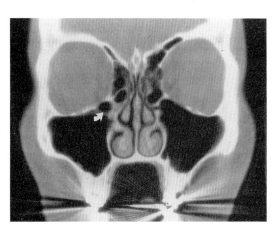

Figure 5.30 Coronal CT scan showing Haller cells (arrow)

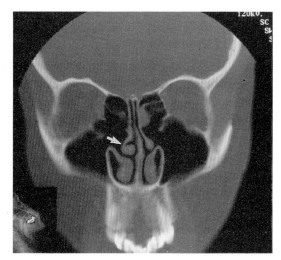

Figure 5.32 Coronal CT scan showing paradoxically bent middle turbinate (arrow)

Table 5.1 Anatomical variants on CT

	Control (%)	Patient (%)
Concha bullosa	14	24
Bent uncinate process	16	21
Paradoxical middle turbinate	17	15
Overpneumatized ethmoid bulla	17	18
Agger nasi cells	3	15
Haller cells	2	13
	$n = 100$	$n = 100$

1988). This includes pneumatization of the middle turbinate, enlargement of the ethmoidal bulla, a paradoxically bent middle turbinate, everted uncinate process and the presence of Haller cells or a septal deflection. The incidence with which these are seen in a 'normal' population may appear to be less frequent than in those individuals with chronic rhinosinusitis but on closer inspection it is clear that it is narrowing of the ostiomeatal complex rather than the existence of the variant which is the important factor (Lloyd, Lund and Scadding, 1991).

Superior meatus

This meatus is again defined by its relationship to the superior turbinate. The posterior ethmoidal cells open into this region.

A *supreme turbinate* is discernible above the superior meatus in 60–67% of subjects (Schaeffer, 1920; Van Alyea, 1939), though is well developed in less than 20% (Lang and Sakals, 1982). Drainage to the corresponding supreme meatus from the posterior ethmoidal system can take place under these circumstances.

Sphenoethmoidal recess

The sphenoethmoidal recess lies medial to the superior turbinate and is the location of the ostium of the sphenoid sinus.

Histology of the lateral wall

The majority of the lateral wall is covered by respiratory ciliated columnar epithelium though there is a small variable area superiorly of olfactory epithelium spreading down from the cribriform plate. Areas of squamous metaplasia are often found on the lateral wall, particularly in areas subject to greatest airflow such as the anterior inferior turbinate.

Blood supply of the lateral wall (Figure 5.33)

The external and internal carotid arteries supply the lateral wall. The sphenopalatine artery (from the maxillary artery and thus external carotid artery) contributes the majority of the supply to the turbinates and meatus. It enters through the sphenopalatine foramen which lies just inferior to the horizontal attachment of the middle turbinate and may be damaged in excessive enlargement of a middle meatal

antrostomy. Its branches to the respective turbinates and meatus enter posteriorly. On the conchae the vessels are partially embedded in deep grooves. In the inferior meatus the sphenopalatine branch dips below the level of the palate to re-emerge anteriorly, leaving the central portion of the meatus relatively avascular (Lund, 1988b). An area anteriorly is supplied by a branch from the facial and part of the lateral wall adjacent to the palate receives blood from the greater palatine. The internal carotid artery contribution is via the ethmoidal arteries which supply the superior lateral wall. There is considerable overlap between the internal and external carotid arterial systems on each side and between the right and left sides which may complicate attempts at arterial ligation in the management of epistaxis (Shaheen, 1987).

The vascular supply to the nose is well-developed and this is enhanced by cavernous plexus found in the lamina propria in particular on the inferior and middle turbinates which is controlled autonomically. The veins of the plexus are between 0.1 and 0.5 mm wide and anastomose with each other. In addition numerous arteriovenous anastomoses are found in the deep mucosa and around the glands (Cauna, 1970). Venous drainage is to the sphenopalatine veins via facial and ophthalmic vessels, intracranially via the ethmoidal veins to veins on the dura and to the superior sagittal sinus via the foramen caecum.

Nerve supply of the lateral wall (Figure 5.34)

Apart from the olfactory supply on the superior concha, the lateral wall receives ordinary sensation from the anterior ethmoidal nerve anterosuperiorly and from branches of the pterygopalatine ganglion and anterior palatine nerves posteriorly. There is a small area innervated by the infraorbital nerve

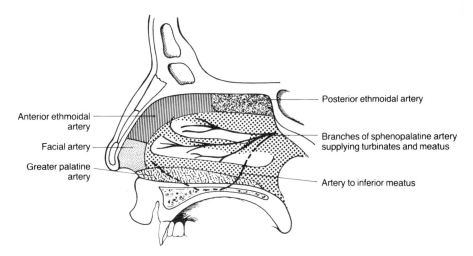

Figure 5.33 Blood supply to the lateral wall of the nose. (From Maran and Lund, 1990 by courtesy of the publisher Georg Thieme Verlag)

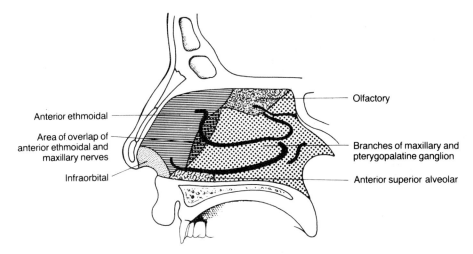

Figure 5.34 Nerve supply to the lateral wall of the nose. (From Maran and Lund, 1990 by courtesy of the publisher Georg Thieme Verlag)

anteriorly and an area of overlap between the ethmoidal and maxillary nerves. The anterior superior alveolar nerve sends a small branch to the anterior inferior meatus which may be damaged in inferior meatal surgery affecting dental sensation (Wood Jones, 1939; Heasman, 1984).

Lymphatic drainage

The lateral wall drains with the external nose to the submandibular nodes anteriorly and to the lateral pharyngeal, retropharyngeal and upper deep cervical nodes posteriorly.

The ethmoid bone and sinuses

Osteology (Figure 5.35)

This complex bone is composed of five parts: two ethmoidal labyrinths suspended either side of a perpendicular plate which forms the upper portion of the bony nasal septum, with an intervening cribriform plate and a superior midline extension, the crista galli. The bone is roughly cruciate in form. All components of the bone are subject to individual variation. The perpendicular plate is quadrilateral in shape and articulates with the nasal spine of the frontal bone and nasal bones, posteriorly with the sphenoid and vomer. The crista ranges in length from 15.1 to 31.4 mm (mean 21.6 mm) and may be pneumatized and/or contain marrow. The cribriform plate divides the nasal cavity from the anterior cranial cavity. The fenestrations in the plate give the area its name, which the olfactory filaments, ethmoidal vessels and nerves and dural prolongations traverse. Two anterior alae complete the foramen caecum, which often transmits an emissary vein to the super-

ior sagittal sinus. The roof of the ethmoidal labyrinths is predominantly completed by the frontal bone. The point at which the frontal and ethmoid bones meet is at a variable height above the cribriform niche (1–17 mm)(Kainz and Stammberger, 1989) and the ethmoid roofs themselves are often asymmetric (10%; Dessi *et al.*, 1994) with the right more often lower than the left.

The *middle turbinate* is crucial to understanding the anatomy of the ethmoid complex. Most anteriorly the turbinate attaches to the maxilla, just anterior to which is the bulge of the agger nasi. The anterior third attaches vertically to the skull base at the lateral border of the cribriform niche with the frontal bone forming the roof of the ethmoids. The posterior third attaches horizontally to the lamina papyracea and medial wall of the maxilla. Between these two portions of the turbinate, there is an obliquely disposed plate of bone, the *basal lamella* of the middle turbinate, attaching laterally to the lamina papyracea. The basal lamella divides the ethmoidal labyrinth into an anterior and posterior group of cells. The basal lamella may be encountered as an obliquely placed plate but is frequently invaginated by anterior cells inferiorly, by posterior cells bulging anteriorly or by the lateral sinus. There are no true middle ethmoidal cells (Figure 5.36).

The ethmoidal labyrinth is a collection of cells and clefts. The lateral walls constitute the orbital plates or lamina papyracea. The lamina is extremely thin and may be dehiscent particularly in the very young or old. The anterior cells are generally smaller and more numerous (2–8) than the posterior group (1–5). The largest and most constant anterior cells form the bulla ethmoidalis, opening directly into the middle meatus.

The posterior cells drain into the superior (or

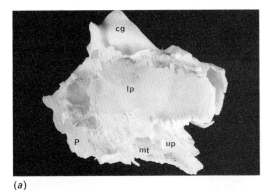

(a)

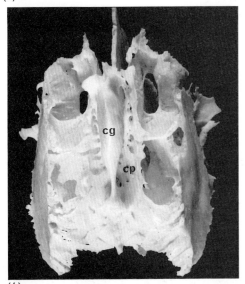

(b)

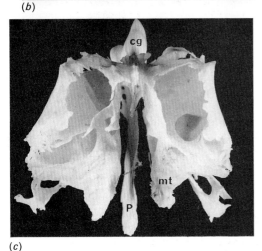

(c)

Figure 5.35 Ethmoid bone. (a) Lateral view; (b) superior view; (c) posterior view. (cg: crista galli, lp: lamina papyracea, mt: middle turbinate, up: uncinate process, P: perpendicular plate of ethmoid, cp: cribriform plate.) (From Maran and Lund, 1990 by courtesy of the publisher Georg Thieme Verlag)

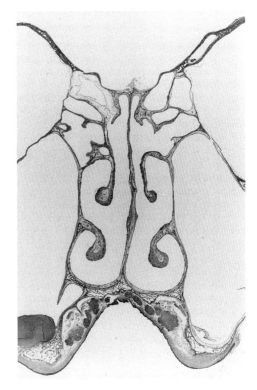

Figure 5.36 Coronal section through an adult midfacial block, showing the lateral (horizontal) attachment of the middle turbinate in posterior part of middle meatus

occasionally supreme) meatus. These cells are large and pyramidal in shape, pointing towards the orbital apex. They are closed posteromedially by the sphenoid bone. The most posterior ethmoidal cell can extend lateral to the sphenoid, up to 1.5 cm posterior to the anterior wall of the sphenoid. This configuration was originally described by Onodi, and bears his name (Onodi, 1903). The optic nerve is particularly vulnerable in such cells and there is considerable ethnic variation in the incidence with which Onodi cells are encountered. The ethmoidal cells may pneumatize the orbital floor, forming Haller cells which can encroach upon the ethmoidal infundibulum (Haller, 1769). Pneumatization proceeds from the anterior system in 70% and from posterior cells in 30%.

Histology

The ethmoidal sinuses are lined by thin ciliated columnar respiratory epithelium. The density of goblet cells is lower than in the maxillary sinus, with a mean of 6500/mm². Tubuloalveolar seromucinous glands are found throughout the mucosa, being more numerous in the ethmoids than in the other paranasal sinuses.

Ethmoidal arteries and veins

The ethmoidal arteries arise from the ophthalmic artery, a branch of the internal carotid. The anterior artery accompanies the nerve and supplies the anterior ethmoidal cells and frontal sinus. It passes through the anterior ethmoidal canal in the medial wall of the orbit, usually at the junction of the frontal bone and lamina papyracea, traverses the roof of the ethmoid, passes through the vertical attachment of the middle turbinate where it abuts the base of skull and reaches the superior surface of the cribriform plate where it gives off an important meningeal branch. The artery then passes down to supply the upper nasal septum and lateral wall of the nose, sending a terminal branch to the nasal dorsum, between the nasal bone and upper lateral cartilages. The artery crosses the roof of the ethmoids just posterior to the frontal recess and may run in a dehiscent canal or in a fold of mucosa. The point where the artery enters the anterior cranial fossa medially may be readily breached. The anterior ethmoidal artery is unilaterally absent in 14%, bilaterally absent in 2%, and multiple in 30% (Shaheen, 1987). If the anterior ethmoidal artery is absent, it is replaced by a branch of the posterior ethmoidal (Lang and Schaefer, 1979).

The smaller posterior ethmoidal artery runs through the canal in the medial wall to supply the posterior ethmoidal cells, and also gives a meningeal branch, and terminates in nasal branches to the septum and lateral wall, anastomosing with the sphenopalatine artery.

Relations

In separating the anterior cranial fossa from the nasal cavity, the ethmoid bone has important relationships with the orbit on either side. The lamina papyracea lies in a vertical plane with the medial wall of the maxillary sinus. It curves 2–3 mm medially as it courses from the orbital apex anteriorly. The posterior cells bear an intimate relationship with the optic nerve. Superiorly the ethmoid labyrinth is closed by the frontal bone and posteromedially by the sphenoid.

Blood, nerves and lymphatic drainage

The vascular supply is derived from the sphenopalatine and ethmoidal (anterior and posterior) arteries and drains by corresponding veins. The ethmoid sinuses are innervated by the anterior and posterior ethmoidal nerves and orbital branches of pterygopalatine ganglion. Lymphatics drain to the submandibular nodes anteriorly and retropharyngeal nodes posteriorly.

The sphenoid bone and sinuses (Figure 5.37)

Osteology

The sphenoid bone is the largest in the skull base and divides the anterior and middle cranial fossa. It is composed of a body (pneumatized to a variable degree), two wings (greater and lesser) and two inferior plates (lateral and medial pterygoid plates). The jugum on the anterior superior surface of the body articulates with the cribriform plate. This surface bears the chiasmatic sulcus connecting the optic canals, the tuberculum sellae, sella turcica and dorsum sellae with related anterior, middle and clinoid processes. The bone slopes away posterior to the dorsum sellae towards the clivus. The lateral surface of the body is grooved by the carotid sulcus on each side as it traverses the cavernous sinus.

The anterior face of the body bears a crest which articulates with the perpendicular plate of the ethmoid. On either side, halfway up the face, lie the ostia of the sinuses. These are large (5–8 mm in diameter) on a macerated skull, but are partially overlapped and closed by the sphenoidal concha and by mucous membrane in life. The sinuses open into

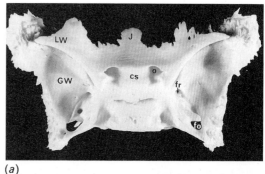

(a)

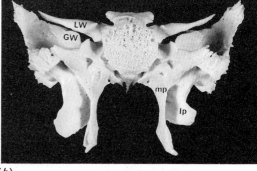

(b)

Figure 5.37 Sphenoid. (a) Superior view; (b) posterior view. (J: jugum, LW: lesser wing, GW: greater wing, cs: chiasmatic sulcus, o: optic canal, fo: foramen ovale, fr: foramen rotundum, mp: medial pterygoid plate, lp: lateral pterygoid plate.) (From Maran and Lund, 1990 by courtesy of the publisher Georg Thieme Verlag)

the sphenoethmoidal recess, superior and medial to the superior (and supreme) turbinate.

The sinus cavities are variable in size and shape. Pneumatization can extend into the greater wing, pterygoid processes and rostrum and may encroach on the basilar part of the occipital bone. Four general forms of pneumatization are described (Elwany *et al.*, 1983):

1 Conchal pneumatization, with only a rudimentary sinus (2–3%).
2 Presellar, in which the sinus is pneumatized as far as the anterior bony wall of the pituitary fossa (11%).
3 Sellar, in which pneumatization extends back beneath the pituitary fossa (59%).
4 Mixed (27%).

The sinuses are divided by a septum which is often paramedian, and there may be diverticula and incomplete septa. It is completely absent in approximately 1% of the population (Grunwald, 1925).

The inferior surface of the body bears the rostrum, which articulates with the vomer. The greater wings contribute to the middle cranial fossa and lateral wall of the orbit. The superior orbital fissure separates it from the lesser wing on each side; the inferior border contributes to the inferior orbital fissure. In addition, the bone is traversed by a number of foramina. The *foramen rotundum* transmits the maxillary nerve, the *foramen ovale* the mandibular nerve, accessory meningeal artery and sometimes the lesser petrosal nerve, and the middle meningeal artery passes through the *foramen spinosum* with a meningeal branch of the mandibular nerve. In 40% of skulls, an emissary venous sphenoidal foramen is found, related to the foramen ovale. The posterior margin of the greater wing contributes to the *foramen lacerum*.

Each pterygoid process consists of a lateral and medial plate which diverge around the pterygoid fossa. The process is pierced superiorly by the *pterygoid canal* which transmits the pterygoid nerve and artery and which may invaginate the floor of the sphenoid sinus. The lateral pterygoid muscle arises in part from the lateral surface of the lateral pterygoid plate, the medial pterygoid muscle from its medial surface. The medial pterygoid plate ends in a hamulus, around which the tendon of the tensor veli palatini hooks.

Although the most posterior ethmoidal cell is closed by the sphenoidal concha, the sphenoid sinus does not simply lie behind. The portion of the sphenoid is usually quite small with the posterior cell often running lateral to the sphenoid sinus and thus the latter may only be entered safely through the most inferior and medial portion of the posterior ethmoid cell.

The optic nerve and internal carotid artery produce variable prominences in the lateral and posterior walls of the sinus, with an intervening cleft which can be deep. The bone overlying these structures is extremely thin or dehiscent in a significant proportion of the population (internal carotid artery: 25%; optic nerve: 6%).

Histology

The goblet cell population of the respiratory epithelium lining the sphenoid sinuses is similar in number to that found in the ethmoids ($6200/mm^2$) though the seromucinous glands are least numerous ($0.06/mm^2$) (Tos and Morgensen, 1979).

Relations

Anterior: posterior ethmoid cell and spheno-ethmoidal recess
Posterior: occipital bone, basilar artery and brain stem
Lateral: cavernous sinus extending from superior orbital fissure to apex of petrous temporal bone. Internal carotid artery, with associated sympathetic plexus, abducent, oculomotor, trochlear nerves, and ophthalmic and maxillary divisions of the trigeminal nerve
Inferior: roof of nasopharynx
Superior: olfactory tracts, frontal lobes, optic chiasma, pituitary gland.

Blood, nerves and lymphatic drainage

The sphenoid sinuses are supplied by the posterior ethmoidal vessels and nerves, with additional supply from the orbital branches of the pterygopalatine ganglion. Lymphatics drain to the retropharyngeal nodes.

The frontal bone and sinuses (Figure 5.38)

Osteology

The frontal bone forms the forehead and orbital roof and is pneumatized to a variable degree. It forms the roof of the ethmoidal sinuses, which produce indi-

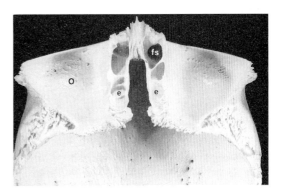

Figure 5.38 Frontal bone, inferior view. (fs: frontal sinus, O: orbital roof, e: ethmoid roof.) (From Maran and Lund, 1990 by courtesy of the publisher Georg Thieme Verlag)

vidual impressions upon the frontal bone, the *fovea ethmoidales ossis frontalis*. The bone is relatively thick in this region, and much thinner in the orbital roofs, where dehiscences may be present. The anterior calvarium increases in thickness from a mean of 4 mm in the newborn to 16 mm in the adult.

The shape and size of the frontal sinuses vary from person to person. In 1% of the British population they are absent. When present, the sinus is usually 'L'-shaped, composed of a horizontal and a vertical compartment but, in addition, diverticula, supernumerary sinuses and incomplete septa are frequently encountered. An intersinus septum is usually present, but may be paramedian and is partially dehiscent in 9%. The sinus drains into the frontal recess, usually by an hour-glass narrowing rather than by any definable 'duct'. Accessory channels are found in 12% of the population and there may be accessory connections to the ethmoidal system. Direct continuity of drainage between the frontal and maxillary sinus may be found depending on the attachment of the uncinate process.

Histology

The frontal sinus respiratory epithelium has a small number of goblet cells ($5900/mm^2$) and a few seromucinous glands ($0.08/mm^2$).

Relations

　Inferior: orbit, ethmoid labyrinths and nasal cavity
　Superior: anterior cranial fossa, olfactory niche, bulbs and tracts
　Medial: cribriform plate and olfactory niche.

Blood, nerves and lymphatic drainage

The supraorbital and anterior ethmoidal arteries supply the frontal sinuses. Venous drainage includes accompanying veins, diploic veins draining into the sagittal and sphenoparietal sinuses and an anastomotic vein in the supraorbital notch connecting the supraorbital and superior ophthalmic vessels.

The nerve supply is derived from the supraorbital nerve and the lymphatics drain to the submandibular gland.

The maxillary bone and sinus (Figures 5.39, 5.40; see also Figure 5.26)

Osteology

The maxilla is the second largest facial bone, forming the majority of the roof of the mouth, the lateral wall and floor of the nasal cavity and the floor of the orbit. The body is usually described as a quadrilateral pyramid, and contains the maxillary sinus. The bone has four processes: zygomatic, frontal, palatine and alveo-

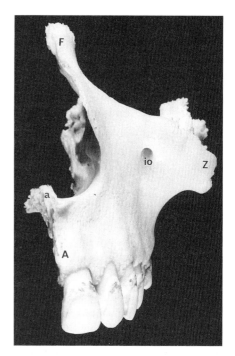

Figure 5.39 Maxilla, anterior view. (a: anterior nasal spine, A: alveolar process, F: frontal process, Z: zygomatic process, io: infraorbital foramen.) (From Maran and Lund, 1990 by courtesy of the publisher Georg Thieme Verlag)

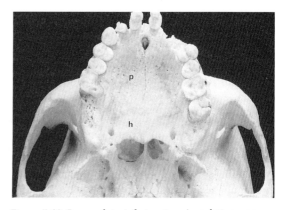

Figure 5.40 Bony palate, inferior view. (p: palatine process of maxilla, h: horizontal process of palatine bone)

lar. It articulates with eight bones; the opposite maxilla, zygoma, frontal, palatine, ethmoid, lacrimal, inferior concha and nasal bones. The anterior surface bears a number of elevations and depressions, related to the dentition which may be named after the adjacent tooth, e.g. canine fossa. The infraorbital foramen is situated above the canine fossa and transmits the infraorbital artery and nerve. The anterior surface is also characterized by the nasal notch and anterior nasal spine.

The maxillary sinuses are relatively symmetrical and only rarely absent.

The roof of the maxillary sinus forms most of the orbital floor. It is traversed by the infraorbital canal, which may be dehiscent. It is indented antero-medially by the lacrimal notch which is related to the lacrimal sac. The posterior edge contributes to the inferior orbital fissure. Inferiorly the floor of the sinus is generally thicker, but can be encroached upon by the roots of teeth, e.g. second premolar and all three molar teeth.

The posterior, infratemporal surface of the bone is convex and grooved by the posterior superior alveolar nerves. Inferiorly it bears the maxillary tuberosity, from which the medial pterygoid muscle takes a small attachment. The medial nasal surface forms the floor of the pyramid and contains a large defect, the maxillary hiatus. This is completed in life by a number of bones and mucous membrane leaving the natural maxillary ostium at the base of the ethmoidal infundibulum. Anterior to the maxillary hiatus is an oblique ethmoidal crest which articulates with the anterior edge of the middle turbinate and agger nasi. The lacrimal canal is created between the maxilla, the lacrimal bone and inferior concha, through which the nasolacrimal duct passes to the anterior part of the inferior meatus. Anterior to the lacrimal notch is the conchal crest to which the inferior concha is attached. Posteriorly, the greater palatine canal is formed between the perpendicular plate of the palatine and maxilla.

When the two maxillae are articulated, the alveolar processes form the alveolar arch. The frontal process bears the anterior lacrimal crest, to which the medial palpebral ligament is attached. The palatine process contributes a large portion of the nasal cavity floor and roof of the mouth, articulating with its opposite number in the midline and forming the incisive canal just posterior to the incisors. This transmits the greater palatine arteries and nasopalatine nerves in separate channels to each side of the nose. Posteriorly the palatine process articulates with the horizontal plate of the palatine bone to complete the hard palate. The inferior surface of the palatine process is pitted by Sharpey's fibres from the palatal periosteum, by vascular foramina and indentations from small salivary glands.

Histology

The maxillary sinus is lined by ciliated columnar epithelium which contains the highest density of goblet cells compared to the other paranasal sinuses (median: 9700/mm^2). The seromucinous glands are relatively infrequent, but again more common in the maxillary sinus and concentrated around the ostium.

Relations

Superior: infraorbital artery and nerve, orbit
Inferior: upper dentition and hard palate
Posterior: pterygopalatine and infratemporal fossae
Anterior: cheek with skin, fat and facial musculature.

Blood, nerves and lymphatic drainage

Small branches of the facial, maxillary, infraorbital and greater palatine arteries and veins supply the maxilla. Venous drainage is to the anterior facial vein and pterygoid plexus. The maxillary division of the trigeminal nerve supplies sensation via the infraorbital, superior alveolar (anterior, middle and posterior) and greater palatine nerves. Near the midpoint of the infraorbital canal, a small branch, the anterior superior alveolar nerve arises which passes in its own canal, the canalis sinusus, to the anterior wall of the maxilla. It passes anterior to the inferior turbinate and reaches the nasal septum in front of the incisive foramen. It supplies the anterior wall of the maxillary sinus, the pulps of the canine and incisor teeth, the anteroinferior quadrant of the lateral nasal wall, the floor of the nose and a small portion of the anterior nasal septum.

The posterior superior alveolar nerves arise from the maxillary nerve in the pterygopalatine fossa and enter the maxilla through the posterior wall to supply the adjacent mucosa and molar teeth. The middle superior alveolar nerve, when present, arises from the infraorbital nerve in its canal and supplies the lateral wall of the sinus and upper premolar teeth. The posteromedial wall of the sinus is supplied by the greater palatine nerve and the roof by perforating branches from the infraorbital nerve.

Lymphatic drainage is relatively poor, but follows predominantly into the pterygopalatine fossa and to the submandibular nodes.

Related anatomy

The orbit

Osteology (Figure 5.41)

The orbits are quadrilateral pyramids lying either side of the nose between the cranium and facial skeleton. The bases of the pyramids face forwards, laterally and slightly inferiorly. They contain the globe, extraocular muscles, nerves, vessels and some associated structures such as the lacrimal apparatus. There is considerable individual and ethnic variation in the dimensions but the adult Caucasian orbit has a mean volume of 30 ml and quite small increases in orbital contents will result in marked proptosis. The *orbital margin* is quadrilateral, on average 41.3 mm wide and 34.4 mm in height, though the female orbit is generally more elongated and larger than that of the male. It is well-ossified at birth, providing protection to its contents.

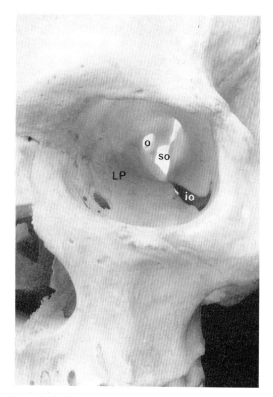

Figure 5.41 Orbit (o: optic canal, so: superior oblique fissure, io: inferior oblique fissure, LP: lamina papyracea)

The orbit has the following relations:
superior: the anterior cranial fossa, with meninges and frontal lobes, frontal and ethmoid sinuses to a variable degree
inferior: maxillary sinus, ethmoidal cells (Haller)
medial: the lateral wall of the nose, ethmoidal infundibulum, ethmoid and sphenoid sinuses, optic nerve
lateral: temporal fossa, middle cranial fossa and temporal lobe.

Seven bones contribute to the orbit: frontal, zygoma, sphenoid, palatine, ethmoid, lacrimal, and maxilla. The *superior* wall or *roof* is triangular and gently concave, composed of the orbital plate of the frontal and the lesser wing of the sphenoid. The orbital part of the lacrimal gland is found in a deep fossa at its anterolateral corner, and the trochlear fovea lies medially. The superior margin has a supra-orbital notch or foramen, transmitting the respective vessels and nerves, and in 50% of the population a frontal notch, lying more medially. Pneumatization of the roof from the frontal or ethmoid sinuses is sometimes found. At the posterior junction of the roof with the medial wall lies the optic canal, which contains the optic nerve (with dura and pia-arachnoid) and ophthalmic artery.

The *medial* wall is composed of the frontal process of the maxilla, the lacrimal bone, the lamina papyra-cea of the ethmoid and the body of the sphenoid. It is consequently extremely thin in parts and may be naturally dehiscent. Anteromedially lies the fossa for the lacrimal sac, demarcated by anterior and posterior lacrimal crests, from the latter of which the lacrimal part of orbicularis oculi takes origin. Through the fronto-ethmoid suture, where it joins the roof, foramina for the anterior and posterior ethmoidal vessels and nerves are located. Their position is variable, but a rule of '24–12–6' has been suggested, based respectively on the average distance in millimetres from the anterior lacrimal crest to the anterior ethmoidal foramen, from the anterior to the posterior ethmoidal foramen, and from the posterior ethmoidal foramen to the optic canal (Rontal, Rontal and Guilford, 1979). This is very much a rough guide as 16% of individuals have no anterior ethmoidal foramen, 30% have multiple foramina and 4.6% have none (Shaheen, 1987).

The *inferior* wall or *floor* is composed of the orbital plate of the maxilla, the orbital surface of the zygoma and the orbital process of the palatine. The infra-orbital sulcus runs forwards from the inferior orbital fissure and at a variable point converts into a canal, which emerges on the anterior face of the maxilla, 4–7 mm beneath the orbital rim. It transmits the infraorbital vessels and nerve, from which the anterior superior alveolar branch arises and in 34% of individuals, a middle superior alveolar branch is also found (Wood Jones, 1939). Anteromedially is the nasolacrimal canal, lateral to which is a small pit marking the origin of the inferior oblique muscle in 91% of individuals (Harrison, 1981). The floor is generally thin (0.5–1 mm) and the infraorbital canal is the commonest site for blow-out fractures.

The *lateral* wall is composed of the greater wing of the sphenoid, the orbital surface of the zygoma, the zygomatic process of the frontal bone. The sphenoidal portion is separated from the roof and floor by the superior and inferior orbital fissures respectively. A small bony projection on the inferior margin of the superior orbital fissure gives origin to the lateral rectus muscle and a tubercle on the orbital surface of the zygomatic bone (the lateral orbital tubercle of Whitnall) gives attachment to the check ligament of the lateral rectus, the suspensory ligament of the eyeball and the aponeurosis of the levator palpebrae superioris.

The *superior orbital fissure* lies between the greater and lesser wings of the sphenoid. It is divided into three by the common tendinous ring, which attaches superomedially round the margin of the optic canal. The lacrimal, frontal and trochlear nerves pass through it superolaterally; the superior division of the oculomotor, nasociliary, sympathetic root of the ciliary ganglion, the inferior division of the oculomotor and abducent nerves pass through the ring centrally; and a branch of the superior ophthalmic vein passes most inferomedial to the ring.

The *inferior orbital fissure* lies between the lateral and inferior orbital walls, communicating with the pterygopalatine fossa medially and infratemporal fossa laterally. In life it is filled by a membrane which transmits the infraorbital vessels and nerves, zygomatic nerves and veins draining the orbit into the pterygoid plexus.

The *optic canal* or *foramen* lies at the apex of the orbit, surrounded by strong bone of the sphenoid and connecting the orbit with the middle cranial fossa. Attached to its margin is the *common tendinous ring* (*of Zinn*) which gives origin to the straight extraocular muscles. It transmits the optic nerve (with dura and pia-arachnoid), the ophthalmic artery and sympathetic plexus. It is intimately related to the most posterior ethmoidal and sphenoid sinuses.

The orbital contents are bound and supported by condensations of fascia. The *periorbita* is the periosteal lining of the socket to which it is loosely attached. It is firmly adherent to the orbital margins, sutures, foramina, fissures and lacrimal crest, enclosing the fossa and duct as far as the inferior meatus. It is also continuous with the periosteum of the facial bones and with the dura surrounding the optic nerve. Areas of thickening are present around the trochlea and lacrimal sac and septa pass into the orbital fat. Inferiorly it forms a definable suspensory ligament (of Lockwood) which is strengthened by the lateral margins of the sheaths of the medial, lateral and inferior recti and by the medial and lateral check ligaments. This forms a retinaculum 15 mm long and 3–4 mm wide which will effectively support the orbit after sub-total maxillectomy.

The *orbital septum* is a fibrous sheet stretching across the entrance to the orbit. It is related to the posterior surface of orbicularis oculi, attaches to the margin of the orbit and is continuous with the periosteum. It strengthens the lids and contains the fat within the orbit. The *bulbar sheath* (Tenon's capsule) is a thin fibrous sheath around all but the corneal part of the orbit. It is perforated by the optic nerve, the ciliary vessels, vorticose veins and tendons of the bulbar muscles. The orbital fascia ensheaths the bulbar muscles as they pass to the orbital wall and around the medial and lateral recti form well-defined condensations, the *check ligaments*.

The *trochlea* is a connective tissue sling anchoring the tendinous part of the superior oblique muscle to the orbit. The fovea for the trochlea is a small depression lying close to the orbital margin. In about 10% of individuals, the ligaments attaching the pulley are ossified. The tendon is enclosed in a synovial sheath within the pulley.

The *medial and lateral palpebral* (*canthal*) *ligaments* attach the tarsal plates to the orbital wall. The medial ligament is a strong triangular band which runs towards the root of the nose. It divides into anterior and posterior limbs, embracing the lacrimal sac and attaching to the anterior and posterior lacrimal crests. The lateral palpebral ligament attaches to the orbital tubercle on the zygomatic bone 11 mm below the frontozygomatic suture. It is less defined than the medial ligament.

The teeth

See Chapter 8.

Pterygopalatine fossa

This small space, the shape of an inverted pyramid, contains the vascular and nerve supply to the upper jaw. The apex is the pterygopalatine canal and its relations are:

posterior: greater wing of sphenoid
anterior: posterior wall of maxilla
superior: inferior surface of body of sphenoid
medial: perpendicular plate of palatine
lateral: infratemporal fossa via pterygomaxillary fissure.

The space connects with five regions of the skull:

anterior: via the inferior orbital fissure with the orbit transmitting infraorbital vessels, nerves and ascending branches of pterygopalatine ganglion
posterior: via foramen rotundum with the middle cranial fossa transmitting the maxillary nerve and via the pterygoid canal extending to the foramen lacerum
medial: via the sphenopalatine foramen to the nasal cavity
lateral: via the pterygomaxillary fissure to the infratemporal fossa, transmitting maxillary vessels and superior alveolar nerves
inferior: via the greater palatine canal to the roof of the mouth, transmitting the anterior, middle and posterior palatine nerves and greater and lesser palatine vessels.

The *pterygoid* (*Vidian*) *canal* lies inferior and medial to the foramen rotundum. It transmits the pterygoid nerve (and artery) which passes via the pterygopalatine fossa to the sphenopalatine ganglion. The pterygoid nerve is composed of the greater and lesser petrosal nerves which carry respectively preganglionic parasympathetic fibres from the superior salivatory nucleus and postganglionic sympathetic fibres from the cervical sympathetic chain (Figure 5.42). The *sphenopalatine foramen* is formed superiorly by the body of the sphenoid which closes the sphenopalatine notch of the palatine bone and transmits the respective vessels and nerves.

The contents of the pterygopalatine fossa may be divided into a neural compartment composed of

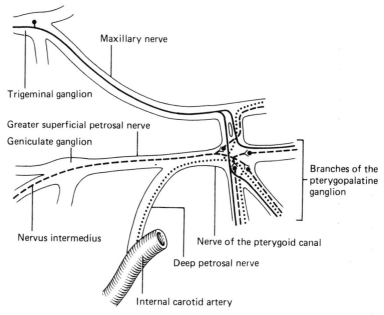

Figure 5.42 Connections of the pterygopalatine ganglion. Each branch contains sensory fibres from the maxillary nerve (—), sympathetic postganglionic fibres which traverse the ganglion (· · · ·) and postganglionic parasympathetic fibres which relay in the ganglion (– – – –)

pterygopalatine ganglion and maxillary nerve, and a vascular compartment containing the terminal part of the maxillary artery and its branches.

Infratemporal fossa

This irregular space lies beneath the base of the skull between the side wall of the pharynx and the ascending ramus of the mandible. Its relations are:

anterior: posterior wall of maxilla
posterior: styloid apparatus, carotid sheath and prevertebral fascia
superior: continuous with the temporal fossa
inferior: continuous with the parapharyngeal space
medial: the lateral pterygoid plate.

The roof is formed by the infratemporal surface of the greater wing of the sphenoid, perforated by the foramina ovale and spinosum, and by a small part of squamous temporal bone. The anterior and medial walls are separated superiorly by the pterygomaxillary fissure, through which the infratemporal and pterygopalatine fossae communicate. The infratemporal fossa communicates with the orbit via the inferior orbital fissure.

The fossa contains the medial and lateral pterygoids, branches of the mandibular nerve, maxillary artery and the pterygoid venous plexus within the lateral pterygoid muscle. The maxillary artery is di-

vided into three parts by its relation to the lateral pterygoid muscle and each of these parts gives five branches.

Anterior cranial fossa (Figure 5.43)

The anterior cranial fossa is formed by the orbital plate of the frontal bone, the cribriform plate of the ethmoid, and the lesser wings and anterior part of the body of the sphenoid. The configuration and thickness of the bone is variable, though it has an

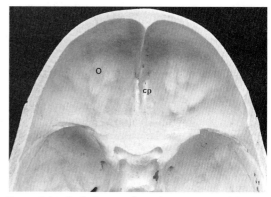

Figure 5.43 Skull, showing floor of anterior cranial fossa (O: orbital roof, cp: cribriform plate)

average length medially to the optic foramen of 47.7 mm and laterally of 35 mm (Lang, 1989). It supports the frontal lobes and associated olfactory bulbs and lies at a higher level than the other cranial fossae. It is lined by dura which forms the *falx cerebri*, arching between the frontal lobes and attaching to the crista and frontal crest. The *superior sagittal sinus* occupies the attached convex margin of the falx, receiving venous drainage from the nose via the foramen caecum. The frontal sinus impinges on the fossa anteriorly and medially, as may superior anterior ethmoidal cells. The jugum of the sphenoid articulates with the cribriform plate anteriorly, and posteriorly it is grooved by the chiasmatic sulcus, connecting the optic canals. The crista galli lies in the midline. It varies in size and shape and may be pneumatized or contain marrow. Anteriorly lies the foramen caecum. The cribriform plate transmits olfactory fibres with dural prolongations, and is related to the ethmoidal vessels. The length of the plate and the depth of the cribriform niche is also subject to considerable individual variation. Up to the age of 9 years the plate lengthens, but shortens relatively thereafter due to overgrowth of the planum sphenoidale. The average length is 20.8 mm (range 15.5–25.8 mm (Lang, 1983)).

References

BOURNE, G. H. (1972) *The Chimpanzee*. Basel: Karger. pp. 153–192

CAUNA, N. (1970) The fine structure of the arteriovenous anastomosis and its nerve supply in the human nasal respiratory mucosa. *Anatomical Record*, 168, 9–22

CAVE, A. J. E. (1973) The primate nasal fossa. *Journal of the Linnean Society*, 5, 377–387

CAVE, A. J. E. and WHEELER HAINES, R. (1939) The paranasal sinuses of the anthropoid ape. *Journal of Anatomy*, 74, 493–523

DESSI, P., MOULIN, G., TRIGLIA, J. M., ZANARET, M. and CANNONI, M. (1994) Difference in the height of the right and left ethmoid roofs. *Journal of Laryngology and Otology*, 108, 261–262

DIEULAFE, L. (1906) Morphology and embryology of the nasal fossae of vertebrates. *Annals of Otology, Rhinology and Laryngology*, 15, 1–60, 267–349, 513–584

ELWANY, S., YACOUT, Y. M., TALAAT, M., EL-NAHAAS, M. and GUNIED, A. (1983) Surgical anatomy of the sphenoid sinus. *Journal of Laryngology*, 97, 227–241

GHERARDI, F. (1939) Contributo alla conoscenza della irrorazione sanguinea della mucosa del detto nasale. *Otorhinolaryngologica Italiano*, 9, 132–148

GRUNWALD, L. (1925) Anatomie und Entwicklungsgeschichte. In: *Handbuch der Hals-Nasen-Ohrenheilkunde*. Band 1; *Die Krankheiten der Luftwege und Mundhohle*, edited by H. Denker and O. Kahler. Berlin: Springer J; Munchen: Bergmann J. F. pp. 1–95

GRYMER, L. and MELSEN, B. (1989) The morphology of the nasal septum in identical twins. *Laryngoscope*, 99, 642–646

HALLER, A VON. (1769) Elementa physiologiae corporis humani. Tumus Quintus: Sensus extreni interni. Lausannae, MDCCLXIX

HAMILTON, W. J. and MOSSMAN, H. W. (eds) (1972) *Human Embryology*. Cambridge: Heffer

HARRISON, D. F. N. (1981) Surgical approaches to the medial orbital wall. *Annals of Otology, Rhinology and Laryngology*, 90, 415–419

HARRISON, D. F. N. (1987) Preliminary thoughts on the incidence, structure and function of the mammalian vomeronasal organ. *Acta Otolaryngologica*, 105, 163–171

HEASMAN, P. (1984) Clinical anatomy of the superior alveolar nerves. *British Journal of Oral and Maxillo-facial Surgery*, 6, 439–447

HINCK, V. C. and HOPKINS, C. E. (1965) Concerning growth of the sphenoid sinus. *Archives of Otolaryngology*, 82, 62–66

JOHNSON, A., JOSEPHSON, R. and HAWKE, M. (1985) Clinical and histological evidence for the presence of the vomeronasal organ in adult humans. *Journal of Otolaryngology*, 14, 71–79

KAINZ, J. and STAMMBERGER, H. (1989) The roof of the anterior ethmoid; a place of least resistance in the skull base. *American Journal of Rhinology*, 4, 191–199

KOELLIKER, A. VON (1882) Der Lobus olfactorius und die Nervi olfactorii bei jungen menschlichen Embryonen. Wurzburg: S.-B Phys.-Med Gest. pp. 68–72

LANG, J. (1983) *Clinical Anatomy of the Head*. Berlin: Springer Verlag, p. 70

LANG, J. (1989) *Clinical Anatomy of the Nose, Nasal Cavity and Paranasal Sinuses*. Stuttgart: Georg Thieme Verlag, a–f:pp. 7,15,19,20,32,37

LANG, J. and SAKALS, E. (1982) Uber den Recessus sphenoethmoidalis, die Apertura nasalis des Ductus nasolacrimalis und den Hiatus semilunaris. *Anatomischer Anzeiger*, 152, 393–412

LANG, J. and SCHAEFER, K. (1979) Arteriae ethmoidales: Ursprung, Verlauf, Versorgungsbiete und Anastomosen. *Acta Anatomica (Basel)*, 104, 183–197

LLOYD, G. A. S., LUND, V. J. and SCADDING, G. K. (1991) Computerised tomography in the pre-operative evaluation of functional endoscopic sinus surgery. *Journal of Laryngology and Otology*, 105, 181–185

LOOSEN, J. VAN, VERWOERD-VERHOEF, H. L. and VERWOERD C. D. A. (1988) The nasal septal cartilage in the newborn. *Rhinology*, 26, 161–165

LUND, V. J. (1987) Anatomical considerations in the aetiology of fronto-ethmoidal mucocoeles. *Rhinology*, 25, 83–88

LUND, V. J. (1988a) The maxillary sinus in the higher primates. *Acta Otolaryngologica*, 105, 163–171

LUND, V. J. (1988b) Inferior meatal antrostomy. Fundamental considerations of design and function. *Journal of Laryngology and Otology*, Suppl. 15, 1–18

MARAN, A. G. D. and LUND, V. J. (1990) *Clinical Rhinology*. Stuttgart: Georg Thieme Verlag

MOORE, K. L. (1982) *The Developing Human*. Philadelphia: W. B. Saunders. pp. 197–206

MOORE, W. J. (1981) *The Mammalian Skull*. Cambridge: Cambridge University Press. pp. 240–279

NAPIER, J. R. and NAPIER, P. H. (1967) *Handbook of Living Primates*. London: Academic Press

NEGUS, J. R. (1958) *The Comparative Anatomy and Physiology of the Nose and Paranasal Sinuses*. Edinburgh: E. S. Livingstone. pp. 286–327

ONODI, J. (1903) Das Verhaltnis des Nervus opticus zu der Keilbeinhohe unde insbesondere zu der hintersten Siebbeinzelle. *Archiv fur Laryngologie*. Band XIV und XV

OSMAN HILL, W. C. (1970) *Primates; Comparative Anatomy and Taxonomy.* Edinburgh: University Press, vols I–VIII

PIRSIG, W. (1977) Septoplasty in children: influence on nasal growth. *Rhinology*, **15**, 193–204

PROETZ, A. W. (1953) *Essays on the Applied Physiology of the Nose*, 2nd edn. St Louis: Annals Publishing Co

RHYS EVANS, P. (1992) The paranasal sinuses and other enigmas: an aquatic evolutionary theory. *Journal of Laryngology and Otology*, **106**, 214–225

RITTER, F. N. (1973) *The Paranasal Sinuses – Anatomy and Surgical Technique.* St Louis: C. V. Mosby Co

RONTAL, E., RONTAL, M. and GUILFORD, F. T. (1979) Surgical anatomy of the orbit. *Annals of Otology, Rhinology and Laryngology*, **88**, 382–386

SARNAT, B. G. and WEXLER, M. R. (1966) Growth of the face and jaws after resection of the septal cartilage in the rabbit. *Journal of Anatomy*, **118**, 755–768

SASAKI, C. T. and MANN, D. G. (1976) Dilator naris function; a useful test of facial integrity. *Archives of Otolaryngology*, **102**, 365–367

SCHAEFFER, J. P. (1920) *The Nose, Paranasal Sinuses, Nasolacrimal Passageways and Olfactory Organ in Man.* Philadelphia: Blakiston

SCHULTZ-COULON H. J. and ECKERMEYER, L. (1976) Zum postnatalen Wachstum der Nasenscheidewand. *Acta Otolaryngologica*, **82**, 131–142

SCOTT J. H. (1953) The cartilage of the nasal septum. *British Dental Journal*, **95**, 37–44

SCOTT, J. H. (1956) Growth at facial sutures. *American Journal of Orthodontics*, **42**, 381–387

SCOTT, J. H. (1957) Studies in facial growth. *Dental Practitioners and Dental Records*, **7**, 344–345

SCOTT, J. H. (1958) The growth of the human skull. *Journal of the Dental Association of South Africa*, **13**, 133–142

SCOTT, J. H. (1959) Further studies on the growth of the human face. *Proceedings of the Royal Society of Medicine*, **52**, 263–268

SCOTT, J. H. (1963) The analysis of the facial growth from fetal life to adulthood. *Angle Orthodontics*, **33**, 110–113

SHAHEEN, O. H. (1987) Epistaxis In: *Scott-Brown's Otolaryngology*, 5th edn. vol 4, edited by I. S. Mackay and T. R. Bull. London: Butterworths, pp. 272–282

STAMMBERGER, H. (1991) *Functional Endoscopic Sinus Surgery. The Messerklinger Technique.* Philadelphia: B. C. Dekker. p. 62

STAMMBERGER, H. and KENNEDY, D. W. (1995) Paranasal sinuses: anatomic terminology and nomenclature. *Annals of Otology, Rhinology and Laryngology*, **104**, Supplement 167, 7–16

STREETER, G. L. (1945) Developmental horizons in human embryos; description of group XIII, embryos about 4 or 5 millimetres long. *Contributions to Embryology at the Carnegie Institution*, **198**, 27–64

THEILE, F. W. (1855) Die Asymetrien der Nase und des Nasenskelettes. *Zeitschrift für Rationale Medizinische*, **6**, 242

TOS, M. and MORGENSEN, C. (1979) Mucus production in the nasal sinuses. *Acta Otolaryngologica*, Suppl. 360, 131–134

VAN ALYEA, O. E. (1939) Ethmoid labyrinth. *Archives of Otolaryngology*, **29**, 881–902

VERWOERD, C. D. A., URBANUS, N. A. M. and NIJDAM, D. C. (1979) The effects of septal surgery on the growth of the nose and maxilla. *Rhinology*, **27**, 53–63

VIRCHOW, H. (1912) Die anthropologische Untersuchung der Nase. *Zeitschrift Ethnologie*, **44**, 289–337

WARBRICK, J. C (1960) The early development of the nasal cavity and upper lip in the human embryo. *Journal of Anatomy*, **94**, 351–362

WARWICK, R. and WILLIAMS, P. I. (eds) (1973) *Gray's Anatomy*, 35th edn. London: Longman, pp. 299–300

WOOD JONES, F. (1939) The anterior superior alveolar nerve and vessels. *Journal of Anatomy*, **73**, 583–591

ZINREICH, S. J., KENNEDY, D. W. and GAYLER, B. W. (1988) CT of nasal cavity, paranasal sinuses: an evaluation of anatomy in endoscopic sinus surgery. *Clear Images*, **2**, 2–10

ZUCKERKANDL, E. (1893) *Normale und pathologische Anatomie der Nasenhohle und interpneumatischen Anhage.* Leipzig: W. Braumuller

6

The physiology of the nose and paranasal sinuses

Adrian Drake–Lee

Physiology is the science of the normal function and phenomena of living things and their parts. Whereas most works on the physiology of the nose spend considerable time on the pathophysiology, this chapter concentrates on the normal nose and its homeostatic reactions. The development of medical sciences has led to considerable overlap between physiology, biochemistry, microanatomy and immunology and so any work on the physiology of an organ will include some details of other subjects, e.g. the humidification of the air is facilitated by the specialized endothelial cells of the nasal capillaries. The ultrastructure of these shows that there are pores facing the surface epithelium.

The role of the otolaryngologist is to distinguish patients with a normal nose from those who have a pathological condition. This can be very difficult in some cases where factors in the environment modify the normal response. The variable blockage of the nasal cycle may be exaggerated by the patient's response to the dry air produced by underfloor heating or to irritant chemicals in the furniture or flooring but no pathological process is present. An understanding of the physiology of the normal nasal functions will prevent unnecessary surgery to the septum and turbinates.

Although the nose is a paired structure divided coronally into two chambers it acts as a functional unit. The paranasal sinuses are mirror images of each other. The relative importance of the sinuses in the physiology of the upper airway appears to be small. When their function is questioned more deeply no single use can be found. They seem to be like the appendix, although phylogenetically the latter was useful, they are both notable only when diseased.

The nose contains the organ of smell as well as that of respiration. The nose warms, cleans and humidifies the inspired air, and cools and removes water from the expired air, it also adds quality to speech production. A brief summary of nasal physiology can be seen in Table 6.1.

Table 6.1 Physiological functions of the nose

Respiration
    Heat exchange
    Humidification
    Filtration
    Nasal resistance
    Nasal fluids and ciliary function
    Nasal neurovascular reflexes
    Voice modification

Olfaction

Respiration

Respiration provides oxygen for metabolism and removes carbon dioxide from the body. Most of the transfer takes place in the alveoli of the lungs and it is the function of the nose to modify air so that it is ideal for this purpose and exchange is achieved without damaging the alveoli. The nose performs three functions: humidification, heat transfer and filtration. The nose can be bypassed during exercise because there is such a great reserve of function within the respiratory tract. Because of its ability to transfer heat, the nose may be more important in temperature regulation than respiration.

The humidity and temperature of the ambient air in the home is changed by central heating of various types and by air conditioning. The inspired gases themselves are non-irritant but contain pollutants, such as diesel particles, the oxides of nitrogen and sulphur which are irritant, and carbon monoxide, which affects the oxygen carrying capacity of haemoglobin. The inspired air contains not only domestic dust particles and pollen but also industrial products, bacteria and viruses. Diesel particles can affect cellular function and the increase in allergy, particularly seasonal allergic rhinitis, may be due to these acting on antigen processing cells. Many people burden their respiratory tract further by smoking tobacco. Since an adult will inspire over 10^4 litres of air a day, it is surprising that the nose is not diseased more frequently.

Heat exchange

The temperature of the inspired air can vary from $-50\ °C$ to $50\ °C$ and the nose in different racial groups has become modified to suit the local ambient temperatures. Most work on heat exchange has been performed on Europeans in temperate or Mediterranean climates.

Conduction, convection and radiation

Heat may be transferred by conduction, convection or radiation. When conduction takes place alone there must be no flow and heat is transferred by increased molecular movement. A temperature gradient in gases results in convection currents; these affect airflow in the nose and cause turbulence. The gases in the nose are in motion so forced convection will occur. Empirically a formula to express this can be applied:

$$F_H = h(T_{wall} - T_f)$$

where F_H is the heat flux in J/m per s, T_f is the bulk temperature and h is the heat transfer coefficient in J/m per s per °C.

How well the system functions can be expressed by the heat transfer coefficient (Prandtl number):

$$Pr = (C_p\,\eta)/K_H$$

where C_p is the heat capacity of the gas in J/g per °C, η is the viscosity and K_H is the thermal conductivity in J/m per °C.

The nose may be considered as a heat exchange system where two 'fluids' are in thermal but not direct contact. One of the fluids is the inspired air, the other is the blood supply of the nose. The main blood supply is derived from the sphenopalatine artery and its branches run forward in the nose particularly over the turbinates. During inspiration the airflow is opposite or countercurrent to blood flow, thus it is more efficient in warming the inspired air. The efficiency of the system can be measured by comparing the temperature difference of the two 'fluids' at one end ΔT_1 with the difference between them (blood and air) at the other end ΔT_2. A log mean temperature difference is used to express the relationship

$$\Delta T_{LM} = \frac{\Delta T_1 - \Delta T_2}{\log \Delta T_1 - \log \Delta T_2}$$

Radiation does not play much part in warming the inspired air, but the process is complicated by humidification. The surface membrane of the nose is cooled by vaporization. The energy required to vaporize water is 2.352×10^9 J/kg.

The temperature in the nasopharynx varies 2–3°C between inspiration and expiration in temperate climates and the temperature of the expired air on expiration is core temperature (Swift, 1982). Since humidification and temperature changes in the respired gases are complementary, further changes of temperature will be considered under humidification.

Humidification

Inspiration

Saturation of the inspired air rapidly follows the temperature rise. Energy is required for two functions: raising the temperature of the inspired air and the latent heat of evaporation. These functions require about 2100 kJ every day in the adult, and of this, only one-fifth is used to raise the temperature (Cole, 1982). The amount of energy is dependent on the ambient temperature and the relative humidity of the inspired air. Because the process is inefficient in humans, over 10% of the body heat loss takes place through the nose. In some animals, particularly dogs, who do not sweat, loss through respiration is the main source of heat loss and body cooling. Despite variations in temperature of the inspired air, the air in the postnasal space is about 35°C and is 95% saturated.

Expiration

The temperature of the expired air at the back of the nose is slightly below body core temperature and is saturated. As the temperature drops along the nose, some water condenses onto the mucosa. The temperature in the anterior nose at the end of expiration is 32°C and approximately 30°C at the end of inspiration. About one-third of the water required to humidify the inspired air is recovered this way. People who breathe in through the nose and out through the mouth will dry their nasal mucosa.

Water production

It is generally assumed that the water from humidification comes directly from the capillaries through the surface epithelium, however, fluorescent studies showed that except during acute inflammation little water comes directly through the surface epithelium (Ingelstedt and Ivskern, 1949). Water comes from the serous glands which are extensive throughout the nose. Humidification is reduced by atropine probably acting on the glands rather than the vasculature.

During the nasal cycle there is a reduction of secretions which occurs on the more obstructed side. Additional water is extracted from the expired air, the nasolacrimal duct and the oral cavity.

Airflow

It is important to distinguish between airflow and the sensation of airflow which are very different entities. Complaints about the latter, nasal obstruction, may be due to a reduction of the former. The nasal airflow is very different between rest and exercise; most studies have been performed on quiet respiration.

For the purpose of explaining how air flow takes place, the nose may be considered as a tube. Most of the work of heat and mass transport has been performed on simple structures with constant cross-sections. Mathematical formulae have been derived to describe behaviour (Swift, 1982).

$$\text{Airflow: } VA = \text{constant}$$

where V is the average velocity in m/s and A is the cross-sectional area in m^2.

It follows that if the cross-section is decreased then the velocity increases. Gases flow faster through the anterior and posterior choanae than in the rest of the nasal cavity. The magnitude and direction of velocity also change if the shape of the tube changes. This is seen most easily when dye is photographed in fluids and has been applied to casts of the nasal passages.

The flow is maximal at the centre of the tube and drops towards the edge. Near the interface, the viscosity of the medium retards the flow further and at the edge it is zero. Energy is used in overcoming viscosity so the drop in pressure is irreversible.

If there is a change in velocity then the pressure will also alter. This is reversible and is described by Bernoulli's equation:

$$P + 1/2\rho V^2 = \text{constant}$$

where ρ is the density.

However, because some viscous forces are always active in the nose, the Bernoulli equation is not strictly applicable. The nose has a variable cross-section and so the pressure and velocity will alter continuously within the system. The pressures of the respiratory cycle also vary independently. The inspiratory phase lasts approximately 2 seconds and reaches a pressure of -10 mmH$_2$O and expiration lasts about 3 seconds and reaches a pressure of 8 mmH$_2$O. The respiratory rate is between 10–18 cycles a minute in adults at rest.

Laminar and turbulent airflow

In circular tubes, the change between laminar and turbulent flow is denoted by changes in the Reynolds number, Re:

$$\text{Re} = \frac{dv\rho}{\eta}$$

where d is the diameter in m, v is the average velocity in m/s, ρ is the 'fluid' density in g/m and η is the viscosity in g/s per m.

When the Reynolds number varies between 2000–4000, the flow changes from laminar to turbulent.

Initial studies by Proetz (1953) were performed on models made from liquid latex cast at post mortem. Although there is considerable variety of nasal shape, Swift and Proctor (1977) showed that the characteristics of airflow were similar in different noses. These studies used one side of the nose and, more recently, a technique using cast wax has been developed to study the flow in both sides together (Collins, 1985). Studies on flow performed this way do not take into account the variation in the nasal lumen produced by alterations of the blood flow within the nasal mucosa.

Inspiration

During inspiration the airflow is directed upwards and backwards from the nasal valve initially, mainly over the anterior part of the inferior turbinate. It then splits into two, below and over the middle turbinate, rejoining in the posterior choana. Air reaches the other parts of the nose to a lesser degree (Figure 6.1). The velocity at the anterior valve is 12–18 m/s during quiet respiration and is considered laminar for rhinomanometry, although in practice it is turbulent producing eddies in the olfactory region even in quiet respiration.

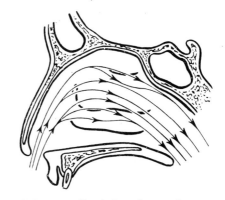

Figure 6.1 Diagram of inspiratory air currents

Expiration

Expiration lasts longer than inspiration and flow is more turbulent (Figure 6.2). Extrapulmonary airflow is turbulent because the direction changes, the calibre of the airway varies markedly and the walls of the nasal cavity are not smooth. The surface area is enlarged by both the turbinates and the microanatomy of the epithelium. The Reynolds number is exceeded.

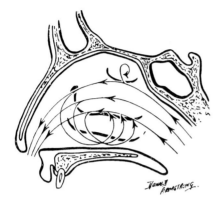

Figure 6.2 Diagram of expiratory air currents

Nasal resistance

The nose accounts for up to half the total airway resistance. It is produced by two resistors in parallel and each cavity has a variable resistance value as a result of the nasal cycle. The resistance is made up of two elements. The first is the bone, cartilage and attached muscles, while the second is the mucosa. The narrowest part of the nose is the nasal valve, which physiologically, is less well defined than the anatomical structures which constitute it. It comprises the lower edge of the upper lateral cartilages, the anterior end of the inferior turbinate and the adjacent nasal septum, together with the surrounding soft tissues.

Electromyographic studies show contraction of the dilator naris alone during inspiration (van Dishoek, 1965). Active dilation takes place during exercise which reduces the airway resistance and can be mimicked by voluntary dilation (Rivron and Sanderson, 1991). Loss of innervation can result in alar collapse even in quiet respiration. As the anterior valve is the narrowest part of the airway, it is one of the main factors in promoting turbulent air flow since it is the largest resistor in the whole airway (Bridger and Proctor, 1970).

In quiet respiration, airflow is more laminar in quality so that the resistance may be calculated by dividing the pressure by the flow rate. When the flow is turbulent, because the nose is an irregular tube, the resistance is then inversely proportional to the square of the flow rate (Otis, Fenn and Rahn, 1950).

The nasal resistance is high in infants as they are obligate nose breathers at least initially. Adults breathe preferentially through the nose at rest even though significant resistance occurs there. Work is required to overcome the resistance. The resistance is important during expiration since the positive pressure is transmitted to the alveoli and keeps the lungs expanded. Removal of this resistance by tracheostomy is a mixed blessing because although it reduces the dead space, it does allow a degree of alveolar collapse. It may result in reduced alveolar ventilation and a degree of right to left shunting of the pulmonary blood.

The morphology of the nose between different racial groups may alter the resistance, but studies on Negroes and Caucasians (of different ethnic origins) show no differences (Babatola, 1990; Calhoun *et al.*, 1990). Technical reasons make it difficult to sample pressures by rhinomanometry in Japanese.

Nasal cycle

The airflow and the nasal resistance are modified by mucosal changes. These changes are produced by vascular activity particularly by the veins of the pseudoerectile tissue of the nose (capacitance vessels). Cyclical changes take place every 4–12 hours; they are constant for each person. The cycle consists of alternate nasal blockage between passages and is unnoticed by the majority of people. The cycle has been recognized since antiquity although Kayser (1895) gave it its first physiological description.

The nasal cycle can be demonstrated in over 80% of adults, but it is more difficult to record in children. It has been shown to be present in early childhood (Van Cauwenberge and Deleye, 1984; Mennella and Beauchamp, 1992). The cycle has been demonstrated by rhinomanometry and, more recently, by thermography (Canter, 1986). The physiological significance is uncertain but, in addition to a resistance and flow cycle, the flow of nasal secretions is also cyclical with an increase in secretions in the side with the greater airflow (Ingelstedt and Ivskern, 1949).

A number of factors may overcome or modify the nasal cycle; these include allergy, infection, exercise, hormones, pregnancy, fear and emotions which include sexual activity. The nasal cycle is controlled by the autonomic nervous system and vagal overactivity causes nasal congestion. High levels of CO_2 in the inspired air produced by rebreathing may also reduce the nasal resistance. This is reversible by hyperventilation (Series *et al.*, 1989).

Drugs which block the action of noradrenalin may cause nasal congestion as do hypotensive agents. The anticholinergic effects of antihistamines block parasympathetic activity and produce relative increase of sympathetic tone, hence an improved airway. Times of hormonal change such as puberty and pregnancy also effect the nasal mucosa. These are probably mediated directly on the blood vessels.

Oestrogens are actively concentrated in nasal tissue

and levels up to a thousand times the serum level have been demonstrated (Reynolds and Foster, 1940). They also inhibit the function of acetylcholinesterase and so may affect the autonomic sensitivity of the nose as well (Michael *et al.*, 1972).

Rhinomanometry

Nasal airflow is usually measured as a volume flow in litres/minute and plotted against pressure (Figure 6.3). Quiet respiration is studied and a sample point of the flow at 150 pascals pressure is the standard reference (Clement, 1984). The details of rhinomanometry are considered elsewhere in this volume.

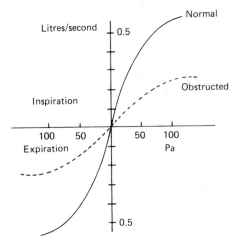

Figure 6.3 The pattern of quiet nasal breathing showing flow (l/s) against pressure (mmH$_2$O)

A number of newer and more practical techniques has been developed to measure nasal resistance as at least one-third of subjects are not able to perform rhinomanometry adequately. Thermography of the expired air has been used and the sounds of nasal respiration have been analysed either directly or by the forced random noise technique (Fullton *et al.*, 1984).

Acoustic rhinometry

Pulsed sound may be reflected (sonar) and the pattern of reflection is determined by the cross-sectional area of the nose. It is more accurate nearer the nasal valve than elsewhere in the nose.

Protection of the lower airway: mechanical and chemical

Protection of the lower airway is one of the major functions of the nose. The nose is able to remove particles of 30 μm or more from the inspired air. This includes most pollen particles which are among the smallest particles deposited on the nasal mucosa and accounts for the nose being the predominantly affected site in hay fever. Other characteristics of smaller particles, such as shape and surface smoothness, may determine whether they are deposited in the nose.

The morphology of the nose causes air to change direction. The inspired air changes direction by 180° in passage through the nose and during this time the velocity decreases considerably as a consequence of the nasal valve. Turbulence encountered in the flow increases the deposition of particles.

Particles in motion tend to persue the same direction; the larger the mass the greater the tendency. Resistance to change in velocity is greater in irregularly shaped particles because of their larger surface area and number of facets or surfaces. Nasal hairs only stop the largest particles and are only relevant to other organisms.

Nasal secretions

Nasal secretions are composed of two elements, glycoproteins and water with its proteins and ions. Most information on the nature and action of the mucus has been obtained from samples acquired from the lower respiratory tract. The glycoproteins are produced by the mucus glands and the water and ions from the serous glands and also indirectly from transudation from the capillary network. The nasal mucus film is in two layers, one upper more viscous layer, and a lower more watery layer in which the cilia can move freely. The tips of the cilia have small hooks which enter the viscous layer and facilitate its movement. There are two secretory cell types in the mixed nasal glands, mucus and serous cells. The glycoproteins found in mucus are produced by the two cell types, the goblet cells within the epithelium and the glandular mucus cells.

Glandular mucus and goblet cells contain large secretory granules which can be seen as lucent areas on electron microscopy and contain the acidic glycoproteins (Lamb and Reid, 1970) (Figures 6.4 and 6.5). Serous cells contain discrete electron dense granules. The granules contain material of two different densities, the core being of a greater density (Figure 6.6). These granules contain neutral glycoproteins, enzymes such as lysozymes and lactoferrin as well as immunoglobulins of the IgA class.

The IgA dimers are conjugated with a secretory piece which is produced in the serous cells. The submucosal glands are almost always mixed and are arranged around ducts. The anterior part of the nose contains serous glands only in the vestibular region. These produce a copious watery secretion when stimulated. The sinuses have fewer goblet cells and mixed glands.

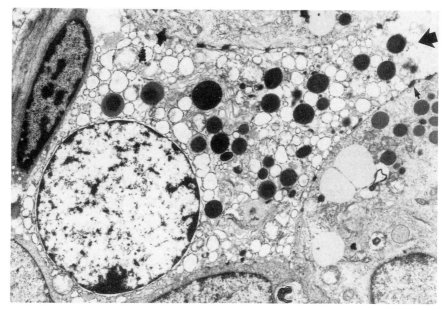

Figure 6.4 Holocrine cell. The large arrow points to the opening and shows the contents being discharged directly. The small arrow shows the tight junctions. (× 10 000)

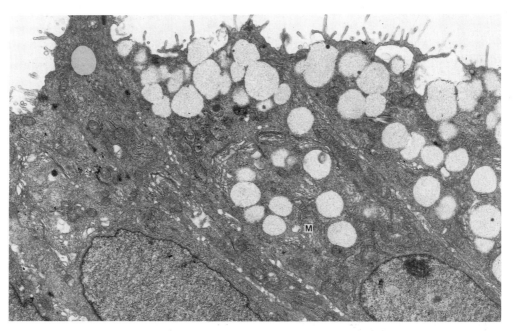

Figure 6.5 Goblet cells. The mucus is removed during preparation. Note the large number of mitochondria (M). (× 10 900)

Composition of mucus (Table 6.2)

Although some of the water, ions and enzymes may come from outside the nose, e.g. tears, the majority are produced in the nasal cavity. The watery layer in

mucus merges gradually into the more viscous upper layer. It is, however, more practical to consider mucus as two layers, a sol layer and a gel layer. Desiccation by the flow of dryer inspired air may help to develop a more viscous gel layer. The gel layer

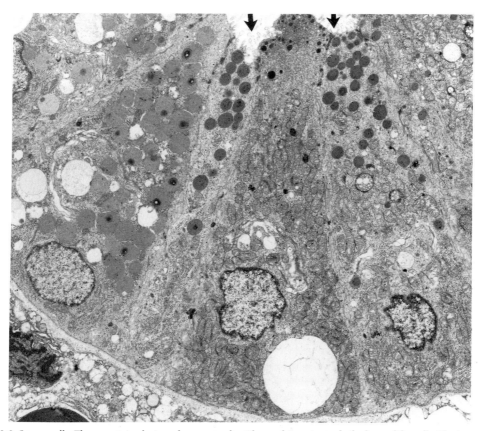

Figure 6.6 Serous cells. These contain electron dense granules. The nuclei are towards the base of the cells. The lumen is arrowed. Several cell types are found. (× 8545)

Table 6.2 Nasal secretions

Water and ions from transudation

Glycoproteins: sialomucins, fucomucins, sulfomucins

Enzymes: lysozymes, lactoferrin

Circulatory proteins: complement, α_2-macroglobulin, C reactive protein

Immunoglobulins: IgA, IgE, IgG, IgM, IgD

Cells: surface epithelium, basophils, eosinophils, leucocytes

contains more of the glycoproteins from which many of the properties of mucus are derived. The glycoproteins form about 80% of the dry weight of mucus (Masson and Heremans, 1973). Each consists of a single sugar side chain linked covalently to a polypeptide chain. These units are polymerized by disulphide linkages. Complexes in secretions may weigh up to 10^6 daltons. These hydroscopic polymers interact with water and ions to form a gel. Analysis leads to dissolution and as a result some properties are altered.

Hydroxyamino acids form up to 70% of the amino acids of which serine is the most abundant in nasal mucus (Boat *et al.*, 1974). The glycoproteins are classified as acidic or neutral. The acid is either sialic acid (sialomucins) or a sulphate group (sulphomucins). The neutral glycoproteins contain fucose (fucomucins). Sialomucins can be subdivided into those that are digested by sialidases and those that are not. Secretory cells may contain a mixture of different mucins.

Rheology of mucus

Glycoproteins give mucus its two most commonly measured properties, viscosity and elasticity. The role of mucus in covering the nasal mucosa and the action of the cilia upon it are dependent on its elastic properties as the ciliary beat frequency is between 10 and 20 Hz (Widdicombe and Wells, 1982). The viscosity and elasticity are easier to measure but adhesiveness and fluidity may be more important properties.

The viscosity of mucus is lowered by reducing the ionic content. The temperature of the nasal cavity is fairly constant and so does not have much effect on flow characteristics. However, the temperature of the nasal cavity is lower than in the tracheobronchial tree, although both the constituents and flow have yet to be compared between the two types of mucus. In conclusion the rheology of nasal mucus requires further study.

The other compounds such as immunoglobulins and albumin, do not add much to the flow characteristics of mucus. Most of the protein structures help to defend the host from the environment, whereas the water and ions have a role in the respiratory function.

Proteins in nasal secretion

These are derived either from the circulation or are produced within the mucosa or the surface cells. Comparison of levels within the plasma or serum with oedema fluid or nasal secretions suggest local production; some compounds such as lactoferrin are present only in nasal secretions. Many of the proteins are involved in the immunological responses of the nose and will be considered briefly later.

Lactoferrin

This is present in the secretions of the body, is not present in serum and is produced by the glandular epithelium, mainly the serous cells. It acts by binding divalent metal ions, as does transferrin, in the circulation; transferrin is not found in any quantity in secretions. They bind two divalent metal ions, particularly iron, and have a molecular weight of 76–77 000 daltons. By removing heavy metal ions, lactoferrin prevents the growth of certain bacteria, particularly *Staphylococcus* and *Pseudomonas*.

Lysozymes

These are produced by secretion from the serous glands in the nose, but some come from tears which gain entry via the nasolacrimal duct. They are also produced from leucocytes which are found in nasal secretions and mucosa. The action of lysozymes is non-specific and depends on the absence of bacterial capsules for effect.

Antiproteases

A number of different antiproteases have been demonstrated. They increase with infection and their role remains uncertain. They include α-antitrypsin, α_1-antichymotrypsin, α_2-macroglobulin and other antiproteases produced by leucocytes.

Complement

All components of complement have been identified. C3 is produced by the liver and also locally by macro-phages. It is activated by both non-specific and specific immunological responses through the alternative and classical pathways. It has a variety of functions, including the lysis of microorganisms and enhancement of neutrophil function as well as leucotaxis.

A number of other proteins and macromolecules have been identified from plasma and are probably present as a result of capillary leakage.

Lipids

Phospholipids and triglycerides are present, their exact function is unknown.

Ions and water

Evaporation may account for a part of the hyperosmolarity of Na^+ and Cl^- in mucus but active ion transport also contributes (Widdicombe and Welsh, 1980). This takes place mainly within the serous glands which produce the major proportion of the water in nasal secretions.

Immunoglobulins

Immunoglobulins are part of the immune system and all classes have been found in nasal secretions. Since the nose is a mucosal surface, the two immunoglobulins involved with mucosa defence, IgA and IgE, have been found to be present in greater quantities than in serum. IgA accounts for 50% of the total protein content. The immune system will be considered later.

Cilia

Ultrastructure

Cilia are found on the surface of the cells in the respiratory tract. They propel mucus backwards towards the nasopharynx. The nasal cilia are relatively short (5 μm) and over 200 are present on each cell. They are ultrastructurally identical to other cilia, each having a surface membrane which encloses nine paired outer microtubules which encircle a single inner pair of microtubules. Adjacent outer paired microtubules are linked by nexin and also to the inner pair of microtubules in a spoke-like fashion. The outer pairs of microtubules also have inner and outer dynein arms which consist of an ATPase. These are absent in patients with Kartagener's syndrome. At the base of the cilia, the microtubules blend into the basal body of the cell; the outer pairs of microtubules become triplets and the inner pair disappears completely. Each triplet of microtubules is structurally similar to the centrioles of mitotic cells and it has been suggested that centrioles migrate to the cell surface to form these structures (Sleight, 1974) (Figures 6.7 and 6.8).

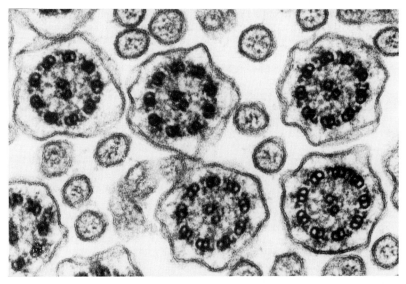

Figure 6.7 Ultrastructure of cilia. The nine plus two structure is clearly seen. The inner and outer dynein arms may be seen occasionally. The radial links may just be inferred. The smaller structures are microvilli

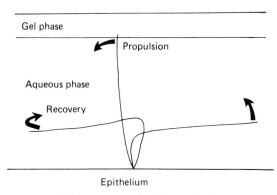

Figure 6.8 The beat pattern of a cilium, only the tip is in the gel layer

Ciliary action

The beat frequency of the cilia is between 10 and 20 Hz at body temperatures with a mean of around 14 Hz. It remains fairly constant between 32°C and 40°C and does not appear to be temperature dependent within this range. Each beat consists of a rapid propulsive stroke followed by a slow recovery phase. During the propulsive phase the cilium is straight and the tip engages the viscous layer of the mucus blanket; whereas during the recovery phase the cilium is bent over and lies in the aqueous layer. The energy for this is produced by the conversion of ATP to ADP by the ATPase of the dynein arms and the reaction is Mg^{2+} ion dependent. ATP is generated by the mitochondria near the cell surface next to the basal bodies of the cilia. Motion is produced by each

pair of outer microtubules sliding in relation to the next.

The mucous blanket is propelled backwards by metachronous movement of the cilia. In other words, only those at right angles to the direction of mucus flow are in phase and all the other cilia are slightly out of phase until the cycle of movement is complete. Initiation of ciliary movement is by mechanical action, a reversible domino effect, or the Mexican wave in the nose! Mucus flows from the front of the nose posteriorly. Mucus from the sinuses joins the stream on the lateral wall of the nasal cavity. This stream of mucus passes mainly through the middle meatus and then around the eustachian orifice before being swallowed.

Factors affecting ciliary action

The nose is a remarkably constant environment and changes in it affect ciliary function. Drying stops ciliary action. This may be reversible if dried only for a short period. Large changes in temperature also affect function with cessation of ciliary beating below 10°C and above 45°C. Consequently, *in vitro* ciliary beat frequency is measured on a microscope with a warmed stage.

Isotonic saline preserves ciliary activity, but solutions above 5% and below 0.2% cause paralysis. K^+ ions have no effect on ciliary function unless outside what would be considered to be a physiological range (Robson, Smallman and Drake-Lee, 1992). Similarly, cilia will beat above pH 6.4 and will function in slightly alkaline fluids of pH 8.5 for long periods. The commonest *in vivo* factor affecting ciliary function is infection. In this state the epithelium may be damaged to such a degree that the surface cells slough away.

Drugs

Neurotransmitters affect ciliary beat frequency (CBF). Acetylcholine increases the rate while adrenalin decreases it. The effects of α- and β-agonists and antagonists are variable. For adrenalin, the effects are reversible and dose dependent below a concentration of 1:1000. Topically active drugs such as ephedrine have not been shown to affect function.

High concentrations of the α_1-agonist, phenylephrine, decrease ciliary beat frequency whereas lower doses increase it *in vitro*. Propranolol (β-antagonist) decreases ciliary beat frequency in a dose-dependent fashion (Robson, Smallman and Drake–Lee, 1992). Cocaine hydrochloride causes immediate paralysis in solutions above 10%. Following one week's therapy with corticosteroids, the rate of saccharin clearance is reduced, the implication being that this is secondary to a change in ciliary beat frequency (Holmberg and Pipkorn, 1985).

Protection of the lower airways: immunological

The effect of altering the direction and velocity of the inspired air is to deposit particles on the surface epithelium. If the particles are not inert, there has to be a mechanism which prevents these particles from damaging the host. Mucus is the barrier for the respiratory mucosa which otherwise would not be as effective as skin in protecting the internal environment from invasion. Mucus contains a number of different compounds which are able to neutralize antigenically active compounds. It may do this by innate mechanisms or by acquired immunological responses. The two main surface immunoglobulins are IgA and IgE. IgM and IgG immunoglobulins are activated if the mucosa is breached. These mechanisms cope with a number of bacterial antigens, however, for several other bacteria and viruses, protection of the host is achieved by activation of cell-mediated immune responses.

Lymphocytes are conveniently classified into B and T types, the latter being further subdivided by surface markers into suppressor, helper and killer cells respectively. T and some B cells interact with macrophages which have specific and non-specific immunological properties. Antigens are presented to T lymphocytes by macrophages, certain lymphocytes and Langerhans' cells. Some feel that the Langerhans' cells in the nasal mucosa are an important component of the allergic response (Fokkens *et al.*, 1991).

The lymphatic system has been subdivided into two components based on the class of immunoglobulin produced, the unencapsulated and encapsulated systems. The unencapsulated system includes the tonsils, adenoids, Peyer's patches, aggregations of lymphoid tissue within the respiratory and gastrointestinal tracts. It is broadly classified as the gut or mucosal associated lymphoid tissue (GALT or MALT). Plasma cells at these sites mainly produce IgA and IgE. The encapsulated system is activated if this system is overcome in the nose. It is situated in the lymph nodes and the spleen and produces IgG and IgM. Certain respiratory diseases can affect a lymphocyte cell type, e.g. the virus responsible for infectious mononucleosis replicates in B lymphocytes and may produce tonsillar hypertrophy, lymphadenopathy and splenomegaly (Table 6.3).

Table 6.3 Nasal immune system

Surface properties
Mechanical
　Physical characteristics of mucus

Innate immunity
Bacteriocidal activity in mucus
　Proteins: lactoferrin, lysozymes, α_2-macroglobulin, C
　reactive protein, complement system
　Cellular: polymorphs and macrophages

Acquired immunity
Surface IgA, IgM, IgE and IgG
　Primed macrophages
　Submucosa macrophages IgM, IgG, T and B
　Lymphocytes – mucosal associated lymphoid tissue

Distant sites
Adenoids, lymph nodes and spleen

Non-specific immunity

Lactoferrin, lysozymes, complement, antiproteases and other macromolecules interact with a number of bacteria, particularly those without capsules, to give an innate non-specific immunity. The actions of polymorphic leucocytes and reaction of macrophages result in phagocytosis and destruction of foreign material. Many organisms and viruses are resistant and so specific reactions are required.

Acquired immunity

Acquired immunity may be produced by the immunoglobulins and interferon. Viruses and mycobacteria initiate cell-mediated immunity. Two different types of immunoglobulin may be produced as a first line of defence in the nose. First, IgA, which produces insoluble complexes in mucus and binds with immunologically primed surface active cells, which are capable of phagocytosis. Since IgA is found in considerable quantities in nasal secretions its production will be considered further. Second, IgE, which is implicated in acute allergic reactions. As the nose is the commonest site for allergic reactions to take place, a few comments will be included here as well.

IgA

IgA is divided into two subgroups IgA_1 and IgA_2. The former is a monomer and more plentiful in serum, while the latter is a dimer and more common in nasal secretions. IgA accounts for as much as 70% of the total protein in nasal secretions. The monomer has a molecular weight of 160 000 daltons and two units are joined by a junctional chain (molecular weight 16 000 daltons). These units are produced in the same plasma cells so that antigenically similar IgAs are linked together. The IgA dimer is then transferred passively through the interstitial fluid and is actively taken up by the seromucinous glands and the surface epithelium. In the epithelium, a secretory piece is attached to the IgA dimer which makes it stable in mucus. It forms an insoluble complex when it reacts with an antigen which is swallowed and destroyed by acid in the stomach. IgA does not activate complement.

IgE

IgE is the main immunoglobulin to cause allergic reactions and was first identified by Ishizaka and Ishizaka (1967). It is mainly produced in lymphoid aggregates such as the tonsil and adenoid, and also within the submucosa. IgE becomes firmly attached to mast cells and basophils. Two molecules of allergen specific IgE must occupy adjacent receptor sites on mast cells to cause degranulation. IgE has a molecular weight of 190 000 daltons and does not activate complement. It is usually directed against intestinal parasites.

Surface cells

In addition to its molecular components, mucus also contains cells. These consist of epithelial cells, leucocytes, basophils, eosinophils, mast cells and macrophages. Leucocytes and macrophages migrate through the interstitium from the circulation and are important for surface phagocytosis. They may also help to prevent bacterial or viral invasion. Cytological examination of the nasal secretions can assist diagnosis.

Nasal vasculature and nerve supply

Comparisons between the nose, trachea and bronchial tree have limitations. The nose is a rigid box which is devoid of a constricting smooth muscle wall. Changes in its resistance to airflow are produced by alterations in the blood flow to its lining and in the amount of blood within the blood vessels; in other words by controlled changes in capacitance and the resistance vessels. The arrangement of the blood vessels is complex and varies at different sites within the nose (Figure 6.9). It is best developed where the airflow is maximum, which is over the

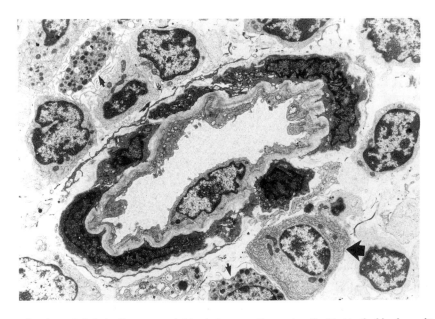

Figure 6.9 Arteriole. The endothelial cell is surrounded by darker smooth muscle cells. Next to the blood vessel is a plasma cell identified by the larger arrow. The two smaller arrows point to mast cells. (× 4000)

turbinates and part of the nasal septum and is less well developed in the sinuses and floor of the nose. The vascular anatomy was described extensively by Burnham (1935) and the microanatomy has been further studied by Cauna (1970). The blood supply is derived from deep vessels traversing through the bone.

Figure 6.10 shows the arrangement of the blood vessels within a turbinate. In general, the arteries and arterioles produce the resistance and the venules and sinusoids the capacitance. Shunting of blood between the arteries and veins deep within the mucosa bypasses the surface vessels and reduces the amount of blood within the system. Anastomotic arteries spiral upward through the cavernous plexus of veins where most of the shunting takes place. Towards the surface, the arteries ramify and give rise to arterioles which lack an elastic lamina and end in capillaries which run parallel and just below the surface epithelium. They also encircle the mucous glands. The capillaries are fenestrated with more 'holes' towards the epithelium (Cauna, 1970). This facilitates transudation and the parallel course of vessels permits maximum heat exchange. The capillaries drain into a superficial venous system which is most highly developed immediately proximal to venous sinusoids.

The venous sinusoids are a cavernous plexus of large tortuous anastomotic veins which lack valves and receive both arterial and venous blood. Drainage of blood from the sinusoids is regulated by cushion or throttle veins which have a longitudinal muscle coat. They do not close the lumen completely but are able to regulate the flow into the bone through the deep venous plexus. About 60% of the blood flow is shunted through arteriovenous anastomosis in cats (Anggard, 1974) and the actual blood flow per cubic millimetre is greater than muscle, brain or liver (Drettner and Aust, 1974).

Although the arterial supply is derived from a number of different sources, the main supply is from the maxillary artery. The direction of arterial blood flow is forwards through the nose against the flow of inspired air. The vascular arrangement within the turbinates is often called pseudoerectile because of the similarities to the blood supply of the penis.

Blood flow

Measurement of the nasal blood flow is difficult because instruments introduced into the nose reflexly alter the nasal resistance if they touch the mucosa. Blood flow may be inferred by:

1 Changes in the colour of the mucosa
2 Photoelectric plethysmography
3 Alteration in the temperature.

Since the nasal resistance is related to blood flow, rhinometry may be used to assess blood flow. Capillary leakage may be gauged by the appearance of labelled albumin in nasal secretions following intravenous injection or by the xenon wash-out method.

Subtle changes in arterial blood flow, arteriovenous shunting and venous pooling allow almost unlimited permutations of mucosal perfusion. In clinical practice three main patterns are recognized:

1 Hyperaemia with both shunting and venous congestion
2 Reduced arterial perfusion with no shunting which results in venous congestion
3 Ischaemia.

Control of vascular flow is by the autonomic nervous system and influenced by local inflammatory reactions.

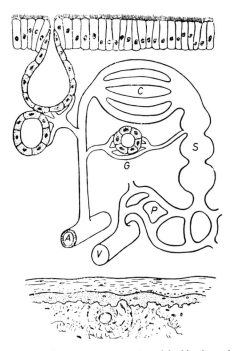

Figure 6.10 Schematic representation of the blood supply of the turbinates. It shows the arteriole (A) supplying the subepithelial capillaries (C), the glandular capillaries (G) which drain into the sinusoids (S) and the venous plexus (P)

The nasal autonomic nervous system

The autonomic nervous system controls the vascular reflexes in the nose and its distribution is shown schematically in Figure 6.11. The afferent and final efferent pathway of these reflexes is the trigeminal nerve through its ethmoid and sphenopalatine branches respectively.

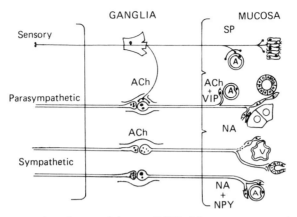

Figure 6.11 The autonomic nerve supply to the nose. Substance P (SP) of the sensory nerves acts on arterioles. The action of acetylcholine (ACh) and vasoactive intestinal peptide (VIP) on the vessels and glands is shown. Noradrenalin (NA) and neuropeptide Y (NPY) act on the venules (V) in addition to the arterioles

Sympathetic nerve supply

The sympathetic nerve supply is derived from the lateral horn of the grey matter of the spinal cord at the level of the first and second thoracic vertebrae. Preganglionic axons run through the anterior nerve roots, anterior primary rami and white rami and communicate to the sympathetic chain. They synapse in the superior cervical ganglion. Postganglionic fibres hitch hike along the carotid to the deep petrosal and vidian nerves. They continue through the sphenopalatine ganglion and pass into the nerves of the nasal cavity.

Parasympathetic nerve supply

The preganglionic fibres have their cell bodies in the superior salivary nucleus in the pons. They proceed via the intermediate branch of the facial nerve to the geniculate ganglion through which they pass. After continuing along the greater superficial petrosal nerve, the deep petrosal nerve and the nerve of the pterygoid canal they synapse in the sphenopalatine ganglion. Postganglionic fibres then pass to the nasal mucosa.

Sensory nerves

The main sensory nerve supply is mediated through the ophthalmic and maxillary divisions of the trigeminal nerve. Sneezing is mediated through the vidian nerve (Malcolmson, 1959). It is uncertain precisely to which modalities the nasal mucosa may be sensitive, but temperature, pain (or discomfort) and touch or irritation can be appreciated. Thermoreceptors are limited to the nasal vestibule. Proprioception does not appear to be present. It may be impossible to define nasal nerve endings in the same manner as in

skin and the locomotor system. There is some evidence that sensory nerve endings have H_1 receptors (Mygind and Lowenstein, 1982). Olfaction is considered later in this chapter.

Airflow appears to be detected by cold receptors and there are more nerve endings near the nasal vestibule (Tsubone, 1989; Clarke and Jones, 1992). There is little contribution from tactile receptors and the rate of cooling is also important. Receptors can be stimulated by the l-menthol isomer giving rise to an apparent increase in air flow (Eccles, Lancashire and Tolley, 1987).

Neurotransmitters

Both parasympathetic and sympathetic nerve fibres supply the vasculature and glandular epithelium. Postganglionic fibres have been shown to have more than one neurotransmitter which may account for the discrepancy in behaviour between expected experimental responses and *in vivo* reflexes. Classic cholinergic antagonists do not block parasympathetic vasodilation completely (Eccles and Wilson, 1973) and in this respect there is a similarity to mast cell reactions, where antihistamines do not block reactions completely either as there is more than one cellular mediator.

In addition to acetylcholine and noradrenalin, immunofluorescent techniques have demonstrated neuropeptides in sympathetic, parasympathetic and sensory nerves (Uddman *et al.*, 1978; Anggard *et al.*, 1979; Lundberg *et al.*, 1982).

The main transmitter in the *parasympathetic* supply is acetylcholine but vasoactive intestinal polypeptide (VIP) is also present in postganglionic fibres. There are specific receptors for this on the blood vessels but not within the glandular epithelium. The transmitters probably act in combination. Acetylcholine results in widespread vasodilation and increased glandular activity. If the rate of nerve impulses is low, acetylcholine probably acts alone on blood vessels. At higher rates, VIP causes vasodilation which is atropine resistant but, in this state, acetylcholine may cause suppression of VIP release by negative feedback (Uddman, Malm and Sundler, 1980). Acetylcholine is secretor motor for glandular tissue alone, but the effects of VIP on neighbouring blood vessels may indirectly affect secretion.

The transmitter to postganglionic *sympathetic* fibres is acetylcholine and the main postsynaptic transmitter is noradrenalin. Two neuropeptides may also be found, namely neuropeptide Y (NPY) and pancreatic polypeptide. Neuropeptide Y is probably the more effective of the two. Unlike noradrenalin, which causes both arterial, arteriole and venous constriction, NPY causes only arteriolar constriction (Lundberg and Tatemoto, 1982). Avian pancreatic polypeptide is similar morphologically to substance P and shares its action of vasodilation (Lundberg *et al.*, 1980).

A number of nasal *sensory* neurons has been shown to contain the neuropeptide substance P. They are present in the sphenopalatine ganglion, near blood vessels and under the surface epithelium (Anggard *et al.*, 1979). Substance P causes vasodilation and is found in C fibres.

Reflexes

These may be mediated through the brain stem but axon reflexes may take place through the sensory nerves alone.

Axon reflexes

The newer neuropeptide, substance P, has been shown to be a transmitter in the antidromic reflex. It may be initiated by mechanical irritation or by mast cells which produce histamine. In addition to histamine causing the reflex, substance P is also able to liberate histamine from mast cells. The concept of neurovascular reflexes and mast cell reactions being separate entities may need to be revised.

Reflexes from nasal stimuli

Chemical irritation, temperature change and physical stimulation of the nose may all cause widespread cardiovascular and respiratory responses. The degree of the response depends on the intensity of the stimulus and ranges from mere sneezing to cardiorespiratory arrest (Berger, Nolte and Reichenhall, 1979). Sneezing is associated with facial movements, lacrimation, nasal secretions and vascular engorgement.

More usually a change in respiratory rate with closure of the larynx and a variable cardiovascular response also happens.

Animal studies have shown that sensory stimulation of the nose can result in intense vasoconstriction of skin, muscles and visceral arteries and is accompanied by a lowered cardiac output. This is a modification of the submersion reflex which diverts blood away from the skin to the brain and explains why passage of an endotracheal tube through the nose may give rise to a bradycardia.

Nasopulmonary reflexes

Increased airflow through one side of the nose is associated with an increased ventilation of the homolateral lung. This reflex change has been shown to follow the nasal cycle. Blowing air through a nostril causes the bronchial muscle to relax on the same side and increase its respiratory activity (Samzelius–Lejdstrom, 1939).

Reflexes acting on the nose

The resistance of the nose may vary because of changes in the metabolic requirements of the individual. Exercise, emotion and stress may all cause vasoconstriction. These are mediated by increased sympathetic tone and are abolished by a stellate ganglion block. An increase in arterial CO_2 mediated by chemoreceptors results in nasal vasoconstriction. Hypoxia has the same effect while hyperventilation causes the opposite effect, nasal congestion.

Cutaneous stimulation

Heating the skin of parts of the body, such as the feet, arms or neck produces an increase in nasal resistance. Cooling will result in vasoconstriction (Cole, 1954). Adaptation to both develops and is followed by rebound. Pressure to the axilla or lying causes nasal blockage on the dependent side (Davies and Eccles, 1985).

Central control

The hypothalamus controls the cardiorespiratory responses. Stimulation causes marked nasal vasoconstriction. Exercise, fight and flight reflexes and reflexes following emotional change are coordinated by the hypothalamus. The relationship between the rhinencephalon and nasal function needs further evaluation.

Drugs acting on the vascular tissue of the nose

Four groups of drugs that act on the nasal vasculature have clinical importance (Table 6.4):

1 Sympathomimetics and their antagonists
2 Parasympathomimetics and their antagonists
3 Histamine and antihistamines
4 Local anaesthetics.

Remarkably, the modes of action of these groups have not been evaluated fully in man. Our knowledge of behavioural changes induced by some drugs, particularly the antihistamines, is based on studies in cats and dogs.

Sympathomimetics and their antagonists

The two natural sympathomimetics, noradrenalin and adrenalin, act on the nose mainly through α_1-receptor sites, although it has been suggested that there may be some α_2-receptors which have a physiological role in the nose. Compounds which act on α_1-receptors cause vasoconstriction, whereas agonists such as isoprenaline which act on α_2-receptors, cause vasodilation. There are many sympathomimetics, related to ephedrine, that are used for vasoconstriction; some such as neosynephrine hydrochloride, are very strong and cause prolonged vasoconstriction. The main nasal complication of the use of sympathomimetics is rebound hyperaemia which is associated with rhinorrhoea.

Although essentially a local anaesthetic, cocaine blocks the uptake of noradrenalin and so potentiates its local vasoconstrictive action. Drugs used in the treatment of hypertension may cause nasal obstruction by blocking sympathetic activity. Reserpine, which is no longer used, was the worst offender. Methyldopa and β-blockers may all give rise to nasal symptoms.

Parasympathomimetics and their antagonists

Intravenous pilocarpine and carbachol cause nasal congestion, vasodilation and watery secretions. These actions are blocked by atropine and are a cholinergic effect. As mentioned earlier, atropine resistant vasodilation is recognized and is mediated by VIP. Other mediators, such as histamine, are present in normal nasal secretions and may also cause vasodilation.

Histamine and antihistamines

The pharmacology of histamine is complex and both H_1 and H_2 receptors have been demonstrated in the nasal mucosa, H_1 receptors being predominant. Histamine acts on the smooth muscle of the vasculature causing vasodilation and the capillary endothelium which shrinks to promote leakage through its walls. It is also irritant to the sensory nerve endings and stimulates sneezing. Histamine has been shown to be present only in mast cells and basophils. Although not as powerful as other inflammatory mediators derived from mast cells, histamine is produced in much larger amounts. The actions of histamine, therefore, account for only some of the mast cell reactions.

Antihistamines are widely used in medicine and are a heterogeneous group of compounds. They have a number of properties which include blockage of H_1 receptors, anticholinergic activity, local anaesthesia and sedation. Not all actions are present in each compound and the newer antihistamines such as terfenadine and astemizole have little in the way of a sedative effect which makes them safer. Although antihistamines are effective for clinical use, one study would suggest that they do not have any action against histamine in the nose (Bentley and Jackson, 1970).

Local anaesthetics

Local anaesthetics work by stopping nerve conduction through the effect of their amide group which

Table 6.4 Drugs acting on the nasal mucosa

Group	Examples
Sympathomimetics and their antagonists	Adrenalin and synthetic analogues Antihypertensives particularly β-blockers
Parasympathomimetics and their antagonists	Atropine, pilocarpine Antihistamines with this activity
Histamine and antihistamines	Mainly H_1 blockers Sedative and non-sedative
Local anaesthetics	Cocaine, lignocaine
Hormones	Sex hormones, thyroxine, corticosteroids

blocks transmembrane channels and affects ion exchange. The two main groups of local anaesthetics are lignocaine or its derivatives and cocaine. Cocaine is also a powerful vasoconstrictor as it prevents the recycling of noradrenalin by blocking its reuptake into sympathetic nerve endings. Lignocaine has an effect on the precapillary sphincters which it dilates and so, by contrast to cocaine, is a mild vasodilator. Consequently, a sympathomimetic should be added to the solution to prolong its effect. All local anaesthetics, if given in high concentration, have systemic effects on the heart and central nervous system.

Hormones

A close link exists between the anterior pituitary and the hypothalamus by way of the hypothalamohypophyseal tract. A complex interrelationship is present between emotional states, the autonomic nervous system and the hormones of the body. In all animals, olfaction is part of sexual behaviour and will be considered in more detail later.

Sex hormones

The nasal mucosa is susceptible to sex hormones particularly oestrogens which it can concentrate. Conditions where oestrogen levels are high are associated with nasal obstruction and with rhinorrhoea. There are changes in nasal function during menstruation, pregnancy and puberty in both sexes. High dose oestrogen contraceptives have been associated with rhinitis in some women.

Thyroxine

Hyperthyroidism may give rise to rhinitis, though the exact mechanism is unclear. Hypothyroidism is associated with nasal obstruction due to the deposition of mucopolysaccharides in the extracellular spaces of the submucosa, which is similar to the condition found in the larynx and elsewhere.

Corticosteroids

Glucocorticosteroids affect nasal function indirectly by stabilizing cell membranes. They also stabilize the mast cell surface membrane and make the vascular endothelium less permeable. Fluticasone may have a direct action on the smooth muscle of nasal arterioles causing vasoconstriction.

Adrenal medulla

The sympathomimetics cause vasoconstriction by a direct effect and have been discussed earlier.

Emotional states

Three different responses can be recognized: fight or flight, which causes vasoconstriction; sexual behaviour, which produces a number of different responses; and stress, which causes vagal hypertonia. In the abdomen it may precipitate duodenal ulceration, while in the nose it results in prolonged congestion and nasal obstruction. Stress may also precipitate migraine which, by way of the hypothalamus, can also be associated with nasal symptoms, usually congestion and clear rhinorrhoea.

The nose and the voice

The voice is produced by modifying the vibrating column of air from the larynx. The larynx produces the vowel sounds and the pitch of the voice. The fundamental voice frequencies are under 1000 Hz (F_1 300–400 Hz, F_2 500–1900 Hz, F_3 1800–2600 Hz). High frequency sounds, the consonants, are added by the pharynx, tongue, lips and teeth. The nose adds quality to this by allowing some air to escape through it. The sound resonates within the nose and mouth; if too little air escapes from the nose then rhinolalia clausa results, if too much then rhinolalia aperta ensues. The nose is most effective when resonating at the laryngeal F_1 frequencies. It is doubtful whether the sinuses have any effect on modifying voice although they may help with auditory feedback. Transmission of sound through the facial skeleton helps monitor voice quality. Many nasal conditions affect the quality of the voice by blocking the passage of air in expiration. Alteration is commonly heard in allergic rhinitis, the common cold and nasal polyps.

Olfaction

Olfaction initiates and modifies behaviour in many creatures. Man minimizes its importance by concentrating on the audiovisual aspects of behaviour. Despite this, much money is spent each year on modification of body odours which are intended to make the wearer less offensive and more attractive to the opposite sex.

Odours are a complex mixture of different compounds, each one at a low concentration. Studies in olfaction concentrate on single compounds or mixtures with two or three chemicals. Olfactory compounds must contact the nasal mucosa in order to produce a smell and have to be soluble in water and lipids. Man is able to discriminate between a large number of different smells. The olfactory mucosa and pathway is rapidly fatigued but recovers quickly.

Sniffing

Maximum exposure of the olfactory area to smells is achieved by sniffing which causes turbulent air flow. Animal studies suggest that the olfactory stimulus is augmented by increasing the velocity of airflow (Ottoson, 1956).

Olfactory area

The area of the olfactory epithelium varies between species. Dogs and rabbits have larger olfactory areas than man. The human has 200–400 mm² of sensory epithelium with a cellular density of about 5×10^4 receptor cells/mm². These receptor cells have modified cilia which increase their surface area and project like normal cilia into the mucus.

Stimulus

Odours are absorbed into the water fraction of mucus and the lipid reacts with the lipid bilayer of the receptor cells at specific sites. This causes K^+ and Cl^- to flow out and thereby depolarize the sensory cells (Takagi *et al.*, 1968). After a latent period of up to 400 ms a slow compound action potential may be recorded from the olfactory mucosa which Ottoson (1956) called the electro-olfactogram (EOG). The speed of the rising phase varies with the intensity of the stimulus and the recovery or falling phase is an exponential decay with a time constant of 0.9–1.45 ms.

Receptors

Olfaction appears to be mediated by G-protein coupled receptors in the cells. These interact with a specific adenyl cyclase (type 111) within the neuroepithelium (Bakalyar and Reed, 1990). It has been found that adrenergic and muscarinic antagonists block some odour responses in the olfactory receptor neurons, whereas glutamine antagonists do not. This suggests that there is some degree of specificity (Firestein and Shepherd, 1992).

Threshold

The olfactory response exhibits variation in threshold and adaptation. The threshold concentration can vary by 10^{10} depending on the chemical nature of the stimulus. The threshold of perception is lower than identification; i.e. a smell is sensed before it is recognized. Threshold values vary widely between studies and they reflect the nature of smell and the different methods of detection. Smell does not have an absolute threshold but depends, to a large extent, on the level of inhibitory activity generated by the higher centres. Some animals, particularly dogs, have a much lower threshold than man.

Adaptation

The olfactory response shows marked adaptation, the threshold increases with exposure and recovery of the electro-olfactogram is rapid when the stimulus is withdrawn.

$$R = a + bc^t$$

where R is the perceived intensity, a is the asymptote, b is a constant and c is the rate of decline which is a function of time (t).

Adaptation is both a peripheral and central phenomenon. Cross-adaptation is present between odours at high concentrations, whereas cross-facilitation develops near threshold values.

Other factors affecting threshold

Changes in the nasal mucus and its pH will alter olfactory perception. Threshold decreases with age and is both increased and altered by hormones, particularly the sex hormones. In man some genetic variation is present which is similar to colour blindness: there is a familial lack of perception to certain odours which is more common in males.

Discrimination

Man appears to be better at detecting the pleasantness of an odour rather than recognizing it. The pleasantness is largely cultural and is therefore learned. If two odours are mixed the resulting intensity is always less than the sum of the two individually perceived intensities and is dominated by the stronger component.

Pathways

There is no interaction between the individual receptor cells. Each receptor cell is connected to the olfactory bulb by non-myelinated nerve fibres. These fibres terminate and synapse on olfactory glomeruli, each of which receives about 25 000 fibres and acts as an integrator. The conduction time between the receptor cells and the glomerulus is just 50 ms, for even though the fibres are slow, they are short. The glomerulus fires with an all or none response into the mitral or tufted cells whose axons transport the signal through the lateral olfactory tract. Inhibition is derived from feedback from the high cortical centres.

Higher centres

The anterior olfactory nucleus sends impulses to the opposite bulb and also to the ipsilateral forebrain through the anterior commissure. The primary olfactory cortex lies rostral to the telencephalon and includes the olfactory tubercle, the prepyriform and preamygdaloid areas. There are projections to the thalamus where they are integrated with taste fibres, and there are also projections to the hypothalamus. Communication from the receptor cell to the brain stem is achieved with only two synapses.

Perceived intensity

Perception of smell is a complex activity which involves both the pathways and the higher centres which have learned to recognize the smell. It is possible to determine a mathematical relationship between the perceived intensity of the stimulus, R, and the stimulus concentration, S:

$$R = CS^n$$

where C is a constant and the value of n is below one. Since n is below one the system attenuates, particularly at high concentrations.

Trigeminal input

Most smell is independent of the trigeminal nerve but at high concentrations irritation develops and this is a factor in detecting the intensity of certain compounds such as butyl acetate and may account for 30% of the odour intensity (Cain, 1974). Anosmic patients can only distinguish between sweet, sour, salt and bitter and whether a compound is irritant. The irritant effect cannot be bypassed in normal people and does contribute to the nature of smell. It is important when testing olfaction to use compounds which are not irritant.

Classification of odours

There is no satisfactory classification of odours, but Amoore (1969) has suggested that there are as many as 30 primary odours which are recognized by humans, basing his theory on the stereochemistry of compounds and variations of anosmia to substances which are present in man. The human being has difficulty in detecting and recognizing variation in intensity of more than 17 odours. Furthermore, because humans do not rely on conscious detection of odour, only its quality, training is necessary for scientific experiments and for occupations which require a 'good nose'. An obvious discriminatory mechanism has not been found in the nose at the receptor site or in the olfactory bulb. Some cells in the olfactory bulb increase their discharge rate while others decrease their rate of discharge on stimulation.

Theories of smell

It is a general scientific rule that if there is no single theory of function then no one really knows or has proven the mechanism involved. However, there is a number of hypotheses which have been advanced to explain the nature of smell.

Molecular structure

Moncrieff (1967) suggested that molecular structure is important, however, no stereospecific olfactory receptors have been demonstrated.

Electrochemical reactions

Some cells contain carotenoids similar to the eye and these could give rise to photochemical reactions similar to those that take place in the eye (Briggs and Duncan, 1962).

Stereospatial patterns

Certain receptors could have a stereospatial, lock and key form, and receptor cells fire when the surface membrane is altered (Mozell, 1970).

Molecular properties

A modification of the previous theory would hold that basic molecular properties account for receptor specificity and include molecular volume at boiling point, proton affinity and donation, and local polarization within the molecule (Laffort, Patte and Etcmeto, 1974). Theoretical thresholds correlate with experimental values.

Olfactory mucosa morphology

The pattern of the stimulus within the mucosal configuration of receptor cells detects the nature of the smell. This theory of discrimination is based partly on specific receptor sites and partly on their position within the olfactory mucosa (Holley and Doving, 1977). Olfaction may well be an analogue system. A number of different combinations from a few receptor sites could give rise to a large number of different smells.

Olfaction and behaviour

Olfaction is important in regulating behaviour in all animals and insects including man. The degree of development depends on the species. Smell is used in four main areas of behaviour: the detection and consumption of food, recognition, territorial markings and sexual behaviour. In humans eating and sexual behaviour are particularly important.

Eating

Olfaction is related to two aspects of eating, the recognition of food types and the initiation of digestion. The initiation of digestion is mediated via the lateral and ventromedial hypothalamus; it causes salivation and increases the output of gastric acid and enzymes.

Sexual behaviour

Pheromones were first described in insects. The term describes chemicals which are produced by glands and are sexually attractive. They have been encountered widely in all animals. Three types of pheromone have been described: releaser pheromones, primer pheromones and imprinting pheromones. Releaser pheromones produce an immediate and reversible response and act through the nervous systems, whereas primer pheromones require prolonged stimulation and act on the anterior pituitary where they cause hormones to be released. Imprinting pheromones are chemicals which are encountered during development, modify behaviour and may subsequently initiate a response.

The degree of involvement in human behaviour is uncertain but the influence of smell is probably underestimated since most activity takes place at the subconscious level.

The nasovomeral organ

The nasovomeral organ is vestigial in man. It is important in reptiles where molecules are presented to it by the tongue – hence the flicking tongue in snakes. It is an accessory organ of smell but differs from the olfactory area in that it has no pigment within the epithelium. Its function may be more related to taste. It can be found as a small pit on the nasal septum in about 20% of the population and has no neurological connections with the central nervous system. There appears to be no correlation between its presence and human behaviour.

The paranasal sinuses

The physiological role of the paranasal sinuses is uncertain. They are a continuation of the respiratory cavity and are covered by respiratory mucosa. They share certain features with the nose but the responses are much less marked on account of the relatively poorly developed vasculature and nerve supply. In man, they assume importance in the diseased state only and this is outside the scope of this chapter, being discussed elsewhere.

The development of the sinuses takes up to 25 years: the ethmoids and maxillary sinuses are rudimentary at birth, the frontal sinuses develop after the age of 6 years but may be completely absent; the sphenoid sinus differs considerably in the degree of development. It holds true that whatever physiological role they play, it is not essential and of only minor importance.

Mucosa

The mucosa runs in continuity from the nose and is respiratory in type; however, there are differences between the nose and the sinuses. Goblet cells and cilia are less numerous in sinus mucosa but increase in frequency near the ostia; the blood supply is less well developed with no cavernous plexus, which gives the mucosa a pale almost translucent appearance. As the nerve supply is less well developed, the sinus mucosa is able to give only a weak vasomotor response and increase mucus production on parasympathetic stimulation.

Drainage

Mucociliary clearance in the maxillary sinus is spiral, towards the natural ostium (Toremalm, Mercke and Reimor, 1975). Drainage of the frontal and sphenoid sinuses is downwards, aided by gravity. Ciliary motion remains normal if the blood supply is adequate. If the blood supply is impaired then ciliary activity is reduced and stasis of secretions results. The secretions join the nasal mucus in the middle meatus and may contribute to both the total amount and effectiveness of the nasal mucus.

Oxygen tension

The Po_2 is lower in the maxillary sinuses than in the nose and it is lower still in the frontal sinuses. The oxygen tension drops further if the ostium becomes blocked.

Ostium size

Blockage of the natural sinus ostium results in a reduction of ventilation and stasis of secretions. If the ostium size is below 2.5 mm, it predisposes to the development of disease (Aust, Drettner and Hemmingsson, 1976).

Pressure changes

The pressure in the maxillary sinus varies with respiration but lags behind by 0.2 s. There is little fluctuation when the nose is patent, and the variation of pressure during quiet respiration is $+/-4$ mmH$_2$O which reaches 17–20 mmH$_2$O on exercise. Pressure fluctuations are much more marked if the nose is blocked. Barotrauma is five times less common than in the ear and is most frequently seen in the maxillary sinuses, particularly in divers.

Physiological functions of the sinuses

The possible functions of the sinuses are listed below:

Vocal resonance and diminution of auditory feedback
Air conditioning
Pressure damper
Reduction of skull weight
Flotation of skull in water
Mechanical rigidity
Heat insulation
Increasing the olfactory area
No function.

The volume of the largest sinus is under 50 ml and, therefore, contributes little to air conditioning. Similarly, a pressure damper has to have a large volume to be effective. The reduction of weight is small compared to the overall weight of the skull and flotation would appear to be irrelevant as man has long ceased to be an amphibian. Most of the cranial activity is away from the sinuses so they play little part in insulating the brain. It has been held that the development of the sinuses is phylogenetically important in order to increase the olfactory area. However, many smaller animals do not have well developed sinuses but their sense of smell is very acute. Larger animals, such as the dog, have an ethmoturbinal system which is a complex convoluted arrangement which increases the surface area but does not contain true sinuses. Both man and other animals use scent soon after birth to recognize their parents and to initiate behaviour, well before the sinuses are developed. Olfaction would appear to be fully developed at birth, but recognition and learning come later, probably after the age of 2 years in humans. In other words, the sense of smell is fully developed well before the sinuses achieve their maximum dimensions. It is probable that, apart from mucus production and some strengthening of the facial bones, the paranasal sinuses have little or no physiological function.

References

AMOORE, J. (1969) A plan to identify most primary odors. In: *Olfaction and Taste*, edited by C. Pfaffman. New York: Rockerfeller University Press. pp. 158–171

ANGGARD, A. (1974) Capillary and shunt blood flow in the nasal mucosa of the cat. *Acta Otolaryngologica*, 78, 418–422

ANGGARD, A., LUNDBERG, J. M., HÖKSELT, T., NILSSON, G., FAHRENKRUG, J, and SAID, S. (1979) Innervation of cat nasal mucosa with special reference to relations between peptidergic and cholinergic neurones. *Acta Physiologica Scandinavica*, Suppl. 473, 50, abstract 143

AUST, R., DRETTNER, B. and HEMMINGSSON, A. (1976) Elimination of contrast medium from the maxillary sinus. *Acta Otolaryngologica*, 81, 468–474

BABATOLA, F. (1990) Nasal resistance values in the adult Negroid Nigerian. *Rhinology*, 28, 269–273

BAKALYAR, H. and REED, R. (1990) Identification of a specialized adenyl cyclase that may mediate odorant detection. *Science*, 250, 1403–1406

BENTLEY, A. and JACKSON, R. (1970) Changes in patency of the upper nasal passage induced by histamine and antihistamines. *Laryngoscope*, 80, 1859–1870

BERGER, D., NOLTE, D. and REICHENHALL, B. (1979) On nasobronchial reflex in asthmatic patients. *Rhinology*, 17, 193–198

BOAT, T. F., KLEINEMAN, J. I., CARLSON, D. M., MALONEY, W. H. and MATTHEWS, L. W. (1974) Human respiratory tract secretions. 1 Mucous glycoproteins secreted by cultured nasal polyp epithelium from subjects with allergic rhinitis and with cystic fibrosis. *American Review of Respiratory Diseases*, 110, 427–441

BRIDGER, G. P. and PROCTOR, D. P. (1970) Maximum nasal inspiratory flow and nasal resistance. *Annals of Otology*, 79, 481–488

BRIGGS, M. and DUNCAN, B. (1962) Pigment and olfactory mechanism. *Nature*, 195, 1313–1314

BURNHAM, A. H. (1935) An anatomical investigation of blood vessels of the lateral nasal walls and their relation to turbinates and sinuses. *Journal of Laryngology and Otology*, 50, 569–593

CAIN, W. S. (1974) Contribution of the trigeminal nerve to perceived odor magnitude. *Annals of the New York Academy of Science*, 237, 28–34

CALHOUN, K., HOUSE, W., HOKANSON, J. and QUINN, F. (1990) Normal nasal airway resistance in noses of different sizes and shapes. *Otolaryngology, Head and Neck Surgery*, 103, 605–609

CANTER, R. (1986) A non-invasive method of demonstrating the nasal cycle using flexible liquid crystal thermography. *Clinical Otolaryngology*, 11, 329–336

CAUNA, N. (1970) Electron microscopy of the nasal vascular bed and its nerve supply. *Annals of Otorhinolaryngology*, 79, 443–450

CLARKE, R. and JONES, A. (1992) Nasal airflow receptors: the relative importance of temperature and tactile stimulation. *Clinical Otolaryngology*, 17, 388–392

CLEMENT, P. (1984) Committee report on standardisation of rhinomanometry. *Rhinology*, 22, 151–155

COLE, P. (1954) Respiratory mucosal vascular responses, air conditioning and thermoregulation. *Journal of Laryngology and Otology*, 68, 613–622

COLE, P. (1982) Modification of inspired air. In: *The Nose: Upper Airway Physiology and the Atmospheric Environment*, edited by D. Proctor and I. Anderson. Amsterdam: Elsevier, pp. 351–375

COLLINS, M. P. (1985) A practical guide to the construction of a 'cire perdue' model of the human nose. *Rhinology*, 23, 71–78

DAVIES, A. and ECCLES, R. (1985) Reciprocal changes in nasal resistance to airflow caused by pressure applied to the axilla. *Acta Otolaryngologica*, 99, 154–159

DRETTNER, B. and AUST, R. (1974) Plethysmographic studies of the blood flow in the mucosa of the human maxillary sinus. *Acta Otolaryngologica*, 78, 259–263

ECCLES, R. and WILSON, H. (1973) The parasympathetic nerve supply of the nose of the cat. *Journal of Physiology*, 230, 213–223

ECCLES, R., LANCASHIRE, B. and TOLLEY, N. (1987) Experimental studies on nasal sensation of airflow. *Acta Otolaryngologica*, 103, 303–306

FIRESTEIN, S. and SHEPHERD, G. (1992) Neurotransmitter antagonists block some odor responses in olfactory receptor neurons. *Neuroreport*, 3, 661–664

FOKKENS, W., BROEKHUIS-FLUITSMA, D., RIJNTJES, E., VROOM, T. and HOEFSMIT, E. (1991) Langerhans cells in the nasal mucosa of patients with grass pollen allergy. *Immunobiology*, **182**, 135–142

FULLTON, J., FISCHER, N., DRAKE, A. and BROMBERG, P. (1984) Frequency dependence of effective nasal resistance. *Annals of Otology, Rhinology and Laryngology*, **93**, 140–145

HOLLEY, A. and DOVING, K. (1977) Receptor sensitivity, acceptor distribution, convergence and neural coding in the olfactory system In: *Olfaction and Taste VI*, edited by J. Le Magna and P. Macleod. London: Information Retrieval. pp. 113–128

HOLMBERG, K. and PIPKORN, U. (1985) Mucociliary transport in the human nose. The effect of topical glucocorticoid treatment. *Rhinology*, **23**, 181–186

INGLESTEDT, S. and IVSKERN, B. (1949) The source of nasal secretion in normal conditions. *Acta Otolaryngologica*, **37**, 446–450

ISHIZAKA, K. and ISHIZAKA, T. (1967) Identification of E antibodies as a carrier of reaginic activity. *Journal of Immunology*, **99**, 1187–1198

KAYSER, R. (1895) Die exacte Messung der Luftdurchangiklit der Nase. *Archives of Laryngology*, **3**, 101–210

LAFFORT, P., PATTE, F. and ETCMETO, O. (1974) Olfactory coding in the basis of physiochemical properties. *Annals of the New York Academy of Science*, **237**, 193–208

LAMB, D. and REID, L. (1970) Histochemical and autoradiographic investigation of the serous cells of the human bronchial glands. *Journal of Pathology*, **100**, 127–138

LUNDBERG, J. and TATEMOTO, K. (1982) Pancreatic polypeptide family (APP, BPP, NPY and PYY) in relation to sympathetic vasoconstriction resistant to α-adrenoceptor antagonists. *Acta Physiologica Scandinavica*, **116**, 393–402

LUNDBERG, J., ANGGARD, A., FAHRENKRUG, T., HONFELT, T. and MUTT, V. (1980) Vasoactive intestinal polypeptide in cholinergic neurones of exocrine glands: functional significance of coexisting transmitters for vasodilation and secretion. *Proceedings of the National Academy of Science, USA*, **77**, 1651–1655

LUNDBERG, J. M., HOKFELT, T., ANGGARD, A., TERENIUS, L., ELDE, R., MARKEY, Y. *et al.* (1982) Organisational principles in the peripheral sympathetic nervous system. *Proceedings of the National Academy of Science, USA*, **79**, 1303–1307

MALCOLMSON, K. G. (1959) The vasomotor activities of the nasal mucous membrane. *Journal of Laryngology and Otology*, **73**, 73–98

MASSON, P. L. and HEREMANS, J. F. (1973) Sputum proteins. In: *Sputum: Fundamentals and Clinical Pathology*, edited by M. J. Dulfano. Springfield, Illinois: Charles C Thomas. pp. 412–474

MENNELLA, J. and BEAUCHAMP, G. (1992) Developmental changes in nasal airflow patterns. *Acta Otolaryngologica*, **112**, 1025–1031

MICHAEL, R. P., ZUMPE, D., KEVERNE, D. B. and BONSALL, R. W. (1972) Neuroendocrine factors in the control of primate behaviour. *Recent Progress in Hormone Research*, **28**, 665–706

MONCRIEFF, R. (1967) *The Chemical Senses*. London: Leonard Hill

MOZELL, M. (1970) Evidence for a chromatographic model of olfaction. *General Physiology*, **56**, 46–63

MYGIND, N. and LOWENSTEIN, H. (1982) Allergy and other environmental factors In: *The Nose: Upper Airway Physiology and the Atmospheric Environment*, edited by D. F. Proctor and I. Anderson. Amsterdam: Elsevier. pp. 377–397

OTIS, A., FENN, W. and RAHN, H. (1950) The mechanics of breathing in man. *Journal of Applied Physiology*, **2**, 597–607

OTTOSON, D. (1956) Analysis of the electrical activity of the olfactory epithelium. *Acta Physiologica Scandinavia*, Suppl. 122, 1–83

PROTETZ, A. W. (1953) *Applied Physiology of the Nose*, 2nd edn. St Louis: Mosby

REYNOLDS, S. R. M. and FOSTER, F. (1940) Acetylcholine equivalent content of the oestrogen nasal mucosa in rabbits and cats, before and after administration. *American Journal of Physiology*, **131**, 422–425

RIVRON, R. and SANDERSON, R. (1991) The voluntary control of nasal airway resistance. *Rhinology*, **29**, 181–184

ROBSON, A., SMALLMAN, L. and DRAKE-LEE, A. (1992) Factors affecting ciliary function in vitro: a preliminary study. *Clinical Otolaryngology*, **17**, 125–129

SAMZELIUS-LEJDSTROM, I. (1939) Respiratory movements. *Acta Otolaryngologica*, Suppl. 35, 3–104

SERIES, F., CORMIER, Y., DESMEULES, M. and LA-FORGE, J. (1989) Influence of respiratory drive on upper airway resistance in normal men. *Journal of Applied Physiology*, **66**, 1242–1249

SLEIGHT, M. (1974) *Cilia and Flagella*. London: Academic Press

SWIFT, D. L. (1982) Physical principles of airflow and transport phenomena influencing air modification. In: *The Nose: Upper Airway Physiology and the Atmospheric Environment*, edited by D. F. Proctor and I. Anderson. Amsterdam: Elsevier. pp. 337–349

SWIFT, D. L. and PROCTOR, D. F. (1977) Access of air into the respiratory tract. In: *Respiratory Defense Mechanisms*, edited by D. Brain, D. F. Proctor and L. M. Reid. New York: Dekker. Vol 1, Ch. 3

TAKAGI, S. F., WYSE, G. A., KITAMURA, H. and ITO, K. (1968) The roles of sodium and potassium ions in the generation of the electro-olfactogram. *Journal of General Physiology*, **1**, 552–578

TOREMALM, N., MERCKE, U. and REIMOR, A. (1975) The mucociliary activity of the upper respiratory tract. *Rhinology*, **13**, 113–120

TSUBONE, H. (1989) Nasal 'flow' receptors of the rat. *Respiratory Physiology*, **75**, 51–64

UDDMAN, R., ALUMETS, J., DENSERT, O., HAKANSSON, R. and SUNDER, P. (1978) Occurrence and distribution of VIP nerves in the nasal mucosa and tracheobronchial wall. *Acta Otolaryngologica*, **85**, 448–555

UDDMAN, R., MALM, L. and SUNDLER, F. (1980) VIP increases in nasal venous blood after stimulation of the vidian nerve. *Acta Otolaryngologica*, **87**, 304–308

VAN CAUWENBERGE, P. B. and DELAYE, L. (1984) Nasal cycle in children. *Archives of Otolaryngology*, **110**, 108–110

VAN DISHOEK, H. A. G. (1965) The part of the valve and turbinate in total nasal resistance. *International Rhinology*, **3**, 19–26

WIDDICOMBE, J. and WELSH, M. (1980) Ion transport by dog tracheal epithelium. *Federation Proceedings*, **39**, 3062–3066

WIDDICOMBE, J. G. and WELLS, U. K. (1982) Airway secretions. In: *The Nose: Upper Airway Physiology and the Atmospheric Environment*, edited by D. F. Proctor and I. Anderson. Amsterdam: Elsevier. pp. 215–244

7

Pathophysiology of the ears and nasal sinuses in flight and diving

Joseph C. Farmer and Cameron A. Gillespie

The ear and the paranasal sinuses are the most common organs injured by exposure to altered barometric pressures. Vestibular injuries can result in fatalities, which are fortunately infrequent. Other damage such as middle and inner ear barotrauma, are often encountered in general otolaryngological practice. It is, therefore, essential to be knowledgeable about the pathophysiology of this type of injury.

The evolution of the air-containing organs of hearing and balance and the paranasal sinuses has helped adapt air-breathing creatures for terrestrial life with small variations in ambient pressure. The air-containing external and middle ears overcome, to a remarkable degree, the impedance mismatch of the transmission of sound from air to water. While these structures usually adapt to gradual and small changes in ambient pressure, the relatively rapid and marked changes encountered in diving and, to a lesser extent, with altitude exposure can present significant problems and, in these circumstances, the existence of such air-containing organs becomes a liability.

The authors of this chapter have written previously on these subjects, and the reader is referred to these works for a more detailed historical perspective and alternative subject organizations (Farmer, 1990; Farmer, 1993; Farmer and Gillespie, 1988). For those principles related to flight, the reader should consult the flight surgeons' manuals of the military services.

Physical principles of altered environmental pressures and gases

The reference units for measurement of pressure are either absolute vacuum, zero pressure, or the actual pressure in one's geographic location, which is known as gauge pressure. At sea level, the absolute pressure (ATA) is 1 atmosphere (1.0 ATA) and the gauge pressure is zero. Conversions to various unit systems in measuring pressure are:

$$
\begin{aligned}
1 \text{ atmosphere} &= 14.7 \text{ lb/in}^2 \\
&= 1.033 \text{ kg/cm}^2 \\
&= 1.013 \text{ bars} \\
&= 101 \text{ kPa (kilopascals)} \\
&= 760 \text{ mmHg or } 760 \text{ torr.}
\end{aligned}
$$

When diving, each additional 33 feet (10 metres) in depth of sea water (34 feet in fresh water) results in an increase in pressure of 1 atmosphere. Thus, at a sea water depth of 66 feet (approximately 20 metres) the actual pressure is 3 atmospheres absolute (ATA) or 2280 mmHg with a gauge pressure of 2 atmospheres or 1520 mmHg.

The mass of the earth's atmosphere constantly results in an ambient pressure on the earth's surface (one ATA at sea level). With ascent from the surface, the density of the atmospheric gas and surrounding pressure decrease; with descent, gas density and ambient pressure increase. Ascent or descent in denser aqueous media results in significantly greater pressure changes per unit distance travelled than those encountered with altitude alterations in the less dense gaseous atmosphere. The maximum pressure change possible with altitude or aerospace exposure is 14.7 lb/in^2 or 760 mmHg, whereas divers encounter greater and/or more rapid pressure changes, especially with exposures deeper than 33 feet (10 metres) of sea water. Recent diving exposures have exceeded depths of 2000 feet of sea water and pressures approaching 70 ATA.

Pressure-volume relationship: Boyle's law

At a constant temperature, the volume of a gas is inversely proportional to the absolute pressure:

$$P_1 V_1 = P_2 V_2$$

For example, 5 litres of gas at sea level pressure (1 ATA) will be compressed to one-half volume or 2.5 litres at a sea water depth of 33 feet (2 ATA); to one-third volume or 1.67 litres at 66 feet (3 ATA), to one-quarter volume or 1.25 litres at 99 feet (4 ATA), and to one-fifth volume or 1.0 litres at 132 feet (5 ATA) (Figure 7.1). With altitude exposure, 5 litres of gas at sea level pressure (1 ATA) will occupy a volume of 10 litres at a pressure of 0.5 ATA (approximately 380 mmHg) at 18 000 feet; a volume of 15 litres at a pressure of 0.33 ATA (252 mmHg) at an altitude of 27 000 feet; and a volume of 20 litres at a pressure of 0.25 ATA (190 mmHg) at an altitude of 34 000 feet (Figure 7.2). Pressure equilibration in the paranasal sinuses and middle ear during diving and altitude exposure is accomplished by gas movement through the eustachian tubes and paranasal sinus ostia.

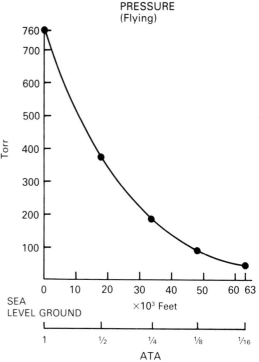

Figure 7.2 Relationship between barometric pressure and altitude. The greatest pressure changes for any change in altitude takes place near sea level. Thus, barotrauma is more common during the latter stages of descent and landings and during take-offs and early ascent. (From: Farmer, J. and Gillespie, C. Exposures to aerospace, diving, and compressed gases. In: *Otologic Medicine and Surgery*, edited by P. W. Alberti and R. J. Ruben, Churchill Livingstone, New York, (1988) pp. 1753–1802. Reprinted by permission)

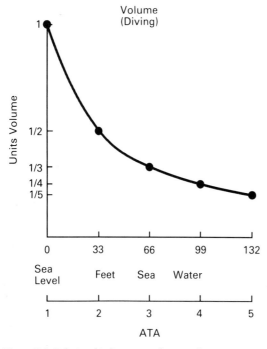

Figure 7.1 Relationship between volume and sea water depth and pressure. The greatest volume changes take place nearest the surface. Thus, barotrauma is sustained more frequently near the surface. (From: Farmer, J. and Gillespie, C. Exposures to aerospace, diving, and compressed gases. In: *Otologic Medicine and Surgery*, edited by P. W. Alberti and R. J. Ruben, Churchill Livingstone, New York, (1988) pp. 1753–1802. Reprinted by permission)

Pressure-volume relationships in diving and flying

In diving and flying, the biggest volume and pressure changes per distance travelled with ascent or descent develop near the surface. For example, the change in

volume in diving from the surface to 33 feet of sea water is one-half of the original volume and from 33 feet to 66 feet of sea water is one-third of the original volume (see Figure 7.1). In flight, the pressure change is one-half that of sea level (380 mmHg) during ascent to an altitude of 18 000 feet; the pressure change travelling to an altitude of 34 000 feet is one-half again (190 mmHg), and one-half again (95 mmHg) on rising to 48 000 feet. Thus, changes in pressure during altitude changes are much greater nearer sea level than at great heights (see Figure 7.2).

Temperature and volume relationship: Charles' law

At a constant pressure, the volume of any gas varies directly with the absolute temperature expressed in degrees Kelvin (°C + 273):

$$V_1/T_1 = V_2/T_2$$

This law accounts for the heating of equipment with pressurization and its cooling with depressurization.

Universal gas relationship

Boyle's and Charles' laws are combined to form the universal gas relationship:

$$P_1V_1/T_1 = P_2V_2/T_2$$

with temperature again expressed in degrees Kelvin. Increases and decreases in temperature can cause marked alteration in the pressures of gases contained in rigid cylinders. In some cases, increases in temperature cause pressure rises greater than the maximum design pressure and result in catastrophic consequences. Conversely, the pressure in a rigid cylinder will decrease as the cylinder is cooled.

Partial pressure and gas mixtures: Dalton's law

The total pressure of a mixture of gases is the sum of the pressures of each of the constituent gases in the mixture.

Each gas exerts a pressure known as the partial pressure which is equal to that which would be exerted by the gas if it were alone and occupied the same volume. The partial pressure is proportional to the number of molecules of that gas, to the number of molecules in the total volume and to the total pressure of the mixture. Thus air, containing 80% nitrogen and 20% oxygen, has a total pressure of 760 mmHg at 20°C and one atmosphere absolute (sea level); the nitrogen partial pressure is approximately 80% of 760 mmHg or 608 mmHg; the oxygen partial pressure is about 20% of 760 mmHg or 152 mm Hg. At 3 ATA and 20°C, the total pressure is 2280 mm Hg with nitrogen and oxygen partial pressures of 1824 mmHg and 456 mmHg respectively; at an altitude of 18 000 feet (20°C), with a pressure of 0.5 ATA (about 379 mmHg), nitrogen and oxygen partial pressures would be 303 mmHg and 76 mmHg respectively.

Paschal's principles

During the usual pressure alterations encountered in sports scuba diving and altitude exposures, the volume of the fluid-filled body spaces remains constant since fluids are virtually incompressible. However, these pressure changes follow the universal gas laws, particularly Boyle's law in the air-containing body spaces. Exposure of the ears and sinuses to greater pressures does not result in damage if the pressure in the gas-filled spaces is equal to the external pressure of the surrounding environment. With pressure differences, barotrauma to the ear and si-

nuses may be sustained. Similarly, pulmonary barotrauma can also happen if the pressure in the lung alveoli becomes greater than the external pressure acting upon the chest wall; gas may escape into the pleural or mediastinal spaces or into the bloodstream with the formation of gas emboli.

Henry's law of dissolved gases

The amount of a gas dissolved in a liquid or body tissue at a given temperature is directly proportional to the local partial pressure and the solubility coefficient of that gas in the particular liquid or tissue.

Exposure to increased gas partial pressures in diving results in increased amounts of dissolved nitrogen with compressed air or nitrox diving, or dissolved helium with heliox diving.

General pathophysiology in diving and flying

A complete review and more detailed discussion of these topics is found in Bennett and Elliott (1993), Bove and Davis (1990), and Edmonds, Lowry and Pennefather (1992).

Decompression sickness

During decompression in diving, dissolved inert gas comes out of solution into the gaseous phase. This also takes place with decompression in aerospace prior to extravehicular activity in low pressure space suits. With rapid reductions in pressure, a supersaturated condition develops and inert gas bubbles may form in tissues and body fluids rather than in the lung alveoli. This may result in mechanical disruption of tissue, obstruction of blood vessels, increased capillary permeability with leakage of fluid into the tissues, haemoconcentration, decreased vascular volume, increased platelet adhesiveness and intravascular coagulopathy.

To avoid bubble formation in inappropriate body tissues, it is necessary to slow the rate of decompression in order to avoid exceeding a critical difference between the decreasing ambient pressure and the pressure of dissolved gases in different tissue compartments. It is also necessary to determine the maximum rate of removal of gas molecules from the 'slowest' tissues, a complex problem that is altered by many factors such as surrounding temperature changes in the limbs, changes in microvascular perfusion, cardiac output, solubility coefficients, local tissue pressures, blood viscosity and ambient pressure changes. Current decompression schedules try to take all of these factors into account and use computers to estimate the amount of dissolved gas by recording the various exposure times to different ambient pressures; however, as noted above, there may be frequent changes in local tissue physiology and variations between individuals. Perfect decompression tables for each individual do not exist. Recompression, administration of hyperoxic breathing gases, intravascular fluid replacement and salicylate administration to counteract platelet agglutination are the essential components of decompression sickness treatment.

Diving-related nitrogen narcosis

Nitrogen becomes narcotic when subjected to increased atmospheric pressures. The symptoms are similar to those experienced when breathing nitrous oxide at atmospheric pressure and include euphoria and a decrease in the ability to assess one's surroundings in a realistic manner. Divers suffering from nitrogen narcosis have been seen to perform bizarre and dangerous manoeuvres such as removal of the scuba mouthpiece and continuing their descent to dangerous depths. Fatalities have been recorded. Most healthy individuals will show some signs and symptoms of nitrogen narcosis at depths in excess of 50 feet of sea water.

Martini's law of diving states that each 50 feet of depth is equal to the effects of consuming one gin and martini. Obviously, this is quite variable; most individuals do not appear to show obvious or overt symptoms until depths greater than 80–100 feet are reached. Nitrogen narcosis becomes a major limiting factor for deeper diving; thus, divers at extreme depths require non-narcotic mixtures of helium and oxygen.

Oxygen toxicity

Breathing increased partial pressures of oxygen (> 380 mmHg or 50% oxygen at 1 ATA) for a prolonged period will result in pulmonary oxygen toxicity. This most often causes pulmonary oedema but pleural effusions and atelectasis can also develop. Demonstrable reductions in vital capacity have been seen breathing 100% oxygen at 1 atmosphere absolute for greater than 4 hours or for shorter exposures at greater pressures.

Central nervous system oxygen toxicity also develops when breathing increased partial pressures of oxygen. Its onset is rapid and can happen in some healthy individuals breathing 100% oxygen at a depth of 66 feet of sea water (3 ATA). Variation in individual susceptibility and manifestations is seen. The initial signs may include muscle twitching, irregular respiration, nausea, dizziness, incoordination, paraesthesia, light headedness, euphoria or confusion with frank convulsions. A generalized convulsion may be the first sign encountered. Individuals with a history of seizures in the absence of exposure to increased amounts of oxygen have a much greater susceptibility to CNS oxygen toxicity. Oxygen toxicity during deep mixed gas diving is prevented by decreasing the oxygen percentage of the mixture to less than 380 mmHg (0.5 ATA) yet maintaining a physiological partial pressure of oxygen greater than 150 mmHg (0.20 ATA). For example, a heliox mixture suitable for diving to 19.18 ATA (600 feet) would have about 1.7% oxygen and about 98.3% helium with an oxygen partial pressure of about 248 mmHg. The percentage of oxygen must decrease to 1.7% during descent and increase to 21% on ascent, maintaining oxygen partial pressures in these ranges.

The high pressure nervous syndrome

Because of the limiting effect of nitrogen narcosis with compressed air diving, mixed gas diving using non-narcotic helium is usually performed by commercial and military divers going to depths below 120 feet. However, during compression while breathing helium-oxygen at depths generally deeper than 600 feet, the high pressure nervous syndrome is noted with tremors, dizziness, anorexia, periods of microsleep and decrements in psychomotor performance. Animals compressed at deeper depths, around 3000 feet, breathing helium-oxygen mixtures suffer convulsions (Brauer, 1968; Buhlmann *et al.*, 1970; Bennett and Towse, 1971). Some investigators (Adolfson, Goldberg and Berghage, 1972; Braithewaite, Berghage and Crothers, 1974) have demonstrated decrements in postural equilibrium and standing steadiness during the high pressure nervous syndrome. However, these investigators, plus Farmer *et al.* (1974) and Gauthier (1976), revealed that high pressure nervous syndrome was not associated with sustained nystagmus. Ocular tremor and dysmetria together with symmetrical increases in the vestibulo-ocular reflex were noted to accompany the decrements of postural equilibrium. Farmer *et al.* (1974) postulated that the high pressure nervous syndrome was the result of an equal decrease in the usual cerebellar inhibitory modulation of the brainstem vestibular nuclei. This raised firing rates with a resultant increase in the vestibulo-ocular reflex, ocular tremor and dysmetria. Studies by Bennett (1982) showed that additions of small amounts of nitrogen to the helium-oxygen mixtures (Trimix) caused a reduction of the signs of the high pressure nervous syndrome. This supported the theory that the mechanism of action of anaesthetic gases and also nitrogen at pressure, was due to swelling of synaptic membranes which decreases synaptic transmission. However, exposure at great depths, breathing helium and oxygen, causes a short-circuit in synaptic transmission from hydrostatic compression of synaptic membranes. More normal membrane thickness and synaptic transmission can be achieved by the addition of small amounts of nitrogen to the high pressure helium-oxygen atmosphere, thereby counteracting the compression effect.

Pathophysiology of the organs of hearing and balance and the paranasal sinuses in diving and flying

Otological changes due to increased gas density

Fluur and Adolfson (1966) reported increased air-conducted hearing thresholds of between 30 and 40 dB in the middle frequency range of 26 experienced divers compressed in chambers to simulated sea depths of 330 feet (100 m) in hyperbaric air. No changes in bone conduction were noted. The thresholds decreased to pre-dive levels upon return to surface pressure. Prior to this, Lester and Gomez (1898) had noted increased air and bone conduction in humans exposed to compressed air 3.0–3.5 ATA. As these hearing impairments persisted for 1–2 days after the hyperbaric exposures, otological barotrauma was suspected to be the cause. Fluur and Adolfson (1966) observed an absence of barotrauma and therefore postulated that the conductive hearing losses were related to increased impedance of the middle ear transformer from denser gas. Farmer, Thomas and Preslar (1971) and Thomas, Summitt and Farmer (1974) measured hearing in divers exposed to heliox while pressurized in a chamber to pressures equal to those encountered at 600 to 100 feet of sea water. Calibrated transducers were used, and the divers did not have any evidence of barotrauma. At depth, reversible air-conduction threshold elevations of 26 dB were noted in the lower frequencies with a decreased threshold or improved auditory sensitivity at 6 kHz. Cochlear function, as measured by sensory acuity levels and frequency different limens, was not altered. These findings were felt to be related to an increase in the resonant frequency of the ear associated with the increased speed of sound in helium. This had previously been suggested by Waterman and Smith (1970), who also noted improvement in hearing at 8 kHz while breathing 80% helium and 20% oxygen at 1 ATA. The findings at the lower frequencies by Farmer, Thomas and Preslar (1971) and Thomas, Summitt and Farmer (1974) in divers compressed and breathing heliox were felt to indicate a conductive hearing loss due to the increased density of the helium-oxygen atmospheres versus air at 1.0 ATA. These losses were not as great as those noted in air by Fluur and Adolfson (1966) which would be expected since the hyperbaric helium mixtures were of a lesser density than an equal pressure of hyperbaric air.

Auditory thresholds are technically more difficult to measure under water than in dry pressure chambers. The function of the eardrum and ossicles for sound transformation, as well as impedance matching, is very significantly altered when water fills the external auditory canal and creates water to tissue to air interfaces in addition to a mass which loads the eardrum. Also, the stimulus must be presented as a sound field stimulus rather than using earphones and this increases the problems with acoustic patterns and scatter in water. In spite of these difficulties, several investigators (Silvian, 1943; Hamilton, 1957; Wainwright, 1958; Montague and Strickland, 1961; Brandt and Hollien, 1967) have reported threshold shifts ranging from 44 to 80 dB in water depths ranging from 10 to 105 feet. No significant differences were noted between thresholds at 12 feet and 105 feet.

The relative densities of heliox, air and water would suggest that the smallest threshold changes due to increased gas density might be expected to be detected in pressurized helium, with greater changes in hyperbaric air and the greatest changes in water. Interestingly, Brandt and Hollien (1969) failed to record any significant differences in underwater hearing thresholds with or without air bubbles in the external auditory canals. Because these changes in impedance did not seem to alter hearing thresholds, underwater hearing was postulated to be achieved primarily by bone conduction.

Several groups of authors (Roger, Cabarrou and Gastaut, 1955; Bennett and Glass, 1961; Bennett, 1964; Bennett, Ackles and Cripps, 1969; Bennett and Towse, 1971; Bevan, 1971) have noted reversible decreases in the amplitude of the auditory and visual evoked responses and in spontaneous EEG activity under hyperbaric mixtures of nitrogen and argon. No such changes have been recorded with hyperbaric helium mixtures. Impaired neural synaptic transmission in the central nervous system due to nitrogen narcosis was hypothesized to account for these changes; however, none of the studies involving auditory stimuli took into account the reversible depth-related conductive hearing loss as seen by others (Fluur and Adolfson, 1966; Farmer, Thomas and Preslar, 1971; Thomas, Summitt and Farmer, 1974). Thus, the alterations in the auditory evoked responses could be related to a decrease in stimulus strength under hyperbaric conditions.

Effects of immersion

Balance alterations

In terrestrial environments, humans perceive spatial orientation, position and motion by the central nervous system integration of sensory inputs from the visual, proprioceptive and vestibular systems. Water, which may frequently be murky or cloudy, and buoyancy alter visual and proprioceptive inputs; thus, spatial orientation and motion perception become more dependent upon the peripheral vestibular system. As in most diving situations, if the vestibular end organs are stimulated appropriately and equally, vertigo does not develop. However, vestibular dysfunction and injury may happen in multiple phases of diving; also, such changes, including sensory input mismatch, can develop in flight and aerospace. The resultant vertigo or disequilibrium together with nausea and vomiting may be life-threatening, especially underwater or while piloting a high-performance aircraft.

Transient balance disturbances during diving and flying have also been associated with nitrogen narcosis, hypercarbia, hypoxia, alcohol ingestion, hyperventilation and breathing contaminated gas. However, the disequilibrium with these problems is probably related to the direct effects of these conditions upon the cardiovascular, respiratory and central nervous systems and not directly to primary ear or neural dysfunction.

Caloric vertigo in divers

Edmonds, Lowry and Pennefather (1992) have described caloric vertigo in divers caused by cold water entering their ear canals, either with unequal amounts of cold water in each ear or unequal responses to equal amounts of cold water. It has been particularly noted when divers were in a position where the horizontal semicircular canal was vertical in orientation: supine with the head elevated 30° or prone with the head flexed or depressed 30°. It has also been seen in divers who have partial obstruction of one canal with cerumen, foreign bodies, exostosis, etc., or a tympanic membrane perforation with resulting unequal responses to the entry of cold water into both ears. Divers usually describe this phenomenon while swimming in a prone position with the head flexed 30°. Resumption of an upright position results in termination of the vertigo. This problem should be prevented by trying to avoid more than brief placement of the horizontal semicircular canals in a vertical orientation while underwater and by pre-diving physicals which note those conditions that may predispose divers to caloric stimulation, such as canal obstructions or eardrum perforations. Marine and flight motion sickness are discussed elsewhere in this chapter.

Otitis externa

Otitis externa is the second most common medical problem affecting divers after middle ear barotrauma. It is related to the effects of moisture and/or humid atmospheres upon cerumen in the canal skin. Fatty acids in cerumen are dissolved or diluted causing a shift in pH towards the alkaline side. This, together with skin desquamation in the moist environment produces a perfect medium for the growth of bacteria. Contributing factors may include collections of ceruminous debris, local trauma, seborrhoeic dermatitis, poorly fitting and improperly cleaned ear plugs or swimming in polluted water. Exostoses of the bony external canal may also contribute to otitis externa.

These hard lumps in the bony ear canal are not uncommon in swimmers and divers and are believed to be due to repeated cold water exposure. Presumably, the very thin tissue overlying the periosteum renders the bony external ear canal susceptible to ischaemic cold injury with reactive hyperaemia and repair by exostosis formation.

Common organisms to cause otitis externa in divers include *Pseudomonas* and *Proteus* species in addition to staphylococci. Other organisms found include diphtheroids, streptococci, *Aerobacter*, and *Escherichia coli*. Fungi such as *Aspergillus* and *Candida* are usually only found after prolonged treatment with topical antibacterial agents.

The treatment of this condition is dealt with elsewhere but does not differ from that used in non-diving situations. Prevention is important and includes proper cleaning of ear canals, avoidance of local trauma, the acidification of the ear canal in humid and aqueous environments with a buffered 2% acetic acid solution. Alcohol and alcohol-boric acid preparations, as well as ear drops containing antibiotics, have not been particularly successful. This has been noted by divers compressed for prolonged periods in chambers which tend to contain high ambient humidity. Alcohol solutions may dissolve fat soluble fatty acids, which may be protective, and can also be irritating to the ears. Antibiotic-containing solutions are usually ineffective or simply increase the chance of infection with resistant organisms.

Pathophysiology of barotrauma

Comparison of aerospace and diving otological barotrauma

The greatest potential for barotrauma is during ascent or descent at low altitude in unpressurized aircraft and during shallow diving. The maximum theoretical pressure change with altitude exposure is 760 mmHg or 1.0 ATA; conversely, a change of this magnitude is achieved by only a 33 foot alteration in sea water depth.

During ascent in both diving and flying, the ambient pressure decreases and the volume of gas in a body cavity expands. In the middle ear, this pushes the tympanic membrane laterally with a slight increase in the middle ear volume. With further ascent, a rise in middle ear pressure develops and the eustachian tube usually opens, allowing a release of gas which limits any increase in pressure. Otic barotrauma during ascent in both diving and flying is infrequent unless there is pre-existing eustachian tube dysfunction.

Pathophysiology of middle ear barotrauma

The cartilaginous eustachian tube is normally closed. It opens during swallowing primarily due to the contraction of the levator veli palati muscle together with some activity of the tensor veli palatini and the salpingopharyngeus muscles. There is a wide individual variation in the ability of persons to undergo ambient pressure changes without difficulty. Developmental narrowing, inflammation or oedema of the tubal mucosa compromises its patency and predisposes to inadequate middle ear pressure equilibration usually during descent in flying and diving. The development of barotrauma is dependent upon the rate of descent or the rate of increase of ambient pressure in contrast to the rate of increase of middle ear pressure. The latter is affected by the patency of the lumen and by the degree, frequency and duration of eustachian tube opening (Dickson and King, 1954; Miller, 1965).

During descent, the middle ear pressure becomes negative relative to the increasing ambient and adjacent tissue pressure. The pathophysiology is demonstrated in Figure 7.3 which describes the pressure changes in the temporal bone spaces and in the nasopharynx during descent in sea water without eustachian tube opening. At a depth of 2.6 feet, a pressure differential of 60 mmHg causes mucosal congestion, oedema, and microscopic haemorrhages (Figure 7.3b). This narrows the eustachian tube lumen and, because of the nasopharyngeal valve effect, there is a decreased ability to open and ventilate the middle ear by increasing nasopharyngeal pressure. The tympanic membrane and round window bulge into the middle ear and there is inward displacement of the stapes footplate. A diver may notice pain and pressure in his ear with a conductive hearing loss and sometimes vertigo. With further descent to a depth of approximately 3.9 feet and a 90 mmHg pressure differential (Figure 7.3c), it is usually impossible to open the eustachian tube by increasing nasopharyngeal pressure. This is due to a valve effect from pressure on the tubal cartilage together with further mucosal haemorrhage which may also be seen in the middle ear. Ruptures of the tympanic membrane have been sustained at pressure differentials ranging from 100 to 400 mmHg or depths at sea equivalent to 4.3 to 17.4 feet (Figure 7.3e) (Keller, 1958). With a forceful, modified, Valsalva manoeuvre under these conditions, CSF and inner ear pressures increase, and the existing pressure differential between the inner ear and middle ear becomes greater. In this situation the round window may rupture (Figure 7.3d) with consequent leakage of perilymph and the inner ear membrane may break and/or be disrupted by haemorrhages (see inner ear barotrauma in a following section). Animal studies have demonstrated round window ruptures when, at 1.0 ATA, CSF pressure has been increased by 120–300 mmHg (Harker, Norante and Rzu, 1974).

An important point is that significant narrowing of the eustachian tube can develop with descents of 1–2 feet without equilibration of middle ear pressure.

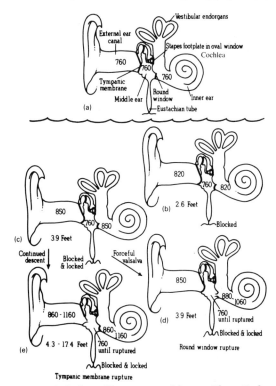

Figure 7.3 Otological barotrauma of descent. Theoretical pressure changes and tissue trauma in the right ear of a diver who does equilibrate middle ear pressure during descent. Pressures are shown in mmHg. (*a*) Surface condition with equal pressures throughout and patent eustachian tube with normally closed nasopharyngeal ostium. Actual inner ear perilymph pressure is 1–2 mmHg higher than ambient pressure. (*b*) Depth of 2.6 feet with a pressure difference of 60 mmHg. Tympanic membrane and round window are bulging into the middle ear. Mucosal changes have occurred as described in the text. (*c*) Depth of 3.9 feet with a 90 mmHg pressure difference and blocked and locked eustachian tube. (*d*) A forceful Valsalva manoeuvre or straining leads to increased CSF and inner ear pressure with an increased inner ear-middle ear pressure difference and round window rupture. (*e*) Eardrum ruptures occur at variable pressures and depths. (From: Farmer, J. and Thomas, W. Ear and sinus problems in diving. In: *Diving Medicine*, edited by R. Strauss, Grune and Stratton, New York. (1976) p. 118. Reprinted by permission)

Thus, subsequent descents and pressure equilibration become more difficult. This is especially troublesome for novice divers attempting to descend with a 2–4 foot sea swell.

Most authorities feel that significant middle ear and eustachian tube mucosal oedema with microscopic haemorrhages develop with negative middle pressures as little as 30–35 mmHg. This is well within the 196 mmHg pressure change usually encountered with the 8000 feet descent in a pressurized passenger aircraft flying at altitudes greater than 25 000 feet where the cabin is usually pressurized to 8000 feet. Brief ear canal pressure changes of 200–300 mmH$_2$O, equal to 147–22 mmHg, encountered in tympanometry, do not produce barotrauma. The changes of middle ear barotrauma require a greater pressure differential for longer durations.

Delayed middle ear barotrauma after flying

This entity was originally described by Comroe *et al.* (1945). Barotrauma was noted to develop several hours after the completion of long flights that involved breathing 100% oxygen. Commonly, affected fliers had no symptoms immediately after such flights, but noted ear fullness or blockage upon awakening. Minimal otoscopic signs are usually present. This entity has been attributed to the breathing and replacement of middle ear gas with 100% oxygen. The oxygen is absorbed while an individual is asleep during which time there is decreased swallowing and eustachian tube opening. A negative middle ear pressure and, frequently, a serous transudate develop. This mechanism has been supported by research which has indicated a faster rate of middle ear pressure change when filled with oxygen rather than air (Jones, 1959).

Manoeuvres to equilibrate middle ear pressure during diving and flying

Four common manoeuvres have been recommended to equilibrate middle ear pressure:

1 The *modified Valsalva manoeuvre* is a controlled expiration with the lips closed and nose obstructed by digital compression. This manoeuvre must be used with some caution, as the accompanying increased intrathoracic pressure decreases venous return to the heart and lowers cardiac output and syncope has been recorded (Duvoisin, Kruse and Saunders, 1962). Also, as noted previously in Figure 7.3d, a modified Valsalva manoeuvre may contribute to inner ear barotrauma with labyrinthine window rupture.
2 The *Frenzel manoeuvre* consists of closing the glottis, mouth, and nose while simultaneously contracting the muscles of the floor of the mouth and the superior constricture muscles. This manoeuvre is independent of intrathoracic pressure and can be performed in any phase of respiration. Research has indicated that the mean tubal opening pressure achieved with the Frenzel manoeuvre is 6 mmHg compared with a mean opening pressure of 33 mmHg with the modified Valsalva technique. During this manoeuvre, the tensor palatini muscle contracts and aids opening of the eustachian tubes (Chunn, 1960).
3 The *Toynbee manoeuvre* is performed by swallowing

with a closed nose. This was described in 1853 and involves an initial small, positive nasopharyngeal pressure which quickly becomes negative. Its effectiveness is debated but presumably some benefit might be derived by opening a 'locked' eustachian tube in the presence of a negative middle ear pressure (Thomsen, 1958).
4 The simplest way to equilibrate middle ear pressure is a modified yawn or swallow, accomplished by thrusting the lower jaw anteriorly and slightly opening the jaw while maintaining the mouth closed and the nasal passageways open. This manoeuvre requires a period of learning and practice and may not be effective if a significant pressure differential exists.

Clinical considerations of middle ear barotrauma

Middle ear barotrauma is the most common medical problem encountered in divers. The initial symptom may be a sensation of ear fullness or blockage and is usually noted early during descent. With further descent and greater pressure differentials, ear pain is experienced. The presence, severity and sequence of these symptoms in indivuals are variable. A conductive hearing loss is always present but usually either evades recognition or is not the primary complaint as the diver is in an aqueous environment. Mild tinnitus and vertigo, when there is a difference in pressure between the right and left middle ears (see alternobaric vertigo below), have been described. If hearing loss, tinnitus and vertigo are severe, especially after a non-decompression dive, possible inner ear barotrauma should be suspected.

The presence of nasal dysfunction, such as congestion and discharge, increases the likelihood of inadequate eustachian tube function and subsequent middle ear barotrauma during descent in diving and flying. Similarly, a history of otitis media, middle ear or mastoid inflammatory disease, a previous mastoid and/or middle ear surgery is suggestive of inadequate eustachian tube function in the absence of the usual atmospheric pressure changes encountered in diving. Affected individuals are much more likely to have inadequate eustachian tube function with exposure to the greater pressure changes encountered in flight and particularly in diving. In addition, divers who descend rapidly and do not attempt to equilibrate middle ear pressures every 1–2 feet of descent, as noted above (see Figure 7.3), are more likely to acquire changes in the mucosa of the eustachian tube with resultant narrowing and be affected by middle ear barotrauma during subsequent dives. This can be a particular problem when diving in a sea with swells higher than 3 feet. A common history is that of recreational divers who have no difficulty with middle ear pressure equilibration during the first dive of a week-long diving trip only to develop increasing difficulty with subsequent dives.

Physical signs of middle ear barotrauma

Otoscopic examination reveals changes which include oedema and haemorrhage in the middle ear mucosa as well as inflammation and collections of serous fluid and/or blood in the middle ear cleft. Six grades of diving related middle ear barotrauma have been described (Edmonds *et al.*, 1973).

Grade 0   symptoms without otoscopic signs
Grade I   diffuse redness and retraction of the tympanic membrane
Grade II   grade I changes plus slight haemorrhage within the tympanic membrane
Grade III   grade I changes plus gross haemorrhage within the tympanic membrane
Grade IV   dark and slightly bulging tympanic membrane due to free blood in the middle ear; a fluid level might be present
Grade V   free haemorrhage into the middle ear with tympanic membrane perforation. Blood can frequently be seen in the ear canal.

While these grades describe the pathological alterations seen, the otoscopic findings in middle ear barotrauma frequently include a combination of changes assigned to different grades. Scarred eardrums from previous disorders or surgery together with diving related middle ear disease can obscure the otoscopic appearance. Also, the treatment of middle ear barotrauma is not completely dependent upon which of these grades is present.

Treatment of middle ear barotrauma

The most important aspect of the management of middle ear barotrauma is prevention. Adequate pre-flying or diving otolaryngological examinations which emphasize nasal and eustachian tube function in addition to otological aspects are necessary. Particular attention should be given to those individuals who have a pre-existing history, symptoms or signs of middle ear or mastoid disease.

Other factors in the prevention of middle and possible inner ear barotrauma while diving include the avoidance of diving with significant nasal congestion and discharge, refraining from diving in rough seas with swells in excess of 2 feet, discontinuing descent without adequate middle ear pressure equilibration every 1–2 feet, slow, feet first descents, and avoiding performing a forceful modified Valsalva manoeuvre at depth. Divers and fliers should be aware of the manoeuvres to equilibrate middle ear pressure. The pre-dive or pre-flight use of topical long-acting nose drops (0.05% oxymetazoline) can be helpful. Systemic decongestants and/or antihistamines may also be helpful; however, undesired adrenergic side effects may be seen with these oral medications.

The first step in the examination of a patient with middle ear barotrauma is to exclude inner ear injury.

The presence of loud tinnitus, dizziness, vertigo, nystagmus, or nerve deafness suggest possible inner ear barotrauma and the need for a more complete clinical examination, which should include auditory and vestibular testing (see inner ear barotrauma below).

Once inner ear injury has been excluded, the treatment principles of middle ear barotrauma depend upon the degree of injury and the presence or absence of tympanic membrane perforation.

Three types of such injury are described:

Type I middle ear barotrauma

This type includes cases with symptoms immediately after diving or flying but with minimal otoscopic signs such as small haemorrhages around the annulus and over the malleolar processes. The recommended treatment is:

1 Avoid further diving and flying until pre-existing nasal and ear symptoms have cleared and the individual can easily autoinflate both ears at the surface. This may be accomplished in 24–48 hours and then diving using the recommended preventative precautions might be resumed.
2 Systemic and/or long-acting, topical nasal decongestants may be useful.

Type II middle ear barotrauma

This type includes symptoms plus more obvious otoscopic findings such as diffuse haemorrhages, serous middle ear effusions, and/or haemotympanum, but without eardrum perforation. The recommended treatment is:

1 Rest and avoid further diving until complete resolution is apparent and the ear can be easily autoinflated. This usually takes 7–21 days depending upon the severity of the injury.
2 Systemic and topical nasal decongestants are usually beneficial. Short courses of systemic steroids have been reported to help if there is no individual contraindication to their use.
3 Systemic antibiotics may be used prophylactically. This is controversial as eustachian tube function is frequently inadequate because of significant middle ear and tubal mucosal inflammation or swelling, which increases the risk of secondary bacterial infection. Of course, if purulent nasal discharge and/or cough with purulent sputum production are present, systemic antibiotics are indicated.
4 With an intact eardrum, topical ear drops are of no benefit at all as these substances do not readily cross the tympanic membrane. An inert, oily preparation such as Auralgan warmed to body temperature may be instilled into the ear canal to provide pain relief.

Type III middle ear barotrauma

This includes symptoms and the above otoscopic findings together with perforation of the eardrum. The recommended treatment is:

1 Avoid further diving until a complete otological evaluation has been performed and the middle ear damage has resolved with healing or surgical repair of the eardrum. Most perforations heal spontaneously and surgical repair is not necessary. Persistent poor eustachian tube function and/or middle ear inflammation from secondary infection will impede healing. Post-healing audiometry should be performed. If vertigo and/or nystagmus are present, vestibular testing should be undertaken. Further sports diving is not recommended if there is inner ear dysfunction.

2 Solutions containing alcohol or acids and most commercial antibiotic ear drop preparations which contain drugs that are ototoxic should not be instilled into the ear. If ear canal cleaning is needed, this is best done by binocular microscopic suctioning.

3 Systemic and topical nasal decongestants plus antibiotics should be employed as described for type II cases. Many clinicians recommend the use of prophylactic antibiotics in the absence of purulent discharges because of the increased possibility of secondary middle ear infection in the presence of a perforated eardrum.

4 If the eardrum does not heal after appropriate therapy, surgical repair may be needed. Pre- and post-repair audiometry should be performed and further diving or flying should be avoided until the eardrum has healed and adequate middle ear ventilation is present. Other diving audiometric standards are recommended in a subsequent section of this chapter.

External ear canal barotrauma (reverse ear squeeze)

Blockage of the external ear canal during diving results in pressure within the canal becoming negative during descent or positive during ascent relative to ambient middle ear pressures. This causes congestion and haemorrhage within the middle ear, displacement and possible rupture of the eardrum as well as swelling and inflammation of the skin of the bony external ear canal. The usual causes of the ear canal obstruction are the use of tight-fitting diving hoods or ear plugs and the presence of osteomas or impacted cerumen. The treatment of external ear canal barotrauma is similar to that described for the management of otitis externa in the above section. If eardrum rupture has occurred, ototoxic ear drops should be avoided. The best treatment is prevention with care being taken to ensure external ear canal patency during pressure changes. Accumulations of wax should be removed and the use of tight-fitting diving hoods, solid ear plugs or head phones which can completely seal the eardrum should be avoided.

Alternobaric vertigo

Transient vestibular dysfunction related to asymmetrical middle ear pressure equilibration in divers has been described (Lundgren, 1965; Terry and Dennison, 1966; Vorosmarti and Bradley, 1970). This entity is considered as another consequence of middle ear barotrauma with mucosal congestion and swelling due to inadequate middle ear pressure equilibration during descent. Thus, the eustachian tube becomes obstructed and expanding middle ear gas cannot readily escape during ascent. An asymmetric or unilateral increase in middle ear pressure can cause unequal vestibular end organ stimulation. A typical history consists of fullness developing in one ear together with vertigo while ascending, usually at the end of a dive. The vertigo is transient and usually disappears with the sudden hissing of air in one ear, either spontaneously or upon stopping ascent and descending again. Further work by Tjernstrom (1973) and Ingelstedt, Ivarsson and Tjernstrom (1974), using a technique for indirectly measuring middle ear pressure changes with simultaneous electronystagmographic recordings, has shown vestibular nystagmus with an over-pressure in one middle ear during decompression in a pressure chamber.

The exact frequency of alternobaric vertigo is unknown. Lundgren, Tjernstrom and Ornhagen (1974) performed a questionnaire survey of over 2000 Swedish divers and recorded that 453 had experienced vertigo during diving and that all were likely to have had alternobaric vertigo. In 97% the vertigo lasted from a few seconds up to 10 minutes. Those individuals who had experienced vertigo reported a higher frequency of middle ear pressure equilibration problems during diving, with these problems being more prominent in one ear. Sports divers who experience alternobaric vertigo should not dive. Vertigo with nausea and vomiting together with spatial disorientation can be quite hazardous and may explain some of the previously unexplained deaths of experienced scuba divers. Diving should be avoided if difficulties with ear clearing exist or if a modified Valsalva manoeuvre produces vertigo on the surface. It cannot be emphasized too strongly that divers should take precautions to equilibrate middle ear pressure every 1–2 feet of descent; if any ear fullness, blockage, or vertigo is experienced the descent should be halted. If vertigo is noted during ascent, and if gas supplies and other conditions permit, the ascent should be stopped and the diver should descend until the symptoms disappear and a slower ascent can be performed. Diving with a trained companion and the avoidance of delaying an ascent until gas supplies are almost depleted are excellent rules that should never be violated.

Inner ear barotrauma related to diving

Inner ear injuries acquired after relatively shallow diving or when the otological symptoms began during the compression phase of deeper diving have been termed inner ear barotrauma. These injuries were first documented by Freeman and Edmonds (1972) and have been related to labyrinthine window ruptures (Edmonds, Freeman and Tonkin, 1974; Freeman, 1978). These reports described divers who had difficulty with ear clearing during descent and/or otoscopic evidence of middle ear barotrauma after dives in which decompression sickness was unlikely. Sensorineural deafness with and without varying degrees of vestibular dysfunction were noted. Goodhill (Goodhill, 1972; Goodhill, Harris and Brockman, 1973) proposed that diving as well as non-diving-related inner ear injuries were secondary to oval and/or round window ruptures and postulated implosive and explosive mechanisms for such damage.

Pathophysiology of inner ear barotrauma

The explosive mechanism is depicted in Figure 7.3*d*. Negative middle ear pressure associated with inadequate middle ear pressure equilibration during descent becomes negative relative to perilymph pressure as well as ambient pressure. A modified Valsalva manoeuvre or other physical strain causes increased CSF pressure. This is transmitted to the inner ear with a further increase in the pressure differential between the labyrinth and the middle ear. Rupture of the round or oval windows with the development of a perilymph fistula and/or injury to the membranous labyrinth is produced.

The implosive mechanism suggests that a sudden and/or forceful Valsalva manoeuvre results in a rapid increase in middle ear pressure due to vascular congestion of the middle ear mucosa and/or forcing a sudden bolus of air through the eustachian tube. This rapid pressure increase causes a rupture of the round or oval window with possible entry of air into the intralabyrinthine space. Another, more likely, implosive mechanism in diving involves the subluxation of the stapes footplate into the labyrinth from inward displacement of the eardrum and ossicular chain in the presence of negative middle ear pressure developing during descent. Indeed, inadequate eustachian tube opening during descent, with subsequent negative middle ear pressure, is thought to be more common in divers. However, there are cases in which inner ear injury and middle ear barotrauma took place after shallow water diving in which the symptoms were not noted until reaching the surface. These cases, together with observations regarding alternobaric vertigo, suggest another possible implosive mechanism for inner ear barotrauma. This mechanism involves window ruptures due to overpressure developing in the middle ear during ascent

from eustachian tube obstruction, itself related to asymptomatic mucosal congestion and further swelling developing with inadequate middle ear pressure equilibration during descent.

Parell and Becker (1985) noted that inner ear barotrauma in association with diving-related middle ear barotrauma may be acquired without a persistent labyrinthine window rupture or fistula. Animal studies by Vail (1929) described haemorrhage into the basal turn of the cochlea without labyrinthine window ruptures. Kelemen (1983) found haemorrhage into the middle and inner ears of the temporal bones of two drowning victims without inner ear membrane tears or labyrinthine window ruptures. Simmons (1968, 1978) suggested that the pressure changes encountered with inadequate middle ear pressure equilibration during diving caused intralabyrinthine membrane break, more frequently than labyrinthine window rupture. This was supported by Gussen (1981) who described the temporal bone of a woman who suffered severe ear pain with subsequent hearing loss, tinnitus and vertigo after an aeroplane trip. A break in Reissner's membrane without labyrinthine window rupture was seen.

Parell and Becker (1985) classified 14 cases of inner ear barotrauma related to scuba diving into those with inner ear haemorrhage, labyrinthine membrane tears, and perilymph fistulae. Those that had absent or transient vestibular symptoms and moderate nerve deafness with complete hearing recovery were felt to have suffered inner ear haemorrhages. Those who had similar symptoms and recovered without surgery, except for a persistent hearing loss at one or two frequencies were felt to have had labyrinthine membrane tears. The four patients observed to have labyrinthine window fistulae exhibited persistent vestibular symptoms together with nerve deafness. In one patient the fistula was found in a round window that was more vertical in orientation. This finding was previously noted by Pullen, Rosenberg and Cabeza (1979) and by Singleton (1986). Most reported labyrinthine window ruptures associated with diving have involved the round window; few have been recorded in the oval window (Caruso *et al.*, 1977). This is directly contrary to non-diving labyrinthine window fistulae, where the oval window is the most commonly reported site.

Money *et al.* (1985) described a unique case, the temporal bones of an experienced diver who died after pulmonary barotrauma caused by ascent while breath holding. They found blood in the middle and inner ear with rupture of the round window membrane in one temporal bone, the other being entirely normal.

Animal studies by Nakashima *et al.* (1988) have supported the observations that inner ear barotrauma may take place without labyrinthine window rupture. Guinea-pigs exposed to 2 atmospheres were found to have actual damage to the organ of Corti in association with a hearing loss, but no labyrinthine window ruptures. Weisskopf, Murphy and Merzenich (1978) and Nishokia and Yanaghiara (1986) found that removal or rupture of the round window membrane alone in guinea-pigs did not result in alteration of the cochlear microphonic or nerve action potentials. Alterations in these functions were noted only after air bubbles entered the cochlea, as happens with increased middle ear pressure. However, it should be noted that guinea-pigs have patent cochlear aqueducts whereas most humans do not. Thus, inner ear damage may be less likely where cerebrospinal fluid can rapidly replace leaking perilymph or impede the entrance of air into the scala tympani or vestibuli.

Inner ear barotrauma during flight

Inner ear barotrauma related to altitude or hypobaric exposures has been less frequently documented than that during diving. Benson and King (1979) mentioned oval window injury in aircraft crew. Tingley and MacDougal (1977) suggested that round window ruptures may account for some cases of alternobaric vertigo in fliers. Rayman (1972) discussed oval window ruptures in individuals who underwent altitude exposure after stapedectomy and it was suggested that, if certain criteria were followed, flying after stapedectomy may not be hazardous.

The mechanism of inner ear barotrauma acquired in flight would seem similar to that related to diving. It involves the development of inadequate middle ear pressure equilibration and middle ear barotrauma, with or without a forceful modified Valsalva manoeuvre or physical straining. Rupture of the labyrinthine window membrane due to alterations in inner ear fluid pressures, or displacement of the eardrum and ossicles including the prosthesis, may be the initial injury which results in inner ear haemorrhage and/or labyrinthine membrane tears.

Treatment of inner ear barotrauma

Any diver or flier who develops symptoms or signs of inner ear injury – vertigo with or without sensorineural hearing loss and tinnitus – after dives in which decompression sickness is unlikely, or after flights, should be suspected of having inner ear barotrauma and possible labyrinthine window rupture. Unless other clinical signs and findings suggest pulmonary overpressure accidents, with possible CNS air embolism and/or CNS decompression sickness, such divers should not be subjected to recompression therapy since this treatment exposes the diver to the same middle ear pressure changes that contributed to the otological injury. If there appears to be CNS gas-bubble disease requiring recompression therapy, such therapy should proceed promptly with, possibly, a myringotomy being undertaken first to prevent further inner ear injury during the recompression treatment.

Patients with suspected inner ear barotrauma should be treated with bed rest and head elevation. Care should be taken to ensure that CSF and inner ear fluid pressures are not increased by the avoidance of Valsalva manoeuvres, coughing, nose-blowing and straining. Medications which supposedly increase intracranial and inner ear blood flow are usually not effective and may result in a decrease of the axial circulation. Anticoagulants are potentially harmful because of possible haemorrhage in the inner ear. Ear drops containing ototoxic antibiotics are not indicated. A complete otological examination which includes audiometric and vestibular testing, as well as a neurological examination, is required.

The timing and need for exploratory tympanotomy in the management of inner ear barotrauma is controversial. Some authors have advocated immediate exploratory surgery in all suspected cases of labyrinthine window fistula (Pullen, Rosenberg and Cabeza, 1979; Caruso *et al.*, 1977). However, as noted above, inner ear barotrauma may not be associated with an active perilymph fistula. Also, animal studies have suggested that most fistulae quickly seal and heal without treatment. Some surgeons have suggested reserving surgery for those who exhibit progressive deterioration of inner ear function or who do not improve after 48–72 hours of bed rest with head elevation (Goodhill, Harris and Brockman, 1973; Singleton *et al.*, 1978). Others have advised that an initial trial of medical management with the avoidance of any manoeuvres which may increase CSF and inner ear fluid pressures should be undertaken; exploratory surgery being reserved for those who demonstrate no improvement after 5–10 days or if inner ear function deteriorates in the interim (Althaus, 1981; Love and Waguespack, 1981).

Indeed, the diagnosis of an active perilymph fistula in cases not related to diving or altitude exposure is difficult and controversial. Seltzer and McCabe (1986) noted a wide variety of signs and symptoms ranging from unilateral tinnitus and aural fullness to profound sensorineural deafness, roaring tinnitus, and whirling vertigo in 91 patients with documented perilymph fistulae. Twenty-three per cent were associated with head trauma, barotrauma, direct ear trauma, or acoustic trauma. Kohut, Hinojosa and Budetti (1986) suggested that the persistence of the following criteria in an otherwise healthy ear would indicate the presence of an active perilymphatic fistula:

1 A fluctuating or rapidly progressive sensorineural hearing loss
2 A positive Hennebert's sign
3 Disequilibrium with loud noise exposure or physical exertion
4 Positional nystagmus
5 Constant disequilibrium of varying severity between attacks of vertigo.

The authors of this chapter feel that most barotrauma-related labyrinthine window fistulae heal spontaneously and that persistent inner ear dysfunction results from the inner ear membrane tears, trauma or haemorrhages associated with the original trauma. Therefore, the more appropriate method of management would seem to include initial conservative therapy with exploratory surgery reserved for those who demonstrate worsening function or who have no improvement after 72 hours.

Returning to diving after inner ear barotrauma

Divers who have persistent inner ear deficits should not dive again. Further inner ear injury to the same ear may be more likely and could, as stated earlier be exceptionally dangerous. Also, an injury to the opposite inner ear could result in significant disability for other activities. The persistence in either ear of a pure tone audiometric threshold greater than 25 dB in the frequency ranges of 500 Hz–2 kHz, a speech discrimination score of less than 90%, or electronystagmographic findings suggestive of inner ear vestibular dysfunction should disqualify the individual from further diving. Those individuals who undergo surgical repair of a labyrinthine window fistula should avoid flying for at least 6 weeks to allow for complete healing. Decisions about future diving should await audiometric and vestibular test results (see otological standards for diving and flying below).

Facial nerve barotrauma

Unilateral facial paralysis in association with ipsilateral middle ear overpressure during ascent has been seen in divers (Molvaer, 1979; Becker, 1983) and fliers (Bennett and Liske, 1967). They were accompanied by an overpressure in the ear on the same side as the facial paralysis. The divers also experienced alternobaric vertigo. In each case, the paralysis subsided within 1 hour of onset. It was postulated (Becker, 1983) that the middle ear overpressure during ascent compressed the horizontal portion of the facial nerve through a dehiscent bony facial nerve canal. Another theoretical mechanism suggested that the excessive middle ear pressure during ascent resulted in gas bubbles entering a non-dehiscent facial nerve canal through the fenestra of the chorda tympani nerve. Facial nerve barotrauma is rare and, as it is usually only transient, even less frequently described. The possibility of more unreported cases exists.

The best treatment is prevention and should focus upon equilibration of middle ear pressure and measures to prevent inadequate ear clearing during exposures to altered atmospheric pressures. These methods are described above.

Intracranial complications of otological barotrauma

In 1986, Goldmann described a 26-year-old healthy male scuba diving instructor who, while ascending to the surface after a 60-foot fresh water dive, noted left ear pain. The pain suddenly disappeared after reaching the surface, to be replaced by a left-sided vertex headache. After several hours on the surface, he dived again to 60 feet and noticed that the headache improved at depth. With ascent from this dive, the headache returned and was more severe. He went to his local emergency room where physical examination showed signs of left middle ear barotrauma. Skull X-rays revealed a pneumocephalus on the left side of the cranium; this was confirmed by a CT scan. A magnetic resonance scan 16 days later revealed a small amount of blood in the left epidural space near the base of the skull with blood in both mastoid cavities, but more so on the left side. After conservative treatment with prophylactic antibiotics, his headache gradually resolved and a follow-up CT brain scan one month later was normal. This case is felt to represent expansion of gas in the middle ear during ascent after the development of middle ear barotrauma and blockage of the eustachian tube from mucosal swelling, congestion, and haemorrhage during descent. It would seem that the expanding gas entered the cranium through the roof of the attic or the petrosquamous suture. Indeed, the bony roof of the attic is frequently thin with dehiscence in approximately 22% of normal human temporal bones (Ferguson *et al.*, 1986).

Inner ear decompression sickness

Decompression sickness related to altitude exposures usually involves the joints and muscles (type I decompression sickness). Inner ear and central nervous system decompression sickness (type II) is associated with diving but has not, thus far, been reported with altitude exposures. Otological decompression injuries were described a long time ago by Smith (1873), Alt (1897), Alt *et al.* (1896) and Vail (1929). These workers suggested that inner ear injuries during decompression were possibly related to nitrogen bubble formation in the labyrinth. Diving-related inner ear injuries were discounted until the 1960s when the frequency of exposure to deeper depths began to increase and isolated inner ear decompression sickness was described. Buhlmann and Waldvogel (1967), in a description of 82 incidences of decompression sickness in a series of mixed gas chamber dives of depths ranging from 11 to 23 ATA, said that the only neurological symptoms of the entire series were otological and consisted of vertigo, nausea, vomiting, and tinnitus in 11 divers with hearing loss in two. Rubenstein and Summitt (1971) described 10 cases of isolated inner ear decompression sickness after diving. Farmer *et al.* (1976) included these 10 cases and added 13 more instances of isolated inner ear decompression sickness during or shortly after decompression from four air and 19 helium oxygen dives. None of these dives was associated with middle ear barotrauma, central nervous system decompression sickness, or air emboli to explain the otological symptoms and findings. Ten of the divers had vestibular symptoms only, seven had cochlear symptoms, and six exhibited both cochlear and vestibular dysfunction. A significant correlation between prompt recompression treatment and recovery was noted; the 11 divers who were recompressed within 42 minutes after symptom onset obtained relief of symptoms during recompression and no subsequent residual inner ear dysfunction. Three divers were recompressed within 60–68 minutes of the onset of their symptoms. One obtained relief while the other two did not and demonstrated residual inner ear dysfunction. All divers whose recompression treatment was omitted or delayed longer than 68 minutes after the onset of their symptoms experienced persistent inner ear deficits.

Thirteen of the 19 helium-oxygen dives in this series involved a change to an air atmosphere at depths ranging from 60 to 100 feet during the latter stages of decompression. Farmer *et al.* (1976) suggested this was related to formation of helium gas bubbles in the inner ear due to the sudden decrease in the helium partial pressure associated with the air switch during decompression. Another possible mechanism was to the formation of gas bubbles in inner ear tissue boundaries caused by the counterdiffusion of two different dissolved inert gases between inner ear fluid compartments. This is similar to the counter-diffusion mechanism suggested by Graves *et al.* (1973) and by Lambertsen and Idicula (1975) to explain inner ear injuries at stable but extreme depths after changes between two different inert gases with different solubility coefficients.

Animal studies of inner ear decompression sickness

Animal studies of inner ear decompression sickness have produced interesting findings. McCormick *et al.* (1973, 1975) demonstrated that guinea-pigs subjected to rapid decompression in helium-oxygen had bubble formation and haemorrhages in the labyrinthine fluid spaces and reduced cochlear potentials which could be minimized by pre-dive treatment of the animals with heparin. This suggested that a mechanism of inner ear decompression sickness may be platelet agglutination and hypercoagulation as described by Philp (1974). Landolt *et al.* (1980) in Toronto, subjected squirrel monkeys to heliox decompression and demonstrated inner ear injuries by electronystagmographic recordings and post-dive histological studies. Temporal bones obtained within a few days after the dives showed varying degrees of haemorrhage and blood/protein exudates in the inner ear fluid spaces. The inner ears of monkeys obtained 38–383 days following decompression revealed progressive new growths of connective tissue and bone that tended to obliterate the damaged regions of the semicircular canals.

In the sections obtained early after decompression, breaks and displacement of the endosteal bone layer into the canal lumen were noted. This was postulated to be related to bubble enucleation and growth during decompression within the osteoclastic cell cavities of the endosteal bone. This produced pressure differentials between these bony osteoclastic spaces sufficient to cause an implosive fracture of the endosteal layer into the canal space. The implosive force was also speculated to cause a perilymph pressure wave bolus to move rapidly along the canal, with tearing of the endosteum and loosening of the attachment of the membranous semicircular ducts to the canal wall and bleeding. These changes provided the stimuli for subsequent canal fibrosis and new bone growth.

These findings in monkeys by Landolt *et al.* (1980) were further supported in a report by Money *et al.* (1985) in which they described similar changes in the left lateral semicircular canal of a professional diver who died of an unrelated cause 56 days after suffering inner ear decompression sickness during a heliox dive. He had not responded to prompt recompression therapy and was noted to have a persistent loss of left vestibular function and a partial left sensorineural deafness. At autopsy, which fortunately included the temporal bone study, ectopic bone growth and fibrosis were found in the left lateral semicircular canal. The histological appearance was very similar to that of the squirrel monkeys sacrificed 38 days or longer after inner ear decompression sickness.

Management of inner ear decompression sickness

As a result of human experience and animal investigations, the following principles for the management of inner ear decompression sickness were suggested by Farmer *et al.* (1976) and thus far appear to be appropriate:

1 Cochlear and/or vestibular symptoms beginning during or shortly after the decompression phase of dives in which decompression sickness is possible should be considered as representing inner ear decompression sickness and should be recompressed promptly. Otolaryngologists seeing such divers should have appropriate diving tables to consult or be prepared to consult with diving medical specialists.
2 It is suggested to diving medical authorities that divers who experience inner ear symptoms during or shortly after a change to an air environment during decompression from a deep helium-oxygen exposure, should be returned to the helium-oxygen atmosphere and recompressed promptly.
3 The optimum treatment depth, or depth of recompression, for inner ear decompression sickness has not been well established. Theoretically, the optimum recompression depth is the lesser of the depth

of relief and of the bottom depth. However, the animal studies described earlier and the one human temporal bone available suggest that, at least in some cases, inner ear structural deformities will take place which are not likely to be reversed, even though an adequate depth of recompression to drive residual bubbles into solution is achieved. Also, returning to the bottom depth in some diving situations may be hazardous or impractical. Therefore, it has been suggested that the optimum treatment depth should be at least 100 feet deeper than the depth of symptom onset (Farmer *et al.*, 1976). Until we have greater experience in the treatment of this type of injury, this recommendation still stands. All cases of inner ear decompression sickness should be promptly recompressed to the lesser of the depth of relief or the maximum depth during the previous 24 hours. When the latter is not feasible, attempts should be made to recompress the diver at least 3 atmospheres deeper than the symptom onset depth.

4 Drugs which supposedly increase intracranial and inner ear blood flow are, in general, not effective in this regard and can result in shunting of blood to the periphery. Also, anticoagulants after the injury has occurred may result in additional intracochlear bleeding and may be potentially harmful.

5 Antivertigo drugs, such as diazepam, given parenterally have been noted to provide relief from vertigo, nausea, and vomiting in acute vestibular disorders as well as otological decompression sickness. Monitoring of respiratory rate and blood pressure is recommended after parenteral administration of diazepam. Fluid replacement and other measures, such as the administration of oxygen enriched gases, which are advocated in the treatment of general decompression sickness, are indicated. The use of steroids and salicylates in the management of inner ear decompression sickness is controversial. If significant inner ear haemorrhage has taken place, the use of salicylates may not be desirable.

6 A complete otological examination as soon as possible after recompression therapy is necessary. This includes a complete history, physical examination, neurological examination, audiometry, and electronystagmography.

7 Divers who suffer permanent inner ear dysfunction should not dive again for the same reasons as those given in the section on inner ear barotrauma. The same criteria apply for disqualification to dive.

Differential diagnosis of inner ear barotrauma and inner ear decompression sickness

In most instances, the differential diagnosis of inner ear barotrauma and inner ear decompression sickness is easily made. However, in some cases this differentiation can be difficult. The symptoms of difficulty with middle ear pressure equilibration during descent may not be noticed by some individuals. For them, only an overpressure in the middle ear and subsequent inner ear injury are apparent during ascent, particularly during the latter stages close to the surface. Also, the determination of whether the dive involved an exposure in which decompression sickness is possible is made more difficult by the use of dive computers, a more frequent event in the sports diving population. If there are no signs of middle ear barotrauma, the bottom depths and times are not known, and/or the dives were close to the limits requiring staged decompression, the differentiation of inner ear barotrauma and decompression sickness can be very difficult indeed. An accurate, prompt diagnosis is important; the pathophysiology of such injuries as described above indicates that recompression is an inappropriate treatment for inner ear barotrauma and potential labyrinthine window rupture. A repeat exposure to pressure may result in further intratemporal bone pressure differentials and additional injury. Conversely, bed rest and possible middle ear surgery are inappropriate for cases of inner ear decompression sickness, where delays only increase the likelihood of permanent inner ear dysfunction (Farmer *et al.*, 1976) and may increase the possibility of more extensive CNS decompression sickness.

In order to differentiate inner ear barotrauma from inner ear decompression sickness, the medical staff must first have the knowledge that such injuries can take place while diving and be familiar with the likely pathological mechanisms. They must also be able to obtain an accurate history, physical otoscopic and neurotological examination. In those cases in which the differential diagnosis is still difficult, it is recommended that a diving medical specialist be consulted and that all of the following factors be considered:

1 The time of otological symptom onset – inner ear barotrauma is more likely to be present in divers who noted the onset of symptoms of middle ear barotrauma during compression. Alternatively, decompression sickness is more likely if otological symptom onset developed during the latter stages of, or shortly after, decompression. However, one must note that some cases of middle and inner ear barotrauma have been recorded in divers who did not experience otological symptoms until after reaching the surface from dive profiles in which decompression sickness was not felt to be likely.

2 Knowledge of the dive profile is important. Divers surfacing with otological dysfunction from shallow dives or dives which do not approach the accepted limits requiring staged decompression, are unlikely to have decompression sickness but should be suspected of having inner ear barotrauma. Likewise, dive profiles containing rapid descents are more

likely to result in inadequate middle ear pressure equilibration during compression and subsequent inner ear barotrauma, especially with inexperienced divers. Most of the cases of inner ear barotrauma have been associated with air diving, but this entity can happen also with helium diving. Isolated inner ear decompression sickness appears to be more common during decompression from helium dives, but also happens with air diving. Deep dives requiring, or close to the limits of, staged recompression in which there was a rapid ascent, increase the likelihood of decompression sickness. In addition, all dives associated with rapid ascents raise the possibility of pulmonary overpressure accidents and CNS air embolism. The CNS manifestations in these cases are usually those involving the cortical areas such as loss of consciousness, signs of upper motor neuron and/or cortical sensory injuries.

3 The presence or absence of associated symptoms must be noted. Ear pain, blockage, or fullness during compression are more likely to be associated with inner ear barotrauma. This was emphasized by Freeman (1978) who described a series of labyrinthine window ruptures in which the common history given by the divers was difficulty with middle ear pressure equilibration during descent. Alternatively, symptoms suggestive of decompression sickness involving other organs or tissues should suggest that divers who exhibit inner ear symptoms during or shortly after decompression are more likely to have inner ear decompression sickness. Such symptoms would include those suggesting sensory loss, motor weakness, bowel or bladder difficulties associated with spinal cord, type II decompression sickness, or pain in the bones, joints, or muscles associated with type I decompression sickness. A combination of type I and II symptoms may be encountered.

4 The presence or absence of other associated physical findings must be noted. Signs of middle ear barotrauma, such as a retracted, haemorrhagic or ruptured eardrum are more likely to suggest that the inner ear symptoms are related to barotrauma. Other signs of decompression sickness such as spinal cord deficits would suggest that the otological symptoms are the result of inner ear decompression sickness.

In instances where an accurate differential diagnosis is difficult, it is suggested that major consideration should be given to factors such as the likely maximum dive duration and depth, the breathing mixture used, and the presence or absence of other decompression sickness signs or symptoms, especially those involving the CNS. If it is felt that decompression sickness or a pulmonary overpressure accident is likely, it is recommended that immediate recompression therapy at an appropriately staffed recompression chamber facility is arranged. A myringotomy prior to recompression may prevent further inner ear injury if associated inner ear barotrauma has taken place.

Hearing loss related to excessive noise exposure

Hearing loss due to excessive noise exposure, usually from loud engines, in flight crews and aircraft maintenance workers has been often described in the aerospace medical literature. Hearing loss from noise exposure in divers has not been recorded as often. Several studies (Schilling and Everley, 1942; Haines and Harris, 1946; Taylor, 1959; Coles and Knight, 1961; Brady, Summitt and Berghage, 1976) have concluded that hearing in divers was no different from that of a population of non-divers, similar in various other respects such as age, degrees of cardiovascular disease, and non-diving noise exposures. However, Zannini, Odaglia, and Giorgio (1975) found more instances of high frequency hearing loss in professional divers than in the general Italian population. These were postulated to be related to 'vasomotor problems' encountered in diving. Edmonds (1985) performed an audiometric survey of professional abalone divers and described excessive high frequency sensorineural hearing losses in over 60%. These losses satisfied the criteria for disqualification set out in the Australian standards for diving. Allowing for age, compensatable hearing losses according to Australian standards were found in over 70%. It was further noted that these divers were of a low average age, 37.5 ± 7.7 years, were rarely in diving chambers or did not wear diving helmets, had no history of excessive noise exposure, and were felt more likely to have suffered decompression sickness and middle ear barotrauma than other professional divers. Therefore, it was concluded that these hearing losses could not be entirely explained on the basis of diving and non-diving noise exposure, and that high frequency hearing loss was an occupational disease of compressed air divers. Findings suggestive of a higher incidence of sensorineural hearing loss in professional divers has also been noted by Norwegian investigators (Molvaer and Albrektsen, 1990).

Support that noise-induced hearing loss may be acquired in diving conditions was provided by Murray (1970) and by Summitt and Reimers (1971) who demonstrated noise levels in pressure chambers and diving helmets that, according to acceptable surface damage risk criteria in the USA (Eldredge and Miller, 1969), may result in noise-induced hearing loss with exposure times as short as 15 minutes. Summitt and Reimers (1971) demonstrated significant temporary threshold shifts, the initial manifestation of cochlear hair cell injury, and inner ear damage from excessive noise exposure following a 190-foot, 64 minute air dive and a 60-foot, 53 minute air dive. The hearing returned to pre-dive levels within 24–48 hours after the dives. These changes could not be accounted for on the basis of middle ear barotrauma or decompression sickness. Further support for this was found in a study by Curley and Knafelc (1987) who described potentially excessive noise levels in diving helmets and temporary hearing threshold shifts in divers after surfacing from dives of various depths and durations.

These studies, demonstrating the temporary threshold shifts, suggest that the previously noted reversible and depth-related conductive hearing losses secondary to decreased sound transmission by the eardrum and ossicles in compressed gases (Fluur and Adolfson, 1966; Thomas, Summitt and Farmer, 1974) may not be sufficient to provide attenuation from excessive noise exposure during diving with helmets or in chambers. Smith (1983) at the US Naval Submarine Medical Research Laboratory in New London indicated that auditory threshold shifts are smaller during noise exposures at depth than comparable noise exposures on the surface. Thus, some protective attenuation, though probably insufficient, is gained from the temporary conductive hearing losses caused by a compressed gas environment.

Paranasal sinus barotrauma

Paranasal sinus barotrauma in aviators has been described thoroughly by Campbell (1945) and by Wright and Boyd (1945). Further studies by Dickson and King (1954) suggested that the incidence of middle ear and paranasal sinus barotrauma had a frequency ratio of 5:2. King (1965) noted involvement of the frontal sinuses in 80% and the maxillary sinuses in 29%. Ten per cent had both frontal and maxillary sinus involvement. Paranasal sinus barotrauma has been reported in divers by Idicula (1972) and by Fagan, McKensie and Edmonds (1976).

The mechanisms and pathophysiology of paranasal sinus barotrauma appear similar in both diving and flying except that the magnitude of the pressure changes in diving are much greater. The basic mechanism relates to inadequate pressure equilibration between the air-containing sinus cavities during ascent or more commonly during descent. This, in turn, is frequently due to chronic nasal inflammatory disease which is commonly related to allergy, chronic irritation from smoking or fume exposure, mechanical obstruction from internal nasal deformities or lesions. This results in blocking of the paranasal sinus ostia from swollen and inflamed mucosa. Cysts or polyps either within the nose or within the sinus cavity can also block the sinus ostia and may produce a one-way valve effect during descent or ascent.

With paranasal sinus ostial obstruction during descent, an intrasinus vacuum develops with swelling, engorgement, and inflammation of the sinus mucosa together with haemorrhage into the submucosal layers and sinus cavities, similar to the pathological changes which take place in the ear with middle ear barotrauma. Paranasal sinus barotrauma during ascent has been related to blockage of the sinus ostium by inflammatory mucosal changes. These have been precipitated by barotrauma during descent or by pre-existing cysts or polyps in the sinus cavities caused by unrelated rhinosinusitis. In this condition, pressure equilibration can be impaired during ascent but unimpaired or less impaired during descent.

Fagan, McKensie and Edmonds (1976) described 50 consecutive cases of documented paranasal sinus barotrauma in divers and recorded that 68% developed symptoms during or immediately after descent with 32% noting the onset of symptoms during or immediately after ascent. The most common symptom was pain over the involved sinus being felt with every descent and in 75% of the cases beginning during ascent. Epistaxis was the second most common symptom which was experienced by 58% of the cases. Additional symptoms included pain in the upper teeth. As had been described previously in aviators by King (1965), the frontal sinus was most commonly involved. In those affected, there was a prior history of previous paranasal sinus barotrauma in one-third and a history of recent upper respiratory tract infections or chronic nasal and sinus inflammatory disease in one-half (Fagan, McKensie and Edmonds, 1976). At the time of their study, there were also signs of associated middle ear barotrauma in almost one-half of the patients. X-rays showed abnormalities in 75% of the cases; mucosal thickening being the most common finding and an air-fluid level was present in 12%. Neuman *et al.* (1975) noted paraesthesias and decreased sensation in the distribution of the infraorbital nerve in a patient who had maxillary sinus barotrauma.

Treatment of paranasal sinus barotrauma involves the use of topical and systemic decongestants. If purulent nasal discharge is present, cultures and appropriate antibiotics should be used. Further diving should be avoided until complete recovery which usually takes place within 5–10 days, although complete reversal of the mucosal changes may take 2–4 weeks. Intranasal or intrasinus cysts or polyps contributing to the problem usually require surgical intervention. Because of the possibility of such lesions, paranasal sinus X-rays or CT scans should be obtained to determine the most appropriate management of paranasal sinus barotrauma. Fortunately, most cases of paranasal sinus barotrauma do not require surgery and recover with conservative therapy. Not one of the cases reported in the series reported by Fagan, McKensie and Edmonds (1976) required surgery.

Otological and nasal-paranasal sinus standards for diving and flying

Appropriate medical standards for diving have been covered in diving medicine texts by Bennett and Elliott (1993), Bove and Davis (1990), and Edmonds, Lowry and Pennefather (1992). This subject is also alluded to in the above sections concerning middle and inner ear barotrauma and inner ear decompression sickness. It has also been reviewed in our previous publications (Farmer, 1990) and by Neblett (1985). Those related to ear and paranasal sinus injuries in diving and flying are summarized here.

Otological standards

Otological history

A history of previous middle ear inflammatory disease or tympanomastoid surgery suggests inadequate eustachian tube function in the absence of barometric pressure changes. In these subjects there is increased likelihood of middle ear barotrauma during barometric pressure changes. Frequent or chronic respiratory tract inflammatory disease, for example allergic rhinitis and bronchitis, a history of chronic nasal blockage, congestion, or purulent nasal discharge also increases the likelihood of middle ear barotrauma and inner ear barotrauma with diving and flying.

Individuals who have previously had a simple myringoplasty or type I tympanoplasty might be considered for diving if the eardrum has remained healed for at least 12 months and if the ear can be easily autoinflated and cleared at the surface. Their initial diving exposures should be slow descents in an upright condition in a swimming pool. Initial altitude exposures should be as a passenger in a commercial aircraft descending slowly from a cruising cabin altitude of 8000 feet. Difficulties with middle ear pressure equilibration during such altitude descent should be considered as likely to disqualify the individual from diving and as a pilot of an aircraft. Those who have undergone previous canal wall up mastoidectomy that has healed well and who appear to have adequate eustachian tube function and good middle ear ventilation at the surface or with a slow descent in the upright position in a swimming pool can usually equilibrate middle ear pressure with flying and can be considered for diving. However, such potential divers should observe slow, feet first descents with adequate, non-forceful attempts to equilibrate middle ear pressure every 1–2 feet. They should be instructed to stop the dive and ascend if such equilibration is not possible.

Patients who have undergone a canal wall down mastoidectomy should not dive. Water is more likely to enter such a cavity and elicit a caloric response. The subsequent vertigo, nausea and possible vomiting could cause drowning. Also, those who have had a modified radical mastoidectomy with a small air-containing middle ear space are more likely to have poor eustachian tube function. This state disqualifies from diving and possibly also from piloting an aircraft.

Patients who have undergone stapedectomy or stapedotomy surgery should not dive because of the increased risks of an oval window fistula or inner ear injury with middle ear pressure changes. Some other form of recreational activity should be sought and encouraged. Rayman (1972) has suggested that if certain criteria are followed, flying after stapedectomy may not be hazardous. It is the first author's opinion that patients who undergo stapedectomy or stapedotomy should avoid flying for the first 4–6 weeks or until such time that the surgeon is reasonably certain that middle ear ventilation is adequate to avoid significant dysbarism with altitude exposure.

Patients who have a history suggestive of Menière's disease or endolymphatic hydrops should not undertake diving because of the possibility of vertigo with nausea and vomiting which might cause drowning. Also, the presence of pathological changes in the inner ear may increase the likelihood of inner ear injury while diving. These are appropriate contraindications even if the audiometric and vestibular testing results do not fall into the disqualification categories.

Otological physical examination

The prerequisites of a physical examination for diving include an intact tympanic membrane and the ability to autoinflate each ear easily as seen by movement of the tympanic membrane with a gentle, modified Valsalva or Toynbee manoeuvre. The presence or need for ventilation tubes indicates inadequate eustachian tube function in the absence of barometric pressure changes and would disqualify such an individual from diving. Tympanosclerotic plaques do not disqualify if the eardrum is intact, moves well, and the patient can easily autoinflate. A thin, flaccid eardrum with or without shallow retraction pockets indicates poor eustachian tube function and an increased likelihood of eardrum perforation, worsening retraction, further drum thinning, as well as barotrauma with diving and flying. The existence of cholesteatoma suggests chronic middle ear disease and poor eustachian tube function. It is a contraindication for diving and usually also for an aircraft pilot. Stenosis of the external ear canal and acute otitis externa should also be contraindications for diving and flying. Impacted wax should be removed before diving and flying.

Audiometric and electronystagmographic standards

The presence in either ear of a pure tone audiometric threshold greater than 25 dB in the frequency range of 500 Hz–2.5 kHz and/or speech discrimination score of less than 90% should disqualify an individual from diving. Flying in aircraft with noise levels exceeding safe exposure limits should be discouraged. Electronystagmographic findings of gaze nystagmus, significant positional nystagmus, optikokinetic or sinusoidal tracking anomalies, unilateral weakness, failure of suppression of caloric-induced nystagmus, all of which indicate vestibular dysfunction, should disqualify an individual from diving and piloting aircraft. Inner ears with these audiometric and electronystagmographic abnormalities may be more susceptible to future inner ear injury during diving; also, injury to the opposite inner ear could result in significant disability. Some individual consideration is needed to determine the suitability for diving or flying, especially after injury. For example, a sports scuba diver or aircraft pilot who suffers inner ear injury should not return to this activity and should consider some other form of recreation or hobby. On the other hand, an avid diver, professional diver or pilot, who has complete recovery of hearing except for a high-frequency hearing loss above 2.5 kHz, normal electronystagmographic results, who can adequately equilibrate middle ear pressures during pressure alterations which could be expected to be encountered, may consider returning to diving or flying after 3 months of convalescence, provided his practices can be altered so that future middle ear and/or inner ear barotrauma is rendered less likely. These alterations would include adequate middle ear pressure equilibration every 2 feet of descent for divers with termination of the dive if this cannot be accomplished. Fliers should equilibrate their middle ear pressures frequently and avoid rapid descents. Both aviators and divers should only perform gentle modified Valsalva manoeuvres to clear the ears, and avoid diving and flying with active upper respiratory tract inflammation.

Individuals who have inner ear dysfunction can usually safely fly as passengers or in commercial aircraft provided they are not suffering acute vestibular symptoms, have no recent past history or physical findings suggesting active middle ear disease, and can equilibrate middle ear pressure on descent. Pilots of aircraft require stricter otological standards which include the absence of middle ear pressure equilibration problems during rapid descents, no history of sudden attacks of vertigo, normal hearing and vestibular test results.

Nasal-paranasal sinus standards

Pre-diving physical examinations should focus on both the upper and lower respiratory tracts. Divers and fliers who have experienced paranasal sinus or otological barotrauma should be warned that these conditions must be adequately managed before diving and flying, especially piloting, can be safely undertaken. Individuals who are unable to maintain appropriate middle ear or sinus ventilation in the absence of barometric pressure exposures should not be expected to be able to ventilate them during such exposures, especially during the large barometric pressure changes encountered in diving.

Systemic and topical adrenergic agents can im-

prove paranasal sinus and middle ear ventilation and are often used prophylactically for diving or flying. Cautions concerning the use of such agents are needed and should include discussions regarding rebound phenomena and the possibility of developing rhinitis medicamentosa. In addition, other concerns include tachycardia, possible coronary artery spasm, elevated blood pressure, excessive drying of the respiratory tract mucosa, and the sedatory effect of some antihistamines.

Nasal and paranasal sinus history

Patients who have a history suggestive of upper or lower respiratory tract disease such as nasal obstruction, discharge, past history of nasal or sinus surgery, chronic cough with sputum production, haemoptysis, shortness of breath, etc., should be suspected of being susceptible to barotrauma during diving or with rapid descent from altitude exposures. Patients who require frequent or chronic use of decongestants, antihistamines, steroids, or antibiotics for such symptoms are more likely to develop barotrauma while diving or flying. Active bronchial asthma is a contraindication for diving and piloting an aircraft. Similarly, a past history of nasal, sinus or cleft palate surgery should make the examiner suspicious that adequate ventilation of the ears and sinuses may not be possible during diving or rapid descents while flying.

Nasal and paranasal sinus examination

Potential divers and fliers who exhibit upper airway mucosal oedema and inflammation, significant internal and external nasal deformities, or intranasal/nasopharyngeal mass lesions such as polyps or other growths should have these treated before being considered fit to fly or dive. These conditions all make it less likely that they can equilibrate intrasinus or middle ear pressures with barometric pressure changes, especially those of the magnitude encountered with diving. Persistent nasal and paranasal sinus inflammatory disease, in spite of treatment, is a contraindication for diving and is likely to prohibit a pilot from flying an aircraft safely.

Oropharyngeal, laryngeal and dental standards

Oropharyngeal

A history of cleft palate repair or the finding of a cleft palate increases the likelihood of inadequate eustachian tube function and otological barotrauma with diving and flying.

Laryngeal

Patients who have intermittent chronic aspiration indicating gastro-oesophageal reflux or an incompetent larynx should not be allowed to dive. A laryngo-coele should also disqualify a patient from diving until the problem is corrected. It goes without saying that a tracheostomy is an absolute contraindication to swimming as well as diving.

Dental standards (Benson and King, 1987; Edmonds, Lowry and Pennefather, 1992)

Dental barotrauma is common in diving and flying, having been noted in up to 20% of US Air Force fighter pilots (Ashley, 1977). During flight, it is most troublesome in ascent, and in diving during descent. It has been postulated that the cause is trapped gas beneath restorations or areas of caries which can expand or contract and thereby apply pressure to the sensitive dental pulp.

The dental standards for divers and pilots of aircraft include dental checks every 6 months with X-rays at least yearly, avoidance of diving and piloting aircraft until complete healing after oral surgery including dental extractions. Pre-diving and flying examinations should include a dental evaluation with X-rays. Barometric pressure changes should be avoided until adequate treatment of active dental disease has been completed.

Motion sickness (Benson and King, 1987; Farmer and Gillespie, 1988)

Motion sickness may be induced on an aeroplane, boat, ship, car, or domesticated animal and can be the normal response of a healthy individual to unfamiliar, unhabituated movement. If the provocative motion is severe and prolonged, the absence of symptoms may be considered abnormal, since those without functioning labyrinths do not suffer from motion sickness (James, 1882; Miller and Goodson, 1960). Thus, the term '*kinetosis*' may be preferred.

The *sopite syndrome* is a form of kinetosis in which the sole expression of the motion sickness is drowsiness, lethargy, a reduced interest in ongoing events, and a performance decrement (Graybiel and Knepton, 1976).

Symptoms and signs of motion sickness

The predominant and usual initial symptom of motion sickness is nausea followed by the signs of pallor, diaphoresis, and vomiting. A feeling of increased body warmth, excessive salivation, eructation, and flatulence are common in the initial phase. Frontal headache, an alteration of respiratory rhythm with sighing and yawning, and, in those particularly anxious, hyperventilation may develop. An ill-defined tinnitus and dizziness, or light-headedness may also be described, apathy and depression may be noted. Drowsiness develops and is often ignored; it may

persist for hours after the provocative motion has ceased. Significant and sometimes dangerous performance decrements can happen in pilots.

Theories of the aetiology of motion sickness

The neural mismatch theory as elaborated by Reason (1970) and by Reason and Brand (1975) has as its basic premise that motion sickness ensues when there is an unexpected or unlearned correlation of sensory information from the eyes, the vestibular apparatus and proprioceptors. Within the central nervous system there is a memory bank linked to a comparator where sensory receptor signals and stored neural signals are correlated. If the input signals do not match with the expected and stored information, there is an error or signal mismatch which triggers the motion sickness syndrome and later a modification of the stored material to accommodate the new input pattern. Sustained or strong mismatch signals are more likely to have both effects; whereas a weak mismatch signal, if sustained, can allow adaptation to take place without the more obvious symptoms of motion sickness, although some drowsiness and lethargy of the sopite syndrome may be noted.

Two main types of mismatches of motion sensory data can be identified:

1 Visual-vestibular mismatch
2 Canal-otolith or intravestibular mismatch (Benson and King, 1987; Farmer and Gillespie, 1988).

Visual-vestibular mismatch

There are two types of visual-vestibular mismatches: simultaneous, incongruous, visual and vestibular inputs, and isolated and uncoupled visual and vestibular inputs.

Type I visual-vestibular mismatch

Both the visual and vestibular systems simultaneously signal motion, but of an unlearned and incompatible kind. An example would be the sickness suffered by an observer who directly observes the passing landscape from the side window of a vehicle that is changing direction or speed. Another example is that of an individual in a helicopter who observes the ground with binoculars; the relative movements seen through the binoculars fail to correlate with the motion of the observer's head and the vestibular cues.

Type II visual-vestibular mismatch

Type II visual-vestibular mismatches may be further subdivided into two types: type IIa, visual motion cues present without the expected vestibular cues, e.g when piloting a fixed simulator in which the usual visual surroundings are presented to the occupant without the linear and angular accelerations that would be expected. Conversely, there may be a type IIb mismatch, with vestibular cues unaccompanied by visual cues, commonly noted when a passenger looks only at a stable visual scene in a moving and turbulent vehicle. This is characteristic of any vehicle in which the passenger or operator has no view of the outside world such as in a hatchless ship's cabin.

Intravestibular mismatch

Intravestibular (semicircular canal-otolith organ) mismatch takes place when the head is moved, actively or passively, in a vehicle which itself is undergoing angular and/or linear acceleration or is subject to an abnormal, other than 1.0 g, force environment. Input signals from the canals and otolith organs differ from those that were learned and are generated when the same head movements are made in a stable normogravic environment. Two types of intravestibular mismatch may be identified: type I is experienced when both the semicircular canals and otolith organs signal motion, and type II when one of these receptor systems signals motion in unexpected isolation from stimulation of the other.

Type I intravestibular mismatch

Type I intravestibular mismatch happens when an angular movement of the head is made in a vehicle which is turning simultaneously. If the planes of the head motion and turning vehicle differ, a cross-coupled or Coriolis stimulus develops (Figure 7.4). If the movement of the head is made after the start of the turn, then the cross-coupled stimulus does not evoke any inappropriate sense of angular motion (Guedry and Benson, 1976). If the head movement is made during angular deceleration from a sustained turn or if vehicular rotation is sustained for more than 5 seconds, then the rotation signalled by the canals will not correspond with the imposed rotation or the head movement. Upon completion of the head movement, the deflected cupulae of the stimulated canals will take 10 or more seconds to return to their neutral position. During this persistent cupula deflection with altered angular accelerometer firing rates, the otoliths will provide correct information about the attitude of the head with regard to gravity. Canal-otolith mismatch and its sequelae will take place.

In addition to Coriolis stimulation, this type of intravestibular mismatch may develop when a head movement is made in an abnormal gravitational field and the otolithic cues about the change of orientation of the head relative to the abnormal gravitational force vector differ from those of the same head move-

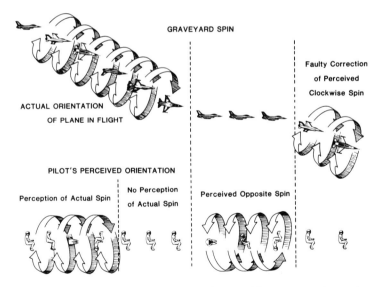

Figure 7.4 Graveyard spin. The pilot initially perceives the spin as the aircraft begins its angular acceleration. Then, the pilot loses this spin perception when a constant spin velocity is reached and the cupulae return to neutral positions. A perception of an opposite spin develops when the aircraft recovers to straight and level flight. The pilot then makes a faulty and hazardous correction that gives him the sensation of normalized flight while he is actually returning to the original spin. (From: Farmer, J. and Gillespie, C. Exposures to aerospace, diving, and compressed gases. In: *Otologic Medicine and Surgery*, edited by P. W. Alberti and R. J. Ruben, Churchill Livingstone, New York (1988) pp. 1753–1802. Reprinted by permission)

ment learned in the normogravic environment. For example, during the rapid transition from the hypergravity of space vehicle launch to the zero gravity of orbital flight, the semicircular canals are little influenced by the linear accelerations and correctly signal the angular movements of the head. This is a mismatch situation in which the otolithic organ information is constantly changing and does not correspond with learned sensory inputs.

Type II intravestibular mismatch

Two types of type II intravestibular mismatch can be identified:

a The canals signal rotation in the absence of the expected otolithic signal
b The otoliths indicate movement with no corresponding canal signal.

Type IIa, may be the mechanism of space motion sickness where the regular head movements in microgravity will be correctly sensed by the canals without a corresponding change in afferent discharge rate from the macular receptors. If, however, the angular movement is rapid, significant transient linear acceleration of the otoliths will result in atypical stimulation and generate a type I intravestibular mismatch (Benson, 1977).

When a pilot is exposed to linear oscillation or sustained rotation about a non-vertical axis, type IIb intravestibular mismatch takes place. If a pilot, executing a prolonged roll, establishes a steady rate of roll, there will be no further semicircular canal stimulation but strong otolithic cues of continued rotation.

Linear accelerations experienced in an aircraft flying through turbulent air are often responsible for motion sickness. The incidence of motion sickness appears to relate inversely to the frequency of oscillation in swing experiments (Fraser and Manning, 1950), vertical oscillator studies (O'Hanlon and McCauley, 1974; McCauley, Royal and Wylie, 1976), and in modified lift experiments (Alexander, summarized by Baker, 1966). Kennedy *et al.* (1972) observed that aircraft with a high frequency of oscillation (0.8–0.9 Hz) produced less motion sickness than those responding at a lower frequency (0.4 Hz) when flying through turbulent air. This may have to do with the sensory inputs learned and stored during the usual walking locomotor activities, with frequencies higher than 0.5 Hz not usually encountered. At lower frequencies, a change in head position will be signalled by the otolith organs acting in a non-kinetic position-sensing role, and will normally be associated with a vertical semicircular canal signal. If this canal message does not arise during linear oscillation, a type IIb intravestibular mismatch and motion sickness develops.

Tolerance to motion sickness

Tolerance to motion varies widely among individuals. Susceptible persons may appear to be in the minority; however, motion sickness will affect most people if the sensory input mismatches are of a sufficient kind, intensity and duration (Gillies, 1965). While susceptibility to sea sickness may not necessarily mean susceptibility to air sickness, Money (1970) noted that there was considerable evidence that those who were prone to sickness in one motion environment tended to have a low threshold in other environments. Interestingly, in space motion sickness, there seems to be an inverse relationship between motion sensitivity on earth and in weightless orbital flight (Thornton *et al.*, 1985).

Multiple factors, including age, sex, physical condition, emotional state, have been indicated as influencing motion sickness susceptibility. The peak ages of susceptibility have been reported between the ages of 2 and 12 years, with a steady decline in susceptibility thereafter. By the age of 50 years, motion sickness is rare (Reason and Brand, 1975). Reason (1970) noted that females seem more susceptible to motion sickness than males of the same age. Since susceptibility seems increased during pregnancy and menstruation, hormonal factors have been implicated as the cause of this susceptibility. Fear or anxiety appear to increase susceptibility to motion sickness. In military air transport, Littbauer (1943) reported that 80% of troops became sick. This, of course, resulted in serious military operational liabilities. Introverts, as assessed by the Eysenck Personality Inventory, have more frequent and pronounced symptoms with provocative movement and adapt more slowly than do extroverts (Kennedy, 1975). Susceptibility also correlates with the perceptual style of the individuals (Barrett and Thornton, 1968).

Reason (1970) suggested that the wide intersubject variations in susceptibility are attributable to two constitutional factors, receptivity and adaptability, which relate to the manner in which the individual processes sensory information. A given physical stimulus evokes a greater subjective experience in a person of high receptivity than in a person of low receptivity. Thus, a person of high receptivity will have a more intense mismatch signal than a person of low receptivity, and be more likely to suffer from motion sickness. Slow adapting individuals are more likely to suffer from motion sickness since slow adaptability results in more prolonged rearrangement of the neural store and a delay in attenuation of the mismatch signal. Although high receptivity and low adaptability may increase susceptibility, these two factors appear to be independent of one another (Reason and Graybiel, 1972).

Space motion sickness

Space motion sickness has been reported within minutes of reaching orbit and is most severe during the first day in weightlessness (Graybiel, Miller and Homick, 1974). Gemini flights with small restrictive cabins and use of in-flight pressure suits were relatively free of space motion sickness, as compared to present-day Shuttle flights which permit free movement about the cabin in light-weight clothing. Usually, adaptation without recurrence takes place in 2–4 days. The time scale for adaptation to space flight seems similar to that described for sea sickness (Groen, 1960) and for subjects living in a rotating room (Graybiel *et al.*, 1965).

Graybiel (1972, 1980) has distinguished between two categories of vestibular side effects in space flight. The first comprises a great variety of 'immediate reflex motor responses' such as postural illusions, sensations of rotation, nystagmus, and dizziness or vertigo; the second is a delayed epiphenomenon, superimposed on the reflex motor responses. Symptoms of motion sickness are usually elicited when the transition from one motion environment to another has been rapid (Money, 1970). That the primary or essential aetiological factor is vestibular is confirmed by the observation that those without vestibular function do not become sick (Kellogg, Kennedy and Graybiel, 1965).

Vestibular tests in microgravity

Vestibular testing by the astronauts revealed no definite abnormalities (NASA, 1977). The tests performed included tests for postural equilibrium. The results were correlated with age, history of motion sickness, and the Coriolis sickness susceptibility index (Miller and Graybiel, 1970). Canal thresholds of response were within normal limits for the nine subjects. Two of the nine had directional preponderances on modified Fitzgerald–Hallpike manoeuvres. The low values observed for ocular counter-rolling, a test of macular function, confirmed the predicted decrease in macular responses in microgravity. The Coriolis sickness susceptibility indices noted during weightless phases of parabolic flight were predictive of motion sickness susceptibility in orbit in only 22% of the subjects. Results of provocative tests for motion sickness before, during, and after orbital flight indicated that susceptibility was lower in orbital flight than on the ground, where pre- and post-flight testing readily elicited symptoms. This decreased susceptibility could not be quantified, because the maximum limits of the rotating chair test were reached. This difference in susceptibility to motion sickness with provocative movement appears related to the decreased macular function with possible decreases in touch, pressure and kinesthetic receptor system inputs in microgravity, since the stimulation of the canals was the same in orbital flight as on the ground.

Thornton *et al.* (1985) correlated a physician's in-flight examination, and electronystagmography tests in orbiting astronauts. With electronystagmography

testing, no abnormal eye movements or pathological nystagmus responses were noted. During space motion sickness, saccadic and visual pursuit systems showed no evidence of abnormality. Tracking of head-synchronized targets was also normal, indicating probably normal cervical and vestibular inputs. The head oscillation test, despite having the limitations of a single angular rate, poor control of that rate, contamination by volitional and cervical inputs, and differing eye target distances, revealed no gross disturbances. More extensive ENG studies including cold air calorics, more feasible than cold water calorics in the weightlessness of orbit are planned for future orbital flights. Studies during parabolic flight have indicated that thermally induced nystagmus declined and disappeared during the weightless phase (Graybiel *et al.*, 1981). This is the expected finding since gravity would be needed to produce a nystagmus response from a thermal alteration of endolymph density.

Prevention of motion sickness

Manning and Stewart (1949) noted that head support and body restraint reduced the frequency of motion sickness. Johnson *et al.* (1951) found that head immobilization, restricting both active and passive head movements, also lowered the incidence of motion sickness. The absence of reported space motion sickness in the USA space programme until the Apollo missions, which used larger vehicles, has been attributed to the greater opportunity in these space craft for free-floating activities and to the reduced use of couch restraints and helmets in orbit (Graybiel, Miller and Homick, 1975). Soviet investigators, in addition to other space motion sickness counter-measures, such as lower body negative pressure to reduce cephalad fluid shifts, have recommended the use of a head cap that restricted head movements and simultaneously provided a force stimulus to the cervical antigravity muscles (Matsnev, 1980).

Other preventative measures include providing aviators or passengers with a good forward view from the cabin. This offers visual cues which are more likely to fit with previously programmed inputs. If no visual external reference is possible, closing the eyes and sitting or lying results in reduced mismatch and symptoms. Guedry (1970) noted decreased susceptibility to motion sickness with involvement in operational tasks and mental activity. This was also noted in Skylab II astronauts (Graybiel, Miller and Homick, 1975; Graybiel, 1980).

Ground-based desensitization therapy has been found to be of benefit to aircrew or student aircrew who do not develop sufficient adaptation during the course of their normal flying duties (Dowd, 1972; Dobie, 1974; Cramer, Graybiel and Oosterveld, 1976). This has also been recommended for the prevention of space motion sickness (Homick, 1980). Ground-based training involves graded incremental exposure to cross-coupled (Coriolis) stimulation. The subject, while rotating on a turntable, is required to move or be moved in pitching or rolling motions.

The rapidity and success of adaptation training appear related not only to the receptivity and adaptability of the individual to the training stimuli, but also to his retentivity. Retention of adaptation varies widely between individuals and is not correlated well with receptivity or adaptability (Reason and Brand, 1975). Graybiel and Lackner (1983) have compared acquisition and retention of adaptation effects in three motion environments and found that an individual's rates of acquiring and losing adaptations are quite consistent even in very different situations. They developed an index of susceptibility to motion sickness that documents each individual's rate of acquisition and decay of adaptation. Motion sickness screening procedures have gained much significance for both US and Soviet space programmes (Homick, 1980; Iakloveva *et al.*, 1982), because of its clearly significant operation implications.

Medication recommended for the prevention of motion sickness tends to be empirical. A large number of drugs has been assayed (Wood and Graybiel, 1968; Lukomskaya and Nikol'skay, 1971), but relatively few have been noted to show high efficacy and specificity. A review of the literature on the subject is confusing, because of variations in drug end-point, equivalent dosages, time of onset and duration of action. With all of the drugs suggested to prevent motion sickness, there are side effects which substantially limit usefulness in the aerospace environment. Antihistamines (like promethazine and dimenhydrinate) and the parasympatholytics (like hyoscine) are central depressants and should not generally be taken by flight crew or divers.

Duration of exposure to provocative motion, and individual differences in tolerance to side effects and effectiveness of the specific agent, determine the choice of prophylactic drug (Graybiel *et al.*, 1975). L-hyoscine hydrobromide, in a single oral dose of 0.3–0.6 mg, acts in 0.5–1 hour and provides protection for about 4 hours. Longer parasympatholytic action is provided by the scopolamine patch. Promethazine hydrochloride (25 mg oral dose) and meclizine hydrochloride (50 mg oral dose) require 1–2 hours to act and are effective for 12 hours or longer. Dimenhydrinate (50 mg oral dose) and cyclizine hydrochloride (50 mg oral dose) are both useful antihistaminics, and are absorbed at the same rate as promethazine but have a shorter duration of action. Thus for short exposures, oral L-hyoscine is to be preferred; scopolamine patches and the other oral long-acting medications are of use for more prolonged exposures. Repeated doses of L-hyoscine can result in cumulative and disturbing side effects including hallucinations and so caution should be observed with long-term use.

Wood and Graybiel (1968) demonstrated that D-amphetamine and ephedrine increased subjects' tolerance to cross-coupled stimulation; these agents were combined with L-hyoscine and the antihistamines for synergistic prophylactic effects and reduction of side effects (notably drowsiness). Skylab II and Skylab III astronauts carried anti-motion sickness capsules containing L-scopolamine 0.35 mg + D-amphetamine 5 mg; in addition to this drug, the Skylab IV crew had a drug combination of promethazine hydrochloride 25 mg + ephedrine sulphate 50 mg, which were found to be effective under experimental and operational conditions. This combination raised the stimulus thresholds for eliciting motion sickness and is effective in many motion environments.

Spatial disorientation in flight

In 1919, Anderson noted that with poor visibility in dense cloud formations at night, during powered flight, pilots rapidly became disoriented and failed to maintain the desired attitude and direction of flight. These disorientations lessened as instrumentation improved, beginning with the development of turn and bank indicators and leading to the current vast array of position, attitude, and altitude indicators. Still, accidents happen because of a pilot's false perceptions of position or attitude with respect to the surface of the earth (Nuttall and Sanford, 1959). A common cause of fatal general aviation accidents is continuation of a flight from visual flight rules (VFR) in clear weather to instrument flight rules (IFR) in bad weather conditions, with subsequent loss of aircraft control caused by spatial disorientation due to inadequate use of the aircraft position, attitude and altitude instruments.

The task of spatial orientation in flight is inherently more difficult than on the ground, for in the air there are six degrees of freedom (three in linear movement and three in rotation), while on the ground only five degrees of freedom are involved (two in linear movement and three in rotation). During the abnormal static and kinetic environments of flight the orientation cues of terrestrial life are at times misleading. Also, terrestrial man orients himself with respect to the direction of the force of gravity, which he believes to be vertical to the surface of the earth. In flight, however, linear and angular accelerations, especially in high performance aircraft, may stimulate the receptors of the vestibular end organ in such a manner that false perception of the true directions of motion and gravity is effected with a resulting inappropriate control and manoeuvre of the aircraft.

Spatial disorientation in flight related to the limitations of the semicircular canal functions include the graveyard spin, the graveyard spiral, the leans, and the Coriolis illusion. Those related to limitations of the utricle and saccule include the oculogravic illusion, the inversion illusion, and the elevator illusion (Figures 7.5–7.10 and see Figure 7.4).

Semicircular canal illusions

Graveyard spin (see Figure 7.4)

The graveyard spin starts with the production of an appropriate sensation of spinning as an aircraft angularly accelerates into a spin. Once a constant spin angular velocity is reached, the perception of the spin ceases as the cupulae return to neutral positions. During the initial phase of aircraft recovery from the spin, there is angular deceleration and a false sensation of spinning in the opposite direction. If the pilot allows this false perception to determine his behaviour, he will put the aircraft back into a spin in the original direction, eliminating the false sensation but actually losing control of the aircraft. Modern all-weather pilots, educated in the vestibular illusions of flight, are trained to use their instruments to override their own sensations; yet in earlier, less sophisticated, days this illusion was often fatal.

Graveyard spiral (Figure 7.5)

The restoration of the cupulae to their neutral positions during a protracted constant angular velocity is also responsible for the vestibular illusion known as the graveyard spiral. During a continuous banked turn, the net gravitoinertial force becomes perpendicular to the floor of the aircraft and not toward the centre of the earth. The semicircular canal cupulae

return to neutral and the angular acceleration forces are no longer perceived. After flying for some time in a turn, a novice pilot can become confused about the direction of the true vertical. Since an airplane in a bank cannot maintain its altitude with the same power setting and stick position for level flight, the pilot, not recognizing the illusion, will add power and pull back on the stick to make up the lost altitude, thereby tightening the turn and worsening the situation with a fatal spiral into the ground. If the pilot heeds the level flight indicator, he will stop the turn and return to level flight. Yet, on stopping the turn the endolymph will be accelerated, the cupulae deviated, and the perception of turning in the opposite direction will falsely arise. This perception must be ignored and the instruments relied upon until straight and level flight has been maintained long enough for the false sensation to dissipate (see Leans, type 1 below). If these steps are not undertaken and there is no visual fix on the horizon, the pilot will resume turning and tightening his graveyard spiral until he crashes.

The leans, types 1 and 2 (Figures 7.6 and 7.7)

The most common vestibular illusion in flight is the leans, types 1 and 2.

Type 1

An aircraft flying in poor visibility can gradually develop a subthreshold rotation and bank to one side. The pilot notes that the bank is present by consulting the flight level indicator and rotates the aircraft in the opposite direction to return to level flight. Only this correcting rotation is perceived by the vestibular accelerometers. Reflexly, the pilot leans in the direction of the original unperceived bank but usually retains control of the aircraft.

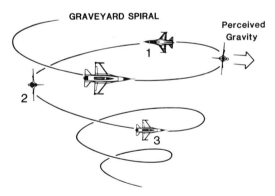

Figure 7.5 Graveyard spiral. In a coordinated banked turn without 'slip', the net gravitoinertial force is perpendicular to the aircraft floor, not the centre of the earth. The aircraft naturally loses altitude during a bank turn, and the pilot will add power and pull back on the stick to regain the lost altitude. This only tightens the turn, and progressively worsens the problem. (From: Farmer, J. and Gillespie, C. Exposures to aerospace, diving, and compressed gases. In: *Otologic Medicine and Surgery*, edited by P. W. Alberti and R. J. Ruben, Churchill Livingstone, New York, (1988) pp. 1753–1802. Reprinted by permission)

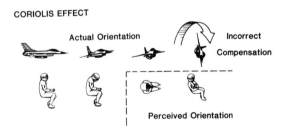

Figure 7.6 Leans Type 1. A slow, gradual and unperceived roll to the left, with a rapid instrument-guided correction to the right results in the sensation of a right roll. Reflexly the pilot leans left but is usually able to retain control of the aircraft. (From: Farmer, J. and Gillespie, C. Exposures to aerospace, diving, and compressed gases. In: *Otologic Medicine and Surgery*, edited by P. W. Alberti and R. J. Ruben, Churchill Livingstone, New York, (1988) pp. 1753–1802. Reprinted by permission)

LEANS TYPE I

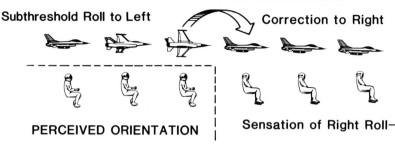

ACTUAL ORIENTATION

Subthreshold Roll to Left   **Correction to Right**

PERCEIVED ORIENTATION | **Sensation of Right Roll–**

Pilot Leans Left

Figure 7.7 Leans Type 2. During a long banked turn to the left, the perception of the turn is lost. On recovery to straight flight by rolling to the right, the pilot perceives a right roll. He will then lean to the left, usually while retaining control of the aircraft. (From: Farmer, J. and Gillespie, C. Exposures to aerospace, diving, and compressed gases. In: *Otologic Medicine and Surgery*, edited by P. W. Alberti and R. J. Ruben, Churchill Livingstone, New York, (1988) pp. 1753–1802. Reprinted by permission)

Type 2

During a long banked turn the perception of the angular acceleration is lost and down is perceived as perpendicular to the aircraft floor. With recovery to level flight the pilot perceives a roll opposite to the turn bank. He then leans to the left, yet retains aircraft control.

Coriolis illusion (Figure 7.8)

The Coriolis illusion is very dangerous for novice pilots. It happens when the aircraft is in a turn, commonly during the final approach turn just before landing; the pilot rotates his head to check for something in the cockpit. He is likely to experience a potent sensation of turning which differs from the

LEANS TYPE II

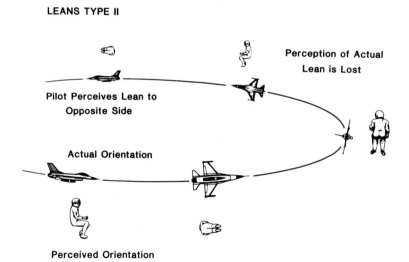

Perception of Actual Lean is Lost

Pilot Perceives Lean to Opposite Side

Actual Orientation

Perceived Orientation

Figure 7.8 Coriolis illusion. If the pilot's head turns downward during a constant yawing turn to the right, the semicircular canals are thrust into new planes. Angular momentum will be gained by the canal close to the plane of constant velocity and lost by those in other planes. In this example, the pilot will perceive a (clockwise) roll to the right and make faulty (counterclockwise) roll to the left, endangering his aircraft. (From: Farmer, J. and Gillespie, C. Exposures to aerospace, diving, and compressed gases. In: *Otologic Medicine and Surgery*, edited by P. W. Alberti and R. J. Ruben, Churchill Livingstone, New York, (1988) pp. 1753–1802. Reprinted by permission)

true motion of the aircraft. To orient himself, he has to refer quickly to his instruments or to the external scene and in consequence must again move his head, evoking further false sensations. A series of fatal accidents in aircraft where the pilot had to turn his head downward and to the right to adjust the radio during an instrument flight turn was attributed to the Coriolis illusion by Nuttall (1958). To understand the mechanism of this illusion, the principles of the conservation of angular momentum must be considered. Rotating at a constant angular velocity in a given spatial plane, the endolymph in the semicircular canals has a certain angular momentum in that plane. If the head is rotated in a spatial plane that cuts across the plane of the constant angular velocity, angular momentum is suddenly withdrawn from the semicircular canals that were in the plane of the constant rotation; yet the endolymph continues to rotate in the new semicircular canal spatial plane. The associated cupulae will remain deviated until the angular momentum is dissipated by friction and the cupular restoring force. The resulting sensation will be in the new plane of the semicircular canals, which is neither in the plane of the original constant angular velocity nor in the plane of the head movement. The semicircular canals that were not in the plane of the constant angular velocity, but are thrust into that plane by the head movement immediately gain angular momentum in the new plane. Here, too, the resulting sensation in these ducts will not be in the plane of the head movement. In general, the net result of stimuli in the six semicircular canals during a head movement in a plane that cuts across a plane of constant angular velocity will be a sensation of rotation in a plane perpendicular to the planes of the other rotations. Thus, if the head is pitched down during a constant turn to the left, the pilot will perceive a counterclockwise roll. If this takes place at a critical phase of flight prior to landing, with high ground speed and low altitude, and the pilot reacts, the aircraft will roll upside down in response to a Coriolis illusion. The pilot may not have time or altitude sufficient to recover his error, and the false roll may cause the aircraft to crash.

The receptors of the semicircular canals, although normally stimulated only by angular accelerations, in certain susceptible individuals, can be stimulated by rapid middle ear pressure changes. Approximately 10% of a group of pilots interviewed by Jones (1957) experienced vertigo immediately after equilibration of middle ear pressure. This vertigo was of sudden onset, preceded by a click as air entered or left the middle ear, and decayed rapidly over 15–20 seconds. There may be a transient blurring of vision or an apparent movement of objects in the visual field, presumably caused by brief nystagmus. This may represent unequal middle ear pressure equilibration and different tympanic membrane, ossicle, and endolymph motion,

similar to diving alternobaric vertigo described earlier. The illusory sensation of the aircraft turning is usually in the yawing or rolling plane and is consistent in any one individual.

Otolithic organ illusions (Figures 7.9 and 7.10)

Illusions related to the otolithic organs are the inversion illusion and the elevator illusion.

The inversion illusion

In flight, the resultant of the force of gravity, which is always directed to the centre of the earth, and of the inertial force may be erroneously perceived. One type of inversion illusion is shown in Figure 7.9. A pilot levelling an aircraft off after a rapid climb will perceive that the nose has gone up and over or in a direction that results from the combination of inertial and centrifugal forces with the force of gravity. The faulty response felt needed is to throw the nose down which would result in a rapid inappropriate dive. Another form of inversion illusion is perceived with acceleration in level flight where the resultant of the inertial force (opposite to the acceleration force) and the gravitational force shifts from the vertical to a point downward and toward the tail. The pilot perceives this as still vertical and that the nose has risen. An erroneous pointing of the nose down with an inappropriate dive may result. The opposite may happen with deceleration in level flight; i.e. perceived lowering of the nose and the need to point the nose up.

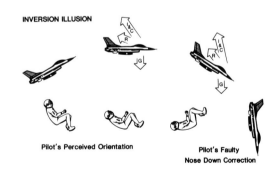

Figure 7.9 One type of inversion illusion. Levelling off from a rapid climb produces inertial (I) and centrifugal (C) forces that counter the gravitational force (G) to form a resultant force (R) that is perceived as going up and over. The faulty response is to throw the nose down, and a rapid, inappropriate dive results. (From: Farmer, J. and Gillespie, C. Exposures to aerospace, diving, and compressed gases. In: *Otologic Medicine and Surgery*, edited by P. W. Alberti and R. J. Ruben, Churchill Livingstone, New York, (1988) pp. 1753–1802. Reprinted by permission)

The elevator illusion

The elevator illusion happens in turbulent weather conditions, when vertical linear accelerations cause vestibulo-ocular reflexes in which the eyes move up or down. This results in temporary displacements of the perceived horizontal. From an aerospace safety standpoint, the significance of this has not been established.

The otolith system is inadequate to correct visual misconceptions – a pilot flying over a sloping cloud formation may be convinced that the cloud deck is horizontal (Figure 7.10). Likewise, a dark sky and an ocean may not be visually separable, and the pilot may perceive the shoreline as the horizon. In such ambiguous situations, the visual system will dominate the vestibular system. Although the vestibular system suffices in the normal terrestrial environment, in aerospace travel it must be supplemented with visual and instrument input.

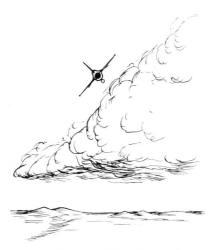

Figure 7.10 Visual illusion of flight. After spending a long time flying over a cloud formation that has gradually changed its slope, the pilot may think that flight parallel to the clouds is being truly horizontal. In ambiguous situations the vision dominates the vestibular system. (From: Farmer, J. and Gillespie, C. Exposures to aerospace, diving, and compressed gases. In: *Otologic Medicine and Surgery*, edited by P. W. Alberti and R. J. Ruben, Churchill Livingstone, New York, (1988) pp. 1753–1802. Reprinted by permission)

References

ADOLFSON, J. A., GOLDBERG, L. and BERGHAGE, T. E. (1972) Effects of increased ambient air pressures on standing steadiness in man. *Aerospace Medicine*, **43**, 520–524

ALEXANDER, as summarized by BAKER, C. H. (1966) Motion and human performance: review of literature. *Technical Report* **770–1**. Goleta, CA: Human Factors Research, Inc.

ALT, F. (1869) Ueber apoplectiforme labyrintherkrankungen bei caissonarbeitern. *Monatsschrift für Ohrenheilkunde*, **30**, 341–349

ALT, F., HELLER, R., MAGER, W. and VONSCHROTTER, H. (1897) Pathologie der Luftdruckerkrankkungen des Gehororgans. *Monatsschrift für Ohrenheilkunde*, **21**, 229–242

ALTHAUS, S. R. (1981) Perilymph fistulas. *Laryngoscope*, **91**, 538–562

ANDERSON, G. H. (1919) *Medical and Surgical Aspects of Aviation*. London: Hodder & Stoughton

ASHLEY, K. F. (1977) Aerodontalgia – pain felt in the teeth during flight. *Medical and Dental Newsletter*, **26**, 15–17

BARRETT, G. V. and THORNTON, G. L. (1968) Relationships between perceptual style and simulator sickness. *Journal of Applied Physiology*, **52**, 305–308

BECKER, G. D. (1983) Recurrent alternobaric facial paralysis resulting from scuba diving. *Laryngoscope*, **93**, 596–598

BENNETT, D. and LISKE, E. (1967) Transient facial paralysis during ascent to altitude. *Neurology*, **17**, 194–198

BENNETT, P. B. (1964) The effects of high pressures of inert gases on auditory evoked potentials in cat cortex and reticular formation. *Electroencephalography and Clinical Neurophysiology*, **17**, 388–397

BENNETT, P. B. (1982) The high pressure nervous syndrome in man. In: *The Physiology and Medicine of Diving*, 3rd edn, edited by P. B. Bennett and D. H. Elliott. London: Bailliere Tindall. p. 262

BENNETT, P. B. and ELLIOTT, D. H. (1993) *The Physiology and Medicine of Diving*, 4th edn. London: Bailliere Tindall

BENNETT, P. B. and GLASS, A. (1961) Electroencephalographic and other changes induced by high partial pressures of nitrogen. *Electroencephaloraphy and Clinical Neurophysiology*, **13**, 91–98

BENNETT, P. B. and TOWSE, E. J. (1971) Performance efficiency of men breathing oxygen-helium at depths between 100 ft and 1500 ft. *Aerospace Medicine*, **42**, 147–156

BENNETT, P. B., ACKLES, K. N. and CRIPPS, V. J. (1969) Effects of hyperbaric nitrogen and oxygen on auditory evoked responses in man. *Aerospace Medicine*, **40**, 521–525

BENSON, A. J. (1977) Possible mechanisms of motion and space sickness. In: *Life-Sciences Research In Space*. Report **SP-130**, 101–108. Paris: European Space Agency

BENSON, A. J. and KING, P. F. (1979) The ears and nasal sinuses in the aerospace environment. In: *Scott-Brown's Diseases of the Ear, Nose, and Throat*, 4th edn., edited by J. Ballantyne, and J. Groves. London: Butterworths

BENSON, A. J. and KING, P. F. (1987) Physiology of the ears and nasal sinuses in the aerospace environment. In: *Scott-Brown's Otolaryngology*, 5th edn., edited by A. G. Kerr, vol. 1 *Basic Sciences*, edited by D. Wright. London: Butterworths

BEVAN, J. (1971) The human auditory response and contingent negative variation in hyperbaric air. *Electroencephalography and Clinical Neurophysiology*, **30**, 198–204

BOVE, A. A. and DAVIS, J. C. (eds) (1940) *Diving Medicine*, 2nd edn. Philadelphia: W. B. Saunders

BRADY, J. L., SUMMITT, J. K. and BERGHAGE, T. E. (1976) An audiometric survey of navy divers. *Undersea Biomedical Research*, **3**, 41–47

BRAITHWAITE, W. R., BERGHAGE, T. E. and CROTHERS, J. C. (1974) Postural equilibrium in vestibular response at 49.5 ATA *Undersea Biomedical Research*, **1**, 309–323

BRANDT, J. F. and HOLLIEN, H. (1967) Underwater hearing

thresholds in man. *Journal of the Acoustical Society of America*, **42**, 966–971

BRANDT, J. F. and HOLLIEN, H. (1969) Underwater hearing thresholds in man as a function of water depth. *Journal of the Acoustic Society of America*, **46**, 893–897

BRAUER, R. W. (1968) Seeking man's depth level. *Ocean Industry*, **3**, 28–33

BUHLMANN, A. and WALDVOGEL, W. (1967) The treatment of decompression sickness. *Helvetica Medica Acta*, **33**, 487–491

BUHLMANN, A. A., MATTHYS, H., OVERRATH, H. G., BENNETT, P. B., ELLIOTT, D. H. and GRAY, S. P. (1970) Saturation exposures at 31 ATA in a helium-oxygen atmosphere with excursions to 36 ATA. *Aerospace Medicine*, **41**, 394–402

CAMPBELL, P. (1945) Aerosinustis, a resume. *Annals of Otology, Rhinology and Laryngology*, **54**, 69–83

CARUSO, B. G., WINKELMANN, P.E., CORREIA, M. J., MILTEN-BERGER, G. E. and LOVE, J. T., (1977) Otologic and otoneurologic injuries in divers: clinical studies on nine commercial and two sport divers. *Laryngoscope*, **87**, 508–521

CHUNN, S. P. (1960) A comparison of the efficiency of the Valsalva manoeuvre and the pharyngeal pressure test and the feasibility of teaching both methods. *ACAM Thesis.* Brooks, AFB, TX; USAF School of Aerospace Medicine

COLES, R. A. A. and KNIGHT, J. J. (1961) *Aural and Audiometric Survey of Qualified Divers and Submarine Escape Training Instructors.* Medical Research Council (UK) Report RNPL 61/1011. London: MRC

COMROE, J. H., DRIPPS, R. D., DUMKE, R. R. and DEMING, M. (1945) Oxygen toxicity; effect of inhalation of high concentrations of oxygen for 24 hours on normal men at sea level and at simulated altitude of 18,000 feet. *Journal of the American Medical Association*, **128**, 710–717

CRAMER, D. B., GRAYBIEL, A. and OOSTERVELD, W. J. (1976) Successful transfer of adaptations acquired in a slow rotation room to motion environments in Navy flight training. In: *Recent Advances in Space Medicine*, Conference Proceedings 203. AGARD, Neuilly sur Seine: NATO

CURLEY, M. D. and KNAFELC, M. E. (1987) Evaluation of noise within the MK 12 SSDS helmet and its effect on divers' hearing. *Undersea Biomedical Research*, **14**, 187–204

DICKSON, E. D. D. and KING, P. F. (1954) The incidence of barotrauma in present day Service flying. *Flying Personnel Research Committee Report* no. 881. London: Air Ministry

DOBIE, T. G. (1974) Air sickness in aircrew. Report AG 177, AGARD, Neuilly sur Seine: NATO

DOWD, P. J. (1972) The USAFSAM selection test and rehabilitation program of motion-sick pilots in predictability of motion sickness in the selection of pilots. Conference Proceedings 109. AGARD, Neuilly sur Seine: NATO

DUVOISIN, R. C., KRUSE, F. and SAUNDERS, D. (1962) Convulsive syncope induced by Valsalva manoeuvre in subjects exhibiting low G tolerance. *Aerospace Medicine*, **33**, 92–96

EDMONDS, C. (1985) Hearing loss with frequent diving (deaf divers). *Undersea Biomedical Research*, **12**, 315–319

EDMONDS, C., FREEMAN, P. and TONKIN, J. (1974) Fistula of the round window in diving. *Transactions of the American Academy of Ophthalmology and Otolaryngology*, **78**, 444–447

EDMONDS, C., LOWRY, C. and PENNEFATHER, J. (1992) *Diving and Subaquatic Medicine*, 3rd edn. Oxford: Butterworth–Heinemann Ltd

EDMONDS, C., FREEMAN, P., THOMAS, R., TONKIN, J. and BLACK-

WOOD, F. A. (1973) *Otological Aspects of Diving.* Sydney: Australian Medical Publishing

ELDREDGE, D. H. and MILLER, J. D. (1969) Acceptable noise exposures-damage, risk criteria. In: *Noise as a Public Health Hazard*, edited by W. D. Ward and J. E. Fricke. ASHA Report No. 4. pp. 110–120

FAGAN, P., MCKENSIE, B. and EDMONDS, C. (1976) Sinus barotrauma in divers. *Annals of Otology, Rhinology and Laryngology*, **85**, 61–64

FARMER, J. C. JR (1990) Ear and sinus problems in diving. In: *Diving Medicine*, edited by A. A. Bove and J. C. Davis. Philadelphia: W. B. Saunders. pp. 200–222

FARMER, J. C. JR (1993) Otological and paranasal sinus problems in diving. In: *The Physiology and Medicine of Diving*, 4th edn, edited by P. B. Bennett and D. H. Elliott. London: W. B. Saunders. pp. 267–300

FARMER, J. C. and GILLESPIE, C. A. (1988) Otologic medicine and surgery of exposures to aerospace, diving, and compressed gases. In: *Otologic Medicine and Surgery*, Vol. 2 edited by P. W. Alberti and R. J. Ruben. New York: Churchill Livingstone. pp. 1753–1802

FARMER, J. C., THOMAS, W. G. and PRESLAR, M. J. (1971) Human auditory responses during hyperbaric helium-oxygen exposures. *Surgery Forum*, **22**, 456–458

FARMER, J. C., THOMAS, W. G., SMITH, R. W. and BENNETT, P. B. (1974) Vestibular function during HPNS. *Undersea Biomedical Research*, **1**, A–11(abstract)

FARMER, J. C., THOMAS, W. G., YOUNGBLOOD, D. G. and BENNETT, P. B. (1976) Inner ear decompression sickness. *Laryngoscope*, **86**, 1315–1326

FERGUSON, B. J., WILKINS, R. H., HUDSON, W. R. and FARMER, J. C. (1986) Spontaneous CSF otorrhea from tegmen and posterior fossa defects. *Laryngoscope*, **96**, 635–644

FLUUR, E. and ADOLFSON, J. (1966) Hearing in hyperbaric air. *Aerospace Medicines*, **37**, 783–785

FRASER, A. M. and MANNING, G. W. (1950) Effect of variation of swing radius and arc on the incidence of swing sickness. *Journal of Applied Physiology*, **2**, 580–584

FREEMAN, P. (1978) Rupture of the round window membrane. *Otolaryngology Clinics of North America*, **11**, 81–93

FREEMAN, P. and EDMONDS, C. (1972) Inner ear barotrauma. *Archives of Otolaryngology*, **95**, 556–563

GAUTHIER, G. M. (1976) Alterations of the human vestibulo-oculo reflex in a simulated dive at 62 ATA. *Undersea Biomedical Research*, **3**, 103–112

GILLIES, J. A. (ed.) (1965) *A Textbook of Aviation Physiology.* New York: Pergamon Press

GOLDMANN, R. W. (1986) Pneumocephalus as a consequence of barotrauma. *Journal of the American Medical Association*, **255**, 3154–3156

GOODHILL, V. (1972) Letter to the editor: Inner ear barotrauma. *Archives Otolaryngology*, **95**, 558

GOODHILL, V., HARRIS, I. and BROCKMAN, S. (1973) Sudden deafness in labyrinthine window ruptures. *Annals of Otology, Rhinology and Laryngology*, **82**, 2–12

GRAVES, D., IDICULA, J., LAMBERTSEN, C. and QUINN, J. (1973) Bubble formation in physical and biological systems: a manifestation of counterdiffusion in composite media. *Science*, **179**, 582–584

GRAYBIEL, A. (1972) Structural elements in the concept of motion sickness. *Astronaut Acta*, **17**, 5–25

GRAYBIEL, A. (1980) Space motion sickness: Skylab revisited. *Aviation, Space and Environmental Medicine*, **51**, 814–822

GRAYBIEL, A. and LACKNER, J. R. (1983) Motion sickness: acquisition and retention of adaptation effects compared

in three motion environments. *Aviation Space and Environmental Medicine*, **54**, 307–311

GRAYBIEL, A. and KNEPTON, J. (1976) Sopite syndrome; a sometimes sole manifestation of motion sickness. *Aviation Space and Environmental Medicine*, **47**, 873–882

GRAYBIEL, A., MILLER, E. F. and HOMICK, J. L. (1974) Experiment M-131. Human vestibular function. I. Susceptibility to motion sickness. Proceedings of Skylab Life Sciences Symposium, Report TMX-58154, NASA, Houston, TX. **1**, 169

GRAYBIEL, A., MILLER, E. F. and HOMICK, J. L. (1975) Individual differences in susceptibility to motion sickness among six Skylab astronauts. *Acta Astronaut*, **2**, 155–174

GRAYBIEL, A., KENNEDY, R. S., KNOBLOCK, E. C., GUEDRY, F. E., MERTZ, W., MCLEOD, M. E. *et al.* (1965) The effects of exposure to a rotating environment (10 rpm) on four aviators for a period of twelve days. *Report No.* **923**. Pensacola, Fl: US Naval School of Aviation Medicine and National Aeronautics and Space Administration

GRAYBIEL, A., O'DONNELL, R. D., FLUUR, E., NAGABA, M. and SMITH, M. J. (1981) Mechanisms underlying modulations of thermal nystagmic responses in parabolic flight. *Acta Otolaryonologica*, Suppl. 378, 1–16

GRAYBIEL, A., WOOD, C. D., KNEPTON, J., HOCHE, J. P. and PERKINS, G. F. (1975) Human assay of antimotion sickness drugs. *Aviation Space and Environmental Medicine*, **46**, 1107–1108

GROEN, J. J. (1960) Problems of the semicircular canal from a mechanico-physiological point of view. *Acta Otolaryngologica*, Suppl. 163, 59–60

GUEDRY, F. E. (1970) Conflicting sensory orientation cues as a factor in motion sickness. In: *Fourth Symposium on the Role of the Vestibular Organs in Space Exploration* Report SP-187. Washington, DC: NASA. p. 45

GUEDRY, F. E. and BENSON, A. J. (1976) Coriolis cross coupling effects: disorienting and nauseogenic or not? *Aviation Space and Environmental Medicine*, **49**, 29–35

GUSSEN, R. (1981) Sudden hearing loss associated with cochlear membrane rupture. *Archives of Otolaryngology*, **107**, 598–600

HAINES, H. L. and HARRIS, J. D. (1946) Aerotitis media in submariners. *Annals of Otology, Rhinology and Laryngology*, **55**, 347–371

HAMILTON, P. M. (1957) Underwater hearing thresholds. *Journal of the Acoustical Society of America*, **29**, 792–794

HARKER, L., NORANTE, J. and RZU, J. (1974) Experimental rupture of the round window membrane. *Transactions of the American Academy of Ophthalmology and Otolaryngology*, **78**, 448–452

HOMICK, J. L. (1980) Space motion sickness: selection, prediction, and training methods. *Paper at XI Meeting US/ USSR Joint Working Group on Space Biology and Medicine*, October, 1980, Moscow

IAKLOVEVA, I. Y. A., KORNILOVA, T. N., TARASOV, I. K. and ALEKSEEV, V. N. (1982) Results of studying the vestibular function and spatial perception function of cosmonauts. *Kosmicheskaia Biologiia i Aviakosmicheskaia Meditsina*, **1**, 20

IDICULA, J. (1972) Perplexing case of maxillary sinus barotrauma. *Aerospace Medicine*, **43**, 891–892

INGELSTEDT, S., IVARSSON, A. and TJERNSTROM, O. (1974) Vertigo due to relative overpressure in the middle ear: an experimental study in man. *Acta Otolaryngologica*, **78**, 1–14

JAMES, W. (1882) The sense of dizziness in deaf-mutes. *American Journal of Otology*, **4**, 239–254

JOHNSON, W. H., STUBBS, R. A., KELK, G. F. and FRANKS, W. R. (1951) Stimulus required to produce motion sickness. *Journal of Aviation Medicine*, **22**, 365–374

JONES, G. M. (1957) Report No. 1021. London: Flying Personnel Research Committee. Air Ministry

JONES, G. M. (1959) Pressure changes in the middle ear after simulated flights in a decompression chamber. *Journal of Physiology*, **147**, 43p–44p

KELEMEN, G. (1983) Temporal bone findings in cases of salt water drowning. *Annals of Otology, Rhinology and Laryngology*, **92**, 134–136

KELLER, A. P. (1958) A study of the relationship of air pressures myringopuncture. *Laryngoscope*, **68**, 2015–2029

KELLOGG, R. S., KENNEDY, R. S. and GRAYBIEL, A. (1965) Motion sickness symptomatology of labyrinthine defective and normal subjects during zero gravity maneuvers. *Aerospace Medicine*, **36**, 315–318

KENNEDY, R. S., MORONEY, W. F., BALE, R. M., GREGOIRE, H. G. and SMITH, D. G. (1972) Motion sickness symptomatology and performance decrements occasioned by hurricane penetrations in C-121, C-130, and P-3 Navy aircraft. *Aerospace Medicine*, **43**, 1235–1239

KENNEDY, S. (1975) Motion sickness questionnaire and field independence scores as predictors of success in Naval aviation training. *Aviation Space and Environmental Medicine*, **46**, 1349–1352

KING, P. F. (1965) Sinus barotrauma. In: *A Textbook of Aviation Physiology*, edited by J. A. Gillies. London: Pergamon Press. pp. 112–121

KOHUT, R. I., HINOJOSA, R. and BUDETTI, J. A. (1986) Perilymph fistula: a histopathologic study. *Annals of Otology, Rhinology and Laryngology*, **95**, 466–471

LAMBERTSEN, C. J. and IDICULA, J. (1975) A new gas lesion syndrome in man, induced by 'isobaric gas counter-diffusion'. *Journal of Applied Physiology*, **39**, 434–443

LANDOLT, J. P., MONEY, K. E., TOPLIFF, E. D., NICHOLAS, A. D., LAUFER, J. and JOHNSSON, W. H. (1980) Pathophysiology of inner ear dysfunction in the squirrel monkey in rapid decompression. *Journal of Applied Physiology*, **49**, 1070–1082

LESTER, J. C. and GOMEZ, V. (1898) Observations made in the caisson of the new East River bridge as to the effects of compressed air on the human ear. *Archives of Otolaryngology*, **27**, 1–19

LITTBAUER, D. I. (1943) 6th Meeting, Sub-Committee on Motion Sickness. Washington, DC: National Research Council

LOVE, J. T. and WAGUESPACK, R. W. (1981) Perilymph fistulas. *Laryngoscope*, **91**, 1118–1128

LUKOMSKAYA, N. Y. and NIKOL'SKAY, M. I. (1971) In search for drugs against motion sickness. In: *Evolutionary Physiology of Biochemistry*, edited by M. Y. Mikhel'son. Leningrad. 1971 (English translation, published by Defence and Civil Institute of Environmental Medicine, Downsview, Ontario, Canada, 1974)

LUNDGREN, C. E. G. (1965) Alternobaric vertigo – a diving hazard. *British Medical Journal*, **2**, 511–513

LUNDGREN, C., TJERNSTROM, O. and ORNHAGEN, H. (1974) Alternobaric vertigo and hearing disturbances in connection with diving: an epidemiologic study. *Undersea Biomedical Research*, **1**, 251–258

MCCAULEY, M. E., ROYAL, J. W. and WYLIE, C. D. (1976) Motion sickness incidence: exploratory studies of habituation, pitch, and roll, and the refinement of a mathematical model. *Technical Report* **1733**–2. Goleta, Ca: Human Factors Research Inc.

MCCORMICK, J. G., HOLLAND, W. B., BRAUER, R. W. and HOLLEMAN, I. L. (1975) Sudden hearing loss due to diving and its prevention with heparin. *Otolaryngology Clinics of North America*, **8**, 417–430

MCCORMICK, J. G., PHILBRICK, T., HOLLAND, W. and HARRILL, J. A. (1973) Diving induced sensorineural deafness: prophylactic use of heparin and preliminary histopathology results. *Laryngoscope*, **83**, 1483–1501

MANNING, G. W. and STEWART, W. G. (1949) Effect of body position on incidence of motion sickness. *Journal of Applied Physiology*, **1**, 619–628

MATSNEV, E. I. (1980) Mechanisms for vestibular disorders in space flight: facts and hypotheses. Translation of report presented at *11th Joint Soviet-American Working Group on Space Biology and Medicine*, Moscow, October, 1980 (NASA Tech. Memo. 76479). Washington, DC: NASA

MILLER, E. F. II, and GRAYBIEL, A. (1970) A provocative test for grading susceptibility to motion sickness yielding a single numerical score. *Acta Otolaryngologica*, Suppl. 274, 1–20

MILLER, G. R. JR (1965) Eustachian tubal function in normal and diseased ears. *Archives of Otolaryngology*, **81**, 41–48

MILLER, J. W. and GOODSON, J. E. (1960) Motion sickness in a helicopter simulator. *Aerospace Medicine*, **31**, 204–212

MOLVAER, O. I. (1979) Alternobaric facial palsy. *Medicine Aeronautica Spatial and Medicine Subaquatique Hyperbare*, **18**, 249–250

MOLVAER, O. I. and ALBREKTSEN, G. (1990) Hearing deterioration in professional divers: an epidemiologic study. *Undersea Biomedical Research*, **17**, 231–246

MONEY, K. E. (1970) Motion sickness. *Physiology Review*, **50**, 1–38

MONEY, K. E., BUCKINGHAM, I. P., CALDER, I. M., JOHNSON, W. H., KING, J. D., LANDOLT, J. P. *et al.* (1985) Damage to the middle and the inner ear in underwater divers. *Undersea Biomedical Research*, **12**, 77–84

MONTAGUE, W. E. and STRICKLAND, J. F. (1961) Sensitivity of the water immersed ear to high and low level tones. *Journal of the Acoustical Society of America*, **33**, 1376–1381

MURRAY, T. (1970) *Noise Levels Inside Navy Diving Chambers During Compression and Decompression*. US Navy Submarine Med. Center Report no. 643. Groton, Connecticut

NAKASHIMA, T., ITOH, M., WATANABE, Y, SATO, M. and YANAGITA, N. (1988) Auditory and vestibular disorders due to barotrauma. *Annals of Otology, Rhinology and Laryngology*, **97**, 146–152

NATIONAL AERONAUTICS AND SPACE ADMINISTRATION (1977) Scientific and Technical Information Office. Biomedical Results from Skylab. Washington. pp. 74–79

NEBLETT, L. M. (1985) Otolaryngology and sport scuba diving: update and guidelines. *Annals of Otology, Rhinology and Laryngology*, **94** (suppl. 115), 2–12

NEUMAN, T., SETTLE, H., BEAVER, G. and LINAWEAVER, P. G. (1975) Maxillary sinus barotrauma with cranial nerve involvement: a case report. *Aviation Space and Environmental Medicine*, **46**, 314–315

NISHOKIA, I. and YANAGHIARA, N. (1986) Role of air bubbles in the perilymph as a cause of sudden deafness. *American Journal of Otology*, **7**, 430–438

NUTTALL, J. and SANFORD, W. (1959) Spatial disorientation in operational flight. In: *Medical Aspects of Flight Safety*, edited by NATO Aeromedical Panel. London: Pergamon Press. p. 73

NUTTALL, J. B. (1958) The problem of spatial disorientation. *Journal of the American Medical Association*. **166**, 431–438

O'HANLON, J. F. and MCCAULEY, M. E. (1974) Motion sickness as a function of the frequency of vertical sinusoidal motion. *Aerospace Medicine*, **45**, 366–369

PARELL, G. J. and BECKER, G. D. (1985) Conservative management of inner ear barotrauma resulting from scuba diving. *Otolaryngology – Head and Neck Surgery*, **93**, 393–397

PHILP, R. B. (1974) A review of blood changes associated with compression-decompression: relationship to decompression sickness. *Undersea Biomedical Research*, **1**, 117–150

PULLEN, F. W., ROSENBERG, G. J. and CABEZA, C. H. (1979) Sudden hearing loss in divers. *Laryngoscope*, **89**, 1373–1377

RAYMAN, R. B. (1972) Stapedectomy: a threat to flying safety? *Aerospace Medicine*, **43**, 545–550

REASON, J. T. (1970) Motion sickness: a special case of sensory rearrangement. *Advances in Science*, **26**, 386–393

REASON, J. T. and BRAND, J. J. (1975) *Motion Sickness*. London: Academic Press

REASON, J. T. and GRAYBIEL, A. (1972) Factors contributing to motion sickness susceptibility: adaptability and receptivity in predictability of motion sickness in the selection of pilots. Conference Proceedings 109. AGARD, Neuilly sur Seine: NATO

ROGER, A., CABARROU, P. and GASTAUT, H. (1955) EEG changes in humans due to changes of surrounding atmospheric pressure. *Electroencephalography and Clinical Neurophysiology*, **7**, 152

RUBENSTEIN, C. J. and SUMMITT, J. K. (1971) Vestibular derangement in decompression. In: *Underwater Physiology*, Proceedings of the Fourth Symposium on Underwater Physiology, edited by C. J. Lambertsen. New York: Academic Press. pp. 287–292

SELTZER, S. and MCCABE, F. (1986) Perilymph fistula: the Iowa experience. *Laryngoscope*, **94**, 37–49

SHILLING, C. W. and EVERLEY, I. A. (1942) Auditory acuity in submarine personnel. *Naval Medical Bulletin*, **40**, 664–686

SIMMONS, F. B. (1968) Theory of membrane breaks in sudden hearing loss. *Archives of Otolaryngology*, **88**, 41–48

SIMMONS, F. B. (1978) Fluid dynamics in sudden sensorineural hearing loss. *Otolaryngology Clinics of North America*, **11**, 55–61

SINGLETON, G. T. (1986) Diagnosis and treatment of perilymph fistulas without hearing loss. *Otolaryngology – Head and Neck Surgery*, **94**, 426–429

SINGLETON, G. T., KARLAN, M. C., POST, K. N. and BOCK, D. G. (1978) Perilymph fistulas: diagnostic criteria and therapy. *Annals of Otology, Rhinology and Laryngology*, **87**, 797–803

SIVIAN, L. J. (1943) On hearing in water vs. hearing in air, with some experimental evidence. *Report no. 6.1–N DRC–838*. London: Office of Scientific Research and Development, National Defence Research Committee, Division 6, Section 6.1

SMITH, A. H. (1873) *The Effects of High Atmospheric Pressure, including the Caisson Disease*. Brooklyn: Eagle Print. pp. 1–53

SMITH, P. F. (1983) Development of hearing conservation standards for hazardous noise associated with diving operations. *Naval Submarine Medical Center Report No. 1029*

SUMMITT, J. K. and REIMERS, J. D. (1971) Noise: a hazard to

divers and hyperbaric chamber personnel. *Aerospace Medicine*, **42**, 1173–1177

TAYLOR, G. D. (1959) The otolaryngologic aspects of skin and scuba diving. *Laryngoscope*, **69**, 809–858

TERRY, L. and DENNISON, W. L. (1966) Vertigo amongst divers. *US Navy Submarine Medical Center Special Report*, No. 66–2. Groton, Connecticut

THOMAS, W., SUMMITT, J. and FARMER, J. (1974) Human auditory thresholds during deep saturation helium-oxygen dives. *Journal of the Acoustic Society of America*, **55**, 810–813

THOMSEN, K. A. (1958) Investigation on Toynbee's experiment in normal individuals. *Acta Otolaryngologica*, **140**, 263–268

THORNTON, W. D., BIGGERS, W. P., THOMAS, W. G., POOL, S. L. and THAGARD, N. E. (1985) Electronystagmography and auditory evoked potentials in space flight. *Laryngoscope*, **95**, 924–932

TINGLEY, D. R. and MACDOUGAL, J. A. (1977) Round window tear in aviators. *Aviation Space and Environmental Medicine*, **48**, 971–975

TJERNSTROM, O. (1973) On alternobaric vertigo – experimental studies. *Forsvarsmedecin*, **9**, 410–415

VAIL, H. H. (1929) Traumatic conditions of the ear in workers in an atmosphere of compressed air. *Archives of Otolaryngology*, **10**, 113–126

VOROSMARTI, J. and BRADLEY, J. J. (1970) Alternobaric vertigo in military divers. *Military Medicine*, **135**, 182–185

WAINWRIGHT, W. N. (1958) Comparison of hearing thresholds in air and in water. *Journal of the Acoustical Society of America*, **30**, 1025–1029

WATERMAN, D. and SMITH, P. F. (1970) An investigation of the effects of a helium-oxygen breathing mixture on hearing in naval personnel. *US Navy Submarine Medical Center Memorial Report 70–7*. Groton, Connecticut

WEISSKOPF, A., MURPHY, J. T. and MERZENICH, M. M. (1978) Genesis of the round window rupture syndrome; some experimental observations. *Laryngoscope*, **88**, 389–397

WOOD, C. D. and GRAYBIEL, A. (1968) Evaluation of sixteen anti-motion sickness drugs under controlled laboratory conditions. *Aerospace Medicine*, **39**, 1341–1344

WRIGHT, B. and BOYD, H. (1945) Aerosinusitis. *Archives of Otolaryngology*, **41**, 193–203

ZANNINI, D., ODAGLIA, G. and GIORGIO, S. (1975) Auditory changes in professional divers. In; *Proceedings of the Vth Symposium on Underwater Physiology*, edited by C. J. Lambertsen. Bethesda, Md.: Federation of the American Societies of Experimental Biology. pp. 675–684

8

The mouth and related faciomaxillary structures

David W. Proops

The mouth is not only the province of the sister speciality of dentistry, but has enormous social importance to man. All creatures eat to live, but humans have transformed this energy acquiring necessity into the focus of much of their social life.

The development of conceptual thought and the ability to express this through speech is what has most separated the human being from the rest of the animal kingdom. The physiological complexities of speech, as with eating, demand the attention of the speciality. Diseases of the mouth will interfere with these most vital activities.

To the otolaryngologist, therefore, the mouth is not only the route to the pharynx and beyond, but increasingly a meeting ground for the disciplines of oral and maxillofacial surgery, dental surgery and speech therapy. A thorough knowledge of this region, combined with an understanding of modern practices, is therefore essential.

The mouth or oral cavity extends from the lips and cheeks externally to the pillars of the fauces internally. Its boundaries are the lips anteriorly, the cheeks laterally, the hard and soft palate superiorly and the floor of the mouth inferiorly.

The mouth is divided into the vestibule outside the teeth, the alveolar arches, and the oral cavity proper within the dental arcades, which contains the tongue.

Developmental anatomy

The primitive oral cavity or *stomatodaeum* is first apparent in the 4-week old embryo as a slit-like space, bounded by the brain above and the pericardial sac below. The *buccopharyngeal membrane* at the back of the cavity forms a thin septum between the stomatodaeum and the foregut, which later breaks down

so that the mouth cavity becomes continuous with the developing pharynx (Figure 8.1). The branchial arches originate from a number of mesodermal condensations in the lateral wall and floor of the pharynx. Between the arches, successive clefts on the pharyngeal aspects are matched by corresponding clefts in the overlying ectodermal surface.

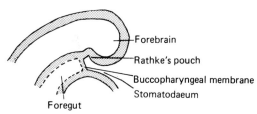

Figure 8.1 Sagittal section of human embryo showing early development of oral cavity

Within these mesodermal condensations, differentiation produces a cartilaginous bar and branchial musculature together with a branchial arch artery (Paten, 1953). Each arch receives an afferent and an efferent nerve to supply the skin, the musculature and the endodermal lining of the arch concerned. In addition, each arch receives a branch from the nerve of the succeeding arch. The branch from its own arch is known as the *post-trematic branch* and the second branch from the succeeding arch is called the *pretrematic branch*. The mandibular division of the trigeminal nerve is the post-trematic nerve of the first branchial arch. The *pretrematic* nerve to the first arch is represented by the chorda tympani branch of the facial nerve.

The facial nerve itself is the post-trematic branch of the second arch, while the pretrematic branch of this arch is derived from the tympanic branch (Jacobson's nerve) of the glossopharyngeal nerve. The glossopharyngeal is the post-trematic nerve of the third arch. The nerves of the remaining arches (fourth and sixth) are derived from the vagus and accessory nerves by their superior and inferior (recurrent) laryngeal branches and from the pharyngeal branches.

By the sixth week of embryonic life, the two mandibular processes, which have arisen from the lateral aspect of the developing head, have met and fused in the midline, to form the tissue of the lower jaw. Meanwhile, the maxillary processes develop as buds from the mandibular process, and grow forward on each side of the face beneath the developing eyes to make contact with the lower ends of the descending nasal processes (Figure 8.2).

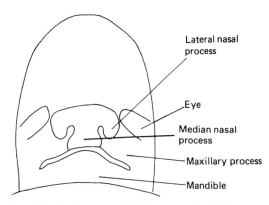

Figure 8.2 Development of the face in 7-week-old fetus

The fusion of the maxillary processes both creates the primary palate and separates the primitive nasal cavity from the primitive oral cavity. The inwardly directed extensions of each maxillary process produce tissues which later form the nasal septum and secondary palate, and which fuse following the descent of the developing tongue (Figure 8.3) (Kraus, Kitamura and Latham, 1966; Sperber, 1976).

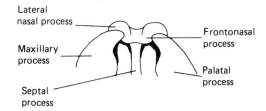

Figure 8.3 View from below of developing palate in 6-week-old embryo

Anomalies of development

Normal development depends upon the crucially timed convergence of tissue processes from different origins. Failures result in anomalies along the lines of normal fusion. The most common of the orofacial clefts is that of the secondary palate, followed by lip clefts and then clefts of the primary palate. The embryological basis for these is failure of fusion of the palatal shelves of the maxillary process, and the medial and lateral limbs of the frontonasal process, respectively. Failure of the tongue to descend in consequence of abnormal embryonic head flexion has been postulated as a cause, although genetic factors do play a part in some cases (Poswillo, 1975). Less common clefts are oblique facial clefts, midline clefts and congenital macrostomia or microstomia, which represent failures in the earlier stages of development (Figure 8.4).

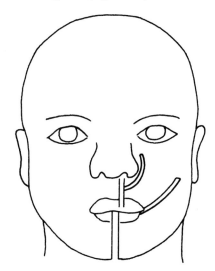

Figure 8.4 The major facial clefts

Other common abnormalities, such as developmental cysts and fistulae, result from the entrapment of epithelium along the lines of fusion, and these include nasolabial, globulomaxillary, median alveolar and median palatal cysts which usually do not present until adult life (Figure 8.5).

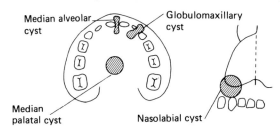

Figure 8.5 Developmental cysts of the maxilla

Development of the tongue

The tongue develops in two parts: the anterior part arises from the mandibular arches, in the form of paired eminences and, from a midline structure, the tuberculum impar in the floor of the mouth; the posterior part is derived from the *hypobranchial eminence* of the third visceral arch which grows forward over the second arches to become continuous with the anterior part of the tongue (Figure 8.6). The V-shaped *sulcus terminalis* lies posterior to the site of union of the two parts. At the apex of this V, just behind the row of *circumvallate* papillae, there is a small median pit in the dorsum of the adult tongue, the *foramen caecum*. This is a vestige of invagination from the floor of the pharynx which gives rise to the thyroid gland. By using the foramen caecum as a landmark, it becomes apparent that the mucosal covering of the body of the tongue arises from the first arch tissue and thus its sensory innervation is derived from the lingual branch of the *trigeminal* nerve, which is the nerve to the first arch.

dense fibrocellular tissue on the lateral side of Meckel's cartilage undergoes ossification and traps the associated mandibular arch nerves (Figure 8.7). Thus the inferior alveolar nerve comes to lie in the inferior dental canal after entering the mandible through the mandibular foramen, and the mental nerve to the lower lip and chin exits through the mental foramen. The two bony halves are united anteriorly by connective tissue, but bony union of this suture takes place before the end of the first year of life. All of Meckel's cartilage, except for the spheno-mandibular ligament, the malleus and the malleolar ligament, disappears.

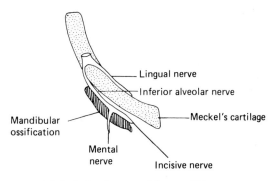

Figure 8.7 Early development of the mandible

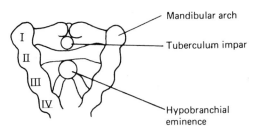

Figure 8.6 Development of the tongue. Floor of the mouth in 9-mm fetus

The sensory innervation to the part of the tongue posterior to the sulcus terminalis is derived from the third arch and hence its innervation is by the *glossopharyngeal* nerve.

Trapped between these two parts of the tongue is some tissue from the second arch, and this tissue is innervated by the nerve to the second arch, the seventh or facial nerve. In fact, the function of the nerve supply is gustatory and served by the *chorda tympani* branch of the facial nerve.

During the early part of its development, the tongue lies partly within the nasal cavity, and a delay in its descent may impede the fusion of the palatal folds, thereby producing clefts in the secondary palate (Brand and Isselhard, 1994).

Development of the mandible

The mandible is formed in the lower or deeper part of the first visceral arch. It is preceded there by *Meckel's cartilage* which represents the primitive vertebrate mandible. The dorsal end of this unbroken rod of cartilage gives rise to the malleus of the middle ear, but Meckel's cartilage itself plays little direct part in the development of the bony mandible. A band of

Surface anatomy
The lips

The lips are covered externally by skin and internally by mucous membrane. The vermilion border of the lips is a characteristic of the human species, and the red zone in the upper lip protrudes in the midline to form the *tubercle*. From the midline to the corners of the mouth the lips widen and then narrow. In the midline of the upper lip is the *philtrum* and the corners of the lips, known as the *commissures*, lie adjacent to the canine teeth. The skin surrounding the lips in the adult male is hirsute, a secondary sexual characteristic. At rest, the lips are lightly closed together when they are said to be *competent*.

The oral vestibule

The oral vestibule is a slit-like space between the lips and cheeks, and the teeth and alveolus. When the teeth are occluded, the vestibule is a closed space which communicates with the oral cavity proper only in the retromolar regions. The reflection of the mucosa from the alveolus to the lips and cheeks is the *fornix of the vestibule*. The upper and lower labial *frenula* are consistent folds of mucosa running from lip to the alveolus.

The cheeks

The cheeks extend from the labial commissures anteriorly to the ascending ramus posteriorly, and are bounded superiorly and inferiorly by the upper and lower vestibular *sulci*. Yellow granules on the mucosal surface are ectopic sebaceous glands known as *Fordyce granules*. The parotid salivary duct drains into the cheek opposite the maxillary second molar tooth. In front of the pillar of the fauces, a fold of mucosa containing the pterygomandibular raphe extends from the upper to the lower alveolus.

The palate

The palate is divided into the bony anterior hard palate and the mobile posterior soft palate. Immediately behind the anterior teeth, the mucosa of the hard palate shows the distinct prominence of the *incisive papilla*. Extending posteriorly to this is the midline raphe and the irregular folds of bound mucosa known as the palatal *rugae*. The junction of the hard and soft palate can be discerned, without palpation, by the change of colour from the pink of the hard palate to the yellow-red of the soft palate. In the middle of the free posterior edge of the soft palate is the *uvula*.

The floor of the mouth

The floor of the mouth is divided into two parts by the lingual frenulum which extends up to the base of the tongue. On either side of the frenulum are the sublingual papillae which mark the entry into the mouth of the ducts of the submandibular glands. On either side of this duct are the sublingual folds overlying the sublingual salivary glands.

The tongue

The tongue has both a dorsal and a ventral surface. The dorsal surface is divided by the V-shaped groove or the *sulcus terminalis* into the larger palatal and smaller posterior pharyngeal parts. Just anterior to these lie the large *circumvallate papillae*, while the remainder of the dorsum is covered with numerous white, conical elevations, the *filiform papillae*, between which are interspersed isolated reddish prominences, the *fungiform papillae*. On the posterolateral aspect of the tongue are the leaf-like *foliate papillae*, which can cause much anxiety when first discovered by the cancerophobic patient (Figure 8.8).

The ventral surface of the tongue is covered by a smooth mucous membrane through which vessels are clearly visible. It is divided into two by the lingual frenulum, on either side of which are fringed folds of

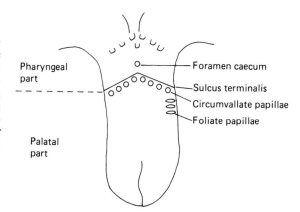

Figure 8.8 Dorsum of the tongue

mucous membrane, the *fimbriated folds* (Liebgott, 1982).

Bony anatomy
Maxilla

The right and left maxillae are the principal bones of the facial skeleton and superior aspect of the mouth. Each maxilla consists of a body and four processes, the frontal, palatine, zygomatic and alveolar, the first three of which articulate with separate bones of the same name while the alveolar process supports the maxillary teeth. In the midline, the two maxillae meet at the intermaxillary suture which is continuous with the suture between the two palatal processes (Figure 8.9).

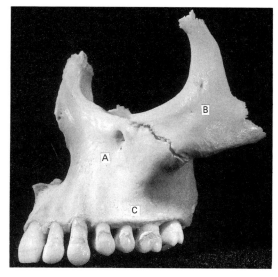

Figure 8.9 The maxilla and the zygoma. A: maxilla; B: zygoma; C: alveolar process

Each maxilla is hollowed by the paranasal sinuses and contains the following foramina: the posterior superior dental, incisive, palatine canal (with palatine bone), nasolacrimal canal (with lacrimal and inferior turbinate bones), infraorbital groove canal and foramen, and ostium to the maxillary antrum (Scott and Symons, 1977).

Growth of the maxilla

The maxilla develops in the fetal maxillary process as a membranous ossification. At birth, the infant maxilla differs from the adult maxilla in having small alveolar processes and rudimentary maxillary sinuses. Growth is by bone apposition, but the forward and downward growth of the mid-third of the facial skeleton also depends on endochondral growth at the *spheno-occipital synchondrosis* (Goose and Appleton, 1982).

The zygoma

The zygoma is an important element in the facial buttress system. It is a paired bone, triradiating into a maxillary, frontal and temporal process (see Figure 8.9). Clinically, this bone, the malus or malar bone, can undergo fracture dislocation following trauma. This may result in an inability to close the mouth because the coronoid process of the mandible impinges on the medially displaced zygoma. Reduction is achieved by passing an instrument under the zygoma from above using the fascia of the temporalis muscle as a guide.

The palatine bone

The horizontal plates of these paired bones articulate with each other and with the palatal process of the maxilla to form the posterior aspect of the bony palate (Figure 8.10).

The mandible

The mandible consists of a horizontal horseshoe-shaped component, the *body* of the mandible, and two vertical plates, the *rami*, which form the body at an obtuse angle. The two lateral halves of the mandible fuse in the midline soon after birth and the lower half of this forms the mental protuberance or chin. The upper border of the ramus carries two processes, the coronoid process anteriorly, and the condyloid process posteriorly, the latter of which articulates with the temporal bone at the *temporomandibular* joint.

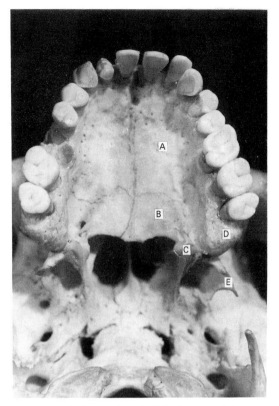

Figure 8.10 The bony palate. A: Palatal process of the maxilla; B: horizontal process of the palatine bone; C: pterygoid hamulus; D: tuberosity of maxilla; E: lateral pterygoid plate

The upper border of the mandible is the alveolar margin which contains the sockets for the roots of the mandibular teeth (Figure 8.11).

On the medial side of each ramus is the inferior dental foramen, opening into the inferior dental canal which runs through the body of the mandible to terminate laterally at the mental foramen.

On the medial aspect of the body of the mandible, the transverse mylohyoid ridge runs anteriorly almost to the genial tubercles at the midline (Figure 8.12) (Berkovitz and Moxham, 1988).

In the retromolar region, a fold of mucosa containing the pterygomandibular raphe extends from the upper to the lower alveolus. The pterygomandibular space, in which the lingual and inferior alveolar nerves run lies lateral to this fold and medial to the ridge produced by the mandibular ramus. The retromolar triangle is important in two ways, first, it is the superficial landmark for the inferior alveolar nerve when local anaesthetic nerve blocks are being undertaken, second, this region has a sinister reputation being the site of silent carcinomas which quickly spread deeply.

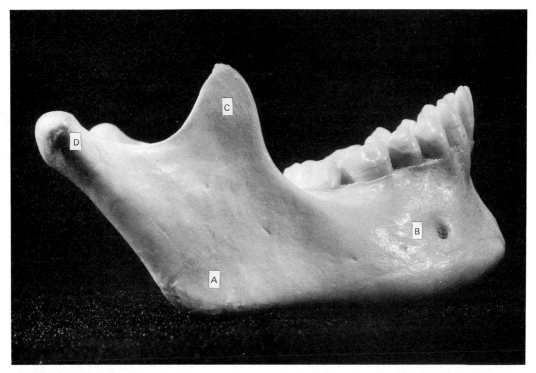

Figure 8.11 Lateral view of mandible. A: Ramus; B: body; C: coronoid process; D: condyloid process

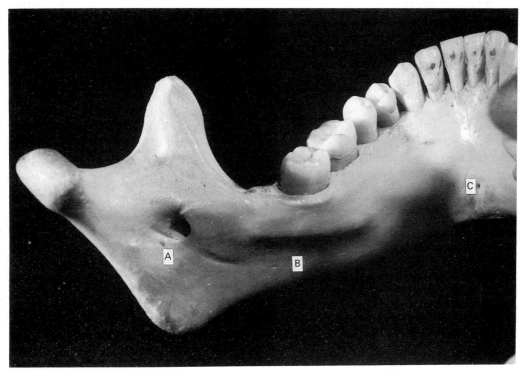

Figure 8.12 Medial view of mandible. A: Mandibular foramen; B: mylohyoid ridge; C: genial tubercles

Growth of the mandible

The ramus of the mandible is composed largely of bone, with the exception of the condyloid process which differentiates into a cone-shaped mass of cartilage. This zone of cartilage beneath, and separate from, the articular cartilage persists until the end of the second decade of life and, by its continued proliferation and endochondral ossification, is responsible for the growth in length of the mandible. Damage to this cartilage will result in failure in growth of the mandible.

Renewed activity by this centre after completion of growth accounts for the prognathism of acromegaly. The change in width and general architecture of the mandible is produced by the remodelling process of resorption and apposition to which all bones are subject. During life the mandible changes in shape. At birth, there is a wide mandibular angle, the ramus is small compared to the body and the chin is poorly developed. By the end of life, if all the teeth have been prematurely lost, the mandible once again approaches its fetal form (Figure 8.13) (Scott, 1967; Ranly, 1988).

Clinical aspects of the facial skeleton

Trauma to the facial skeleton is common, and is usually the result of either a road traffic accident or violent assault. Many combinations of fracture of the mandible are seen but most fractures involve, either singly or in combination, the body, the ramus or the neck of the condyle of the mandible. Treatment of most fractures requires the application of intermaxillary fixation, although fractures distal to the tooth-bearing areas may require additional techniques. Injuries to the mandibular condyle should be mobilized early to prevent ankylosis of the temporomandibular joint (Figure 8.14).

Fractures of the maxilla and facial skeleton were classified by Le Fort at the turn of the century. Le Fort 1 fractures involve the maxilla alone, Le Fort 2 fractures involve the orbits, and Le Fort 3 fractures consist of a separation of the maxilla, nose and ethmoids from the base of the skull (Figure 8.15).

Severe disproportion between the mandible and the maxilla or between these and the face can be treated surgically by maxillary or mandibular osteotomies,

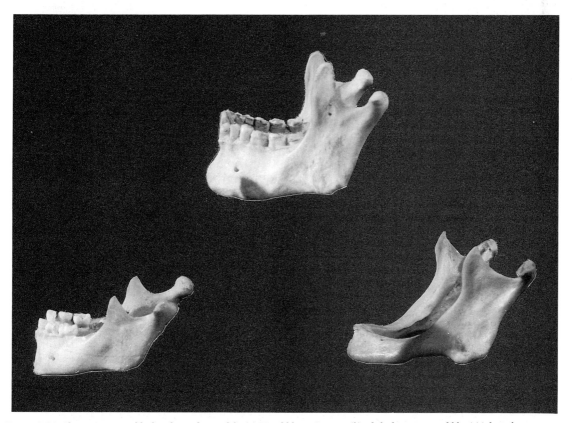

Figure 8.13 Changes in mandibular shape during life. (*a*) Mandible at 6 years; (*b*) adult dentate mandible; (*c*) edentulous mandible

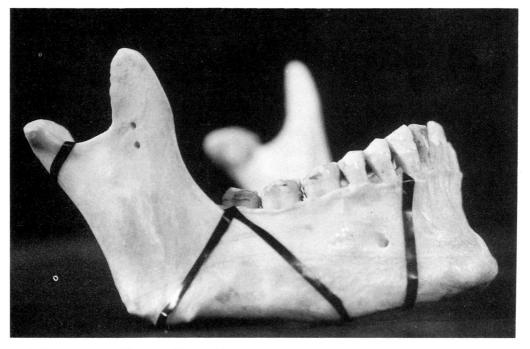

Figure 8.14 Common sites of fractures of the mandible

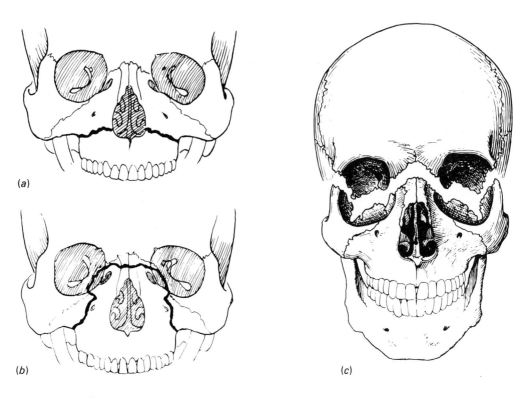

Figure 8.15 Le Fort classification of facial fractures. (*a*) Le Fort 1; (*b*) Le Fort 2; (*c*) Le Fort 3

a branch of maxillofacial surgery now called *orthognathic surgery* (Killey, 1971; Archer, 1978; Laskin, 1980; Mathog, 1984).

The temporomandibular joint

The mandible can be thought of as a single long bone, articulated at both ends. However, both joints must act simultaneously with movement, which is unique in the body.

The temporomandibular joint is a synovial articulation between the head of the mandible and the glenoid fossa of the temporal bone. The joint cavity is divided into two compartments by the intervening articular disc. The movement in the lower compartment is that of a hinge joint, but in the upper compartment some anterior and posterior gliding up and down the articular eminence takes place with wider degrees of jaw opening (Figure 8.16).

A strong joint capsule, which is strengthened laterally and medially by sturdy collateral ligaments, is also present. The lateral ligament is called the temporomandibular ligament, which not only prevents backward displacement of the condyle but which tightens at extreme opening, thus preventing subluxation. Two accessory ligaments of the temporomandibular joint are the sphenomandibular ligament, which runs from the spine of the sphenoid to the lingula of the mandible, and the stylomandibular ligament, which runs from the styloid process to the angle of the mandible; neither of these accessory ligaments, however, is thought to contribute significantly to the stability of the joints (Figure 8.17). The articular disc or meniscus is an important component of the temporomandibular joint. It consists of dense connective fibrous tissue and is moulded to the bony joint surfaces, which makes it thinner centrally than laterally, and it fills the gap produced by the disproportion between the head of the condyle and the glenoid fossa. Some fibres of the lateral pterygoid muscle are inserted into the anterior margin of the meniscus which is thus pulled forward with mandibular opening. Failure of coordinated movement of the articular disc may, on wide opening of the mouth, result in the head of the condyle slipping off the disc anteriorly, producing the familiar symptom of the clicking temporomandibular joint. The posterior aspect of the articular disc is rich in nerve endings concerned with proprioception in the joints (Sarnat and Laskin, 1976).

The movements of the mandible may be described as follows:

Protrusion Both mandibular condyles move forward onto the articular eminences and the teeth remain in gliding contact.

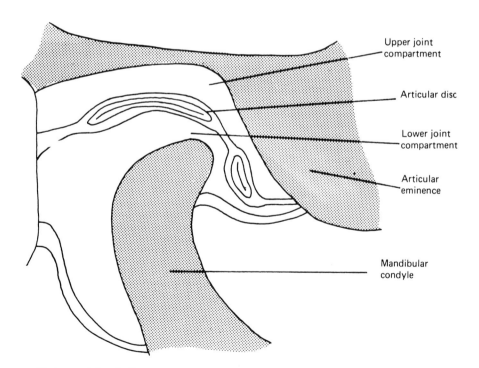

Figure 8.16 Mandibular condyle in half-open position

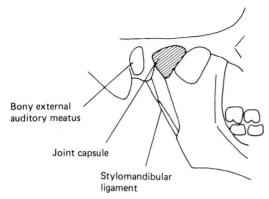

Figure 8.17 Ligaments of the temporomandibular joint

Bony external
auditory meatus

Joint capsule

Stylomandibular
ligament

Retrusion (retraction) This is the reverse process.

Opening This is partly a hinge movement and partly the result of the condyles being drawn on to the articular eminences. The mandible rotates around a horizontal axis so that, as the condyles move forward, the angles of the mandible move backwards and the chin is depressed.

Closing In this movement, the jaw may close in any number of positions. Closure in protrusion with the heads of the condyles remaining on the articular eminences, so that the lower incisors bite edge to edge with the upper incisors, is called incision. Closure with the condyles in the most backward position in the glenoid fossa, so that the teeth meet in normal occlusion, is called trituration.

Mastication requires side-to-side movements of the occlusal surfaces of the molar teeth. The condyle remains in the posterior position in the glenoid fossa on the side to which the chin is moving, and is held there by the tonic contractions of the muscle on that side; on the other side, the condyle is drawn forward and then back by the muscles of mastication on that side. The process is then repeated on the other side.

Myofacial pain dysfunction syndrome

Although the clinical symptoms associated with jaw dysfunction have long been recognized, it is only in the last 20 years that a condition previously referred to as Costen's syndrome or temporomandibular joint syndrome has been shown to be neither a primary joint disorder nor generally caused by occlusal abnormalities. Rather, it is now believed that masticatory muscle spasm is the primary factor responsible for the symptoms, for which the major causative factor is psychological stress (Bell, 1989).

The patient's symptoms are usually those of a unilateral dull ache in the ear or preauricular region that frequently radiates to the temple, to the angle of the mandible or the adjacent cervical region, or to the occiput. The pain is relatively constant but may be worse in the morning, and is exacerbated by use of the mandible.

The signs are fourfold. First, there is tenderness of the masticatory muscles to palpation; this can be elicited over the temporalis muscle but is most marked when the thumb is placed into the retromolar triangle and pressed upwards and backwards into the pterygoid muscles. Second, there is tenderness to firm palpation of the temporomandibular joint itself. Third, there is limitation of mandibular movement and, fourth, there is clicking of the joint. The latter two are lesser cardinal signs.

Treatments of this condition are various but most patients can be reassured that the majority of cases resolve spontaneously over a few weeks. Persistent problems require a dental opinion. Occlusal adjustments and the fitting of bite-raising appliances have been the mainstay of treatment. A very few cases may need referral to an oral surgeon for joint surgery.

The myofacial pain syndrome is commonly seen in otological practice, but the diagnosis should be entertained only after ear pathology has been eliminated following experienced examination.

Mandibular posture

At rest, there remains a gap of a few millimetres between the occlusal surfaces of the teeth, the so-called 'freeway space'. Following speech, mastication or swallowing the mandible returns to this physiological rest position (Lavelle, 1988). However, psychological states are known to interfere with this mechanism and the anxious individual with teeth tightly clenched is well recognized.

When establishing the occlusion of the edentulous patient for the provision of dentures, it is important to establish the physiological freeway space. An over-opened occlusion on the denture produces discomfort and a 'horsey' appearance, whereas too great a freeway space produces overclosure, resulting in the sagging and falling in of the soft tissues of the face, thereby mimicking or enhancing the ageing process of the face.

There has for some time been debate as to whether the temporomandibular joint is stress bearing (Hekneby, 1974). It is felt that most of the considerable stresses engendered by mastication are dispersed through the teeth and then through the well-recognized stress pathways of the facial skeleton to the skull. Some of these forces, however, must be directed through the glenoid cavity and into the temporal bone itself.

The muscles of mastication

Although other muscles also act upon the mandible, the term 'muscles of mastication' is used to describe the temporalis, the masseter and the lateral and medial pterygoid muscles. These muscles all receive their innervation from the mandibular division of the trigeminal nerve, indicating their origin from the musculature of the first branchial arch.

The *temporalis muscles* are fan-shaped muscles which take origin from the lateral aspect of the skull up to the inferior temporal line. The muscle fibres converge towards their tendinous insertions on the coronoid process of the mandible.

The *masseter muscles* may be divided into superficial and deep parts. The superficial parts arise from the lower border of the zygomatic arch and pass downwards and backwards to be inserted into the lower half of the lateral surface of the mandibular ramus. The deep parts arise from the inner surface of the lower part of the zygomatic arch and pass vertically downwards to be inserted into the mandibular ramus above the insertion of the superficial parts of the muscle.

The *lateral pterygoid muscle* has two heads, each with a separate origin: the inferior head arises from the lateral surface of the lateral pterygoid plate, and the superior head from the infratemporal surface of the greater wing of the sphenoid. The muscle fibres are inserted into the neck of the condyle and into the disc and capsule of the temporomandibular joint.

The *medial pterygoid muscle* also has two heads. The anterior head arises from the pyramidal process of the palatine bone and the posterior head from the medial surface of the lateral pterygoid plate.

Actions of the muscles of mastication

The muscles of mastication, in conjunction with other muscles, such as the mylohyoid, buccinator and digastric, initiate the movements of the mandible. The movements may be summarized as follows, with the major actions of the muscle indicated:

Elevation is produced by the masseter, medial pterygoid and anterior fibres of temporalis.
Depression is produced by the lateral pterygoids.
Protrusion is produced by the lateral and medial pterygoids.
Retraction is produced by the posterior fibres of temporalis.
Lateral excursions are produced by the medial and lateral pterygoids of both sides acting alternately (Jenkins, 1978).

Muscles of the cheeks and lips

The cheeks and lips contain some of the muscles of facial expression which are primarily muscles control-ling the degree of opening and closing of the orifices of the face. The expressive functions of the facial musculature have developed secondarily.

The muscles of the face are all derived embryologically from the mesenchyme of the second branchial arch; and therefore, the motor innervation is that to the second arch, the facial nerve.

The muscle of the lip is the *orbicularis oris*, the fibres of which are divided into four parts which correspond to the four quadrants of the lips. Muscle fibres in the philtrum insert into the nasal septum. The range of movements produced by this muscle include lip closure, protrusion and pursing. The muscles which radiate from the orbicularis oris can be divided into the superficial muscles of the upper and lower lips.

Two muscles extend to the corner of the mouth, the *risorius* and the *buccinator* muscles. The risorius which lies superficial to the buccinator stretches the angle of the mouth laterally. The buccinator, which arises from the pterygomandibular raphe, inserts mostly into the mucous membrane covering the cheek, and its main function is to maintain the tension of the cheek against the teeth during mastication.

Numerous minor salivary glands line the inner surfaces of the lips and cheeks. The parotid duct pierces each buccinator muscle after passing around the anterior margin of the masseter muscle, with its orifice lying opposite the second upper molar tooth.

The soft palate

The soft palate is a fibrous aponeurosis, the shape and position of which is altered by the tensor palati muscles, the levator palati muscles, the palatoglossus and the palatopharyngeus muscles.

The tensor palati muscle arises from the scaphoid fossa of the sphenoid bone and from the lateral side of the cartilaginous part of the eustachian tube. The muscle fibres converge towards the pterygoid hamulus where they become tendinous, and bend at right angles around the hamulus to become the palatine aponeurosis. When the tensor palati muscles contract, the palatine aponeurosis becomes taut. The motor innervation is derived from the mandibular division of the trigeminal nerve.

The levator palati muscle takes origin from the petrous temporal bone and the medial side of the cartilaginous part of the eustachian tube. The muscle curves downwards, forwards and medially to form a muscular sling which, when acting against the stiffened aponeurosis, produces an upward and backward movement of the soft palate. The nerve supply to the levator palati is derived from the cranial part of the accessory nerve (Figure 8.18).

The paired *palatopharyngeus* muscles extend from

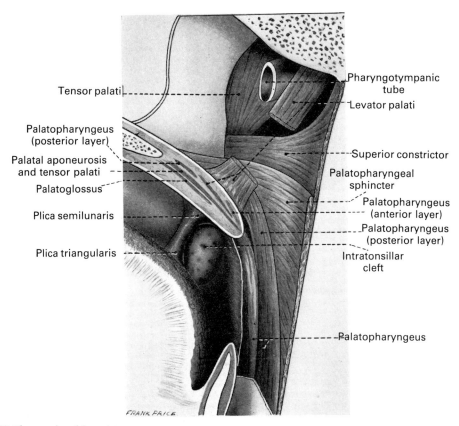

Tensor palati

Palatopharyngeus
(posterior layer)

Palatal aponeurosis
and tensor palati

Palatoglossus

Plica semilunaris

Plica triangularis

Pharyngotympanic
tube

Levator palati

Superior constrictor

Palatopharyngeal
sphincter

Palatopharyngeus
(anterior layer)

Palatopharyngeus
(posterior layer)

Intratonsillar
cleft

Palatopharyngeus

FRANK PRICE

Figure 8.18 The muscles of the palate

the palate down the lateral pharyngeal walls, where they form the posterior pillars of the fauces to insert into the posterior border of the thyroid cartilage. The action of these muscles is to elevate the larynx and pharynx but they also arch the relaxed palate and depress the tensed palate. The nerve supply is from the cranial accessory nerve.

The paired *palatoglossus* muscles arise from the palatine aponeurosis and descend as the anterior pillar of the fauces to insert into the lateral margin of the tongue. Their action is to raise the tongue and narrow the oropharyngeal isthmus. They are innervated by the cranial part of the accessory nerve.

Passavant's muscle is a sphincter-like muscle which encircles the pharynx at the level of the palate. The contraction of this muscle forms a ridge against which the soft palate is elevated, and in this way the oropharynx can be shut off from the nasopharynx during swallowing and speech.

The muscles of the tongue

The muscles of the tongue are paired, and are grouped into an *intrinsic* and *extrinsic* set. The intrin-

sic muscle fibres of the tongue can be divided into three groups, namely the transverse, longitudinal and vertical. Their function is to alter the shape of the tongue and they are innervated by the *hypoglossal* nerve. The extrinsic muscles of the tongue are composed of four groups, namely the *genioglossus, hyoglossus, styloglossus* and *palatoglossus* (Figure 8.19).

The genioglossus is a fan-shaped muscle which arises from the upper genial tubercle and is inserted into the tongue from its tip to its root. When these muscles act together as a pair, they protrude the tongue.

The hyoglossus is a flat quadrilateral muscle arising from the greater cornu of the hyoid bone passing upwards to be inserted into the side of the tongue. When this muscle contracts, the side of the tongue is depressed.

The styloglossus arises from the styloid process and passes downwards and forwards to be inserted into the side of the tongue. The contraction of this muscle causes the tongue to be drawn upwards and backwards.

The palatoglossus arises from the aponeurosis of the soft palate and descends to the tongue as the

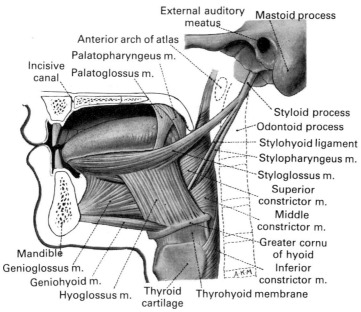

External auditory meatus
Mastoid process
Anterior arch of atlas
Palatopharyngeus m.
Incisive canal
Palatoglossus m.
Styloid process
Odontoid process
Stylohyoid ligament
Stylopharyngeus m.
Styloglossus m.
Superior constrictor m.
Middle constrictor m.
Greater cornu of hyoid
Inferior constrictor m.
Mandible
Genioglossus m.
Geniohyoid m.
Hyoglossus m.
Thyroid cartilage
Thyrohyoid membrane

Figure 8.19 The muscles of the tongue

anterior pillars of the fauces. Its action is to raise the tongue and narrow the oropharyngeal isthmus. In contrast to the other extrinsic muscles of the tongue which are innervated by the hypoglossal nerve, the palatoglossus is innervated by the cranial part of the accessory nerve.

The clinical importance of the tongue in articulation, eating and deglutition is well recognized. Loss of sensation of the tongue is an unpleasant feeling which most adults are familiar with following visits to the dental surgeon. Luckily, however, this anaesthesia is of short duration but if there is damage to the lingual nerve permanent anaesthesia may result.

Loss of motor function to the side of the tongue gives remarkably few symptoms and many patients are unaware that they have a hypoglossal nerve palsy. The sign of a hypoglossal nerve palsy is, of course, the tongue pointing to the side of the lesion on protrusion and a loss of muscle bulk on the affected side of the tongue.

Fixation of the tongue due to malignant infiltration causes slurred speech. Loss of substance of the tongue from surgery can grossly impair both speech and mouth cleaning. However, so long as a tongue tip is preserved it is remarkable how much can be removed without too much disability being apparent.

Blood supply

The arterial supply of the head and neck is very rich and the major branches overlap and collateralize. In addition, a good cross-over exists in the midline so that the external carotid artery, which is the main supply, can be ligated without fear. The face is supplied by the facial artery which anastomoses with the vessel on the other side and also with the other vessels supplying the region – the superficial temporal artery, the infraorbital and mental branches of the maxillary artery and the nasal branch of the ophthalmic artery.

The maxilla and mandible are supplied by branches of the maxillary artery and the tongue by the lingual artery, both of which are branches of the external carotid artery.

The palate derives its blood supply from the greater and lesser palatine branches of the maxillary artery.

The veins in the head and neck have few, if any, valves. This has the advantage of allowing bidirectional flow between deep maxillary veins and intercranial venous sinuses, but has the disadvantage of also allowing bacterial emboli from superficial septic foci to enter the cranial cavity by reverse flow.

The internal jugular vein is the largest channel, beginning at the jugular foramen as a continuation of the sigmoid dural sinus. Much of the drainage from the maxilla and mandible passes backwards, by way of the pterygoid plexus of veins, into the internal jugular system.

The superficial venous system is, however, quite variable, but the facial vein draining the superficial and anterior face usually joins with the retromandibular vein to form the common facial vein. This enters the internal jugular vein and finally drains into the brachiocephalic.

Lymphatic drainage

In general, the lymph from the anterior part of this region drains into the submental and submandibular nodes on the ipsilateral side and then into the deeper jugulodigastric node, whereas lymph from the posterior part drains directly into the jugulodigastric node.

The lymphatic drainage of the tongue, however, is a little more complex. Lymphatics from the anterior two-thirds of the tongue may be divided into the marginal and central vessels. The marginal vessels drain into the submandibular nodes on the same side; the central vessels at the tip of the tongue drain into the submental nodes and from further back into ipsilateral and contralateral submandibular lymph nodes. Lymphatics from the posterior third of the tongue drain directly into the jugulodigastric group of nodes (Figure 8.20).

The deep cervical plexus of lymphatic channels is the final common pathway for all head and neck drainage, terminating in the thoracic duct on the left and the junction of the internal jugular and subclavian veins on the right.

Nerve supply

The whole system, from the oropharynx forward, receives its sensory supply from the maxillary and mandibular division of the trigeminal nerve. The mandible, mandibular teeth, gingivae, and floor of the mouth and tongue are supplied by inferior dental, buccal, mylohyoid and lingual branches of the mandibular division.

The maxilla and maxillary teeth are served by the maxillary nerve, and by the infraorbital, pterygopalatine and anterior, middle and posterior dental nerves of the maxillary division.

The anterior hard palate is supplied by the nasopalatine nerve and the rest by the anterior and posterior palatine nerves from the maxillary division of the trigeminal nerve.

The anterior two-thirds of the tongue are supplied by the lingual nerve; the posterior one-third by the glossopharyngeal nerve (Figure 8.21).

The motor innervation of this region has been described previously.

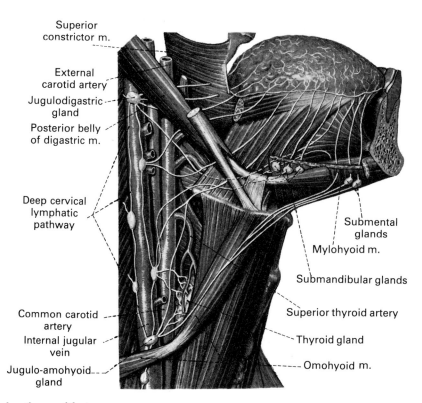

Superior constrictor m.
External carotid artery
Jugulodigastric gland
Posterior belly of digastric m.
Deep cervical lymphatic pathway
Common carotid artery
Internal jugular vein
Jugulo-amohyoid gland
Submental glands
Mylohyoid m.
Submandibular glands
Superior thyroid artery
Thyroid gland
Omohyoid m.

Figure 8.20 Lymph pathways of the tongue

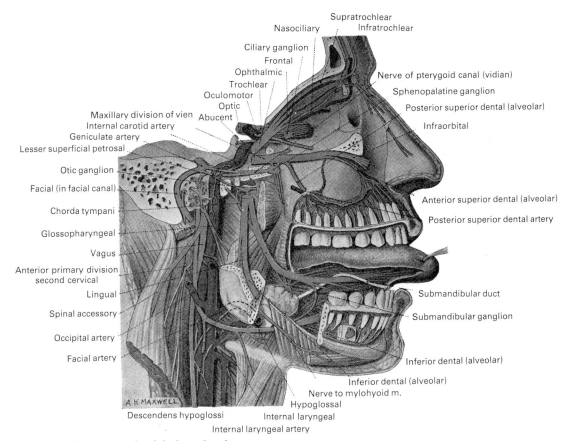

Figure 8.21 The trigeminal and the hypoglossal nerves

The fascial spaces of the head

Within the head there are anatomical spaces bounded by fascial layers, muscle, bone, skin or mucous membrane. Contained within these spaces are vessels, nerves, lymphatics and lymph nodes, and filling the unoccupied space is loose connective tissue (Figures 8.22 and 8.23).

These spaces or potential spaces are important because they determine the spread of infection and, to a lesser extent, of neoplasms in these areas. The most important of these spaces are:

The superficial facial compartment is bounded superficially by the buccinator muscle, the facial surfaces of the maxilla and mandible, and the outer surface of the masseter muscle. It is limited above by the zygomatic arch, behind by the parotid compartment, and below by the lower border of the mandible. It communicates deep to the mandibular ramus with the pterygoid space. It contains the buccal pad of fat, the duct of the parotid gland, the facial artery and vein, the buccal lymph nodes, the mental and infraorbital fora-

mina, branches of the trigeminal and facial nerves, and the muscles of facial expression.

The sublingual compartment is bounded by the lingual surface of the body of the mandible, the mucous membrane of the floor of the mouth and the upper surface of the mylohyoid muscle. It contains the submandibular salivary gland, the sublingual salivary glands, and the lingual and hypoglossal nerves.

The submandibular space is bounded by the body of the mandible, the lower surface of the mylohyoid muscle above and the superficial layer of deep cervical fascia below. It contains the superficial part of the submandibular salivary gland, the anterior belly of the digastric muscle and the submandibular and submental lymph nodes.

The parotid compartment is bounded by the posterior border of the ramus of the mandible, the styloid process and its muscles, the sternomastoid and the posterior belly of the digastric muscle. It contains the parotid salivary gland and its lymph nodes.

The pterygoid space is bounded by the ramus of the mandible and the deep surface of the masseter on the lateral side, the skull base above and the pharynx

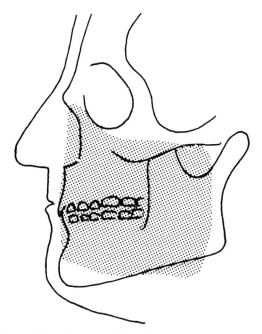

Figure 8.22 The superficial facial compartment

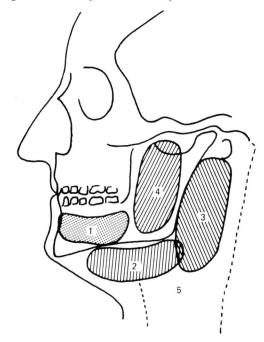

Figure 8.23 The deep fascial spaces. (1) Sublingual space; (2) submandibular space; (3) parotid space; (4) pterygoid space; (5) parapharyngeal space

medially. It contains the pterygoid muscles, the pterygoid venous plexus, the maxillary artery and the mandibular division of the trigeminal nerve.

The parapharyngeal space is bounded by the pharyngeal wall and vertebral column medially, and the deep cervical fascia and sternomastoid muscle laterally. It contains the carotid artery, the jugular vein, cranial nerves IX, X, XI and XII, and the deep cervical lymph node chain.

The paratonsillar space is between the wall of the pharynx and the mucous membrane of the fauces, and extends up into the soft palate.

Taste

Taste buds, which open directly on to the lingual surface of the tongue, are present in *fungiform papillae* which cover the anterior two-thirds of the dorsum of the tongue. These papillae are circular, red, between 1 and 4 mm in diameter and number between 20 and 60. These slightly raised fungiform papillae are surrounded by the more numerous *filiform papillae* which do not contain taste buds. Up to eight taste buds are present within these fungiform papillae, which also contain specialized pressure, tactile and temperature receptors.

Over the posterior third of the tongue, just anterior to the V-shaped *sulcus terminalis*, lie between 8 and 20 *circumvallate papillae* which project above the surrounding lingual tissue (Figure 8.24). Taste buds, in numbers up to 100, are present in both the papillae and the crypts which surround these papillae. In the bottom of the crypts surrounding the circumvallate papillae are the Von Ebner's glands, and encircling the openings of these glands are cilia which propel the secretions into the crypts. A few taste buds may be found on the palate and lips and have even been demonstrated in the upper third of the oesophagus (Henkin, 1976).

Taste buds are made up of between 20 and 50 cells, tightly joined together by desmosomal attachments. These cells are of epithelial origin and migrate into the bud; under neural salivary influence, they differentiate into one of three cell types which undergo constant renewal. All cell types have processes which extend up into the pore region of the bud, and nerves enter and leave the taste bud through its base (Figure 8.25).

For normal function, the taste bud receptors are exposed to the oral environment and are thought to respond to four primary stimuli: salt, sweet, sour and bitter. Differentiation of discrimination from within the various parts of the oral cavity has been observed, but the greatest number of buds respond to sweet stimuli.

Decreased taste activity is called *hypogeusia* and total loss of taste ability is known as *ageusia*. Abnormalities in the production of saliva, which is necessary for taste – such as occurs in Sjögren's syndrome, in the surgical removal of salivary glands, or after radiotherapy of the head and neck area – lead to a

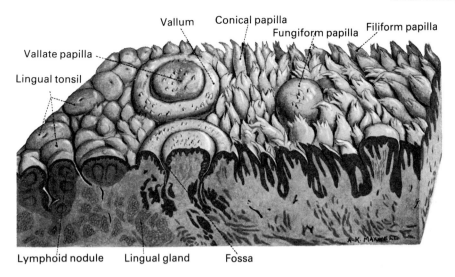

Vallum   Conical papilla   Fungiform papilla   Filiform papilla
Vallate papilla
Lingual tonsil
Lymphoid nodule   Lingual gland   Fossa

Figure 8.24 Surface view of the tongue

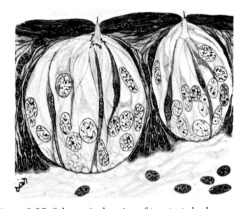

Figure 8.25 Schematic drawing of two taste buds

reduction in saliva flow and also to pathological changes in the taste buds.

Among the many pathological processes known to affect taste are vitamin deficiency, especially that of vitamins A and B_{12} and zinc deficiency. Endocrine disturbances such as hypothyroidism and Cushing's syndrome, as well as numerous drugs, such as amitriptyline and some cytotoxic agents, have been implicated.

Damage to the facial nerve in Bell's palsy, or deliberate section of the *chorda tympani* during middle ear surgery, are well known to the otolaryngologist, but one of the commonest causes of altered or lost taste sensation is postcoryzal or postinfluenzal damage, which may be accompanied by a loss of sense of smell.

Dental anatomy
Dentition

Man has two generations of teeth, namely the deciduous and the permanent.

The deciduous dentition begins to appear in the mouth at about 6 months of age, and the complete set of 20 teeth has erupted by about 2 years.

The permanent dentition starts to appear in the mouth at about 6 years and the last of the deciduous teeth is shed at about 13 years. The permanent dentition is not complete until the third permanent molar teeth (also known as wisdom teeth) erupt at about 18–21 years. The complete permanent set of teeth numbers 32 (Figure 8.26).

The teeth of both dentitions are arranged in upper and lower arches, and in each arch the teeth are arranged symmetrically on either side of the median plane. The teeth are identified according to their anatomical location within each of the four quadrants. In man, the deciduous dentition has five teeth in each quadrant, comprising two incisors, one canine and two molars. The permanent dentition has eight teeth in each quadrant, comprising two incisors, one canine, two premolars and three molar teeth.

Difference between the deciduous and permanent dentitions

The deciduous teeth are smaller than their permanent successors and the crowns are more bulbous with less robust roots. The deciduous teeth are whiter than the permanent teeth, and the enamel is softer and more easily worn.

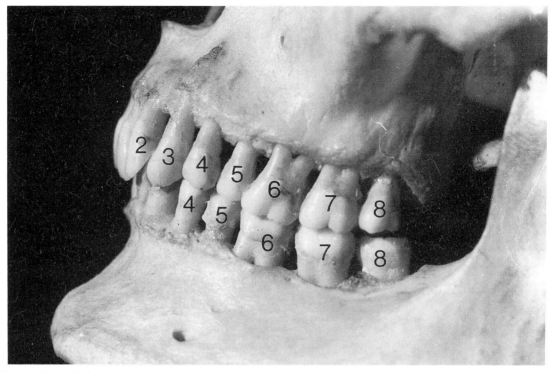

Figure 8.26 Adult dentition in normal occlusion

Each deciduous tooth is finally shed following the resorption of its root by the pressure of its erupting successor.

A dental shorthand is used for tooth identification. The deciduous teeth in each quadrant are labelled a to e and the permanent teeth in each quadrant numbered 1 to 8.

The symbols for the quadrants are derived from an imaginary cross superimposed upon the dentition when looking at the subject.

Upper right	Upper left
Lower right	Lower left

Thus the maxillary left second molar is $\underline{7}$ and the mandibular right deciduous first incisor is $\overline{a|}$.

Definition of terms in description of tooth form

Crown That portion of the tooth visible in the oral cavity.

Root That portion of the tooth which lies within the alveolus.

Occlusal surface The biting surface of a molar or premolar tooth.

Incisal margin The cutting edge of the anterior teeth.

Cusps The elevation in the occlusal surface of the teeth.

Fissure Longitudinal cleft between cusps.

Buccal surface That surface of a premolar or molar adjacent to the cheek.

Labial surface That surface of canine or incisor which is positioned immediately adjacent to the lips.

Palatal surface That surface of the maxillary teeth adjacent to the palate.

Lingual surface That surface of the mandibular teeth adjacent to the tongue.

Mesial That surface of the tooth that faces the median line.

Distal That surface of the tooth that faces away from the median line.

Chronology of tooth eruption

Deciduous dentition

Lower incisors	$\overline{\text{b a}|\text{a b}}$	6–9 months
Upper incisors	b a|a b	8–10 months
Upper and lower first molars	d|d d|d	12–16 months
Deciduous canines	c|c c|c	16–20 months
Upper and lower second molars	e|e e|e	20–24 months

Permanent dentition

First molars	$\frac{6|6}{6|6}$	6–7 years
Central incisors	$\frac{1|1}{1|1}$	6–8 years
Lateral incisors	$\frac{2|2}{2|2}$	7–9 years
First premolars	$\frac{4|4}{4|4}$	10–12 years
Canines	$\frac{3|3}{3|3}$	10–12 years
Second premolars	$\frac{5|5}{5|5}$	10–12 years
Second molars	$\frac{7|7}{7|7}$	10–13 years
Third molars	$\frac{8|8}{8|8}$	17–21 years

Eruption times in the tables are approximate, and variations of up to 6 months either way are not unusual. The permanent dentition tends to be more advanced in girls than in boys (Duterloo, 1991).

The form of the teeth

The incisors

There are two incisors in each quadrant, upper and lower, in both deciduous and permanent dentitions. In each quadrant, the tooth nearest the midline of the dental arch is known as the central incisor and the second tooth as the lateral incisor (Figure 8.27). These single rooted teeth are adapted for biting and the incisal edge undergoes attrition with age. The upper incisor region is a common site for supernumerary teeth and the lower incisors are the most common teeth to exhibit crowding. A gap between the central incisors is called a *diastema*.

The canines

The name is derived from the Latin word for dog because in the dog this type of tooth is very prominent. The canines are less prominent in the human being but are still the longest rooted teeth and the crown has a sharply pointed cusp. They are the first teeth of the true maxilla, as both incisors are carried in the premaxilla.

The premolars

There are two premolars in each quadrant and they replace the deciduous molars.

The upper premolars have a larger buccal cusp and a smaller palatal cusp. The first premolar has two roots and the second premolar has a single root. The first premolar is the tooth most usually sacrificed to create space before orthodontic treatment. The lower premolars have a less prominent lingual cusp and are usually single rooted.

The molars

These teeth are adapted for crushing and grinding food and are multicuspid and multirooted. Upper molars have three roots and lower molars two. They decrease in size from the largest first molar to the smallest third molar. This third molar or wisdom tooth is the most likely to be congenitally missing, and 25% of the population have one or more missing.

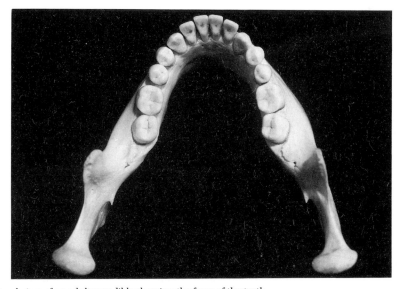

Figure 8.27 Occlusal view of an adult mandible showing the form of the teeth

In Caucasians, there is frequently insufficient room for the third molar to erupt so it may become impacted against the second molar in varied stages of eruption. The inability to clean the partly buried tooth, together with the sepsis that may ensue in the gingival pockets, produces discomfort in the young adult so that extraction is often necessary. Removal of these teeth, especially mandibular impacted wisdom teeth, often requires a surgical approach because of difficult access and the need to remove overlying bone. The apices of the roots of lower molars are usually in close relationship to the inferior alveolar nerve which may even occasionally perforate the root.

The roots of the upper molar teeth, especially those of the first molars, are in very close proximity to the antrum. When viewed from within the antrum, these roots can be seen as elevations of the antral floor.

Periapical abscesses on these molar teeth can therefore lead to sinusitis, although this is rarely seen in present times. Certainly, as part of the treatment of maxillary sinusitis, any carious teeth or infected roots should be appropriately treated.

The bone of the floor of the antrum, which lies between the roots of the molar teeth, is thin and is therefore commonly removed still attached to the roots during dental extraction. The iatrogenic production of oroantral fistulae is certainly more common than is generally recognized. Large oroantral fistulae should be dealt with by immediate surgical closure. However, many of the unrecognized oroantral fistulae heal spontaneously, and the most important determinant is the organization of a healthy blood clot within the socket. Sepsis within the clot will cause lysis and will produce a localized osteitis in the bone. This painful condition of 'dry socket' will predispose to the formation of an oroantral fistula.

Congenital absence of all teeth is known as total anodontia and absence of some of the teeth is known as partial anodontia, although a better term is 'hypodontia'. After the wisdom teeth, the most commonly congenitally absent tooth is the upper lateral incisor. Teeth which are found in excess of the normal number are called *supernumerary* teeth (Van Beek, 1983).

Dental occlusion

Dental occlusion is the relationship of the dental arcades, set upon their bony bases, to each other. There is a recognized ideal relationship of the upper and lower dental arches which is called normal occlusion.

The guidelines for assessing the occlusion are the comparative relationships of the first permanent molars and of the upper and lower incisor teeth. To a large extent, this relationship depends on the relative sizes of the maxilla and mandible. A small set back mandible will give a distocclusion or class II relation-

ship. A large prognathic mandible produces the opposite effect, or mesiocclusion, more commonly called a class III relationship (Figure 8.28).

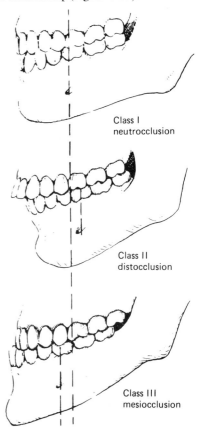

Figure 8.28 Assessment of occlusion

Superimposed upon these bony bases, there may also be a relative dentoalveolar disproportion, more commonly known as dental crowding. In the class I malocclusion, the bony bases are in harmony, but there is a relative crowding so that individual teeth are forced out of the dental arch.

The position that the upper incisors finally assume depends also on a balance of forces between the tongue, which tends to push them outwards, and the lower lip which counterbalances and tends to pull them back. Any 'incompetence of the lips' to become securely sealed at rest may result in the upper teeth becoming proclined outside the control of the lower lip. This produces the characteristic deformity of class II, division I. Alternatively, any overactivity of the musculature of the lower lip will tend to retrocline the upper anterior teeth, producing the deformity of class II, division II.

Treatment of these malocclusions is by means of removable or fixed appliances. These apply light but continuous forces which move the teeth through the bone. This form of treatment is called orthodontics.

Severe malocclusions may have a significant adverse affect on mastication; the majority of orthodontic treatments are, however, undertaken for cosmetic reasons during early adolescence.

The development of teeth

A local proliferation of the oral epithelium in the 7-week-old embryo gives rise to the *dental lamina*. At intervals along its length, small round swellings develop which are the primitive *enamel organs* of the deciduous teeth. The primordia of the permanent dentition develop later by budding off from the deciduous enamel organs. Adjacent to the enamel organ, the mesodermal tissue proliferates to form a dense mass which becomes the *dental papillae*. The enamel organ becomes a bell-shaped structure with the dental papillae now in the hollow of the enamel organ. The inner aspect of the ectodermal enamel organ differentiates, and provokes further differentiation in the dental papilla, to form *odontoblasts*, and it begins depositing enamel upon the recently laid down dentine. The entrapped dental follicle differentiates into the dental pulp (Figure 8.29).

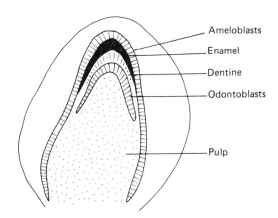

Figure 8.29 Developing human tooth

When the formation of enamel is complete, the enamel epithelium extends below the cervical margin to become a two-layered structure called the *sheath of Hertwig* and this maps out the shape of the roots (Bhaskar, 1986).

When the structure of the crown is complete, the ameloblast layer atrophies to become the reduced enamel epithelium protecting the ectodermal enamel from the mesodermal tissue in which it is buried. During eruption of the tooth, this epithelium finally unites with the epithelium of the alveolus, ensuring continuing epithelial continuity of the mucosa in spite of the eruption of the teeth (Figure 8.30).

An abnormal proliferation of odontogenic epithelium, which does not produce teeth, may occur. The

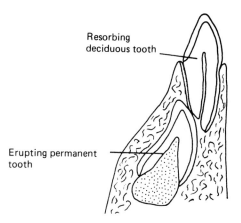

Figure 8.30 Resorption of deciduous incisor by erupting successor

proliferations may remain cellular, resulting in an *ameloblastoma*, or may lead to the production of single or multiple masses of the calcified dental tissues arranged in irregular and haphazard ways. These are known as *complex composite* and *compound composite* odontomes, respectively.

Finally, areas of epithelial dental lamina which do not differentiate into enamel organs may lie entrapped and dormant within the alveolus. These are called the *epithelial rests of Mallasez* (Ham and McCormack, 1979). Later in life, cystic conditions may occur which originate from these remnants of the dental epithelium. Among these are *cysts of eruption*, *dental cysts* and *dentigerous cysts*.

Structure of the teeth

In the human being, each tooth is composed of three calcified tissues, namely enamel, dentine and cementum, and contains a centrally situated soft pulp, which is the nutritive and sensory organ of the tooth.

Enamel forms the outer covering of the crown. It is grey or bluish-white in colour – its colour being modified by that of the underlying dentine – and is semitranslucent. It is the hardest substance in the body, so that it can well withstand masticatory stress, but is somewhat brittle. Enamel is highly mineralized, being 96% inorganic material, mainly in the form of hydroxyapatite crystals, 3% water and 1% organic matter. It has a crystalline prismatic structure, and each prism is the product of one ameloblast. It is ectodermal in origin, and hence no more enamel can be formed once the tooth has erupted.

Particular attention has recently been paid to the surface regions of enamel as it has been discovered that carious lesions within the enamel can be reversed and thereupon can reharden. Surface enamel differs both physically and chemically from subsurface enamel, in that the former is harder and less soluble. Surface enamel is rich in many trace elements, including fluorine, and it is believed that the fluoride ion incorporated in water supplies and tooth pastes has contributed to the rapid decline in the prevalence of dental caries in recent years.

Dentine, which forms the bulk of the tooth, and cementum, which covers the root, are both mesodermal in origin, that is living and capable of repair.

Dentine is composed of cells, the odontoblasts, and an intercellular substance. It is permeated by minute tubes, dentinal tubules, which contain the protoplasmic processes of the odontoblasts; the odontoblasts themselves always form a layer on the surface of the dentine. Dentine is a tissue highly sensitive to stimulation, as is commonly experienced, and although nerve fibres have been demonstrated in dentine, the odontoblasts themselves are believed to take part in the transmission of painful stimuli.

The pulp is composed of loose connective tissues richly supplied with blood vessels and nerves. The pulp is continuous with the connective tissue of the periodontal ligament and, functionally, is nutritive and sensory to the dentine. Any agent which opens up the dentinal tubules produces a reaction in the pulp. As the pulp is contained within unyielding walls of dentine, the hyperaemic and exudative changes accompanying inflammation lead to an increase in pressure inside the pulp cavity which compromises the vessels entering through the apical foramina and may result in infarction of the pulp.

The periodontium

The periodontium is the unique attachment of the teeth to the bony bases, and includes the cementum of the tooth root, the alveolar bone and the intervening collagenous bundles of the periodontal ligament.

The most important elements of the periodontal ligament are the oblique fibres that pass from the cementum on the tooth substance to the lamina dura of the tooth socket. By the arrangement of these fibres, the tooth is suspended in its socket, and pressure upon a tooth is transformed into tension on the walls of the socket (Figure 8.31).

Teeth maintain their position in the arch because of a balance of the various forces acting upon each individual tooth. However, the plasticity of the alveolar bone means that teeth can move, as in eruption, or be moved by steady light pressure, and this property of the periodontium is the basis of orthodontics.

The alveolar bone, which houses the developing tooth germ and, later, the root of the tooth, is normal bone. When the teeth are lost, this bone is gradually resorbed; a process which may cause early problems with the fit of dentures and, with the reduction in face height, produces the ageing effect of the premature loss of the natural dentition.

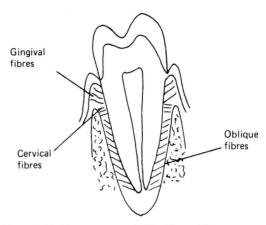

Figure 8.31 The arrangement of the fibres of the periodontal ligament

The pink mucous membrane, immediately related to the teeth and firmly bound down to the alveolar bone, is called the gingiva. The gingiva follows the cervical margin of the teeth; with age, however, it physiologically moves towards the root, exposing more of the crown of the tooth, hence the expression 'getting long in the tooth'. This process is referred to as passive eruption.

At the junction of the gingiva and the tooth, known as the gingival margin – representing the unique feature of a hard mineralized structure protruding through the surface integument of the body – there is a reflection of epithelium in close contact with the crown of the tooth which provides a seal at this point. Damage to this delicate seal, caused by the soft deposits of dental plaque and the calcific deposits of calculus or tartar, initiates and promotes an inflammatory process, resulting ultimately in periodontal disease, which is still the chief reason for tooth loss in adult life.

Age changes

With increasing age, the teeth undergo attrition; the enamel is worn away and the underlying dentine is exposed. The alveolar bone is progressively reduced and remodelled in those areas where the teeth have been prematurely lost. The edentulous mandible changes shape and the angle between the ramus and the body becomes more obtuse. The mental foramen comes to be closer to the upper border of the mandible where it is vulnerable to pressure.

Developmental dental disorders and diseases

Developmental dental disorders and related diseases are often seen. The most common and those of particular interest to the otolaryngologist are mentioned below.

Supernumerary teeth: the most common anomaly, usually found in either the midline or as extra molars. *Odontomes*: tumourous anomalies of calcified dental tissue. Mere exaggerations of cusps in their simplest form, they may, in more complex varieties present as haphazard masses of dental tissue. *Cementoma*; a localized excrescence of cementum which deforms a root. It may make dental extraction more difficult. *Enamel dysplasia* is often the hallmark of a forgotten childhood illness, presenting as pitted imperfections of the tooth surface. *Fluorosis*: excessive amounts of fluoride in the drinking water or increased consumption may result in mottling of the enamel, which can be unsightly. *Tetracycline stains*: the enamel may also be stained by the incorporation of tetracycline administered during calcification of the developing enamel.

Other systemic diseases may also leave their mark on the developing tooth germ. The most well known of these is *congenital syphilis* in which the incisor teeth are notched (Hutchinson's incisors) and the molar teeth resemble mulberries.

Conditions more familiar to the otolaryngologist include *amelogenesis imperfecta*, a genetically determined disease, in which the enamel fails to form properly and sometimes hardly at all. *Dentinogenesis imperfecta* is a genetic condition related to osteogenesis imperfecta, in which the dentine is soft and rapidly obliterates the pulp chamber. The attachment of enamel is poor and so, even though structurally normal, it splits off to leave the dentine completely exposed. When present with osteogenesis imperfecta, the stapes footplate is often fixed. The *otodental syndrome* is a rare condition in which there is globodontia and a high frequency hearing loss. *Mandibulofacial dysostosis* (Treacher Collins syndrome) often has associated dental deformity, e.g. a small mandible, dental crowding, sometimes absent teeth and even a cleft.

Conclusions

As a result of changing attitudes in the UK, and of the increasing availability of innovatory methods of treatment, a greater percentage of the population retain their teeth for life.

Nevertheless, a substantial number of the senior adult population are edentulous and rely upon prostheses or dentures to restore form and function.

Dental extraction is, however, still common practice and may occasionally be necessary in the course of surgical procedures undertaken by the otolaryngologist.

Surgical trainees would do well to acquaint themselves with the surgical techniques of exodontia.

References

ARCHER, W. H. (1978) *Oral and Maxillofacial Surgery*. Philadelphia: W. B. Saunders

BELL, W. E. (1989) *Orofacial Pain*. Chicago: Year Book

BERKOVITZ, B. K. B. and MOXHAM, B. J. (1988) *A Colour Atlas and Textbook of Oral Anatomy*. London: Wolfe

BHASKAR, S. N. (1986) *Orban's Oral Histology and Embryology*. St Louis: C. V. Mosby

BRAND, R. W. and ISSELHARD, D. E. (1994) *Anatomy of Orofacial Structures*. St Louis: Mosby

DUTERLOO, H. S. (1991) *An Atlas of Dentition in Childhood*. London: Wolfe

GOOSE, D. H. and APPLETON, J. (1982) *Human Dentofacial Growth*. Oxford: Pergamon

HAM, A. W. and MCCORMACK, D. H. (1979) *Histology*, 8th edn. Philadelphia: J. P. Lippincott & Co

HEKNEBY, M. (1974) The load on the temporo-mandibular joint; physical calculations and analyses. *Journal of Prosthetic Dentistry*, **31**, 303–312

HENKIN, R. I. (1976) Taste. In: *Scientific Foundations of Otolaryngology*, edited by R. Hinchcliffe and D. F. N. Harrison. London: Heinemann. pp. 468–483

JENKINS, G. N. (1978) *The Physiology and Biochemistry of the Mouth*. London: Blackwell

KILLEY, H. C. (1971) *Fractures of the Mandible*, 2nd edn. Bristol: Wright

KRAUS, B. S., KITAMURA, H. and LATHAM, R. A. (1966) *Atlas of Developmental Anatomy of the Face*. New York: Harper Row

LASKIN, D. M. (1980) *Oral and Maxillofacial Surgery*. St Louis: C. V. Mosby

LAVELLE, C. L. B. (1988) *Applied Oral Physiology*, 2nd edn. London: Butterworth. pp. 1–21

LIEBGOTT, B. (1982) *The Anatomical Basis of Dentistry*. Philadelphia: W. B. Saunders

MATHOG, R. (1984) *Maxillo-facial trauma*. Baltimore: Williams & Wilkins

PATEN, B. M. (1953) *Human Embryology*. London: McGraw Hill

POSWILLO, D. (1975) Causal mechanisms of cranio-facial deformity. *British Medical Bulletin*, **31**, 101

RANLY, D. M. (1988) *A Synopsis of Craniofacial Growth*, 2nd edn. Norwalk: Appleton & Lange

SARNAT, B. G. and LASKIN, D. M. (1976) *The Temporo-Mandibular Joint*. Springfield: C. C. Thomas

SCOTT, J. H. (1967) *Dento-facial Development and Growth*. Oxford: Pergamon

SCOTT, J. H. and SYMONS, N. B. B. (1977) *Introduction to Dental Anatomy*, 8th edn. London: Churchill Livingstone

SPERBER, G. H. (1976) *Cranio-facial Embryology*, 2nd edn. Bristol: Wright

VAN BEEK, G. C. (1983) *Dental Morphology*. Bristol: Wright

9

Anatomy and physiology of the salivary glands

Roderick Cawson and Michael Gleeson

It would not be unreasonable to say that, in the past, most surgeons' interest in salivary glands has been limited to the treatment of primary tumours, duct obstruction and recurrent infections. Yet disturbances of salivary gland function or inability to cope with normal salivary flow can have a devastating effect on the quality of life not only for our patients but also their relatives. For example, the dry mouth of patients with Sjögren's syndrome can lead them to despair, while drooling secondary to cerebral palsy may make them social outcasts and precipitate placement in institutional care.

Over the past decade there has been an explosion in the biotechnology of diagnostic tests. Clinical practice is in the process of change. A wide variety of tests, once almost exclusively confined to the examination of blood and urine can now be undertaken as precisely and accurately on other body fluids, e.g. sweat, tears and saliva. While the collection of saliva may lack the drama of venepuncture, the sincerity of sweat or the emotional appeal of tears, it is at the least readily accessible (Mandel, 1990). Samples can be reliably collected by the patients themselves at home or in their workplace and, unlike blood, samples do not clot or carry the risk of needle-stick injury. Antibodies to both viruses and bacteria can be detected and monitored from salivary samples (Brown and Mestecky, 1985; Smith *et al.*, 1985; Archibald *et al.*, 1986; Parry, Perry and Mortimer, 1987), as can drug and hormone levels (Read *et al.*, 1984; Cone and Weddington, 1989; Kirschbaum and Helhammer, 1989; Schramm *et al.*, 1991, 1992). There is little doubt that our knowledge of saliva, its production and modulation will grow. The next generation of surgeons will require a much more thorough knowledge of salivary gland anatomy and physiology which this chapter attempts to address.

Anatomy

Development

The epithelium of human salivary glands appears to be derived from ectoderm of the oral cavity or from endoderm in the case of von Ebner's glands, which surround the circumvallate papillae, and extraoral (nasopharyngeal) salivary tissue. The anlage develops as a solid bud from the oropharyngeal epithelium at about 6 weeks *in utero* for the parotid glands and 7 weeks *in utero* for the submandibular glands. The club-shaped terminal bulb soon undergoes dichotomous branching and a lumen develops, initially in the main branch. At the same time there is condensation of mesenchyme round the terminal bulbs to form a capsule and, later, the inter- and intralobular septa. The stroma of the parotid glands is rich in lymphocytes which eventually form the intra- and paraparotid lymphoid tissue. The primitive ducts consist of an inner layer of cuboidal cells and an outer layer of flattened myoepithelial cells. As secretory units differentiate, myoepithelial cells become confined to the acini and distal ductal components. In the parotid glands, the striated ducts cannot be reliably identified until after birth. Functional maturation follows establishment of feeding. The facial nerve becomes engulfed by embryonic glandular parenchyma between the 16th and 21st weeks of fetal life.

Distribution

There are three pairs of major salivary glands, the parotid, submandibular and sublingual, each situated outside the oral cavity but connected to it by a duct or system of ducts. In addition to these, there are collections of salivary tissue just below or within the oral mucosa itself. This tissue is collectively termed the minor salivary glands but is classified into groups, strictly on an anatomical basis, for clinical convenience. These are referred to as the palatal, buccal, labial, lingual, glossopalatine and retromolar glands.

The parotid glands

Gross morphology

Each parotid gland is a slender, lobulated, lozenge-shaped structure which has been likened to an inverted pyramid (Figure 9.1). It has a small superior surface and much larger anteromedial, posteromedial and superficial faces. Its anterior border overlies and is densely adherent to the posterior part of the masseter muscle. Superiorly this border is limited by the zygomatic arch, whereas the inferior extent is more variable and, on occasion, reaches as far as the carotid triangle. Its posterior border abuts onto the tragal cartilage superiorly and extends inferiorly to overlap the upper part of the sternomastoid muscle, to which it is only loosely attached. The superior surface is related to the external auditory meatus and the posterior aspect of the temporomandibular joint, while its anteromedial surface is attached to the masseter muscle, posterior border of the mandibular ramus and the medial pterygoid muscle. The posteromedial surface is grooved by the posterior belly of the digastric muscle, styloid process and its attached muscles and ligaments.

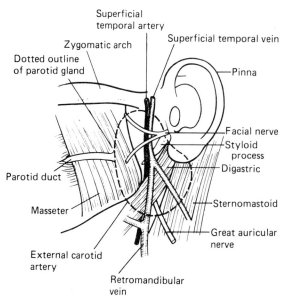

Figure 9.1 The parotid gland is outlined to show its relationship to adjacent structures, associated vessels and nerves

The capsule

The superficial surface of the parotid gland is covered by skin and fascia. Inferiorly it is also covered by the posterior border of the platysma muscle. The fascia condenses immediately over the gland to form its capsule, which for the most part is thick, tough and inelastic, although anteriorly it becomes thinner. This covering is an extension of the deep cervical fascia, continuous posteriorly with the fascial envelope of the sternomastoid muscle and anteriorly with that of the masseter. It sends off fibrous septa into the substance of the gland, some of which are continuous with the connective tissue surrounding the facial nerve. At the anterior and posterior borders of the gland there is a medial extension of the outer fascial covering which becomes progressively thinner as it passes medially. The posteromedial extension blends with the styloid process and, deep to it, the carotid sheath. It condenses into a strong and unyielding band from the styloid process to the angle of the mandible – the stylomandibular ligament.

Within the capsule are the superficial parotid lymph nodes and the greater auricular nerve, which is derived from the cervical plexus and provides sensory innervation to the lower two-thirds of the pinna. Just before the greater auricular nerve enters the parotid capsule, it gives off a slender posterior branch which passes up into the postauricular region. Some surgeons endeavour to preserve this branch while mobilizing the gland during the initial phases of parotidectomy in the mistaken belief that this lessens the sensory deficit acquired by the pinna. In reality, it is usually technically impossible and even if lost does not seem to make much difference to the patient.

The tough and inelastic nature of the parotid capsule accounts for the severe pain associated with parotid gland swelling and the delay encountered before raised parotid tension is recognized as clinical enlargement. Absence of a definite fascial barrier on the deep aspect of the parotid gland encourages infection to spread medially into the parapharyngeal space. In contrast, the stylomandibular ligament proves a very efficient barrier to medial extension of tumours developing in the superficial lobe of the gland. Tumours arising in the parotid gland, either between the mandible and stylomandibular ligament or immediately adjacent to it, can extend in either direction, but are constrained or restricted in the tunnel formed by the ligament and mandible. These tumours assume a dumb-bell shape.

Contained structures and blood supply

Several structures run through the gland and are of considerable surgical importance, the most notable of which is the facial nerve. It is this structure, described in detail later, that divides the gland into its surgical subdivisions, the larger superficial and smaller deep lobes. The external carotid artery enters the postero-medial surface of the gland before dividing into the maxillary artery and the superficial temporal artery. The latter gives off the transverse facial artery before emerging from the superior surface, while the maxillary artery leaves the gland from its anteromedial surface. The retromandibular vein is formed in the gland by the union of the maxillary and superficial temporal veins and leaves its inferior extremity to join the posterior auricular vein and become the external jugular vein. However, the retromandibular vein divides within the gland and its anterior division courses forwards to emerge from the anterior border of the gland as the posterior facial vein. These veins are exceptionally easy to image with ultrasound. They lie immediately deep to the plane of the facial nerve and are used by radiologists to determine whether a tumour lies deep or superficial to the facial nerve. From a surgical standpoint the posterior facial vein is a useful landmark for location of the mandibular branch of the facial nerve which crosses it superficially as it emerges from the gland.

The parotid duct

Within the parotid, the tree-like tributary ducts join near the anterior border of the gland and leave it to pass forward over the superficial surface of the masseter along an imaginary line drawn from the angle of the mouth to the attachment of the earlobe. The duct, Stenson's duct, passes obliquely forwards through the buccinator muscle after turning medially at the anterior border of the masseter muscle to open into the mouth at the parotid papilla, opposite the upper second premolar tooth. Small accessory glands sometimes lie along the line of the parotid duct.

The parotid lymphoid tissue

As described earlier, lymph nodes are present both in the capsule, periparotid nodes, and also within the gland parenchyma, where in addition to nodes there are also small, less well organized aggregates of lymphoid tissue. In an autopsy study, mainly on elderly persons, McKean, Lee and McGregor (1985) plotted the distribution of these nodes. Using strict anatomical criteria for defining the nodes and excluding small lymphoid aggregates, they found 193 intra-parotid nodes in 10 cadavers. Virtually all of these nodes were superficial to the facial nerve and only 16 were in the deep lobe. Most of the latter were superficial to the retromandibular vein.

These nodes and aggregations of lymphoid tissue form part of the mucosa-associated lymphoid tissue (MALT), itself a component of the much larger gut-associated lymphoid tissue (GALT). They produce secretory IgA, an immunoglobulin dimer joined by a secretory piece protein formed by the epithelial cells of the duct system. The relative amounts of IgA secreted by the different glands varies widely. Its apparent function is to form a barrier to the adhesion of bacteria, in particular, to the oral tissues. Within the parotid gland, the lymphoid tissue usually has a well-defined capsule and a peripheral sinus, but at the hilum the lymphoid tissue often merges with the gland parenchyma. Conversely, salivary gland tissue can often be found in intra- and periparotid lymph nodes and also in lymph nodes in the upper cervical chain.

The intraparotid facial nerve

The branching patterns of the facial nerve are varied, complex and hence have been inadequately or inaccurately described in classical anatomical texts. The location and variations of these branches can be of immense surgical significance. In the vast majority of cases the facial nerve leaves the skull as a single trunk through the stylomastoid foramen then splits within the substance of the parotid gland into zygomaticotemporal and cervicomandibular divisions. The terms 'zygomaticofacial' and 'cervicofacial' respectively are sometimes used for these divisions. Each division further subdivides to produce five major branches – temporal, zygomatic, buccal, mandibular and cervical. Katz and Catalano (1987) in a study of the facial nerve's anatomy in 100 patients undergoing parotidectomy, observed double-trunked nerves in three individuals and cautioned surgeons that unless they were aware of this anomaly, unnecessary damage to the facial nerve could result. Others in equally large or larger series have failed to encounter this variant. However, detailed studies of the intratemporal course of the facial nerve have demonstrated both bifurcation and trifurcation of the main trunk within its mastoid segment and therefore the double-trunked, extratemporal, facial nerve must exist, though perhaps less frequently than Katz and Catalano suggested.

Division of the facial nerve within the temporal bone is frequently associated with congenital abnormalities of the pinna or inner ear. An abnormally formed ear or congenital hearing loss should therefore alert the surgeon to this possibility. When present, the minor trunk of the facial nerve is said to enter the zygomaticotemporal division of the main trunk.

The pattern of branching of the facial nerve within the parotid gland is also variable. Although not the first to study the detailed ramifications of the nerve in cadavers, Davis *et al.* (1956) were probably the most thorough. They performed dissections on 350 cervicofacial halves and classified the branching patterns of the facial nerve into six types. Miehlke, Stennert and Chilla (1979) studied the operation records of 100 patients at their institute and grouped the branching patterns into eight types. The more recent study of Katz and Catalano (1987) reclassified these patterns into only five types. This study has the advantage that it was derived from contemporary operative findings rather than cadaver dissections and, as a result, incorporated functional information and the postoperative significance of damage to some of the fine branches. It is, therefore, this classification that is given here.

The five types of branching patterns of the facial nerve are illustrated in Figure 9.2 and are as follows:

Type 1 (25%): This pattern lacks anastomotic links between the main branches of each division. However in one subtype, there is splitting and subsequent reunion of the zygomatic branch while in the other, the mandibular branch splits and reunites
Type 2 (14%): In this type subdivisions of the buccal branch fuse distally with the zygomatic branch
Type 3 (44%): There are major communications between the buccal branch and others
Type 4 (14%): In this type there is a complex branching and anastomotic pattern between the major divisions
Type 5 (3%): The facial nerve leaves the skull as more than one trunk.

The nature of any given pattern in a particular patient is quite unpredictable preoperatively and it is clearly impossible to take account of all possible patterns during parotid surgery. The most important consideration therefore, is to be aware that many possible variations exist and to define the facial nerve and its branches as precisely as possible by taking into account its most frequently found patterns.

Autonomic nerve supply

The secretomotor fibres to the parotid gland emerge from the otic ganglion which is closely related to the auriculotemporal nerve. Preganglionic fibres reach the ganglion from the inferior salivary nucleus via the glossopharyngeal nerve, tympanic plexus and lesser petrosal nerve. The sympathetic supply reaches the gland from the superior cervical ganglion via the neural plexus surrounding the major blood vessels.

The submandibular glands

Gross morphology

The submandibular salivary gland consists of a large superficial and a smaller deep lobe which are continuous around the posterior border of the mylohyoid muscle (Figure 9.3). It fills the submandibular triangle of the neck. The medial aspect of the superficial part lies on the inferior surface of the mylohyoid muscle; the lateral surface is covered by the body of the

mandible, while its inferior surface rests on both bellies of the digastric muscle. Its inferior surface is covered by the platysma muscle, deep fascia and skin. The anterior facial vein runs over the surface of the gland within this fascia and is joined superiorly by the facial artery, which is for the most part related to the deep surface of the gland. Posteriorly, the submandibular and parotid glands are separated by a condensation of deep cervical fascia – the stylohyoid ligament. The deep part of the gland lies on the hyoglossus muscle where it is related superiorly to the lingual nerve and inferiorly to the hypoglossal nerve and deep lingual vein. The capsule of the gland is well defined and derived from the deep cervical fascia which splits from the greater cornu of the hyoid bone to enclose it.

The submandibular duct

The submandibular duct, Wharton's duct, is formed by the union of several tributaries and is about 5 cm in length. It emerges from the middle of its deep surface and runs in the space between the hyoglossus and mylohyoid muscles to the anterior part of the floor of the mouth, where it opens onto a papilla to the side of the lingual fraenum. In its anterior part it is related laterally to the sublingual glands and may receive many of their ducts. During its course on the hyoglossus muscle it is crossed from its lateral side by the lingual nerve.

Blood supply and lymphatic drainage

The submandibular gland receives its blood supply from branches of the facial and lingual arteries. Venous drainage accompanies these vessels. There are several lymph nodes immediately adjacent to the superficial part of the gland; these drain the latter as well as adjacent structures.

Autonomic nerve supply

The parasympathetic supply to the submandibular gland is from the superior salivary nucleus via the nervus intermedius, facial nerve, chorda tympani, lingual nerve and submandibular ganglion. Multiple parasympathetic secretomotor fibres are distributed from the submandibular ganglion which hangs from the lingual nerve. The sympathetic nerve supply is derived from the superior cervical ganglion via the plexus on the walls of the facial and lingual arteries.

The sublingual glands

The sublingual salivary glands lie in the anterior part of the floor of the mouth, between the mucous membrane, the mylohyoid muscle and the body of the mandible close to the symphysis, where each

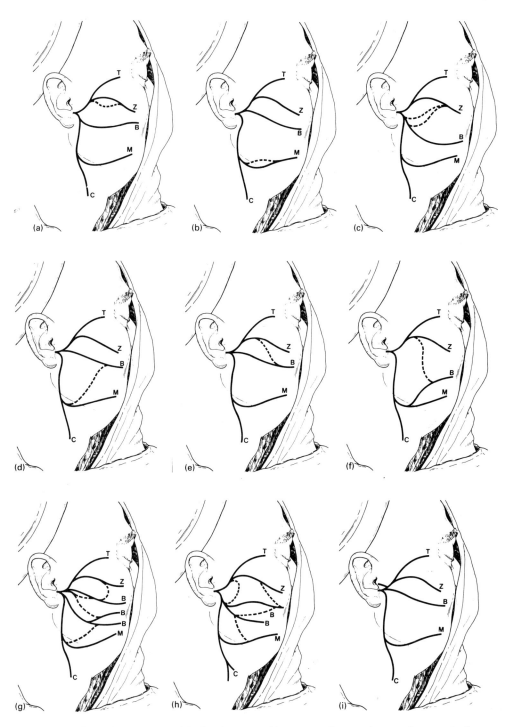

Figure 9.2 Intraparotid branching patterns of the facial nerve. (*a*, *b*) Type 1: in this type there is splitting and subsequent reunion of the zygomatic or mandibular branches. (*c*) Type 2: in this type subdivisions of the buccal branch fuses with the zygomatic branch peripherally. (*d*, *e*, *f*) Type 3: in this type there are major communications between the buccal branch and others. (*g*, *h*) Type 4: there are complex branching and anastomotic patterns between the major divisions in this type. (*i*) Type 5: in this type the facial nerve leaves the skull as more than one trunk. T: temporal branch; Z: zygomatic branch; B: buccal branch; M: mandibular branch; C: cervical branch

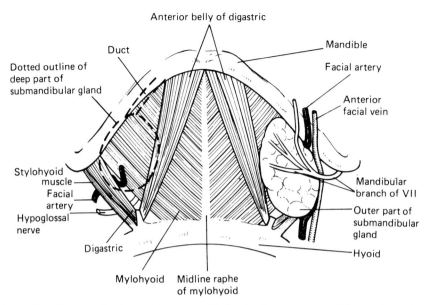

Figure 9.3 Relationships of the superficial part of the submandibular gland. The deep part of the gland together with the duct is outlined

may produce a small depression – the sublingual fossa. The gland has numerous excretory ducts which either open directly onto the mucous membrane or into the terminal part of the submandibular duct.

Microscopic anatomy

Each major gland is enclosed by a fibrous capsule which also contains some elastic tissue as well as blood vessels, autonomic nerve fibres and IgA-secreting plasma cells. As stated previously, the capsule is well defined in the parotid and submandibular glands, but less well developed in the sublingual and minor glands. The glands are split into lobules of variable size by fibrous septa derived from the capsule.

The parenchyma of the glands consists of varying proportions of serous and mucous cells and ducts. The serous acini consist of wedge-shaped secretory cells with basal nuclei surrounding a lumen which forms the origin of an intercalated duct. Myoepithelial cells lie between the basal lamina of the acinar cells and the basal membrane of the acinus. These cells contain microfilaments of actomyosin, which run parallel to the outer surface together with glycogen granules and lipofuscin. Pinocytic vesicles, indicative of active transport of materials between the intra-and extracellular spaces, are also present. The cytoplasm of the serous cells is densely packed with heavily basophilic secretory granules which are predominantly amylase. At the ultrastructural level, these cells contain densely packed endoplasmic reticulum in addition to the secretory granules and other cytoplasmic organelles (Figure 9.4). The mucous

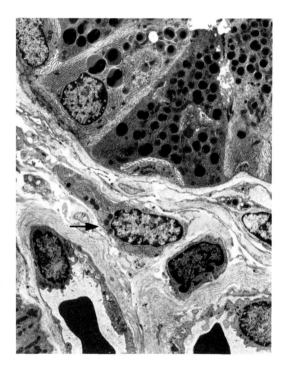

Figure 9.4 Transmission electron micrograph of the parotid gland showing a segment of an acinus surrounded by a myoepithelial cell (arrowed). The cytoplasm of the secretory cells contains granules and there is abundant endoplasmic reticulum

acinar cells have almost clear cytoplasm consisting of vacuoles containing sialomucins, and have flattened basal nuclei. In contrast to serous cells, the mucous cells contain relatively little endoplasmic reticulum. In mixed glands, e.g. the submandibular gland, the mucous cells have caps of basophilic, granular serous cells – serous demilunes.

The parotid glands are almost exclusively serous, the submandibular glands mixed, though mainly serous, and the sublingual glands predominantly mucous. The minor glands of the tongue, lips and buccal mucosa are seromucinous while those of the palate, glossopharyngeal area, retromolar pad and lateral borders of the tongue tend to be largely mucous.

Each acinus is drained by a short intercalated duct. These ducts are lined by a single layer of cuboidal epithelium surrounded by myoepithelial cells. The intercalated duct cells have relatively large, central nuclei and contain few organelles. They actively secrete fluid. The intercalated ducts are continuous with the striated ducts which have a brush border (microvilli) on their luminal face and parallel finger-like cytoplasmic extensions from the opposite pole (Figure 9.5). Ultrastructurally, the parallel infolding of the basal lamina is conspicuous as are the many mitochondria. These cells actively secrete bicarbonate, regulate the water content of saliva and can secrete trace elements and iodine. The duct system also actively secretes or reabsorbs sodium, potassium, chloride and other ions. The striated ducts run into the interlobular duct system which has a simple transport function. Mucous cells are an occasional finding in striated ducts.

Groups of sebaceous glands are scattered throughout the parotid gland parenchyma. Fat is also a conspicuous component of the parotid glands and tends to increase in amount with age.

Physiology of salivary secretion

The amount of saliva secreted and, to a large extent, its composition are normally controlled by the autonomic nervous system. Other factors can also interfere with function, e.g. drugs which affect autonomic responses, deficiency of fluid, and disease or destruction of the gland parenchyma.

Autonomic control of salivary secretion

Much animal experimentation has been undertaken to establish the effects of autonomic stimulation on salivary flow (Garrett, 1987). Normal reflex secretion of saliva depends on centrally coordinated parasympathetic and sympathetic activity. Parasympathetic activity evokes most of the fluid secreted by causing variable degrees of exocytosis from the secretory cells and vasodilatation within the gland. It also induces contraction of the myoepithelial cells. Sympathetic stimulation of the salivary glands tends to be more intermittent and is also directed at the cells that receive parasympathetic impulses. It tends to modulate the composition of saliva by increasing exocytosis from certain cells. Some sympathetic fibres exercise tonic effects on blood vessels; these fibres are likely to be under separate central control and not involved directly in the reflex secretory pathway.

Mechanisms of salivary secretion

The mechanisms of saliva secretion have been reviewed in detail by Baum (1993) who emphasized that much of the information presented below comes from study of rat salivary glands. Little is known of the mechanisms of human salivary secretion but

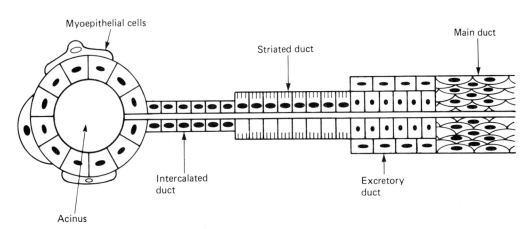

Figure 9.5 Diagrammatic representation of the salivary unit and duct system

such data as exist generally conform to the broad principles discussed here.

As Baum (1993) has described, saliva is produced only in response to neurotransmitter stimulation. Neurotransmitters probably bind to specific receptors in the basolateral region of the acini. Noradrenalin binds to both α- and β-adrenergic receptors while acetylcholine binds to cholinergic receptors. These receptors depend on G protein (guanine nucleotide-binding regulatory protein) for transduction of the neurotransmitter stimuli. The G proteins that carry the stimuli into the acinar cells are heterotrimeric molecules consisting of α, β and γ subunits. The α subunit is the site of guanine nucleotide binding and probably conveys the functional specificity to a G protein. Binding of a neurotransmitter to a receptor greatly strengthens the ability of a receptor to associate with a G protein. The association with a G protein stimulates in turn, replacement of GDP by GTP at the nucleotide binding site and promotes dissociation of the heterotrimer into a free α subunit and a $\beta\gamma$ complex. The α subunit can then activate the appropriate receptor molecule. Activation continues until the GTP is broken down into GDP by endogenous enzymic (GTPase) activity in the α subunit. The GDP bound to the α subunit then unites with the $\beta\gamma$ complex to regenerate the heterotrimeric molecule. There is also some evidence to suggest that the $\beta\gamma$ complex, or even the β subunit alone, may be able to activate some receptor molecules directly. The best recognized signal transduction processes in salivary glands are first, generation of cAMP as a result of β-adrenergic receptor stimulation and second, formation of 1,4,5-inositol triphosphate (IP_3) after acetylcholine receptor stimulation. The latter leads to calcium ion mobilization and, as a consequence, fluid secretion.

The specific mechanism by which cAMP acts as an intermediary in protein exocytosis remains unclear. Typically, cAMP elicits a response by activation of cAMP-dependent protein kinase and protein phosphorylation. In rat salivary glands, β-adrenergic receptor stimulation leads to a rise in cAMP levels, activation of the A kinase, phosphorylation or dephosphorylation of several cellular proteins and thus, amylase or glycoprotein secretion by the parotid or submandibular glands respectively. Indeed, treatment of rat parotid and submandibular gland cells with cAMP analogues also leads to protein secretion. Kinetic analyses suggest that the 24–26 kD species protein is the most probable candidate for phosphorylation though its function in protein exocytosis is unknown. Moreover, the role of a kinase-dependent phosphorylation in rat parotid gland protein secretion has become somewhat controversial.

It is well established that Ca^{++} plays a central role in fluid secretion by acinar cells in response to acetylcholine receptor stimulation. Activation of this receptor leads to fluid-related signal transduction via

coupling to a G protein often designated G_p. The latter is probably a member of the $G_{q/11}$ family which is known to couple to phospholipase C. Activation of phospholipase C results in hydrolysis of a minor membrane phospholipid, phosphatidylinositol 4,5-bisphosphate, and formation of second messengers IP_3 and diacylglycerol. IP_3 is the main mediator of Ca^{++} mobilization and thus of fluid secretion, but diacylglycerol can promote activation of protein kinase C and lead to stimulation of a minor exocytic pathway.

IP_3 binds to a receptor protein located on an intracellular Ca^{++} storage pool that is probably related to, or part of, the endoplasmic reticulum. The IP_3 receptor also functions as a Ca^{++} release channel and allows stored Ca^{++} to move down a concentration gradient into the cytoplasm. These Ca^{++} levels quickly rise approximately 10-fold as a consequence of acetylcholine receptor stimulation. This reaction triggers a cascade of events which include sustained Ca^{++} entry and activation of specific ion transport pathways. Generation of fluid in the acinar lumen is the final result, by mechanisms discussed in detail by Turner (1993).

Extracellular Ca^{++} and entry of Ca^{++} sustain high levels of salivary fluid secretion over long periods. However, mechanisms of Ca^{++} entry into acinar cells which are non-excitable and not voltage activated, are poorly understood. Possible mechanisms for Ca^{++} entry into acinar cells include a direct receptor-gated Ca^{++} channel, a G protein-activated Ca^{++} channel, and a second messenger-activated Ca^{++} channel. However, there is little evidence for the involvement of the first two of these mechanisms and only a few reports have suggested that Ca^{++} entry may be activated by the synergistic action of IP_3 and its metabolite 1,3,4,5-inositol tetrakisphosphate (IP_4).

Currently, the most favoured explanation of the mechanism of Ca^{++} entry is one termed 'capacitative Ca^{++} entry'. This suggests that depletion of the Ca^{++} storage pool provides the driving force for sustained Ca^{++} entry. Support for this theory comes from studies that have shown that graded depletion of the Ca^{++} store have led to similarly graded Ca^{++} entry. Use of non-receptor activation by, for example thapsigargin, to deplete the Ca^{++} store also leads to Ca^{++} entry. Though the exact mechanism by which depletion of Ca^{++} stores causes Ca^{++} entry is uncertain, it is clear that it can be modulated by extracellular pH and cytoplasmic Ca^{++}.

Acinar cells are responsible for production of the fluid component of saliva and most of the proteins that it contains. The acinar cells are water-permeable and derive fluid from the surrounding blood vessels. The fluid is carried by the duct system which is impermeable to water. During passage through the ducts, there is exchange of electrolytes. Most of the sodium and chloride ions are removed, but some potassium and bicarbonate ions as well as a little protein, are added.

Mechanisms of primary fluid secretion in salivary acini

As in all secretory epithelia, fluid transport in salivary gland cells is thought to be driven osmotically by transepithelial salt gradients. Turner (1993) has explained that studies on rat and rabbit salivary glands have suggested three mechanisms for primary salivary fluid secretion. Unexpectedly, these mechanisms do not appear to be alternative explanations for salivary fluid secretion, but appear to operate concurrently within the same gland or possibly within the same acinar cells.

The first mechanism, of which the other two can be regarded as variations, is that fluid secretion depends on the combined action of four membrane transport systems, namely:

1 An Na^+-K^+-$2Cl^-$ cotransporter that is located in the basolateral membrane of the acinar cells
2 A basolateral Ca^{++}-activated K^+ channel
3 An apical conductive pathway for Cl^- which is presumably a Ca^{++}-activated Cl^- channel
4 The Na^+/K^+ ATPase.

In the resting state, both K^+ and Cl^- are concentrated in the acinar cell above electrochemical equilibrium, with K^+ being concentrated by Na^+/K^+ ATPase and Cl^- by Na^+-K^+-$2Cl^-$ cotransporter. As discussed earlier, secretagogue stimulation leads to a rise in intracellular Ca^{++} concentration and, in turn, opening of the basolateral Ca^{++}-activated K^+ channel and the apical Cl^- channel. Increases in K^+ and Cl^- conductance allow KCl to flow out of the cell and this results in accumulation of Cl^- ions and their associated negative electrical charge in the acinar lumen. As a consequence, electrical attraction causes Na^+ to leak from the interstitium through the tight junctions to follow Cl^-. The resulting osmotic gradient for NaCl causes transepithelial movement of water from the interstitium to the lumen. Continued influence of an agonist results in a transepithelial chloride flux and concomitant fluid secretion. This is sustained by Cl^- entry via the Na^+-K^+-$2Cl^-$ cotransporter and exit via the apical Cl^- channel. Removal of the stimulus is followed by a fall in intracellular calcium concentration to resting levels, closure of the K^+ and Cl^- channels and return of the cell to its resting state.

The second mechanism is similar except that the basolateral Na^+-K^+-$2Cl^-$ cotransporter is replaced by a Cl^-/HCO_3 exchanger acting in parallel with an Na^{++}/H^+ exchanger. A fall in intracellular chloride concentration as a result of secretagogue KCl loss, thus leads to entry of more Cl^- in exchange for HCO_3^-. Acidification of the cytoplasm that results from this bicarbonate loss is buffered by the Na^{++}/H^+ exchanger, which uses the extracellular-to-intracellular sodium gradient generated by Na^+/K^+ ATPase, to drive protons out of the cell.

Unlike the first two mechanisms in which chloride is the secreted ion, the third involves acinar bicarbonate secretion. In this last mechanism, CO_2 enters the acinar cell across the basolateral membrane and is converted to HCO_3^- plus a proton, by intracellular carbonic anhydrase. HCO_3^- is lost across the apical membrane via an anion channel which is possibly the same as that involved in chloride secretion. The proton is expelled by the basolateral Na^{++}/H^+ exchanger.

Factors affecting salivary flow

Even in the absence of parenchymal salivary gland disease, function can be abnormal and, when diminished, result in xerostomia. Although xerostomia is usually a complaint of late middle-aged women, it should not be assumed that ageing itself causes deterioration of salivary gland function. Several studies have been carried out and have yielded somewhat conflicting results. In the most recent study, Ship, Patton and Tylenda (1991) found that normal postmenopausal women, the main group thought to be at risk, had no deterioration of salivary gland function.

In clinical practice, drugs are the most common cause of decreased salivary gland function. Tricyclic antidepressants and phenothiazine neuroleptics are among the most troublesome as they have particularly strong antimuscarinic effects and are generally used over long periods. Formerly, ganglion-blocking drugs had the same effect but are now generally regarded as obsolete for the routine management of hypertension. A list of commonly used drugs which affect salivary flow is shown in Table 9.1.

Depression and anxiety states are often associated with a dry mouth. Busfield and Wechsler (1961) measured the rate of salivary secretion in 42 untreated depressed patients and found it to be decreased in comparison with non-depressed hospital patients and healthy controls. No correlation was found between the degree of xerostomia and the assessed severity of depression, nor was there any difference found in secretion rates in a later study by Busfield, Wechsler and Barnum (1961), between the different categories of depression or between those who complained of dry mouth and those who did not.

The fact that decreased salivary flow is associated with sympathetic overactivity, as in anxiety states, or caused by sympathomimetic drugs and can be relieved by β-blockers would seem to suggest that the sympathetic supply to the salivary glands is inhibitory in humans. However, sympathetic inhibitory fibres have not been found and, until they are, the generally

Table 9.1 Drugs liable to cause xerostomia

Drugs with antimuscarinic activity
Atropine and analogues (hyoscine, ipratropium etc.)
Tricyclic antidepressives
Monoamine oxidase inhibitors
Phenothiazines and related neuroleptics
Orphenadrine, benzhexol and related antiparkinsonian agents
Antihistamines
Ganglion blockers and clonidine
Antiemetics (antihistamines, hyoscine and phenothiazines)

Drugs with sympathomimetic activity
'Cold cures' and decongestants containing ephedrine or phenylpropylamine
Bronchodilators (isoprenaline, orciprenaline etc.)
Appetite suppressants, particularly amphetamines and diethylpropion

accepted hypothesis for the mechanism of anxiety-induced xerostomia is that of central inhibition from higher centres which act on the salivary nuclei in the brain stem and suppress reflex activity.

Drying of the mouth is virtually inevitable in dehydration and is a consequence of haemorrhage, diarrhoea, chronic vomiting, polyuria secondary to diabetes mellitus, restricted fluid intake or overdose of diuretics.

A detailed discussion of the salivary gland diseases that cause xerostomia is outside the scope of this chapter. Nevertheless, it is worth noting some of the more common conditions, if only for further reference, namely autoimmune sialadenitis, HIV infection, radiation damage, graft-versus-host disease, sarcoidosis, iron overload, amyloidosis and type V hyperlipoproteinaemia.

Collection of saliva

Saliva may need to be collected to determine the flow rate, to confirm or discard a clinical complaint of xerostomia or to provide a sample for assays of any type. Many methods have been devised and may be summarized as follows:

1 Unstimulated flow of whole (mixed) saliva
2 Stimulated flow of whole saliva
3 Stimulated or unstimulated flow from individual glands.

Salivary stimuli

Over the years a variety of stimulants to salivary secretion has been used. These are either systemic or local sialagogues. The main systemic sialagogue that has been used is the parasympathomimetic pilocarpine. Though effective, it does not precisely reproduce the balance of sympathetic and parasympathetic activity responsible for normal secretion. One consequence is that it can alter the concentrations of normal constituents, particularly sodium and potassium. Pilocarpine can also cause systemic cholinergic effects such as colic, diarrhoea, bradycardia and sweating which may be troublesome.

Local sialagogues are convenient and generally more satisfactory. A good example is 5% citric acid solution, which is a potent sialagogue and does not interfere with the composition of the final specimen. Five drops of this solution can be delivered from a pipette or disposable syringe onto the dorsum of the tongue. This may be used as a preliminary measure before collecting unstimulated saliva. The purpose of this manoeuvre is to flush out stagnant secretions that confuse the analysis. Thus, citric acid is applied to the tongue and saliva is collected for 15 minutes to eliminate rest transients.

Stimulated or unstimulated saliva can then be collected for periods of 15–30 minutes as necessary. However, Ericson (1969) has pointed out that the results obtained by different sialometric methods are not necessarily comparable because individuals with a vigorous secretory response to one stimulus do not necessarily have a similar response to another.

Collection of mixed whole saliva

There is a variety of methods of collecting saliva from individual glands or collecting mixed whole saliva. Many of these methods require specially made equipment and are mainly suitable for research purposes. Mason and Chisholm (1975) described the following methods:

1 Spitting
2 Drainage
3 Suction
4 Cotton wool rolls.

More recently Navesh (1993) has reviewed methods for collecting saliva.

Spitting and drainage methods

The patient is put into a comfortable sitting position with the head inclined forward and encouraged to spit at 1-minute intervals or to allow saliva to drain out of the mouth into a funnel draining into a sterile collecting vessel.

Suction

This method requires the equipment associated with a dental chair. The patient is put into a similar position as before to allow saliva to collect into the anterior floor of the mouth. A saliva ejector is placed behind the lower incisor teeth and the secretion is trapped in a bottle intervening between the ejector and the drainage system.

Cotton wool rolls and other absorbent devices

Pre-weighed cotton wool rolls are placed under the tongue for a 2-minute period then taken out and re-weighed. This method allows quantitation only. More recently proprietary devices such as OraSure have been introduced to simplify saliva collection and pre-serve it for analysis. Its use has been reported by Thieme *et al.* (1994) who collected saliva for determination of measles, mumps and rubella immunization status. OraSure is a cotton-fibre pad which can absorb 1 ml of oral fluid. In manufacture, it is saturated with hypertonic saline solution, dried and mounted on a plastic handle. In clinical practice, it is placed between the gingiva and buccal mucosa for 2 minutes, then withdrawn and placed in an antiseptic transport medium. In the laboratory, the saliva specimen is recovered by centrifugation.

While there appear to be advantages to the OraSure system for gathering oral fluid, it must be appreciated that by virtue of the filtering effect of the cotton-fibre pad, it does not collect whole saliva. Cordeiro, Turpin and McAdams (1993) found that the levels of IgG in OraSure oral fluid were three to four times higher than those of saliva and amylase levels were two to four times higher. They suggested that the cotton-fibre pad might promote passage of crevicular gingival exudate and stimulate secretion of amylase as a result of the pad's buffer solution. However, North *et al.* (1993) found that the OraSure system provided a reliable index of tobacco usage by means of continuous salivary assay.

Collection of parotid gland saliva

Pure parotid gland saliva can be collected by cannulating the parotid duct with a polythene catheter or using a suction cup. Catheterization of the duct allows collection of uncontaminated saliva but is uncomfortable for the patient and the tube has to be held in place. For suction, the most widely used devices are the Carlson-Crittenden or Lashley cups, the centre of which are placed over the parotid pa-pilla. Each cup consists of a central chamber into which the saliva flows and an outer chamber to which suction is applied to cause the cup to adhere to the buccal mucosa (Figure 9.6).

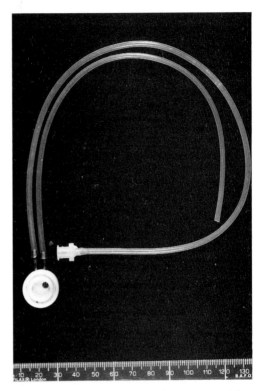

Figure 9.6 A Lashley collecting cup. The cup consists of a central chamber into which the saliva flows and an outer chamber to which suction is applied so that it adheres to the buccal mucosa

Collection of submandibular gland saliva

In the past particularly, submandibular gland saliva was collected by catheterizing the submandibular duct after dilatation. This technique is neither very simple nor comfortable for the patient. Segregator appliances require to be purpose-made to fit the patient's mouth and function in the same way as the Carlson-Crittenden cup. The device, which fits the anterior floor of the mouth, has a central collecting chamber, isolated from the outer suction chambers by a surrounding ridge.

Advantages and disadvantages of the different methods

The choice of method depends on the type of investigation being carried out. If for example, the aim is to investigate viral shedding from the parotid gland then catheterization of the duct has to be carried out or a Carlson-Crittenden cup used.

Mandel (1980) has listed the variations in concentrations of sodium, potassium, calcium, magnesium, bicarbonate and phosphate in the secretions of individual glands and whole saliva. But his findings suggested that collection of whole saliva is satisfactory for such chemical measurements.

For straightforward measurement of salivary flow rate for confirmation of the diagnosis of Sjögren's syndrome, for example, then the simple spitting method for unstimulated saliva over a period of 10 or 15 minutes, requires minimal equipment and is satisfactory. In the past it was thought that, since the parotid glands were predominantly affected by this disease, it was necessary to collect parotid gland saliva. However, the total activity of all salivary glands including the minor glands makes a greater contribution to the amount of saliva produced under normal conditions. Stimulated parotid gland flow is unsatisfactory because of difficulties that some patients have with the collection devices and because the variety of stimulants used has caused confusion as to what is meant by abnormal flow rates. Speight, Kaul and Melson (1992) found that a whole unstimulated salivary flow rate of 0.1 ml per minute or less was 81%

predictive of Sjögren's syndrome if other causes of xerostomia could be excluded. Saliva was collected by encouraging the patients to spit gently or drool into a beaker for 15 minutes. Though controversy persists about methods of saliva collection and whether or not sialagogues should be used, there is a growing body of opinion that collection of unstimulated mixed saliva best reflects the normal resting state. The European Community Study Group on Diagnostic Criteria for Sjögren's Syndrome (Vitali, Moutosopoulos and Bombardieri, 1994) have also concluded that collection of whole unstimulated saliva is the best method for confirming the degree of xerostomia.

Radioisotope salivary function tests

Various isotopes have been used to visualize a number of organs and their ability to concentrate a particular isotope can be used to indicate function. ^{99m}Tc pertechnitate has been used for the study of salivary gland function and, with scintigraphy, an objective measure of its uptake, concentration and excretion can be made (Figure 9.7). This method of

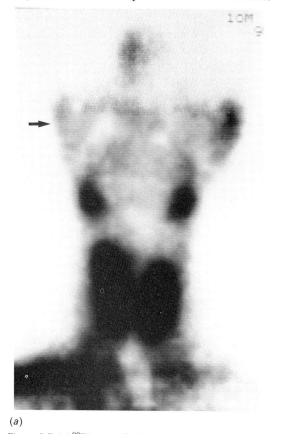

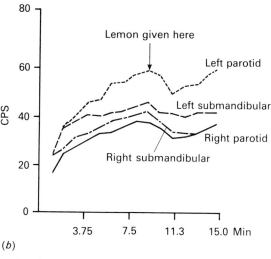

(a)   (b)

Figure 9.7 (a) ^{99m}Tc pertechnitate study undertaken in a patient with early Sjögren's syndrome. There is poor tracer accumulation in the right parotid gland (arrowed) when compared to the left parotid. (b) Following the administration of lemon drops, there is a brisk discharge of activity from the left parotid gland and the right submandibular gland, but less response from the left submandibular gland. CPS: counts per second

investigation has the advantage that both the parotid and submandibular glands can be studied at the same time. Although available for some time, this method of investigation has not met with much clinical enthusiasm.

Sialochemistry

The composition of saliva changes in disease states, particularly those causing xerostomia and these changes have been reviewed by Mandel (1990). It must be emphasized that most studies on the composition of saliva have been based on relatively few subjects and may therefore be biased. Differences in laboratory methods may also result in discrepancies in the results which are not in fact real. Other complications are the presence of enzymes which are probably of bacterial origin.

The composition of saliva in health provides a baseline for variations resulting from disease or drug administration. Unfortunately, even in healthy persons, many variables such as the following can affect the composition of saliva:

- Flow rate
- Source: saliva specifically collected from the major glands differs in composition from whole saliva which includes that secreted by the minor glands
- Diurnal variation
- Duration and type of stimulus
- Rest transients: the concentration of a molecule such as potassium may vary according to whether the saliva sample is taken shortly after stimulation or after the flow has been allowed to continue for several minutes
- Age and gender differences: findings on differences in salivary flow, and hence salivary composition, according to the age or gender of the subjects have been conflicting. Findings that, for example, salivary flow rates are lower in older women than men could conceivably be biased by the presence of unsuspected Sjögren's disease in the women
- Plasma levels: the concentration of many molecules in saliva is related to and varies with their plasma levels
- Diet: findings suggesting that a predominantly carbohydrate diet, for example, leads to higher concentrations of salivary amylase or that high protein diets lead to higher concentrations of salivary amylase have not been widely confirmed or are conflicting
- Drugs: any drug which affects salivary flow rates can affect the concentration of salivary constituents that are flow-dependent. Important drugs which affect salivary flow rates are shown in Table 9.1
- Hormonal effects: mineralocorticosteroids affect both plasma and salivary concentrations of molecules such as sodium and bicarbonate. It has also been suggested that the concentration of some salivary constituents such as calcium and sodium may fall and potassium levels rise at the time of ovulation.

The major constituents of saliva are shown in Table 9.2 but in view of the comments already made,

Table 9.2 Composition of mixed saliva

Substance	Unstimulated		Stimulated	
	Mean ± s.d.	Range	Mean ± s.d.	Range
Protein (g/l)		1.4–6.4	2.8	1.8–4.2
IgA (mg/l)	194.0			
IgG (mg/l)	14.4			
IgM (mg/l)	2.1			
Amylase (g/l)	0.38 ± 0.08			
Lysozyme (mg/l)			108.9 ± 129.1	3.7–625
Carbonic anhydrase (K/l)			2100	
Histamine (mg/l)	0.15	0.11–0.18		
Glucose (mmol/l)	0.55 ±	0.048	0.056	0.02–0.17
Urea (mmol/l)	3.22 ± 2.5	2.33–12.5	2.17	0.1–4.8
Creatinine (mg/l)	0.09	0.05–0.18		
Cholesterol (mg/l)	0.2	0.07–1.3		
Sodium (mmol/l)	6.2 ± 0.46		26.4 ± 11.8	
Potassium (mmol/l)	21.6 ± 1.2		19.7 ± 3.9	
Calcium (mmol/l)	1.56 ± 0.06		1.48 ± 0.04	
Magnesium (mmol/l)	0.21 ± 0.01		0.15 ± 0.04	
Phosphate (mmol/l)	6.2			
Chloride (mmol/l)	17.4 ± 1.4		29.0 ± 8.8	
Iodide (μmol/l)	0.8	0 –3		1–3
Fluoride (μmol/l)	15 ± 0.68	0.5–3	0.56 ± 0.25	0.25–1.2

1/9/14 *Anatomy and physiology of the salivary glands*

these figures should be accepted with caution. Changes in the concentration of inorganic ions have been documented in the following conditions (Mandel, 1980):

- Sialadenitis: raised Na^+, K^+, Ca^{++} and P^+ levels
- Radiation damage: raised Na^+, Ca^{++}, Mg^{++} and Cl^- levels
- Sjögren's syndrome: raised Na^+, Cl^- and P^+ in parotid gland saliva
- Cystic fibrosis: raised Na^+, Ca^{++} and P^+ levels. Mandel (1980) suggested that the combined Ca^{++} and P^+ concentrations formed a useful diagnostic index
- Aldosteronism: depressed Na^+ but raised K^+ levels. Mandel (1980) suggested that the product Na^+/K^+ could form a useful diagnostic index
- Hypertension: depressed Na^+ levels
- Alcoholic cirrhosis: raised K^+ levels
- Hyperparathyroidism: raised Ca^{++} levels
- Diabetes mellitus: raised Ca^{++} levels
- Chronic pancreatitis: depressed HCO_3^- levels
- Psychiatric illness: possibly raised Na^+ levels
- Digitalis intoxication: raised Na^+ and K^+ levels. Mandel (1980) suggested that the product, $Na^+ \times K^+$, could form a useful diagnostic index.

Changes in the concentration of the organic components have been found in the following:

- Sjögren's syndrome: raised total protein and β_2 microglobulin levels in parotid gland saliva
- Cystic fibrosis: raised total proteins, amylase, lysozyme in submandibular gland saliva and glycoproteins in parotid gland saliva
- Cirrhosis: raised total protein and amylase in parotid gland saliva
- Hyperparathyroidism: raised total protein
- Diabetes mellitus: raised total protein, IgA, IgG and IgM and raised glucose levels
- Sarcoidosis: depressed amylase and lysozyme levels.

Two diseases that have been studied in terms of sialochemistry in particular detail are Sjögren's syndrome and cystic fibrosis.

Sjögren's syndrome

Considerable difficulties are sometimes found in confirming the diagnosis of Sjögren's syndrome because of the great variability in the abnormalities that may be detected. The problem is well illustrated by the necessity to institute the European Community Study Group on Diagnostic Criteria for Sjögren's Syndrome (Vitali, Moutosopoulos and Bombardieri, 1994). The Group concluded in its 1994 report, that unstimulated whole saliva flow rate and minor salivary gland

biopsy are two of the most valuable diagnostic tests. Neither involves exposure to X-rays nor scintigraphy.

Mandel (1990) has noted that salivary function changes, in addition to a lowered secretion rate, include raised sodium and chloride but lowered phosphate; raised lactoferrin; raised β_2 microglobulin; raised kallikrein concentrations; and a 20-fold elevation in the concentration of phospholipids. Parotid gland lysozyme was also found to be raised in primary but not in secondary Sjögren's syndrome. Such changes could be useful as screening tests that could indicate whether labial gland biopsy or other tests were indicated but perhaps more important, for monitoring disease progress.

Cystic fibrosis

Although all exocrine gland function is affected, the clinical effects on salivary gland function are minimal, but there are significant changes in salivary composition. In particular there are dramatic elevations in salivary protein and calcium concentrations. The complexing of these substances leads to obvious turbidity of the saliva. This is such as to obstruct the excretory ducts of the minor salivary glands. Their greatly depressed secretion rate can be measured in the accessible labial glands with a capillary tube.

Antibacterial substances in saliva

The function of substances such as lysozyme and lactoferrin secreted by the salivary epithelium and which have antibacterial activity *in vitro* is unclear. Other factors which might affect bacterial activity in the oral cavity are the pH and buffering capacity of saliva and its content of immunoglobulins.

Despite the presence of these substances, the oral cavity supports a flourishing population of microbes including a great variety of pathogens. Dental caries is usually also active on a high sugar diet and periodontal disease is likely to progress unless a high standard of oral hygiene is maintained. Despite great efforts to show protection against these diseases by saliva, the findings have been unconvincing. Moreover salivary mucins for example, may have harmful effects by promoting adhesion of bacteria to the teeth. That aside, putative effects of protective substances are difficult to substantiate in humans because of the difficulty of performing the critical experiments.

It is clear that the oral cavity has a high level of local immunity. The large bony wounds resulting from extraction of teeth normally heal rapidly despite contamination by the vast and pathogenic flora that proliferates in periodontal pockets. However, this fortunate outcome is likely to result from local tissue immunity rather than from salivary components.

Another factor which may affect the nature of the bacterial flora of the mouth is bacterial competition for nutrients in their individual ecological niches. The bacterial flora of the mouth is undoubtedly affected by low salivary flow rates which, in particular, promote cariogenic activity and the proliferation of *Candida* species. Nevertheless, xerostomia does not appear to promote periodontal disease.

The only aspect of saliva production that can be reliably related to protection against infection is that of the overall flow rate. In conditions of xerostomia, the oral bacterial flora changes and in particular *Candida albicans* and staphylococci are likely to flourish. Dental caries activity and mucosal infections are promoted. From the clinical viewpoint therefore, the main contribution of saliva to defence against infection appears to be the largely mechanical effect of its flow washing down microbes into the gastric acid.

Salivary assays in diagnosis

Saliva is undoubtedly a valid medium for many diagnostic assays. Collection of saliva is non-invasive, painless and obviates the risk of needle-stick injuries. Nevertheless, most clinicians are unused to collecting saliva but practised in collecting blood which can usually be achieved more quickly. Moreover, most laboratories use equipment for handling blood and are unused to dealing with saliva with its mucins and other constituents or contaminants which may affect the assays. With regard to drug assays, few current pharmacology texts even mention the possibility of using saliva.

Hormone monitoring

Lipid-soluble, unconjugated steroids pass readily into saliva and their concentrations are proportional to the concentrations of free, unbound steroids in plasma as discussed by Ferguson (1987). Read (1993) has discussed the current status of salivary oestrogen and androgen measurement. An informative light on the limitations of salivary hormone measurements is cast by the problems of salivary dehydroepiandrosterone sulphate assay (DHA-S). The salivary concentration of this hormone is only about 0.1% of that in plasma and is a poor predictor of plasma levels in an individual or a particular plasma sample. The inconsistencies arise from the fact that the concentration in parotid gland fluid is particularly low. Most salivary DHA-S probably therefore comes from blood in gingival exudate. The fall in DHA-S

concentrations with high salivary flow rates helps to confirm this possibility. If this is the case, concentrations of DHA-S in saliva depend largely on the degree of contamination and, as has been shown, are affected by the oral conditions in the person being tested and the method of saliva collection. Read (1993) concluded that salivary assays for testosterone in men, androstenedione and oestriol in particular, were valuable but considered that the value of salivary testosterone and oestradiol in women remained unproven.

Ellison (1993) has considered certain technical aspects of salivary progesterone assay and their interpretation, and reviewed the utility of these assays for clinical purposes, particularly for the diagnosis and treatment of infertility. Salivary progesterone levels are valid indicators of plasma levels and Ellison (1993) concluded that their assay was particularly valuable because of the ease of obtaining serial samples from the same individual. On a shorter time scale, salivary monitoring could provide samples at short intervals for characterization of pulsatile progesterone patterns without the inconvenience and expense of hospitalization. The ability to adapt salivary progesterone monitoring under field conditions has also made possible basic research on a wide scale into human reproductive biology. Ellison's (1993) concerns were the need for standardized laboratory procedures, methods of data reduction and analysis, recognized reference ranges, and statistics on diagnostic efficiency. Further, the low absolute levels of steroids in saliva placed a premium on an unusually high level of quality control in the laboratory.

Testosterone is a hormone that may, in addition, affect social behaviour. Assay of testosterone in saliva provides a valuable method for field studies. Dabbs (1993) has summarized the preliminary findings on differences in salivary testosterone levels both between and within individuals. Studies on individual differences are being carried out in relation to violent and antisocial behaviour, occupational achievement and everyday behaviour. Studies on changing testosterone levels have been undertaken on winning sports contests, winning non-athletic events, winning political contests, 'winning' games of sex, and vicarious winning (sports spectators). Broadly speaking, it appeared that salivary testosterone levels fell in losers and were unchanged or rose in winners according to the importance of the victory. While animal studies confirmed elevations of testosterone with real or anticipated sexual activity, there were considerable difficulties in obtaining samples at appropriate times in humans. However, it appeared that testosterone levels were higher on evenings when there was sexual activity, particularly in females, and low in its absence. Studies on salivary testosterone levels under conditions of abuse, depression and suicide are also in progress.

Drug monitoring in saliva

Jusko and Milsap (1993) have discussed the pharma-cokinetics of drug distribution in saliva. They showed that the primary properties of a drug which determined its entry into saliva were molecular size, lipid solubility, pK_a, and protein binding. However, salivary flow rates, the time of sampling and disease states which altered saliva composition could affect the results.

Haeckel (1993) has summarized some of the reasons for the failure to use saliva to any great extent for therapeutic drug monitoring as follows:

1 Blood has to be sampled anyhow for other electrolytes
2 There are technical difficulties with sampling saliva
3 There are existing difficulties with the interpretation of salivary drug concentrations.

The remaining applications for saliva sampling were therefore:

1 When sampling at home is required
2 Special cases where the sample is taken only for the monitoring of a particular drug
3 Circumstances where the sample volume is critical, e.g. in newborns.

Nevertheless, if a constant saliva/plasma ratio can be established, use of saliva for therapeutic drug monitoring becomes a clinically useful possibility and Siegel (1993) has pointed out that the saliva/plasma ratios for at least 170 drugs have been established experimentally. Drugs which can be monitored in saliva include digitalis, phenytoin, primidone, ethosuximide, carbamazepine, theophylline, caffeine, lithium, methadone, cyclosporin, marijuana, cocaine and alcohol.

A related use for salivary drug monitoring is for detection of drugs of abuse as described by Cone (1993) who reviewed the findings for alcohol, amphetamines, barbiturates, benzodiazepines, caffeine, cocaine, inhalants such as general anaesthetic agents as well as solvents, LSD, marijuana, opioids, phencyclidine and tobacco.

Salivary monitoring of microbial antigens and antibodies

Viral hepatitis

In view of the hazard to surgeons, a simple method of detecting carriers of hepatitis viruses has obvious benefits. The presence of hepatitis B antigen in saliva was demonstrated by Brodersen *et al.* (1974). Shikata *et al.* (1985) were able to detect the surface antigen (HBsAg) and the core antigen in hepatocytes, but could not detect it in parotid gland parenchymal cells. However, in the patient with the highest serum titre of HBsAg, immunoreactivity was detected in the vascular wall and luminal fluid of the parotid gland. Piacentini *et al.* (1993) have reported high sensitivity and specificity in the diagnosis of hepatitis A, B and C using the OraSure collection system, and that the samples had titres of antibodies to viral hepatitis that were similar to those of the serum.

HIV infection

Malamud (1992) has made a strong plea for use of saliva as a diagnostic fluid for the detection of antibodies to HIV, among other purposes. For detection of carriage of antibodies to HIV, saliva testing is a simple non-invasive method and presents enormous advantages. It removes the risk of needle-stick injuries and the emotional connotations of blood sampling in this alarming disease. Salivary sampling has special advantages when investigating children because of the great ease of collection. Archibald *et al.* (1993) have described the practical applications for saliva testing for perinatal HIV diagnosis. Only a minority of infants born to HIV-positive mothers develop HIV infection, but in the neonatal period, usually carry passively transferred antibodies to HIV from the mother. However, it is believed that IgA and IgM antibodies do not cross the placenta. To assess the value of an IgA-specific Western blot assay, Archibald *et al.* (1993) collected blood and saliva from 95 infants and children born to HIV-infected women. Saliva samples from infants were collected by gentle aspiration from the buccal sulcus. The total sensitivity of the salivary assay for detecting antibodies to HIV gp160 antigens was 50% of infants less than 12 months old and 97.3% for infants over 12 months. The earliest age for detection of serum IgA antibodies to HIV is believed to be 2 months. Salivary IgA antibodies were detected by Archibald *et al.* (1993) in an infected infant at 6 months but had been negative at 4 months. Reliable salivary detection of HIV infection in the immediate neonatal period awaits more sensitive methods. However, if these can be found, saliva sampling for antibodies to HIV, particularly for infants and children is a potentially valuable method. Saliva collection does not require skilled personnel, avoids the need for repeated venepunctures and is ideal for studies in developing countries.

Monitoring of immunization status

Thieme *et al.* (1994) have used salivary sampling for measles, mumps and rubella immunization status. Saliva was collected using the OraSure system. Antibodies in oral fluid specimens correlated with levels of sensitivity and specificity to the following degree: measles 97% and 100% respectively; mumps 94% and 94% respectively and rubella 96% and 98% respectively.

References

ARCHIBALD, D. W., ZON, L., GROOPMAN, J. E., MCLANE, M. F. and ESSEX, M. (1986) Antibodies to human T-lymphotrophic virus type III (HTLV-III) in saliva of acquired immunodeficiency syndrome (AIDS) patients and in persons at risk for AIDS. *Blood*, 67, 831–834

ARCHIBALD, D. W., FARLEY, J. J., HEBERT, C. A., HINES, S. E., NAIR, P. and JOHNSON, J. P. (1993) Practical applications for saliva in perinatal HIV diagnosis. *Annals of the New York Academy of Science*, 694, 195–201

BAUM, J. B. (1993) Principles of saliva secretion. *Annals of the New York Academy of Science*, 694, 17–23

BRODERSEN, M., STEGMANN, S., KLEIN, K. H., TRÜLZSCH, D. and RESHSCH, P. (1974) Salivary HBAg detected by radioimmunoassay. *Lancet*, i, 675–676

BROWN, T. A. and MESTECKY, J. (1985) Immunoglobulin A subclass distribution of naturally occurring salivary antibodies to microbial antigens. *Infection and Immunity*, 49, 459–462

BUSFIELD, B. J. and WECHSLER, H. (1961) Studies of salivation in depression. *Archives of General Psychiatry*, 4, 10–15

BUSFIELD, B. J., WECHSLER, H. and BARNUM, W. J. (1961) Studies of salivation in depression. *Archives of General Psychiatry*, 5, 76–81

CONE, E. J. (1993) Saliva testing for drugs of abuse. *Annals of the New York Academy of Science*, 694, 91–127

CONE, E. J. and WEDDINGTON, W. W. JR (1989) Prolonged occurrence of cocaine in human saliva and urine after chronic use. *Journal of Analytical Toxicology*, 13, 65–68.

CORDEIRO, M. L., TURPIN, C. S. and MCADAMS, S. A. (1993) A comparative study of saliva and OraSure oral fluid. *Annals of the New York Academy of Science*, 694, 330–331

DABBS, J. M. JR (1993) Salivary testosterone measurements in behavioral studies. *Annals of the New York Academy of Science*, 694, 177–183

DAVIS, R. A., ANSON, B. J., BUDINGER, J. M. and KURTH, R. E. (1956) Surgical anatomy of the facial nerve and parotid gland based upon a study of 350 cervicofacial halves. *Surgery, Gynecology and Obsterics*, 102, 385–412

ELLISON, P. T. (1993) Measurements of salivary progesterone. *Annals of the New York Academy of Science*, 694, 161–176

ERICSON, S. (1969) An investigation of human parotid saliva secretion rate in response to different types of stimulation. *Archives of Oral Biology*, 14, 591–594

FERGUSON, D. B. (1987) Current diagnostic uses of saliva. *Journal of Dental Research*, 66, 420–424

GARRETT, J. R. (1987) The proper role of nerves in salivary secretion: a review. *Journal of Dental Research*, 66, 387–397

HAECKEL, R. (1993) Factors influencing the saliva/plasma concentration of drugs. *Annals of the New York Academy of Science*, 694, 128–142

JUSKO, W. J. and MILSAP, R. L. (1993) Pharmacokinetic principles of drug distribution in saliva. *Annals of the New York Academy of Science*, 694, 36–47

KATZ, A. D. and CATALANO, P. (1987) The clinical significance of the various anastomotic branches of the facial nerve. *Archives of Otolaryngology – Head and Neck Surgery*, 113, 959–962

KIRSHBAUM, C. and HELHAMMER, D. (1989) Response variability of salivary cortisol under psychological stimulation *Journal of Clinical Chemistry and Clinical Biochemistry*, 27, 237

MCKEAN, M. E., LEE, K. and MCGREGOR, I. A. (1985) The distribution of lymph nodes in and around the parotid gland: an anatomical study. *British Journal of Plastic Surgery*, 38, 1–5

MALAMUD, D. (1992) Saliva as a diagnostic fluid. Second now to blood? *British Medical Journal*, 305, 207

MANDEL, I. D. (1980) Sialochemistry in diseases and clinical situations affecting salivary glands. *CRC Critical Reviews of Clinical and Laboratory Science*, 12, 321–366

MANDEL, I. D. (1990) The diagnostic uses of saliva. *Journal of Oral Pathology and Medicine*, 19, 119–125

MANDEL, I. D. (1993) Salivary diagnosis: Promises, Promises. *Annals of the New York Academy of Science*, 694, 1–10

MASON, D. K. and CHISHOLM, D. M. (1975) *Salivary Glands in Health and Disease.* London: W. B. Saunders

MIEHLKE, A., STENNERT, E. and CHILLA, R. (1979) New aspects in facial nerve surgery. *Clinical Plastic Surgery*, 6, 451–454

NAVESH, M. (1993) Methods for collecting saliva. *Annals of the New York Academy of Science*, 694, 72–77

NORTH, L. M., GAUDETTE, N. D., CORDEIRO, M. L., FITCHEN, J. H., DAVIDSON, S. L. and HIDAHL, M. S. (1993) Detection of cotinine in oral fluid recovered with the OraSure collection system. *Annals of the New York Academy of Science*, 694, 332–333

PARRY, J. V., PERRY, K. R. and MORTIMER, P. P. (1987) Sensitive assays for viral antibodies in saliva: an alternative to tests on serum. *Lancet*, ii, 72–75

PIACENTINI, S. C., THIEME, T. R., BELLER, M. and DAVIDSON, S. L. (1993) Diagnosis of hepatitis A, B and C using oral samples. *Annals of the New York Academy of Science*, 694, 334–336

READ, G. F. (1993) Status report on measurement of salivary estrogens and androgens. *Annals of the New York Academy of Science*, 694, 146–159

READ, G. F., WILSON, D. W., HUGHES, I. A. and GRIFFITHS, K. (1984) The use of salivary progesterone assays in the assessment of ovarian function in post menarcheal girls. *Journal of Endocrinology*, 102, 265–268

SCHRAMM, W., ANNESLEY, T. M., SIEGEL, G. J., SACKELLARES, J. C. and SMITH, R. H. (1991) Measurement of phenytoin and carbamazepine in an ultrafiltrate of saliva. *Therapeutic Drug Monitoring*, 13, 452–460

SCHRAMM, W., SMITH, R. H., CRAIG, P. A. and KIDWELL, D. A. (1992) Drugs of abuse in saliva: a review. *Journal of Analytical Toxicology*, 16, 1–9

SHIKATA, H., SUZUKI, K., HENMI, A., USHIYAMA, H., UCIDA, T., UTSUMI, N. *et al.* (1985) Localization of hepatitis B surface antigen in the human parotid gland. *Oral Surgery, Oral Medicine and Oral Pathology*, 59, 58–62

SHIP, J. A., PATTON, L. L. and TYLENDA, C. A. (1991) An assessment of salivary gland function in healthy premenopausal and postmenopausal females. *Journal of Gerontology*, 46, M11–13

SIEGEL, I. A. (1993) The role of saliva in drug monitoring. *Annals of the New York Academy of Science*, 694, 86–90

SMITH, D. J., EBERSOLE, J. L., TAUBMAN, M. A. and GADALLA, L. (1985) Salivary IgA antibody to *Actinobacillus actinomycetemcomitans* in a young adult population. *Journal of Periodontal Research*, 20, 8–11

SPEIGHT, P. M., KAUL, A. and MELSON, R. D. (1992) Measurement of whole unstimulated salivary flow in the diagnosis of Sjögren's syndrome. *Annals of the Rheumatic Diseases*, 51, 499–502

THIEME, T. R., PIACENTINI, S., DAVIDSON, S. and STEINGART, K. (1994) Determination of measles, mumps and rubella immunization status using oral fluid samples. *Journal of the American Medical Association*, **272**, 219–221

TURNER, R. J. (1993) Mechanisms of secretion by salivary glands. *Annals of the New York Academy of Science*, **694**, 24–35

VITALI, C., MOUTOSOPOULOS, H. M., BOMBARDIERI, S. and THE EUROPEAN COMMUNITY STUDY GROUP (1994) Diagnostic criteria for Sjögren's syndrome. *Annals of the Rheumatic Diseases*, **53**, 637–647

10

Anatomy of the pharynx and oesophagus

P. Beasley

Embryological development

During the development of the embryo, a process of cephalocaudal and lateral folding takes place with the result that part of the endoderm-lined cavity of the secondary or definitive yolk sac is incorporated into the embryo to form the primitive gut. In the cephalic part of the embryo, the primitive gut forms a blind ending tube, the foregut, separated from the ectodermally lined stomatodaeum by the buccopharyngeal membrane (Figure 10.1). Towards the end of the first month (23–25 days, 10–14 somite stage), the foregut comes to lie dorsal to the developing

heart tube and to the developing septum transversum (developing diaphragm). Shortly afterwards (26–27 days, 20 somite stage), the buccopharyngeal membrane ruptures and the stomatodaeum becomes continuous with the foregut. The approximate relationship between the age of the embryo, and the number of somites is given in Table 10.1.

Table 10.1 Approximate relationship between age of embryo and number of somites

Approximate age (days)	No. of somites	Approximate age (days)	No. of somites
20	1–4	25	17–20
21	4–7	26	20–23
22	7–10	27	23–26
23	10–13	28	26–29
24	13–17	30	34–35

The endodermal lining of the foregut differentiates into a number of different structures which can be summarized as follows:
1 Part of the nasal cavities
2 The endodermally lined part of the buccal cavity
3 The pharynx, together with the glands and other structures derived from it, namely the anterior lobe of the pituitary gland, the thyroid, thymus and parathyroid glands, the ultimobranchial body, the pharyngotympanic (eustachian) tube, the middle ear and the tonsils
4 The submandibular and sublingual salivary glands
5 The larynx, trachea, bronchi and lungs
6 The oesophagus
7 The stomach
8 The duodenum as far as the liver diverticulum.

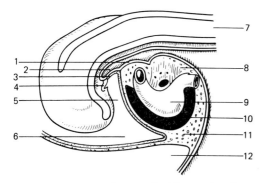

Figure 10.1 A diagram of a sagittal midline section of a 23–25 day (14 somite) embryo to show the position of the foregut and stomatodaeum, separated by the buccopharyngeal membrane

1 Tracheobronchial diverticulum	6 Amniotic cavity
2 Foregut	7 Neural tube
3 Buccopharyngeal membrane	8 Mesocardium
4 Rathke's pouch	9 Heart tube
5 Stomatodaeum	10 Pericardial cavity
	11 Septum transversum
	12 Yolk sac

The development of the cephalic portion of the primitive gut and its derivatives will be discussed in two sections: (1) the pharyngeal gut or pharynx extending from the buccopharyngeal membrane to the tracheobronchial diverticulum; (2) the foregut, lying caudal to the tracheobronchial diverticulum from which the oesophagus develops.

Pharynx (pharyngeal gut)

The development of the branchial or pharyngeal arches in the fifth week provides one of the most characteristic external features of the head and neck region of the embryo. They consist initially of bars of mesenchymal tissue separated by deep clefts known as branchial or pharyngeal clefts. At the same time as the arches and clefts develop on the outside, a number of depressions (the pharyngeal pouches) appear within the pharyngeal gut along the lateral wall. The pouches and clefts gradually penetrate the surrounding mesenchyme but, in spite of there being only a small amount of mesenchyme between the ectodermal and endodermal layers, open communication is not established. Therefore, although these developments resemble the formation of gill slits in fishes, in the human embryo real gills, or branchia, are not formed and the term 'pharyngeal arches' rather than branchial arches has been used in this description (Sadler, 1990). The pharyngeal arches contribute not only to the formation of the neck and pharynx, but to the development of the head (see Chapters 5 and 8). By the end of the fourth week, the stomatodaeum is surrounded by the first pair of pharyngeal arches in the form of the mandibular swellings caudally, and the maxillary swellings laterally, which are the dorsal portion of the first arch. The development of the pharyngeal arches, pouches and clefts, with their derivatives, is discussed separately.

Pharyngeal arches

Each pharyngeal arch is made up of a core of mesodermal tissue covered on the outside by surface ectoderm and on the inside by epithelium derived from endoderm. The core of the arch has, in addition to local mesenchyme, substantial numbers of crest cells which migrate into the arches to contribute to the skeletal components of the face. The original mesoderm of each arch differentiates into a cartilaginous bar and muscular component together with an arterial component. Each arch receives afferent and efferent nerves to supply the skin, musculature and endodermal lining. The muscular components of each arch have their own nerve and, wherever the muscular cells migrate, they carry their own cranial nerve component (Figure 10.2). In addition, each arch receives a branch from the nerve of the succeeding arch. The arrangement of the nerve supply to each

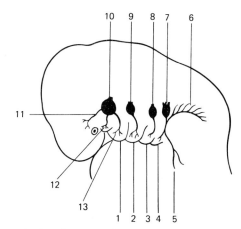

Figure 10.2 A diagram to show the cranial nerve supply to the pharyngeal arches. (Modified from Sadler, T.W., 1990, *Langman's Medical Embryology*, 6th edn, Williams and Wilkins by courtesy of the publisher)

1 First arch (mandibular)	8 Glossopharyngeal
2 Second arch (hyoid)	nerve
3 Third arch	9 Facial nerve
4 Fourth arch	10 Trigeminal nerve and
5 Vagus nerve	ganglion
6 Spinal root of	11 Ophthalmic branch of V
accessory	12 Maxillary branch of V
7 Cranial root of	13 Mandibular branch of
accessory nerve	V

arch is a relic of the pattern found in vertebrates at a time when the nerve to the gill region was distributed cranial and caudal to the corresponding gill cleft. As a result, in man and in mammals generally, each arch receives a branch, called the post-trematic, from the nerve of its own arch; and a second branch, called the pre-trematic, from the succeeding arch. This is illustrated in Table 10.2.

Table 10.2 Arch and nerve arrangement

Arch	Post-trematic nerve	Pre-trematic nerve
1st	Mandibular nerve (V)	Chorda tympani branch of VII
2nd	Facial nerve (VII)	Tympanic branch of IX (Jacobson's nerve)
3rd	Glossopharyngeal (IX)	
4th 5th 6th	Vagus (X) and accessory (XI) nerves via superior and recurrent laryngeal and pharyngeal branches	Pretrematic nerves not well defined in man

At the end of the first month (30–32 days, 34–35 somites), the floor of the foregut shows a number of elevations produced by the mesodermal condensations and separated by depressions (Figure 10.3). The first arch of each side forms an elevation in the side wall of the foregut and the elevations meet in the midline. A small medial elevation, the tuberculum impar, is seen immediately caudal to the middle part of the mandibular swelling. Caudal to the tuberculum impar is a small median depression, the foramen caecum, which marks the site of the invagination which will give rise to the median primordium of the thyroid gland. The second arch of each side is continuous across the midline of the foregut floor. Immediately caudal to the second arch, a second and larger medial swelling develops, the hypobranchial eminence. The third and fourth arches fail to reach the midline owing to the presence of this eminence. The fifth arch makes a transitory appearance only. Caudal to the hypobranchial eminence, a tracheobronchial groove develops in the midline, the lateral boundary of which is the rudimentary sixth arch. From this groove, there develops the lining epithelia and associated glands of the larynx, trachea, bronchi and, possibly, the respiratory epithelium of the alveoli.

The development of the tongue is described in Chapter 8. In the course of this development, there is a caudal migration of the hypobranchial eminence and a relative reduction in its size. At the same time, it comes to be more transversely placed behind the developing tongue, but still remains attached to the side wall of the pharynx by part of the third arch tissue, which becomes the lateral glossoepiglottic fold of the adult. The groove between the dorsum of the tongue and the epiglottis, the glossoepiglottic groove is divided into the two valleculae by the appearance of a median glossoepiglottic fold. The poorly developed swellings which lie each side of the tracheobronchial diverticulum become the arytenoid swellings.

First pharyngeal arch

The cartilage of the first pharyngeal arch consists of a dorsal portion known as the maxillary process, and a ventral portion, the mandibular process or Meckel's cartilage (Figure 10.4). As development proceeds, both the maxillary process and Meckel's cartilage disappear except for small portions at their dorsal ends which form the incus and malleus respectively, together with the sphenomandibular ligament (Figure 10.5). Membranous ossification subsequently takes place in the mesenchyme of the maxillary process to give rise to the premaxilla, maxilla, zygomatic bone and part of the temporal bone. The mandible is formed in a similar way by membranous ossification in the mesenchymal tissue surrounding Meckel's cartilage.

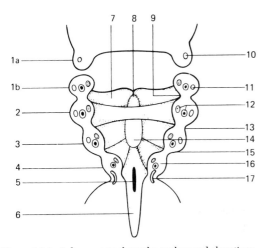

Figure 10.3 A diagram to show the arches and elevations on the floor of the foregut

1a First arch, maxillary process
1b First arch, mandibular process
2 Second pharyngeal arch
3 Third pharyngeal arch
4 Fourth pharyngeal arch
5 Tracheobronchial diverticulum
6 Oesophagus
7 Endodermal lining
8 Tuberculum impar

9 First pharyngeal pouch
10 Maxillary nerve
11 Mandibular nerve
12 Cartilage and artery
13 Second pharyngeal cleft
14 Hypobranchial eminence
15 Ectodermal covering
16 Mesenchyme in fourth arch
17 Superior laryngeal nerve

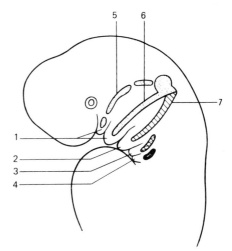

Figure 10.4 A diagram to illustrate the cartilages of the pharyngeal arches. Derivatives are indicated in Figure 10.5. (Modified from Sadler, T.W., 1990, *Langman's Medical Embryology*, 6th edn, Williams and Wilkins, by courtesy of the publisher)

1 First arch
2 Second arch
3 Third arch
4 Fourth arch

5 Maxillary process
6 Meckel's cartilage
7 Reichert's cartilage

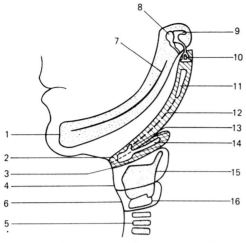

Figure 10.5 A diagram to show the derivatives of the pharyngeal arch cartilages. (Modified from Sadler, T.W., 1990, *Langman's Medical Embryology*, 6th edn, Williams and Wilkins, by courtesy of the publisher)

1 First arch cartilage	11 Styloid process
2 Second arch cartilage	12 Stylohyoid ligament
3 Third arch cartilage	13 Lesser horn and upper
4 Fourth arch cartilage	body of hyoid bone
5 Tracheal rings	14 Greater horn and
6 Sixth arch cartilage	lower body of hyoid
7 Meckel's cartilage	bone
8 Malleus	15 Thyroid cartilage
9 Incus	16 Cricoid cartilage
10 Stapes	

The musculature of the first pharyngeal arch develops to form the muscles of mastication (temporalis, masseter, medial and lateral pterygoids), as well as the anterior belly of the digastric, the mylohyoid, the tensor tympani and tensor palati. Although the muscles are not always attached to the bony or cartilaginous components of their own arch, because of migration into surrounding regions, the arch of origin can always be traced by way of the nerve supply which comes from the original arch. In the case of the first arch, this nerve supply is provided by the mandibular branch of the trigeminal nerve (see Figure 10.2). The same nerve provides an afferent or sensory supply to the skin and endodermal lining of this arch.

Second pharyngeal arch

The cartilage of the second or hyoid arch (Reichert's cartilage) (see Figure 10.4) gives rise to the stapes, the styloid process of the temporal bone, the stylohyoid ligament and, ventrally, the lesser horn and the upper part of the body of the hyoid bone (see Figure 10.5). The muscles of this arch are the stapedius, the stylohyoid, the posterior belly of the digastric, the auricular muscles and the muscles of facial expres-

sion. They are supplied by the facial nerve which is the nerve of this arch.

Third pharyngeal arch

The cartilage of the third arch gives rise to the lower part of the body and the greater horn of the hyoid bone (see Figures 10.4 and 10.5). The caudal part of the arch cartilage disappears. The muscle of the arch is the stylopharyngeus supplied by the glossopharyngeal nerve, the nerve of the third arch.

Fourth and sixth pharyngeal arches

The remaining anterior parts of the cartilages of the fourth and sixth arches fuse to form the thyroid, cricoid, arytenoid, corniculate and cuneiform cartilages of the larynx (see Figure 10.5). The fifth arch only makes a transitory appearance as indicated previously. The muscles of the fourth arch are the cricothyroid, the levator palati and the constrictors of the pharynx. They are innervated by the vagus nerve, the nerve of the fourth arch, through its superior laryngeal branch and its contribution to the pharyngeal plexus. The recurrent laryngeal branch of the vagus, the nerve of the sixth arch, innervates the intrinsic muscles of the larynx.

Pharyngeal pouches

In the human embryo, there are five pairs of pharyngeal pouches, although the last one of these is often considered as part of the fourth. Each pouch has a ventral and dorsal section. The epithelial endodermal lining of the pouches gives rise to a number of derivatives that have functions very different from those of primitive gill slits.

First pharyngeal pouch

The dorsal part of the first pouch, with the adjacent pharyngeal wall and part of the dorsal portion of the second pouch, produces a diverticulum, the tubotympanic recess, which comes into contact with the ectodermal epithelial lining of the first pharyngeal cleft, the future external auditory meatus (Figure 10.6). The distal portion of the tubotympanic recess widens to form the primitive tympanic or middle ear cavity, whereas the proximal, stalk-like part, forms the pharyngotympanic (eustachian) tube. The ventral part of the first pouch is obliterated by the development of the tongue.

Second pharyngeal pouch

As indicated previously, only a portion of the dorsal part of the second pouch takes part in the development of the pharyngotympanic tube. The remainder of this portion is absorbed into the dorsal pharyngeal

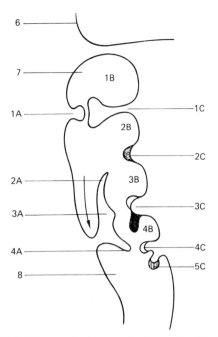 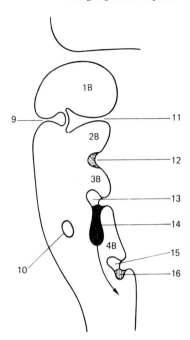

Figure 10.6 A diagram to show the development and derivatives of the pharyngeal pouches and clefts. Note the way in which the second, third and fourth clefts are buried and, if not obliterated, form the cervical sinus. (Modified from Sadler, T.W., 1990, *Langman's Medical Embryology*, 6th edn, Williams and Wilkins, by courtesy of the publisher)

1A First cleft	3C Third pouch	9 External auditory meatus
1B First arch	4A Fourth cleft	10 Superior parathyroid gland
1C First pouch	4B Fourth arch	11 Pharyngotympanic tube
2A Second cleft	4C Fourth pouch	12 Palatine tonsil
2B Second arch	5C Fifth pouch	13 Inferior parathyroid gland
2C Second pouch	6 Maxillary process	14 Thymus
3A Third cleft	7 Mandibular process	15 Superior parathyroid gland
3B Third arch	8 Epicardial ridge	16 Ultimobranchial body

wall. The ventral portion of the second pouch is almost completely obliterated by the proliferation of its endodermal epithelial lining which forms buds that penetrate into the surrounding mesenchyme. These buds are secondarily invaded by mesodermal tissue forming the primordium of the palatine tonsil (Figure 10.6). Part of the pouch persists as the intra-tonsillar cleft or fossa. During the third to fifth months, the tonsil is gradually invaded by lymphocytes which have either arisen *in situ* or have been derived from the blood stream. A similar invasion of the endoderm of the dorsal pharyngeal wall by lymphatic tissue forms the nasopharyngeal tonsil (adenoid). The lingual tonsil is formed by aggregations of lymphatic tissue in the dorsum of the tongue (second and third arch) and the tubal tonsil by aggregations of mesenchymal cells that are later invaded by lymphocytes.

Third pharyngeal pouch

In the fifth week, the endodermal epithelium of the dorsal section of the third pouch differentiates into parathyroid tissue which will form the inferior parathyroid gland. The ventral section of the pouch gives rise to the thymus gland (see Figure 10.6). The primordia of both these glands lose their connection with the pharyngeal wall when the thymus migrates in a caudal and medial direction, taking the parathyroid with it (Figure 10.7). The main portion of the thymus gland fuses with its counterpart from the opposite side when it takes up its final position in the thorax. The tail portion becomes thin and eventually disappears, although sometimes parts of it persist either within the thyroid gland or as isolated thymic cysts.

The parathyroid tissue of this pouch takes up its final position on the posterior surface of the thyroid gland as the inferior parathyroid gland.

Fourth pharyngeal pouch

The endodermal epithelium of the dorsal section of this pouch gives rise to the superior parathyroid gland. When this gland loses its contact with the wall of the pharynx, it attaches itself, while migrating

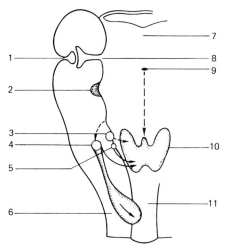

Figure 10.7 A diagram to show the migration of the thymus, parathyroid glands, and ultimobranchial body. The thyroid gland originates at the foramen caecum and descends to the level of the first tracheal ring. (Modified from Sadler, T. W., 1990, Langman's *Medical Embryology*, 6th edn, Williams and Wilkins, by courtesy of the publisher)

1 External auditory meatus
2 Palatine tonsil
3 Superior parathyroid gland from 4th pouch
4 Inferior parathyroid gland from 3rd pouch
5 Ultimobranchial body
6 Thymus
7 Ventral side of pharynx
8 Pharyngotympanic tube
9 Foramen caecum
10 Thyroid gland
11 Foregut

caudally, to the thyroid gland, and reaches its final position on the posterior surface of the thyroid as the superior parathyroid gland (Figure 10.7). The fate of the ventral section of this pouch is uncertain, although it is believed to give rise to a small amount of thymus tissue which disappears soon after its formation.

Fifth pharyngeal pouch

This is the last pharyngeal pouch to develop and is usually considered to be the ventral section of the fourth pouch. It produces the ultimobranchial body which is later incorporated into the thyroid gland (Moseley *et al.*, 1968). The cells of the ultimobranchial body give rise to the parafollicular or C cells of the thyroid gland which secrete calcitonin in the adult, a hormone involved in the regulation of the calcium level in the blood. Occasionally, the ultimobranchial body may persist and give rise to cysts.

Pharyngeal clefts

At about 5 weeks, four pharyngeal clefts can be seen on the external surface of the embryo. The dorsal section of the first cleft penetrates the underlying mesoderm and gives rise to the external auditory meatus (see Figures 10.6 and 10.7). The ectodermal epithelial lining of this cleft makes contact with the endodermal lining of the first pharyngeal pouch and participates in the formation of the tympanic membrane. The mesoderm of the second arch actively proliferates and moves caudally to overlap the third and fourth arches and intervening clefts before finally fusing with the epicardial ridge in the lower part of the neck (Figure 10.8 and see Figure 10.6). The second, third and fourth clefts then lose contact with the outside and form a temporary cavity lined with ectodermal epithelium, the cervical sinus.

Lateral cysts and fistulae of the neck (branchial cysts and fistulae)

The cervical sinus usually disappears completely, but if it does not do so, a cervical or branchial cyst persists. If the second arch fails to fuse completely with the epicardial ridge, the cervical sinus will remain in contact with the surface and be seen as a branchial fistula. These fistulae are found on the lateral aspect of the neck anteriorly to the sternomastoid muscle. It is rare for the cervical sinus to be in communication with the pharynx internally as an internal branchial fistula. The opening of this fistula is in the tonsillar region and normally indicates that there has been a rupture of the membrane between the second pharyngeal pouch and cleft (see Figure 10.8).

Foregut and oesophagus

At about 4 weeks, a small diverticulum appears on the ventral wall of the foregut at its junction with the pharyngeal gut (see Figure 10.3). This is the respiratory or tracheobronchial diverticulum. It is gradually separated from the dorsal part of the foregut, the developing oesophagus, by the formation of a partition known as the oesophagotracheal septum (Figure 10.9). The developing oesophagus comes to lie dorsal to both the developing heart and the septum transversum (diaphragm), as a result of the folding of the anterior part of the embryo. It is embedded in visceral mesoderm without any true mesentery.

The oesophagus is at first a short tube extending from the tracheobronchial diverticulum to the fusiform dilatation of the foregut, which is to become the stomach. As the heart and lungs descend caudally, the oesophagus rapidly lengthens. The muscular coat of the oesophagus is formed from the surrounding mesenchyme and in its upper two-thirds is striated and innervated by the vagus. In the lower third, the muscle coat is smooth and innervated by the splanchnic plexus. The oesophageal endodermal lining is initially of the columnar type, but this is gradually replaced by stratified squamous epithelium.

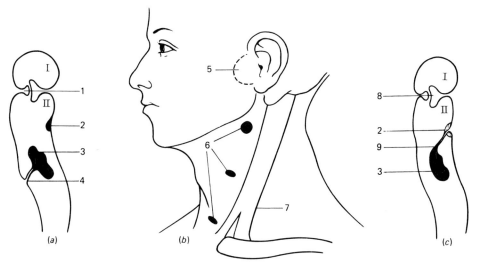

Figure 10.8 (*a*) A diagram to show a lateral cervical (branchial) cyst opening onto the surface as a fistula. (*b*) Location of cysts and fistulae anterior to the sternocleidomastoid muscle. (*c*) Internal opening of a fistula by the palatine tonsil. (Modified from Sadler, T.W., 1990, *Langman's Medical Embryology*, 6th edn, Williams and Wilkins, by courtesy of the publisher)

1 External auditory meatus
2 Palatine tonsil
3 Lateral cervical (branchial) cyst

4 External branchial fistula
5 Region of preauricular fistulae
6 Region of lateral cervical cysts and fistulae

7 Sternocleidomastoid muscle
8 Tubotympanic recess
9 Internal branchial fistula

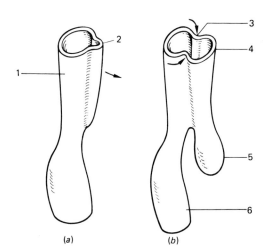

Figure 10.9 The development of the tracheobronchial (respiratory) diverticulum and oesophagus. (*a*) Laryngotracheal groove appearing in the ventral aspect of the foregut. (*b*) The lips of the groove closing in to form the oesophagotracheal septum separating the respiratory tract from the alimentary canal

1 Foregut
2 Laryngotracheal groove
3 Oesophagotracheal septum

4 Trachea
5 Lung bud
6 Stomach

Atresia of the oesophagus and oesophagotracheal fistula are thought to occur either from a spontaneous deviation of the oesophagotracheal septum in a posterior direction, or from some other mechanical factor pushing the dorsal wall of the foregut anteriorly. The most common variety is for the proximal oesophagus to end in a blind sac and for the distal part to be connected to the trachea by a narrow canal which joins it just above the bifurcation. Occasionally, the fistulous canal is replaced by a ligamentous cord. It is very unusual for both portions of the oesophagus to open into the trachea. If the oesophageal lumen is obstructed, amniotic fluid cannot pass into the intestinal tract and thus it accumulates in the amniotic sac. This is called poly-hydramnios and causes enlargement of the uterus. Once the fetus is born, atresia of the oesophagus becomes evident when drinking, resulting in over-flow into the trachea and lungs.

The pharynx
General description

The pharynx forms the crossroads of the air and food passages (Figure 10.10). Each major road from the pharynx can be closed by a muscular sphincter. The number in Table 10.3 corresponds to that in Figure 10.10.

There is a smaller passage each side from the nasal

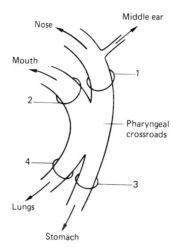

Figure 10.10 Diagram to show the pharynx as a crossroads with entrances and exits controlled by sphincters

1 Nasopharyngeal	3 Cricopharyngeal
2 Oropharyngeal	4 Laryngeal

Table 10.3 Muscles controlling the muscular sphincters in the pharynx

Sphincter	Muscles directly involved
1 Nasopharyngeal	Levator palati Superior constrictor
2 Oropharyngeal	Palatoglossus Horizontal intrinsic muscle of tongue
3 Cricopharyngeal (upper oesophageal)	Cricopharyngeus (normally closed)
4 Laryngeal	Oblique portion of interarytenoid and aryepiglottic muscles

airway, above the nasopharyngeal sphincter, leading to the middle ear; it is the pharyngotympanic or eustachian tube. This tube is normally closed, as is the cricopharyngeal or upper oesophageal sphincter.

The cavity of the pharynx is perhaps best considered as a tube flattened from front to back and with varying widths. Changes in its capacity at different levels in the resting state are best demonstrated by cross-sectional anatomy, which can now be shown by means of computerized tomographic (CT) scanning (see Chapter 17). The pharynx extends from the base of the skull to the level of the sixth cervical vertebra, a distance of about 12 cm, where it joins the oesophagus at the lower level of the cricoid cartilage (Figure 10.11). The junction is marked by the cricopharyngeus muscle which normally holds the upper oesophageal sphincter closed. The lateral and posterior walls

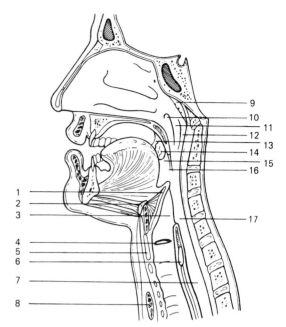

Figure 10.11 A drawing of a sagittal section through the head showing the nasal cavity, pharynx and larynx in the adult

1 Epiglottis	10 Pharyngotympanic tube
2 Hyoid bone	11 Salpingopharyngeal fold
3 Aryepiglottic fold	12 Nasopharynx
4 Vocal cord	13 Palatoglossal fold
5 Thyroid cartilage	14 Palatine tonsil
6 Cricoid cartilage	15 Oropharynx
7 Oesophagus	16 Palatopharyngeal fold
8 Thyroid isthmus	17 Hypopharynx
9 Nasopharyngeal tonsil (adenoid)	

of the pharynx are made up of muscular and fibrous tissue attached to the base of the skull superiorly. The pharynx can be in communication with the air and food passages both anteriorly and inferiorly, as indicated previously. From above downwards, these routes of communication are: the nasal cavities through the posterior nasal apertures; the middle ears through the pharyngotympanic tubes; the mouth through the oropharyngeal isthmus; the larynx through the glottis; and the oesophagus through its upper sphincter.

The interior of the pharynx and its subdivisions

The subdivisions of the pharynx described below are based on those set out in the TNM system for classification of malignant tumours published by the International Union Against Cancer (UICC) (Hermanek and Sobin, 1992; Hermanek *et al.*, 1993). Where the division differs from the purely anatomical one, this has been noted.

Nasopharynx (postnasal space)

The nasopharynx or postnasal space lies behind the nasal cavities and above the soft palate (see Figure 10.11). The anterior wall is formed by the openings into the nasal cavities which allow free communication between the nose and nasopharynx each side of the posterior edge of the nasal septum. Just within these openings lie the posterior ends of the inferior and middle turbinates.

The posterosuperior wall of the nasopharynx extends from the base of the skull, at the superior end of the posterior free edge of the nasal septum, down to the level of the junction of hard and soft palates. Anatomically, this lower level is often considered as being at the free edge of the soft palate. This posterosuperior wall is formed by the anteroinferior surface of the body of the sphenoid bone and basilar part of the occipital bone. These two together are termed the 'basisphenoid'. The bony wall extends as far as the pharyngeal tubercle, but below this the wall is formed by the pharyngobasilar fascia lying in front of the anterior arch of the atlas. A collection of lymphoid tissue, the nasopharyngeal tonsil, is found in the mucous membrane overlying the basisphenoid. When the nasopharyngeal tonsil is enlarged, it is commonly referred to as 'the adenoids'. The nasopharyngeal tonsil has a rectangular shape, similar to a truncated pyramid, dependent from the roof of the nasopharynx. Its surface is deeply grooved in a longitudinal way in line with the airflow across it. The anterior edge of this block of tissue is vertical and in the same plane as the posterior nasal aperture. The posterior edge gradually merges into the posterior pharyngeal wall: the lateral edges incline toward the midline.

On each lateral wall of the nasopharynx is the pharyngeal opening of the pharyngotympanic tube. It lies about 1 cm behind the posterior end of the inferior turbinate just above the level of the hard palate. The medial end of the cartilage of the tube forms an elevation shaped like a comma, with a shorter anterior limb and a longer posterior one. Behind and above the tubal cartilage lies the pharyngeal recess (fossa of Rosenmüller). This recess passes laterally above the upper edge of the superior constrictor muscle and corresponds to the position of the sinus of Morgagni. From the posterior edge of the tubal opening the salpingopharyngeal fold, produced by the underlying salpingopharyngeus muscle, passes downwards and fades out on the lateral pharyngeal wall. A less well-defined fold passes from the anterior edge of the tubal opening on to the upper surface of the soft palate, and is caused by the underlying levator palati muscle.

The inferior wall of the nasopharynx is formed by the superior surface of the soft palate. In the midline of this wall, there is an elevation caused by the two uvular muscles on the dorsum of the palate.

Oropharynx

The TNM system, noted previously, describes the oropharynx as extending from the junction of the hard and soft palates to the level of the floor of the valleculae. Anatomical texts describe it as extending from the lower edge of the soft palate to the tip of the epiglottis or to the laryngeal inlet. In terms of physiology, it is easier to describe the oropharynx as extending from the oropharyngeal isthmus to the level of the floor of the valleculae which is also the level of the hyoid bone. The oropharyngeal isthmus is the boundary between the buccal cavity and the oropharynx and is marked on each side by the palatoglossal fold formed by the underlying palatoglossus muscle passing from the undersurface of the palate to the side of the tongue (Figure 10.12). The paired palatoglossal muscles together with the horizontal intrinsic tongue musculature form the oropharyngeal sphincter.

The anterior wall of the oropharynx is, at its upper end, in free communication with the buccal cavity. Below this, the glossoepiglottic area is formed by the posterior one-third of the tongue posterior to the vallate papillae (base of tongue). At the lower part of this anterior wall are found the paired valleculae (Figure 10.13). The valleculae are separated from

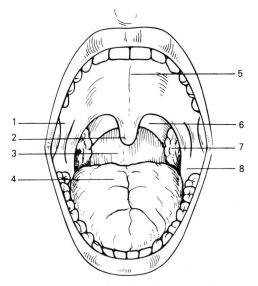

Figure 10.12 The mouth and oropharynx seen from in front

1 Pterygomandibular raphe	5 Soft palate
2 Uvula	6 Palatopharyngeal fold
3 Posterior pharyngeal wall	7 Palatine tonsil
4 Tongue	8 Palatoglossal fold

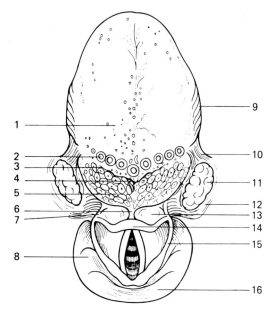

Figure 10.13 The base of tongue and valleculae from above

1 Tongue	8 Pyriform fossa
2 Vallate papillae	9 Folia linguae
3 Sulcus terminalis	10 Palatoglossal fold
4 Foramen caecum	11 Palatine tonsil
5 Base of tongue	12 Palatopharyngeal fold
(pharyngeal part)	13 Vallecula
6 Median glossoepiglottic	14 Epiglottis
fold	15 Aryepiglottic fold
7 Lateral glossoepiglottic	16 Posterior pharyngeal
fold	wall

each other in the midline by the median glossoepiglottic fold passing from the base of the tongue to the anterior or lingual surface of the epiglottis. Laterally, each is bounded by the lateral glossoepiglottic fold. The TNM system incorporates the anterior or lingual surface of the epiglottis into the oropharynx. The anterior boundary of the lateral wall of the oropharynx is drawn by the palatoglossal fold and underlying palatoglossus muscle described previously. Behind this, from the lower edge of the soft palate, the palatopharyngeal fold passes downwards and a little backwards to the side wall of the pharynx, where it fades away. Like the palatoglossal fold, this is caused by an underlying muscle, the palatopharyngeus. In the triangular space between these two folds lies the palatine or faucial tonsil. The pharyngeal surface of the tonsil is oval in shape and demonstrates a variable number of pits or crypts. Towards the upper pole of the tonsil, but within its substance, is found the intratonsillar cleft which is much deeper than the other pits and may extend well down the deep surface of the tonsil within its capsule. A more detailed description of the structure of the tonsil and its anatomical relationships is given later.

Two folds of mucous membrane are usually de-

scribed in connection with the tonsil. A thin triangular fold of mucous membrane passes backwards from the palatoglossal fold to the base of the tongue covering the lower border of the tonsil to a variable extent. A further semilunar fold of mucous membrane passes from the upper part of the palatopharyngeal fold towards the palatoglossal fold. There is wide variation in the extent to which the tonsil is set back between the palatoglossal and palapharyngeal folds. In some cases, the tonsil seems to be very much on the surface of the lateral wall of the oropharynx giving the false impression that it is large; in other instances, it is set deeply between the folds and appears very much smaller even though its volume may be the same in both cases. Tonsils that stand out into the oropharynx are better described as prominent rather than large. The palatoglossal and palatopharyngeal folds are often called the anterior and posterior faucial pillars. Between the tonsil and the base of the tongue lies the glossotonsillar sulcus.

The posterior wall of the oropharynx is formed by the constrictor muscles and overlying mucous membrane. The superior wall of the oropharynx is formed by the inferior surface of the soft palate and uvula. The soft palate is described in detail later.

Hypopharynx (laryngopharynx)

The hypopharynx is that part of the pharynx which lies behind the larynx and partly to each side, where it forms the pyriform fossae or sinuses. It is continuous above with the oropharynx and below with the oesophagus, at the lower border of the cricoid cartilage, through the cricopharyngeal sphincter.

In the anterior wall of the hypopharynx lies the larynx itself with its oblique inlet. The inlet is bounded anteriorly and superiorly by the upper part of the epiglottis, posteriorly by the elevations of the arytenoid cartilages, and laterally by the aryepiglottic folds. Below the laryngeal inlet, the anterior wall is formed by the posterior surfaces of the paired arytenoid cartilages and the posterior plate of the cricoid cartilage. To each side of the larynx lie the pyriform fossae (Figure 10.14). They are bounded laterally by the thyroid cartilage and medially by the lateral surface of the aryepiglottic fold, the arytenoid and cricoid cartilages. They extend from the lateral glossoepiglottic fold (pharyngoepiglottic fold) to the upper end of the oesophagus. Deep to the mucous membrane of the lateral wall of the pyriform fossa lies the superior laryngeal nerve, where it is accessible for local anaesthesia.

The TNM system describes the posterior wall of this section of the pharynx as extending from the level of the floor of the valleculae to the level of the cricoarytenoid joint. This wall is formed by the constrictor muscles and overlying mucous membrane. The region below this, down to the inferior border of the cricoid cartilage is called the pharyngo-oesophageal

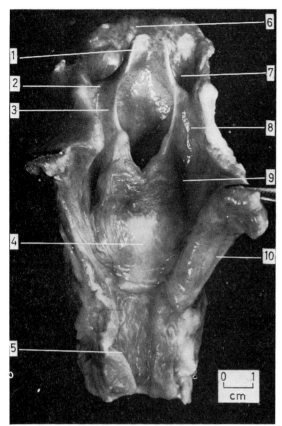

Figure 10.14 The lower pharynx, opened from behind, to show the valleculae, pyriform fossae and postcricoid regions. Note the shallow upper and deeper lower parts of the pyriform fossae

1 Epiglottis	6 Base of tongue
2 Lateral glossoepiglottic fold	7 Vallecula
	8 Upper pyriform fossa
3 Aryepiglottic fold	9 Lower pyriform fossa
4 Postcricoid region	10 Posterolateral pharyngeal wall
5 Cervical oesophagus	

junction (postcricoid area) and is bounded anteriorly by the posterior plate of the cricoid cartilage and encircled by the cricopharyngeus muscle which forms the upper oesophageal sphincter.

The soft palate

The soft palate is a mobile, flexible partition between the nasopharyngeal airway and the oropharyngeal food passage, and it can be likened to a set of points on a railway track, movement of which opens one line and closes another. It extends posteriorly from the edge of the hard palate, and laterally it blends with the lateral walls of the oropharynx. The soft

palate forms the roof of the oropharynx and the floor of the nasopharynx. It lies between two sphincters: the nasopharyngeal which pulls the palate up and back to close the nasopharyngeal airway and the oropharyngeal which pulls it down and forwards to close the oropharyngeal isthmus.

Structure of the soft palate

The basis of the soft palate is the palatine aponeurosis formed by the expanded tendons of the tensor palati muscles which join in a median raphe (Figure 10.15). The aponeurosis is attached to the posterior edge of the hard palate and to its inferior surface behind the palatine crest. It is thicker in the anterior two-thirds of the palate but very thin further back. Near the midline, it splits to enclose the uvular muscle; all the other muscles of the soft palate are attached to it. The anterior part of the soft palate is less mobile and more horizontal than the posterior part and it is principally on this part that the tensor palati acts. From the posterior edge of the soft palate hangs the uvula in the midline. From the base of the uvula on each side, a fold of mucous membrane containing muscle fibres sweeps down to the lateral wall of the oropharynx (Figure 10.16); this is the palatopharyn-

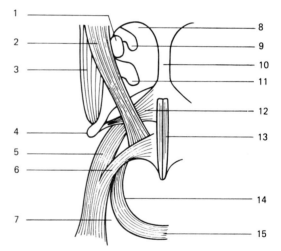

Figure 10.15 The muscles acting on the left side of the soft palate viewed from behind. (Modified from McMinn, R. M. H. and Hobdell, M. H., 1974, *Functional Anatomy of the Digestive System*, p. 25, Figure 2.16, London: Pitman Medical, by courtesy of the authors and publisher)

1 Pharyngotympanic tube	8 Posterior nasal opening
2 Levator palati	9 Middle turbinate
3 Tensor palati	10 Nasal septum
4 Pterygoid hamulus	11 Inferior turbinate
5 Palatopharyngeus – anterior bundle	12 Palatine aponeurosis
	13 Uvular muscle
6 Palatopharyngeus – posterior bundle	14 Palatoglossus
7 Tonsillar fossa	15 Transverse intrinsic tongue muscle

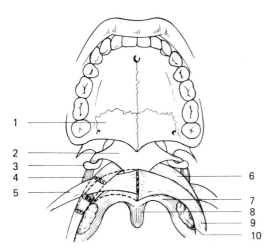

Figure 10.16 A diagram to show the five paired muscles of the soft palate from the oral (inferior) aspect. (Modified from Montgomery, W. W., 1989, *Surgery of the Upper Respiratory System*, Vol. 2, 2nd edn, Philadelphia: Lea and Febiger, by courtesy of the publisher)

1 Palatine bone	7 Palatopharyngeus – posterior bundle
2 Palatine aponeurosis	
3 Pterygoid hamulus	8 Uvular muscles
4 Tensor palati	9 Palatoglossus
5 Levator palati	10 Palatine tonsil
6 Palatopharyngeus–anterior bundle	

geal fold, and the two folds together form the palatopharyngeal arch. More anteriorly, a smaller fold, also containing muscle fibres, passes from the soft palate to the side of the tongue. This is the palatoglossal fold and, with its opposite number, it forms the palatoglossal arch which marks the junction of the buccal cavity and the oropharynx, the oropharyngeal isthmus. The term 'isthmus of the fauces' is sometimes used to describe both the palatal arches together.

The soft palate contains numerous mucous glands and lymphoid tissue, chiefly on the inferior aspect of the palatal aponeurosis and towards its posterior edge (Figure 10.17). The palate also contains the fibres of those muscles acting on it which will be described in detail later.

The mucous membrane on the superior or nasopharyngeal aspect of the palate is pseudostratified ciliated columnar in type, often known as 'respiratory epithelium'. On the inferior or oropharyngeal aspect, the epithelium is of the non-keratinized stratified squamous variety. The lamina propria is very vascular and contains many elastic fibres.

Muscles of the soft palate

The muscles of the soft palate are activated by swallowing, breathing and phonation (Fritzell, 1976). Deglutition is described in detail in Chapter 11.

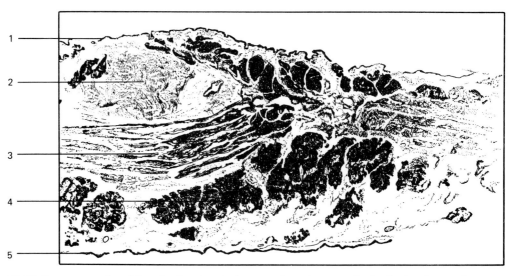

Figure 10.17 Transverse section of the soft palate showing large numbers of mucous glands, chiefly inferior to the aponeurosis and muscles

1 Pseudostratified columnar epithelium on superior (nasopharyngeal) surface	2 Transverse muscle fibres 3 Longitudinal muscle fibres 4 Mucous glands	5 Non-keratinizing stratified squamous epithelium on inferior (oral) surface

Tensor palati

The tensor palati muscle is a thin triangular muscle which arises from the scaphoid fossa of the pterygoid process of the sphenoid bone, the lateral lamina of the cartilage of the pharyngotympanic tube and the medial aspect of the spine of the sphenoid bone (Figure 10.18). As it descends on the lateral surface of the medial pterygoid plate, its fibres converge to form a small tendon which passes round the pterygoid hamulus of the medial plate before piercing the attachment of the buccinator to the pterygomandibular raphe and spreading out to form the palatine aponeurosis described previously (see Figure 10.15). There is a small bursa between the tendon and the pterygoid hamulus. The two tensor palati muscles, acting together, tighten the soft palate, primarily in its anterior part and depress it by flattening its arch. Acting alone, one tensor palati muscle will pull the soft palate to one side. This muscle is also the principal opener of the pharyngotympanic tube, assisted by the levator palati, through its attachment to the lateral lamina of the tubal cartilage.

All the muscles of the soft palate, except the tensor palati, belong to the same group as the superior constrictor and have the same nerve supply by way of the pharyngeal plexus (Table 10.4). The tensor palati, however, is an immigrant muscle which at one time played a part in mastication. Its nerve supply comes from the mandibular division of the trigeminal nerve.

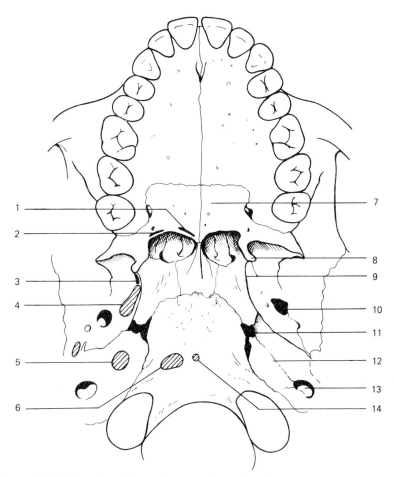

Figure 10.18 The base of the skull seen from below to show muscle attachments

1 Uvular muscle
2 Palatopharyngeus and
  palatine aponeurosis
3 Superior constrictor
4 Tensor palati
5 Levator palati
6 Longus capitis
7 Palatine bone
8 Pterygoid hamulus
9 Medial pterygoid plate
10 Foramen ovale
11 Foramen lacerum
12 Apex of petrous part of
   temporal bone
13 Carotid canal
14 Pharyngeal tubercle

Table 10.4 Main nerves and branches supplying the pharynx and oesophagus

Nerve supply	Area supplied
Facial nerve (VII)	
geniculate ganglion	
greater petrosal nerve	
pterygopalatine ganglion	Palatal muscles – motor
	Mucosal glands – parasympathetic secretomotor
	Taste – sensory
Glossopharyngeal nerve (IX)	
pharyngeal brances	
pharyngeal plexus	Sensory to mucosa
tonsillar branch	Sensory to mucosa
stylopharyngeus branch	Motor supply
Vagus nerve (X)	
superior laryngeal nerve	
internal laryngeal nerve	Sensory to vallecular
external laryngeal nerve	
recurrent laryngeal nerve	
oesophageal branches	
Cranial root of accessory nerve (XI) via vagus nerve	
pharyngeal branches to pharyngeal plexus	
	All soft palate muscles except tensor palati (V)
	All pharyngeal muscles except stylopharyngeus (IX)

Levator palati

The levator palati is a cylindrical muscle arising by a small tendon from a rough area on the inferior surface of the petrous temporal bone immediately in front of the lower opening of the carotid canal (see Figure 10.18). It also arises by a few fibres from the inferior surface of the cartilaginous part of the pharyngotympanic tube. At its origin, the muscle lies inferior rather than medial to the pharyngotympanic tube and crosses to the medial side of the tube only at the level of the medial pterygoid plate. The muscle passes downwards, forwards and inwards over the upper edge of the superior constrictor muscle where it pierces the pharyngobasilar fascia, and descends in front of the salpingopharyngeus muscle to be inserted into the upper surface of the palatine aponeurosis between the two bundles of the palatopharyngeus muscle (Figure 10.19 and see Figure 10.15). The muscle fibres blend with those of the levator palati from the opposite side. The action of the muscle is to raise the soft palate upwards and backwards. Its action, coupled with that of some of the upper fibres of the superior constrictor, described later, plays an important role in the closure of the nasopharyngeal isthmus during deglutition. It also assists in opening the pharyngotympanic tube by elevating the medial lamina of the tubal cartilage, but not until after the age of 7 years or so (Holborow, 1970, 1975).

Palatoglossus

The palatoglossus is a small fleshy bundle of muscle fibres arising from the oral surface of the palatine aponeurosis where it is continuous with the muscle of the opposite side (see Figure 10.16). It passes anteroinferiorly and laterally in front of the tonsil where it forms the palatoglossal arch. It is inserted into the side of the tongue where some of its fibres spread over the dorsum of the tongue while others pass more deeply into its substance to intermingle with the transverse intrinsic muscle fibres. The action of the two muscles, together with the horizontal intrinsic fibres of the tongue, is to close the oropharyngeal isthmus by approximation of the palatoglossal arches and elevation of the tongue against the oral surface of the soft palate.

Palatopharyngeus

The palatopharyngeus arises in the palate as two bundles separated by the levator palati (see Figure 10.15). The anterior bundle, which is the thicker of the two, arises from the posterior border of the hard palate and from the palatine aponeurosis. It passes back between the levator and tensor palati. The posterior bundle is thinner and arises from beneath the mucous membrane of the palate and passes medial to the levator palati. The two bundles unite at

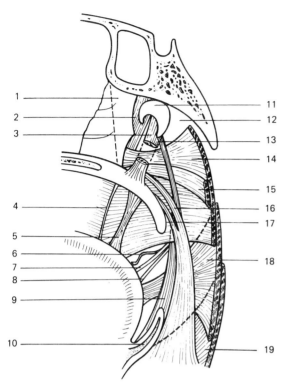

1 ——————
2 ——————
3 ——————

—————— 11
—————— 12

—————— 13

—————— 14

—————— 15
4 —————— —————— 16
—————— 17

5 ——————
6 ——————
7 ——————
8 ——————
9 ——————

—————— 18

10 ——————
—————— 19

Figure 10.19 Right lateral wall of the pharynx, seen from inside, to show the muscles of the palate and pharyngeal wall with associated structures

1 Medial pterygoid plate	11 Pharyngotympanic
2 Tensor palati	tube
3 Levator palati	12 Pharyngobasilar fascia
4 Pterygomandibular	13 Salpingopharyngeus
raphe	14 Superior constrictor
5 Palatoglossus	15 Palatopharyngeal
6 Tonsillar branch of	sphincter
facial artery	16 Palatopharyngeus –
7 Glossopharyngeal	anterior bundle
nerve	17 Palatopharyngeus –
8 Stylohyoid ligament	posterior bundle
9 Stylopharyngeus	18 Middle constrictor
10 Epiglottis	19 Inferior constrictor

the posterolateral aspect of the palate to descend in the palatopharyngeal fold before spreading out to form the inner vertical muscle layer of the pharynx and to be inserted into the posterior edge of the lamina of the thyroid cartilage (Figure 10.20 and see Figure 10.19). The action of the muscle is to pull the walls of the pharynx upwards, forwards and medially, so shortening the pharynx and elevating the larynx during deglutition. Acting together, the two muscles approximate the palatopharyngeal arches to the midline and direct food and fluid down into the lower part of the oropharynx.

Uvular muscle

This is a small paired muscle arising from the palatine aponeurosis just behind the hard palate (see Figure 10.15). Its fibres lie adjacent to the midline between the two laminae of the aponeurosis. It passes backwards and downwards to be inserted into the mucous membrane of the uvula. Its action is to pull up and shorten the uvula and to add bulk to the dorsal surface of the soft palate which assists in closure of the nasopharyngeal opening (velopharyngeal closure) in speech and deglutition (Pigott, 1969; Azzam and Kuehn, 1977).

Nerve supply of the soft palate

All the muscles of the soft palate, except the tensor palati, are supplied by way of the pharyngeal plexus (Broomhead, 1951) with an additional supply from the facial nerve (Nishio *et al.*, 1976a, b; Ibuki *et al.*, 1978). The cell bodies of these motor nerves are found in the nucleus ambiguus and leave the brain stem in the cranial root of the accessory to join the vagus nerve and pass by its pharyngeal branch to the pharyngeal plexus (see Table 10.4). The cell bodies of the facial nerve innervation arise in the facial nucleus and pass through the geniculate ganglion, greater petrosal nerve and pterygopalatine ganglion before reaching the palatal muscles. The tensor palati is supplied by the trigeminal nerve through the nerve to the medial pterygoid, a branch of the mandibular nerve. The fibres pass through, but do not synapse, in the otic ganglion.

The sensory supply to the palate is derived from the greater and lesser palatine branches of the maxillary division of the trigeminal nerve which pass on to the surface of the palate through the greater and lesser palatine foramina. These nerves appear to be branches of the pterygopalatine ganglion but have no synaptic connection in the ganglion, the cell bodies of the sensory fibres being in the trigeminal ganglion. A sensory supply is also provided by pharyngeal branches of the glossopharyngeal nerve. The small number of taste buds on the palate are supplied by the same palatine branches, and the fibres pass up through the pterygopalatine ganglion, without synapsing, into the nerve of the pterygoid canal and the greater petrosal nerve to reach the geniculate ganglion of the facial nerve where the cell bodies are situated. The central processes enter the brain stem by way of the nervus intermedius portion of the facial nerve and end in the nucleus of the tractus solitarius. Sympathetic fibres reach the palate on the blood vessels supplying it and are derived from the superior cervical ganglion.

Blood supply of the soft palate

The blood supply of the soft palate is provided by the palatine branch of the ascending pharyngeal artery

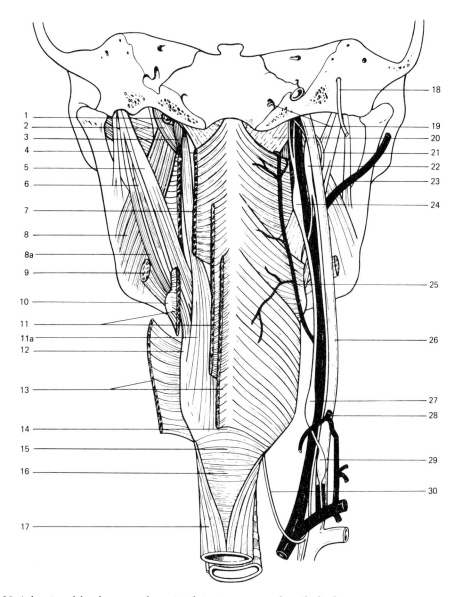

Figure 10.20 A drawing of the pharynx and associated structures as seen from the back

1 Pharyngotympanic tube	11a Palatopharyngeus muscle	20 Pharyngobasilar fascia
2 Tensor palati	12 Superior horn of thyroid cartilage	21 Accessory nerve
3 Levator palati		22 Inferior ganglion of vagus nerve
4 Stylohyoid ligament	13 Inferior constrictor muscle – thyropharyngeus	23 External carotid artery
5 Stylopharyngeus muscle		24 Superior cervical sympathetic ganglion
6 Styloglossus muscle	14 Killian's dehiscence	
7 Superior constrictor muscle	15 Inferior constrictor muscle – cricopharyngeus	25 Ascending pharyngeal artery
8 Medial pterygoid muscle	16 Circular oesophageal muscle coat	26 Internal jugular vein
8a Stylohyoid muscle	17 Longitudinal oesophageal muscle coat	27 Middle cervical sympathetic ganglion
9 Posterior belly of the digastric		28 Inferior thyroid artery
10 Greater horn of hyoid bone	18 Facial nerve	29 Inferior cervical ganglion
11 Middle constrictor	19 Hypoglossal nerve	30 Right recurrent laryngeal nerve

Table 10.5 Main arteries and branches supplying the pharynx and oesophagus

Arterial supply	Area supplied
External carotid artery	
superior thyroid artery	
infrahyoid artery	
superior laryngeal artery	
cricothyroid artery	
ascending pharyngeal artery	
palatine and pharyngeal branches	Palate, constrictors, stylopharyngeus
lingual artery	
dorsal lingual arteries	Tongue base, palatoglossal arch, tonsil, soft palate
facial artery	
ascending palatine artery	Soft palate, tonsil
tonsillar artery	Tonsil, posterior lingual muscles
maxillary artery	
greater (descending) palatine artery and lesser palatine arteries	Soft palate, tonsil
pharyngeal artery	Nasopharynx
artery of the pterygoid canal	Mucous membrane of upper pharynx
Subclavian artery	
thyrocervical trunk	Inferior pharyngeal constrictor
inferior thyroid artery	
ascending cervical artery	Inferior pharyngeal constrictor
muscular branches	Lower pharynx
pharyngeal branches	Oesophagus
oesophageal branches	

which curls over the upper edge of the superior constrictor muscle before being distributed to the palate (Table 10.5). The ascending palatine branch of the facial artery provides an additional supply, as do the lesser palatine branches of the descending palatine branch of the maxillary artery; it runs upwards on the side wall of the pharynx and may, together with the ascending pharyngeal artery, send a branch over the upper edge of the superior constrictor muscle to the palate.

The venous drainage of the palate is to the pterygoid plexus and thence through the deep facial vein to the anterior facial vein and internal jugular vein.

Lymphatic drainage of the soft palate

The lymphatic drainage of the soft palate is partly by way of the retropharyngeal nodes, but chiefly direct to the upper deep cervical group of nodes.

The pharyngeal wall

The pharyngeal wall consists of four layers which, from the inner layer outwards, are as follows:

1 Mucous membrane
2 Pharyngobasilar fascia
3 Muscle layer
4 Buccopharyngeal fascia.

Mucous membrane

The epithelial lining of the pharynx varies in accordance with differing physiological function. The nasopharynx is part of the respiratory pathway and normally only traversed by air. It is lined by a pseudostratified columnar ciliated epithelium as far as the level of the lower border of the soft palate. The oropharynx and hypopharynx are part of the alimentary tract and subject to the abrasion caused by the passage of food. These two areas have an epithelial lining of non-keratinizing stratified squamous epithelium. In the border zone between the nasopharynx and oropharynx, there may be a narrow zone of stratified columnar epithelium. Immediately beneath the epithelium, there is a connective tissue lamina propria that contains a large amount of elastic tissue and which takes the place of the muscularis mucosae found in the oesophagus.

The respiratory type of epithelium in the nasopharynx contains goblet cells. Elsewhere, the mucous membrane is pierced by ducts from glands that lie deep to it in the submucosa. These may be mucous, serous, or mixed.

The pharynx has a large amount of subepithelial or gut-associated lymphoid tissue encircling both its alimentary and respiratory openings forming Waldeyer's ring (Figure 10.21). There are three large aggregations of this tissue and three smaller ones. The larger are the two palatine tonsils in the oropharynx,

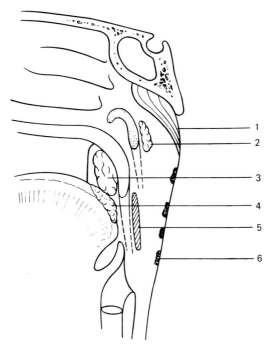

Figure 10.21 Diagram of the right lateral wall of the pharynx to show the aggregations of gut-associated lymphoid tissue that form Waldeyer's ring

1 Nasopharyngeal tonsil (adenoid)
2 Tubal tonsil in fossa of Rosenmüller
3 Palatine tonsil
4 Lingual tonsil on base of tongue
5 Lateral pharyngeal band of lymphoid tissue behind palatopharyngeal fold
6 Lymphoid nodules on posterior pharyngeal wall

and the nasopharyngeal tonsil on the roof of the nasopharynx. The three smaller aggregations are the tubal tonsil, above and behind the pharyngeal opening of the pharyngotympanic tube, the lingual tonsil, and the two lateral bands which run down posterior to the palatopharyngeal fold. The pharyngeal lymphoid tissue is described in more detail later.

Pharyngobasilar fascia

A fibrous intermediate layer lies between the mucous membrane and the muscular layers in place of the submucosa. It is thick above, where the muscle fibres are absent, and is firmly connected to the basilar region of the occipital bone and petrous part of the temporal bone medial to the carotid canal, bridging below the pharyngotympanic tube, and extending forwards to be attached to the posterior border of the medial pterygoid plate and the pterygomandibular raphe (see Figure 10.19). The pharyngobasilar fascia bridges the gap between the superior border of the

superior constrictor and the base of the skull (see Figure 10.20). In this region it is firmly united to the buccopharyngeal fascia, forming a single layer. This fibrous layer diminishes in thickness as it descends. It is strengthened posteriorly by a strong fibrous band which is attached above to the pharyngeal tubercle on the undersurface of the basilar portion of the occipital bone, and passes downwards as a median raphe (the pharyngeal raphe), which gives attachment to the constrictors (see Figure 10.20). Although the pharyngeal muscles are usually described as lying external to the fibrous layer, it is formed, in reality, from the thickened, deep epimysial covering of these muscles, and the thinner external layer of the epimysium constitutes the buccopharyngeal fascia.

Muscle layer

The muscles of the pharyngeal wall are arranged into an inner longitudinal layer and an outer circular layer. The inner layer is formed by three paired muscles, namely:

1 Stylopharyngeus
2 Palatopharyngeus
3 Salpingopharyngeus.

The outer layer also has three paired muscles, namely:

1 Superior constrictor
2 Middle constrictor
3 Inferior constrictor.

Each of the constrictor muscles is a fan-shaped sheet arising on the lateral wall of the pharynx and sweeping round to be inserted into the median raphe posteriorly (Figure 10.22 and see Figure 10.20). The muscles overlap each other from below upwards. Although together they form an almost complete coat for the side and posterior walls of the pharynx, their attachments anteriorly separate the edges, and it is through these intervals that structures can pass from the exterior of the pharynx towards its lumen. The interval between the upper border of the superior constrictor and the base of the skull is sometimes called the sinus of Morgagni. During deglutition, the constrictor muscles contract in a coordinated way to propel the bolus through the oropharynx into the oesophagus. The longitudinal muscles elevate the larynx and shorten the pharynx during this movement.

The superior constrictor muscle

This muscle arises from above downwards from the posterior border of the lower part of the medial pterygoid plate, the pterygoid hamulus, the pterygomandibular raphe, the posterior end of the mylohyoid line on the inner surface of the mandible, and by a few fibres from the side of the tongue (see Figure 10.22).

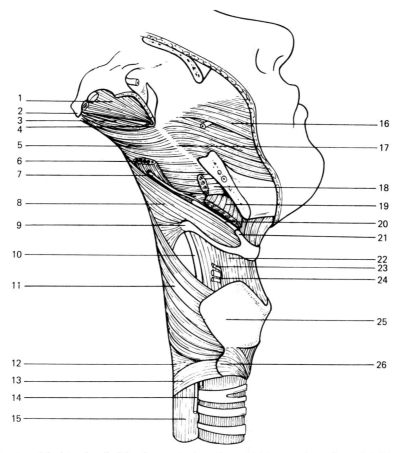

Figure 10.22 A drawing of the lateral wall of the pharynx to show the constrictor muscles and associated structures. (Modified from Williams, P. L. and Warwick, R., 1989, *Gray's Anatomy*, 37th edn, p. 1325, Figure 8.99. Churchill Livingstone, courtesy of the publishers)

1 Tensor palati
2 Spine of sphenoid
   bone
3 Levator palati
4 Pterygoid hamulus
5 Superior constrictor
6 Stylopharyngeus
7 Glossopharyngeal
   nerve
8 Middle constrictor
9 Greater horn of hyoid
   bone
10 Lateral thyrohyoid
   ligament

11 Thyropharyngeus
   part of inferior
   constrictor
12 Killian's dehiscence
13 Cricopharyngeus part
   of inferior constrictor
14 Right recurrent
   laryngeal nerve
15 Oesophagus
16 Buccinator
17 Pterygomandibular
   raphe
18 Styloglossus
19 Geniohyoid

20 Stylohyoid ligament
21 Lesser horn of hyoid
   bone
22 Thyrohyoid
   membrane
23 Internal laryngeal
   nerve
24 Superior laryngeal
   vessels
25 Oblique line on
   thyroid cartilage
26 Fascial bridge over
   cricothyroid muscle

The fibres pass backwards in a largely quadrilateral sheet to be inserted into the median pharyngeal raphe and, by an aponeurosis, to the pharyngeal tubercle on the basilar part of the occipital bone (see Figure 10.18). A band of muscle fibres arises from the anterior and lateral part of the upper surface of the palatine aponeurosis and sweeps backwards, lateral to the levator palati, to blend with the internal surface of the superior constrictor near its upper border (Whillis, 1930). This band is termed the 'palatopharyngeal sphincter' (see Figure 10.19). It produces a rounded ridge on the pharyngeal wall, known as Passavant's ridge, which is seen when the nasopharyngeal sphincter contracts (Calnan, 1958).

The middle constrictor muscle

This muscle arises from the posterior edge of the lower part of the stylohyoid ligament and lesser horn of the hyoid bone, as well as from the whole length of the upper border of the greater horn (see Figure 10.22). The fibres spread in a wide fan-shape upwards and downwards as they pass backwards to be inserted into the whole length of the median pharyngeal raphe (see Figure 10.20). As the upper fibres ascend, they overlap the superior constrictor; the middle fibres pass horizontally backwards, and the lower fibres descend, deep to the inferior constrictor, as far as the lower end of the pharynx.

The inferior constrictor muscle

This is the thickest of the constrictors and consists of two parts: thyropharyngeus and cricopharyngeus. The thyropharyngeus part arises from the oblique line on the lateral surface of the lamina of the thyroid cartilage, from a fine tendinous band across the cricothyroid muscle, and from a small area on the lateral surface of the cricoid cartilage at the lower edge of the above band (see Figure 10.22). There is also a small slip from the inferior horn of the thyroid cartilage. These fibres pass backwards to be inserted into the median pharyngeal raphe, the upper ones ascending obliquely to overlap the middle constrictor (see Figure 10.20). The cricopharyngeus part of the inferior constrictor arises from the side of the cricoid cartilage in the interval between the origin of the cricothyroid in front and the articular facet for the inferior horn of the thyroid cartilage behind. These fibres pass horizontally backwards and encircle the pharyngo-oesophageal junction to be inserted at the same site on the opposite side of the cricoid cartilage. They are continuous with the circular fibres of the oesophagus. Posteriorly, there is a small triangular interval between the upper edge of the cricopharyngeus and the lower fibres of the thyropharyngeus. This interval is sometimes referred to as Killian's dehiscence (see Figure 10.20). It is occasionally described as a point of 'weakness' in the pharyngeal wall, but this is incorrect as it is a feature of the normal anatomy of this region. However, when there is incoordination of the pharyngeal peristaltic wave, and the cricopharyngeus does not relax at the appropriate time, pressure may temporarily build up in the lower part of the pharynx, in which case the most likely place for a diverticulum to form is at Killian's dehiscence, where the additional support of the constrictor muscles is deficient.

The stylopharyngeus muscle

This muscle arises from the medial side of the base of the styloid process of the temporal bone and descends along the side of the pharynx, passing between the superior and middle constrictors, after which its fibres spread out beneath the mucous membrane, some of them merging into the constrictors and the lateral glossoepiglottic fold while others are inserted, with the palatopharyngeus, into the posterior border of the thyroid cartilage (see Figures 10.19 and 10.20). The muscle is long and slender with a cylindrical shape above, flattening out below within the pharynx. It is supplied by a branch of the glossopharyngeal nerve, which winds around its posterior border before entering the pharynx alongside it to reach the tongue.

The palatopharyngeus muscle

This muscle, with its covering of mucous membrane, forms the palatopharyngeal fold or posterior faucial pillar. It arises as two bundles within the soft palate. The anterior bundle, the thicker of the two, arises from the posterior border of the hard palate and from the palatine aponeurosis. It passes backwards, first anterior and then lateral to the levator palati, between the levator and the tensor palati, before descending into the pharynx. The smaller posterior and inferior bundle arises in contact with the mucous membrane covering the surface of the palate, together with the corresponding bundle of the opposite side in the median plane (see Figure 10.15). At the posterolateral border of the palate, the two bundles of muscle unite and are joined by the fibres of salpingopharyngeus. Passing laterally and downwards behind the tonsil, the palatopharyngeus descends posteromedial to, and in close contact with, the stylopharyngeus muscle and is inserted with it into the posterior border of the thyroid cartilage (see Figure 10.19). Some of its fibres end in the side wall of the pharynx attached to the fibrous coat, and others pass across the median plane to decussate with those of the opposite side.

Salpingopharyngeus

This muscle arises from the posteroinferior corner of the cartilage of the pharyngotympanic tube near its pharyngeal opening. The fibres pass downwards and blend with the palatopharyngeus muscle (see Figure 10.19).

Buccopharyngeal fascia

This thin fibrous layer forms the outer coat of the pharynx and, as already indicated, probably represents the thinner external epimysial covering of the constrictor muscles. It is a coat of areolar tissue and contains the pharyngeal plexus of nerves and veins. Posteriorly, it is loosely attached to the prevertebral fascia covering the prevertebral muscles and, at the sides, is loosely connected to the styloid process and its muscles, and to the carotid sheath.

Structures entering the pharynx (see Figure 10.22)

Above the superior constrictor

The cartilaginous part of the pharyngotympanic tube and the tensor and levator palati muscles pass through the pharyngobasilar fascia to reach the lateral wall of the pharynx and palate respectively. The palatine branch of the ascending pharyngeal artery curls over the upper edge of the superior constrictor.

Between the middle and superior constrictor muscles

The stylopharyngeus muscle enters the pharynx at this level, as described previously, before it blends with fibres from the palatopharyngeus. It is accompanied by the glossopharyngeal nerve which supplies it before passing forward to the tongue.

Between the middle and inferior constrictor muscles

The internal laryngeal nerve and superior laryngeal vessels pierce the thyrohyoid membrane and come to lie submucosally on the lateral wall of the pyriform fossa, where the nerve is accessible for local anaesthesia.

Below the inferior constrictor

The recurrent laryngeal nerve and inferior laryngeal artery pass between the cricopharyngeal part of the inferior constrictor and the oesophagus behind the articulation of the inferior horn of the thyroid cartilage with the cricoid cartilage.

Nerve supply of the pharynx

The motor, sensory and autonomic nerve supply of the pharynx is provided through the pharyngeal plexus, which is situated in the buccopharyngeal fascia surrounding the pharynx (see Table 10.4). The plexus is formed by the pharyngeal branches of the glossopharyngeal and vagus nerves together with sympathetic fibres from the superior cervical ganglion. The cells of origin of the glossopharyngeal and vagal motor branches that supply the muscles are in the rostral part of the nucleus ambiguus. The fibres leave the brain stem with the glossopharyngeal nerve and with the cranial root of the accessory nerve which joins the vagus at the level of its superior ganglion. The pharyngeal branch of the vagus carries the main motor supply to the pharyngeal plexus. All the muscles of the pharynx, with the exception of stylopharyngeus, are supplied by the pharyngeal plexus. The stylopharyngeus is supplied by a muscular branch of the glossopharyngeal nerve as it passes round the muscle to enter the pharynx with it. It is the only muscle supplied by the glossopharyngeal which is otherwise a sensory nerve. The cricopharyn-geus part of the inferior constrictor has an additional supply from the external laryngeal nerve and receives parasympathetic vagal fibres from the recurrent laryngeal nerve.

The sensory nerve supply to the pharynx is also provided by branches of the glossopharyngeal and vagus nerves, chiefly through the pharyngeal plexus. The glossopharyngeal nerve provides the supply to the upper part of the pharynx, including the surface of the tonsil, which is also supplied by the lesser palatine branch of the maxillary nerve. The posterior third of the tongue, including the vallate papillae, is supplied for both ordinary sensation and taste by the glossopharyngeal nerve. The tongue in front of the valleculae and the valleculae themselves are supplied by the internal laryngeal nerve, a branch of the superior laryngeal nerve of the vagus. A small part of the nasopharynx behind the opening of pharyngo-tympanic tube receives a sensory supply from the pharyngeal branch of the maxillary nerve. These fibres pass through the pterygopalatine ganglion without synapsing and their cell bodies are in the trigeminal ganglion.

The afferent sensory fibres of the glossopharyngeal nerve have their cell bodies in the superior and inferior ganglia of the nerve. The central processes of the unipolar nerve cells in these ganglia are received in the nucleus of the tractus solitarius for taste, and probably in the nucleus of the spinal tract of the trigeminal nerve for common sensation. In the case of the vagus nerve, the sensory fibres synapse in the inferior vagal ganglion before being received in the above brain-stem nuclei.

The parasympathetic secretomotor supply to the glands of the pharyngeal mucosa, which are mainly in the nasopharynx, comes by way of the pterygopalatine ganglion. The cell bodies are in the superior salivary nucleus, and the fibres leave the brain stem in the nervus intermedius. They pass through the geniculate ganglion of the facial nerve without synapsing and leave it by the greater petrosal nerve, passing by way of the nerve of the pterygoid canal to reach the pterygopalatine ganglion. Here they synapse with the postganglionic cell bodies whose axons reach the pharyngeal mucosa by the nasal, palatine, and pharyngeal branches from the ganglion.

Sympathetic fibres are derived from the superior cervical ganglion of the cervical sympathetic trunk. The preganglionic cell bodies are in the lateral grey column of spinal cord segments T1–T3. Their axons pass up in the sympathetic trunk to synapse in the cervical ganglia from which postganglionic fibres leave and reach the pharynx by running with its blood vessels.

The cricopharyngeal sphincter has a double autonomic innervation. Parasympathetic vagal fibres reach the muscle in the recurrent laryngeal nerve and postganglionic sympathetic fibres come from the superior cervical ganglion. Stimulation of the vagus causes relaxation and sympathetic excitation causes contraction of the sphincter.

Blood supply of the pharynx

The ascending pharyngeal artery arises from the medial side of the external carotid artery just above its origin (see Table 10.5). It passes upwards behind the carotid sheath and immediately against the pharyngeal wall. Branches are distributed to the wall of the pharynx and the tonsils. Its palatine branch passes over the upper free edge of the superior constrictor muscle to supply the inner aspect of the pharynx and the soft palate. A small branch supplies the pharyngotympanic tube. The pharynx receives a further supply of blood from the ascending palatine and tonsillar branches of the facial artery and the greater palatine and pterygoid branches of the maxillary artery. The dorsal lingual branches of the lingual artery provide an additional small contribution.

The veins of the pharynx are arranged in an internal submucous and an external pharyngeal plexus with numerous communicating branches, not only between the two plexuses but with the veins of the dorsum of the tongue, the superior laryngeal veins, and the oesophageal veins. The pharyngeal plexus drains to the internal jugular and anterior facial veins. It also communicates with the pterygoid plexus.

Lymphatic drainage of the pharynx

All the lymph vessels of the pharynx drain into the deep cervical group of lymph nodes, either directly from the tissues themselves, or indirectly after passing through one of the outlying groups of nodes. The efferents from the deep cervical group form the jugular trunk which, on the right side, may end in the junction of the internal jugular and subclavian veins or may join the right lymphatic duct. On the left side, the jugular trunk usually enters the thoracic duct although it may join either the internal jugular or the subclavian vein.

The deep cervical group of nodes lies along the carotid sheath by the internal jugular vein and is divided into superior and inferior groups. The superior group is adjacent to the upper part of the internal jugular vein, mostly deep to the sternocleidomastoid. Within this superior group, a smaller group consisting of one large and several small nodes is particularly to be noted. It lies in the triangular region bounded by the posterior belly of the digastric above, the facial vein, and the internal jugular vein. It is termed the 'jugulodigastric group'.

The inferior group of deep cervical lymph nodes is also partly deep to sternocleidomastoid and extends into the subclavian triangle. It is closely related to the brachial plexus and the subclavian vessels.

Within this group, one lies on, or just above, the intermediate tendon of omohyoid. It is called the juguloomohyoid node. The superior group of nodes drains into the inferior group. In addition to the pharynx, all of the lymph vessels of the head and neck drain into this group. The upper part of the pharynx, including the nasopharynx and the pharyngotympanic tube, drains first into the retropharyngeal lymph nodes which comprise a median and two lateral groups lying between the buccopharyngeal fascia covering the pharynx and the prevertebral fascia. These nodes are said to atrophy in childhood. Efferent vessels from them pass to the upper deep cervical nodes.

The lymphatic vessels of the oropharynx pass to the upper deep cervical group of nodes and, in particular, to the jugulodigastric group described previously. Vessels from the tonsil pierce the buccopharyngeal fascia and the superior constrictor and pass between the stylohyoid and internal jugular vein to the jugulodigastric node.

The hypopharynx drains chiefly to the inferior deep cervical group of nodes, but may also drain to paratracheal nodes which lie alongside the trachea and oesophagus beside the recurrent laryngeal nerves. Efferents from these nodes pass to the deep cervical group.

The lymphoid tissue of the pharynx

A full account of basic immunology appears in Chapter 18. This section discusses some anatomical and histological aspects of the lymphoid tissue in the pharynx.

The walls of the alimentary and respiratory tracts contain large amounts of unencapsulated lymphoid tissue, the lymphoid nodules, and these are collectively termed the 'epitheliolymphoid' or 'gut-associated lymphoid' tissue. They form part of the peripheral lymphoid organs, the other parts being the lymph nodes and similar tissues in the bone marrow and spleen. Lymphoid nodules are particularly prominent in the pharynx and include the nasopharyngeal, tubal, palatine and lingual tonsils. Further down the alimentary tract, nodules occur in the wall of the oesophagus and large groups in the small intestine (Peyer's patches) and the vermiform appendix. There are also nodules in the trachea and bronchial tree. The prominent nodules just described, together with some less easily seen, form a ring of gut-associated lymphoid tissue around the entrance to the respiratory and alimentary tracts, known as Waldeyer's ring (see Figure 10.21).

In general, lymphoid nodules are situated in the lamina propria just beneath the epithelium, although when active they may extend more deeply into the submucosa and be diffused through neighbouring tissue. Although the precise form of the nodules depends on their location, there are certain features common to all sites. It is possible to distinguish within them numerous rounded follicles, similar to those seen in lymph nodes, which have germinal centres. The latter are particularly noticeable when the follicles are actively stimulated with antigens. Between the follicles lie less closely packed parafollicular lymphocytes. The follicles and intervening tissue, together with many macrophages, are supported by a fine mesh of reticulin fibres and associated fibroblasts. In some of the larger nodules, such as the palatine tonsil, there are coarser connective tissue trabeculae. In the case of the tonsil, these arise from the capsule. The surface facing the lumen is covered with epithelium pierced by glandular or other diverticula which penetrate deeply into the aggregations of lymphocytes.

The nodules have an extensive vascular network of blood vessels branching from the surrounding connective tissue to supply the follicles with a capillary plexus, which drains into postcapillary venules. This network allows free movement of lymphocytes to and from the blood stream. The lymphatic vessels associated with the lymph nodules are exclusively efferent and drain into the general network of lymphatic channels serving the area in which they are found.

Immunofluorescent studies have demonstrated that the rounded follicles contain the B lymphocytes, and the parafollicular areas contain the T lymphocytes. These cells can move either into the lymphatic system and rejoin the blood stream, or they may move out into adjacent tissues; in the case of non-stratified epithelia, they may eventually pass into the lumen of the alimentary or respiratory tracts.

The B lymphocytes are concerned with the synthesis of secretory antibodies of the IgA class, whereas T lymphocytes, are concerned with cell-mediated immunity, i.e. they are able to kill cells infected by viruses and fungi, or neoplastic cells.

There continues to be much discussion about the exact role of the lymphoid nodules in the total lymphoid system of the body. It seems likely that these regions provide areas in which B and T lymphocytes can proliferate and act as reservoirs of defensive cells that can infiltrate the surrounding tissue to provide local defences. As already indicated, the B lymphocytes are important in the synthesis of the antibodies of the IgA class which are present in the secretions of the alimentary tract. In the lamina propria, migrating B lymphocytes are often seen to have become transformed into plasma cells, and it is these cells that secrete the antibodies in the intercellular spaces of the unicellular epithelia and into subepithelial glands. Where the epithelial lining is of the stratified squamous type, the subepithelial glands are of particular importance in enabling the antibodies to reach the lumen. In this case, certain varieties of glandular cell appear to take up the antibodies which are then modified to form the final secretory form of IgA. The role of these antibodies is of great importance in dealing with pathogenic organisms within the various tracts in which they are found.

Pathogens which have already penetrated the epithelium are dealt with by other types of antibody, IgM and IgG, secreted by plasma cells of the lamina propria. In order that this system can work efficiently, there must be a mechanism in which the lymphocytes within the lymphoid nodules can detect antigens present on the outer luminal side of the epithelium. Specialized phagocytic cells have been demonstrated in the epithelum overlying lymphoid follicles, and these appear to be capable of passing particulate material to the lymphoid tissue beneath, thus providing a route for antigens to reach the immune system (Brockmann and Cooper, 1973; Owen and Jones, 1974). The longitudinal clefts of the nasopharyngeal tonsil seem to be a way of presenting a bigger surface area to the incoming air in the same way as the crypts of the palatine tonsil increase the surface area presented to food and fluid passing through the pharynx. In the case of the palatine tonsil, an additional mechanism exists which may have some significance in enabling it to undertake 'sampling'. As deglutition takes place, contraction of the pharyngeal musculature, in particular that of the two palatopharyngeus muscles, draws the tonsils towards the midline and turns them forward so that the bolus travels across the surface.

The palatine tonsil

The palatine tonsil has already been briefly described, but is dealt with in more detail here because of the importance of its surgical applied anatomy.

The tonsil is an oval mass of specialized subepithelial lymphoid tissue situated in the triangular tonsillar fossa between the diverging palatopharyngeal and palatoglossal folds (see Figure 10.12). The medial surface of the tonsil is free and projects to a variable extent into the oropharynx, depending partly on its size but, probably more importantly, on the degree to which it is embedded into the tonsillar fossa. In late fetal life, a triangular fold of mucous membrane extends back from the lower part of the palatoglossal fold to cover the anteroinferior part of the tonsil. In childhood, however, this fold is usually invaded by lymphoid tissue and becomes incorporated into the tonsil. It is not usually possible to distinguish it clearly. A semilunar fold of mucous membranes passes from the upper part of the palatopharyngeal arch towards the upper pole of the tonsil and separates it from the base of the uvula. The extent to which this fold is visible depends upon the prominence of the tonsil.

The appearance of the tonsil, on examination of the throat, may give a misleading estimate of its size, as indicated previously. Some tonsils appear to lie very much on the surface of the throat with only a shallow tonsillar fossa; others are much more deeply buried in a deep tonsillar fossa. The upper pole of the tonsil may extend up into the soft palate and the lower pole may extend downwards beside the base of the tongue (Figure 10.23). At this point, the lymphoid tissue of the tonsil is continuous with the subepithelial lymphoid tissue on the base of the tongue, the lingual tonsil. A sulcus usually separates the tonsil from tbe base of the tongue, the tonsillolingual sulcus. The tonsil is larger in childhood, when it is more active, and gradually becomes smaller during puberty.

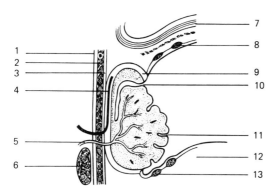

Figure 10.23 A diagram of a coronal section through the palatine tonsil to show local relationships

1 Buccopharyngeal fascia	7 Soft palate
2 Superior constrictor	8 Lymphoid follicles
3 Pharyngobasilar fascia	9 Tonsil capsule
4 Paratonsillar vein	10 Intratonsillar cleft
5 Tonsillar artery	11 Tonsillar crypt
6 Styloglossus	12 Base of tongue
	13 Lingual tonsil

Structure of the tonsil

The tonsil consists of a mass of lymphoid follicles supported in a fine connective tissue framework (Figure 10.24). The lymphocytes are less closely packed in the centre of each nodule, which is described as a germinal centre, because multiplication of the lymphocytes takes place in this situation. The medial surface of the tonsil, facing the lumen, is characterized by 15–20 openings, irregularly spaced over the surface, leading into deep, narrow, blind-ended recesses termed the 'tonsillar crypts'. These may penetrate nearly the whole thickness of the tonsil and distinguish it histologically from other lymphoid organs. The mucous membrane covering the luminal surface is of the non-keratinizing stratified squamous type and is continuous with that of the remainder of the oropharynx. It also dips down to line the crypts. The crypts may contain desquamated epithelial debris and cells. These plugs of debris are usually cleared from the crypts, but may occasionally remain and become hardened and yellow in appearance.

In the upper part of the tonsil, there is a deep intratonsillar cleft, much larger than the tonsillar crypts, extending laterally and inferiorly toward the lower pole of the tonsil within its capsule. This cleft lies within the substance of the tonsil. It is thought to represent a persistent part of the ventral portion of the second pharyngeal pouch. Some authorities, however, believe that the site of this part of the pouch is represented by the supratonsillar fossa, which is the area of mucous membrane above the tonsil between the palatoglossal and palatopharyngeal folds.

The deep surface of the tonsil, i.e. all that part not covered by mucous membrane, is covered by a fibrous capsule which is separated from the wall of the

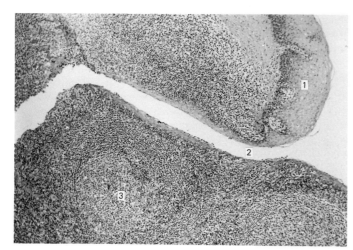

Figure 10.24 A histological section of the palatine tonsil to show mucous membrane, crypts and associated lymphoid follicles. The lymphoid tissue is slightly reactive and germinal centres can clearly be seen. Haematoxylin and eosin, × 40. (Photograph kindly provided by Dr R. H. Simpson, Senior Lecturer in Histopathology, Exeter University)

1 Non-keratinizing squamous epithelium on the luminal surface
2 Crypt lined by similar epithelium
3 Germinal centre of lymphoid follicle

oropharynx by loose areolar tissue. This separation makes dissection of the tonsil relatively easy provided that inflammatory disease has not obliterated this space. Suppuration in this space leads to the formation of a peritonsillar abscess.

Relationships of the tonsil

The medial surface of the tonsil is free and faces towards the cavity of the oropharynx. In the act of swallowing, contraction of the musculature in this region, particularly that of the palatopharyngeus, moves the tonsil medially and turns it towards the buccal cavity.

Anteriorly and posteriorly, the tonsil is related to the palatoglossus and palatopharyngeus muscles lying within their respective folds (Figure 10.25). The muscles have already been described in connection with the soft palate. Some muscular fibres of the

palatopharyngeus are found in the tonsil bed and are attached to the lower part of the capsule, as are fibres of the palatoglossus. Inferiorly, the capsule is firmly connected to the side of the tongue. Superiorly, the tonsil extends to a variable degree into the edge of the soft palate.

Laterally, the floor of the tonsillar fossa is formed by the pharyngobasilar fascia deep to which, in the upper part of the fossa, is the superior constrictor muscle, and below it the styloglossus muscle passing foward into the tongue. Lateral to the superior constrictor is the buccopharyngeal fascia. The glossopharyngeal nerve and stylohyoid ligament pass obliquely downwards and forwards beneath the lower edge of the superior constrictor in the lower part of the tonsillar fossa. A large palatine vein, the external palatine or paratonsillar vein, descends from the soft palate across the lateral aspect of the capsule of the tonsil before piercing the pharyngeal wall to join the

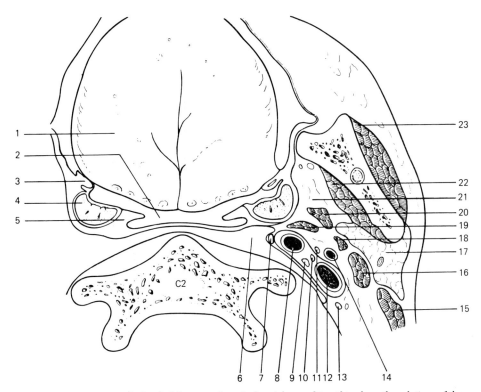

Figure 10.25 Transverse section at the level of the second cervical vertebra and tonsil to show the relations of the oropharynx including the parapharyngeal and retropharyngeal spaces

1 Tongue	9 Vagus nerve	17 Parotid gland
2 Cavity of oropharynx	10 Hypoglossal nerve	18 Stylohyoid muscle
3 Palatoglossus muscle	11 Glossopharyngeal nerve	19 Stylopharyngeus muscle
4 Palatine tonsil	12 Internal jugular vein	20 Styloglossus muscle
5 Palatopharyngeus muscle	13 Accessory nerve	21 Parapharyngeal space
6 Retropharyngeal space	14 External carotid artery	22 Medial pterygoid muscle
7 Sympathetic ganglion	15 Sternocleidomastoid muscle	23 Masseter muscle
8 Internal carotid artery	16 Posterior belly of digastric	

pharyngeal plexus. The tonsillar artery, a branch of the facial artery, pierces the superior constrictor and immediately enters the tonsil accompanied by two small veins. It is at this point of vascular supply that, in the course of a dissection tonsillectomy, a fibrous band will be noted between the tonsil capsule and the tonsil bed.

More distant, lateral relations of the lower part of the tonsil, outside the pharyngeal wall, are the posterior belly of the digastric muscle and the submandibular salivary gland, with the facial artery arching over them. Further laterally still are the medial pterygoid muscle and the angle of the mandible.

Nerve supply of the tonsil

The sensory nerve supply to the tonsillar region is mainly by the tonsillar branch of the glossopharyngeal nerve (see Table 10.4). The cell bodies of these fibres are in the glossopharyngeal ganglia. The upper part of the tonsil nearest to the soft palate is supplied by the lesser palatine nerves, branches of the maxillary division of the trigeminal nerve received by way of the pterygopalatine ganglia. The cell bodies of these fibres are in the trigeminal ganglion. There is no synapse in the pterygopalatine ganglion. Sympathetic fibres reach the tonsil on the arteries supplying it and are derived from the superior cervical ganglion.

Blood supply of the tonsil

The main artery of the tonsil is the tonsillar branch of the facial artery which enters the tonsil near its lower pole by piercing the superior constrictor just above the styloglossus muscle (see Table 10.5). A further arterial supply reaches the tonsil from the lingual artery, by way of the dorsal lingual branches, from the ascending palatine branch of the facial artery, and ascending pharyngeal vessels. The upper pole receives an additional supply from greater palatine vessels of the descending palatine branch of the maxillary artery.

Venous drainage of the tonsil is to the paratonsillar vein, and vessels also pass to the pharyngeal plexus or facial vein after piercing the superior constrictor. There is communication with the pterygoid plexus and drainage is eventually into the common facial and internal jugular veins.

Lymphatic drainage of the tonsil

Lymphatic vessels from the tonsil pierce the buccopharyngeal fascia and pass to the upper deep cervical group of nodes, in particular to the jugulodigastric group situated just below the posterior belly of the digastric muscle. The tonsil has no afferent lymphatic vessels.

Relationships of the pharynx

There are two important potential spaces in relation to the posterior and lateral aspects of the pharynx, and a description of these will precede an account of the other structures related to the pharynx. These spaces provide possible pathways for the spread of infection once it has entered them.

Retropharyngeal space

The potential space, known as the retropharyngeal space, lies between the prevertebral fascia posteriorly and the buccopharyngeal fascia covering the constrictor muscles, anteriorly (see Figure 10.25). (The prevertebral fascia is also known as the prevertebral lamina of the cervical fascia.) The space is filled with loose areolar tissue and may contain the retropharyngeal group of lymph nodes which are present in infancy but disappear as the child grows older. The space is closed above by the base of the skull and on each side by the carotid sheath, which is a condensation of the cervical fascia in which the common and internal carotid arteries, the internal jugular vein, the vagus nerve and constituents of the ansa cervicalis are embedded. It is thicker around the arteries than the vein. Inferiorly, it is possible to pass into the superior mediastinum. A median partition has been described connecting the prevertebral fascia with the buccopharyngeal fascia and dividing the retropharyngeal space into two lateral spaces. However, during deglutition and movement of the head, the pharynx must be free to move and the areolar tissue that fills the space does not tether it.

Posteriorly, the prevertebral fascia covers the prevertebral muscles, longus capitis and longus cervicis, which separate it from the body and transverse processes of the cervical vertebrae. In the midline, the anterior longitudinal ligament of the vertebral column is just beneath the fascia.

Suppuration in a retropharyngeal lymph node, with the formation of pus, may push the posterior pharyngeal wall forward and present as a retropharyngeal abscess. As indicated previously, this normally occurs only in infants. It is possible, however, for such infection to spread downwards into the superior mediastinum. Infection with suppuration behind the prevertebral fascia presents laterally in the posterior triangle of the neck.

Parapharyngeal space

The potential space, filled with areolar tissue and fat, known as the parapharyngeal space and also as the lateral pharyngeal space, lies lateral to the pharynx on each side (see Figure 10.25). It extends from the base of the skull above, where it is widest, downwards towards the superior mediastinum. Its medial wall is formed by the buccopharyngeal fascia overlying the

constrictor muscles. Its posterior wall is the prevertebral fascia. The lateral wall is formed posteriorly by
the parotid gland and anteriorly by the medial pterygoid muscle overlying the angle of the mandible. The
styloid process and its muscles separate, to some
extent, this space from the carotid sheath, which is
more posteriorly situated. In the lower part of the
neck, the lateral wall is formed by the sternomastoid
muscle and the infrahyoid muscles of the neck within
their fascial envelope. The space contains the deep
cervical group of lymph nodes. Infection may enter
the space through lymphatic vessels coming to these
nodes and may extend downwards toward the superior mediastinum or by way of veins to the internal
jugular vein. Infection is prevented from spreading
into the retropharyngeal space by the condensation
of fascia around the carotid sheath.

Lateral relationships of the pharynx

The chief lateral relation running alongside the pharynx is the carotid sheath with its associated arteries,
veins and nerves, together with their branches.
Closely associated with the sheath are the muscles
and ligament arising from the styloid process. More

laterally, the angles of the mandible and pterygoid
muscles are related to the upper part of the pharynx
anteriorly, and with the parotid gland and posterior
belly of the digastric muscle more posteriorly (see
Figure 10.25). At a lower level, the sternocleidomastoid muscle covers the carotid sheath, with the infrahyoid muscles more anteriorly and the lateral lobes
of the thyroid gland interposed (Figure 10.26).

In particular, the superior constrictor has on its
lateral surface the lingual and inferior alveolar
branches of the mandibular nerve, the ascending pharyngeal artery, the ascending palatine branch of the
facial artery, the stylohyoid ligament, the styloglossus
and stylopharyngeus muscles and, more laterally,
the medial pterygoid muscle deep to the angle of the
mandible. The maxillary artery runs anteriorly to
enter the pterygopalatine fossa.

The middle constrictor has on its outer surface the
lingual artery, the hyoglossus muscle and the hypoglossal nerve with the tendon of the posterior belly
of the digastric muscle.

The inferior constrictor has on its lateral surface
the external laryngeal nerve, the thyroid gland and
the sternothyroid and sternohyoid muscles together
with the omohyoid.

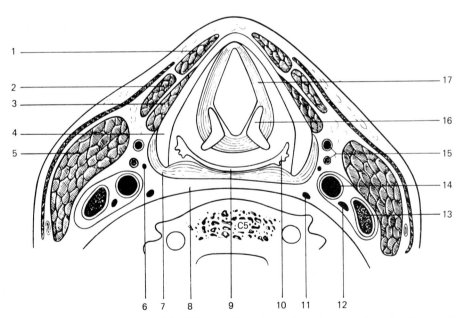

Figure 10.26 Transverse section at the level of the fifth cervical vertebra and vocal cords to show the relations of the
hypopharynx and pyriform fossae

1 Sternohyoid	7 Inferior constrictor muscle	13 Internal jugular vein
2 Omohyoid	8 Retropharyngeal space	14 Internal carotid artery
3 Thyrohyoid	9 Hypopharynx	15 Superior thyroid artery
4 Thyroid cartilage	10 Pyriform fossa	and vein
5 Sternocleidomastoid	11 Cervical sympathetic ganglion	16 Arytenoid cartilage
6 External laryngeal nerve	12 Vagus nerve	17 Vocal fold

The oesophagus

General description

The oesophagus is a muscular tube, about 25 cm in length, connecting the pharynx to the stomach. It extends from the lower border of the cricoid cartilage at the level of the sixth cervical vertebra, where it is continuous with the pharynx, to the cardiac orifice of the stomach at the side of the body of the eleventh thoracic vertebra. In passing from the pharynx to the stomach, it traverses the neck and then the superior and posterior parts of the mediastinum before piercing the diaphragm, after which it has a short abdominal course before joining the stomach.

In the newborn infant, the upper limit of the oesophagus is found at the level of the fourth or fifth cervical vertebra and it ends higher, at the level of the ninth thoracic vertebra. At birth, the length of the oesophagus varies between 8 and 10 cm, but by the end of the first year it has increased to 12 cm. Between the first and fifth years, it reaches a length of 16 cm, but growth after this is slow as it measures only 19 cm by the fifteenth year.

The diameter of the oesophagus varies according to whether or not a bolus of food or fluid is passing through it. At rest, in the adult, the diameter is about 20 mm, but this may increase to as much as 30 mm. At birth, the diameter is about 5 mm, but this dimension almost doubles in the first year, and by the age of 5 years it has attained a diameter of 15 mm. In its course from the pharynx to the stomach, the oesophagus presents an anteroposterior flexure, corresponding to the curvature of the cervical and thoracic parts of the vertebral column. It also presents two gentle curves in the coronal plane. The first begins a little below the commencement of the oesophagus and continues with a deviation to the left through the cervical and upper thoracic parts of its course, until it returns to the midline at the level of the fifth thoracic vertebra. The second coronal curve is formed as the oesophagus bends to the left to cross the descending thoracic aorta, to pierce the diaphragm and then to join the stomach.

The oesophagus is the narrowest region of the alimentary tract, except for the vermiform appendix, and it has three constrictions or indentations in its course. These are found:

1 At 15 cm from the upper incisor teeth where the oesophagus commences at the cricopharyngeal sphincter, which is normally closed
2 At 23 cm from the upper incisor teeth where it is crossed by the aortic arch and left main bronchus
3 At 40 cm from the upper incisor where it pierces the diaphragm and where the lower 'physiological' oesophageal sphincter is sited.

The oesophageal wall

The wall of the oesophagus has four layers (Figure 10.27) which are, from within outwards:

1 Mucous membrane
2 Submucosa
3 Muscle coat
4 Outer fibrous layer.

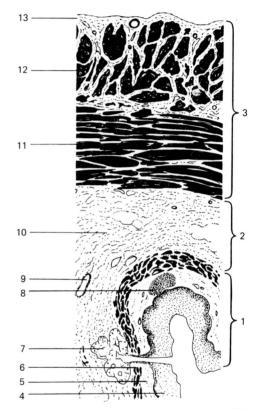

Figure 10.27 Drawing of a transverse section through the oesophageal wall. (From Hamilton, W. J., 1976, Editor, *Textbook of Human Anatomy*, 2nd edn, Figure 469, p. 359. London: The Macmillan Press Limited, by courtesy of the publishers)

1 Mucous membrane	8 Lymphoid nodule
2 Submucosa	9 Blood vessel
3 Muscle coat	10 Submucosa
4 Epithelium	11 Circular muscle
5 Lamina propria	12 Longitudinal muscle
6 Muscularis mucosae	13 Fibrous layer
7 Oesophageal gland	

Mucous membrane of the oesophagus

The oesophagus is lined by a non-keratinizing stratified squamous epithelium which is continuous with that of the pharynx. At the junction with the stomach, however, there is an abrupt change to the columnar epithelium of that organ.

The epithelium of the oesophagus has the typical basement membrane beneath which is a loose connective tissue lamina propria containing a very fine network of elastic fibres and lymphoid nodules. At rest the mucous membrane is thrown into longitudinal folds which disappear when the organ is distended by the passage of a bolus. They can be clearly seen on a normal barium swallow (Chapter 17). Although the pharynx contains no muscularis mucosae, this layer of visceral muscle cells makes its appearance soon after the oesophagus begins. Towards the lower end of the oesophagus, this layer becomes thicker than in any other part of the alimentary tract and because of this thickening, it is sometimes mistakenly identified in histological preparations as part of the muscular wall.

In early embryonic life, the epithelium of the oesophagus is composed of columnar epithelium many of the cells of which are ciliated. At the time of birth, the ciliated cells are isolated in small groups and eventually disappear. The oesophagus is now lined with stratified squamous epithelium five to six cell layers in thickness. Soon after birth, the epithelium thickens rapidly to assume its adult appearance.

The submucosa of the oesophagus

The submucosa loosely connects the mucous membrane and the muscular coat. It contains the larger blood vessels and Meissner's nerve plexus of postganglionic parasympathetic fibres, as well as the oesophageal glands which are small, compound racemose glands of the mucous type. Each gland opens into the lumen by a long duct which pierces the muscularis mucosae. These glands secrete the mucus that lubricates the passage of food through the oesophagus. The glands are distributed irregularly throughout the oesophagus. In the abdominal part of the oesophagus, near to its junction with the stomach, other glands are found which do not penetrate the muscularis mucosae and which, because structurally they resemble the cardiac glands of the stomach, are called oesophageal 'cardiac' glands. They are also found at the upper end of the oesophagus where they continue to be called 'cardiac' glands. The distal part of the duct of the oesophageal glands is lined with three or four layers of stratified squamous epithelium. Proximally, at the junction of the duct with the gland, there is a gradual transition from this stratified epithelium to a low cuboidal epithelium.

The muscular coat of the oesophagus

The muscular layer of the oesophagus is composed of an outer longitudinal and an inner circular coat. The longitudinal fibres form a complete covering for nearly the whole of the oesophagus, but at the upper end, at a point between 3 and 4 cm below the cricoid cartilage, the fibres diverge from the median plane posteriorly and form two longitudinal fasciculae which incline upwards and forwards to the front of the oesophagus where they are attached to the posterior surface of the lamina of the cricoid cartilage through a small tendon. In general, the longitudinal muscular coat of the oesophagus is thicker than the circular muscular coat.

The fibres of the circular coat are continuous superiorly with the fibres of the cricopharyngeus part of the inferior constrictor. Anteriorly, these fibres are inserted into the lateral margins of the tendon, already described, of the longitudinal fibres. Inferiorly, the circular muscle fibres are continuous with the oblique fibres of the stomach. At the lower end of the oesophagus, the circular fibres form one component of a 'physiological' sphincter which will be described later.

In the upper third of the oesophagus, the muscle fibres of both coats are striated. In the middle third, there is a gradual transition to non-striated muscle, and the lower third contains only non-striated muscle.

Fibrous layer of the oesophagus

The fibrous layer consists of an external adventitia of irregular, dense connective tissue containing many elastin fibres. The arrangement of this tissue allows expansion during swallowing and maintains the position of the oesophagus in relation to adjacent structures. In the abdominal segment of the oesophagus there is an additional covering of peritoneum. At the diaphragmatic opening, the fibrous layer attaches the oesophagus to the margins of the opening and this attachment is known as the phreno-oesophageal ligament.

The presence of this adventitial layer makes it possible for the oesophagus to be mobilized by blunt finger dissection during operations from above and below without the chest being opened. It can then be withdrawn from the thorax as, for example, in the operation of pharyngolaryngo-oesophagectomy.

Nerve supply of the oesophagus

The striated muscle in the upper third of the oesophagus is supplied by the recurrent laryngeal branches of the vagus (see Table 10.4). The cell bodies for these fibres are in the rostral part of the nucleus ambiguus. However, the chief motor supply to the non-striated muscle is parasympathetic, and the cell bodies for these fibres are in the dorsal nucleus of the vagus. They reach the oesophagus by way of the oesophageal branches of the vagus itself and through its recurrent laryngeal branches, and synapse in the oesophageal wall in the ganglia of the submucosal plexus (Meissner's) and myenteric plexus (Auerbach's), which is between the outer longitudinal and inner circular muscle layers. From these cell bodies, short postganglionic fibres emerge to innervate the muscle fibres.

The cell bodies of the preganglionic sympathetic motor fibres are found in the lateral grey column of the spinal cord in thoracic segments 2 to 6 (chiefly 5 and 6). The fibres pass out in the anterior nerve roots and reach the sympathetic trunk by way of white rami communicantes. They then run upwards to the cervical ganglia where they synapse. From these ganglia, postganglionic fibres pass down into the thorax by the superior, middle, and inferior cardiac nerves to join the cardiac plexus, which they traverse without synapsing to reach the oesophagus. Some sympathetic fibres take a more direct route to the oesophagus by way of the thoracic ganglia 2 to 6, where the synapses are situated. The cervical oesophagus receives its sympathetic supply by means of a plexus around the inferior thyroid artery. The thoracic oesophagus has branches from the sympathetic trunks which form a plexus around the blood vessels supplying this section. In the abdominal oesophagus, the plexuses form around the left gastric and inferior phrenic arteries.

Afferent fibres from the oesophagus run with the branches of the vagus and have their cell bodies in the inferior vagal ganglion from where impulses reach the dorsal vagal nucleus and nucleus of the tractus solitarius. Some of the afferent fibres that run with the sympathetic nerves convey pain sensation.

Oesophageal pain

From cervical cardiac nerves and sympathetic trunk ganglia, fibres enter the thoracic spinal nerves by way of grey rami communicantes. Although any one of the thoracic nerves may be involved, most of the pain fibres have their cell bodies in the dorsal root ganglia of thoracic spinal nerves 5 and 6. After entering the spinal cord, the fibres synapse with cell bodies in the gelatinous substance and posterior horn. The impulses are then conveyed by the lateral spino-thalamic tract to the thalamus. The stimulus which seems to initiate oesophageal pain is tension in the muscular wall, resulting from either distension or muscular spasm. The mucosa is sensitive to heat and cold but not to touch. Chemical stimulation by reflux of gastric acid may, under certain conditions, cause pain.

Oesophageal pain is poorly localized and is referred to other areas. It can be severe and, if retrosternal, resembles cardiac pain. Pain produced by experimental oesophageal distension is localized anteriorly in the midline of the body in the region of the sternum. The area of reference to which the pain is projected corresponds roughly with the level of the part of the oesophagus being distended. Pain from the upper oesophagus is referred to the suprasternal region; that from the middle of the oesophagus to the retro-sternal region; and that from the lower end of the oesophagus to the epigastrium.

Another variety of oesophageal pain, commonly called heartburn, is a burning, hot sensation felt under the lower part of the sternum and radiating up into the neck and jaw. The sensation may be accompanied by regurgitation of acid fluid into the throat. This pain is often ascribed to irritation of the oesophageal mucosa by acid regurgitation from the stomach. However, heartburn has been reported in patients with achlorhydria, and instillation of acid into normal oesophagus may not cause this sensation. On the other hand, a burning sensation similar to heartburn has been produced by inflation of a balloon introduced into the lower oesophagus in normal subjects. Furthermore, radiological studies have shown that during an attack of heartburn, the whole oesophagus is often in spasm. This suggests that the cause of heartburn sensation is not primarily acid reflux, but a prolonged spastic contraction of muscle comparable to that causing the pain of intestinal colic. In some patients, where there is inflammation of the oesophageal mucosa, the pain threshold may be lowered and reflux of gastric acid may well precipitate heartburn. It is still possible, however, that the mechanism of the pain production is that the acid irritates the lower oesophageal mucosa causing muscle spasm.

Blood supply of the oesophagus

The oesophagus obtains its blood supply from adjacent vessels (see Table 10.5). In the cervical part, this is from the inferior thyroid arteries which arise from the thyrocervical trunks of the subclavian artery. In addition, a supply is obtained from the left subclavian artery. In its thoracic part, the oesophagus is supplied segmentally, either directly from the descending thoracic aorta, or by way of branches of the bronchial or upper posterior intercostal arteries. In its abdominal part, the oesophagus is supplied by the left gastric branch of the coeliac trunk and the left inferior phrenic artery direct from the abdominal aorta.

An extensive venous plexus is formed on the exterior of the oesophagus and drains in a segmental way similar to the arterial supply. In the neck, the veins drain into the inferior thyroid veins; in the thorax they drain to the azygos and hemi-azygos system; and in the abdomen into the left gastric vein. This vein is a tributary of the portal system, whereas the other veins are part of the systemic system. The lower end of the oesophagus is a site of major importance for portal–systemic anastomoses and there is free communication between the two systems. When there is portal obstruction, the multiple, small thin-walled subepithelial veins in this region become varicose and may break down and bleed heavily into the lumen.

At the upper end of the oesophagus, longitudinal submucosal oesophageal veins enter the pharyngeal/

laryngeal plexus situated on the posterior and anterior walls of the pharynx at the level of the cricoid cartilage.

Lymphatic drainage of the oesophagus

Two networks of lymphatic vessels are found in the oesophagus. There is a plexus of fairly large vessels in the mucous membrane which is continuous above with those of the pharynx and below with those of the gastric mucosa. The second plexus of finer vessels is present within the muscular coat and, although this may be independent of the mucosal plexus, it drains by the same collecting vessels. The latter leave the oesophagus in two ways, either piercing the muscular coat immediately and draining into neighbouring nodes, or ascending and descending beneath the mucosa. The efferent vessels from the cervical part of the oesophagus drain into the lower group of deep cervical nodes and into the paratracheal nodes. Vessels from the thoracic part drain into the posterior mediastinal nodes and the tracheobronchial nodes. Vessels from the abdominal part pass to the left gastric nodes. Some vessels may pass directly to the thoracic duct.

The oesophageal sphincters

A full account of the working of the oesophageal sphincters in the course of deglutition is given in Chapter 11. This section deals with some anatomical aspects of the sphincters.

The upper oesophageal sphincter

The upper oesophageal sphincter is provided by the cricopharyngeus part of the inferior constrictor which encircles the oesophageal entrance, being attached to each side of the cricoid cartilage. This muscle has no posterior median raphe. Its fibres are continuous with the circular muscle coat of the oesophagus below. It is described in more detail above, where its nerve supply is also detailed.

This sphincter is always closed, and manometric studies demonstrate a region of raised pressure over about 3 cm in length. The pressure profile in this region shows a 1-cm zone of rising pressure proximally followed by 1 cm of peak pressure reaching about 35 mmHg. This region of peak pressure corresponds to the position of the cricopharyngeus. Beyond this is a distal 1 cm in which the pressure decreases to atmospheric pressure. These recordings demonstrate the existence of a tonic sphincter that is very competent.

The lower oesophageal sphincter

It is not possible to demonstrate a lower oesophageal sphincter histologically, on account of there being no thickening of the circular muscle coat. Manometric studies demonstrate a zone of raised pressure about 3 cm in length at the oesophagogastric junction extending above and below the diaphragm. The mean pressure here is approximately 8 mmHg higher than the intragastric pressure. Although this pressure is only slightly in excess of that in the stomach, regurgitation of gastric contents does not normally occur. This 'sphincter' region of the oesophagus, with an intraluminal pressure higher than the rest of the oesophagus or stomach, is regarded as one component of a 'physiological' sphincter at the oesophagogastric zone. Radiological studies show that swallowed food is momentarily held up at the lower end of the oesophagus, before entry into the stomach. The possible components of this sphincter mechanism are as follows:

1 An intrinsic sphincter. Present in the circular muscle fibres of the oesophagus, described previously.

2 Pinch-cock effect of the diaphragm. The fibres of the right crus of the diaphragm split to encircle the oesophageal opening and may play an auxiliary role in achieving an effective lower oesophageal sphincter.

3 Mucosal folds. These have been described at the lower end of the oesophagus and have been thought to exert a valvular effect (Figure 10.28). They may be thrown into prominence by contraction of the muscularis mucosae.

4 Oblique muscle fibres of the stomach. The portion of the stomach adjacent to the oesophageal opening has a definite collar of muscle which is part of the innermost oblique muscle layer of the stomach. The fibres sweep up from the lesser curvature to encircle the terminal oesophagus. They may help to preserve the angle between the left edge of the oesophageal opening and the fundus of the stomach, the cardiac notch.

5 Thoracoabdominal pressure gradient. The thoracic part of the oesophagus is subject to a negative pressure as opposed to the abdominal oesophagus which has a positive pressure applied to it. It is felt that this pressure differential may collapse the lower end of the oesophagus like a mechanical flutter valve, preventing reflux. Food and fluid passing down the oesophagus would open this valve, but it would otherwise remain closed.

6 Oesophagogastric junction angle. It has been suggested that the sharp angle at which the left edge of the oesophagus meets the fundus of the stomach forms a fold that can act as a mechanical flap valve. A rise of intragastric pressure will compress the adjacent part of the terminal oesophagus and prevent a reflux. The higher the pressure in the stomach, the more securely will this flap valve be closed. The angle of entry of the oesophagus into the stomach is, however, very variable in humans, and patients appear to suffer reflux despite a normal oesophagogastric angle.

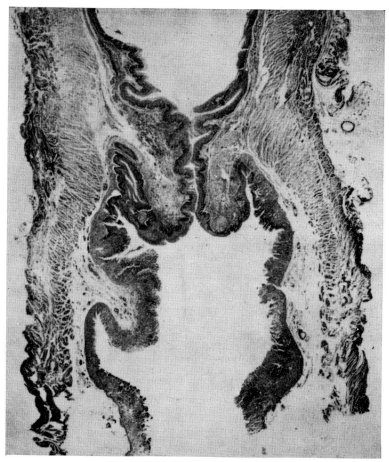

Figure 10.28 Section of oesophagogastric junction showing mucosal folds forming a valve. (From Creamer, 1955, reproduced by courtesy of the Editor of *The Lancet*)

The way in which a competent lower oesophageal sphincter is achieved remains uncertain, but it seems that a number of mechanisms may act in concert to accomplish this (Figure 10.29).

Relationships of the oesophagus

The relationships of the cervical, thoracic and abdominal parts of the oesophagus will be dealt with separately. They are illustrated from anterior and lateral aspects in Figures 10.30–10.32 and in cross-section at different levels in Figures 10.33–10.40.

The cervical part of the oesophagus

In the neck, the trachea lies anterior to the oesophagus attached by loose connective tissue. The recurrent laryngeal nerves ascend on each side in the groove between the trachea and oesophagus (Figures 10.30 and 10.33). Posteriorly, the oesophagus rests on the prevertebral fascia covering the C6–C8 vertebral bodies and the prevertebral muscles. The thoracic duct passes upwards behind the left border of the oesophagus and, at the level of C6, the duct arches laterally between the carotid and vertebral systems before opening into the junction of the left internal jugular and left subclavian veins. Laterally, on each side, lie the corresponding parts of the carotid sheath together with its contents, with the lower poles of the lateral lobes of the thyroid gland between.

Thoracic part of the oesophagus

In the superior mediastinum, the oesophagus lies between the trachea and the vertebral column, slightly to the left of the median plane. It passes behind and to the right of the aortic arch and enters the posterior mediastinum at the level of the fourth thoracic vertebra (Figures 10.30–10.32). It is related anteriorly to the trachea and posteriorly to the third

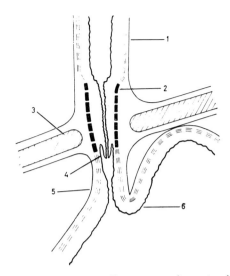

Figure 10.29 A diagram to illustrate some factors involved in the prevention of oesophagogastric reflux

1 Negative intrathoracic pressure
2 Intrinsic muscular sphincter
3 Pinch-cock effect of right crus of diaphragm
4 Mucosal folds
5 Positive intra-abdominal pressure
6 Oesophagogastric angle

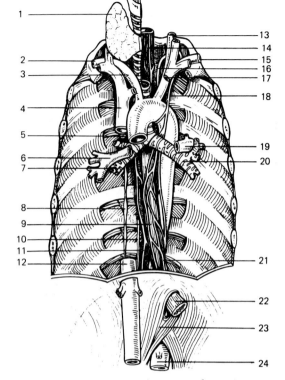

Figure 10.30 Anterior view of superior and posterior mediastinal structures to show course and relations of the oesophagus

1 Right lobe of thyroid
2 Right subclavian artery
3 Brachiocephalic artery
4 Superior vena cava
5 Azygos vein
6 Right pulmonary artery
7 Right principal bronchus
8 Sympathetic trunk
9 Right vagus nerve
10 Azygos vein
11 Thoracic duct
12 Inferior vena cava
13 Left common carotid artery
14 Left recurrent laryngeal nerve
15 Left subclavian artery
16 Thoracic duct
17 Left brachiocephalic vein
18 Left vagus nerve
19 Left pulmonary artery
20 Left principal bronchus
21 Left vagus nerve
22 Abdominal oesophagus
23 Right crus of diaphragm
24 Abdominal aorta

to fourth thoracic vertebrae (Figures 10.34–10.36). The left recurrent laryngeal nerve is in the groove between the oesophagus and trachea on the left. The thoracic duct is behind the left oesophageal border.

Laterally, adjacent to the left border of the oesophagus, is the arch of the aorta passing from before backwards and slightly to the left, with the vagus nerve crossing the arch on its outer side and giving rise to the left recurrent laryngeal branch, which hooks beneath the ligamentum arteriosum to reach the groove between the oesophagus and the trachea. The left subclavian artery is immediately to the left of the oesophagus as the vessel arises from the aortic arch. On the right side, adjacent to the right margin of the oesophagus, is the azygos vein arching from posterior to anterior over the lung root to enter the superior vena cava. The mediastinal pleura of both sides is in contact with the oesophagus, separated on the right by the azygos vien and on the left by the aortic arch and left subclavian artery.

In the posterior mediastinum, anterior to the oesophagus, the trachea bifurcates at the level of the fifth thoracic vertebra and below this the fibrous pericardium comes into contact with the anterior surface of the oesophagus (Figures 10.30–10.40). At the bifurcation of the trachea, the oesophagus is crossed anteriorly by the left principal bronchus passing into the left lung root beneath the aortic arch. It may indent the oesophagus anteriorly on the left.

The right pulmonary artery crosses the oesophagus immediately below the tracheal bifurcation. The inferior tracheobronchial lymph nodes are interposed between the bifurcation of the trachea and the oesophagus. Below this, it is the left atrium of the heart that lies in front of the oesophagus, separated only by the pericardium and its oblique sinus. Lower still, the diaphragm is in front until the oesophagus enters the abdomen.

Posteriorly, in the posterior mediastinum, are the

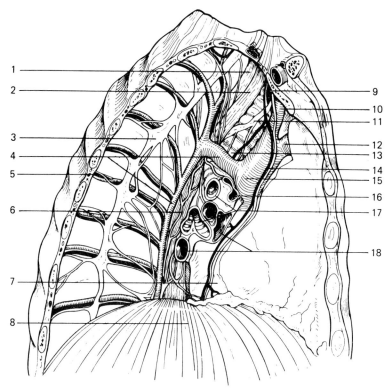

Figure 10.31 The right side of the mediastinum to show the course and relations of the oesophagus (Modified from Augur, 1991, *Grant's Atlas of Anatomy*, 9th edn, p. 40, Figure 1.43)

1 Longus colli muscle	7 Inferior vena cava	13 Trachea
2 Oesophagus	8 Dome of diaphragm	14 Phrenic nerve
3 Sympathetic trunk	9 Brachiocephalic artery	15 Superior vena cava
4 Azygos vein	10 Right brachiocephalic vein	16 Right pulmonary artery
5 Intercostal vessels and nerve	11 Right vagus nerve	17 Right principal bronchi
6 Nerve plexus on oesophagus	12 Left brachiocephalic vein	18 Right pulmonary veins

vertebral column and the long cervical muscles. The right posterior intercostal arteries arising from the descending thoracic aorta pass toward the right across the vertebral column. The thoracic duct enters the thorax through the right side of the aortic opening in the diaphragm and runs up behind the right margin of the oesophagus until, at the level of the fifth thoracic verebra, it crosses obliquely to come to lie behind the left margin as described previously. The two hemi-azygos veins intervene between the oesophagus and the vertebral column, at the level of the seventh and eighth thoracic vertebrae, as they pass across to join the azygos vein on the right. Inferiorly, near the diaphragm, the aorta passes behind the oesophagus as the latter curves toward the left and turns forward to pass through the diaphragm to the stomach.

On the left side, in the posterior mediastinum, the oesophagus is related to the descending thoracic aorta and left mediastinal pleura (see Figure 10.32). On the right side, the oesophagus is related to the right pleura separated only by the azygos vein (see Figure 10.31). The left and right vagus nerves, having branched to form the cardiac and pulmonary plexus, come together again as the oesophageal plexus on the oesophageal wall and then form single or multiple nerve trunks that descend with the oesophagus through the same opening in the diaphragm (see Figure 10.30). The left vagal fibres usually lie on the anterior surface of the oesophagus and those on the right posteriorly.

Abdominal part of the oesophagus

After the oesophagus emerges from the right crus of the diaphragm, slightly to the left of the median plane at the level of the tenth thoracic vertebra, it comes to lie in the oesophageal groove on the posterior surface of the left lobe of the liver. It curves sharply to the left to join the stomach at the cardia

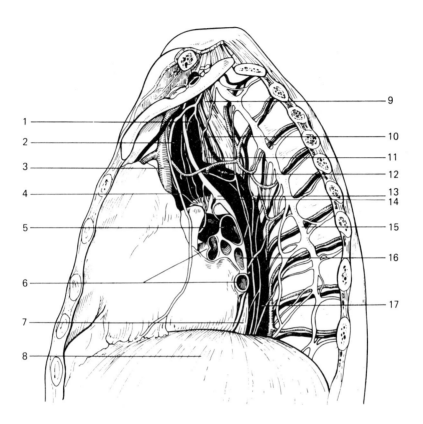

Figure 10.32 The left side of the mediastinum to show the course and relations of the oesophagus (Modified from Augur, 1991, *Grant's Atlas of Anatomy*, 9th edn, p. 41, Figure 1.44)

1 Left subclavian artery	7 Oesophagus	13 Vagus nerve
2 Left common carotid artery	8 Dome of diaphragm	14 Left recurrent laryngeal nerve
3 Left brachiocephalic vein	9 Longus colli muscle	15 Sympathetic nerve trunk
4 Left phrenic nerve	10 Thoracic duct	16 Left principal bronchi
5 Left pulmonary artery	11 Oesophagus	17 Descending thoracic aorta
6 Left pulmonary veins	12 Aortic arch	

(see Figure 10.30). The right border of the oesophagus continues evenly into the lesser curvature of the stomach, while the left border is separated from the fundus of the stomach by the cardiac notch. This short abdominal section of the oesophagus is covered with the peritoneum of the greater sac anteriorly and on its left side, and with the lesser sac on the right. It is contained in the upper left portion of the lesser omentum and the peritoneum, reflected from its posterior surface to the diaphragm, is part of the gastrophrenic ligament in which the oesophageal branches of the left gastric vessels pass to the oesophagus. Behind the oesophagus at this level are the left crus of the diaphragm and the left inferior phrenic artery.

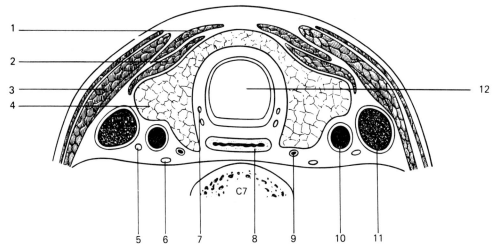

Figure 10.33 Transverse section at the level of the seventh cervical vertebra and commencement of the trachea and oesophagus to show the relations of the latter

1 Sternohyoid muscle	5 Left vagus nerve	9 Inferior thyroid artery
2 Sternothyroid muscle	6 Cervical sympathetic ganglion	10 Common carotid artery
3 Sternocleidomastoid muscle	7 Left recurrent laryngeal nerve	11 Internal jugular vein
4 Thyroid gland	8 Oesophagus	12 Trachea

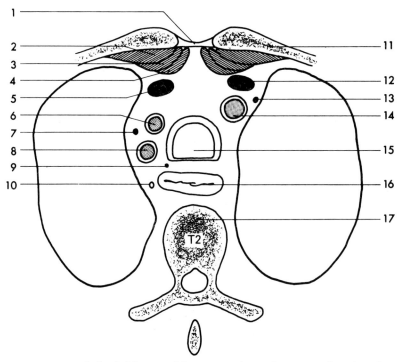

Figure 10.34 Transverse section at the level of the second thoracic vertebra and suprasternal notch to show the relationships of the lower cervical oesophagus

1 Suprasternal notch	7 Left vagus nerve	13 Right vagus nerve
2 Sternocleidomastoid muscle	8 Left subclavian artery	14 Brachiocephalic artery
3 Sternohyoid muscle	9 Left recurrent laryngeal nerve	15 Trachea
4 Sternothyroid muscle	10 Thoracic duct	16 Oesophagus
5 Left brachiocephalic vein	11 Right clavicle	17 Second thoracic vertebra
6 Left common carotid artery	12 Right brachiocephalic vein	

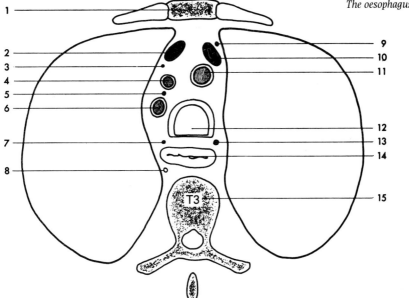

Figure 10.35 Transverse section at the level of the third thoracic vertebra just above the level of the aortic arch to show relationships of the oesophagus in the superior mediastinum

1 Manubrium sterni
2 Left brachiocephalic vein
3 Left phrenic nerve
4 Left common carotid artery
5 Left vagus nerve
6 Left subclavian artery
7 Left recurrent laryngeal nerve
8 Thoracic duct
9 Right phrenic nerve
10 Right brachiocephalic vein
11 Brachiocephalic artery
12 Trachea
13 Right vagus nerve
14 Oesophagus
15 Third thoracic vertebra

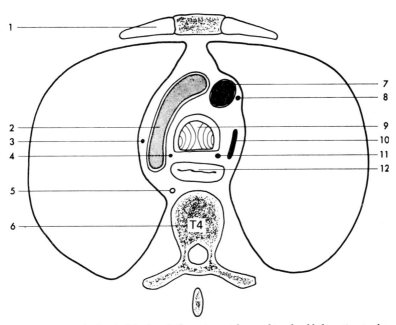

Figure 10.36 Transverse section at the level of the fourth thoracic vertebra and tracheal bifurcation to show relationships of the oesophagus at the junction of superior mediastinum with posterior mediastinum

1 Second costal cartilage
2 Aortic arch
3 Left vagus nerve
4 Left recurrent laryngeal nerve
5 Thoracic duct
6 Fourth thoracic vertebra
7 Superior vena cava
8 Right phrenic nerve
9 Tracheal bifurcation
10 Azygos vein
11 Right vagus nerve
12 Oesophagus

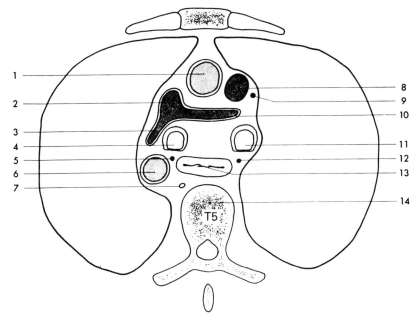

Figure 10.37 Transverse section at the level of the fifth thoracic vertebra approximately 3 cm distal to the tracheal bifurcation and just above the heart to show relationships of the oesophagus in the posterior mediastinum

1 Ascending aorta	6 Descending thoracic aorta	11 Right principal bronchus
2 Pulmonary trunk	7 Thoracic duct	
3 Left pulmonary artery	8 Superior vena cava	12 Right vagus nerve
4 Left principal bronchus	9 Right phrenic nerve	13 Oesophagus
5 Left vagus nerve	10 Right pulmonary artery	14 Fifth thoracic vertebra

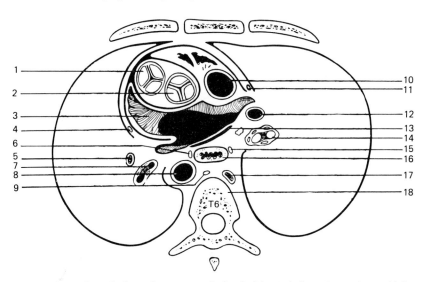

Figure 10.38 Transverse section through the mediastinum at the level of the sixth thoracic vertebra and left atrium, to show the relationships of the oesophagus in the posterior mediastinum

1 Pulmonary valve	7 Left principal bronchus	13 Oblique sinus
2 Aortic valve	8 Descending thoracic aorta	14 Right principal bronchus
3 Left atrium	9 Thoracic duct	15 Right vagus nerve
4 Left phrenic nerve	10 Superior vena cava	16 Oesophagus
5 Left pulmonary artery	11 Right phrenic nerve	17 Azygos vein
6 Left vagus nerve	12 Right pulmonary artery	18 Sixth thoracic vertebra

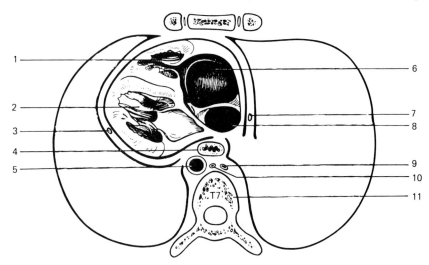

Figure 10.39 Transverse section at the level of the seventh thoracic vertebra and left ventricle to show the relationships of the oesophagus to the heart in the lower posterior mediastinum

1 Right ventricle
2 Left ventricle
3 Left phrenic nerve
4 Oesophagus with nerve plexus

5 Descending thoracic aorta
6 Right atrium
7 Right phrenic nerve
8 Inferior vena cava

9 Azygos vein
10 Thoracic duct
11 Seventh thoracic
   vertebra

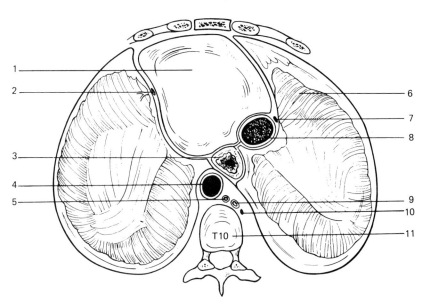

Figure 10.40 Transverse section at the level of the tenth thoracic vertebra showing the relationships of the oesophagus at the diaphragm (Modified from Augur, 1991, *Grant's Atlas of Anatomy*, 9th edn, p. 42, Figure 1.45)

1 Pericardial sac
2 Left phrenic nerve
3 Oesophagus
4 Descending aorta

5 Thoracic duct
6 Dome of diaphragm
7 Right phrenic nerve
8 Inferior vena cava

9 Azygos vein
10 Splanchnic nerve
11 Tenth thoracic vertebra

References

AUGUR, A. M. R. (1991) *Grant's Atlas of Anatomy*, 9th edn. London: Williams and Wilkins

AZZAM, N. A. and KUEHN, D. R. (1977) The morphology of musculus uvulae. *Cleft Palate Journal*, **14**, 78–87

BROCKMANN, D. E. and COOPER, M. D. (1973) Pinocytosis by epithelium associated with lymphoid follicles in the bursa of Fabricius, appendix and Peyer's patches. An electron microscopic study. *American Journal of Anatomy*, **136**, 455–477

BROOMHEAD, I. W. (1951) The nerve supply of the muscles of the soft palate. *British Journal of Plastic Surgery*, **4**, 1–15

CALNAN, J. (1958) Modern views on Passavant's ridge. *British Journal of Plastic Surgery*, **10**, 89–113

CREAMER, B. (1955) Oesophageal reflux and the action of carminatives. *Lancet, i*, 590–592

FRITZELL, B. (1976) Palatal function. In: *Scientific Foundations of Otolaryngology*, edited by R. Hinchcliffe and D. Harrison. London: William Heinemann. pp. 484–493

HAMILTON, W. J. (ed.) (1976) *Textbook of Human Anatomy*, 2nd edn. London: Macmillam Press Limited

HERMANEK, P. and SOBIN, L. H. (eds) (1992) *TNM Classification of Malignant Tumours*, 4th edn. Berlin: Springer Verlag

HERMANEK, P., HENSON, D. E., HUTTER, R. V. P. and SOBIN, L. H. (1993) *TNM Supplement 1993*. Berlin: Springer Verlag

HOLBOROW, C. A. (1970) Eustachian tubal function. *Archives of Otolaryngology*, **92**, 624–626

HOLBOROW, C. A. (1975) Eustachian tubal function, changes throughout childhood and neuromuscular control. *Journal of Laryngology and Otology*, **89**, 47–55

IBUKI, K., MATSUYA, T., NISHIO, J., HAMAMURA, Y. and MIYAZAKI, T. (1978) The course of the facial nerve innervation for the levator palatini muscle. *Cleft Palate Journal*, **15**, 209–214

MCMINN, R. M. H. and HOBDELL, M. H. (1974) *The Functional Anatomy of the Digestive System*. London: Pitman Medical

MONTGOMERY, W. W. (1989) *Surgery of the Upper Respiratory Tract*, 2nd edn, Vol. 2. Philadelphia: Lea and Febiger

MOSELEY, J. M., MATHEWS, E. W., BREED, R. H., GALANTE, E., TSE, A. and MACINTYRE, I. (1968) The ultimobranchial origin of calcitonin. *Lancet, i*, 108–110

NISHIO, J., MATSUYA, T., MACHIDA, J. and MIYAZAKI, T. (1976a) The motor nerve supply of the velopharyngeal muscles. *Cleft Palate Journal*, **13**, 20–30

NISHIO, J., MATSUYA, T., IBUKI, K. and MIYAZAKI, T. (1976b) Roles of the facial, glossopharyngeal and vagus nerves in velopharyngeal movement. *Cleft Palate Journal*, **13**, 201–214

OWEN, R. L. and JONES, A. L. (1974) Epithelial cell specialisation within human Peyer's patches. An ultrastructural study of intestinal lymphoid follicles. *Gastroenterology*, **66**, 189–203

PIGOTT, R. W. (1969) The nasendoscopic appearance of the normal palatopharyngeal valve. *Plastic and Reconstructive Surgery*, **43**, 19–24

SADLER, T. W. (1990) *Langman's Medical Embryology*, 6th edn. Baltimore: Williams and Wilkins

WHILLIS, J. (1930) A note on the muscles of the palate and the superior constrictor. *Journal of Anatomy*, **65**, 92–95

WILLIAMS, P. L., WARWICK, R., DYSON, M. and BANNISTER, L. H. (1989) *Gray's Anatomy*, 37th edn. London: Churchill Livingstone

11

Deglutition

Alan Johnson

Deglutition is the act of swallowing. It can be defined as the mechanism which transmits liquids or solids from the mouth to the stomach via the pharynx and oesophagus without entering the respiratory tract. It is initiated voluntarily, but once triggered it becomes an involuntary process, relying on complex neuromuscular interaction.

In this chapter, the main emphasis is on the physiology of the swallowing process in humans, from the lips to the entrance of the oesophagus. In clinical practice, otolaryngologists see patients with many different swallowing disorders, but the medical and surgical management of swallowing disorders related to intrathoracic and distal oesophageal disease is largely undertaken by other specialties.

Evolution of the upper aerodigestive tract

Some single-celled organisms have a swallowing mechanism. The protozoon, *Paramecium*, has a mouth and a cytopharynx. The alimentary tract developed further in the most primitive multicellular organisms, in some there is the mechanism to propel ingested materials from the 'mouth' to the area where digestion takes place. In itself, this is a primitive form of swallowing.

Terrestrial invertebrates have respiratory systems which are separate from their alimentary tracts, so there is no conflict of function in the alimentary tract during swallowing seen in higher animals. In aquatic vertebrates, water for respiration and food both enter through the mouth; the water is exhaled through the gills while the food is swallowed. Conflict of function is limited as during respiration water is sucked in through the mouth and pumped out across the gill surfaces where gas exchange happens. When the creature swallows food, it is sucked into the mouth but then directed down the oesophagus.

By the time vertebrates left their aquatic environment, respiratory function had evolved dramatically so that gaseous exchange could take place between air and circulating blood. Gill systems would have resulted in a major loss of water through evaporation and their delicate surfaces, imperative for adequate gas exchange, would have required support and protection. To overcome this, amphibians exchange gases through their skins, but the capacity to achieve this is restricted if the skin is toughened to protect against dehydration and injury, as found in those that lead a more terrestrial existence. Thus in higher forms a respiratory diverticulum is seen, arising from the upper digestive tract. The requirement was a large moist surface, very permeable to gases and, therefore, very thin and delicate – quite unlike the tough impermeable surface of the upper alimentary tract. Thus, an invaginated system developed which avoided dehydration, protected the delicate respiratory tissues and allowed gases to be pumped in and out – the lungs. With the evolution of warm-blooded creatures, the rise in metabolic rate increased the need for gas exchange and more complex lungs evolved to meet this need.

A protective mechanism to stop ingested material entering the respiratory organ evolved – the larynx – a sphincter to protect the lung during deglutition. Examples of this evolutionary process are fascinating. For example, the climbing perch developed a diverticulum above its gills which allowed it to stay out of water briefly – a valveless breathing system. The lungfish evolved a sphincter which retains air in its lung on re-entering the water and allows it to survive in times of drought. The Mexican axolotl has evolved lateral laryngeal cartilages which assist in the sphincteric action of the primitive larynx (Negus, 1949).

The complexity of the larynx increased as higher

animals evolved with thoracic skeletons and a muscular diaphragm to facilitate inhalation and exhalation of air. In these, the larynx not only closes off the respiratory tract during swallowing but also has to remain open when subjected to the negative pressure of inspiration, in other words, acquire a degree of rigidity. In evolutionary terms the respiratory and protective functions of the larynx preceded its phonatory function by a very long time. Phonation is only an important function in higher animals which communicate by sound. The secondary nature of sound production is best illustrated by birds, in which the function of airway protection and sound production are anatomically separated. The airway in birds is protected by the rima glottidis in the floor of the mouth, while sound is produced by the syrinx which is situated just above the bifurcation of the trachea. In mammals, the larynx performs both functions and phonation has probably reached its highest form in human languages (Negus, 1949).

Relationship between deglutition and respiration

The physiology of swallowing and respiration are inextricably linked because the oropharynx and laryngopharynx have the dual function of respiratory and alimentary passages. In herbivores, the larynx is close to the back of the nose which permits continued respiration during swallowing, the food bolus skirting round the raised laryngeal inlet into the oesophagus. In carnivores, the larynx is not placed so cranially, but the nasolaryngeal connection is achieved by an elongated epiglottis which reaches up as far as the edge of the soft palate. The same arrangement exists in the human neonate which is an obligatory nasal breather for the first 4–6 months of its life. This arrangement allows suckling using tongue and cheeks while respiration continues. However, respiration has to be interrupted when swallowing.

In larger children and adults the larynx lies lower in the neck, and the epiglottis is well below the free margin of the soft palate, but preparation of food by chewing and mixing can still continue without having to stop respiration. This is achieved by the tongue base and palate being held together until swallowing is initiated. Once swallowing is initiated, respiration has to cease in order to avoid aspiration. Laryngeal function is critical because it protects the airway from material destined for the stomach and beyond and if it fails to do so, the consequences are dire. Although less critical, the soft palate also protects the nose and nasopharynx from food and liquid during swallowing.

The role of the larynx during deglutition

Passive valvular effect of the larynx

The structure of the larynx has a passive valve effect on respiration and aspiration. The false cords act as a valve which blocks exhalation and it has been estimated that they offer a resistance of 30 mmHg to tracheal pressure, while the true vocal cords act as a valve in the opposite direction and present a resistance of up to 140 mmHg. Both these effects combine to minimize the risk of aspiration during inspiration.

Active functional effect of the larynx

The larynx acts mainly as a sphincter during swallowing, but also has a sensory capacity to detect material entering it which should be progressing down the oesophagus. Sasaki and Isaacson (1988) demonstrated in the cat that below the anterior commissure, in the midline, there is a diamond-shaped area which is bilaterally innervated through branches of the external division of the superior laryngeal nerve. The concentration of sensory nerve endings is greatest in the laryngeal inlet, the laryngeal surface of the epiglottis having the highest level of innervation, while the true cords are more densely innervated posteriorly than anteriorly. Chemical and thermal receptors are limited to the supraglottic larynx.

The importance of laryngeal sensation during deglutition is clearly that of a safety mechanism. As explained later, under normal conditions the glottic closure reflex effects laryngeal closure and elevation in the second stage of swallowing. Because of this, ingested material rarely comes into contact with the supraglottis. However, when oral or pharyngeal function is so impaired that ingested material reaches the hypopharynx without the second stage of swallow being triggered properly, good sensation of the larynx becomes a vital mechanism to prevent aspiration. The trachea is also exquisitely sensitive to touch, which evokes a powerful cough reflex, as seen when a suction catheter is passed through a tracheostomy tube.

Protective laryngeal reflexes

The glottic closure reflex

This reflex causes laryngeal closure during swallowing. Electrical stimulation of a superior laryngeal nerve produces an evoked action potential in the adductor fibres of the recurrent laryngeal nerve. The latency of the response indicates that it is a polysynaptic brain stem reflex (Sasaki and Isaacson, 1988). In humans, the adductor response only takes place on the side which is stimulated, thus differing from some animals where unilateral stimulation causes a bilateral response. This implies that injury to one superior laryngeal nerve in humans might cause aspiration if that side of the larynx fails to close properly during deglutition, even though both recurrent laryngeal nerves are normal.

The closure produced by this reflex is achieved at three levels within the larynx: the aryepiglottic folds, the false cords and the true cords. The passive valve effect of the true cords and the muscular effect of the lower division of the thyroarytenoid muscle make this the most powerful level of the sphincter. In experiments, stimulation of the recurrent laryngeal nerve in the dog demonstrated that the thyroarytenoid muscle was one of the fastest contracting muscles in the entire body (nearly as fast as the medial rectus of the eye) responding at 14 ms, compared with 40 ms for the cricothyroid muscle and 44 ms for the posterior cricoarytenoid. This speed of response is an important factor at this site.

The glottic closure reflex develops in line with maturation of the nervous system and myelination of the peripheral nerves after birth. This has been demonstrated in the pup and it might explain the lesser ability of the newborn's larynx to protect the lungs, which in turn may contribute to the risk of sudden infant death syndrome.

Laryngospasm is a well-recognized demonstration of the glottic closure reflex which, in surgical practice, is usually caused by stimulation of the larynx in an unsedated patient by a tube or secretions. Hypoxia, hypercapnia, local anaesthesia and central sedation all reduce the reflex and, by inference, the likelihood of laryngospasm. Superior laryngeal nerve stimulation may also have an inhibitory effect on laryngeal and respiratory function as evidenced by a reduction of posterior cricoarytenoid muscle and phrenic nerve activity. This explains why reflex apnoea may develop at the same time as laryngospasm when the supraglottis is stimulated.

The swallowing process

Swallowing has traditionally been divided into three stages: the oral stage, the pharyngeal stage and the oesophageal stage. This has helped in the clinical analysis of swallowing disorders, a topic in which there has been increased interest recently. There is comforting evidence that patients with dysphagia are greatly helped merely by an accurate diagnosis and explanation of their problem (Gustafsson, Tibbling and Theorell, 1992).

The oral phase

The oral phase of swallowing has been subdivided into preparatory and propulsive stages (Logemann, 1983; Dodds, 1989; Dodds, Stewart and Logemann, 1990).

Preparatory stage

This begins when food or drink is placed in the mouth (Figure 11.1, frame 1). It requires the coordination of lip, buccal, mandibular and tongue move-

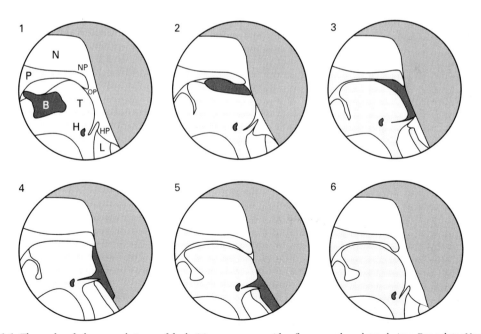

Figure 11.1 The oral and pharyngeal stages of deglutition as seen on video-fluorography – lateral view. P = palate; N = nose; B = bolus; T = tongue; H = hyoid; L = larynx; NP = nasopharynx; OP = oropharynx; HP = hypopharynx

ments, and also closure of the oropharyngeal sphincter so that food or liquid is retained in the mouth until the person is ready to initiate the swallow. Its duration is dependent on the consistency and texture of the food. Liquids require no preparation at all other than to assemble the bolus, while solids need much more. The normal oral preparatory phase is under voluntary control; so the gourmet can savour a special taste or the unwilling child gulp down foul tasting medicine. The cranial nerves involved in this complex coordinated process are the trigeminal (sensation and mastication), facial (lips and buccal movement and control), vagus (oropharyngeal sphincter) and hypoglossal (tongue movement).

Solid food requires chewing to break up the particle size and to mix it with saliva. This action facilitates tasting and also digestion by intimate contact with salivary amylase. The jaws open, close and have a grinding motion, but the pattern of chewing is determined by the consistency of the ingested food. A biphasic pattern with rapid closure is established for hard substances until there is tooth-food-tooth contact, when the speed of jaw closure suddenly decreases but with a simultaneous increase in muscle activity. On the other hand, with soft food there is more anteroposterior tongue movement (Thexton, 1992). It almost goes without saying that the dentition is vital in the preparatory stage for solids. vander-Bilt *et al.* (1993) showed that not only did those who had lost their premolar and molar teeth have to chew more, but they also swallowed larger particles of food. The presence of dentures also alters the function of the lips and facial musculature (Tallgren and Tryde, 1992).

At the end of the oral preparatory phase, a single ball of ingested material, the bolus, is assembled between the tongue and the roof of the mouth. This requires fine accurate tongue movements. The central part of the tongue forms a groove in which the bolus is placed and held against the hard palate at the front of the mouth. The lateral edges of the tongue achieve a seal against the hard palate and the tongue base is kept in firm contact with the soft palate.

Propulsive stage

The propulsive stage begins once the bolus is assembled between the tongue and the hard palate (see Figure 11.1, frame 2). A wave of contraction starts from the tip of the tongue, the superior surface of the tongue pushes up on to the hard palate in a wave from front to back thereby displacing the bolus posteriorly into the oropharynx. The seal between the edges of the tongue and the hard palate is maintained to keep the bolus together. Pressure rises within the bolus as the tongue exerts its force. The pressure developed in large boluses is higher than in smaller ones and so large boluses are vigorously expelled from the mouth, whereas smaller boluses are expelled

with less force. Despite this, the time taken to expel a bolus from the mouth is not dependent on its size (Hamlet, 1989; Kahrilas *et al.*, 1993).

As the wave of contraction progresses, the palatoglossal sphincter relaxes. The soft palate is pulled posterosuperiorly to interrupt nasal respiration and the posterior third of the tongue drops anteroinferiorly to allow the bolus to move into the oropharynx. At the end of the oral stage there should be no significant food or liquid residue in the mouth. The oral stage takes less than a second in normal people, and does not vary with the age of the patient or the consistency of the food (Logemann, 1986).

Pharyngeal stage (see Figure 11.1, frames 3,4,5)

Precisely what initiates the pharyngeal stage is not certain. There is considerable variation in the position of the leading edge of the bolus at the onset of the pharyngeal stage in normal adults. Linden *et al.* (1989) found that the head of the bolus was usually beyond the anterior pillar when the pharyngeal phase was triggered. Similarly, timing the onset of the pharyngeal stage is variable. Palmer *et al.* (1992) timed the onset of this stage in normal subjects from the moment the bolus entered the pharynx and found a range of 0.3 to 6.4 seconds (mean 1.1). They noted that the bolus reached the vallecula in 37% of swallows before the onset of this stage and also found that the onset varied significantly with consistency of the food, being shortest with liquids. When swallowing is observed in normal people, using a nasendoscope, there is a noticeable difference in the triggering of the second stage with food and liquid boluses. With liquids, although some liquid is seen trickling into the oropharynx before the pharyngeal stage is triggered (Wilson, Hoare and Johnson, 1992), the amount of fluid is minimal and, in any case, triggering follows promptly. With more solid boluses, material is often clearly visible on the tongue base for a long time before triggering. From this evidence it seems that the trigger for the pharyngeal stage is not bolus contact with a specific point or area and the action of the tongue assumes importance. Whatever the precise mechanisms, the sensory input must travel via the glossopharyngeal and vagus nerves. From the clinical point of view, the value of the 'gag reflex' is limited as an objective assessment of the second stage trigger mechanism. The gag response is variable in normal individuals, as often observed during mirror examination of the larynx and pharynx, and does not have a consistent relationship to delay of the pharyngeal stage of swallowing. However, there is a correlation between aspiration and a reduced gag reflex in stroke patients (Horner, Massey and Brazer, 1990).

Once triggered, the pharyngeal stage is completed

within 1 second. Although 'pharyngeal peristalsis' used to be considered as the main propulsive force during this stage of swallowing, manofluorographic analysis has demonstrated that the two key elements are in fact the pumping action of the tongue base, the *tongue driving force*, and the elevation of the larynx, which gives rise to the *hypopharyngeal suction pump* (McConnell, Cerenko and Mendelsohn, 1988). Once the bolus has reached the tongue base, it acts like a piston, pumping the bolus posteroinferiorly towards the entrance of the oesophagus. At the same time the suprahyoid muscles pull the larynx antero-superiorly away from the cervical spine. This gives rise to a negative pressure in the entrance of the oesophagus. At this stage of the swallow, the upper oesophageal sphincter has already relaxed (Jacob *et al.*, 1989). The movement of the larynx also holds the cricoid lamina away from the cervical spine which opens the oesophageal approach to receive the bolus.

The upper oesophageal sphincter is the physiological sphincter which holds the entrance to the oesopha-gus shut at rest. It does not correspond exactly with the anatomical position of cricopharyngeus, measures 4–6 cm in length and includes the lower fibres of thyropharyngeus and the upper fibres of the oesophageal musculature as well as cricopharyngeus itself. The pressure in the sphincter is not symmetrical, the anteroposterior pressure being higher than the lateral, a resting pressure of 45 mmHg being recorded. Using manofluorographic techniques it has been shown that there is an initial rise in pressure in the sphincter as the bolus enters the oropharynx followed by a decrease to 0 mmHg which sucks the bolus in. The pressure returns to zero for about half a second after the bolus has passed and then increases to about 90 mmHg before returning to the resting pressure (McConnell, Cerenko and Mendelsohn, 1988). In a small group of patients with cricopharyngeal spasm, cricopharyngeal activity is totally discoordinated during the swallow and this can be shown by manometry (Figure 11.2).

During the pharyngeal stage of deglutition, the laryngeal inlet and nasopharynx are closed to prevent

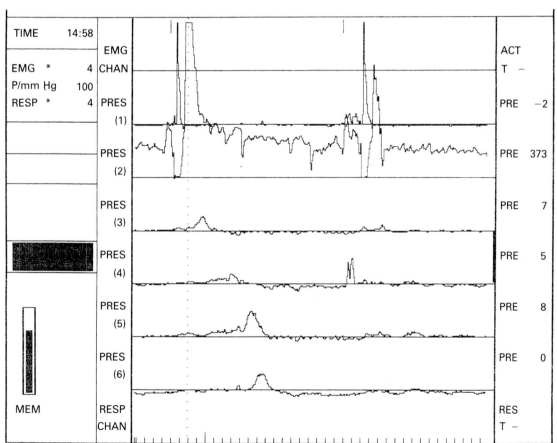

Figure 11.2 (*a*) Manometric recording of a normal subject. Transducer 1 is in the pharynx and transducer 2 is situated at the upper oesophageal sphincter. There is coordinated relaxation and contraction during each swallow. Transducers 3–6 are at 5 cm intervals lower down the oesophagus. The propagation of the peristaltic wave can be seen

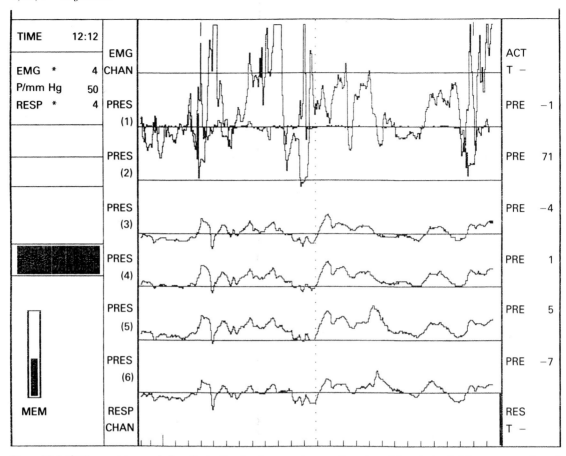

TIME	12:12			ACT	
		EMG		T –	
EMG	*	4	CHAN		
P/mm Hg		50			
RESP	*	4	PRES (1)	PRE	–1
			PRES (2)	PRE	71
			PRES (3)	PRE	–4
			PRES (4)	PRE	1
			PRES (5)	PRE	5
			PRES (6)	PRE	–7
MEM			RESP CHAN	RES T –	

Figure 11.2 (*b*) Manometric record of a patient with cricopharyngeal spasm. Transducer 1 is at the level of the upper oesophageal sphincter and shows continuous pressure changes regardless of swallowing. (Courtesy of Mr W. J. Owen and Mrs A. Anggiansah, Department of Surgery, Guy's Hospital)

aspiration and nasal regurgitation. The larynx closes from below upwards, commencing with the vocal cords, its most powerful sphincter, followed by the false cords and finally the epiglottis, which is pulled down against the cuneiform cartilages. As a result of laryngeal elevation, the epiglottis adopts a horizontal position and its tip is pushed inferiorly over the posterior aspect of the arytenoids by the passing bolus. It is interesting to note that the downfolding of the epiglottis is not seen during breath-holding in spite of contraction of the aryepiglottic muscles. This indicates that the laryngeal elevation and tongue pressure account for the lid effect of the epiglottis during swallowing, not the action of the intrinsic laryngeal muscles (Mendelsohn, 1993).

The soft palate closes the entrance to the nasopharynx by the action of palatopharyngeus and levator palati contracting against the palate, itself stiffened by the tensor palati muscle. The horizontal part of palatopharyngeus, Passavant's muscle, assists in clos-

ing the nasopharyngeal isthmus. The shape and length of the soft palate passively assist the process, which is also aided, to some extent, by the passing bolus.

The bulk of the bolus proceeds rapidly through the relaxed upper oesophageal entrance while the larynx is elevated and closed, pumped by the tongue and sucked by the oesophagus. Gravity assists this process if the individual is upright, but this is not essential. Once this leading edge of the bolus has passed into the oesophagus, the pharyngeal constrictors contract from above downwards and the larynx descends again, stripping any residue out of the pharynx and closing the upper oesophageal sphincter behind the bolus. Once this has happened, the pharyngeal or second stage of swallowing is complete (see Figure 11.1, frame 6). McConnell, Cerenko and Mendelsohn (1988) found that it took 0.835 ± 0.194 seconds for the bolus to pass through the pharynx in 26 normal subjects.

Oesophageal stage

This begins when the bolus enters the oesophagus and ends when it has passed through the lower oesophageal sphincter into the stomach. It lasts 8–20 seconds in normal subjects (Logemann, 1983). During swallowing, peristaltic waves pass down the oesophagus which generate a positive pressure of about 50 mmHg. The form of the wave varies according to the substance being swallowed. With liquids and semisolids, there is an initial negative wave resulting from the elevation of the larynx drawing on the cervical oesophagus, followed by an abrupt positive wave which coincides with the entry of the bolus into the oesophagus. There is then a slow increase in pressure succeeded by a final, large positive pressure wave which rises and falls rapidly, known as the peristaltic stripping wave (Figure 11.3).

Secondary peristaltic waves arise locally in the oesophagus in response to distension, and they complete the transportation of bolus portions which have been left behind after the primary peristaltic wave. Tertiary oesophageal contractions are irregular, non-propulsive contractions involving long segments of the oesophagus, which frequently develop during emotional stress. In the upper part of the oesophagus, peristalsis progresses rapidly; in the lower one-third, the contraction wave is more sluggish. The differences in motor activity are related to the muscular coats being striated in the former situation and unstriated in the latter (Figure 11.4).

At the lower end of the oesophagus there is a zone of raised pressure about 3 cm in length, extending above and below the diaphragm, with a mean pressure of approximately 8 mmHg higher than the intragastic pressure. This region is regarded as the location of the 'physiological sphincter' of the oesophagogastric region. Like the cricopharyngeal sphincter, the oesophagogastric sphincter is normally in tonic contraction and relaxes just before the peristaltic wave reaches it.

The lower oesophageal sphincter

Jewell and Selby (1982) stated that the lower oesophageal sphincter formed the major barrier to gastro-oesophageal reflux. When the muscle of the sphincter is destroyed by disease or surgery, reflux commonly results, e.g. scleroderma and cardiomyotomy for achalasia. The resting sphincter pressure in patients with gastro-oesophageal reflux is often subnormal but there is a wide overlap with the normal range. Many variables govern the actual pressure recorded. Radial asymmetry of pressure is present, with higher pressures being recorded towards the patient's left side (Luckman and Welch, 1977).

Circular muscle fibres from the oesophagogastric junction behave differently from those in the body of the oesophagus, in that they possess a greater resistance to stretch. The cause of the tone of the lower oesophageal sphincter in humans is poorly under-

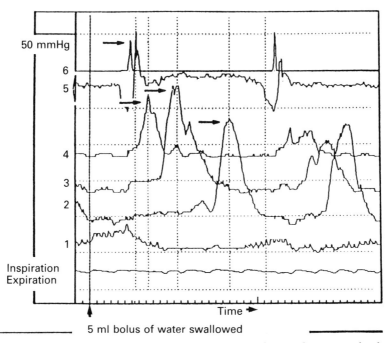

Figure 11.3 Normal manometry showing a typical peristaltic sequence (arrowed). Transducer 6 is in the pharynx, 5 at the cricopharyngeus and 1 is at the lower oesophageal sphincter, which shows normal relaxation. (Courtesy of Mr W. J. Owen and Mrs A. Anggiansah, Department of Surgery, Guy's Hospital)

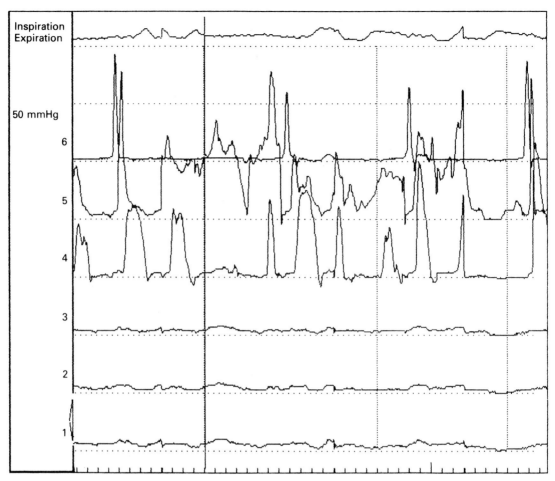

Figure 11.4 Manometric record of a patient with scleroderma. There is no activity in the lower part of the oesophagus as this condition primarily affects smooth muscle. (Courtesy of Mr W. J. Owen and Mrs A. Anggiansah, Department of Surgery, Guy's Hospital)

stood. A number of controlling factors have been suggested which include neural influences, hormonal factors and the intrinsic properties of the muscle fibres themselves. In the opossum, the isolated circular muscle of the sphincter retains its tone after treatment with tetrodotoxin, which blocks all nerve conduction, implying that, in this animal, tone is myogenic in origin (Goyal and Rattan, 1976).

Neural regulation of the lower oesophageal sphincter

The vagus nerve is concerned with the regulation of lower oesophageal sphincter function. Section of the vagus has a variable effect upon the lower oesophageal sphincter in different species. In the dog, high bilateral vagotomy results in oesophageal dilatation and aperistalsis, as might be expected with denervation of striated muscle, and the lower oesophageal sphincter pressure falls (Khan, 1981). The opossum

has much more smooth muscle in the oesophagus and here a transient increase in sphincter pressure follows bilateral vagotomy, while stimulation of the peripheral end of the severed nerve causes the sphincter to relax. Stimulation of the central end causes sphincteric contraction, even when vagotomy is bilateral, which indicates that the efferent pathway for this centrally mediated mechanism lies outside the vagi (Rattan and Goyal, 1974).

In humans, gastro-oesophageal reflux is a common consequence of surgical truncal vagotomy. Resting pressure in the lower oesophageal sphincter falls to the low or low normal range after vagotomy. However, truncal vagotomy does impair the sphincteric response to stress and the increase in sphincter pressure normally seen after an increase in intra-abdominal pressure is inhibited (Angorn *et al.*, 1977). As the vagal nerve supply to the oesophagus and the lower oesophageal sphincter comes from the vagi above the level of section at truncal vagotomy, it seems probable that the operation will have severed the afferent fibres of the reflex concerned in the sphincteric response to the increased abdominal pressure. Patients with gastro-oesophageal reflux who have not undergone previous surgery, show a similar lack of sphincteric contraction in response to a rise in intra-abdominal pressure, and it appears that disruption of this reflex may well be of aetiological importance in reflux.

Much less is known about the role of the sympathetic nerve supply to the oesophagus. No gross disturbance in oesophageal function followed bilateral thoracolumbar sympathectomy when this was employed in the treatment of hypertension. This suggests that the sympathetic nerve supply to the oesophagus is not of vital importance in the regulation of motor activity.

Hormones and the lower oesophageal sphincter

Gastrin causes an increase in lower oesophageal pressure (Giles *et al.*, 1969). This action is mediated through cholinergic mechanisms which can be blocked by atropine. There can be no doubt that this and other alimentary hormones do exert a pharmacological effect upon the sphincter. However, the evidence that these hormones are of physiological importance in the regulation of sphincter tone is much less certain. Changes in serum gastrin levels in health and disease do not correlate closely with changes in sphincteric pressure. In pernicious anaemia, the lower oesophageal sphincter pressure tends to be low, yet the serum gastrin level may be high; and in patients with the Zollinger–Ellison syndrome, the lower oesophageal sphincter pressure is certainly not increased. Although meals influence the lower oesophageal sphincter pressure, and the rise in pressure roughly coincides with increased secretion of gastrin by the antral G cells, it seems more likely that the fluctuations in sphincteric tone are mediated by way of nervous rather than hormonal pathways.

Many other gut hormones have been shown to increase or decrease the tone of the lower oesophageal sphincter. As in the case of gastrin, it is difficult, with the present state of knowledge, to conclude that any of these play a significant part in the physiological regulation of oesophageal motility or in the prevention of gastro-oesophageal reflux. Other agents exert a pharmacological effect on the lower oesophageal sphincter and a number of drugs with anticholinergic actions, notably the tricyclic antidepressants, may aggravate gastro-oesophageal reflux.

The effect of age on swallowing
Infancy

The anatomy and the diet of the newborn are significantly different from those of the adult. As stated above, the larynx lies at a higher level in the infant, the epiglottis reaching as high as the free edge of the soft palate. This helps to close off the mouth from the pharynx. Because the diet is entirely liquid and liquid boluses are more difficult to control in the mouth, good oral function is particularly important. The infant also has to suckle to obtain each bolus before swallowing and this takes time. Infants are, therefore, obligate nasal breathers during feeding and the oropharyngeal sphincter is particularly important to prevent milk trickling into the pharynx before a swallow is made (Kramer and Eicher, 1993).

Old age

Studies have been undertaken to identify any changes in the physiology of swallowing which may develop as a result of age (Perlman, Schultz, VanDaele, 1993; Ren *et al.*, 1993; Shaker *et al.*, 1993). Overall, there is no evidence of significant deterioration in swallowing in otherwise healthy people in their sixth and seventh decades of life. Bolus pressures are said to be higher in the pharyngeal stage in older people when compared to those in their second decade, but the duration of this stage is not lengthened (Perlman, Schultz and VanDaele, 1993; Shaker *et al.*, 1993). Shaker *et al.* (1993) found the resting pressure in the upper oesophageal sphincter to be lower in the elderly, but the response to dilation of the upper oesophagus was unimpaired.

The coordination between laryngeal function and upper oesophageal sphincter function is preserved in the elderly. Ren *et al.* (1993) studied 10 young (23 $\pm$ 2 years) and 10 fit elderly (73 $\pm$ 2 years) subjects by concurrent videoendoscopy, manometry, respirography and submental surface electromyography. The coordination of laryngeal closure and upper oesophageal relaxation were the same in both groups. Bolus volume and temperature did not have any significant effect on the duration of laryngeal closure in either group. However, in both groups, wet swallows significantly shortened the interval between laryngeal closure and upper oesophageal sphincter relaxation as opposed to dry swallows. The authors felt that the shortened interval may be a mechanism which improved the safety of the airway during liquid swallows.

The effect of surgery on swallowing
Tracheostomy

In the tracheostomized patient, the movement of the larynx and upper trachea relative to the skin and soft tissue anterior to these structures is impaired by the tube. Restriction of laryngeal elevation tends to impair swallowing. This often causes a clinical dilemma when it is difficult to be sure whether the dysphagia is due to the condition which required the tracheostomy, the presence of the tube itself, or a combination of both.

An inflated tracheostomy tube cuff in the trachea may cause further problems. There has been a tendency to try to control aspiration by the use of a cuffed tube, but obviously the cuff pressure has to be low. Saliva will accumulate above the cuff of the tube and some may well find a way past it. The inflated cuff also tends to fix the trachea even more and put some pressure on the upper oesophagus, none of which will assist a normal swallow. To avoid these problems, Tippett and Siebens (1991) recommended ventilating suitable patients with the cuff deflated. Even after the tracheostomy has been removed, scarring may impair laryngeal elevation and cause some dysphagia. Biering-Sorensen and Biering-Sorensen (1992) suggested that the use of a minitracheostomy might reduce this complication.

Laryngectomy

Dysphagia secondary to laryngectomy may result from either structural or functional changes in the pharynx. Surgeons tend to concentrate on the structural causes which are usually due to recurrent disease, distortion or stenosis of the pharynx. One of the commonest of these is the formation of a *pseudo-vallecula*, a U-shaped fold of pharynx behind the tongue base. This develops if the pharynx is closed vertically because, when the neck is flexed following this type of closure, the relatively long anterior wall forms a transverse fold. Dysphagia results if food becomes trapped in this fold, but is seldom a serious problem. If treatment is necessary, the band of tissue can be simply divided endoscopically. This particular problem is less likely to develop if a T-shaped or horizontal closure is used.

Stenosis of the pharynx is more common if a partial pharyngectomy has been performed. Management of this problem and that of recurrent cancer are beyond the scope of this chapter.

When the mechanism of swallowing in the laryngectomee is considered, the absence of a larynx can be predicted to cause significant impairment in the pharyngeal stage. As stated earlier, laryngeal elevation is important in opening the upper oesophageal sphincter and helps to generate the negative pressure in the opening of the oesophagus referred to as the hypopharyngeal suction pump (McConnell, Cerenko and Mendelsohn, 1988). In the absence of a larynx, this will be abolished and the passage of the bolus through the hypopharynx is delayed. A second effect is caused by the absence of the descending larynx, which normally squeezes the tail of the bolus into the upper oesophagus. These problems can be compensated by increased pressure from the tongue pump. However, if the bulk or motility of the tongue base has been compromised by surgery, the detrimental effect on swallowing is predictably much greater.

Surgery of the mouth and tongue

The key part played by the tongue in swallowing has already been stressed. Desensitization, fixation or resection of the anterior two-thirds of the tongue causes impairment in the oral stage of swallowing. Tongue mobility is particularly important for preservation of function. Patients can tolerate reduction in the bulk of the tongue better than loss of mobility.

Jaw resection is obviously detrimental to the oral stage too, but particularly to the oral preparatory phase because mastication is disrupted. If continuity of the mandible is maintained, mastication may be better rehabilitated, particularly if dentures can be fitted.

Surgery of the tongue base may also disturb the oropharyngeal sphincter, leading to loss of bolus into the pharynx before the second stage begins. The other effect of surgery to this area is to impair the action of the tongue pump at the beginning of the second stage of swallow. This is one of the most important components of the pharyngeal phase and so impairment of it is likely to have a serious effect on the swallow.

Pharyngeal resection may be well tolerated if the remaining pharynx is large enough, but if total resection and grafting is required, the second stage is totally disrupted. A stomach pull up results in a very wide pharynx and, consequently, dysphagia is an unusual complaint. On the other hand, free jejunal grafts can cause more dysphagia because they do not function physiologically and, if they are too long, kinking can develop which causes hold up at the lower end of the graft.

Neurosurgery

The role of the lower cranial nerves in swallowing is pivotal. The function of the mouth and pharynx during swallowing involves cranial nerves V, VII, IX, X, XI and XII, and the complexity of the muscular anatomy gives some indication of the level of neural and muscular integration and coordination that is required to allow normal swallowing to be achieved. Any surgery which damages these cranial nerves will have a predictably deleterious effect on deglutition. The effect on swallowing is equally devastating if motor or sensory nerves are damaged, whether the site of damage is peripheral or central, and is often seemingly out of proportion to the extent of the deficit.

Investigation of swallowing and swallowing disorders

The importance of taking a history in the assessment of disordered swallowing has already been stated. A thorough structural and functional examination of the patient is equally important. The points to note are summarized in Table 11.1. Many techniques to visualize and document the swallowing process are currently in use. Each offers advantages and has its own drawbacks. None is capable of providing all the information necessary to make a complete assessment.

Contrast nasendoscopy

This technique is a valuable method of assessing deglutition and it is really an extension of the physical examination of the patient. The fibreoptic nasendoscope is an intrinsic part of modern otolaryngology practice and so there is little reason for not using it to assess patients with dysphagia and aspiration (Wilson, Hoare and Johnson, 1992; Mendelsohn, 1993).

The technique is straightforward. It should be undertaken by someone who is experienced in the use of the flexible fibreoptic nasendoscope. One nostril may be anaesthetized to allow comfortable passage of the endoscope, but the anaesthetic has to be used sparingly or the pharynx will be anaesthetized as well and make interpretation of the findings inaccurate. The endoscope is passed through the nose and a preliminary examination of the pharynx made. Any structural abnormality or lesion in the pharynx can be identified; palatal and vocal cord movement can be assessed. The sensitivity of the supraglottic larynx is also tested by gently touching the laryngeal surface of the epiglottis with the tip of the endoscope. Both sides should be tested in stroke patients. This manoeuvre will elicit a brisk response in normal subjects, a reduced response is very significant.

The tip of the endoscope is then withdrawn to the level of the soft palate and the patient is given something to drink. A measured quantity of milk or a suitably coloured safe liquid is given, either from a cup, syringe or straw. The patient is asked to hold this in the mouth. The observer watches the base of the tongue. Even normal subjects can lose a small quantity of liquid into the oropharynx with liquid boluses at this stage but a large quantity of liquid entering the oropharynx indicates poor oral control. If liquid does pour into the pharynx, it is important to observe what happens next. The patient may swallow or the liquid may pool in the vallecula or hypophar-

Table 11.1 Assessment of deglutition

History	
Onset	Sudden or gradual Associated symptoms such as hemiparesis, speech disturbance, or other neurological symptoms
Progress	Gradual deterioration or sudden onset with subsequent improvement
Food consistency	Is the problem greater with a particular consistency – liquids, sloppy food or hard food?
Site of dysphagia	At which stage of the swallow is the delay occurring?
Serious problem?	Is the patient aspirating? Does coughing occur in association with swallowing? Has the patient developed chest infections or pneumonia? Is the patient losing weight?
Aspirating?	Is it before, during or after the pharyngeal stage? Timing of coughing. Is there silent aspiration or significant reflux associated with aspiration?
Examination	
Condition	Nutritional state intellectual state respiratory state
Structure	Teeth Tongue Pharynx Larynx
Function	Motor and sensory assessment of the upper aerodigestive tract – lips, cheeks, jaws, tongue, pharynx and larynx. Sensation, power, range of movement, reflex activity

ynx and then trickle into the larynx. If liquid enters the larynx or trachea, the patient's response must be noted. Some clinicians rely on clinical examination to detect aspiration (Horner, Massey and Brazer, 1990), whereas others recognize its shortcomings (Linden, Kuhlemeier and Patterson, 1993). Any patient who aspirates and does not cough is at severe risk of chest problems; such 'silent aspirators' may go undetected if the clinician relies on clinical examination alone. The author identified four silent aspirators in 20 dysphagia patients using milk nasendoscopy.

The patient is then asked to swallow a bolus. The examiner will lose sight of the pharynx momentarily, but this should be brief. When the view clears, there should be minimal coating of the pharynx with milk and minimal pooling in the vallecula and pyriform fossae. There should be no contrast in the larynx or trachea. A brisk paroxysm of coughing is expected if aspiration has taken place. If there is much coating or pooling, it is important to observe whether the remaining liquid spills into the larynx and what the response is if this should happen. It is also important to ask the patient to swallow again, because good clearance can often be achieved with the second swallow.

The test should be repeated with increasing quantities of liquid and the patient's head position altered from the optimum position, sitting up with the chin down, to any other position. Milk can be channelled down one side of the throat or the other by head tipping or rotation. In stroke patients this is useful because it will show unilateral problems and suggest simple solutions. If nothing abnormal is detected, the 'gulp test' may unmask aspiration. Here the patient is given the cup and asked to drink it down completely as fast as possible.

Solid food is often used also to assess the competence of the swallow. Yoghurt consistency is often the easiest for patients with difficulties in oral control. When endoscoping with solid food, the bolus is frequently seen on the tongue base before the pharyngeal stage is triggered in normal subjects. Food is also given which requires the patient to chew, e.g. biscuit. The tongue base is observed during chewing and if there is difficulty triggering the pharyngeal stage, tongue pumping may be seen.

Some clinicians record their examination with a video system and incoporate a timing device to provide a more objective documentation of the swallowing stages. The test has advantages and disadvantages when compared with videofluorography (Table 11.2) but its main advantages are the low cost, the ease with which it can be performed and its accuracy at detecting aspiration.

Videofluorography

Videofluorography, videofluoroscopy or modified barium swallow are all terms used to describe the

Table 11.2 Comparison of contrast nasendoscopy and videofluorography

	Contrast nasendoscopy	*Videofluorography*
Cost	Endoscope Video-recording Timer	X-ray screening Video-recording Timer
Personnel	Otolaryngologist Assistant	Radiologist Otolaryngologist Speech therapist Radiographer
Hazard	No radiation Readily repeatable	Radiation limits use
Versatility	Portable equipment Bedside use	X-ray department only
Oral stage	Indirect assessment only	Well seen
Pharyngeal stage	Direct assessment Brief loss of view	Well seen
Oesophageal stage	Not seen	Can be observed
Aspiration	Accurate assessment	Accurate assessment
Pharyngeal sensation	Tested	Cannot be tested

technique of observing and recording deglutition using X-rays and recording the results on videotape. It has been used for over a decade and has been well explained and advocated by Logemann (1983, 1986).

The essential requirement for videofluorography is an X-ray screening facility which can be video-recorded with accurate timing on the tape. It is most useful to have sound recording running on the videotape during the test, because this allows the patient's and investigator's comments to be recorded. These are particularly valuable when the videotape is being reviewed. It is also useful to have a special chair for patients, especially those with neurological problems, who are unable to stand or even sit upright. This chair needs to have both chest and head supports, it has to be narrow and manoeuvrable enough to fit into the X-ray machine with the patient in both the anteroposterior and lateral positions, most importantly it has to be radiolucent in these positions.

There is value in having a team approach to videofluorography. The usual members of the team are a speech and language therapist, an otolaryngologist, a radiologist and a radiographer. The therapist and otolaryngologist are the core of the swallowing service; before deciding to perform videofluorography they will have formed an opinion of the nature and severity of the problem from a detailed interview and examination of the patient. With this knowledge, they are able to guide the radiologist and radiographer so that the maximum amount of useful information is obtained from the investigation.

A standard technique is valuable when performing the test. This makes comparisons easier and ensures that no part of the test is omitted. It also facilitates writing a formal report, reviewing the tapes at a future date and comparing results with those of other investigators. The technique described is that used in the author's department, and is based on that advocated by Logemann (1983, 1986).

The field covered during screening must include the whole of the relevant part of the upper aerodigestive tract. This extends from lips and face anteriorly to well behind the posterior pharyngeal wall, from above the hard palate to below the upper oesophageal sphincter. It is particularly important to include the mouth as well as the pharynx. This can cause problems with the lateral view because the area under the chin absorbs no X-rays and it can alter the balance of the image. Masking this area may be necessary to obtain a good image of the whole field.

An explanation is given to the patient about what is going to happen. The patient is first screened in the anteroposterior position and then in the lateral. Unless otherwise indicated, initial screening is with liquids. A measured bolus of liquid is given to the patient, normally starting with 5 ml. This is delivered on a spoon if possible, but if lip control is poor, it can be put into the front of the mouth with a syringe and a quill. The patient is asked to hold the bolus in the mouth until instructed to swallow it. Screening and recording are then begun and oral control observed. The instruction to swallow is given and the process is observed. This is repeated at least once before the bolus size is increased in 5 ml increments up to 20 ml if the swallow is normal or until an abnormality is identified. The posture can be varied if this is likely to contribute to the value of the study. For example, if there is a bulbar palsy on one side, the patient can be tilted in the opposite direction to see if this improves the ability to swallow. Foods of different consistencies can be given according to the patient's ability. Mousse, a paste made with crushed biscuit and solids coated in barium are all useful textures to try. Different investigators use different recipes, but if barium sulphate is incorporated in a recipe, it should not be cooked otherwise it will become toxic.

The principle of starting with small quantities and increasing them is the same with all food consistencies. If one food consistency is particularly troublesome, it is sensible to start with the least troublesome consistency and then select the one which is causing problems. Typically patients with neurological problems find thickened liquids easiest.

All stages of oral and pharyngeal swallow are carefully observed. It is important to be able to review the videotape during the investigation, because this allows any particular event to be seen again on the monitor. A video-recorder with a shuttle button is recommended so that frame by frame analysis can be made. Thus an event which happened very quickly can be analysed slowly, and if more screening is required, it can be designed to give the maximum amount of information. This helps to reduce unnecessary radiation exposure.

If there is any suggestion of an oesophageal disorder, or if reflux may be contributing to the problem, the patient can be stood up, laid down and tipped so that the oesophageal stage can be followed and reflux assessed as part of the study.

Manometry and manofluorography

Manometry has proved a useful method in the investigation of oesophageal physiology and pathophysiology. However, when the function of the pharynx is being assessed by manometry, the capabilities of the manometer have to be quite different. The pharynx generates pressures of 200–400 mmHg, whereas oesophageal pressures reach only 80–140 mmHg. There is also marked asymmetry of pressure in the upper oesophageal sphincter, a greater pressure anteroposteriorly than laterally, so the instrument has to be able to measure pressure in a specific direction. Pharyngeal pressure waves travel at 9–25 cm/s whereas oesophageal waves travel at 4 cm/s, so the response rate of the manometer has to be much faster in the pharynx if accurate results are to be achieved. For this purpose a solid state pressure gauge is required (Figure 11.5). Finally, there is much more movement

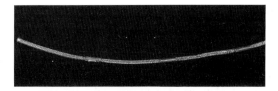

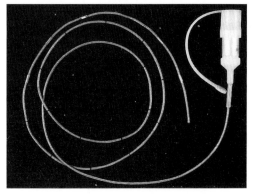

Figure 11.5 (*a,b*) A Gaeltec oesophageal manometer with pressure transducers located at 5 cm intervals along its length. (Courtesy of Mr W. J. Owen and Mrs A. Anggiansah, Department of Surgery, Guy's Hospital)

in the pharynx and upper oesophageal sphincter in which the pressure changes are far more localized than in the oesophagus. It is, therefore, important to know exactly where the manometer is located during the examination. Simultaneous fluorography and manometry provides an accurate, precisely timed, record of information of the pressure changes at precise points in the pharynx and upper oesophagus during deglutition (McConnell, Cerenko and Mendelsohn, 1988).

This method of investigating deglutition is very sophisticated and detects abnormalities that other modalities do not. Although once a research facility it is now firmly established as a routine investigation of swallowing and dysphagia. It has undoubtedly contributed significantly to the understanding of normal and abnormal deglutition.

Oesophageal pH monitoring

This method is valuable in the detection and measurement of reflux in cases where it is thought to contribute to dysphagia and aspiration. Twenty-four-hour monitored records allow accurate documentation of the incidence and duration of episodes of reflux (Figure 11.6).

Other techniques of investigation

Static X-rays

Static imaging with plain X-rays can provide information on structural abnormalities but have little else to contribute to the investigation of swallowing. Static

ACID REFLUX		Total	Upright	Supine	Meal	PostP
Duration	(HH:MM)	22:49	14:19	08:30	01:21	04:00
Number of reflux episodes	(#)	2	2	0	0	0
Number of reflux episodes						
longer than 5.0 minutes	(#)	1	1	0	0	0
Longest reflux episode	(min)	5	5	0	0	0
Total time pH below 4.00	(min)	5	5	0	0	0
Fraction time pH below 4.00	(%)	0.4	0.6	0.0	0.0	0.0

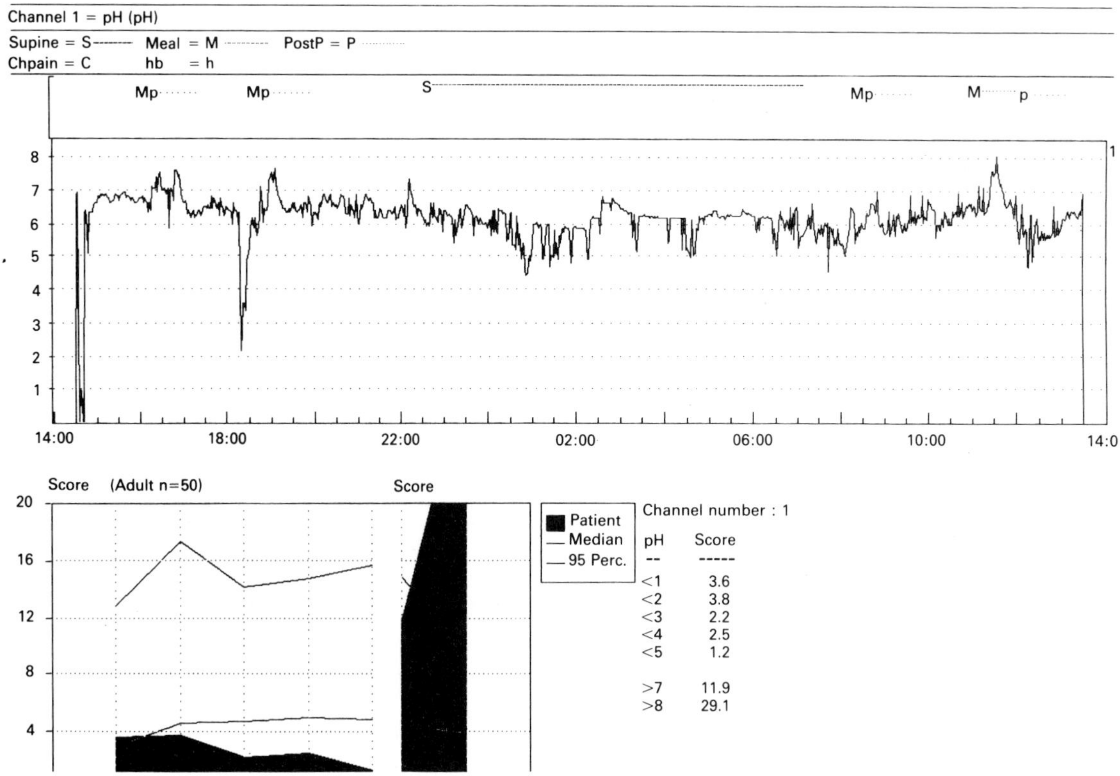

Channel 1 = pH (pH)

Supine = S   Meal = M   PostP = P
Chpain = C   hb   = h

		pH	Score
Patient			
Median		<1	3.6
95 Perc.		<2	3.8
		<3	2.2
		<4	2.5
		<5	1.2
		>7	11.9
		>8	29.1

Channel number : 1

Figure 11.6 (*a*) A normal oesophageal pH tracing with short but brief episodes of reflux. This is reflected in the lower plot, the DeMeester score, which expresses the overall pH result. The lower line represents the median score and the upper line the 95th centile of 50 normal subjects. The black area represents the composite score of the patient throughout pH values 1–8

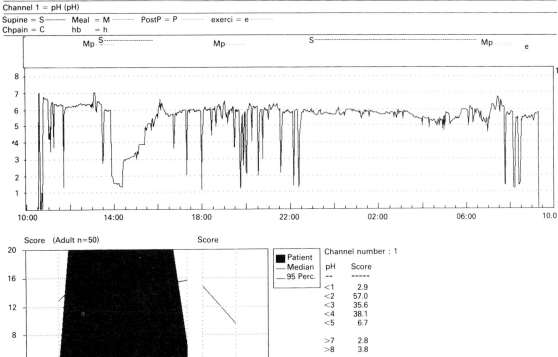

ACID REFLUX		Total	Upright	Supine	Meal	PostP	exerci
Duration	(HH:MM)	22.35	12:45	09.50	00:28	03:00	00:10
Number of reflux episodes	(#)	21	20	2	0	6	0
Number of reflux episodes longer than 5.0 minutes	(#)	2	1	1	0	1	0
Longest reflux episode	(min)	88	6	88	0	11	0
Total time pH below 4.00	(min)	117	28	90	0	17	0
Fraction time pH below 4.00	(%)	8.7	3.6	15.2	0.0	9.7	0.0

Channel 1 = pH (pH)

Supine = S   Meal = M   PostP = P   exerci = e
Chpain = C   hb = h

Channel number : 1	
pH	Score
--	-----
<1	2.9
<2	57.0
<3	35.6
<4	38.1
<5	6.7
>7	2.8
>8	3.8

Figure 11.6 (*b*) An abnormal oesophageal pH tracing with long and frequent periods of reflux in comparison to that of (*a*). (Courtesy of Mr W. J. Owen and Mrs A. Angglansah, Department of Surgery, Guy's Hospital)

views taken during or after a contrast swallow may show part of the normal process or abnormalities such as excess coating of the pharynx or contrast below the vocal cords.

CT and MRI scans

These techniques both have their own strengths in demonstrating structural lesions. Scanning has greatly improved the identification of intracranial pathology in patients with neurological causes of dysphagia. Dynamic scans are available, but videofluorography is still the most popular dynamic radiological method for investigating deglutition.

Scintigraphy

Swallowing a radioactive bolus and observing its progress with a gamma camera is another method of examination which can be used to measure transit times and to detect aspiration. It does not have significant advantages over the methods described above.

Ultrasound

This has been used to study oral function and tongue movement during swallowing by recording with the transducer in the submental region. It avoids any radiation exposure and the tongue muscles can be seen, but the quality of the image is not as easy to interpret as in videofluorography.

References

ANGORN, E. B., DIMOPOULOS, G., HEGARTY, M. M. and MOSHAL, M. G. (1977) The effect of vagotomy on the lower oesophageal sphincter: a manometric study. *British Journal of Surgery*, **64**, 466–469

BIERING–SORENSEN, M. and BIERING–SORENSEN, F. (1992) Tracheostomy in spinal cord injured: frequency and follow up. *Paraplegia*, **30**, 656–660

DODDS, W. J. (1989) Physiology of swallowing. *Dysphagia*, **3**, 171–178

DODDS, W. J., STEWART, E. T. and LOGEMANN, J. A. (1990) Physiology and radiology of the normal oral and pharyngeal phases of swallowing. *American Journal of Roentgenology*, **154**, 953–963

GILES, G. R., MASON, M. C., HUMPHRIES, C. and CLARK, C. G. (1969) Action of gastrin on the lower oesophageal sphincter in man. *Gut*, **10**, 730–734

GOYAL, R. K. and RATTAN, S. (1976) Genesis of basal sphincter pressure: effect of tetrodotoxin on lower oesophageal pressure in opossum in vivo. *Gastroenterology*, **71**, 62–67

GUSTAFSSON, B., TIBBLING, L. and THEORELL, T. (1992) Do physicians care about patients with dysphagia? A study on confirming communication. *Family Practice*, **9**, 203–209

HAMLET, S. L. (1989) Dynamic aspects of lingual propulsive activity in swallowing. *Dysphagia*, **4**, 136–145

HORNER, J., MASSEY, E. W. and BRAZER, S. R. (1990) Aspiration in bilateral stroke patients. *Neurology*, **40**, 1686–1688

JACOB, P., KAHRILAS, P., LOGEMANN, J., SHAH, V. and HA, T. (1989) Upper oesophageal sphincter opening and modulation during swallowing. *Gastroenterology*, **97**, 1469–1478

JEWELL, D. P. and SELBY, W. S. (eds) (1982) Physiology of the oesophagus. In: *Topics in Gastroenterology*. Oxford: Blackwell Scientific Publications. pp. 42–45

KAHN, T. A. (1981) Effect of proximal selective vagotomy on the canine lower oesophageal sphincter. *American Journal of Surgery*, **141**, 219–221

KAHRILAS, P. J., LIN, S., LOGEMANN, J. A., ERGUN, G. A. and FACCHINI, F. (1993) Deglutitive tongue action: volume accommodation and bolus propulsion. *Gastroenterology*, **104**, 152–162

KRAMER, S. S. and EICHER, P. M. (1993) The evaluation of pediatric feeding abnormalities. *Dysphagia*, **8**, 215–224

LINDEN, P., KUHLEMEIER, K. V. and PATTERSON, C. (1993) The probability of correctly predicting subglottic penetration from clinical observations. *Dysphagia*, **8**, 170–179

LINDEN, P., TIPPETT, D., JOHNSTON, J., SIEBENS, A. and FRENCH, J. (1989) Bolus position at swallow onset in normal adults: preliminary observations. *Dysphagia*, **4**, 146–150

LOGEMANN, J. (1983) *Evaluation and Treatment of Swallowing Disorders*. San Diego: College-Hill Press

LOGEMANN, J. A. (1986) *Manual for the Videofluorographic Study of Swallowing*. London: Taylor & Francis Ltd

LUCKMAN, K. and WELCH, R. W. (1977) The significance of lower oesophageal pressure asymmetry in man and its correlation with a new measure of closure strength. *Gastroenterology*, **72**, 1091 (abstract)

MCCONNELL, F. M. S., CERENKO, D. and MENDELSOHN, M. S. (1988) Manofluorographic analysis of swallowing. *Otolaryngologic Clinics of North America*, **21**, 625–635

MENDELSOHN, M. (1993) New concepts in dysphagia management. *Journal of Otolaryngology*, **22**, (suppl. 1)

NEGUS, V. E. (1949) *The Comparative Anatomy and Physiology of the Larynx*. London: Heinemann

PALMER, J. B., RUDIN, N. J., LARA, G. and CROMPTON, A. W. (1992) Coordination of mastication and swallowing. *Dysphagia*, **7**, 187–200

PERLMAN, A. L., SCHULTZ, J. G. and VANDAELE, D. J. (1993) Effects of age, gender, bolus volume, and bolus viscosity on oropharyngeal pressure during swallowing. *Journal of Applied Physiology*, **75**, 33–37

RATTAN, S. and GOYAL, R. K. (1974) Neural control of the lower oesophageal sphincter: influence of the vagus nerve. *Journal of Clinical Investigation*, **54**, 899–906

REN, J., SHAKER, R., ZAMIR, Z., DODDS, W. J., HOGAN, W. J. and HOFFMANN, R. G. (1993) Effect of age and bolus variables on the coordination of the glottis and upper esophageal sphincter during swallowing. *American Journal of Gastroenterology*, **88**, 665–669

SASAKI, C. T. and ISAACSON, G. (1988) Functional anatomy of the larynx. *Otolaryngologic Clinics of North America*, **21**, 595–612

SHAKER, R., REN, J., PODVRSAN, B., DODDS, W. J., HOGAN, W. J., KERN, M. *et al.* (1993) Effect of aging and bolus variables on pharyngeal and upper esophageal sphincter motor function. *American Journal of Physiology*, **264**, G427–432

TALLGREN, A. and TRYDE, G. J. (1992) Swallowing activity of lip muscles in patients with a complete upper and a partial lower denture. *Journal of Oral Rehabilitation*, **19**, 329–341

THEXTON, A. J. (1992) Mastication and swallowing: an overview. *British Dental Journal*, **173**, 197–206

TIPPETT, D. C. and SIEBENS, A. A. (1991) Using ventilators for speaking and swallowing. *Dysphagia*, **6**, 94–99

VAN-DER-BILT, A., OLTHOFF, L. W., BOSMAN, F. and OOSTERHAVEN, S. P. (1993) The effect of missing postcanine teeth on chewing performance in man. *Archives of Oral Biology*, **38**, 423–429

WILSON, P. S., HOARE, T. J. and JOHNSON, A. P. (1992) Milk nasendoscopy in the assessment of dysphagia. *Journal of Laryngology and Otology*, **106**, 525–527

12

Anatomy of the larynx and tracheobronchial tree

Neil Weir

Development of larynx, trachea, bronchi and lungs

During the fourth week of embryonic development, the rudiment of the respiratory tree appears as a median laryngotracheal groove in the ventral wall of the pharynx (Figure 12.1). The groove subsequently deepens and its edges fuse to form a septum, thus converting the groove into a splanchnopleuric laryngotracheal tube. This process of fusion commences caudally and extends cranially but does not involve the cranial end where the edges remain separate, bounding a slit-like aperture through which the tube opens into the pharynx.

The tube is lined with endoderm from which the epithelial lining of the respiratory tract is developed. The cranial end of the tube forms the larynx and the trachea, and the caudal end produces two lateral outgrowths from which the bronchi and right and left lung buds develop. These grow into the pleural coelomas and are thus covered with splanchnic mesenchyme from which the connective tissue, cartilage, non-striated muscle and the vasculature of the bronchi and lungs are developed.

Larynx and trachea

The primitive larynx is the cranial end of the laryngotracheal groove, bounded vertically by the caudal part of the hypobranchial eminence and laterally by the ventral folds of the sixth arches. The arytenoid swellings appear on both sides of the groove and as they enlarge they become approximated to each other and to the caudal part of the hypobranchial eminence from which the epiglottis develops. The opening into the laryngeal cavity is at first a vertical slit or cleft, which becomes T-shaped with the appearance of the

arytenoids. However, the epithelial walls of the cleft soon adhere to each other and the aperture of the larynx is thus occluded until the third month when its lumen is restored. The arytenoid swellings grow upwards and deepen to produce the primitive aryepiglottic folds. This, in turn, produces a further aperture above the level of the primitive aperture which itself becomes the glottis. During the second month of fetal life, the arytenoid swellings differentiate into the arytenoid and corniculate cartilages (derivatives of the sixth arch), and the folds joining them to the epiglottis become the aryepiglottic folds in which the cuneiform cartilages are developed as derivatives of the epiglottis. The thyroid cartilage develops from the ventral ends of the cartilages of the fourth branchial arch, appearing as two lateral plates, each with two chondrification centres. The cricoid cartilage and cartilages of the trachea develop from the sixth branchial arch during the sixth week. The trachea increases rapidly in length from the fifth week onwards.

The branchial nerves of the fourth and sixth arches, namely the superior laryngeal and recurrent laryngeal nerves, supply the larynx (Figure 12.2).

Each visceral arch is traversed by an artery (aortic arch). Each aortic arch connects the ventral and dorsal aortae of its own visceral arch. The primitive recurrent laryngeal nerve enters the sixth visceral arch, on each side, caudal to the sixth aortic arch. On the left side, the arch retains its position as the ductus arteriosus and the nerve is found caudal to the ligamentum arteriosum after birth. On the right side, the dorsal part of the sixth aortic arch and the whole of the fifth arch disappear. The nerve is, therefore, found on the caudal aspect of the fourth aortic arch, which becomes the subclavian artery. Piersol (1930) described the 'complete persistence of the distal portion of the right aortic arch associated with the disappearance of its proximal part'. Here the right sub-

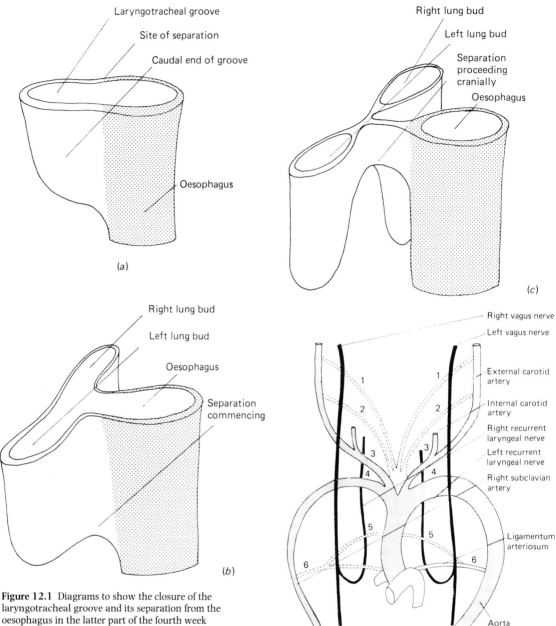

Figure 12.1 Diagrams to show the closure of the laryngotracheal groove and its separation from the oesophagus in the latter part of the fourth week

Figure 12.2 The branchial arteries and recurrent laryngeal nerves

clavian artery originates from the descending aorta and passes right behind the oesophagus. In the absence of the proximal portion of the right fourth aortic arch no structure remains in contact with the right recurrent nerve. Instead of being pulled down into its usual position, the nerve passes directly from the main vagal trunk to enter the larynx (Work, 1941). In this context the nerve is called the *non-recurrent laryngeal nerve*. The incidence is variously reported to be between 0.3% and 1.0%. For a left

non-recurrent nerve to exist there would have to be either a loss of the ductus arteriosus in fetal life or a right-sided aorta. A case of the latter situation was reported by Berlin in 1935.

Bronchi and lungs

The right and left lung buds appear before the laryngotracheal groove is converted into a tube. They grow out into the pleural passages caudal to the common cardinal veins and divide into lobules, three appearing on the right and two on the left.

It is uncertain whether lung budding determines the septal pattern or whether the development of the connective tissue septa controls the final form of the lung (Emery, 1969). Each primary bronchus continues to divide dichotomously until, by birth, some 18–23 generations of divisions have appeared which are not necessarily equal in the individual lobes.

Three periods of development of the lung are described: a 'glandular' period, when the primitive bronchi ramify through the mesenchyme (up to 4 months); a 'canicular' period when the primitive respiratory bronchioles are generated from the terminal bronchi (4–6 months); and an 'alveolar' period from 6 months onwards when further respiratory bronchioles and the terminal alveoli, which will be the functional airspaces with their blood-air barriers, are formed.

There has been considerable discussion concerning how much of the subsequent development of the bronchi and alveoli takes place after birth. The current views are summarized by Reid (1967) in her three 'laws' of lung development:

1 The bronchial tree is fully developed by the sixteenth week of intrauterine life
2 Alveoli, as commonly understood, develop after birth, increasing in number until the age of 8 years, and in size until growth of the chest wall is complete
3 Blood vessels are remodelled and increase in number, certainly while new alveoli are forming.

During the course of their development, the lungs migrate in a caudal direction, so that by birth the bifurcation of the trachea is opposite the fourth thoracic vertebra. As the lungs grow, they become enveloped in pleura derived from the splanchnic mesenchyme.

For further reading on development of the trachea and lungs, consult O'Rahilly and Boyden (1973) and Reid (1976).

The larynx

Comparative anatomy and modification for olfaction and deglutition

The prime reason for the existence of the larynx is not to make phonation possible, but to provide a protective sphincter at the inlet of the air passages. This can be seen in a lung fish, where the larynx takes the form of a simple muscular sphincter surrounding the opening of the air passage in the floor of the pharynx. In birds, the rima glottidis in the floor of the mouth shuts to close the air inlet but it makes no sound; phonation is produced from a dilatation, the syrinx, at the lower end of the trachea just above its bifurcation.

The first breathers of air, the amphibia, do however phonate. They achieve this by 'swallowing air' which, as there is no separate nasal cavity, is drawn in through valvular 'nostrils' opening anteriorly into the roof of the mouth. In mammals, a nasal cavity develops with the appearance of a palate. The separation of a respiratory and olfactory chamber from the mouth has considerable advantages: predatory mammals can still breathe while the mouth is obstructed by prey, and herbivorous prey can still sense warning odours while feeding. In aquatic vertebrates, such as crocodiles, dolphins and whales, an intranarial larynx has been developed where the inlet of the larynx is suspended within the nasopharynx and clasped by the sphincter of the nasopharyngeal inlet (the palatopharyngeus). Thus respiration and olfaction can continue at the water surface even with the mouth submerged, open and ready for prey.

The larynx of humans is still an essential sphincter, preventing the entry of swallowed food and other foreign bodies, and providing a blockade to build up pressure for coughing or for aiding extreme muscular efforts. However, humans differ from other mammals in the ability to produce speech by the highest integrations of the nervous and locomotive systems.

Descriptive anatomy

The larynx is situated at the upper end of the trachea; it lies opposite the third to sixth cervical vertebrae in men, while being somewhat higher in women and children. The average length, transverse diameter and anteroposterior diameter are, in the male, 44 mm, 43 mm and 36 mm, and, in the female, 36 mm, 41 mm and 26 mm, respectively.

There is little difference in the size of the larynx in boys and girls until after puberty when the anteroposterior diameter in the male almost doubles.

The skeletal framework of the larynx (Figures 12.3 and 12.4) is formed of cartilages, which are connected by ligaments and membranes and are moved in relation to one another by both intrinsic and extrinsic muscles. It is lined with mucous membrane which is continuous above and behind with that of the pharynx and below with that of the trachea.

The infantile larynx is both absolutely and relatively smaller than the larynx of the adult. The lumen is therefore disproportionately narrower. It is more funnel-shaped and its narrowest part is at the junction of the subglottic larynx with the trachea. A very slight swelling of the lax mucosa in this area may thus produce a very serious obstruction to

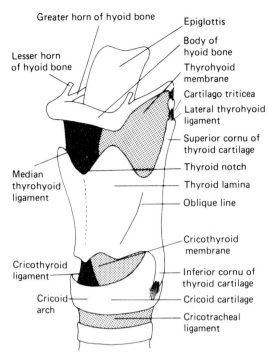

Figure 12.3 The cartilages and ligaments of the larynx

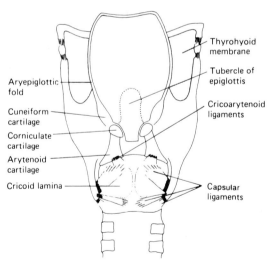

Figure 12.4 Ligaments, membranes and cartilages of the larynx seen from behind

breathing. The laryngeal cartilages are much softer in the infant and therefore collapse more easily in forced inspiratory efforts. The infantile larynx starts high up under the tongue and with development assumes an increasingly lower position.

Laryngeal cartilages

The thyroid cartilage

The shield-like cartilage (see Figures 12.3 and 12.4) is the longest of the laryngeal cartilages and consists of two laminae which meet in the midline inferiorly, leaving an easily palpable notch, the thyroid notch, between them above. The angle of fusion of the laminae is about 90° in men and 120° in women. In the male, the fused anterior borders form a projection, again easily palpable, which is the laryngeal prominence or 'Adam's apple'. A small narrow strip of cartilage, the intrathyroid cartilage, separates the two laminae anteriorly in childhood. Posteriorly, the laminae diverge and the posterior border of each is prolonged as two slender processes, the superior and inferior cornua. The superior cornu is long and narrow and curves upwards, backwards and medially, ending in a conical extremity to which is attached the lateral thyroid ligament. The inferior cornu is shorter and thicker and curves downwards and medially. On the medial surface of its lower end there is a small oval facet for articulation with the cricoid cartilage.

On the external surface of each lamina, an oblique line curves downwards and forwards from the superior thyroid tubercle, situated just in front of the root of the superior horn, to the inferior thyroid tubercle on the lower border of the lamina. This line marks the attachments of the thyrohyoid, sternothyroid and inferior constrictor muscles. The inner aspects of the laminae are smooth and are mainly covered by loosely attached mucous membrane. The thyroepiglottic ligament is attached to the inner aspect of the thyroid notch, and below this, and on each side of the midline, the vestibular and vocal ligaments, and the thyroarytenoid, thyroepiglottic and vocalis muscles are attached. The fusion of the anterior ends of the two vocal ligaments produces the anterior commissure tendon which is of importance in the spread of carcinoma.

The superior border of each lamina gives attachment to the corresponding half of the thyrohyoid ligament. The inferior border of each half is divided into two by the inferior tubercle. The cricothyroid membrane is attached to the inner aspect of the medial portion of the inferior border of the thyroid cartilage.

The cricoid cartilage

The cricoid cartilage (see Figures 12.3 and 12.4) is the only complete cartilaginous ring present in the air passages. It forms the inferior part of the anterior and lateral walls and most of the posterior wall of the larynx. Likened to a signet ring, it comprises a deep broad quadrilateral lamina posteriorly and a narrow arch anteriorly. Near the junction of arch and lamina, an articular facet is present for the inferior cornu of the thyroid cartilage. The lamina has sloping shoulders, which carry articular facets for the arytenoids. These joints are synovial with capsular ligaments. Rotation of the cricoid cartilage on the thyroid cartilage can take place about an axis passing transversely through the joints. A vertical ridge in the midline of the lamina gives attachment to the longitudinal muscle of the oesophagus and produces a shallow concavity on each side for the origin of the posterior cricoarytenoid muscle. The entire surface of the cricoid cartilage is lined with mucous membrane.

The arytenoid cartilages

The two arytenoid cartilages (see Figure 12.4) are placed close together on the upper and lateral borders of the cricoid lamina. Each is an irregular three-sided pyramid with a forward projection, the vocal process, attached to the vocal folds, and also a lateral projection, the muscular process, to which are attached the posterior cricoarytenoid and lateral cricoarytenoid muscles. Between these two processes is the anterolateral surface which is irregular and divided into two fossae by a crest running from the apex. The upper triangular fossa gives attachment to the vestibular ligament and the lower to the vocalis and lateral cricoarytenoid muscles. The apex is curved backwards and medially and is flattened for articulation with the corniculate cartilage to which is attached the aryepiglottic folds. The medial surfaces are covered with mucous membrane and form the lateral boundary of the intercartilaginous part of the rima glottidis. The posterior surface is covered entirely by the transverse arytenoid muscle.

The base is concave and presents a smooth surface for articulation, with the sloping shoulder on the upper border of the cricoid lamina. The capsular ligament of this synovial joint is lax, allowing both rotatory and medial and lateral gliding movements. In humans the cylindrical articulating surfaces permit a greater range of gliding than of rotatory movement, and the shape of the open human glottis resembles a V. A firm posterior cricoarytenoid ligament prevents forward movement of the arytenoid cartilage.

The corniculate and cuneiform cartilages

The corniculate cartilages (see Figure 12.4) are two small conical nodules of elastic fibrocartilage which articulate as a synovial joint, or which are sometimes fused, with the apices of the arytenoid cartilages. They are situated in the posterior parts of the aryepiglottic folds of mucous membrane. The cuneiform cartilages are two small elongated flakes of elastic fibrocartilage placed one in each margin of the aryepiglottic fold.

The cartilage of the epiglottis

The epiglottis is a thin, leaf-like sheet of elastic fibrocartilage which projects upwards behind the tongue and the body of the hyoid bone (see Figures 12.3 and 12.4). The narrow stalk is attached by the thyroepiglottic ligament to the angle between the thyroid laminae, below the thyroid notch. The upper broad part is directed upwards and backwards; its superior margin is free.

The sides of the epiglottis are attached to the arytenoid cartilages by the aryepiglottic folds of mucous membrane which, together with the free edge of the epiglottis, form the anterior boundary to the inlet of the larynx. The posterior surface of the epiglottis is concave and smooth but a small central projection, the tubercle, is present in the lower part. The bare cartilage is indented by numbers of small pits into which mucous glands project. The anterior surface of the epiglottis is free and is covered with mucous membrane which is reflected on to the pharyngeal part of the tongue and on to the lateral wall of the pharynx, forming a median glossoepiglottic fold and two lateral glossoepiglottic folds. The depression formed on each side of the median glossoepiglottic fold is the vallecula. An elastic ligament, the hyoepiglottic ligament, connects the lower part of the epiglottis to the hyoid bone in front. The space between the epiglottis and the thyrohyoid membrane is filled with fatty tissue and is named the pre-epiglottic space. The epiglottis is not functionally developed in humans in that respiration, deglutition and phonation can take place almost normally even if it has been destroyed. In neonates and infants, however, the epiglottis is omega-shaped. This long, deeply grooved, 'floppy' epiglottis more closely resembles that of aquatic mammals and is more suited to its function of protecting the nasotracheal air passage during suckling.

Calcification of the laryngeal cartilages

The corniculate and cuneiform cartilages, the epiglottis, and the apices of the arytenoids consist of elastic fibrocartilage, which shows little tendency to calcify. The thyroid, cricoid and greater part of the arytenoids consist of hyaline cartilage which begins to calcify in the person's late teens or early twenties. Calcification of the thyroid cartilage starts in the region of the inferior cornu and proceeds anteriorly and superiorly until the entire rim is involved. A central translucent window persists into old age.

Calcification of the posterior part of the lamina of the cricoid and of the posterior part of arytenoid may be confused at radiology with a foreign body (see also under Applied anatomy of larynx). Calcification of the body and muscular process of the arytenoid takes place later in the fourth decade but the vocal process tends not to ossify.

The ligaments

Extrinsic ligaments

The extrinsic ligaments (Figure 12.5 and see Figures 12.3 and 12.4) connect the cartilages to the hyoid and trachea.

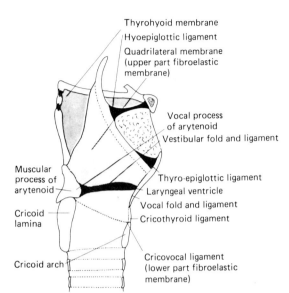

Figure 12.5 Ligaments and membranes of the larynx seen laterally

The thyrohyoid membrane stretches between the upper border of the thyroid and the upper border of the posterior surfaces of the body and greater cornua of the hyoid bone. The membrane is composed of fibroelastic tissue and is strengthened anteriorly by condensed fibrous tissue called the median thyrohyoid ligament. The posterior margin is also stretched to form the lateral thyrohyoid ligament which connects the tips of the superior cornua of the thyroid cartilage to the posterior ends of the greater cornua of the hyoid. The ligaments often contain a small nodule, the cartilago triticea. The membrane is pierced by the internal branch of the superior laryngeal nerve and by the superior laryngeal vessels.

The cricotracheal ligament unites the lower border of the cricoid cartilage with the first tracheal ring.

The hyoepiglottic ligament connects the epiglottis to the back of the body of the hyoid.

Intrinsic ligaments

The intrinsic ligaments (see Figure 12.5) connect the cartilages themselves, and together they strengthen the capsules of the intercartilaginous joints and form the broad sheet of fibroelastic tissue, the fibroelastic membrane, which lies beneath the mucous membrane of the larynx and creates an internal framework.

The fibroelastic membrane is divided into an upper and lower part by the laryngeal ventricle. The upper quadrilateral membrane extends between the border of the epiglottis and the arytenoid cartilage. The upper margin forms the frame of the aryepiglottic fold which is the fibrous skeleton of the laryngeal inlet; the lower margin is thickened to form the vestibular ligament which underlies the vestibular fold or false cord. The lower part is altogether a thicker membrane, containing many elastic fibres. It is commonly called the cricovocal ligament, cricothyroid ligament or, by a more loose term, the conus elasticus. It is attached below to the upper border of the cricoid cartilage and above is stretched between the midpoint of the laryngeal prominence of the thyroid cartilage anteriorly and the vocal process of the arytenoid behind. The free upper border of this membrane constitutes the vocal ligament, the framework of the vocal fold or true cord. Anteriorly, there is a thickening of the membrane, the cricothyroid ligament, which links the cricoid and the thyroid cartilages in the midline. (For laryngotomy, see under Applied anatomy of the larynx.)

The interior of the larynx

The cavity of the larynx extends from the pharynx at the laryngeal inlet to the beginning of the lumen of the trachea at the lower border of the cricoid cartilage and is divided by the vestibular and vocal folds into three compartments. The superior vestibule is above the vestibular folds, the ventricle or sinus of the larynx lies between the vestibular and vocal folds, and the subglottic space extends from the vocal folds to the lower border of the cricoid cartilage (see Figure 12.5). The fissure between the vestibular folds is called the rima vestibuli and that between the vocal folds is the rima glottidis or glottis. The paraglottic and pre-epiglottic spaces, which are of importance in the spread of tumours, lie within the larynx.

The laryngeal inlet is bounded superiorly by the free edge of the epiglottis and on each side by the aryepiglottic folds. Posteriorly, the inlet is completed by the mucous membrane between the two arytenoid cartilages. This region of the larynx was formerly termed the posterior commissure but is now more correctly called the posterior glottis (McIlwain, 1991). There is a plentiful supply of mucous glands in the margins of the aryepiglottic folds.

The superior vestibule lies between the inlet of the larynx and the level of the vestibular folds. It narrows as it extends downwards and the anterior wall, which is the posterior surface of the epiglottis, is much deeper than the posterior wall which is formed by mucous membrane covering the anterior surface of the arytenoid cartilages. The lateral walls are formed by the inner aspect of the aryepiglottic folds.

The pre-epiglottic space is a wedge-shaped space lying in front of the epiglottis and is bounded anteriorly by the thyrohyoid ligament and the hyoid bone. Above a deep layer of fascia, the hyoepiglottic ligament connects the epiglottis to the hyoid bone. It is continuous laterally with the paraglottic space which is bounded by the thyroid cartilage laterally, the conus elasticus and quadrangular membrane medially and the anterior reflection of the pyriform fossa mucosa posteriorly. It embraces the ventricles and saccules.

The laryngeal ventricle and vestibular folds

The middle part of the cavity (and ventricle) lies between the vestibular and vocal folds which cover the ligaments of the same name. On each side, it opens, through a narrow horizontal slit, into an elongated recess, the laryngeal ventricle or sinus. From the anterior part of the ventricle, a pouch, the saccule of the larynx, ascends between the vestibular folds and the inner surface of the thyroid cartilage.

It may extend as far as the upper border of the cartilage; indeed, in some monkeys and apes, it extends even further into the neck, as far as the axilla. In humans, the saccule occasionally protrudes through the thyrohyoid membrane. The mucous membrane lining the saccule contains numerous mucous glands, lodged in submucous alveolar tissue. Fibrous tissue surrounds the saccule and a limited number of muscle fibres pass from the apex of the arytenoid cartilage across the medial aspect of the saccule to the aryepiglottic fold. The muscle is presumed to compress the saccule and to express the secretion of its mucous glands over the surface of the vocal folds.

The vestibular folds are two thick, pink folds of mucous membrane, each enclosing a narrow band of fibrous tissue, the vestibular ligament, which is fixed in front to the angle of the thyroid cartilage, just below the attachment of the epiglottic cartilage, and behind to the anterolateral surface of the arytenoid cartilage, just above the vocal process.

The vocal folds

The vocal folds are defined as two fold-like structures which extend from the middle of the angle of the thyroid cartilage to the vocal processes of the arytenoid cartilages. Each fold is a layered-structure. Figure 12.6 shows the histological structure of a vertical section of the adult human vocal fold at the middle of the membranous portion. The vocal fold is made up of mucosa and muscle. The mucosa is subdivided into epithelium which is of the stratified squamous type and the lamina propria, which consists of superficial, intermediate, and deep layers. The superficial layer of the lamina propria, referred to as Reinke's space, consists of loose fibrous substance which can be likened to a mass of soft gelatin. It is this layer which vibrates most significantly during phonation.

If it becomes stiff due to some pathological state such as inflammation, tumour or scar tissue, its vibrations are disturbed and voice problems result. The intermediate layer, consisting mainly of elastic fibres, and the deep layer, consisting of collagenous fibres rich in fibroblasts, together form the vocal ligament, deep to which is the vocalis muscle which constitutes the main body of the vocal fold.

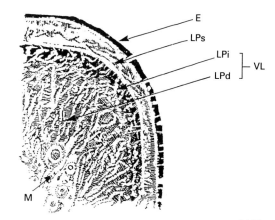

Figure 12.6 Coronal section of an adult human vocal fold. E: epithelium. LPs, LPi, LPd: superficial (Reinke's space), intermediate and deep layers of lamina propria. VL: LPi and LPd together constitute the vocal ligament. M: vocalis muscle. (Illustration by Mrs Jill Richardson Jones)

Around the edge of the vocal fold the elastic and collagenous fibres in the lamina propria, and the muscle fibres of the vocalis muscle run parallel to the edge. The layered structure is not uniform along the length of the vocal fold (Figure 12.7). At the anterior end there is a mass of collagenous fibres which appear to be connected to the inner perichondrium of the thyroid cartilage anteriorly and to the deep layer of the lamina propria posteriorly. Posterior to this mass of collagenous fibres there is another mass of elastic fibres, continuous with the intermediate layer of the lamina propria, called the anterior macula flava. A similar picture is seen at the posterior end of the membranous part of the vocal fold. These structures at both ends of the membranous vocal folds appear to serve as cushions to protect the ends from mechanical damage caused by vocal fold vibration.

The vocal fold is a multilayered vibrator which, from a mechanical point of view, can be reclassified into three layers: the *cover*, consisting of the epithelium and superficial layer of the lamina propria; the *transition*, consisting of the intermediate and deep layers of the lamina propria; and the *body* consisting of the vocalis muscle.

The blood vessels in the mucosa at the edge of the vocal fold run parallel to the edge. All the vessels are very small and therefore do not impede vibration.

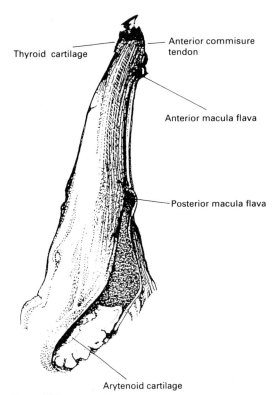

Figure 12.7 Horizontal section of human vocal fold at the anterior and posterior ends of the membranous portion. (After Hirano, 1981, p. 6. Illustration by Mrs Jill Richardson Jones)

Histological variations in structure of the vocal fold in children and the elderly

The structure of the edge of the vocal fold in the newborn differs markedly from its adult form. The main difference is in the lamina propria which is very thick relative to the length of the vocal fold and is uniform in structure. There is no evidence of a vocal ligament as almost the entire lamina propria is loose and pliable. Some fibrous tissue, immature macula flava, is present near the anterior and posterior ends of the membranous vocal fold.

An immature vocal ligament emerges between the ages of 1 and 4 years. Differentiation between the two layers of the vocal ligament starts between 6 and 12 years of age and the ligament becomes thicker. Near the end of adolescence the three-layer structure of the lamina propria is clearly evident.

There is great individual variation in changes in structure of the vocal fold with increasing age. There is a little change in the epithelium but the superficial layer of the lamina propria tends to become oedematous and thicker with age. Elastic fibres in the intermediate layer become loose and atrophied and the layer thus becomes thinner. The collagenous fibres of the deep layer become thicker and denser and the vocalis muscle tends to atrophy with age.

The glottis

The rima glottidis or glottis is an elongated fissure between the vocal folds anteriorly, and the vocal processes and bases of the arytenoid cartilages posteriorly. It is limited behind by the mucous membrane between the arytenoid cartilages with the top portion of the cricoid lamina as its base. The region between the vocal folds accounts for three-fifths of the length of the aperture and is termed the 'intermembranous part'. The remainder lies between the vocal processes and is called the intercartilaginous part. The average length of the glottis varies between 23 mm in men and 16–17 mm in women. In the resting state, the vocal processes are usually 8 mm apart. The glottis alters shape with phonation and respiration.

The subglottis

The lower part of the laryngeal cavity or subglottic space extends from the level of the vocal folds to the lower border of the cricoid cartilage. Its upper part is elliptical in form, but its lower part widens and becomes circular in shape and continuous with the cavity of the trachea. It is lined with mucous membrane, and its walls consist of the cricothyroid ligament above and the inner surface of the cricoid cartilage below.

The muscles

The muscles of the larynx may be divided into extrinsic, which attach the larynx to neighbouring structures and maintain the position of the larynx in the neck and intrinsic, which move the various cartilages of the larynx and regulate the mechanical properties of the vocal folds.

Extrinsic muscles

The extrinsic muscles may be divided into those below the hyoid bone (infrahyoid muscles) and those above the hyoid bone (suprahyoid muscles). The infrahyoid muscles include the thyrohyoid, sternothyroid, sternohyoid and omohyoid.

The thyrohyoid muscle arises from the oblique line of the thyroid lamina and is inserted into the inferior border of the greater cornu of the hyoid bone. It is supplied by C1 fibres by way of the hypoglossal nerve and elevates the larynx if the hyoid is fixed, or depresses the hyoid if the larynx is fixed.

The sternothyroid muscle arises from the posterior surface of the manubrium sterni and from the edge of the first, and occasionally the second, costal cartilage and is inserted into the oblique line on the anterolateral surface of the thyroid lamina. It is supplied by the ansa cervicalis (C2, 3), and depresses the larynx.

The sternohyoid muscle originates from the clavicle and the posterior surface of the manubrium sterni and is inserted into the lower edge of the body of the hyoid bone. It is supplied by a branch of ansa cervicalis (C1,2,3) and depresses the larynx by lowering the hyoid bone.

It is likely that a more significant role of the infrahyoid muscles is to oppose the elevators of the larynx (the suprahyoid muscles) by 'paying out rope' during contraction of the elevators; descent of the larynx after elevation is due to elastic recoil of the trachea.

The suprahyoid muscles include the mylohyoid, geniohyoid, stylohyoid, stylopharyngeus, palatopharyngeus and salpingopharyngeus.

The myelohyoid muscle originates from the mylohyoid line on the inner aspect of the mandible and is inserted into a midline raphe with fibres from the opposite side. The midline raphe and the posterior fibres are attached to the body of the hyoid bone. Its nerve supply is derived from the motor root of the trigeminal nerve by way of the mylohyoid branch of the inferior alveolar nerve and its action is to raise the hyoid bone and pull it anteriorly.

The geniohyoid muscle extends from each inferior genial tubercle to the upper border of the body of the hyoid bone. It is supplied by C1 fibres by way of the hypoglossal nerve and raises and pulls forward the hyoid bone.

The stylohyoid muscle arises from the back of the styloid process. It bifurcates around the intermediate tendon of the digastric muscle and is inserted by two slips into the base of the greater cornu of the hyoid bone. It is supplied by the facial nerve and acts as a retractor and elevator of the hyoid bone, used in swallowing.

The digastric muscle originates from the digastric notch on the medial surface of the mastoid process. Its posterior belly tapers to an intermediate tendon, held beneath a fibrous sling attached near the lesser cornu of the hyoid bone. The anterior belly connects the intermediate tendon to the digastric fossa on the lower border of the mandible. The posterior belly is supplied by the facial nerve, the anterior by the mylohyoid nerve (trigeminal). The anterior belly pulls the hyoid bone anteriorly and raises it whereas the posterior belly pulls the hyoid bone posteriorly and also raises it.

The stylopharyngeus muscle arises from the deep aspect of the styloid process and sloping down crosses the lower border of the superior constrictor and passes down inside the middle constrictor. Here it lies behind the palatopharyngeus and is inserted into the posterior border of the lamina of the thyroid cartilage and the side wall of the pharynx. The muscle is supplied by the glossopharyngeal nerve and helps to elevate the larynx.

The palatopharyngeus muscle is described in Chapter 10. It is inserted into the posterior border of the thyroid ala and cornua. Some of the posterior fibres merge with the surrounding fibres of the inferior constrictor. It is supplied by the accessory nerve through the pharyngeal plexus. Although its main action is to raise and shorten the wall of the pharynx, it probably also helps in tilting the larynx forward, thus enabling food to pass straight into the oesophagus during the act of swallowing.

The salpingopharyngeus muscle arises from the tubal elevation and passes vertically down inside the pharynx to be inserted into the posterior border of the thyroid cartilage and the side wall of the pharynx. It is supplied by the pharyngeal plexus and elevates the larynx and pharynx in the second (involuntary) stage of swallowing.

Intrinsic muscles

The intrinsic laryngeal muscles (Figures 12.8 and 12.9) are of great importance in regulating the mechanical properties of the vocal folds as they control not only position and shape of the vocal folds, but also the elasticity and viscosity of each layer of the vocal fold. They may be divided into: first, those that open and close the glottis, namely the posterior cricoarytenoids, the lateral cricoarytenoids and the transverse and oblique arytenoids; second, those that control the tension of the vocal folds, namely the thyroarytenoids (vocalis) and cricothyroids; and third, those that alter the shape of the inlet of the larynx, namely the aryepiglotticus and the thyroepiglotticus. With the exception of the transverse arytenoid, all these muscles are paired.

The lateral cricoarytenoid arises from the superior border of the lateral part of the arch of the cricoid cartilage and inserts into the front of the muscular process of the arytenoid. It adducts and lowers the tip of the vocal process of the arytenoid by rotating the arytenoid medially. The entire vocal fold is thus adducted, lowered, elongated and thinned. The edge of the vocal fold becomes sharp and all the layers are passively stiffened.

The posterior cricoarytenoid which is the only muscle to open the glottis, arises from the lower and medial surface of the back of the cricoid lamina and fans out to be inserted into the back of the muscular process of the arytenoid cartilage. Its upper fibres are almost horizontal, while its lateral fibres are almost vertical. The horizontal action rotates the arytenoids and moves the muscular processes towards each other, thus separating the vocal processes and abducting the vocal folds. The vertical action (lateral fibres) draws the arytenoids down the sloping shoulders of the cricoid cartilage, thus separating the arytenoids from each other. These actions take place simultaneously, although in humans there is a greater proportion of vertical movement, thus opening the glottis in a V shape. The posterior cricoarytenoid abducts and elevates the tip of the vocal process of the arytenoid cartilage and therefore the entire vocal fold becomes markedly elongated and thin. The edge of the vocal fold is rounded and all the layers are passively stiffened.

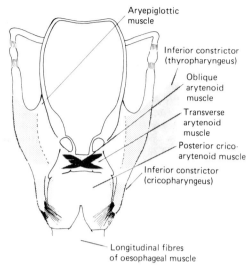

Figure 12.8 Intrinsic muscles of the larynx seen from behind

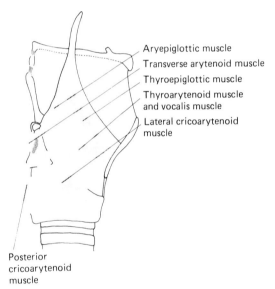

Figure 12.9 Intrinsic muscles of the larynx seen laterally

The weight of the abductor muscles of the larynx is not more than 25% of that of the adductors (Bowden and Sheuer, 1960), which may explain the greater vulnerability of the abductors in the event of partial injury to the recurrent laryngeal nerve. In a study of the intrinsic muscles of 54 normal post-mortem larynges, it was observed that while no significant alterations had developed in the cricothyroid, interarytenoid, lateral cricoarytenoid or thyroarytenoid muscles, all the larynges from patients 13 years old or over revealed microscopical changes in the posterior cricoarytenoid muscle, and in many of

those from patients over 46 years old there had also been some necrosis and associated reactive changes (Guindi *et al.*, 1981). Because the posterior cricoarytenoid muscle is the sole abductor of the vocal folds, the changes may be a manifestation of the continuous activity of this muscle. The changes start with the deposition of coarse lipofuscin granules near the sarcolemma. Similar granules are found in tongue muscle and in myocardial fibres from an early age. Only in the posterior cricoarytenoid muscle, however, does concomitant muscle and other sarcoplasmic change take place.

The interarytenoid muscles comprise the unpaired transverse arytenoid muscle and the paired oblique arytenoid muscles. The transverse arytenoid muscle arises from the posterior surface of the muscular process and outer edge of one arytenoid and passes to similar attachments on the other cartilage. The oblique arytenoid muscles lie superficial to the transverse arytenoid muscle and pass from the posterior aspect of the muscular process of one arytenoid cartilage to the apex of the other thus crossing each other. Some of the fibres pass round the apex of the arytenoid cartilage and are prolonged into the aryepiglottic fold as the aryepiglottic muscle which acts as a rather weak sphincter of the laryngeal inlet. The interarytenoid muscle adducts the vocal fold chiefly at the cartilaginous portion. It controls the position of the vocal fold, but does not significantly affect its mechanical property.

The thyroarytenoid (vocalis) muscle extends from the back of the thyroid prominence and from the cricothyroid ligament to the vocal process of the arytenoid and to the anterolateral surface of the body of the cartilage. Each muscle is in the form of a broad sheet which lies lateral to and above the free edge of the cricovocal ligament (see Intrinsic ligaments). The lower part of the muscle is thicker and forms a distinct bundle called the vocalis muscle, contraction of which adducts the vocal folds, especially at the membranous portions. It lowers, shortens and thickens the vocal fold, causing the edge of the vocal fold to be rounded. The body (muscular layer) of the vocal fold is actively stiffened but the cover and transition layers are passively slackened. Considerable numbers of fibres of the throarytenoid are prolonged into the aryepiglottic fold, some continuing to the margin of the epiglottis as the thyroepiglottic muscle which tends to widen the inlet of the larynx by pulling the aryepiglottic folds slightly apart. Occasionally, there is present a very fine muscle, the superior thyroarytenoid, which lies on the lateral surface of the main mass of the thyroarytenoid and extends obliquely from the angle of the thyroid cartilage to the muscular process of the arytenoid cartilage.

The cricothyroid muscle (Figure 12.10) is the only intrinsic laryngeal muscle which lies outside the cartilaginous framework. It is fan-shaped and arises from

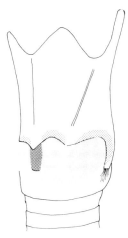

Figure 12.10 The cricothyroid muscle

the lateral surface of the anterior arch of the cricoid cartilage. Its fibres then diverge and pass backwards in two groups. The lower, oblique fibres pass backwards and laterally to the anterior border of the inferior cornu of the thyroid cartilage, and the anterior, straight fibres ascend to the posterior part of the lower border of the thyroid lamina. The cricothyroid muscle rotates the cricoid cartilage about the horizontal axis passing through the cricothyroid joint (Figure 12.11). The question of whether the thyroid cartilage

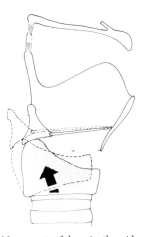

Figure 12.11 Movements of the cricothyroid muscle

moves on a fixed cricoid cartilage, as in phonation when the cricoid cartilage is held immovably against the vertebral column by the action of cricopharyngeus, or whether the cricoid cartilage moves on the thyroid cartilage, as in swallowing, is immaterial because the action of the cricothyroid muscle in each case is to lengthen the vocal folds by increasing the distance between the angle of the thyroid cartilage and arytenoids. When the cricoarytenoid muscle contracts the vocal folds are brought into a line between the anterior commissure and the posterior cricoarytenoid ligament, namely the paramedian position. The level of the vocal folds is lowered and the entire fold is stretched, elongated and thinned. The edge of the vocal fold becomes sharp and all the layers are thereby passively stiffened.

Movements of the vocal folds and the anatomy of speech

The vocal folds usually vibrate at 100–300 Hz during normal conversation, and even at 1000 Hz or more during singing. The observation and interpretation of such vibrations was enhanced by the high-speed film made by the Bell Telephone Laboratories in 1937. This classic film, shot at 4000 frames per second, has been analysed by many observers (Farnsworth, 1940; Pressman, 1942). Other methods of observing vocal fold movements during phonation include frontal tomography (Fink and Kirschner, 1958; Hollien and Curtis, 1960) and stroboscopy (Smith, 1954; Beck and Schönhärl, 1954; Schönhärl, 1960). A schematic presentation of vocal fold vibration is shown in Figure 12.12 (Hirano, 1981) and of the function of the laryngeal muscles in Figure 12.13 (Hirano, 1981). Movement of the vocal folds whether in quiet respiration or in phonation is controlled by the combined activity of all the muscles described above.

In quiet respiration, the intermembranous part of the glottis is triangular, and the intercartilaginous part is rectangular as the medial surfaces of the arytenoids are parallel (Figure 12.14a).

In forced respiration (Figure 12.14b), the vocal folds undergo extreme abduction; the arytenoid cartilages are rotated laterally and their vocal processes move widely apart.

Abduction of the vocal folds (Figure 12.14c) is effected by the pull of the posterior cricoarytenoid muscles. The arytenoids are laterally rotated and thus the glottis becomes triangular.

Preparatory to phonation, the intermembranous and intercartilaginous parts of the glottis are reduced to a linear chink by the adduction of the vocal folds and adduction and medial rotation of the arytenoid cartilages. The crude adduction is effected by the cricothyroid and lateral cricoarytenoid muscles (Figure 12.14d) and the fine tension of the vocal fold is produced by the tonic contraction of the vocalis muscle. The interarytenoid muscles, by pulling the arytenoid cartilages together, complete adduction by closing the posterior glottic chink (Figure 12.14e).

The vocal folds are lengthened by the cricothyroid muscles. Because of the nature of the felted membrane of fibroelastic tissue within the vocal folds, squares of this network are converted into diamonds by increasing the length of the vocal folds without a corresponding increase in tension. The tension of the vocal fold is a function of the tonic contraction of the

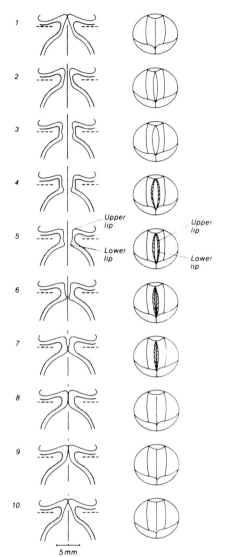

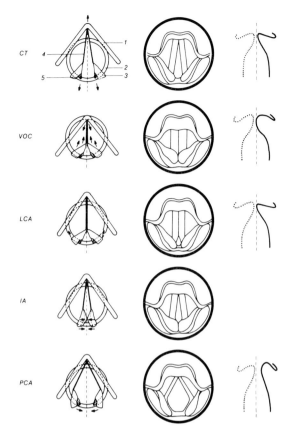

Figure 12.12 Schematic presentation of vocal fold vibration. Left column: frontal section, right column: view from above. (From Hirano, M. (1981) *Clinical Examination of Voice*. New York: Springer-Verlag, p. 44, with permission)

Figure 12.13 A schematic presentation of the function of the laryngeal muscles. The left column shows the location of the cartilages and the edge of the vocal folds when the laryngeal muscles are activated individually. The arrow indicates the direction of the force exerted. 1, The thyroid cartilage; 2, the cricoid cartilage; 3, the arytenoid cartilage; 4, the vocal ligament; 5, the posterior cricoarytenoid ligament. The middle column shows views from above. The right column presents contours of frontal sections at the middle of the membranous portion of the vocal fold. The dotted line shows a control where no muscle is activated. CT, cricothyroid; VOC, vocalis; LCA, lateral cricoarytenoid; IA, interarytenoid; PCA, posterior cricoarytenoid. (From Hirano, M. (1981) *Clinical Examination of Voice*. New York: Springer-Verlag, p. 8, with permission)

vocalis muscle which is well designed to produce a wide range of tension in many small steps (Zenker, 1964).

Changes in length and tension control the pitch of the voice and are produced normally only when the vocal folds are in contact for phonation.

Three forces act to bring the vocal folds in contact with each other. They are: first, the tension in the fold; second, the decrease in subglottic air pressure which happens with each vibratory opening of the glottis; and third, the sucking-in effect of escaping air

(the Bernoulli effect). The result of this rapidly repeating cycle of opening and closing at the glottis is the release of small puffs from the subglottic air column which form sound waves.

Frontal tomography shows that the area of vocal fold surface in contact with its partners varies according to pitch; at low pitches, the cross-sectional area of the vocal folds is large, but as the pitch rises, the folds become thinner (Hollien and Curtis, 1960).

Stroboscopy allows observation and description of fundamental frequency, symmetry of bilateral movements, regularity (periodicity), glottal closure, ampli-

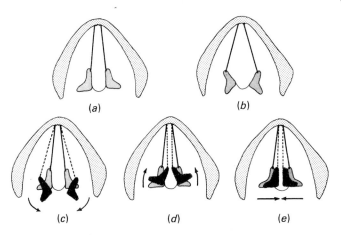

Figure 12.14 Diagrams to show the different positions of the vocal folds and arytenoid cartilages. (*a*) Position at rest in quiet respiration; (*b*) forced inspiration; (*c*) abduction of the vocal folds; (*d*) adduction of the vocal folds; (*e*) closure of the posterior glottic chink

tude, mucosal wave and non-vibrating portions. In the normal vocal fold the mucosal wave travels on the mucosa from its inferior to superior surface. This is observed during vibrations except for falsetto and is a function of the soft and pliant superficial layer of the lamina propria.

The function of the vocal folds is to produce sound varying only in intensity and pitch. This is then modified by various resonating chambers above and below the larynx and is ultimately converted into phonemes by the articulating action of the pharynx, tongue, palate, teeth and lips.

Techniques of spectral analysis of the voice show that the vocal tract (larynx, pharynx, mouth and nasal cavities) acts as an intricately selective filter and resonator which propagates a remarkably similar pattern irrespective of the fundamental frequency. This is essential to speech as it ensures that, in spite of a continuously varying tone of voice, a constant quality or timbre is maintained.

Consonants of speech are associated with particular anatomical sites, from which they usually take their designations in the terminology of phonetics; e.g. 'p' and 'b' are labials, 't' and 'd' are dentals, and 'm' and 'n' are nasals. These sites have two factors in common. They cause a partial obstruction or constriction at some level in the vocal tract, and they produce an aperiodic vibration or noise which is superimposed on or interrupts the flow of laryngeal tones. For example, dental consonants result from apposition of the top of the tongue to the back of the teeth. This momentarily constricts the passage of escaping air, modifies the resonant parameters of the 'vocal tract' and also generates local noise.

The extreme complexity of speech is reflected in the multiplicity of laryngeal, pharyngeal, hyoid, palatal, lingual and circumoral muscular movements which are combined in rapidly changing combinations to produce phonation and articulation.

Mucous membranes of the larynx

The mucous membrane lining the larynx is continuous above with that of the pharynx and below with that of the trachea. It is closely attached over the posterior surface of the epiglottis, over the corniculate and cuneiform cartilages, and over the vocal ligaments. Elsewhere, it is loosely attached and therefore liable to become swollen.

The epithelium of the larynx is either squamous, ciliated columnar or transitional. The upper half of the posterior surface of the epiglottis, the upper part of the aryepiglottic folds and the posterior commissure are covered with squamous epithelium. The vocal folds are also covered with squamous epithelium. The height of the vocal fold diminishes towards the anterior commissure mainly because the inferior edge of the vocal fold slopes upwards. The lower edges of the anterior end of the folds form the apex of the triangular fixed part of the subglottis. Thus a tumour reaching or spreading across the anterior commissure has been found to involve the subglottic space in 50% of post-mortem larynges taken from non-smokers (Stell, Gregory and Watt, 1980).

Mucous glands are freely distributed throughout the mucous membrane and are particularly numerous on the posterior surface of the epiglottis, where they form indentations into the cartilage, and in the margins of the lower part of the aryepiglottic folds, and in the saccules. The vocal folds do not possess any glands, and the mucous membrane is lubricated by the glands within the saccules. The squamous epithelium covering the vocal folds is therefore vulnerable to desiccation. Scanning electron microscopy has demonstrated the existence not only of microvilli, but also of microridges (microplicae) on the surface cells of the epithelium of the folds and elsewhere in the larynx (Andrews, 1975; Tillmann, Peitzch-Rohrscheider and Hoenges, 1977). Such features have been observed in other epithelia subjected to drying out (e.g. the corneal epithelium), and microplicae are regarded as being conducive to the retention of surface secretions.

Some taste buds, similar to those in the tongue, are scattered over the posterior surface of the epiglottis, and in the aryepiglottic folds.

Blood supply

The blood supply is derived from the laryngeal branches of the superior and inferior thyroid arteries and the cricothyroid branch of the superior thyroid artery. The superior thyroid artery arises from the external carotid artery, and the inferior thyroid artery arises from the thyrocervical trunk of the first part of the subclavian artery. On the left side, the thoracic duct is an important relation to the thyrocervical trunk, crossing from medial to lateral side.

The superior laryngeal artery arises from the superior thyroid artery. It passes deep to the thyrohyoid muscle and, together with the internal branch of the superior laryngeal nerve, pierces the thyrohyoid membrane to supply the muscles and mucous membrane of the larynx and to anastomose with branches of its opposite side and with those of the inferior laryngeal artery. The latter arises from the inferior thyroid artery at the level of the lower border of the thyroid gland and ascends on the trachea, together with the recurrent laryngeal nerve. It enters the larynx beneath the lower border of the inferior constrictor muscle and supplies the muscles and mucous membrane. The cricothyroid artery passes from the superior thyroid artery, across the upper part of the cricothyroid ligament and anastomoses with the branch of the opposite side.

The veins leaving the larynx accompany the arteries; the superior vessels enter the internal jugular vein by way of the superior thyroid or facial vein; the inferior vessels drain by way of the inferior thyroid vein into the brachiocephalic veins. Some venous drainage from the larynx is by way of the middle thyroid vein into the internal jugular vein.

Lymphatic drainage

The lymphatics of the larynx are separated by the vocal folds into an upper and lower group. The part of the larynx above the vocal folds is drained by vessels which accompany the superior laryngeal vein, pierce the thyrohyoid membrane and empty into the upper deep cervical lymph nodes; whereas the zone below the vocal folds drains, together with the inferior vein, into the lower part of the deep cervical chain often through the prelaryngeal and pretracheal nodes.

The vocal folds are firmly bound down to the underlying vocal ligaments and this results in an absence of lymph vessels, a fact which accounts for the clearly defined watershed between the upper and lower zones.

Nerve supply

The nerve supply of the larynx is from the vagus by way of its superior and recurrent laryngeal branches.

The *superior laryngeal nerve* arises from the inferior ganglion of the vagus and receives a branch from the superior cervical sympathetic ganglion. It descends lateral to the pharynx, behind the internal carotid and, at the level of the greater horn of the hyoid, divides into a small external branch and a larger internal branch. The external branch provides motor supply to the cricothyroid muscle while the internal branch pierces the thyrohyoid membrane above the entrance of the superior laryngeal artery and divides into two main sensory and secretomotor branches. The upper branch supplies the mucous membrane of the lower part of the pharynx, epiglottis, vallecula and vestibule of the larynx. The lower branch descends in the medial wall of the pyriform fossa beneath the mucous membrane and supplies the aryepiglottic fold and the mucous membrane down to the level of the vocal folds.

The internal branch of the superior laryngeal nerve also carries fibres from neuromuscular spindles and other stretch receptors in the larynx. The nerve ends by piercing the inferior constrictor muscle of the pharynx, and unites with an ascending branch of the recurrent laryngeal nerve. This branch is called Galen's anastomosis or loop and is purely sensory.

The *recurrent laryngeal nerve* on the right side leaves the vagus as the latter crosses the right subclavian artery and then loops under the artery and ascends to the larynx in the groove between the oesophagus and trachea. On the left side, the nerve originates from the vagus as it crosses the aortic arch. It then passes under the arch and the ligamentum arteriosum to reach the groove between the oesophagus and trachea. In the neck, both nerves follow the same course and pass upwards accompanied by the laryngeal branch of the inferior thyroid artery, deep to the lower border of the inferior constrictor, and enter the larynx behind the cricothyroid joint. The nerve then divides into motor and sensory branches.

The motor branch has fibres derived from the cranial root of the accessory nerve with cell bodies lying in the nucleus ambiguus; these supply all the intrinsic muscles of the larynx with the exception of the cricothyroid. The sensory branch supplies the laryngeal mucous membrane below the level of the vocal folds and also carries afferent fibres from stretch receptors in the larynx.

As the recurrent laryngeal nerve curves round the subclavian artery or the arch of the aorta, it gives off several cardiac filaments to the deep part of the cardiac plexus. As it ascends in the neck, it gives branches – which are more numerous on the right than the left – to the mucous membrane and the muscular coat of the oesophagus and trachea, and some filaments to the inferior constrictor.

Applied anatomy of the larynx

Surface anatomy and laryngotomy

In the midline from above downwards, it is possible to palpate the hyoid bone, the thyroid cartilage with the laryngeal prominence (Adam's apple), the cricoid cartilage and the trachea. The level of the vocal folds is approximately at the midpoint of the anterior surface of the thyroid cartilage. By rolling the finger upwards over the cricoid cartilage, it is possible to feel a soft depression between the cricoid and thyroid cartilages. This is the cricothyroid ligament (Figure 12.15) and is the site at which to perform a cricothyrotomy or laryngotomy to relieve upper airway obstruction. This is preferable, as an emergency procedure, to a tracheostomy because of the increased depth of soft tissue associated with an approach to the trachea and the greater likelihood of bleeding from the thyroid isthmus.

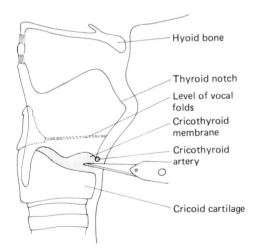

Figure 12.15 The site for cricothyrotomy

Laryngoscopic examination

The larynx and surrounding structures can be examined by either indirect or direct laryngoscopy. With a cooperative patient, indirect laryngoscopy (Figure 12.16), using the laryngeal mirror, will give a good view of the back of the tongue, the valleculae, the epiglottis (which is seen foreshortened), the pyriform fossae and the structures of the larynx. If the patient will not tolerate the laryngeal mirror, there are two options open to the examiner. First, the flexible fibreoptic nasolaryngoscope can be passed along the floor of a previously locally anaesthetized nasal cavity and then suspended above the larynx to give a direct view. This technique affords an excellent view of the nose and nasopharynx as well as of the larynx and adjacent structures. The laryngeal position is natural in that the patient's tongue is not being pulled out, and the examination is well tolerated by the patient. Second, if a pathological lesion is seen or suspected and a biopsy or removal of tissue is required, then direct laryngoscopy with or without microscopy under general anaesthesia is recommended. This technique will afford a better view of the laryngeal ventricles and of the subglottis.

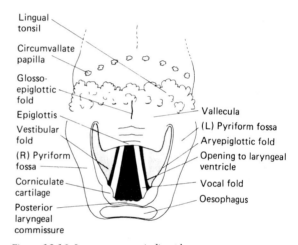

Figure 12.16 Larynx seen on indirect laryngoscopy

Radiology

A good lateral cervical radiograph (Figure 12.17) will give a wealth of information about the state of the upper airway, signs of obstruction or the presence of foreign bodies. Oedema of the epiglottis or supraglottic structures will be visible, as will stenosis of the subglottis or upper trachea. The normal ventricle is seen as a clear horizontal area. Care must be taken not to confuse fine lines of calcification in the arytenoid cartilages or the posterior aspect of the thyroid cartilage with foreign bodies (Figure 12.18). Tomography, scanning, and contrast laryngography can all aid the diagnosis of laryngeal lesions.

Injuries to the laryngeal nerves

There is an intimate and important relationship between the nerves which supply the larynx and the vessels which supply the thyroid gland. In a postopera-

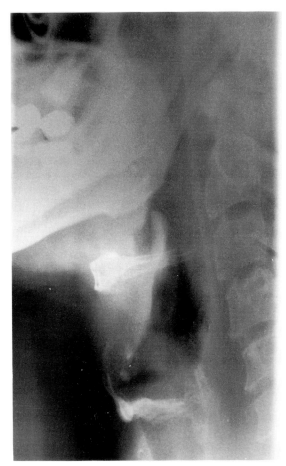

Figure 12.17 Lateral cervical radiograph

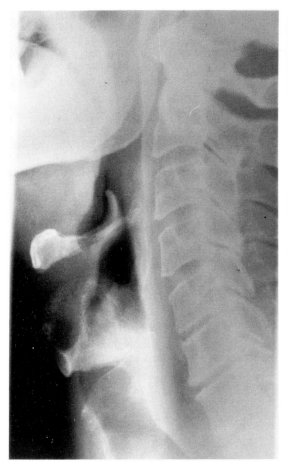

Figure 12.18 Lateral cervical radiograph showing calcification in cartilages not to be confused with foreign bodies

tive study of voice function in 325 patients who had undergone thyroidectomy, Kark *et al.* (1984) found that permanent changes had been sustained by 35 (25%) after a subtotal thyroidectomy, and by 19 (11%) after lobectomy. The commonest cause of voice change appeared to be injury to the external branch of the superior laryngeal nerve on one or both sides. Damage to the recurrent laryngeal nerve, which was routinely identified and protected, was rarely a cause. They found that when the external branch of the superior laryngeal nerve – which descends over the inferior constrictor muscle immediately deep to the superior thyroid artery and vein as these pass to the superior pole of the gland – was identified and preserved, permanent voice changes were recorded in only 5% of cases (Figure 12.19). This was similar to an incidence of 3% in control patients after endotracheal intubation alone. The functional effect of damage to the external laryngeal nerve is a lower pitched, husky voice that is easily fatigued and has a reduced range. The laryngoscopic changes are much less obvious than those which are seen after palsy of

the recurrent laryngeal nerve, and their identification may be helped by the use of a stroboscopic light. The edge of the affected vocal fold may be irregular or wavy and usually lies at a lower level, producing an oblique glottic aperture. Recovery after palsy of the external nerve is poor and prognosis is not good (Arnold, 1962).

The recurrent laryngeal nerve comes into close relationship with the inferior thyroid artery as the latter passes medially, behind the common carotid artery, to the gland. The artery may cross posteriorly or anteriorly to the nerve, or the nerve may pass between the terminal branches of the artery (Figure 12.20). On the right side, there is an equal chance of locating the nerve in each of these three situations; on the left, the nerve is more likely to lie posterior to the artery (Bowden, 1955). Injury to the recurrent nerve is enhanced by its displacement from the normal anatomical location by the diseased thyroid gland.

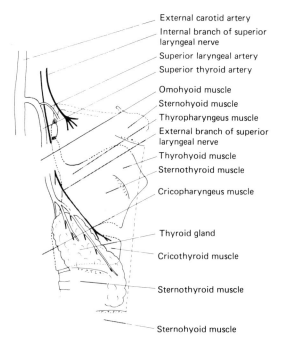

External carotid artery
Internal branch of superior laryngeal nerve
Superior laryngeal artery
Superior thyroid artery
Omohyoid muscle
Sternohyoid muscle
Thyropharyngeus muscle
External branch of superior laryngeal nerve
Thyrohyoid muscle
Sternothyroid muscle
Cricopharyngeus muscle
Thyroid gland
Cricothyroid muscle
Sternothyroid muscle
Sternohyoid muscle

Figure 12.19 Anatomy of the external branch of the superior laryngeal nerve

Apart from injury complicating thyroidectomy, the nerve can also be affected by benign or malignant enlargement of the thyroid gland, by enlarged lymph nodes or by cervical trauma. Paralysis of the left nerve, by virtue of its intrathoracic course, is twice as likely to happen as that of the right. It may be involved by malignant tumours of the lung or oesophagus, by malignant or inflamed nodes, by an aneurysm of the aortic arch, or by left atrial hypertrophy associated with mitral stenosis.

The anomalous position of a non-recurrent laryn-geal nerve predisposes to injury during thyroidectomy and to compression by a thyroid mass. Symptoms range from hoarseness associated with a vocal fold paralysis to a vague pressure sensation over the larynx, a need to clear the throat or a chronic cough. Recognition of this uncommon anomaly, which is usually right-sided, is necessary and no structure passing medially from the carotid sheath, except the middle thyroid vein, should be ligated until the recurrent laryngeal nerve is identified (Friedman *et al.*, 1986).

The functional effect of damage to one recurrent laryngeal nerve is hoarseness, which later resolves itself almost completely in 50% of patients (Watt-Boolsen *et al.*, 1977), either by a return of function on the affected side or by compensatory over-adduction of the opposite normal vocal fold. Bilateral paralysis, however, results in complete loss of vocal power and a marked inspiratory stridor often necessitating tracheostomy. Respiratory obstruction following a thyroidectomy can also result from the collapse of the tracheal cartilages (tracheomalacia) associated with a large goitre or with carcinoma of the thyroid or from external pressure on the trachea from post-operative haemorrhage.

It is generally accepted that the concept embodied in Semon's law, namely that the abductor nerve or muscle fibres are generally more susceptible to injury, is no longer valid. The 'law', after several amendments, stated: 'In the course of a gradually advancing organic lesion of a recurrent nerve or its fibres in the peripheral trunk, three stages can be observed. In the first stage, only abductor fibres are damaged and the vocal folds approximate in the midline and adduction is still possible. In the second stage, additional contracture of the adductors occurs so that the vocal folds are immobilized in the median position. In the third stage, the adductor becomes paralysed and the vocal fold assumes the cadaveric position'.

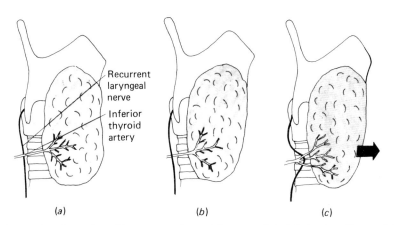

Recurrent laryngeal nerve
Inferior thyroid artery

(a)   (b)   (c)

Figure 12.20 Variations in the relationship of the recurrent laryngeal nerve and the inferior thyroid artery (after Bowden, 1955). (a) The nerve may cross posteriorly to the artery, (b) anterior to the artery, or (c) through the branches of the artery. The lateral lobe of the thyroid has been pulled forward as it would be during thyroidectomy

Descriptions of multiple positions assumed by paralysed vocal folds still cause confusion.

The hypothesis, attributed to Wagner (1890) and Grossman (1897), which states, first, that total paralysis of the recurrent nerve immobilizes the vocal fold in the paramedian position because of the adductive action of the intact cricothyroid muscles, and second, that a 'combined' recurrent laryngeal nerve and superior laryngeal nerve paralysis causes the fold to be immobilized in the intermediate (open or cadaveric) position, is the one preferred by present day laryngologists (Dedo and Dedo, 1980).

This hypothesis is supported by electromyographic and photographic studies of both the human and canine larynx which confirm that the adduction and lengthening effect of an intact cricothyroid muscle is the primary force that holds a paralysed vocal fold in the paramedian position. A vocal fold in the paramedian position is, therefore, paralysed only by a defective recurrent laryngeal nerve, while a vocal fold immobilized in the intermediate position is usually paralysed by a lesion affecting both recurrent and superior laryngeal nerves (Figure 12.21). The apparent small variations of positions can be attributed to compensation provided by the normal vocal fold crossing the midline, or to atrophy and scarring of the paralysed vocal fold.

Kirchner (1982) stated that if the ipsilateral vagus nerve, as well as the recurrent laryngeal nerve, were injured, the vocal fold might assume the intermediate position because of the loss of the adductor function of the cricothyroid muscle brought about by the interruption of vagal afferent fibres originating in pulmonary stretch receptors. These receptors exert a monitoring effect on the respiratory centre which, in turn, allows reflex adjustments of laryngeal resistance in breathing.

Trachea and bronchi

The trachea

The trachea is a cartilaginous and membranous tube, about 10–11 cm in length, which extends from its attachment to the lower end of the cricoid cartilage, at the level of the sixth cervical vertebra, to its termination at the bifurcation at the level of the upper border of the fifth thoracic vertebra, or more easily the second costal cartilage or the manubriosternal angle. The bifurcation moves upwards during the act of swallowing, and downwards and forwards during inspiration, often to the level of the sixth thoracic vertebra. The trachea lies mainly in the median plane, although the bifurcation is usually a little to the right of the midline. The diameter of the air passages increases appreciably during inspiration, and decreases during expiration.

In the child, the trachea is smaller, more deeply placed and more mobile than in the adult, and the bifurcation is at a higher level until the age of 10–12 years.

The trachea is D-shaped in cross-section, with incomplete cartilaginous rings anteriorly and laterally, and a straight membranous wall posteriorly. The rings of the trachea can easily be seen endoscopically in outline beneath the mucosa, as they cause a slight elevation and pallor of the mucosa. The transverse diameter is greater than the anteroposterior (about 20 mm compared with 15 mm in the adult male). Measurements of the internal diameter of the trachea vary from study to study but those given in Table 12.1 (after Engel, 1962) are representative.

The main bronchi and branches

In the adult, the trachea bifurcates into the right and left main bronchi at the level of the second costal cartilage. The main bronchi are separated at their origin by a narrow ridge which, in view of its resem-

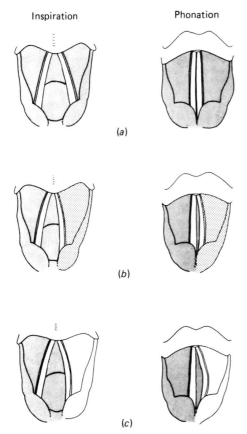

Inspiration   Phonation

(a)

(b)

(c)

Figure 12.21 Vocal fold positions in inspiration and phonation. (*a*) Normal, (*b*) paramedian and (*c*) intermediate

Table 12.1 The internal dimensions of the trachea (after Engel, 1962)

Age	Average length (cm)	Average diameter (mm)	
		Sagittal	Coronal
0–1 month	3.8	5.7	6.0
1–3 months	4.0	6.5	6.8
3–6 months	4.2	7.6	7.2
6–12 months	4.3	7.0	7.8
1–2 years	4.5	9.4	8.8
2–3 years	5.0	10.8	9.4
3–4 years	5.3	9.1	11.2
6–8 years	5.7	10.4	11.0
10–12 years	6.3	9.3	12.4
14–16 years	7.2	13.7	13.5
Adults	9.15	16.5	14.4

blance to the keel of an upturned boat, is called the carina. The carina always contains cartilage, although the actual dividing ridge is frequently membranous.

The right main bronchus

The definition (to be used in this chapter) of the extent of the right main bronchus is that portion from the tracheal bifurcation to the orifices of the right middle lobe bronchus and the apical segment of the right lower lobe. The right main bronchus (Figure 12.22) is about 5 cm in length. It is wider, shorter and more vertical than the left main bronchus. It has a posterior membranous wall and a series of cartilage rings which, although smaller in size, are very similar in structure to those of the trachea. The average angle made by the right main bronchus with the trachea is 25–30°. The coronal diameter of the right main bronchus is about 17 ± 4 mm in men and about 15 ± 4 mm in women; the corresponding diameter on the left side is 2–3 mm less. The right pulmonary artery is at first below and in front of the right main bronchus and the azygos vein arches over it. The right upper lobe bronchus is given off 2.5 cm along the course of the main bronchus which, on entering the hilum of the lung, divides into a middle and lower lobe bronchus.

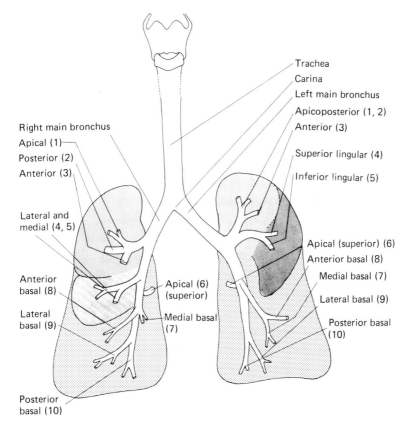

Figure 12.22 Anterior view of trachea, bronchi and bronchopulmonary segments

The right upper lobe bronchus (1, 2 and 3)

The right upper lobe bronchus arises from the right lateral aspect of the parent bronchus about 12–20 mm from the carina. It runs superolaterally to enter the hilum of the lung. It is about 1 cm in length and divides into three segmental bronchi which supply the apical, posterior and anterior segments of the upper lobe (Figure 12.23 and see Figure 12.22). All these can be seen bronchoscopically with a right-angled telescope or with a fibreoptic bronchoscope. This subdivision has a remarkably constant pattern. The most notable of the few variations that are seen is that of an apical segment supplied by a 'tracheal' bronchus which arises from the right lateral aspect of the trachea just above the carina. Its chief clinical importance is that of the confusion it may cause during the resection of a lung, in the case, for example, of carcinoma.

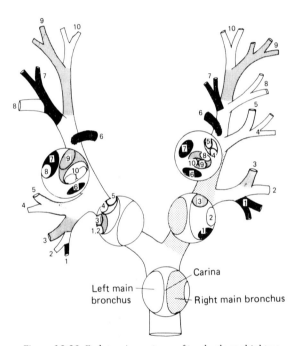

Figure 12.23 Endoscopic anatomy of tracheobronchial tree

The apical segmental bronchus (1) passes upwards. After about 1 cm, it divides into apical and anterior subsegmental branches. The posterior segmental bronchus (2) serves the posterior-inferior part of the superior lobe of the lung and runs backwards and somewhat upwards. It divides into lateral (or axillary) and anterior subsegmental bronchi.

The anterior segmental bronchus (3) runs anteroinferiorly to supply the rest of the superior lobe. After a short distance, it divides into lateral (or axillary) and anterior subsegmental branches.

The right middle lobe bronchus (4 and 5)

The right middle lobe bronchus arises about 2.5 cm beyond the origin of the right upper lobe bronchus from the anterior aspect of the bronchus. It is directed forwards, downwards and laterally, and after a short distance divides into lateral (4) and medial (5) subsegments.

The right lower lobe bronchus (6, 7, 8, 9 and 10)

The right lower lobe bronchus is the continuation of the principal stem beyond the origin of the middle lobe bronchus. It supplies five segments of the lung.

The apical (superior) segmental bronchus (6) arises from the posterior aspect of the termination of the right main bronchus. Its orifice is opposite to and only a short distance lower than that of the right middle lobe. It subsequently divides into medial, superior and lateral branches, the former two usually arising from a common stem.

In over 50% of right lungs, a subapical (subsuperior) segmental bronchus arises from the posterior surface of the right lower lobe bronchus between 1 and 3 cm below the apical (superior) segmental bronchus. This is distributed to the region of lung between the apical (superior) and posterior basal segments.

The medial basal (cardiac) segmental bronchus (7) has a higher point of origin than the other basal bronchi. It runs inferomedially parallel to the right border of the heart. The lower lobe bronchus then divides into an anterior basal segmental bronchus (8) which descends anteriorly, and a trunk which divides into lateral (9) and posterior (10) basal segments.

The left main bronchus

The left main bronchus is 5.5 cm long and, because it supplies the smaller lung, is narrower than the right main bronchus. In order to reach the hilum of the lung, the main bronchus has to extend laterally beneath the aortic arch. Its angle to the trachea averages 45°. The bronchus crosses anterior to the oesophagus, thoracic duct and descending aorta; the left pulmonary artery lies at first anterior and then superior to it. At the level of the sixth thoracic vertebra, it enters the hilum of the lung and divides into the upper and lower lobe bronchus.

The left upper lobe bronchus (1, 2, 3, 4 and 5)

The left upper lobe bronchus arises from the antero-lateral aspect of the parent bronchus about 5.5 cm from the carina. It curves laterally for a short distance and then divides into two bronchi, which correspond to the branches of the right main bronchus to both apical (superior) and middle lobes of the right lung. They are both distributed to the apical (superior) lobe of the left lung, which does not possess a separate

Table 12.2 The bronchopulmonary segments

Right lung		Left lung	
Right upper lobe		Left upper lobe	
apical segment	(1)	apicoposterior	
posterior segment	(2)	segment (1 + 2)	
anterior segment	(3)	anterior segment	(3)
Right middle lobe		Lingula	
lateral segment	(4)	superior segment	(4)
medial segment	(5)	inferior segment	(5)
Right lower lobe		Left lower lobe	
apical segment	(6)	apical segment	(6)
medial basal segment	(7)	medial basal segment	(7)
anterior basal segment	(8)	anterior basal segment	(8)
lateral basal segment	(9)	lateral basal segment	(9)
posterior basal		posterior basal	
segment (10)		segment (10)	

Bronchopulmonary segments

The lung is divided functionally into a series of bronchopulmonary segments, each with its own bronchus and its own blood supply from the pulmonary artery. Each segment is surrounded by connective tissue, continuous with that of the visceral pleura, and forms a separate respiratory unit of the lung. Lung resection surgery, postural drainage and chest radiology are based on the detailed anatomy of these segments (see Applied anatomy of trachea and bronchi).

The segments which have been described in detail previously are summarized in Table 12.2 and also in Figure 12.23. For further details of bronchopulmonary segmentation, consult Brock (1943, 1954), and Boyden (1955).

middle lobe. The cranial division ascends for about 10 mm before giving off an anterior segmental bronchus (3). It then continues upwards for a further 1 cm as the apicoposterior segmental bronchus (1 and 2), which subsequently subdivides into apical and posterior branches.

The caudal division descends anterolaterally to be distributed to the anteroinferior part of the superior lobe of the left lung. This part of the lung is called the lingular area. The lingular bronchus divides into superior lingular (4) and inferior lingular (5) segmental bronchi.

The left lower lobe bronchus (6, 7, 8, 9 and 10)

The left lower lobe is smaller than the right. The apical (superior) segmental bronchus (6) takes its origin posteriorly from the left lower lobe bronchus about 1 cm below the upper lobe orifice. The inferior lobe bronchus continues for a further 1–2 cm before dividing into two stems, an anteromedial and a posterolateral stem. The medial basal segmental bronchus (7) arises in common with the anterior basal segmental bronchus (8) from the former; the lateral basal segmental bronchus (9) arises in common with the posterior basal segmental bronchus (10) from the latter.

There has not always been recognition of the medial basal segmental bronchus on the left side because of its common origin with the anterior basal segment. However, in 10% of lungs it arises independently from the lower lobe bronchus, and in all cases it supplies a territory similar to its opposite number on the right side.

A subapical (subsuperior) segmental bronchus arises from the posterior surface of the left lower lobe bronchus in as many as 30% of lungs.

Structure of trachea and major bronchi

The trachea and extrapulmonary bronchi consist of a framework of incomplete rings of hyaline cartilage, united by fibrous tissue and non-striated muscle. They are lined by mucous membrane (Figure 12.24).

The cartilages

The number of cartilages in the trachea varies from 16 to 20. The cartilages are incomplete rings which stiffen the wall of the trachea both anteriorly and laterally. Behind, where the 'rings' are deficient, the tube is flat and is completed by fibrous and elastic tissue and non-striated muscle fibres. The cartilages measure about 4 mm vertically and 1 mm in thickness. They are placed horizontally one above the other, and are separated by narrow intervals; two or more of the cartilages often unite, partially or completely, and are sometimes bifurcated at their extremities. They are highly elastic, but may become calcified in advanced life. In the extrapulmonary bronchi, the cartilages are shorter, narrower, and rather less regular than those of the trachea, but otherwise they have a similar arrangement.

The first tracheal cartilage is broader than the rest and is sometimes blended with the cricoid cartilages to which it is connected by the cricotracheal ligament. The last tracheal cartilage is thick and broad in the middle where its lower border is prolonged into a triangular process which curves downwards and backwards between the two bronchi forming a bridge called the carina. The C-ring structure persists in the extrapulmonary portion of the bronchial tree where the walls need to be relatively rigid. In the extrapulmonary bronchi, the walls are supported by numerous cartilaginous plates of very varied shape

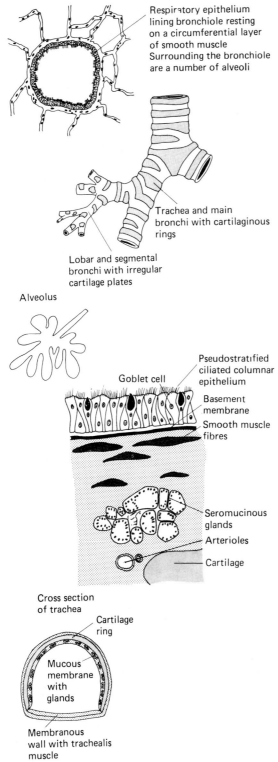

Respiratory epithelium lining bronchiole resting on a circumferential layer of smooth muscle Surrounding the bronchiole are a number of alveoli

Trachea and main bronchi with cartilaginous rings

Lobar and segmental bronchi with irregular cartilage plates

Alveolus

Pseudostratified ciliated columnar epithelium

Goblet cell

Basement membrane

Smooth muscle fibres

Seromucinous glands

Arterioles

Cartilage

Cross section of trachea

Cartilage ring

Mucous membrane with glands

Membranous wall with trachealis muscle

Figure 12.24 Diagrams to illustrate the histological structure of the trachea, bronchus and bronchiole

and size. Here the walls need to be relatively mobile and have less tendency to collapse (Vampeperstraete, 1973).

The fibrous membrane

Each of the cartilages is enclosed in perichondrium. This is continuous with a sheet of dense irregular connective tissue forming a fibrous membrane between adjacent 'rings' of cartilage and, at the posterior aspect of the trachea and extrapulmonry bronchi, where the cartilage is incomplete. The fibrous layer of the perichondrium and the fibrous membrane are composed mainly of collagen intermingled with some elastic fibres. The fibres cross each other diagonally, allowing changes in diameter of the enclosed airway, and the elastic component provides the property of elastic recoil when the membrane is stretched.

Non-striated muscle fibres are present within the fibrous membrane at the back of the tube. Most of these fibres are transverse and are inserted into the perichondrium of the posterior extremities of the cartilages (in the trachea, they are known as the trachealis muscle). Contraction of these fibres, therefore, alters the cross-sectional area of the trachea and bronchi. A few longitudinal muscle fibres lie external to the transverse fibres. The relative thickness of the muscle increases as the branching bronchi become narrower.

The mucous membrane

The mucous membrane is continuous with, and similar to, that of the larynx above and the intrapulmonary bronchi below. It consists of a layer of pseudostratified ciliated columnar epithelium with numerous goblet cells resting on a broad basement membrane. The cilia beat the overlying layer of mucus upwards to the larynx and pharynx. Deep to the epithelium and its basement membrane are: first, a lamina propria, rich in longitudinal elastic fibres; second, a submucosa of loose irregular connective tissue in which are situated larger blood vessels, nerve trunks and most of the tubular glands and patches of lymphoid tissue; and third, the perichondrium and fibrous membrane, lying deep to the submucosa.

The outer fibrous and muscular layer of the trachea and bronchi is continuous with the fascial planes of surrounding muscles and the oesophagus, and also with the loose areolar tissue of the mediastinum.

The structure of the smaller bronchi

With increased branching of the segmental bronchi, the epithelial lining becomes thinner and, ultimately, single-layered. There are fewer goblet cells, on a narrower basement membrane, in the smaller air passages. The cartilage plates also gradually become smaller and fewer in number, and are not found in the cartilages of smaller bronchi. Circular muscle fibres almost completely surround the tube inside the cartilages, replacing the fibroelastic layer found in the trachea. The muscle fibres contain numerous elastic fibres and are arranged in an interlacing network, partly circular and partly diagonal, so that their contraction constricts and shortens the tube.

The branched tubuloracemose glands are less numerous in the smaller bronchi and are not present in the bronchioles. Lymphoid tissue is found diffused throughout the mucosa of the bronchi, often in solitary nodules and particularly at points of bifurcation.

Blood supply

The blood supply of the trachea is derived mainly from branches of the inferior thyroid arteries. However, the thoracic end is supplied by bronchial arteries which anastomose with the inferior thyroid arteries and also supply the oesophagus in this region. The tracheal veins drain into the thyroid venous plexus.

The bronchi, from the carina to the respiratory bronchioles, lung tissue, visceral pleura and pulmonary nodes are all supplied by the bronchial arteries, which are usually three in number, one for the right lung and two for the left. The left bronchial arteries usually arise from the anterior aspect of the descending thoracic aorta. The right is more variable; it may arise from the aorta, the first intercostal artery, the third intercostal artery (which is the first intercostal branch of the aorta), the internal mammary artery, or the right subclavian artery. The arteries lie against the posterior walls of their respective bronchi.

The bronchial veins form two distinct systems (Marchand, Gilroy and Wilson, 1950). The deep bronchial veins commence as a network in the intrapulmonary bronchioles and communicate freely with the pulmonary veins; they eventually join to form a single trunk which terminates in a main pulmonary vein or in the left atrium. The superficial bronchial veins drain the extrapulmonary bronchi, the visceral pleura and the hilar lymph nodes. They terminate in the azygos vein on the right side, and in the left superior intercostal vein or the accessory (superior) hemiazygos vein on the left side. The bronchial veins do not receive all the blood conveyed to the lungs by the bronchial arteries for the reason that some enters the pulmonary veins.

Lymphatic drainage

The tracheal lymphatics drain to the pretracheal and paratracheal groups of nodes.

The lung has an abundant lymphatic supply which exists as two systems. The superficial or pleural system forms a plexus of lymphatics beneath the pleura and is provided with numerous valves. These lymphatics unite and drain into the hilar lymph nodes. The deep or alveolar system accompanies the

pulmonary and bronchial arteries and conveys lymph from the interior of the lung to the hilar nodes. There are few valves, except at points of anastomoses with pleural lymphatics, and at the hilum. The bronchial lymph vessels originate in a plexus beneath the mucous membrane. They then penetrate the muscle coat and form a second plexus in the outer fibrous coat, often incorporating nodules of lymphoid tissue.

The distribution of tracheal and bronchial lymph nodes is shown in Figure 12.25. There are pulmonary groups of nodes around the smaller bronchi, with bronchopulmonary nodes being mainly beneath the points of division of the intrapulmonary air passages, inferior tracheobronchial nodes being beneath the divisions of the larger bronchi, and a subcarinal group of nodes being beneath the bifurcation of the trachea.

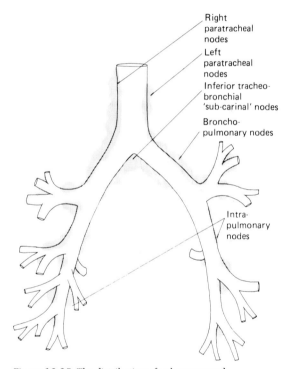

Figure 12.25 The distribution of pulmonary and tracheobronchial lymph nodes

All these nodes subsequently drain to either the right or the left paratracheal nodes by way of the right and left superior tracheobronchial nodes. The right superior tracheobronchial nodes drain the whole of the right lung and also have communications with the left upper lobe. The left superior tracheobronchial nodes drain the greater part of the left lung. The inferior tracheobronchial (subcarinal) group of nodes is important in that these nodes drain lymph from both lungs and, in turn, drain to both right and left paratracheal nodes. Clinically, if these nodes become enlarged, they will cause widening of the carina which should be visible on bronchoscopy.

Lymphatics from the right and left paratracheal nodes unite with vessels from the internal thoracic and brachiocephalic lymph nodes to form the right and left bronchomediastinal trunks which drain either into the right lymphatic duct and left thoracic duct respectively, or independently into the junction of the internal jugular and subclavian veins of their own side.

Nerve supply

The muscle fibres of the trachea, including the trachealis muscle, are innervated by the recurrent laryngeal nerves which also carry sensory fibres from the mucous membrane. Sympathetic nerve fibres are derived mainly from the middle cervical ganglion and have connections with the recurrent laryngeal nerves.

The lungs are supplied from the anterior and posterior pulmonary plexuses situated at the hilum of each lung. The parasympathetic fibres, carried in the vagus nerve, are afferent (cell bodies in the inferior ganglion) and efferent (cell bodies in the dorsal nucleus with relay in the bronchial mucosa). The vagal efferents are bronchoconstrictor to the bronchial muscles, and secretomotor and vasodilator to the bronchial mucous glands. Afferent fibres are involved in the cough reflex. The efferent sympathetic fibres are postganglionic branches of the second to fifth thoracic ganglion, with an occasional contribution from the first (stellate) ganglion. They are dilator (inhibitory)

to the bronchi and pulmonary arterioles. The afferent sympathetic fibres have their cells of origin in the ganglion on the posterior roots of the second to fifth thoracic spinal nerves.

Relations of cervical trachea (Figure 12.26)

Anterior

The central part of the trachea is covered anteriorly by skin, superficial and deep fascia and by the sternohyoid and sternothyroid muscles. The isthmus of the thyroid gland covers a variable number of uppermost rings, usually the second to the fourth. There are thus a large number of layers between skin and trachea that have to be divided in a tracheostomy operation, in spite of the fact that in a thin subject the trachea is easily palpated in the neck. The trachea in the lower part of the neck is crossed by a communicating band between the anterior jugular veins, as well as by the inferior thyroid veins and, when present, by the thyroidea ima artery which ascends from the arch of the aorta or from the brachiocephalic artery.

Lateral

The right and left lobes of the thyroid gland, which descend to the level of the fifth and sixth tracheal cartilages, lie on either side of the trachea, as does the carotid sheath enclosing the common carotid artery, the internal jugular vein and the vagus nerve. The inferior thyroid artery lies anterolaterally.

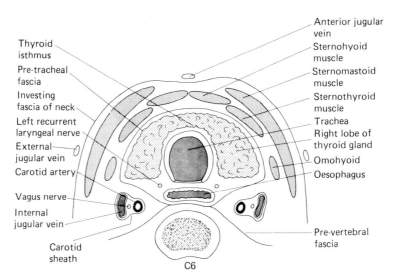

Figure 12.26 Relations of the cervical trachea as shown by transverse section of the neck at the level of the sixth cervical vertebra

Posterior

The oesophagus lies behind the trachea, and in the groove between them is the recurrent laryngeal nerve. Behind the oesophagus are the prevertebral fascia and the vertebral column.

Relations of the thoracic trachea (Figure 12.27)

Anterior

As the trachea descends through the superior mediastinum, it is related anteriorly to the manubrium sterni, the origins of the sternohyoid and sternothyroid muscles and the thymus gland – the latter of which is usually small and insignificant in the adult, but quite large and fleshy in the infant – the inferior thyroid veins, the left brachiocephalic vein, the arch of the aorta, the brachiocephalic and left common carotid arteries, the deep part of the cardiac plexus and a variable number of pretracheal and paratracheal lymph nodes.

It should be noted that in infants the brachiocephalic artery is higher and crosses the trachea just as it descends behind the suprasternal notch. The left brachiocephalic vein may project upwards into the neck to form an anterior relation of the cervical trachea and a potential hazard during tracheostomy.

Lateral

On the left side are the left common carotid and left subclavian arteries, the left vagus nerve and the descending part of the arch of the aorta. The left recurrent laryngeal nerve passes upwards deep to the arch of the aorta and then into the groove between the trachea and oesophagus.

On the right side, the trachea is related to the pleura and upper lobe of the right lung, the right brachiocephalic vein, the superior vena cava, the right vagus nerve and the azygos vein.

Posterior

The trachea is related to the oesophagus and, behind it, to the vertebral column. To the left and posterior to the oesophagus lies the thoracic duct.

Relations of lung root (Figure 12.28)

The root or hilum of the lung transmits the following structures within a sheath of pleura: the pulmonary artery, the two pulmonary veins, the bronchus, the bronchial vessels, the lymphatics, the lymph nodes and the nerves. The bronchi are situated posterior to the pulmonary vessels. The pulmonary arteries lie above the veins. The bronchial vessels hug the posterior surface of the bronchi. All these structures lie between anterior and posterior pulmonary plexuses.

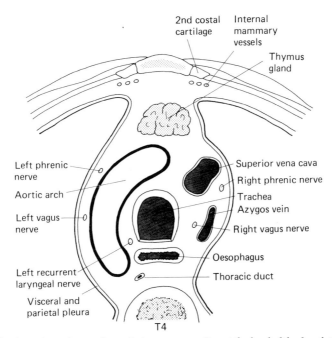

Figure 12.27 Relations of the thoracic trachea as shown in transverse section at the level of the fourth thoracic vertebra

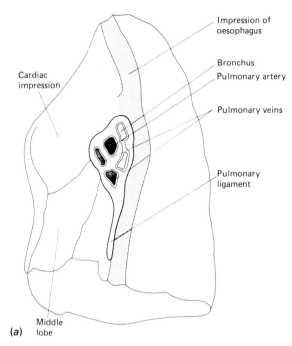

Cardiac
impression

Impression of
oesophagus

Bronchus
Pulmonary artery

Pulmonary veins

Pulmonary
ligament

Middle
(a)   lobe

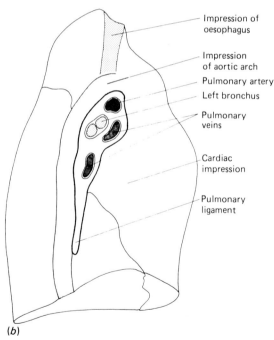

Impression of
oesophagus

Impression
of aortic arch
Pulmonary artery
Left bronchus

Pulmonary
veins

Cardiac
impression

Pulmonary
ligament

(b)

Figure 12.28 (*a*) Root of right lung, (*b*) Root of left lung

The right side differs from the left in one respect, namely that there is an additional upper lobe bronchus which lies above ('eparterial'), but still posterior to, the pulmonary vessels.

The following are the relationships of the lung roots themselves.

Anterior

On the left is the phrenic nerve, and on the right are the superior vena cava and the phrenic nerve.

Posterior

On the left are the descending aorta and vagus nerve, and on the right is the vagus nerve.

Superior

On the left is the aortic arch, and on the right the azygos vein.

Inferior

The pulmonary ligaments are merely a sleeve of slack pleura allowing the necessary freedom of 'dead space' for the structures of the lung root.

Applied anatomy of the trachea and bronchi

Surface anatomy of trachea and main bronchi and relationship to tracheostomy

The trachea, which lies about 2 cm under the skin, extends from the cricoid cartilage almost vertically downwards in the median plane as far as the sternal angle, after which it inclines very slightly to the right. The right main bronchus runs from the lower end of the trachea downwards and to the right for 2.5 cm, to reach the hilum of the lung opposite the sternal end of the right third costal cartilage. The left main bronchus runs at a smaller angle from the lower end of the trachea for 5 cm to the left and downwards to reach the hilum of the lung behind the left third costal cartilage, 3.5 cm from the median plane.

In order to increase the proportion of cervical trachea before a tracheostomy, the head is extended maximally by placing a sandbag between the shoulders. The cricoid cartilage is palpated and the skin incision in the adult is placed approximately 2.5 cm below this level. From the cosmetic point of view, a short collar skin incision is preferable to a vertical one. By staying exactly in the midline, danger to the major vessels in the neck is avoided. The pretracheal muscles are separated and the thyroid isthmus is either displaced upwards, downwards or divided. The trachea is opened between the second and third rings. In the adult, a window is cut out of the front of the trachea by removing a part of the second and third, or the third and fourth rings. In the child, the cartilages are very soft and a vertical incision is sufficient to introduce a tube. Care must always be taken not to damage the first tracheal ring. As mentioned previously, the left brachiocephalic vein may project up into the neck in children, and the close relationship of the brachiocephalic artery to the trachea has led to a sudden profuse haemorrhage in consequence of erosion of the tracheal wall by a tracheostomy tube.

Examination of trachea and bronchi by tracheoscopy and bronchoscopy, and clinical significance of bronchopulmonary segments

Tracheoscopy and bronchoscopy (see Figure 12.23)

Tracheoscopy and bronchoscopy can be performed under local or general anaesthesia using either rigid or fibreoptic instruments. At the present time, the most common method is probably that of fibrescopi instrumentation under local anaesthesia combined with controlled sedation. Examination of the trachea and bronchi enables pathological states to be studied and biopsies for histology to be taken, foreign bodies to be removed, or accumulation of fluid to be aspirated by suction.

Bronchoscopy is an exercise in the practical knowledge of bronchopulmonary segments.

The trachea is a glistening tube which has a white appearance where there are rings of cartilage and a reddish appearance in the areas between them. The tube appears slightly flattened where it is crossed by the aortic arch, and pulsations are visible. The tracheal bifurcation or carina lies slightly to the left of the midtracheal line because of the more vertically placed right main bronchus. It is consequently easier to advance initially down this bronchus. With the aid of the retrograde telescope or, alternatively, by bending the tip of the fibrescope, the orifices of the anterior, posterior and apical branches of the right upper lobe can be seen. Further advance will reveal a horizontal ridge marking the anteriorly placed orifice of the middle lobe bronchus, below which the lower lobe bronchus lies. Posteriorly, the latter's apical branch orifice can be seen; then the medial (cardiac) orifice appears and, finally, placed close together, from above downwards, appear the anterior, lateral and posterior basal orifices. If the instrument is now withdrawn into the trachea and advanced along the left main bronchus, the first impression is that of the greater length of the bronchus before the appearance of the left upper lobe in the lateral wall. The mouth of the lingula bronchus can best be seen through a retrograde telescope or by bending the tip of the fibrescope. The advance along the lower lobe bronchus brings the apical and medial basal branches into view posteriorly and then beyond this, the cluster of orifices of the anterior, lateral and posterior basal bronchi.

Clinical significance of bronchopulmonary segments

The right main bronchus is more nearly in line with the trachea than is the left. It is easier, therefore, for inhaled foreign bodies or fluids, such as gastric contents, to enter the right rather than the left bronchial tree. If the patient is lying on his side, such material enters the lateral (or 'axillary') subsegments of the anterior and posterior segments of the lobe (Figure 12.29a). They are thus a frequent site for the development of inhalational pneumonitis, segmental collapse or of a lung abscess.

If the patient is supine then the apical (superior) segmental bronchus, which arises from the posterior aspect of the right or left lower lobe bronchi, is the most likely part of the lung for aspirated material to collect (Figure 12.29b). It was formerly, also, a not uncommon site for a tubercular cavity.

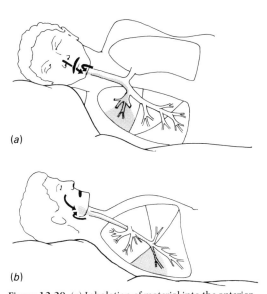

Figure 12.29 (*a*) Inhalation of material into the anterior and posterior segmental bronchi of the right upper lobe by an unconscious patient lying on the right side.
(*b*) Inhalation of material into the apical bronchus of the right lower lobe by an unconscious patient lying in the supine position

When inhaled, foreign bodies may, according to their size, obstruct either a main, lobe, segmental or smaller bronchus.

While pathological conditions, such as bronchiectasis, and certain infective processes may be restricted to one or more bronchopulmonary segments, malignant neoplasms and tuberculosis break through from one segment to adjacent ones.

If appropriate, surgical resection of a single bronchopulmonary segment can be undertaken. More radical procedures include the removal of a number of segments, of a whole pulmonary lobe (lobectomy), or of a complete lung (pneumonectomy).

Acknowledgement

The illustrations for this chapter, unless acknowledged otherwise, were drawn by Mr Stephen Metcalfe, FRCS.

References

ANDREWS, P. M. (1975) Microplicae. *Journal of Cell Biology*, **67**, 11a

ARNOLD, J. E. (1962) Vocal rehabilitation of paralytic dysphonia. *Archives of Otolaryngology*, **75**, 549–570

BELL TELEPHONE LABORATORIES (1937) *High Speed Motion Pictures of the Vocal Cords*. New York: Bureau of Publication Bell Telephone Laboratory

BECK, J. and SCHÖNHÄRL, E. (1954) Ein neus mikrophongesteuertes Lichblitz-Stroboskop. *HNO-Wegweiser*, **4**, 212–214

BERLIN, D. D. (1935) The recurrent laryngeal nerves in total ablation of the normal thyroid gland. *Surgery, Gynecology and Obstetrics*, **60**, 19–26

BOWDEN, R. E. M. (1955) The surgical anatomy of the recurrent laryngeal nerve. *British Journal of Surgery*, **43**, 153–157

BOWDEN, R. E. M. and SHEUER, J. L. (1960) Weight of abductor and adductor muscles of the human larynx. *Journal of Laryngology and Otology*, **74**, 971–980

BOYDEN, E. A. (1955) *Segmental Anatomy of the Lungs*. New York: McGraw-Hill

BROCK, R. C. (1943) Observations on the anatomy of the bronchial tree, with special reference to the surgery of lung abscess. *Guy's Hospital Reports*, **92**, 35–37

BROCK, R. C. (1954) *The Anatomy of the Bronchial Tree*. London: Oxford University Press

DEDO, D. D. and DEDO, H. H. (1980) Vocal cord paralysis. In: *Otolaryngology Volume III*, edited by M. M. Paparella and D. A. Shumrick. Philadelphia: W. B. Saunders. pp. 2489–2503

EMERY, J. (1969) (ed.) *The Anatomy of the Developing Lung*. London: Heinemann

ENGEL, S. (1962) *Lung Structure*. Springfield: Thomas

FARNSWORTH, D. W. (1940) High speed motion pictures of human vocal cords. *Bell Laboratories Records*, **18**, 203–213

FINK, B. R. and KIRSCHNER, F. (1958) Observations on the acoustical and mechanical properties of the vocal folds. *Folia Phoniatrica (Basel)*, **11**, 167–175

FRIEDMAN, M., TORIUMI, D. M, GRYBAUSKAS, V. and KATZ, A. (1986) Nonrecurrent laryngeal nerves and their clinical significance. *Laryngoscope*, **96**, 87–90

GROSSMAN, M. (1897) Experimentelle Beitrage zur Lehre von der 'Posticuslahmung'. *Archiv für Laryngologie und Rhinologie*, **6**, 282–360

GUINDI, G. M., MICHAELS, L., BANNISTER, R. and GIBSON, W. (1981) Pathology of the intrinsic muscles of the larynx. *Clinical Otolaryngology*, **6**, 101–109

HIRANO, M. (1981) *Clinical Examination of Voice*. New York: Springer-Verlag. pp. 5, 6, 8, 44

HOLLIEN, H. and CURTIS, J. (1960) A laminographic study of vocal pitch. *Journal of Speech and Hearing Research*, **3**, 157–165

KARK, A. E., KISSIN, M. W., AUERBACK, R. and MEIKLE, M. (1984) Voice changes after thyroidectomy: role of the external laryngeal nerve. *British Medical Journal*, **289**, 1412–1415

KIRCHNER, J. A. (1982) Semon's law a century later. *Journal of Laryngology and Otology*, **96**, 645–657

MCILWAIN, J. C. (1991) The posterior glottis. *Journal of Otolaryngology*, **20**, (suppl. 2), 1–24

MARCHAND, P., GILROY, J. C. and WILSON, V. H. (1950) Anatomical study of bronchial vascular system and its variations in disease. *Thorax*, **5**, 207–221

O'RAHILLY, R. and BOYDEN, E. A. (1973) The timing and sequence of events in the development of the human respiratory system during the embryonic period proper. *Zeitschrift für Anatomie und Entwicklungsgeschichte*, **141**, 237–250

PIERSOL, G. A. (1930) *Human Anatomy*, 9th edn. Philadelphia: J. B. Lippincott. p. 724

PRESSMAN, J. J. (1942) Physiology of vocal cords in phonation and respiration. *Archives of Otolaryngology*, **35**, 355–398

REID, L. (1967) In; *Development of the Lung* (Ciba Foundation Symposium). London: Churchill. p. 109

REID, L. (1976) Visceral cartilage. *Journal of Anatomy*, **122**, 349–355

SCHÖNHÄRL, E. (1960) *Die Stroboskopie in der praktischen laryngologie*. Stuttgart: G. Thieme

SMITH, S. (1954) Remarks on the physiology of the vibrations of the vocal cords. *Folia Phoniatrica (Basel)*, **6**, 166–171

STELL, P. M., GREGORY, I. and WATT, J. (1980) Morphology of the human larynx. II. The subglottis. *Clinical Otolaryngology*, **5**, 389–395

TILLMAN, B., PEITZCH-ROHRSCHEIDER, I. and HOENGES, H. L. (1977) The human vocal cords surface. *Cell Tissue Research (Berlin)*, **185**, 279–283

VAMPEPERSTRAETE, F. (1973) The cartilaginous skeleton of the bronchial tree. *Advances in Anatomy, Embryology and Cell Biology*, **48**, 3–10

WAGNER, R. (1890) Die medianstellung der stimmbander bei der Rekurrenslahmung. *Archiv für Pathologische Anatomie und Physiologie*, **120**, 437–459

WATT-BOOLSEN, S., BLICHERT-TOFT, M., HENSE, J. B. JORGENSEN, S. J. and BOBERG, A. (1977) Late voice function after injury to the recurrent nerve. *Clinical Otolaryngology*, **2**, 191–197

WORK, W. P. (1941) Unusual position of the right recurrent laryngeal nerve. *Annals of Otology, Rhinology and Laryngology*, **50**, 569

ZENKER, W. (1964) Vocal muscle fibres and their motor endplates. In: *Research Potentials in Voice Physiology*, edited by D. W. Brewer. New York: New York State University Press. pp. 256–271

13

Physiology of respiration

Neil Pride

The primary function of the lungs is to supply oxygen to the blood for distribution to the tissues and to excrete the carbon dioxide produced by metabolism but, for the nose and throat specialist, the most relevant aspect of respiratory function is the conducting airways which are the pathway for ventilation of the lungs. This chapter therefore concentrates on ventilatory and airway function and puts less emphasis on other important aspects of respiratory function, such as pulmonary gas exchange and the pulmonary circulation. The physiology of the extrathoracic airway is covered in more detail in the chapters on nasal physiology, obstructive sleep apnoea, laryngeal control and swallowing (see Chapters 6 and 11, and Volume 4, Chapter 19). More detailed reviews of the practical assessment of respiratory function and of normal values are available (Cotes, 1993; Quanjer, 1993; Gibson, 1995; Pride, 1995).

Respiratory mechanics

Ventilation and respiratory muscles

Ventilation of the lungs is produced by the inspiratory muscles expanding the intrathoracic cavity and lowering the pleural surface pressure. The actual expansion of the lungs achieved then depends on the flow resistance of the intra- and extrathoracic airway and the elasticity of the lungs.

In normal subjects, resting total ventilation is only about 5–6 l/min, a small proportion of the maximum ventilatory capacity which is greater than 100 l/min. Even on strenuous exercise, ventilation does not usually increase above about 80 l/min. In chronic lung diseases, ventilation at rest is usually maintained at

or slightly above the value in healthy subjects, but there is a gross reduction in the ability to increase ventilation during exercise.

At rest in normal subjects the diaphragm is the most important inspiratory muscle, expanding the intrathoracic cavity primarily by its downward piston action. When the diaphragm contracts, there is a reduction in pleural surface and consequently intra-alveolar pressure and an increase in abdominal pressure and outward movement of the abdomen. The increase in abdominal pressure leads to some outward expansion and elevation of the lower rib cage in the area of apposition of the diaphragm against the internal surface of the rib cage. There is also some inspiratory activation of rib cage muscles which slightly expands the rib cage and prevents indrawing of the intercostal spaces due to the reduction in pleural surface pressure. During inspiration, pressure throughout the airways is subatmospheric. For the intrathoracic airways, the pressure around the airways decreases more than the intra-airway pressure, so these airways slightly enlarge during inspiration. In contrast the subatmospheric airways pressure would tend to narrow the compliant extrathoracic airway: in practice activation of muscles of the supralaryngeal oropharyngeal airway slightly precedes the inspiratory activation of the diaphragm and other muscles acting directly on the lungs; this widens the supralaryngeal airway and reduces its compliance, protecting it against the collapsing tendency of the negative intra-airway pressure (Schwartz et al., 1994). There is also abduction of the vocal cords (Brancatisano, Collett and Engel, 1983).

At rest, expiratory flow depends on the passive recoil of the respiratory system without active contraction of the expiratory muscles. Indeed the duration of expiration is much greater than the time needed for passive recoil to return the lungs to the neutral position of the respiratory system (relaxation volume, Vr; which in normal subjects corresponds to the end-tidal volume, functional residual capacity). Braking of expiration is produced by activity of the inspiratory muscles continuing into the first part of expiration, which ensures a smooth transition between the end of inspiration and the early part of expiration, and by narrowing of the glottic aperture throughout expiration (Bartlett, 1986).

When ventilation increases, as during exercise, diaphragmatic and inspiratory intercostal muscle activity increases and accessory muscles such as the scalenes and sternomastoids are recruited; postinspiratory activity of inspiratory muscles and expiratory narrowing of the larynx are reduced and replaced by increasing activity of abdominal and expiratory intercostal muscles. The external oblique muscles are usually recruited before the rectus abdominus muscles. There is further increase in inspiratory activation of the muscles surrounding the extrathoracic airway, widening the alae nasi, oropharynx and larynx which, in combination with positioning of the soft palate, alters the distribution of ventilation between the nasal and oral routes (Niinimaa *et al.*, 1980, 1981). This pattern of recruitment of respiratory muscles as ventilation is increased is stereotyped; in severe obstruction of the airways, the pattern of activation at rest is similar to that of normal subjects during exercise, with contraction of neck muscles during inspiration and abdominal muscles on expiration.

The contractile properties of the respiratory muscles are similar to those of other skeletal muscles, though the respiratory muscles may be less prone to fatigue. The optimum length of the diaphragm for generating tension is at lung volumes around or below the normal resting breathing position and its ability to develop tension decreases considerably at larger lung volumes. Clinical problems with the respiratory muscles may arise in neuromuscular disease (e.g. myasthenia gravis, motor neurone disease, myopathy or polymyositis) but also when the muscles themselves are normal but working at a mechanical disadvantage (Gibson, 1989; Laroche, Moxham and Green, 1989). Examples of the latter group are diseases distorting the rib cage, such as kyphoscoliosis, and airflow obstruction where increase in end-tidal lung volume shortens the initial length of the diaphragm. In severe emphysema the domes of the diaphragm may be flattened so that contraction may narrow rather than widen the lower rib cage on inspiration (Hoover's sign). Respiratory muscle weakness may also become important with cachexia, long-standing illness (including emphysema) or in acute illness which reduce blood levels of potassium, calcium or phosphate.

Airway function

Assessment of airway calibre

Airway calibre is commonly assessed by two distinct types of measurement (Gibson, 1995):

Airflow resistance in which the pressure drop between the alveoli and the airway opening (usually the mouth, but sometimes the nose or even a tracheostomy) is related to the simultaneous flow rate, measured at the airway opening. Measurements are usually made during resting tidal breathing.

Flow, volume and time measurements made during maximum effort vital capacity manoeuvres; spirometry, peak flow or maximum flow versus volume may be measured and provide estimates of maximum capacity.

Because the two types of measurements are so different, perfect correspondence cannot be expected but, in fact, many tests derived from maximum effort manoeuvres, particularly on expiration, depend on the mechanical properties of the lungs and are relatively independent of the muscular force applied.

Total airflow resistance measures the pressure drop through all the airway segments arranged in series. Because of the relative ease with which posterior nasal or pharyngeal pressure can be measured, nasal calibre is usually assessed by one of several resistance methods.

For studying the calibre of intrathoracic airways the reverse is the case. Methods for measuring airflow resistance are not well established outside specialized pulmonary function laboratories. In contrast, peak flow, spirometry and maximum flow-volume curves are simple and widely available and are the usual methods of estimating calibre of the intrathoracic airways. All the tests use flow at the airway opening during maximum effort manoeuvres. This flow can be diminished by narrowing in any part of the airways, but disease of the extrathoracic airway, including the nose, characteristically decreases maximum inspiratory flow disproportionately, while the major effect of intrathoracic airway obstruction is on maximum expiratory flow. These differences have led to recognition of specific patterns of abnormality of maximum flow-volume curves which are useful in the diagnosis of obstruction of the extrathoracic airway.

Airflow resistance

Three techniques for measuring intrathoracic airflow resistance are used in the specialized pulmonary function laboratory – body plethysmography which measures total airway resistance (Raw), the oesophageal balloon-catheter technique which measures total lung resistance (RL = Raw plus resistance of lung tissue) and the forced oscillation technique applied at the mouth which measures total respiratory resistance (Rrs) which is the sum of RL and the flow resistance of the chest wall. All these measurements are usually made with the subject seated and breathing through a large mouthpiece, but all can be modified to measure resistance while breathing via the nose.

Total resistance to airflow is the sum of all the resistances arranged in series in the supratracheal airway, intrapulmonary airways, lung tissue and chest wall (Figure 13.1). Serial components of resistance can be measured by placing needles or catheters appropriately; in practice this is only commonly used to measure nasal airway resistance (Rnaw). Total nasal resistance during tidal breathing normally accounts for about 50% of total resistance during quiet nasal breathing; it can be measured using a pharyngeal catheter to measure transnasal pressure and nasal flow via a pneumotachograph attached to a tight-fitting nasal mask. Alternatively the difference between total respiratory resistance (Rrs) (measured with the forced oscillation technique) when breathing via the mouth and via the nose can be used to calculate nasal airway resistance (Shelton *et al.*, 1990). Other techniques measure resistance of one nostril or the pressure drop when flow is passively supplied to one nares (see Volume 4, Chapter 4). Measurements have also been made of pharyngeal resistance but there is a suspicion that catheters and/or associated local anaesthesia may affect the pressure drop.

Relatively few measurements of intrathoracic resistance, however, are made in clinical practice in the UK, despite their relevance to tidal breathing. Disadvantages are the expense and bulk of equipment (body plethysmography), or the need for intubation (oesophageal pressure measurement), while the forced oscillation technique, which is simpler, has not yet achieved widespread acceptance. Values of resistance vary according to the lung volume at which it is measured, the phase of respiration (inspiration or expiration), the size of the laryngeal aperture, and the flow rate. Consequently the measurement conditions have to be closely controlled making the methods more suitable for research into airway pharmacology than for routine clinical assessment.

Serial distribution of airflow resistance

Nasal airway resistance is the largest single contributor to the total airflow resistance of the respiratory system, typically accounting for about 50% of normal resistance during quiet nasal breathing. Most measurements of airflow resistance however are made with a large diameter mouthpiece which minimizes the oral resistance. Under these circumstances the total resistance of the airways is 1–2 cmH$_2$O/l/s in normal subjects with about one-third of the resistance being offered by the supratracheal airway, another one-third by trachea and conducting airways > 3 mm diameter, and the final one-third by peripheral airways < 3 mm diameter (Hogg, Macklem and Thurl-

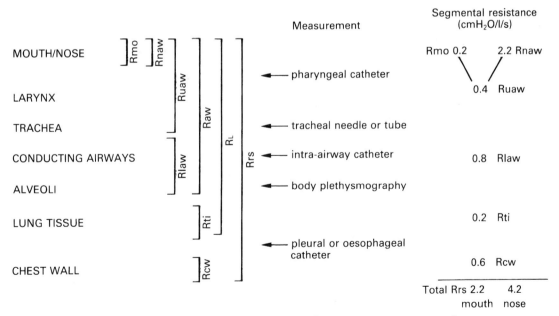

Figure 13.1 Serial distribution of total respiratory resistance. Rmo: oral airway resistance; Rnaw: nasal airway resistance; Ruaw: airway resistance above the upper end of the trachea; Rlaw: airway resistance of intrathoracic airways (alveoli to trachea); Raw: total airway resistance; RL: total pulmonary resistance; Rti: tissue resistance; Rcw flow resistance of chest wall; Rrs: total respiratory resistance. Conversion factor 1kPa $\approx$ 10 cmH$_2$O

beck, 1968). The small contribution of the normal peripheral airways is not intuitively obvious. Intrathoracic airflow resistance is the sum of the resistance of a complex branching system with 20 or more generations of airways arranged in series and with many parallel pathways in the more peripheral airway generations. Because each succeeding airway generation from trachea out to the periphery is smaller in size, the resistance offered by each individual airway of successive generations increases. However, the effect of the diminished calibre of each individual airway is far outweighed by the increase in the total number of airways in each generation which results in the total cross-sectional area available for gas flow at any fixed distance from the trachea increasing dramatically as the alveoli are approached. Because the velocity of gas flow depends on the ratio of bulk flow to cross-sectional area, velocity is at a maximum in the trachea and central airways and slows progressively towards the periphery, so that in the terminal airways gas flow takes place solely by diffusion.

Effects of lung volume

Airways expand as lung volume is increased and are 30–40% larger in diameter at full inspiration (total lung capacity, TLC) than at full expiration (residual volume, RV) (Butler *et al.*, 1960). This results in a significant decrease in airflow resistance, so that airway narrowing can be partially overcome by breathing at a larger lung volume.

Control of airway tone

The calibre of the airways at any lung volume is under the control of the autonomic nervous system (Postema *et al.*, 1985). Most normal subjects have some bronchomotor tone mediated by vagal efferent nerves, which is reduced on exercise and at rest can be removed by β-adrenoceptor agonists or muscarinic antagonists, reducing airflow resistance by about 30%. The role of the sympathoadrenal system in controlling airway tone is less clear; in humans, sympathetic nerves may not directly innervate bronchial muscle, though they probably modulate the activity of the vagal ganglia in the airway wall. The many β-adrenoceptors in normal bronchial muscle probably respond to circulating catecholamines rather than to sympathetic nerve stimulation. The importance of the non-adrenergic, non-cholinergic nervous system which has both excitory and inhibitory actions is probably mainly to modulate vagally induced tone. The role of other factors such as endogenously produced nitric oxide, which is a bronchodilator and may be the mediator of the dilator effects of the non-adrenergic, non-cholinergic system, or leukotrienes, which are bronchoconstrictors, are currently areas of intensive investigation.

Tone of the intrathoracic airways shows a circadian rhythm which peaks at about 04.00 hours and is least in mid-afternoon. This rhythm reflects circadian variations in vagal nerve activity, cortisol secretion and sympathoadrenal activation. Tone can be briefly increased by many inhaled stimuli, such as cold air, inert dust, cigarette smoke, sulphur dioxide and other air pollutants. These stimuli act on irritant or cough receptors situated immediately under the airway epithelium which trigger reflex bronchoconstriction; both afferent and efferent nervous pathways run in the vagus nerve. In some instances the stimuli may also directly induce local release of mediators, leading to mucosal thickening and oedema. There is a wide range of airway responsiveness to exogenous stimuli in healthy, asymptomatic subjects and responsiveness may be increased for some weeks after severe respiratory tract infections and for a shorter period after exposure to environmental pollutants. The 'protective' effects of this response are uncertain. The airway hyperresponsiveness found in asthma is an exaggeration of this normal response, one effect of which is to increase the amplitude of the circadian rhythm in airway calibre: this leads to the characteristic early morning worsening of symptoms.

Variations with breathing route, posture, sleep and exercise

Measurements made under laboratory conditions in resting, seated subjects breathing via a large diameter mouthpiece give a minimum value of airflow resistance. Natural breathing at rest is via the nasal or combined oronasal route with the oral airway smaller and offering a higher resistance. In the supine posture nasal resistance increases (Cole and Haight, 1984), especially in the presence of nasal disease, and resting lung volume is reduced, decreasing intrapulmonary airway dimensions and increasing their resistance (Linderholm, 1963). Nocturnal changes include increased vagal tone of the airways and, with sleep, reduced activation of tongue and pharyngeal muscles with increase in pharyngeal resistance (Skatrud and Dempsey, 1985). All these changes will increase resistance above the value obtained at rest in 'ideal' laboratory conditions. In contrast, during exercise airway dimensions enlarge; there is decongestion of the nasal mucosa, the oral pathway is held open, the supraglottal airway and glottis widen and vagal tone of intrapulmonary airways is reduced. Positioning of the soft palate allows both oral and nasal routes to be used in parallel to accommodate the increased ventilation.

Apart from the decongestion induced by exercise, the nose shows a spontaneous vascular rhythmicity with alternating congestion and decongestion of the nasal mucosa at about 3-hour intervals. In some individuals this rhythm is out-of-phase in the two nostrils, so that total nasal airflow resistance remains constant due to this nasal 'cycle'. The pharyngeal airway and glottis also enlarge with inspiration, in phase with ventilation of the lungs.

Airway responsiveness

Sublaryngeal airways

In subjects with asthma there is an increased tendency for airways narrowing to develop in response to a whole range of stimuli (e.g. exercise, hyperventilation, breathing cold air, hypo- or hyperosmolar aerosols, constrictor drugs such as histamine or cholinergic agonists or mediators such as bradykinin or leukotrienes). This responsiveness may be quantified using an incremental dose–response technique. Most commonly histamine or methacholine is used as the stimulus and the dose increased until a 20% fall in forced expiratory volume in 1 second (FEV_1) is produced. Airway responsiveness is often increased in smokers with chronic airflow obstruction, when it may reflect altered airway geometry and increased thickness of the airway wall (Boushey *et al.*, 1980).

Larynx

Narrowing of the glottic aperture also occurs with many of the same stimuli that lead to narrowing of intrapulmonary airways. The glottal response to histamine is enhanced in subjects with asthma (Higenbottam, 1980).

Nose

Vascular changes can also be induced by a variety of exogenous stimuli, such as topical histamine and methacholine, but the normal range of responsiveness is less wide than with intrathoracic airway responsiveness and there is more overlap between normal subjects and the modestly increased responsiveness found in patients with rhinitis.

Nasobronchial interactions

Transient reflex narrowing of the intrathoracic airways can be provoked by nasal stimulation in normal humans but despite this, remarkably little is known about the biological, and possible clinical, importance of these interactions. Evidence for an effect of bronchoconstriction on nasal patency is less certain in humans (Yap and Pride, 1994), although in animals intrapulmonary stimuli have been shown to lead to nasal vascular changes which alter nasal airflow resistance.

Maximum flow rates and dynamic airway changes

Intrathoracic airways

During quiet breathing, the subatmospheric pleural pressure throughout the breathing cycle slightly distends the airways. With vigorous expiratory efforts, as in a cough, central intrathoracic airways are dramatically compressed by the positive pleural pressures which may exceed +100 cmH$_2$O. Airway closure does not occur because the positive pleural pressure not only compresses the central airways (which increases resistance) but also increases the driving pressure for expiratory flow, alveolar pressure. Above a certain minimum expiratory pressure at lung volumes in the lower 75–85% of the vital capacity, these two tendencies precisely counterbalance each other so that at any given lung volume, expiratory flow via the mouth reaches a maximum plateau value which remains constant with further increases in pressure. The compressed central airways act as the flow-limiting mechanism and the plateau value of maximum expiratory flow provides the physiological basis for the widely used tests of forced expiration and their relative independence from the precise expiratory pressure applied. In the upper 15–25% of the vital capacity, on expiration via the mouth flow still increases as driving pressure is increased in normal subjects because sufficiently large expiratory pressures to achieve plateau conditions cannot be generated. In the presence of intrapulmonary airway narrowing, plateau conditions for expiratory flow may be achieved throughout the vital capacity. On forceful inspiration via the mouth in normal subjects intrathoracic airways are progressively distended by increase in transairway pressure as inspiratory driving pressure is increased so no intrapulmonary airflow limitation develops.

Extrathoracic airway

Transairway pressures in the extrathoracic airway show a completely different pattern on forced manoeuvres because extra-airway pressure is close to atmospheric pressure and is not influenced by inspiratory or expiratory efforts. On expiration airway pressures within the extrathoracic airway are above atmospheric pressure and maintain the airway open; on inspiration the subatmospheric pressure in the extrathoracic airways narrows the airway unless it is supported against collapse by activation of the surrounding muscles. In practice during forceful inspiratory efforts through the mouth held open by a mouthpiece in normal subjects, there is no significant extrathoracic airway narrowing. But pharyngeal pressures are more negative when breathing via the nose due to nasal resistance being higher than oral resistance; these lower pressures, combined with the reduced activation of muscles surrounding the pharyngeal airway during sleep, are responsible for the narrowing that leads frequently to snoring and in extreme cases to obstructive apnoea. When forced inspiratory manoeuvres are made through the nose, the nasal valve acts as a flow-limiting mechanism once about 20 cmH$_2$O driving pressure is developed in the posterior nasopharynx (Bridger and Proctor, 1970). A plateau of maximum inspiratory flow, which is independent of further increases in driving pressure, develops throughout the vital capacity, the level of maximum inspiratory flow being relatively constant throughout the vital capacity (Pertuze, Watson and Pride, 1991). Maximum inspiratory flow through the nose can be increased by decongestants and by stabilization of the alae nasi and anterior nares. Inspiratory flow limitation facilitates clearance of the nose of foreign particles by permitting these to be moved into the posterior nasopharynx by a sniff which generates a burst of high velocity flow through the nasal valve, in a manner analogous to the expiratory action of cough for the intrathoracic airways.

Effects of airway disease

The dyspnoea and wheeze of chronic, persistent asthma and other diseases of the intrathoracic airways have to be distinguished from structural or functional obstruction of the extrathoracic airway. Fortunately extrathoracic obstruction usually leads to distinctive changes in maximum flow-volume curves which indicate the need for endoscopy.

Intrathoracic airways

Many lung diseases diminish the resting calibre of the intrathoracic airways, increasing airflow resistance and reducing maximum expiratory flow. Airway narrowing may result from disease of the airway wall or lumen (as in asthma or the obstructive bronchiolitis of smokers) or from loss of the normal forces distending the airways (as occurs with the alveolar destruction of emphysema). When narrowing of the intrapulmonary airways is present, dynamic narrowing of the central airways and flow limitation occurs on expiration at unusually low flows and pleural pressures, so that reductions in maximum flow and increases in airflow resistance characteristically are much greater on expiration than on inspiration.

The site of intrapulmonary airway narrowing has been particularly studied in smokers with varying combinations of irreversible airway disease and emphysema (chronic obstructive pulmonary disease). Pathological studies suggest that the usual site of fixed disease of the airway wall and lumen leading to increased resistance is in the small peripheral airways of less than 2–3 mm diameter (Hogg, Macklem and Thurlbeck, 1968). Because these airways account for only a small proportion of normal airflow resistance,

considerable disease can develop insidiously in the 'quiet zone' of the lung before obvious increases in total airflow resistance and reductions in maximum expiratory flow are found. The site of airway narrowing in asthma is much less certain, both because it probably varies from patient to patient (and probably within a patient as asthma varies), and because physiological studies cannot be backed up by appropriate pathological evidence.

Extrathoracic airway

Obstruction in the extrathoracic airway may increase airflow resistance and lead to dyspnoea which simulates that due to intrathoracic airway obstruction. The obstruction, as with a rigid tracheal stenosis or laryngeal paralysis, may be similar in inspiration and expiration, but if a dynamic effect develops it is during inspiration, in contrast to the dynamic worsening on expiration found with intrathoracic airway disease. Differences between fixed and dynamic narrowing can be detected by the contour of the maximum inspiratory and expiratory flow-volume curves, breathing via the mouth.

During asthmatic attacks there is also narrowing of the larynx (Lisboa *et al.*, 1980; Collett, Brancatisano and Engel, 1983) and supralaryngeal airways (Collett, Brancatisano and Engel, 1986), but the functional significance of these changes is uncertain.

Tests of forced expiration and inspiration

Breathing via the mouth

The volume expired via the mouth in the first second of a forced expiration commenced from total lung capacity (forced expiratory volume in one second, FEV$_1$) relates well to the maximum voluntary ventilation that could be sustained over 15 s both in subjects with normal lungs and in the presence of many lung diseases. Provided a modest minimum expiratory pressure is achieved, the values obtained do not depend on the pressure applied but only on the mechanical characteristics of the lungs and airways. In contrast, tests of forced inspiration are much more dependent on the applied inspiratory pressures. Both forced expiration and inspiration may be analysed as change in volume versus time (by spirometry) or as change in instantaneous flow rate (usually measured by a pneumotachograph) versus change in lung volume (maximum flow-volume curve) (Figure 13.2). Standard spirometric measurements are the FEV$_1$ and the vital capacity; the latter may be obtained from the forced expiration (forced vital capacity, FVC) or from a separate, slower full expiration. In intrapulmonary airway disease, forced vital capacity may be considerably less than the slow vital capacity. Normally FEV$_1$ is more than 70% of the vital capacity. Two patterns of spirometric abnormality can be distinguished –

'obstructive' in which, although there is usually some reduction in forced vital capacity, FEV_1 is reduced even more so that FEV_1/VC ratio is low, and 'restrictive' in which a small forced vital capacity is associated with normal or even accelerated emptying on forced expiration and a normal or increased FEV_1/FVC ratio. The maximum flow-volume curve (see Figure 13.2) shows that normally, on expiration, flow rapidly rises to a peak value and then declines in an approximately linear fashion. Peak expiratory flow can also be measured simply with a peak flow meter or gauge. The most effort-dependent part of expiration is close to full inflation and therefore in measuring peak expiratory flow the subject must take a full inspiration and make a rapid and forceful start to the subsequent full expiration. For clinical assessment of ventilatory function in intrathoracic disease, FEV_1 and vital capacity (or forced vital capacity) are usually adequate, although these tests will not pick up mild airway disease. In asthma, the value of peak expiratory flow is closely related to the value of FEV_1, and because peak expiratory flow can be measured by simple meters which can be used by patients in the home or at work, this measurement is particularly useful for identifying asthmatic episodes and their response to treatment. The maximum flow-volume curve cannot be used to distinguish different mechanisms of intrapulmonary airway narrowing.

Distinctive patterns in flow-volume curves however are found with obstruction of the extrathoracic airway, which reflect differences in the transmural pressures developed during forceful manoeuvres in the extrathoracic and intrathoracic airways. As already discussed, dimensions of the *intrathoracic* airways at a given lung volume tend to enlarge on forced inspiration, but dynamic compression of central intrathoracic airways develops on forced expiration. In contrast, dimensions of the *extrathoracic* airway are maintained on forced expiration but tend to narrow on inspiration.

A distinction may be made between fixed obstruction of the extrathoracic airways, which leads to a relatively symmetrical pattern of maximum expiratory and inspiratory flow (Figure 13.3) and a pattern where there is dynamic narrowing of the extrathoracic airways which reduces maximum inspiratory flow, but in extreme cases may not affect maximum expiratory flow (Miller and Hyatt, 1969, 1973). Examples of conditions which give a 'fixed' obstruction pattern include tracheal stenosis or laryngeal paralysis; dynamic narrowing may be associated with weakness of the muscles surrounding the supralaryngeal airway,

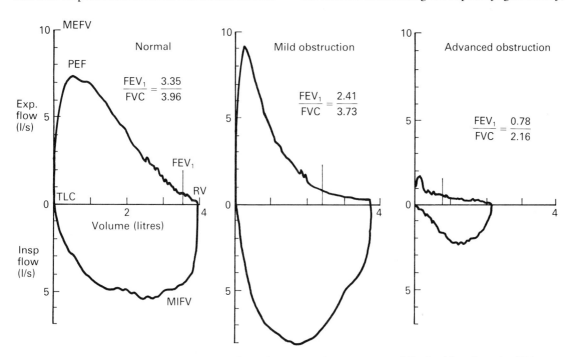

Figure 13.2 Maximum expiratory and inspiratory flow-volume (MEFV/MIFV) curves in (left) a healthy subject, (middle) a subject with mild intrathoracic airway obstruction, (right) advanced intrathoracic airway obstruction. FEV_1 indicated on volume axis by vertical bar. TLC = total lung capacity. RV = residual volume. FVC = forced vital capacity. PEF = peak expiratory flow. Note the development of convexity of flow to volume axis in mild obstruction which gives a diagnostic contour despite preservation of a large peak expiratory flow and FVC and only small reduction in FEV_1/FVC ratio. In advanced disease there is gross shrinkage on both volume and flow axes and expiratory flow during tidal breathing at rest reaches the MEFV curve

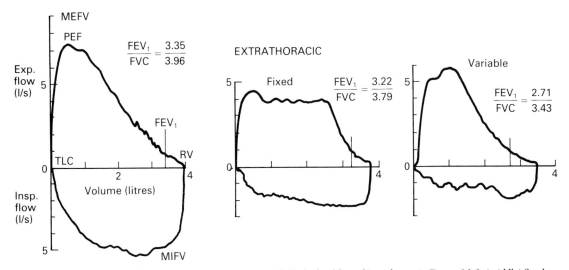

Figure 13.3 Maximum flow-volume (MEFV/MIFV) curves in (left) the healthy subject shown in Figure 13.2, (middle) fixed extrathoracic obstruction pattern as seen in tracheal stenosis with reduction in flow of MEFV and MIFV curves, a distinctive plateau of flow on MEFV curve and preservation of normal FEV_1 and FEV_1/FVC ratio, (right) variable extrathoracic obstruction with dynamic inspiratory narrowing of the upper airway but preservation of a normal MEFV curve, FEV_1 and FEV_1/FVC ratio in a patient with severe obstructive sleep apnoea, studied when awake and seated. TLC = total lung capacity. RV = residual volume. FVC = forced vital capacity. PEF = peak expiratory flow

with laryngeal polyps or tumours and tracheomalacia, either primary or following surgery or intubation.

FEV_1 may be well preserved with extrathoracic airway obstruction; this is because any reduction in maximum expiratory flow is confined to the upper half of the vital capacity (see Figure 13.3, middle) or may even be absent (see Figure 13.3, right). The pattern shown in Figure 13.3 (middle) can be detected by finding a reduction in peak expiratory flow which is greater than the reduction in FEV_1. But the best measurements to make are complete maximum expiratory and inspiratory flow-volume curves.

Functional obstruction of the extrathoracic airway presents a particular problem; it is characteristically episodic and may mimic acute asthma and airway function tests may be highly variable. Two distinct patterns have been described (Cormier, Camus and Desmeules, 1980; Rodenstein, Francis and Stanescu, 1983; Goldman and Myers, 1991). Most commonly, inspiratory stridor is associated with reduction in maximum inspiratory flow throughout the vital capacity and normal maximum expiratory flow; sometimes however there is reduction in both maximum inspiratory and expiratory flow. Limited endoscopic examinations suggest the obstruction is in the larynx. Typically patients are young women, some of whom are repeatedly admitted to hospital with recurrent attacks of noisy acute breathlessness. The second type of functional wheezing is mainly expiratory and is produced by forceful breathing close to residual volume; this is associated with completely normal maximum flow-volume curves; the wheeze probably arises from excessive tidal narrowing of central intrathoracic airways during expiration. Other aspects of lung function such as blood gases, single breath N_2 test, and functional residual capacity are usually normal.

Breathing via the nose

Breathing via the nasal rather than the oral route alters maximum flow-volume curves. Because the nose usually offers a higher resistance than the oral route, significant pressures are dissipated across the nose on forced expiration and intrapulmonary flow limiting conditions with a plateau of flow at a given lung volume are achieved only at smaller lung volumes than when expiring via the mouth, and maximum expiratory flow is reduced at larger lung volumes (Pertuze, Watson and Pride, 1991) (Figure 13.4). The extent of the difference between nasal and oral maximum expiratory flow-volume curves depends on the nasal airflow resistance. In some subjects there are considerable reductions in maximum expiratory flow via the nose, but in others the nasal curve may approach that via the mouth although it never appears to exceed it. On inspiration there is reduction in maximum inspiratory flow on the nasal curve compared with the oral curve at all lung volumes, as would be predicted from the additional

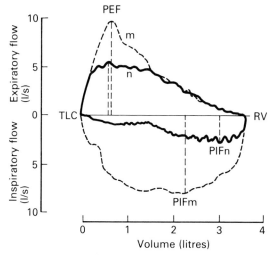

Figure 13.4 Maximum inspiratory and expiratory flow-volume curves of breathing via mouth (m. dashed line) and nose (n, solid line) in a normal subject. PEF, peak expiratory flow; PIF, peak inspiratory flow; TLC, total lung capacity; RV, residual volume. (From Pertuze, Watson and Pride (1991) *Journal of Applied Physiology*, **70**, 1369–1376)

resistance of the nose. But, in addition, the nasal valve acts as a flow-limiting mechanism on forceful inspiration, so that a pressure-independent plateau of maximum inspiratory flow develops throughout the vital capacity, the level of maximum inspiratory flow being relatively constant throughout the vital capacity.

Tests of maximum flow through the nose have been used to a limited extent to assess nasal disease. Because the nose is in series with the lungs and the respiratory muscles, care has to be taken that reduced flows are not due to inadequate driving pressures (poor cooperation or genuinely weak respiratory muscles) or accompanying lung disease (notably asthma accompanying rhinitis). Certainly, if simple tests like peak expiratory or inspiratory flow via the nose are used to monitor nasal obstruction, a useful safeguard is to measure the corresponding peak flows at the mouth.

Other techniques

Obviously methods for imaging the larger airways are advancing rapidly and computerized tomography of the lungs has been used to measure wall thickness of central intrapulmonary airways in asthma. Of particular interest is the acoustic reflection technique in which a sound pulse is generated and propagated in a sound tube before entering the airway (either via the nose or the mouth). The sound pulse is modified by local changes in cross-sectional area of the airway and the reflected signals measured by a microphone in the sound tube; from these signals an area-distance curve can be generated. Reliable signals can be obtained for the nasal cavity, virtually unnoticed by the subject (Hilberg *et al.*, 1989). The technique is more difficult to apply via the mouth and currently involves breathing a helium-oxygen mixture. Nevertheless useful information has been obtained on pharyngeal dimensions in obstructive sleep apnoea (Bradley *et al.*, 1986), and attempts are being made to make the method more robust and extend to subcarinal airways.

Airway protective mechanisms

The airway is potentially exposed to a wide variety of inhaled noxious agents such as dusts, irritant gases, microorganisms and allergens. A variety of protective mechanisms is usually highly effective in excluding particulate matter from, and maintaining sterility within, the sublaryngeal airway. Thus the nose detects foreign substances by smell and irritation and traps large particles such as pollen; these may be expelled by sneezing or carried to the nasopharynx by nasal cilia. Soluble pollutants such as SO_2 are absorbed by the nose, reducing the concentration inhaled to the tracheobronchial tree. Particulates that reach the tracheobronchial tree are trapped in airway secretions which have antimicrobial activity. Secretions and inhaled foreign material are then removed by a combination of mucociliary transport and cough; the latter also acts as a warning of inhaled noxious gases even when there is no particulate matter requiring expulsion. The cough reflex is initiated by stimulation of sensory nerve endings throughout the distribution of the vagus nerve, but usually in the upper and lower airways.

Deposition of inhaled particles

Deposition of particles takes place by three mechanisms – inertial impaction which is important for larger particles in the nose and at the division of major intrapulmonary airways, sedimentation, and diffusion – the latter two mechanisms being important for smaller particles. The nose is an effective filter for particles above 5 μm; once an aerosol reaches the trachea, the airways become increasingly effective filters as particle size increases from 1 to 10 μm. The greatest alveolar deposition is found with particles of 4 μm; smaller particles can be exhaled while larger particles are increasingly filtered out by the airways.

Respiratory tract secretions

Secretions are produced by mucous and serous glands in the submucosa and also by transudation and goblet cells in the airway mucosa which discharge their secretions directly into the airway lumen. Glycoproteins (mucus) are produced by the mucous glands and goblet cells in the nose and tracheobronchial tree; serous cells and transudation are responsible for water, ions, enzymes such as lactoferrin and lysozyme and IgA immunoglobulins. Submucosal glands are found in the nose and the trachea and central conducting airways but become less frequent in the more distal airway generations. Goblet cells are also predominantly located in the central, cartilaginous airways but are found in more peripheral airways in smokers. Clara cells are present in the terminal bronchioles and are believed to be responsible for bronchiolar secretion of surfactant which plays a role in maintaining patency of the bronchioles by reducing the surface forces tending to close them.

The glands are under autonomic nervous control, which determines the volume and modulates the biochemical composition of the secretions. The efferent parasympathetic nerves appear to be the most important component, although cholinergic effects may be modified by co-release of transmitters of the non-adrenergic, non-cholinergic system (Ramnarine and Rogers, 1994). The normal volume of mucus secretion in the tracheobronchial tree is said to be 100 ml a day and this is removed by the mucociliary escalator to the pharynx where it is swallowed without provoking cough. The surface film of secretion lies on top of the cilia and provides a trap for inhaled particles and may diminish water loss from the respiratory tract; it also provides some protection against the proliferation of microorganisms by virtue of its immunoglobulin, antibody, lysozyme and lactoferrin content. The surface lining also moistens and smooths the airway wall reducing the frictional component of airflow resistance.

Ciliary clearance

In the nose the cilia, except in the vestibule where their action is directed anteriorly, carry particles in the mucociliary blanket posteriorly to the pharynx where any aggregated secretions are presumably swallowed or expectorated. Alternatively a sneeze, a violent expiration via the nose, may expel accumulated secretions. A similar mucociliary clearance mechanism exists in the tracheobronchial tree which removes particles from the peripheral airways up to the trachea at an estimated rate of 1–3 cm/minute.

The ciliary beat moves in constant direction and results from shortening, by internal molecular changes, of longitudinally disposed contractile elements. The rapid propulsive stroke may be explained as due to initial shortening of intraciliary contractile elements on one side only, and the recovery stroke as resulting from a later contraction of contractile structures on the opposite side. Ciliary beat frequency is increased by

both β-adrenergic and cholinergic agonists and also by a variety of peptides including bradykinin.

The efficiency of the nasal and tracheobronchial mucociliary mechanisms in removing bacteria from the inspired air is shown by the fact that, in health, the bronchi are free of microorganisms. Effective ciliary motion is dependent on normal composition and viscosity of the mucus; changes in viscosity readily affect ciliary propulsion. Drying causes degeneration and destruction of cilia. Ciliary beating is also inhibited by thermal changes, by changes of pH from the normal, and by hypertonic and hypotonic solutions.

Mucociliary function in the tracheobronchial tree can be assessed by inhaling radionuclide-labelled microspheres and following their clearance from the airways after impaction. Cough needs to be suppressed during the measurement. Ciliary beat frequency, usually 12–15 Hz, can be assessed *in vitro* on specimens obtained by brushing the nasal (or tracheal) mucosa.

Nasal transport of labelled microspheres can also be studied; a simpler test is the time taken to detect the taste of saccharine placed in the anterior nose. Sniffs must be avoided during these measurements.

Cough reflex

A cough is an explosive burst of high velocity expiratory airflow. The reflex is initiated by stimulation of the sensory nerve endings. Afferent impulses are carried via the vagus nerve to the cough centre in the dorsal medulla, where they are subject to cortical influences which can inhibit or indeed initiate cough. The efferent limb involves contraction of abdominal and intercostal muscles to raise intrathoracic pressure, and activation of pharyngeal and laryngeal muscles first to close and then rapidly open the glottis; there is often associated vagal efferent activation resulting in contraction of airway smooth muscle.

Efferent limb

The mechanics of cough involve four phases: inspiration, compression, expiration and cessation (Leith *et al.*, 1986) (Figure 13.5).

In the first phase the glottis is abducted and a variable volume of air inspired. The factors influencing the lung volume from which the expiratory phase is initiated are not well understood. If a large volume is inspired and the expiratory phase is initiated from a large lung volume, the expiratory muscles can generate maximal pressures and the increase in airway size allows the highest flows; this combination generates the highest velocity of flow through the central airways and the most effective clearing of the airway. A disadvantage of inspiring a large volume is that it may expose the airway to further exposure to a noxious stimulus or foreign material; direct entry

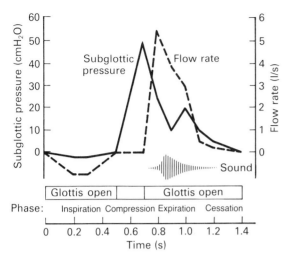

Figure 13.5 Development of subglottic pressure and expiratory flow during a cough. The glottis may close again at the cessation of cough. (Modified from Yanagihara, von Leden and Werner–Kukuk, (1966) *Acta Otolaryngologica*, 61, 495–510)

of foreign material towards the larynx may trigger an immediate cough without prior inspiration.

During the phase of compression, the glottis closes for about 0.2 seconds and the supraglottic airways narrow; during glottal closure the expiratory muscles contract and intrathoracic pressures (pleural surface and alveolar) rise. However, the diaphragm also contracts opposing the full abdominal pressure being transmitted to the thoracic cavity.

The compressive phase is followed by active abduction of the glottis and relaxation of the diaphragm so that intrathoracic pressure rises. This results in an explosive decompressive phase in which subglottic pressure rapidly drops to atmospheric pressure producing a large gradient between alveolar and tracheal pressure which, in turn, generates a large expiratory flow. The combination of high intrathoracic pressure and low intra-airway pressure leads to dynamic compression of central airways, with encroachment on the lumen by the posterior membrane. This leads to high linear velocities of flow through the central airways generating considerable shearing forces at the airway wall and high kinetic energy which clear secretions and/or foreign material.

The extent of dynamic compression of the airways during a forceful expiration is dependent on the position of flow-limiting segments in the airways in normal subjects; these are believed to be in the most central lobar airways at large lung volumes and to move an uncertain distance towards the periphery of the lung as lung volume is reduced. Therefore during a sequence of coughs started at large lung volume, the larger central airways will be cleared first, and smaller airways will be cleared as lung volume is reduced. However, it is unlikely that more peripheral airways can be cleared by the cough mechanism because the velocity of expiratory flow that can be achieved in these airways is very much less than in the central airways.

The expiratory phase is followed by cessation of expiratory muscle activity and is sometimes accompanied by glottal closure.

The effectiveness of the efferent limb of cough is well preserved in airway disease but is diminished when there is inability to generate high abdominal and intrathoracic pressures as happens in quadriplegia, gross muscle weakness or when abdominal muscle contraction is inhibited by pain, as after abdominal surgery.

Central control

Unfortunately, very little is known about the control of the central neurotransmitter and receptor mechanisms which modulate cough. Opiates suppress cough by their central action (Fuller *et al.*, 1988), but little further is known; experiments with α-adrenergic and 5-hydroxytryptamine agonists in animals have shown some effects in suppressing cough but these have not been replicated in humans. By the analogy of drugs which suppress vomiting, it may be possible to develop non-opiate antitussive drugs which have a central action. The cortex can override to a limited extent the reflex mechanisms involved in cough, voluntarily suppressing cough despite the presence of incoming vagal impulses. Cough can also be voluntarily initiated by cortical mechanisms.

Afferent limb

Cough may be initiated by stimulation of sensory nerve endings throughout the distribution of the vagus nerve, usually in the upper or lower airway but occasionally from stimulation of the external auditory meatus, the tympanic membrane or the oesophagus (Fuller and Jackson, 1990). Gastrointestinal reflux is an important cause of persistent nonproductive cough; it has been claimed that chronic inflammation stimulates vagal sensory endings in the lower oesophagus (Irwin, Curley and French, 1990; Ing, Ngu and Breslin, 1994).

Larynx

The larynx has abundant sensory innervation and is critically placed for the initiation of protective reflexes. Five distinct types of laryngeal receptors have been identified. Pressure, drive and cold/flow receptors are activated throughout the respiratory cycle and are probably not involved in cough. Studies in animals suggest rapidly adapting stretch receptors (syn:irritant receptors) play a major role in cough. The role of laryngeal C-fibre receptors is less clear. Inhalation of capsaicin, in animals and humans, causes cough, but it is not certain whether this occurs predominantly via stimulation of laryngeal or tracheobronchial receptors.

Sublaryngeal airways

Four types of receptors have been identified, all of which may be involved in cough.

Slowly adapting stretch receptors

Activity in slowly adapting stretch receptors increases during inspiration and their primary function is probably termination of inspiration and facilitation of expiratory muscle activity (Hering–Breuer reflex). While they do not respond directly to recognized tussigenic stimuli there is some evidence they may facilitate cough. Patients with non-productive cough and a heightened cough reflex sometimes comment that deep inspiration triggers episodes of coughing.

Rapidly adapting stretch receptors

There is convincing evidence supporting a direct role for bronchial rapidly adapting stretch receptors in cough in various animal species and in man. They respond to extremely light mechanical stimuli and to irritants that are known to cause cough in man, such as cigarette smoke and prostaglandins. They are most abundant in the central airways, and are found especially at airway bifurcations where deposition of inhaled particles is greatest. They are situated superficially in airway epithelium and connect to fast-conducting myelinated nerve fibres. Although rapidly adapting stretch receptors can be stimulated by rapid lung inflation and deflation without induction of cough in normal individuals, the bulk of the evidence suggests they have a prominent and direct role in cough.

Bronchial and pulmonary C-fibre endings

C-fibre endings give rise to slowly-conducting, unmyelinated fibres which comprise the majority of vagal fibres originating in the lung. They have been subdivided into bronchial (receiving their blood supply from the bronchial circulation) and pulmonary (J-receptors, receiving their blood supply from the pulmonary circulation) receptors. The two types of C-fibre receptors have different sensitivities to mechanical and chemical stimulation. In humans, intravenous injection of lobeline or capsaicin causes cough, within a time that suggests stimulation of pulmonary C-fibres. There is also some evidence that bronchial C-fibres may play a role in cough. Thus, SO_2 administered by inhalation to animals causes cough in concentrations which stimulate C-fibres but not rapidly or slowly adapting stretch receptors. Inhalation of SO_2 also causes cough in humans. Similarly, inhalation of bradykinin aerosol in concentrations which stimulate C-fibres in animals, consistently elicits cough in humans.

Assessment of cough frequency and responsiveness

The frequency of cough can be monitored by diary cards and more precisely using ambulatory recorders (Hsu et al., 1994) which utilize microphones and upper abdominal surface electromyograms. The efferent mechanism can be assessed by measuring intrathoracic pressure during cough (see Figure 13.5) and less directly by measuring expiratory pressure at the mouth at full inflation during occluded maximum expiratory efforts or by measuring transient peaks of flow measured with a pneumotachograph at the mouth during cough.

The sensitivity of the afferent and central components of the cough reflex can be assessed by inhaling sequential small doses of capsaicin and counting the number of coughs provoked; other stimulants sometimes used are citric acid, hypo- or hyperosmolar solutions or mediators such as bradykinin. Capsaicin cough sensitivity is normal in most patients with productive cough, such as that due to chronic bronchitis and is usually normal in asthma. Sensitivity is enhanced in persistent non-productive cough such as may occur with ACE-inhibitor drugs, variant asthma, following acute respiratory tract infection or associated with gastro-oesophageal reflux (O'Connell et al., 1994). Sensitivity can be reduced peripherally by local anaesthetic or centrally by opiates.

Relation of cough to reflex bronchoconstriction

Cough is one of a number of reflexes protecting the respiratory tract against noxious events. Other examples are sneezing, laryngeal narrowing, stimulation of airway mucus secretion and reflex bronchoconstriction. Many stimuli which induce cough elicit other protective reflexes simultaneously either via the same or different afferent nerves. Thus stimuli such as capsaicin or hypotonic aerosols which induce cough also cause transient bronchoconstriction. As a result some authors have regarded reflex bronchoconstriction as being an integral part of the efferent limb of the cough reflex; in support of this argument, some studies have found reflex cough to be attenuated by treatment with β-adrenergic agonist or muscarinic antagonist aerosols. However, most studies do not find that cough sensitivity is altered by bronchodilators, and there is accumulating evidence that cough and reflex bronchoconstriction are mediated by distinct afferent pathways (Karlsson, Sant'Ambrogio and Widdicombe, 1988) even though the same stimuli can induce both reflexes.

Airway constriction as a protective mechanism

The sublaryngeal airways and sometimes the larynx can narrow in response to a large variety of inhaled stimuli. These effects are usually small in healthy non-asthmatic subjects but are exaggerated and a central feature in asthma and, to a lesser extent, in other diseases of the intrathoracic airways. The extent of the protective action of airway constriction is unclear; ventilation is typically increased in the presence of narrowing. Airway narrowing probably increases the velocity of flow during cough and perhaps leads to a more peripheral location of flow limiting airways so that the efficiency of cough might be enhanced.

Effects of disease on protective mechanisms

Ciliary clearance is reduced in most chronic nasal or pulmonary airway diseases such as rhinitis, asthma, chronic obstructive pulmonary disease and cystic fibrosis. Irritant gases, cigarette smoke, environmental pollution, viral and bacterial infections also depress ciliary clearance and the efficiency of ciliary beating. There is often some loss of cilia but they remain structurally normal and the effects may be confined to nose or bronchus. In contrast primary ciliary dyskinesia, which results in hypomotile cilia, affects nasal, tracheobronchial (and cervical) cilia equally and there are similar ultrastructural defects in nasal and bronchial cilia with defects of dynein arms (Greenstone *et al.*, 1988). Hence nasal cilia obtained by brushing the nasal mucosa can be used to detect these motility defects. In smokers (and also in asthma and chronic irritation by dust and gases) there may be associated hypertrophy of mucus-producing glands in the submucosa of central conducting airways (the volume may increase 25-fold) ('chronic bronchitis') and chronic mucus hypersecretion. Although initially this may have evolved as a protective mechanism against the irritant effects of tobacco smoke, in practice mucus hypersecretion appears to be associated with impaired mucociliary clearance – some of which may be due to replacement of ciliated epithelial cells by goblet cells, although 'overload' cannot be excluded – loss of the normal bacteriological sterility of the sublaryngeal airways and a tendency to repeated bronchopulmonary infections. In contrast the cough mechanism is well preserved, indeed narrowing of the airways, increased dynamic compression of central airways and a more peripheral location of flow limiting airways may all enhance the efficiency of cough in these patients. Surprisingly, perhaps, there is very little suggestion that bronchial infections are more common in patients treated with inhaled corticosteroids; this contrasts vividly with the increased incidence of bronchopulmonary infections in severe hypogammaglobulinaemia or acquired immune deficiency syndrome.

Conditioning of inspired air

Another important role of the airways, particularly the nasal passages and central conducting airways,

is to condition the inspired and expired air. Under normal ambient conditions at rest, heating and humidification of inspired air to body temperature and 100% saturation with water vapour is achieved by the time it reaches the carina. When the volume of inspired air is large, cold and dry and the nose is bypassed (as occurs with strenuous exercise on cold, wintry mornings) or when tracheostomy or endotracheal intubation is performed, conditioning of inspired air may not be complete until it has penetrated further into the lungs. However, because the total mucosal surface area available for air conditioning rapidly increases as the periphery of the lung is approached, it is unlikely that alveolar temperature ever deviates from core body temperature. Central airways cooling and water loss during strenuous exercise is believed to be the immediate stimulus provoking the bronchoconstriction that occurs after strenuous exercise in many asthmatic subjects, but it is not clear precisely how this triggers the generalized airway narrowing as changes in central airway temperature on exercise are similar in asthmatic and normal subjects (Anderson, 1992).

Airway blood flow

Compared to other superficial vascular beds, the vasculature of the airway mucosa has the additional role of conditioning inspired and expired air. Both in the nose and the central sublaryngeal airways there is an extensive subepithelial capillary network with a plexus of deeper vessels in the submucosa. In addition, the nose has an extensive system of distensible blood sinuses which have a major role in controlling nasal airway resistance; this feature is much less prominent in the sublaryngeal airways. In the lower airways the subepithelial capillaries travel longitudinally which may carry locally generated mediators and locally absorbed drugs more peripherally. The strongest neural influence on the airways vessels is the vasoconstrictor action of the sympathetic system, with the parasympathetic system having a lesser vasodilator effect. Additional modulating roles on the sympathetic and parasympathetic systems are played by a variety of neuropeptides. Cooling of the airway surface causes vasodilatation; although this can increase nasal airway resistance, vascular changes in the sublaryngeal airways are unlikely to have much effect on their resistance (Laitinen, Salonen and Widdicombe, 1990).

Airway permeability

Surprisingly little is known about airway permeability to drugs and inhaled gas and noxious substances. Probably airway permeability is increased when there is airway inflammation as in rhinitis and asthma.

The permeability of the nasal mucosa to inhaled substances led to the use of tobacco snuff and, more recently, nicotine sprays as an aid to quitting smoking, and is used for treatment with vasopressin. It also results in the absorption of soluble environmental pollutants, such as SO_2. The largest part of asthma treatment is now given by the inhaled route (e.g. β-adrenergic agonists, muscarinic antagonists and inhaled corticosteroids), but how much of their action is directly at the site of absorption and how much due to dispersal by the airway mucosal circulation is unknown.

Lung volumes and compliance

The elastic recoil of the lungs causes them to collapse to a very small volume when no expanding force is applied. In contrast the chest wall (rib cage-diaphragm) has a relatively large neutral volume. Thus the relaxation volume of the respiratory system (Vr, the volume it adopts when there is no respiratory muscle activity) is determined by the volume at which the tendency of the chest wall to recoil outwards and enlarge exactly balances the tendency of the lungs to collapse inwards to a smaller volume. In young normal subjects at rest relaxation volume and functional residual capacity are identical and in the range 2–3 l, about half the lung volume achieved during a full inspiratory manoeuvre (total lung capacity) (Figure 13.6).

With increasing age there is some increase in functional residual capacity, but no change in total lung capacity so that tidal breathing takes place at slightly larger lung volumes. Measuring total lung capacity and functional residual capacity (Figure 13.6) is particularly useful to find the cause of a reduction in vital capacity. Intrapulmonary airways obstruction consistently leads to a rise in residual volume and functional residual capacity, while total lung capacity is either normal or, in some subjects with emphysema, increased. Even when total lung capacity is increased, the accompanying increase in residual volume is almost always greater, so that there is still a decreased vital capacity.

A reduced total lung capacity ('restrictive lung

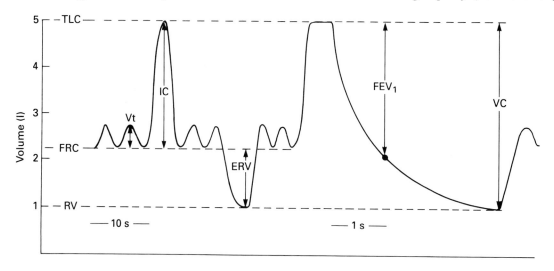

Figure 13.6 Subdivision of lung volumes. Static and dynamic lung volumes indicated as a record of tidal breathing against time followed by an expiratory forced vital capacity manoeuvre for which time scale has been expanded. *Vital capacity (VC)* is the volume expired from full inflation (TLC) to full expiration (residual volume, RV) and can be measured by a spirometer or by integrating flow at the mouth. A reduction in VC can occur with a reduction in TLC or an increase in RV. *Functional residual capacity (FRC) and total lung capacity.* FRC (volume of lungs at end of a tidal expiration) can be measured by (a) gas dilution: a foreign, relatively insoluble gas (usually helium) is allowed to mix with intrapulmonary gas and the volume calculated from the difference between the initial and final concentration of foreign gas. Mixing may take more than 5 minutes in patients with intrapulmonary airway obstruction. (b) Whole body plethysmography: the subject makes panting efforts against a shutter closed at the end of a tidal expiration while seated in a large, air-tight chamber. As mass movement of gas is prevented, changes in alveolar volume during this manoeuvre are due to compression and rarefaction of alveolar gas and allow alveolar volume to be calculated using Boyle's law. For both methods the volume inspired (inspiratory capacity, IC) during a maximum inspiration from FRC is measured with a spirometer to derive TLC. The plethysmographic method often gives higher values than the gas dilution method for FRC in severe intrapulmonary airways disease; this is because plethysmography measures intrathoracic gas which hardly communicates with the airway (bullae and other very poorly ventilated areas). (c) TLC can also be obtained from planimetry of standard posteroanterior and lateral chest radiographs or from computed tomograms taken at full inflation. FEV_1, forced expiratory volume in 1 s; Vt, tidal volume, ERV, expiratory reserve volume

disease') is usually accompanied by a decrease in functional residual capacity and is found either when the lungs have low compliance (reduced volume change per unit change in distending or transpulmonary pressure, usually expressed as ml/cmH_2O) and cannot be expanded normally above their resting volume, or when inadequate expanding forces are applied to the lungs, as with weakness of the inspiratory muscles. Uncoupling of the lung from the chest wall due to air or fluid in the pleural cavity also increases pleural pressure and reduces resting and maximum lung volumes. The elastic properties of the lungs as measured by their compliance represent the number of ventilated units and the combined effects of tissue elasticity and the surface properties of the alveoli in these ventilated units. The surfactant layer lining the alveoli, produced by the type II alveolar cells, greatly reduces surface forces. In lung fibrosis reduced compliance is due to a combination of loss of functioning peripheral lung units and thickening of the alveolar wall and interstitium of surviving ventilated units. Loss of functioning units is the important factor reducing lung compliance when there is fluid filling of the alveoli in pneumonia or pulmonary oedema. Absence of the surfactant lining layer has been shown to be a definite cause of reduced compliance only in the lungs of premature infants with respiratory distress syndrome of the newborn, but surfactant production is inevitably affected in other severe lung diseases which damage type II alveolar cells and are responsible for the adult respiratory distress syndrome.

Lung compliance can be measured either during tidal breathing (dynamic compliance) or during breath holding (static compliance). In either case transpulmonary pressure (difference between oesophageal, which approximates pleural surface, pressure and mouth pressure) is measured by introducing a balloon-catheter into mid-oesophagus, while change in volume is measured at the mouth. Dynamic compliance is measured at points of zero flow at end-expiration and end-inspiration. At functional residual capacity with respiratory muscles relaxed, pleural surface pressure is about 5 cmH_2O below atmospheric pressure. Inspiratory muscle activity reduces this pressure to -8 or -9 cmH_2O below atmospheric pressure during quiet tidal breathing. In normal lungs at rest about 80% of the tidal change in inspiratory pressure is dissipated in overcoming forces attributable to the elasticity of the lungs and only 20% in overcoming airflow resistance. Static measurements are often made over the whole vital capacity range after a full inflation to total lung capacity. Static lung compliance is greatest close to functional residual capacity and declines as the lungs are expanded towards total lung capacity. Increase in static compliance and loss of transpulmonary pressure at a given volume is characteristic of emphysema. Reductions in static and dynamic compliance

and increased transpulmonary pressure at total lung capacity are characteristic of restrictive lung disease. Reductions in dynamic compliance are also found with intrathoracic airway disease, including emphysema, so that the static pressure-volume curve provides a better distinction between obstructive and restrictive lung disease.

Pulmonary gas exchange

Effective pulmonary gas exchange depends on sufficient ventilation to renew oxygen in, and remove carbon dioxide from, the blood (West, 1990; Wagner and Rodriguez–Roisin, 1991). At rest an average tidal inspiration adds 350–500 ml of fresh air to the initial lung volume of about 3 l. The inspired air filling the conducting airways at the end of inspiration makes no contribution to pulmonary gas exchange and is exhaled unchanged at the start of the subsequent expiration. In the normal subject the volume of these conducting airways is about 140 ml (anatomical dead space) so that only about two-thirds of each breath mixes completely with alveolar gas. About half this volume is above the upper third of the trachea and is bypassed by laryngectomy or tracheostomy.

The fall in partial pressure of oxygen as it is transported from ambient air to the tissue via a perfectly homogeneous lung is shown schematically in Figure 13.7. Hypoxia can arise from a decrease in ambient Po_2 or abnormal gradients at any of the subsequent stages, but in practice tissues can metabolize and function at very low levels of Po_2. The most important cause of a low arterial Po_2 in diffuse lung disease however is ventilation-perfusion imbalance and is not shown in Figure 13.7. Inhomogeneity of mechanical properties between different units within the lungs leads to uneven ventilation and widespread differences in local alveolar and end-capillary Po_2 (Figure 13.8); any corresponding changes in perfusion do not fully match the change in ventilation. The resulting ventilation-perfusion imbalance leads to a large difference between arterial and mean alveolar Po_2.

Alveolar Po_2 is always lower than inspired Po_2 and can be estimated from the simplified alveolar air equation:

Alveolar Po_2 = Inspired Po_2 − 1.2 × arterial Pco_2

At sea level when breathing air, inspired Po_2 in tracheal gas is 150 mmHg (20 kPa); if arterial Pco_2 is normal (40 mmHg, 5.3 kPa), alveolar Po_2 is 100 mmHg (13.3 kPa).

If the lungs function as perfect gas exchangers, arterial and alveolar Po_2 and Pco_2 are identical. Inefficiency of gas exchange results in arterial Po_2 being less than alveolar Po_2. In normal lungs this difference is less than 7–10 mmHg (1–1.3 kPa). Thus a low arterial Po_2 may be due to a low alveolar Po_2 or an increased

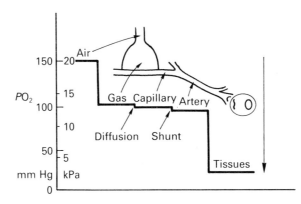

Figure 13.7 Scheme of fall in Po_2 between ambient air and tissues, assuming a perfectly homogeneous lung. (Modified from West (1990) *Ventilation/Blood Flow and Gas Exchange*, 5th edn. Oxford: Blackwell Scientific Publications)

difference between alveolar and arterial Po_2 (or a combination of these two changes) (Table 13.1).

Factors reducing alveolar Po_2 are a low inspired Po_2, as found at altitude, or a rise in alveolar and arterial Pco_2 and fall in alveolar Po_2 as occurs with acute reductions in total ventilation. The most obvious examples of the latter are acute asphyxia following sudden obstruction of the upper airway, overdose of some sedative drugs (or anaesthesia) and acute weakness of respiratory muscles, as may occur in myasthenia gravis. Chronic reduction in total ventilation is very unusual and is essentially confined to patients with chronic respiratory muscle weakness or chest cage deformity or rare patients with abnormal central control of ventilation. In most chronic lung diseases resting ventilation is normal or even slightly increased even when a raised arterial Pco_2 is present, the rise in Pco_2 developing because of the inefficiency of the lungs as gas exchangers. In chronic lung disease the important mechanism of hypoxaemia is an increased alveolar-arterial Po_2 difference. Even in hypercapnic respiratory failure in chronic obstructive pulmonary disease where there is a low alveolar Po_2 much of the hypoxaemia is due to an associated large alveolar-arterial Po_2 difference.

The cause of the increase in alveolar-arterial Po_2 difference in patients with intrapulmonary airways obstruction is ventilation-perfusion imbalance. Some experts think the same mechanism even applies in conditions like asbestosis and fibrosing alveolitis, classically thought to show a diffusion defect or 'alveolar-capillary block'. In practice the distinction between ventilation-perfusion inequality and diffusion defects is not important because in both hypoxae-

Table 13.1 Causes of a low arterial Po_2

Mechanism	Example
*Reduced alveolar Po_2**	
Low inspired Po_2	Altitude
Reduced ventilation with raised Pco_2	Asphyxia Anaesthetic or sedative drugs Gross respiratory muscle weakness
Increased alveolar-arterial Po_2 difference	
Right-to-left shunt	Intracardiac Intrapulmonary, as in adult respiratory distress syndrome
Diffusion defect (difference between alveolar and end-capillary Po_2)	Normal subjects exercising at altitude Fibrosing alveolitis
Ventilation-perfusion imbalance	Asthma, emphysema and chronic airways obstruction

* See text for discussion of the reduced alveolar Po_2 that occurs with a raised alveolar and arterial Pco_2 in chronic lung disease.

mia can be readily corrected by modest increases in inspired O_2. This is not the case when hypoxaemia is due to right-to-left shunts either in the heart or lungs. Shunts in the lungs occur with severe pulmonary oedema and adult respiratory distress syndrome, where extensive fluid-filling of alveoli is accompanied by continuing blood flow through the affected areas.

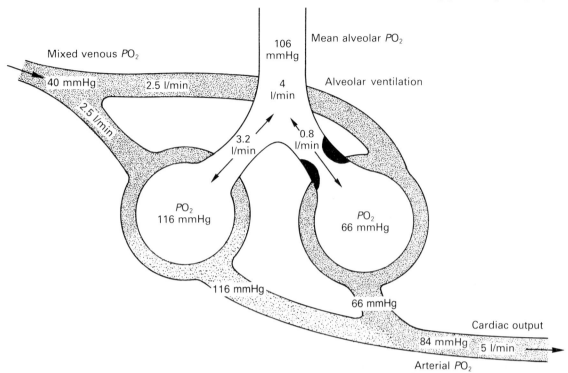

106 mmHg — Mean alveolar PO₂

Mixed venous PO₂

40 mmHg   2.5 l/min

2.5 l/min

4 l/min — Alveolar ventilation

3.2 l/min   0.8 l/min

PO₂ 116 mmHg

PO₂ 66 mmHg

116 mmHg

66 mmHg

Cardiac output

84 mmHg   5 l/min

Arterial PO₂

Figure 13.8 Schematic representation of development of difference between mean alveolar and arterial P_{O_2} illustrated by a two-compartment model in which blood flow is evenly distributed but there is a fourfold difference in ventilation. The increase in alveolar P_{O_2} (116 mmHg) in the well-ventilated compartment does not increase O_2 content in the pulmonary venous blood sufficiently to compensate for the low O_2 content in the pulmonary venous blood leaving the poorly-ventilated compartment. The result is the mixed pulmonary venous (and arterial) blood has a P_{O_2} of 84 mmHg, 22 mmHg less than the mean alveolar P_{O_2} which is determined by the proportionate ventilation of the two compartments. Note that in both compartments the blood P_{O_2} comes into equilibrium with the alveolar P_{O_2}. In practice ventilation-perfusion imbalance results from differences in ventilation between large numbers of parallel lung units and the effect may be reduced by some reduction in blood flow to poorly ventilated units. Conversion of P_{O_2} mmHg to kPa, $\div$ 7.5. (Modified from J. F. Murray (1985) *The Normal Lung*, 2nd edn. Philadelphia: W. B. Saunders)

Relation between arterial P_{O_2}, oxygen saturation and tissue oxygenation

The vast majority of oxygen in the blood is carried as oxyhaemoglobin. At a normal arterial P_{O_2} of 85 mmHg (11.3 kPa) or more, percentage saturation (oxygenation) of haemoglobin is close to 100. Giving normal subjects higher inspired O_2 to breathe has little effect on arterial O_2 saturation; conversely small reductions in arterial P_{O_2} have little deleterious effect, but below an arterial P_{O_2} of about 60 mmHg (8.0 kPa), small falls in arterial P_{O_2} are associated with large falls in O_2 saturation (Figure 13.9).

The O_2 content of arterial blood at a given P_{O_2} will be reduced if there is a reduction in available haem binding sites (anaemia, occupation by carboxyhaemoglobin) or a shift to the right of the O_2 dissociation curve (as happens with an acid pH, increase in P_{CO_2}, temperature or the concentration of 2,3-diphosphoglycerate within the red blood cell).

The difference between arterial P_{O_2} and local tissue P_{O_2} depends critically on cardiac output and local blood flow, so that the combination of a low arterial P_{O_2} with anaemia or seriously impaired cardiac output threatens survival.

Assessment of pulmonary gas exchange

Pulmonary gas exchange at rest is routinely assessed by arterial blood gas analysis; for proper interpretation and for sequential measurements, patients should be breathing either air or a known concentration of inspired air, such as is achieved by Venturi principle masks, but not by nasal cannulae or other types of masks used to deliver additional oxygen. If the inspired gas is air or a precisely known O_2 concentration then the alveolar air equation can be used to estimate the mean alveolar P_{O_2} and hence the alveolar-arterial P_{O_2} difference. Alternatively the

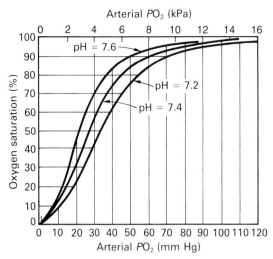

Figure 13.9 The relation between arterial Po_2 and percentage O_2 saturation of haemoglobin at three different pH levels

ratio of inspired O_2/arterial Po_2 can be used to estimate the efficiency of gas exchange. For longer-term monitoring it is desirable to use non-invasive methods; oximeters on the finger or ear can continuously monitor O_2 saturation, but cannot detect small declines in arterial Po_2 (see Figure 13.9). Cutaneous electrodes for measuring local Po_2 or Pco_2 have limited use in adults and the values they record are not close to arterial levels; the best established use is for detecting slowly increasing Pco_2 overnight.

Although the difference between alveolar and arterial Po_2 gives an overall idea of the efficiency of gas exchange in the lung, the absolute value of this difference is influenced by the alveolar Po_2. By making simultaneous measurements of Po_2 and Pco_2 in mixed expired air and in arterial blood, ventilation-blood flow balance can be expressed by a three compartment model comprising lung with normal ventilation-perfusion balance, the proportion of the tidal volume which goes to lung which is ventilated but not perfused (physiological dead space, 'wasted ventilation') and the proportion of pulmonary blood flow which does not come into contact with alveolar gas (venous admixture). In normal subjects physiological dead space is similar to the anatomical dead space, the volume of the major conducting airways, but in lung disease physiological dead space may be as large as 250–300 ml, emphasizing the need to compensate by some increase in resting ventilation. The three compartment model simplifies the real situation in the lungs, where there is a gradation of units which have abnormally high ventilation-perfusion ratios. These are modelled as the equivalent

part of the tidal volume which does not come into contact with pulmonary blood. Likewise venous admixture expresses the total effect of lung units with low ventilation-perfusion ratio as the per cent of pulmonary blood flow *not* in contact with alveolar gas. In fact in airways obstruction, fibrosing alveolitis and many other lung diseases the true shunt through the lungs is very small and almost all the units contributing to venous admixture have some ventilation. This is important in clinical practice because arterial Po_2 then responds well to increases in inspired Po_2 which is not the case with true shunts as seen in adult respiratory distress syndrome.

Arterial blood gases remain normal at rest until lung disease is relatively advanced. Exercise capacity and measurement of saturation with an oximeter during exercise provide useful estimates of the reserves of pulmonary gas exchange; this may be useful in assessing cardiopulmonary fitness for major operations.

Carbon monoxide transfer is widely used in pulmonary function laboratories as an indication of pulmonary gas exchange. It is useful in its own right, and falls at a relatively early stage in the development of restrictive lung disease and emphysema, but does not have a close relation to exercise capacity or maximum O_2 uptake (Forster and Ogilvie, 1983; Cotes, 1993). Carbon monoxide transfer per litre lung volume (transfer 'coefficient') provides useful further information, sometimes being preserved, despite a reduction in total carbon monoxide transfer in face of disease – as with pneumonectomy, restriction due to respiratory muscle weakness and sarcoidosis – and sometimes reduced – as in fibrosing alveolitis and emphysema. The values are reduced in anaemia but may be raised if there is bleeding into the lungs as the extravasated red blood cells provide a considerable sump for the uptake of carbon monoxide.

Regional differences in ventilation and blood flow

In the normal upright position lung blood flow (per unit of lung volume) at rest is much greater at the bases than at the apices of the lungs; there is a similar but smaller gradient of ventilation. These regional differences in ventilation-perfusion imbalance only lead to a small inefficiency in gas exchange in normal lungs estimated as an alveolar-arterial Po_2 difference of 4 mmHg (0.5 kPa). Pulmonary blood flow becomes more evenly distributed through the lung during exercise. In the supine or lateral decubitus position the dependent part of the lung has the greater blood flow and ventilation. At small lung volumes airway closure may occur, reversing the tendency for increased ventilation in dependent zones; this is a particular problem in supine obese subjects in whom resting lung volume is reduced by elevation of the diaphragm by the increased abdominal mass (West, 1990).

O_2 *treatment*

Correct administration of increased inspired O_2 is essential for the treatment of hypoxaemic patients. The dangers of undertreatment are obvious but overtreatment may exacerbate hypercapnia in patients with chronic airflow obstruction, or lead to pulmonary O_2 toxicity in patients with adult respiratory distress syndrome treated in the intensive care unit. Choice of inspired O_2 concentration depends on the acuteness of the problem and the clinical diagnosis. Patients with long-standing chronic hypoxaemia and a good cardiac output can tolerate remarkably low levels of arterial Po_2 which would cause unconsciousness if suddenly applied to a normal subject. In general, patients with hypoxaemia related to airway disease and with no opacification of the lungs on the chest radiograph can be treated with small increases in inspired O_2 (24.5 or 28% O_2 via a ventimask). Precise control of the inspired O_2 concentration is important for the initial 2 days of an acute exacerbation in patients with severe chronic airflow obstruction: later, nasal cannulae with O_2 added at 1–2 1/min provide inspired O_2 in the 25–30% range, but with less precision (Bazuaye *et al.*, 1992). Usually there is time to step up to 24.5% and then, 0.5–1 hour later, to 28%. In severe airflow obstruction increments of about 10 mmHg (1.3 kPa) in arterial Po_2 are expected; a small increase in arterial Pco_2 of about 3–4 mmHg (0.5 kPa) is often found – if increases in Pco_2 are larger further estimates are required to exclude progressive hypercapnia. The modest increases in arterial Po_2 provide a considerable increase in O_2 supply to the tissues (provided cardiac output is maintained), so that a 'safe' arterial Po_2 in patients with severe chronic airflow obstruction is often said to be as low as 50 mmHg (6.7 kPa). The relative ease with which hypoxaemia can be relieved in airway disease contrasts with the difficulty in achieving a satisfactory arterial Po_2 when there is filling of alveoli with fluid (pulmonary oedema, adult respiratory distress syndrome) or extensive consolidation and pneumonia – all conditions which lead to gross radiographic changes. With fluid filling, pulmonary blood flow continues to the affected alveoli resulting in a shunt through the lungs; the effects of increasing concentrations of inspired O_2 on arterial Po_2 are disappointing and concentrations of 50% or more, which are potentially toxic to the lungs, may have to be used. An alternative strategy is to inflate the non-fluid filled parts of the lungs by using positive end-expired pressure.

Respiratory control of acid–base balance

Carbon dioxide entering red blood cells reacts with water to form carbonic acid, most of which dissociates to form hydrogen and bicarbonate ions:

$$CO_2 + H_2O \rightleftharpoons H_2CO_3 \rightleftharpoons H^+ + HCO_3^-$$

The CO_2 produced by cellular respiration is by far the largest source of production of hydrogen ions in the body so the lungs play a major role in controlling blood pH. The amount of CO_2 in the blood can be rapidly regulated in a few minutes by the lungs but adjustment of HCO_3^- which is regulated by the kidneys, is much slower, taking 24–48 hours. The arterial pH depends on the dissociation constant of carbonic acid (which can be represented as a constant, 6.1) and the balance between the two routes of excretion, as indicated by the classical Henderson-Hasselbach equation:

$$\text{Arterial pH} = 6.1 + \log_{10}(HCO_3^-/0.03\ Pco_2\ \text{mmHg*})$$

When there is a chronic elevation of Pco_2 (more than 48 hours), there is usually an associated rise in HCO_3^- so that the pH may return to within the normal range (7.36–7.44). Thus measuring pH as well as Pco_2 in hypercapnic respiratory failure helps to decide whether or not a rise in arterial Pco_2 is acute (Figure 13.10). In acute cardiorespiratory emergencies with inadequate ventilation and cardiac output, the pH may be very low due to the combination of respiratory acidaemia and a metabolic acidaemia due to a rise in lactic acid. Severe metabolic acidaemia, due to diabetes, renal failure, methanol poisoning and other rare causes, leads to increase in ventilation and very low arterial Pco_2; although in theory a metabolic alkalaemia (as used to develop occasionally with neglected and persistent vomiting of gastric acid) can lead to a small 'compensatory' reduction in ventilation and increase in arterial Pco_2, this is a very rare event (Flenley, 1971).

Pulmonary circulation

A major function of the pulmonary circulation is to deliver blood in a thin sheet to the alveolar-capillary membrane for gas exchange. This is achieved with a low mean pulmonary artery pressure, of about 15 mmHg at rest, so allowing gravitational differences in vascular pressure to have large effects on the distribution of pulmonary blood flow. In keeping with this low pressure, the walls of normal pulmonary arteries and arterioles contain little muscle and resistance to blood flow is distributed relatively evenly between arteries, capillaries and veins. In the upright posture, blood flow is very low at the lung apices in the resting normal subject and increases progressively down the lung at least until near the bases. The distribution of flow becomes more even during exercise.

---

* In SI units 0.225 Pco_2 kPa

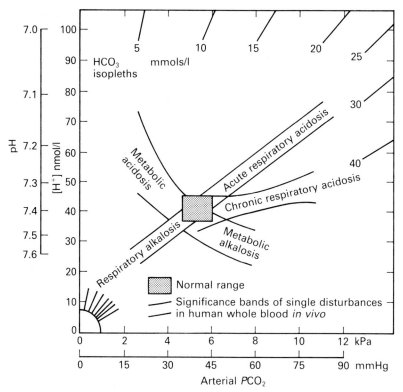

Figure 13.10 Relation between arterial P_{CO_2} (horizontal axis), pH and its reciprocal $[H^+]$ (vertical axis) and HCO_3^- represented by interrupted diagonal lines. Normal values are shown by the hatched square. The five abnormal bands show the effects of acute respiratory acidosis and alkalosis, acute metabolic acidosis and alkalosis, and also the effects of chronic hypercapnia where there is a compensatory metabolic alkalosis with rise in HCO_3^- and nearly normal pH. (From Flenley (1971) *Lancet*, i, 961–965)

In normal lungs the balance between hydrostatic pressure, tending to filter fluid out of the small blood vessels, and osmotic forces which tend to retain fluid in the microcirculation, results in a very small net outflow of fluid which is drained through the interstitium and then via lymph vessels running in the connective tissue sheaths around larger vessels and airways. When the capacity of this drainage system is exceeded, fluid first accumulates in the interstitial space around arteries; when the capacity of the interstitial space is exceeded the excess fluid fills alveoli leading to problems with oxygenation as blood flow usually continues through the fluid-filled alveoli. Increases in pulmonary capillary pressure or increases in permeability of the vascular endothelium predispose to pulmonary oedema.

Pulmonary arterioles constrict and arterial pressure rises in response to overall alveolar hypoxia, as develops on going to altitude. The extent of this vasoconstriction is quite variable between individuals. An acid pH increases the vasoconstrictor effect of hypoxia. With prolonged alveolar hypoxia, pulmonary artery muscle hypertrophies. Local alveolar hy-

poxia also causes some local pulmonary vasoconstriction, which will tend to divert blood away from such hypoxic areas.

Apart from the major function of pulmonary gas exchange, the smaller pulmonary blood vessels act as a filter of emboli and the large area of vascular endothelium plays an important role in the metabolism of a variety of circulating vasoactive (and often bronchoactive) substances. The endothelium converts angiotensin I to angiotensin II by angiotensin-converting enzyme on the luminal surface, but the endothelium is also involved in the inactivation of circulating bradykinin, serotonin, noradrenaline and some prostaglandins; some forms of pulmonary vasodilatation are dependent on relaxing factors produced by the endothelium, such as nitric oxide.

Diagnosis of pulmonary embolism

Primary generalized disorders of the pulmonary circulation without other involvement of the lungs or heart are rare. Local occlusions of the pulmonary arteries are much commoner and are usually due to thrombotic emboli, but occasionally to pulmonary vasculitis, such as Wegener's vasculitis. Acute occlusions may result in pulmonary infarction, haemoptysis and pleuritic pain, particularly if there is accompanying congestive heart failure, but more commonly present as an unexplained increase in breathlessness, sometimes accompanied by a low arterial Po_2 which persists for a day or two, but without local signs in the lungs or abnormality of the chest radiograph. Apart from measuring blood gases and finding an unexplained fall in arterial Po_2, pulmonary function tests are not helpful in diagnosing pulmonary embolism. Scans of regional lung perfusion using radiolabelled microspheres are the best means of diagnosis but interpretation may be complicated by chronic airway disease which is characterized by multiple matched defects of ventilation and perfusion (PIOPED Investigators, 1990). In doubtful cases, pulmonary artery angiography is often recommended, but a common strategy is to treat with anticoagulants and repeat the ventilation and perfusion scans 5–7 days later.

Control of ventilation and breathlessness

The control of the respiratory muscles is complex because a voluntary system has been superimposed on an automatic control system. The automatic control system, situated in the brain stem, is concerned primarily with O_2, CO_2 and acid–base homeostasis. When metabolic requirements are modest, this automatic system can be over-ridden by the voluntary control system, which arises in the cerebral cortex, and the ventilatory system can be used for other activities such as talking, coughing, and singing. In ordinary waking life, breathing is characterized by its disorderliness. Because of this strong behavioural component, there is great difficulty in studying control in humans, except under extreme metabolic stress which over-rides the voluntary system (heavy exercise, breathing hypoxic or hypercapnic mixtures), or during sleep or anaesthesia. Even putting in a mouthpiece and wearing a nose clip increases ventilation.

In all the differing physiological conditions imposed by changes in mechanical load (nose or mouth breathing, increase in resistance during sleep, supine or standing posture) or metabolic load (vigorous exercise may increase O_2 consumption and CO_2 output 10-fold), neurological output in normal man is adjusted to maintain arterial Po_2 and Pco_2 overall within rather narrow limits. The automatic regulation of neurological output from the central pool of neurons controlling respiratory muscles in the pons and medulla is influenced by the degree of respiratory stimulation by the reticular activating system (which is dependent on the state of wakefulness) and three main sensor systems. These are: the peripheral chemoreceptors in the carotid and aortic bodies; the central chemoreceptors on or beneath the ventral surface of the medulla; and mechanoreceptors in the larger airways and lung parenchyma. A low arterial Po_2, high arterial Pco_2, or acid pH all stimulate ventilation, although it is difficult to dissociate the effect of Pco_2 and pH. The effects of hypoxaemia are mediated via the peripheral chemoreceptors, while an increased Pco_2 acts mainly to stimulate central chemoreceptors with a much smaller effect on peripheral chemoreceptors.

The ventilatory response to hypoxaemia or hypercapnia can be studied either by breathing appropriate gas mixtures and achieving a steady state or as a rapid rebreathing test in which progressive hypoxia or hypercapnia is produced while the other gas (carbon dioxide or oxygen) is kept constant. The role of mechanoreceptors is more difficult to define but probably they are particularly important in determining the pattern and timing of breathing. In clinical practice they are assessed by measuring the ventilatory response to an increase in resistance (or sometimes an elastic load) at the mouth.

During sleep a distinctive pattern of recurrent obstruction of the oropharynx may be found in grossly obese patients and some non-obese patients with abnormalities of the upper airway. This appears to be due to a disproportionate reduction in activation of the genioglossus and other pharyngeal muscles compared with the thoracic cage muscles during sleep which allows the subatmospheric airway pressure developed in inspiration to collapse the pharyngeal airway (Remmers *et al.*, 1978). These episodes of apnoea are associated with continued and increasing breathing efforts against the obstructed airways. In most subjects this results in brief arousals, increased activation of the pharyngeal muscles and opening of the upper airway before the whole cycle starts again. The brief arousals fragment sleep (which is often not appreciated by the subject but often is by the partner) and may lead to daytime somnolence and loss of concentration. When the repetitive obstruction becomes established the episodes become longer and are associated with hypoxaemia; eventually, in advanced untreated disease, daytime hypoxaemia and hypercapnia develop together with reduction of the ventilatory responses to oxygen and carbon dioxide (obesity-hypoventilation or 'Pickwickian' syndrome). Sleep studies of varying complexity are required to make the diagnosis: videos and microphones are probably more useful than multiple EMG and EEG leads. Obstructive sleep apnoea tends to occur in subjects with small pharyngeal cross-sectional areas. This can be assessed in awake subjects by complex imaging techniques or by acoustic reflection which provides an area-distance plot of the airway to below the larynx. Direct measurements of pharyngeal resistance using catheters have been made but there is a suspicion that these may stimulate pharyngeal muscle contraction and increase segmental resistance.

Breathlessness

Breathlessness is one of the commonest symptoms of cardiopulmonary disease and may be broadly defined as an awareness that breathing effort is inappropriately high for the task performed. This implies a comparison with the individual's previous experience. Effort may be increased when increased resistance or reduced compliance of the lungs require larger pressures to be generated to sustain a normal ventilation, or when total ventilation is increased but lung mechanics are normal. Breathlessness may also occur when more effort has to be obtained from weak respiratory muscles. Various systems have been developed to score the sensation of breathlessness at rest and during periods of increased ventilation (Mador and Kufel, 1992). These have proved robust and repeatable within an individual but with considerable differences in scaling between individuals. Breathlessness can be improved by successful treatment of mechanical problems in the lungs or respiratory muscles; alternatively attempts may be made to attenuate the cortical awareness of the sensation as is done by prescribing opiates in acute pulmonary oedema. Attempts to use such drugs on a chronic basis to alleviate breathlessness have been largely unsuccessful (Eiser *et al.*, 1991). Appropriate doses usually cause unacceptable sedation, restricting their use to advanced malignancy, such as lymphangitis carcinomatosis.

References

ANDERSON, S. D. (1992) Asthma provoked by exercise, hyperventilation, and the inhalation of non-isotonic aerosols. In: *Asthma: Basic Mechanisms and Clinical Management*, 2nd edn, edited by P. J. Barnes, I. W. Rodger and N. C. Thomson. London: Academic Press. pp. 473–490

BARTLETT, D. (1986) Upper airway motor system. In: *Handbook of Physiology* section 3. *The Respiratory System*. Volume II *Control of Breathing*, Part I. Bethesda: American Physiological Society. pp. 223–245

BAZUAYE, E. A., STONE, T. N., CORRIS, P. A. and GIBSON, G. J. (1992) Variability of inspired oxygen concentration with nasal cannulae. *Thorax*, **47**, 609–611

BOUSHEY, H. A., HOLTZMAN, M. J., SHELLER, J. R. and NADEL, J. A. (1980) State of the art: bronchial hyperreactivity. *American Review of Respiratory Disease*, **121**, 389–413

BRADLEY, T. D., BROWN, I. G., GROSSMAN, R. F., ZAMEL, N., MARTINEZ, D., PHILLIPSON, E. A. *et al.* (1986) Pharyngeal size in snorers, non-snorers, and patients with obstructive sleep apnoea. *New England Journal of Medicine*, **315**, 1327–1331

BRANCATISANO, T., COLLETT, P. W. and ENGEL, L. A. (1983) Respiratory movements of the vocal cords. *Journal of Applied Physiology*, **54**, 1269–1276

BRIDGER, G. P. and PROCTOR, D. F. (1970) Maximum nasal inspiratory flow and nasal resistance. *Annals of Otology, Rhinology and Laryngology*, **79**, 481–489

BUTLER, J., CARO, C. G., ALCALA, R. and DUBOIS, A. B. (1960) Physiological factors affecting airway resistance in normal subjects and in patients with chronic respiratory disease. *Journal of Clinical Investigation*, **39**, 584–591

COLE, P. and HAIGHT, J. S. J. (1984) Posture and nasal patency. *American Review of Respiratory Disease*, **129**, 351–354

COLLETT, P. W., BRANCATISANO, T. and ENGEL, L. A. (1983) Changes in the glottic aperture during bronchial asthma. *American Review of Respiratory Disease*, **128**, 719–723

COLLETT, P. W., BRANCATISANO, T. and ENGEL, L. A. (1986) Upper airway dimensions and movements in bronchial asthma. *American Review of Respiratory Disease*, **133**, 1143–1149

CORMIER, Y. F., CAMUS, P. and DESMEULES, M. J. (1980) Non-organic acute upper airways obstruction and a diagnostic approach. *American Review of Respiratory Disease*, **121**, 147–150

COTES, J. E. (1993) *Lung Function*, 5th edn. Oxford: Blackwell Scientific Publications

EISER, N., DENMAN, W., WEST, E. and LUCE, P. (1991) Oral diamorphine: lack of effect on dyspnoea and exercise tolerance in the 'pink puffer' syndrome. *European Respiratory Journal*, **4**, 926–931

FLENLEY, D. C. (1971) Another non-logarithmic acid base diagram. *Lancet*, i, 961–965

FORSTER, R. E. and OGILVIE, C. M. (1983) The single breath carbon monoxide transfer test 25 years on: a reappraisal. *Thorax*, **38**, 1–9

FULLER, R. W. and JACKSON, D. M. (1990) Physiology and treatment of cough. *Thorax*, **45**, 425–430

FULLER, R. W., KARLSSON, J. A., CHOUDRY, N. B. and PRIDE, N. B. (1988) Effect of inhaled and systemic opiates on responses to inhaled capsaicin in humans. *Journal of Applied Physiology*, **65**, 1125–1130

GIBSON, G. J. (1989) Diaphragmatic paresis: pathophysiology, clinical features and investigation. *Thorax*, **44**, 960–970

GIBSON, G. J. (1995) *Clinical Tests of Respiratory Function*, 2nd edn. London: Chapman and Hall

GOLDMAN, J. and MYERS, M. (1991) Vocal cord dysfunction and wheezing. *Thorax*, **46**, 401–404

GREENSTONE, M., RUTMAN, A., DEWAR, A., MACKAY I. and COLE, P. J. (1988) Primary ciliary dyskinesia: cytological and clinical features. *Quarterly Journal of Medicine*, **67**, 405–423

HIGENBOTTAM, T. (1980) Narrowing of glottis opening in humans associated with experimentally induced bronchoconstriction. *Journal of Applied Physiology*, **49**, 403–407

HILBERG, O., JACKSON, A. C., SWIFT, D. L., and PEDERSEN, O. F. (1989) Acoustic rhinometry, evaluation of nasal cavity geometry by acoustic reflection. *Journal of Applied Physiology*, **66**, 295–303

HOGG, J. C., MACKLEM, P. T. and THURLBECK, W. M. (1968) Site and nature of airway obstruction in chronic obstructive lung disease. *New England Journal of Medicine*, **278**, 1355–1360

HSU, J. Y., STONE, R. A., LOGAN-SINCLAIR, R. B., WORSDELL, M., BUSST, C. M. and CHUNG, K. F. (1994) Cough frequency in patients with persistent cough: assessment using a 24 hour ambulatory recorder. *European Respiratory Journal*, **7**, 1246–1253

ING, A. J., NGU, M. C. and BRESLIN, A. B. X. (1994) Pathogenesis of chronic persistent cough associated with gastroesophageal reflux. *American Journal of Respiratory and Critical Care Medicine*, **149**, 160–167

IRWIN, R. S. CURLEY, F. J. and FRENCH, C. L. (1990) Chronic cough. The spectrum and frequency of causes, key components of the diagnostic evaluation, and outcome of specific therapy. *American Review of Respiratory Disease*, **141**, 640–647

KARLSSON, J. A., SANT'AMBROGIO, G. and WIDDICOMBE, J. (1988) Afferent neural pathways in cough and reflex bronchoconstriction. *Journal of Applied Physiology*, **65**, 1007–1023

LAITINEN, L. A., SALONEN, R. O. and WIDDICOMBE, J. G. (eds) (1990) Tracheobronchial and nasal circulation. *European Respiratory Journal*, **3**, suppl 12, 5535–6845

LAROCHE, C. M., MOXHAM, J. and GREEN, M. (1989) Respiratory muscle weakness and fatigue. *Quarterly Journal of Medicine*, **71**, 373–397

LEITH, D. E., BUTLER, J. P., SNEDDON, S. L. and BRAIN, J. D. (1986) Cough. In: *Handbook of Physiology, vol 3: Mechanics of Breathing*, part 1, edited by P. T. Macklem and J. Mead. Bethesda: American Physiological Society. pp. 315–336

LINDERHOLM, H. (1963) Lung mechanics in sitting and horizontal postures studied by body plethysmographic methods. *American Journal of Physiology*, **204**, 85–91

LISBOA, C., JARDIM, J., ANGUS, E. and MACKLEM, P. T. (1980) Is extra-thoracic airway obstruction important in asthma? *American Review of Respiratory Disease*, **112**, 115–112

MADOR, M. J. and KUFEL, T. J. (1992) Reproducibility of visual analog scale measurements of dyspnea in patients with chronic obstructive pulmonary disease. *American Review of Respiratory Disease*, **146**, 82–87

MILLER, R. D. and HYATT, R. E. (1969) Obstructing lesions of the larynx and trachea: clinical and physiologic characteristics. *Proceedings of the Mayo Clinic*, **44**, 145–161

MILLER, R. D. and HYATT, R. E. (1973) Evaluation of obstructing lesions of the trachea and larynx by flow-volume loops. *American Review of Respiratory Disease*, **108**, 475–481

MURRAY, J. F. (1985) *The Normal Lung*, 2nd edn. Philadelphia: W. B. Saunders

NIINIMAA, V., COLE, P., MINTZ, S. and SHEPHARD, R. J. (1980) The switching point from nasal to oronasal breathing. *Respiration Physiology*, **42**, 61–71

NIINIMAA, V., COLE, P., MINTZ, S. and SHEPHARD, R. J. (1981) Oronasal distribution of respiratory airflow. *Respiration Physiology*, **43**, 69–75

O'CONNELL, F., THOMAS, V. E., PRIDE, N. B. and FULLER, R. W. (1994) Capsaicin cough sensitivity decreases with successful treatment of chronic cough. *American Journal of Respira-*

tory and Critical Care Medicine, **150**, 374–380

PERTUZE, J., WATSON, A. and PRIDE, N. B. (1991) Maximum airflow through the nose in humans. *Journal of Applied Physiology*, **70**, 1369–1376

PIOPED INVESTIGATORS (1990) Value of ventilation/perfusion scan in acute pulmonary embolism. Results of the prospective investigation of pulmonary embolism diagnosis (PIOPED). *Journal of the American Medical Association*, **263**, 2753–2759

POSTMA, D. S., KEYZER, J. J., KOËTER, G. H., SLUITER, H. J. and DE VRIES, K. (1985) Influence of the parasympathetic and sympathetic nervous system on nocturnal bronchial obstruction. *Clinical Science*, **69**, 251–258

PRIDE, N. B. (1995) Lung function testing. In: *Oxford Textbook of Medicine*, 3rd edn, edited by D. Weatherall, J. G. Ledingham and D. A. Warrell. Oxford: Oxford University Press. pp. 2666–2675

QUANJER, P. H. (ed.) (1993) Standardized lung function testing. *European Respiratory Journal*, **6**, suppl. 16, 1–100

RAMNARINE, S. I. and ROGERS, D. F. (1994) Non-adrenergic, non-cholinergic neural control of mucus secretion in the airways. *Pulmonary Pharmacology*, **7**, 19–33

REMMERS, J. E., DE GROOT, W. J., SAUERLAND, E. K. and ANCH, A. M. (1978) Pathogenesis of upper airway occlusion during sleep. *Journal of Applied Physiology*, **44**, 931–938

RODENSTEIN, D. O., FRANCIS, C. and STANESCU, D. C. (1983) Emotional laryngeal wheezing. A new syndrome. *American Review of Respiratory Disease*, **127**, 354–356

SCHWARTZ, A. R., SMITH, P. L., KASHIMA, H. K. and PROCTOR, D. F. (1994) Respiratory function of the upper airways. In: *Texbook of Respiratory Medicine*. 2nd edn, edited by J. F., Murray and J. A., Nadel. Philadelphia: W. B. Saunders. pp. 1451–1470

SHELTON, D. M., PERTUZE, J., GLEESON, M. J., THOMPSON, J., DENMAN, W. T., GOFF, J. *et al.* (1990) Comparison of oscillation with three other methods for measuring nasal airways resistance. *Respiratory Medicine*, **84**, 101–106

SKATRUD, J. B. and DEMPSEY, J. A. (1985) Airway resistance and respiratory muscle function in snorers during NREM sleep. *Journal of Applied Physiology*, **59**, 328–335

WAGNER, P. D., and RODRIGUEZ–ROISIN, R. (1991) Clinical advances in pulmonary gas exchange. *American Review of Respiratory Disease*, **143**, 883–888

WEST, J. B. (1990) *Ventilation/Blood Flow and Gas Exchange*, 5th edn. Oxford: Blackwell Scientific Publications

YANAGIHARA, N., VON LEDEN, H. AND WERNER–KUKUK, E. (1966) The physical parameters of cough: the larynx in a normal single cough. *Acta Otolaryngologica*, **61**, 495–510

YAP, J. C. H. and PRIDE, N. B. (1994) Effect of induced bronchoconstriction on nasal airflow resistance in patients with asthma. *Clinical Science*, **86**, 55–58

14

The generation and reception of speech

Adrian Fourcin, Julian McGlashan and Mark Huckvale

This chapter is designed to give a brief overview of areas of work in the fields of speech sciences and spoken language engineering which are making increasingly important contributions both to practical clinical work and its theoretical foundations. Although the extent of the activity is large and has far reaching commercial and social consequences there is, nevertheless, a relatively small number of basic principles of enduring importance and an attempt has been made to put these essential factors into perspective. The chapter is divided into nine main working sections. The first, *phonetic and linguistic systems*, is concerned with some special aspects of the cognitive processing of speech and language. It introduces practical tools coming from spoken language engineering with regard to computer compatible segmental description and discusses the concepts of normalization and contrast. The second section, *physical factors*, discusses the concept of a system and the range of levels of input and output with which different orders of system complexity can be associated – here from a singly resonant system to the much more complex vocal tract with its many resonances. The third section is concerned with *levels of representation*, going from segmental phonetic descriptions to the brief discussion of individual speech signal parameters. The fourth part of this chapter, *voice excitation*, concentrates on the physical characteristics of voice input to the vocal tract in normal phonation. It refers briefly to the types of data obtainable from the use of stroboscopic, electrolaryngographic and waveform based methods of processing, and it is followed by a section on *voice pathology*. The sixth section discusses *resonance and timbre*, building on the discussions of the earlier sections. Sections seven and eight similarly make use of the work of the earlier sections in discussion of *rehabilitation and habilitation* with regard particularly to interactive visual displays and meth-

ods of signal processing for the extraction of essential speech elements in auditory prostheses. The final section is concerned with *future needs and possibilities*, where a particular view is given of some of the aspects of future development which may be both of clinical consequence and practical possibility.

Phonetic and linguistic systems

All methods of information transmission depend on the use of readily communicable differences. These differences are effective to the extent that they are able to provide the basis for the definition of contrasts. For example in Morse code, where a single dimension is used as a function of time, the presence or absence of a tonality can provide an effective basis for communication. This printed page also makes use of one salient contrastive dimension in respect of the difference between black and white but, in addition, involves the employment of contrastive pattern forms which are used to summarize and indicate the more complex contrasts of speech. All natural languages have the common property that their systems use hierarchically organized contrastive structures. The sound sequences of speech can be regarded as being made up of components which are structured in rule-governed patterned forms. Speech is only acceptable and intelligible and regarded by the users as natural when it is both generated and received according to these pattern-structured rules. It has evolved as a very practical and robust method of communication and this has led to redundancy, over-description, at every level of its organization, so that the lack of information about one part of a sound, or one part of a sound sequence, does not necessarily lead to a failure of information transmission. When due account is taken of these basic rules there can be substantial practical benefits.

Although we perceive and produce speech sound sequences rather than separate sounds, in practice it is helpful to describe what is often a continuous stream of acoustic information in terms of a string of separate component sounds. The 'phone' level is used at this stage of description to give a first approximation to contrastive sound differences and to provide a basis for the definition and discussion of the nature of individual sounds. It is important to distinguish between the physical nature of the sounds of speech, their representation at the phone level and their use to convey meaning. Whereas the phone level is concerned with the nature of the sound itself, the 'phoneme' level is concerned with the use of sounds to convey meaning. Quite different detailed phones, for example as the result of differences in production or speech source, can contribute to establishing the same meaning contrast. Going from the physical nature of sound sequences to phone representations of individual sound, then to phoneme sequences to convey meaning, involves more and more abstract levels of representation which are, however, of great practical importance. For example, in naming a particular object a child, a man and a pathological speaker may all produce linguistically identical phoneme sequences. If they come from the same accent region, the phonetic analysis of each utterance at the level of a phone description might be identical for the child and the man and yet, however, employ different tokens (the sound elements of an individual contrastive system) for the pathological speaker. At the detailed physical level of analysis the three speech sequences will be quite dissimilar. Indeed, at this physical level of description, no two utterances no matter how carefully spoken can ever be identical.

Work in phonetics has provided a structured approach to the description of the sound contrasts of the languages of the world, using sets of production based descriptions which are represented in terms of special sets of printed characters. The complexity of this task has made it necessary to use 'phonetic' fonts which are not ordinarily available. Work in the field of spoken language engineering (SLE) has led to the introduction of a typewriter keyboard-based set of contrastive characters, which can be used within the context of the needs of an increasingly large number of different languages. Table 14.1 illustrates this system of speech sound representation for English with, in each of the two columns, the keyboard character (SAMPA: Speech Assessment Methods Phonetic Alphabet) shown on the left and the corresponding keyword shown on the right. The aim of this Table is to give a basis for a convenient, and accurate, method of clinical representation for the purposes of a particular language. The SAMPA approach is not intended to make it possible to give the detailed phonetic representation which is in principle feasible when the descriptors of the International Alphabet are used. SAMPA, in the form shown here, is between the phone and phoneme levels of description, in the sense that it provides a broad phonetic representation which makes it possible to relate discrete phonetic character sequences to continuous acoustic streams of real data.

Table 14.1 Phonetic representation of English sounds

Vowels and diphthongs		Consonants	
Keyboard character	Keyword	Keyboard character	Keyword
i	bead	N	sing
I	bid	T	thin
e	bed	D	then
{	bad	S	shed
A	card	Z	beige
Q	cod	tS	etch
O	cord	dZ	edge
U	good		
u	food		
V	bud		
3	bird		
@	allow	Consonantal characters	
eI	day	which do not	
@U	know	require special definition	
aI	eye		
aU	cow		
OI	boy		
I@	beer		
e@	bare	p t k b d g m n f v s z r l w j h	
U@	tour		

As an example, the word 'bat' would be represented using Table 14.1 as [b{t] when produced by an individual speaker (the use of square brackets is intended to indicate that the description is at the level of individual sounds rather than necessarily at the level of meaning). In this example three phones are used to represent the individual sound components of this particular utterance. If the speaker had produced the word 'tab' it would be represented here simply as [t{b]. In the present example, broadly transcribed with the help of SAMPA, [b] is phonetically not the same utterance at the beginning of the word as it is at the end. For many practical purposes, the two different phones are grouped together and described as allophones of /b/, where the slanting brackets are simply used to refer to the phonemic level of representation.

The complete inventory of the phonemic classes of a language can be derived by systematically going through possible substitutions in phone sequences. For instance, in addition to the sequence /b{t/, the sequences /b{d/, /b{g/, also occur in which a substitution has been made in the third position in the sequence. Similarly, changes can be made in the first place as in /p{t/, /s{t/, or in the second place as in /bIt/, /bet/. 'Minimal' pairs of this type are also of value in the clinical assessment and detailed evaluation of both production and perception.

Traditionally, the phonetic descriptions of sound classes are based on their means of production. These are summarized in Table 14.2. The Table gives a brief articulatorily based classification of the pure (sustainable) vowels which are represented in Table 14.1. Here, however, the classification is in terms of whether or not the speaker's tongue tends to be humped towards the front or the back of the oral cavity and whether the oral cavity itself is shaped by the tongue being relatively close to or distant from the speaker's palate. This simple but useful classification system has its approximate correlates in roughly corresponding acoustic dimensions (see Figure 14.15c). Table 14.3 provides an articulatory, vocal tract, set of descriptors for the contrastive consonantal classes which appear in Table 14.1. The essential dimensions here are those of 'voice, place and manner'. The 'voice' descriptor is concerned with the presence or absence of vocal fold vibratory activity in the production of the sound. It is important at least to touch on the difference between the periodic regular excitation which is associated with voicing, and the irregular, aperiodic, excitation of the vocal tract which is associated with a turbulent flow of air at a point or points of constriction. The voiced consonants are shown in bold in Table 14.3. The 'place' descriptor refers to the salient positioning of the main articulators, lips, tongue, soft palate, in the temporal evolu-

tion of the sound. 'Manner' refers to the nature of the control of the production of the consonant as a function of time in association with both the movement of the essential articulators and the control of the acoustic excitation of the whole vocal tract. Voice, place and manner do not, however, have readily definable simple acoustic correlates.

Sequences of phonemes rather than individual units are at the heart of communication and the next level of description which is often employed is that of the morpheme. This has a grammatical function. Each type of linguistic unit is distinguished rather by its function than its form. For example, the utterance 'bat' was used in a discussion of phone and phonemic systemic contrasts. In English there are two English morphemes 'bat', one which functions as a noun and the other which functions as a verb. The verb form may have another morpheme added to it, for instance the morpheme 'ing', as in the sentence, 'he's been batting for an hour'. Similarly, the morpheme 'ed' could be used to form the sentence 'he batted for an hour'. The successive processes of using phones to map onto phonemes in order to produce combinations which give morphemes, and morphemes to give words, is a feature of the hierarchical structure of language itself. It is important in regard to the understanding of the acquisition of language by the child and the reacquisition of skills by the adult in the face of pathological handicap. In spoken language engineering this intrinsic economy of language structure is now beginning to be used and this development is likely to be increasingly important in the clinical application of this technology for training, prostheses and eventually diagnosis.

At the morpheme and word levels, the normal language user will have a fairly large vocabulary of units which he can recognize (passive vocabulary) and a more restricted list of units which he will make use of in active speech production. In a similar way, most of the information concerning the sentence level of operation is stored, but now the storage is

Table 14.2 English vowels: tongue shapings within the oral cavity

Phonetic descriptor	Front	Central	Back
Close	i		u
Half-close	I		U
Half-open	e	3, @	O
Open	{	V	A, Q

Table 14.3 English consonants: main places of constriction on closure in the vocal tract and manners of articulation

Manner	Place						
	Bilabial	Labiodental	Dental	Alveolar	Palatal	Velar	Glottal
Approximant	w			r	j		
Lateral				l			
Plosive	pb			td		kg	
Affricative				tS dZ			
				tr dr			
Fricative		fv	TD	sz	SZ		h
Nasal	m			n		N	

The need to use typewriter and computer keyboards in the clinic, in spoken language engineering and for e-mail transmission had led to the widespread use of SAMPA (speech assessment methods phonetic alphabet) notation defined above. Voiced sounds are shown in bold.

primarily in the form of rules for combining words into sequences that are possible and acceptable in language. Sets of rules are intrinsic to the operation of speech communication at every level. Basic to the instructions, which make it possible for the sound sequences of speech to be produced, are the rules which govern the control of the vocal tract in production and the auditory monitoring of its acoustic output.

Physical factors

In all systems which involve the transmission of information, it is often profitable to break down what is often a very complex whole into three essential components – input, system and output. The physical descriptions of both speech production and speech reception certainly benefit from this simplification. Figure 14.1a illustrates the core representation which serves as a basic building block for the discussion and analysis of even the most complex communication systems. In the simplest case, a physical system such as a weight supported by a spring has a natural frequency. If it is moved impulsively from its position of equilibrium it will return to its normal resting position with a gradually diminishing to and fro vibration. This situation is illustrated in Figure 14.1b, where the input to a simple acoustic system is a single pressure pulse and the output consists of a series of oscillatory peaks of pressure. The amplitudes of these peaks of pressure diminish in such a way

that the size of each peak is a constant fraction of that of its predecessor. The complete cycles of oscillation are spaced by equal intervals of time which correspond to the natural period of movement of the system – the time interval for one complete to and fro movement. The reciprocal of this period is the natural frequency of the system.

Reductions in amplitude from period to period take place because the vibrating system loses energy. The time interval over which the vibrations persist after the excitation has been applied depends on energy loss from the system; the process of losing energy in this way is ordinarily referred to as 'damping'. If energy were not lost, the system would continue to vibrate indefinitely with successive peaks of pressure being of equal amplitude and the wave shape being sinusoidal – of pure tone form. If, instead of a pulse of pressure, a pure tone had been applied to this simple system, its maximum response to the pure tone would have happened when the pure tone input had the same frequency as the natural frequency of the vibrating system. Response as a function of frequency is illustrated in the centre part of Figures 14.1b and c. This selective response is referred to as 'resonance'.

The basic factors associated with the nature and response of a simple resonant system are at the heart of all modern descriptions of both speech production and speech perception. In Figure 14.1b, the simple pulse of pressure is shown and its energy/frequency composition is illustrated immediately below in Figure 14.1c. The relatively sharp pulse has energy distributed, as a function of its shape, over a continuous

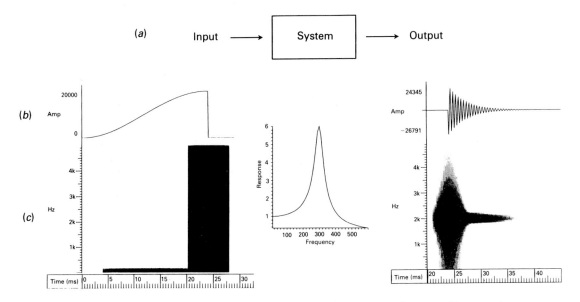

Figure 14.1 Characteristics of a simple resonant system. (a) The essential components of a system; (b) input and output pressure-time waveforms; (c) input and output frequency-time energy distributions corresponding to the waveforms of (b). Note that the frequency response of the system itself is shown in the centre of the figure

range of pure tone frequencies. If it were required to build up or synthesize the pulse from a number of pure tones, these would have to be distributed continuously over frequency and time in order to produce the discontinuous event shown in Figure 14.1*b*. The frequency composition of the output of the system, corresponding to the right hand waveform of Figure 14.1*b*, is shown immediately below it in Figure 14.1*c*. Energy is now distributed over only a very limited frequency range, that corresponding to the response of the vibrating system itself. The real vocal tract provides an example of a vibrating system which has a number of resonators with different natural frequencies, with differing degrees of damping. Vocal tract resonances are called 'formants'.

Figure 14.2 illustrates the relationships between input and output which would be typical for a simple vocal tract system which varies in shape with time. This example is based on an artificial representation of real speech events. It makes use of a computer simulation, and involves only two formant resonances controlled in time and frequency with an artificial input representing laryngeal excitation. Figure 14.2*e* shows two schematic vocal tracts relating to the extremes of the range of variation, on the left with the articulatory configuration for [A] and on the right with the vocal tract articulators set to produce another oral vowel [i].

Controlled change, with time, of the parameters of the system is an essential aspect of the patterned structure of speech production, which is neither simple in regard to its representation in terms of resonant components, nor in respect of its stability with time. The voiced sounds of speech are characterized by having an input to the vocal tract, derived from the quasi-regular pulsatile pressure changes, which are the result of the interruption of the tracheal air stream by the vibrating vocal folds. This is illus-

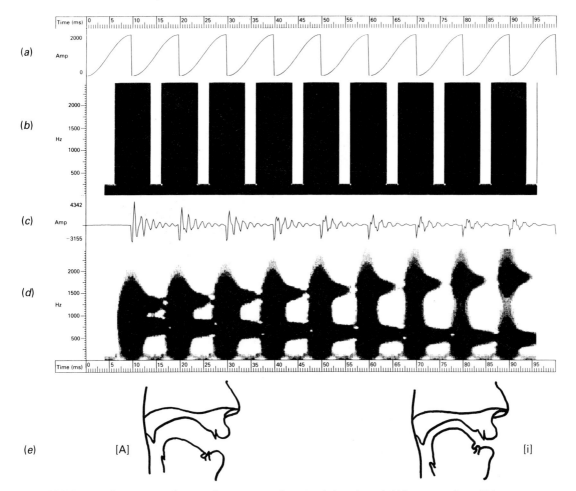

Figure 14.2 Input and output waveforms and spectrograms for a simple 'vocal tract'. (*a*) Input waveform; (*b*) input spectrogram; (*c*) output waveform; (*d*) output spectrogram; (*e*) schematic 'vocal tract' shapes at the beginning and end of the sound

trated in the top of Figure 14.2*a*. Just as in Figures 14.1*b* and *c*, there is also the possibility here of relating pressure-time waveforms to frequency-time distributions. They are simply different ways of representing the same physical events. In Figure 14.2*b* each pulse is associated with a well-defined distribution of energy, shown by the blackness of the marking, as a function of frequency. In Figure 14.2*c*, the vocal tract output pressure response as a function of time is shown corresponding to the evolving articulatory setting. In Figure 14.2*d*, the frequency time plot, called a 'spectrogram', shows how the changing shape of the 'speaker's' vocal tract has altered its resonant structure so that it responds selectively in frequency to the acoustic energy output from the larynx. At the start of the example the resonant responses are set so that they are closely spaced in frequency, for [A], while at the end of the synthetic utterance they are widely separated in frequency, for [i]. Each vertical pair of resonator responses is the result of an individual input pulse. The expressions 'larynx frequency' and 'larynx period' are used here to refer to the rate of vibration of the vocal folds and the time separation between their successive closures. Resonance frequency, on the other hand corresponds to the vertical position of the resonator outputs in

Figure 14.2*d*. Together with these frequency changes in resonator outputs go corresponding changes in the nature of the pressure time waveform responses from the resonators. These are shown for the whole of the utterance in Figure 14.2*c*.

Levels of representation

Figure 14.3 gives a more representative, although more complex, example of the phonetic and acoustic levels of description which would typically be associated with a real speech sequence. At the head of the Figure, the words 'Scott Brown' are represented in the SAMPA notation already discussed, with the individual phonetic characters aligned approximately with the hypothetical speech sounds which they are intended to represent. The very first part of the utterance is made up of the alveolar voiceless fricative [s] produced in following conjunction with the velar voiceless plosive [k]. Here, there is voiceless excitation of the vocal tract. The frequency time representation, or spectrogram (Figure 14.3*b*), has no low frequency energy shown for this part of the complete utterance and the pattern displayed also does not have the regular vertical periodic marking associated with the

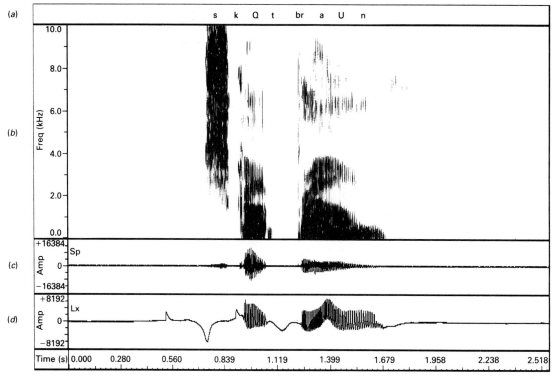

Figure 14.3 Levels of representation for the sequence of sounds in the utterance 'Scott-Brown'. (*a*) Phonetic representation using SAMPA. (*b*) Wide band frequency-time spectrogram. (*c*) Speech pressure (Sp) waveform. (*d*) Electrolaryngograph (Lx) waveform: upward deflection indicates vocal fold closure

regular succession of closures of the speaker's vocal folds which produce voice–larynx frequency excitation. Vocal tract excitation here is due to the random acoustic input derived from turbulent flow at constrictions within the vocal tract. The onset of [Q] is quite different. Here it is possible to see both the vertical striations, each corresponding to a separate closure of the speaker's vibrating vocal folds, and the evolving resonant structures which result from the changing shape of the vocal tract.

Figure 14.3c gives the acoustic speech pressure waveform which is associated with these events. The aperiodicity of the first part of the utterance and the periodicity associated with [Q] are easily seen and so are the differences in amplitude for these different excitations. When this utterance was produced a recording was made not only of the acoustic activity but also of the speaker's associated vocal fold movement by the use of an electrolaryngograph, giving the waveform, Lx, in Figure 14.3d. The electrolaryngograph simply gives an output corresponding to the change of conductance across the speaker's throat, which is associated primarily with vocal fold contact. Since the vocal folds must be abducted in order to allow air flow for the production of voiceless fricatives and consonants, there is no vibratory Lx component for [sk] as there is for [Q]. Similarly, the production of the [t] consonant is associated with a cessation of voice activity before the beginning of the totally voiced sequence associated with the word 'Brown'.

Voice excitation

The essentially regular and controlled vibration of the vocal folds is basic to the production of the voiced sounds of speech, exemplified physically above by the components of Figures 14.3b and c which correspond to the vibratory activity detected in Figure 14.3d. Perceptually, voice can be described as the input to the vocal tract which gives speech its characteristic pitch and enables singing and the contrasts of intonation to be produced. In all languages of the world, the voiced sounds are the most important with regard to the communication load that they carry and the most important in regard to the sequence of development of speaking abilities in the first days and months of life, perhaps even before birth. Figure 14.4 illustrates a sequence of instants in the cycle of vibratory activity for a particular adult male speaker during the sustained production of a neutral vowel sound, [i]. The electrolaryngograph waveform (Lx) was obtained by the use of surface electrodes lightly placed on both sides of the neck at the level of the thyroid alae. A flash X-ray source, operating at approximately 300 kV, with a flash duration time of 1.5×10^{-9} seconds was synchronized by the use of this laryngograph waveform, so that any predetermined instant in the regular vibration of the vocal folds could be used to trigger a frontal irradiation of the speaker's vocal folds. The total dosage for one flash was less than 100 nGy.

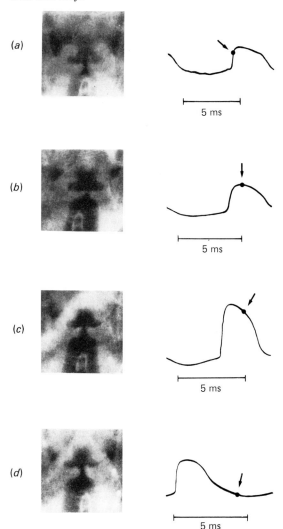

Figure 14.4 Frontal flash X-ray radiograms. Four separately recorded instants in the cycle of vocal fold vibratory activity for a sustained [i] from an adult male speaker. The triggering instants are shown of the Lx waveform: (a) immediately prior to maximum vocal fold contact; (b) point of maximum closure; (c) beginning of separation; (d) mid-open phase

Figure 14.4a shows the vocal folds in their position immediately before complete closure, the ventricular folds are clearly seen above the superior edges of the folds themselves, which are just visible as a result of their anterior downward tilt. The separation of the lower edges is clearly greater than that of the upper.

In Figure 14.4b the closure cycle has been completed with the superior edges of the vocal folds shown in maximum contact. Maximum contact in normal phonation is typically associated with only a modest abuttal of the opposing vocal folds.

In Figure 14.4c the vocal folds can be seen to be separating after the peak of closure.

Finally, in Figure 14.4d the vocal folds are maximally separated, the glottal area is greatest and the output from the laryngograph electrodes is near to its absolute minimum. The Figure shows the precursive shaping of the vocal folds prior to the beginning of a new oscillatory cycle and the inferior edges are already coming closer to the midline.

The essential elements of the vocal fold vibratory cycle may now be briefly summarized. At first, the inferior edges of the folds come closer and then separate as the superior edges once more come rapidly into slight but intimate contact. This rapid contact initiates as a function of the speed and completeness of closure, a new acoustic excitation of the vocal tract. Maximum acoustic output from the vocal tract is then obtained during the subsequent interval of maximum isolation of the supraglottal vocal tract from the damping introduced during the open phase by the subglottal cavities. Although the pitch of the voice has been controlled, each one of these images was taken with a separate production of the vowel by the speaker (who is the same as for Figure 14.3). The images however have the advantage of giving a direct frontal view of the vocal folds during normal voice production.

Light stroboscopy provides a more closely related set of images, although they are not gathered from a single glottal cycle. Figure 14.5 shows two sets of stroboscopic visual images of the vocal folds together with the synchronous electrolaryngographic activity. Each sequence was captured using a videocamera system linked to a computer with a frame grabber. The computer uses the closure phase and period of the electrolaryngograph waveform to determine the stroboscopic flash onset time so that it automatically acquires images of the vocal fold vibratory cycle which are progressively separated by $45°$ intervals. The relevant segment of the synchronously acquired electrolaryngograph trace is displayed under each image together with a vertical marker indicating the exact onset of flash in relation to the trace.

Figure 14.5a shows an asymmetrical larynx in a woman phonating at 312 Hz in falsetto. The stroboscopic images in Figure 14.5b show a woman also phonating at 312 Hz but with oedematous vocal folds and bilateral nodules. The abnormal electrolaryngograph waveform of Figure 14.5b is consistent with the altered vocal fold contact pattern due to the pathological vocal folds and helps in the understanding of the pathophysiological processes. The first work of this type was conducted in conjunction with Rupert Donovan and Peter Roach (using 16 mm film) and this present approach, which builds on and extends this initial work, is by Julian McGlashan and

Darryl de Cunha. The present methods take the earlier work from being a matter of scientific interest to being at the point of daily clinical practical application. It is now possible to make use of the laryngograph information as an additional source of diagnostic input.

Different voice qualities are associated with different acoustic output waveforms and spectra from the speaker's vocal tract. They are also associated with quite different modes of vibration of the speaker's vocal folds and these can, to an appreciable degree, be delineated by the laryngograph. Figure 14.6a gives an example taken from a sustained neutral vowel, the [@] produced by the same speaker as Figure 14.4. The two waveforms Sp (for speech pressure) and Lx have not, for this illustration, been time aligned and are exactly as they were initially obtained. There is a small time interval between the rapid upward movement of the Lx waveform and the rapid upward increase in speech pressure. This interval corresponds to the propagation time (of 1.1 ms) required for the sound to travel along the length of the speaker's vocal tract and from his lips to the recording microphone. The Lx waveform has a very clear closure phase. It is during this closure phase interval, following the initial acoustic excitation produced by the rapid closure of the vocal folds, that the resonances of the vocal tract give their maximum response. Ordinarily, during the open phase of vocal fold movement there is a degree of coupling between the vocal tract and the subglottal cavities, which introduces some additional damping to the resonances of the vocal tract. This process of damping is at its greatest for breathy voice when there is only a relatively brief interval of vocal fold contact and a long open phase. An example of this type of excitation and speech response is given in Figure 14.6b for the voiced fricative [v] again produced by the same speaker. The slower closure of the vocal folds produces a less distinct excitation of the vocal tract resonances. The abduction of the folds allows sufficient air flow to produce adequate frication at the constriction produced by the lower lip and upper incisors. This recording has been produced with little reverberation and the synchrony between the open phase and the parts of the waveform with most frication in speech pressure are clearly visible.

Another important aspect of activities that take place within a complete vocal fold cycle of vibration is shown in Figure 14.7 for a creaky voice quality produced by the same speaker. As before, the lower waveform has been obtained from an electrolaryngograph but the upper waveform has been extracted by a process of signal analysis, applied to the original speech acoustic waveform. This has made it possible to represent the response of just one of the resonances (for the second formant F2) of the speaker's vocal tract, rather than the whole set, as in the complete speech pressure waveform. This gives a particularly

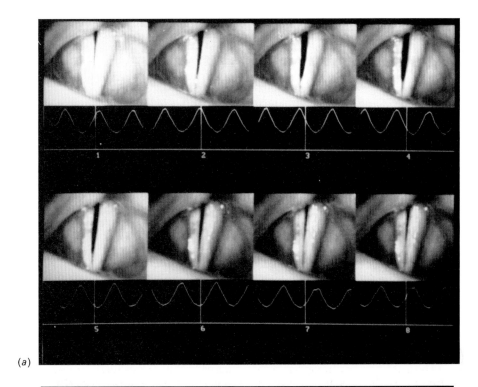

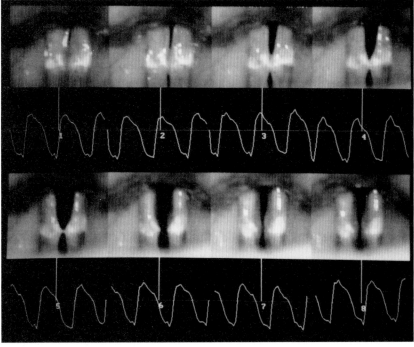

Figure 14.5 Eight sequential stroboscopic images are taken automatically at 45° phase intervals through the complete vibratory cycle. A segment of the synchronously acquired electrolaryngograpic trace is displayed under each picture and is marked with a vertical line to indicate the exact position at which the stroboscopic flash was triggered. (*a*) A subject with an asymmetrical larynx phonating at 312 Hz in falsetto. (*b*) A patient with inflamed vocal folds and bilateral nodules phonating at 312 Hz

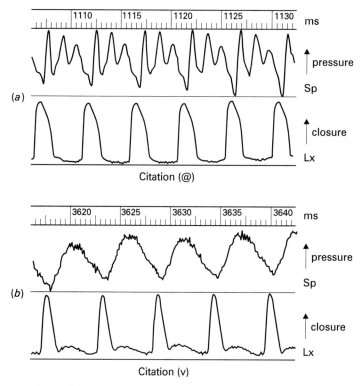

Figure 14.6 Speech pressure (Sp) and electrolaryngograph (Lx) waveforms (*a*) for a purely voiced sound [@], (*b*) for a voiced fricative [v]. The Sp waveform is delayed approximately 1.1 ms relative to the Lx waveform as a result of the transmission time of the acoustic energy from larynx to microphone. (From Singh and Soutar, 1993)

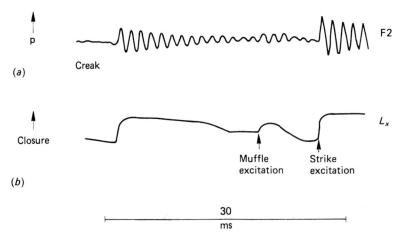

Figure 14.7 Characteristic waveform aspects of 'creaky' voice: (*a*) speech pressure (Sp) waveform for the isolated second formant of [A]; (*b*) the accompanying electrolaryngograph (Lx) waveform. (*a*) and (*b*) are time aligned in this example. (From Singh and Soutar, 1993)

clear indication of the relationship between excitation and response, as in Figure 14.1*b*. The first closure of the vocal folds has initiated a response from this

resonator which has the characteristic damped sinusoidal form associated with a simple single resonating system. The two waveforms are time aligned so that the Lx waveform has been delayed by the propagation time between the vocal folds and the microphone. Creaky voice is characterized by a diplophonic character, the result of two closures, typically of variable periodicity, in each vocal fold cycle and, in this case, the second closure is less pronounced than the first and has been responsible for initiating a correspondingly less well defined acoustic response. The final closure is more rapid than the first and here the response of the vocal tract resonance is correspondingly greater. In creaky voice, the closure of the vocal folds is more prolonged than in other voice qualities and it is the relatively greater isolation of the vocal tract from the subglottal cavities which is responsible for the relatively long period of damped response of this second resonance, F2.

Although breathy voice and creaky voice are both encountered in normal speech, they have some of the essential elements of important pathological conditions. In breathy voice there is both inadequate closure, producing a poor resonance response, and a large open phase producing increased damping of the vocal tract resonant cavities, particularly those adjacent to the glottis. In creaky voice, there is irregularity of vocal tract excitation associated with variability both in periodicity and adequacy of rapidity of closure. Figure 14.8 illustrates two of the important aspects of good quality voice. In Figure 14.8*a* the opposing

vocal folds are shown in contact. It is during this 'hold phase' that the resonances of the vocal tract are best defined, since there is a minimum of internal damping of their response. The speech pressure waveform shows a well-defined response from the vocal tract resonances. In Figure 14.8*b* the vocal folds are shown in their open phase. It is during this open phase that a maximum degree of damping of resonant response as a function of subglottal coupling is present. This corresponds to, but in a less extreme form, the characteristics of breathy voice. Good voice production requires regular vibration of the vocal folds, well defined closure phases of their successive vibrations and a correspondingly small open phase. The open phase is not without importance since it enables rapid adjustment of the vocal tract resonators to be better defined acoustically. The near absence of damping would involve the super-position of successive vocal tract responses onto adjacent cycles of larynx period initiated activity, which would cause acoustic smearing and reduce the listener's ability to perceive controlled changes in resonant structure.

Figures 14.7 and 14.8 give a time-based analytic view of moment-to-moment variation in vocal fold vibration. They provide an insight into different mechanisms of phonation which can have an influence on the overall quality of voice production. In Figure 14.9 the results of a quite different analysis

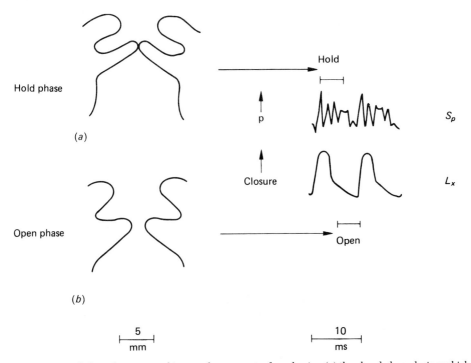

Figure 14.8 Acoustic and electrolaryngographic waveform aspects of good voice: (*a*) the closed phase during which the supraglottic vocal tract is isolated from the trachea; (*b*) the open phase during which there is an acoustic link. (From Singh and Soutar, 1993)

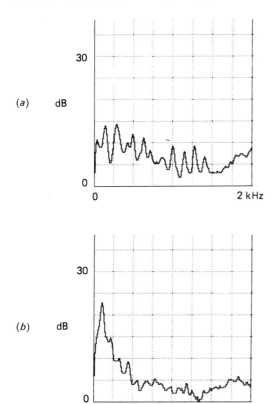

Figure 14.9 Long-term average spectra (200 Hz analysing filter, common dB references) for 1.5 s sentences produced by same adult male speaker as for Figures 14.7 and 14.8, (*a*) with normal voice quality, (*b*) with breathy voice quality. (From Singh and Soutar, 1993)

are shown, one which is made from the whole acoustic signal. A 1.5 second sentence, produced by the same speaker as in Figures 14.7 and 14.8, has been processed by long-term average spectrum (LTAS) analysis so that an overall energy/frequency spectral distribution for the complete utterance is shown. This is exactly as if the analysis of Figure 14.1*b* were presented with only its amplitude and frequency components shown for the whole of its time course and averaged at every point along the frequency axis. Figure 14.9*a* relates to the sentence produced with normal voicing and, over the frequency range shown, there is a relatively uniform distribution of energy with peaks corresponding to the most prominent harmonics contained in this relatively short utterance. Figure 14.9*b* gives the result of processing exactly the same sentence but spoken now with a 'breathy' voice quality. This analysis shows a much greater relative amount of low frequency energy and less well defined harmonics of the fundamental frequency. The particular advantage of analyses of this type is that they are dependent only on the acoustic

signal and may be obtained from a relatively large length of sample (typically many seconds).

Phonetogram analyses are closely related to this simple long-term average spectrum measurement and relate the range of speech energy output, sound intensity level, to the whole of the range of laryngeal frequencies. This gives a dynamic energy/frequency area representation of the distribution and limits to the phonation of the speaker.

Three examples of phonetogram analysis for normal speech are shown in Figure 14.10. A 'continuous phonetogram' is shown at the top of the figure where the intensity of the speech signal in absolute acoustic terms is shown vertically and related to the corresponding fundamental larynx frequency shown horizontally. In this particular analysis the combined acoustic and laryngographic signals have been used. In this way it has been possible to obtain 'instantaneous Fx and Ax' measurements (where Fx refers to the 'instantaneous' frequency of vocal fold vibration measured from each individual period and Ax refers to the maximum amplitude of the speech signal following laryngeal closure), rather than the average values of fundamental frequency, (F0), and intensity which are ordinarily employed. A 2-minute speech sample, based on a read text, has been used and the analysis in Figure 14.10*a* gives a larynx period by period distribution of the range of frequencies and intensities used by the speaker in the whole of the sample. This type of analysis is very useful in helping to define the profile of a speaker's output and is of value not only for the study of normal speech production, but also in pathology at one extreme and in work with singers, who are operating at the peak of their performance and at the other extreme of voice and speech generation.

In Figure 14.10*b*, the phonetogram has been simplified by the use of frequency bins so that the vertical lines, relating to the associated analysis, are regularly spaced at quarter tone intervals along the frequency axis. This frequency binning has made it possible to clarify the presentation and facilitate its use, since the thickness of each of the vertical lines now corresponds to the distribution of amplitudes in the speaker's output at that subrange of larynx frequencies. There is one further advantage to this process of binning, it makes possible another analysis based on the use of a very simple measure of laryngeal regularity. Only those points are included in the printout which are associated with two successive vocal fold periods occurring within the same quarter tone frequency bin. This simple technique of presentation, shown in Figure 14.10*c*, substantially eliminates irregularities from the final display and shows the core phonatory activity which is associated with essentially regular laryngeal vibration in the speaker's output.

In Figure 14.11, the same sample of speech has been used to produce long-term analyses based only on the laryngograph signal. Figure 14.11*a* shows the probability of finding a larynx frequency value in the

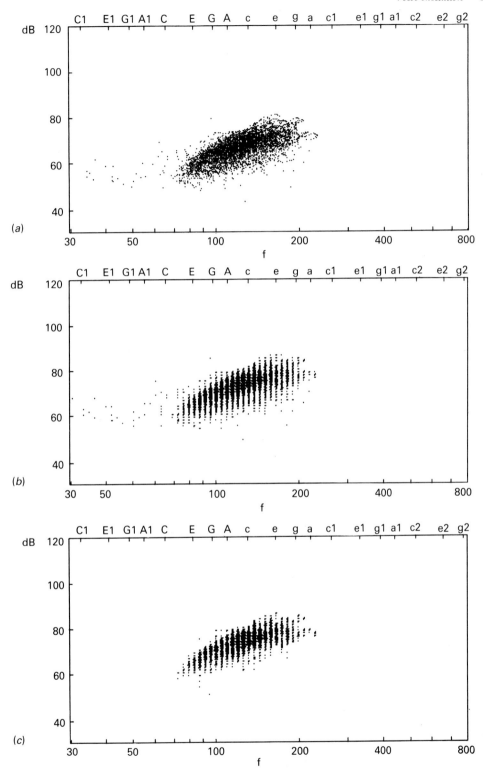

Figure 14.10 Phonetogram analyses for a normal voice. (*a*) The standard phonetogram, in which speech intensity is shown as a function of vocal fold vibration frequency – except that here, the vocal fold frequency is directly obtained from the vocal folds by the use of the laryngograph signal, Lx. (*b*) The first order phonetogram, in which the analysis is based on the use of quarter tone intervals, or bins, spaced along the larynx frequency axis. (*c*) The second order phonetogram, in which are plotted only those pairs of successive speech intensities which have the same larynx frequency bin. This analysis gives an immediate indication of the degree of voice productive regularity

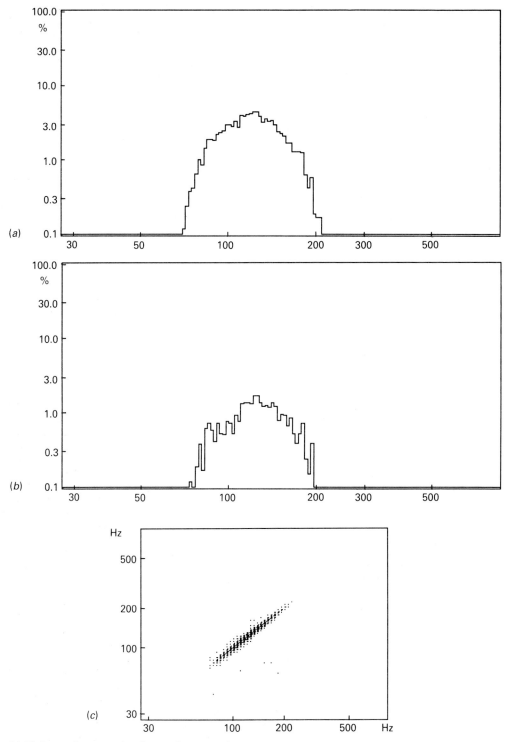

Figure 14.11 Larynx frequency distributions for a normal voice. (*a*) First order histogram, Dx1, based on the measurement of each vocal fold period in isolation (the analysis bins are spaced along the frequency axis by quarter tone intervals). (*b*) Second order histogram, Dx2, based on the occurrence of those successive pairs which both fall into the same frequency analysis bin. (*c*) Cross-plot showing the relation between successive larynx periods for the whole speech sample

analysed sample of Lx. This analysis takes each single vocal fold vibratory period into account. On the basis of this type of quantification the range of larynx frequencies together with the modal and median values of the Fx distribution are readily obtained and ordinarily these are given in an associated statistical printout. Quite long samples of speech can be readily analysed in this way, but for clinical purposes, a sample of not less than 2 minutes is adequate to give a sufficiently realistic basis for the appraisal of the primary larynx frequency characteristics of the speaker's sample output.

Figure 14.11*b* is similar to 14.11*a* except that, as in Figure 14.10*c*, only those laryngeal periods which took place twice in succession are included in the analysis bins. This makes it possible to give an indication of laryngeal regularity with regard to cycle to cycle control of vocal fold vibration. A 'digram' presentation of this type effectively enhances the definition of both mode and effective range; and the difference in probability heights between the distribution shown in Figure 14.11*a* and this digram analysis is an indication of the overall regularity of vocal fold vibration. Another, and more graphic, way of showing the irregularity which may take place from one vocal fold vibratory cycle to its neighbour is given in Figure 14.11*c*. Here successive vocal fold periods are plotted against each other in a period based Fx cross-plot, Cx. Good normal voice is associated with a well defined diagonal distribution of occurrences – each point corresponds to a pair of adjacent vocal fold periods. Any major scatter of points from this diagonal is associated with departure from normality. This plot relates directly to measurements of jitter, but instead of having one global parameter, the nature of the jitter associated with a speech sample can be examined in respect of both its degree and distribution at different larynx frequencies.

Essentially the same method of analysis, as has just been discussed for the distribution of larynx frequencies, can be applied to the distribution of speech acoustic intensities. Figure 14.12 shows the results of larynx synchronous speech amplitude distribution measurement, in which the speech waveform for each larynx cycle is sampled at the point of its maximum amplitude. The distributions in Figures 14.12*a*, *b* and *c* correspond to those of Figures 14.11*a*, *b* and *c*. Here, however, the parameter analysed is that of the epoch dependent measure of intensity, Ax, obtained by measuring the maximum acoustic amplitude of the speech waveform during the closed phase of vocal fold excitation. This is also exactly the measure of intensity which has been used in Figure 14.10 for the phonetogram presentations. The histogram in Figure 14.12*a* shows the speaker's range of intensity over the whole of his larynx frequency range (the same sample has been used here as was employed for the analyses of Figures 14.10 and 14.11). The range of intensities associated with

a degree of period-to-period regularity is shown in Figure 14.12*b* by using the same simple criterion of regularity as for Dx 2 in Figure 14.11. Figure 14.12*c* gives an indication of amplitude variability from period to period. This corresponds to the analysis of shimmer which is ordinarily presented in the form of a single figure, but here there is the possibility of a much greater insight into the nature of shimmer, since it is given as a function of larynx frequency.

All of the speech analysis figures which have been discussed have been derived from a single family of commercially available computer-based programs. Once the basic data have been acquired for the patient, normal speaker, or singer, any of these presentations can be called up for display and examination. The flexibility of present day processing provides a substantial degree of choice in respect of mode of presentation of the data, dependent upon the particular application requirements of the clinician. The especial advantage, which is now available clinically, is that analyses which were previously only possible in the laboratory are now routine and cross-comparisons become readily possible in a disciplined and quantitative fashion as a result of the availability of computer-based files.

Voice pathology

Three broad physical areas of description relate to the effects of different voice pathologies. They are those which are concerned with the range of fundamental frequency used by the speaker; the regularity of vocal fold vibration and the effects of the pathology on voice quality, particularly with regard to adequacy of vocal fold closure. Figure 14.13 gives a particular subset of illustrative examples of the application of the analyses, which were discussed in the last section for normal voice, to the patient of Figure 14.5 with bilateral vocal fold nodules. The speaking range in terms of fundamental frequency is shown by the Dx1 distribution, Figure 14.13*a*. Here a main body of vocal fold vibratory activity is well defined by the main lobe of the distribution, with a central mode associated with the preferred, and rather narrow range of frequencies used by the speaker. The phonetogram analysis (Figure 14.13*b*) shows a similar organization of phonatory activity but now in terms of distributions of speech intensity/amplitude as a function of vocal fold frequency. The overall intensity distribution plot shown by this phonetogram has been produced by the first order binning technique discussed above and indicates a core of phonatory activity which has a narrow frequency range but a normal range of amplitude. It provides a basis for the examination of progress as the result of therapy in this particular instance. Figure 14.13*c* gives an example of the Sp and Lx waveforms taken from a range of frequencies which is in the area of irregular vocal fold vibration for this speaker (from the utterance

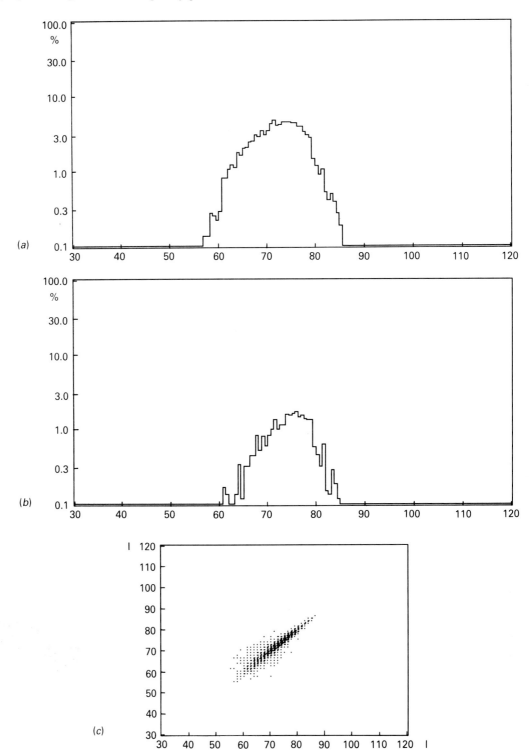

Figure 14.12 Distribution of larynx-synchronous amplitudes for a normal voice. (*a*) First order histogram based on the separate measurement of the amplitude of the speech waveform at the moment of closure indicated by the Lx waveform. (*b*) Second order histogram based on the occurrence of those successive pairs which both fall into the same frequency analysis bin. (*c*) Cross-plot showing the relation between the amplitudes of the speech waveform at successive larynx periods, for the whole speech sample. (x axes: dB)

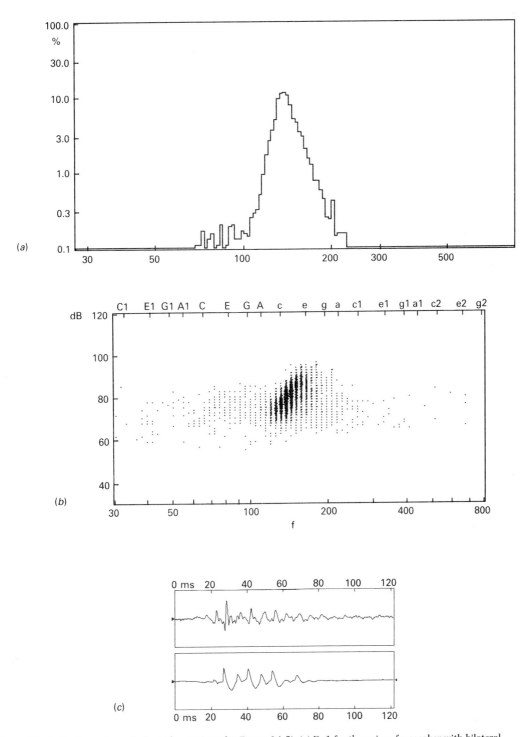

Figure 14.13 Analyses of a pathological voice (see also Figure 14.5). (*a*) Dx1 for the voice of a speaker with bilateral nodules (x axis in Hz); (*b*) first order phonetogram for the same speech sample (x axis in Hz); (*c*) speech pressure (above) and laryngograph waveforms for a small sample of the data

[k@1] in 'Michael'. The variability, both in regard to rate of closure and in respect of intensity of excitation, associated with the vocal fold input to the vocal tract is very clearly seen in Lx as are the consequent perturbations of the speech pressure output.

Figure 14.14 gives a quite different approach to the analysis of voice activity. Voice quality, of course, is a complex concept associated with, among other factors, rate of closure, length of closure duration and appropriate control during ordinary speech. The two Qx plots simply relate to a particular measurement of a physical correlate of voice quality. The previous discussion based on Figures 14.4, 14.5, 14.6, 14.7 and 14.8 showed how the relation of the closed phase duration to the open phase was an important indicator of the acoustic quality of the voice. This Qx measurement has, in consequence, been based on the ratio of the time width of the positive going Lx waveform, at the 80% points below each peak, to the total period of the cycle. The use of Qx, as a percentage of the closed phase relative to the total period in any vocal fold cycle, is a convenient measure which has a direct correlation with the physical basis of voice production. It facilitates the implementation of an analysis which can be immediately understood when comparing one voice condition with another for the same speaker, or as in this case, the normal voice of a woman speaker of 45 years of age with that of a woman of the same age with Reinke's oedema. In other respects the patient, whose Qx analysis is shown here, has essentially normal control with regard to range and detailed contrastive intonation contours. The analyses of Figure 14.13 would not reveal any substantial departure from normality. The Qx distributions, however, show that there is a large and evident difference between the normal and pathological voices.

Resonance and timbre

Acoustic output and auditory input

The vocal tract extends from the larynx to the lips and nostrils. It can be regarded as a set of tubes of irregular shape, varying intrinsically both as a function of the anatomy of the speaker and the setting of the articulators. Although in English the lips, tongue and soft palate are the primary articulators – the means of control of the shape of the vocal tract used by the speaker – in other language environments, additional articulators are employed, e.g. the epiglottis and the body of the larynx itself. In all languages, however, the whole ensemble of the vocal tract can be conveniently regarded as an acoustic filter which operates on the energy coming from an excitation input. So far, the primary discussion in respect of the means of excitation of the vocal tract has been essentially centred on the acoustic energy coming from the larynx as the result of the regular and irregular vibrations of the vocal folds in a normally egressive air stream, but other sources of excitation are also possible. Voiced excitation is the primary source of contrastive linguistic information in all speech systems.

Figure 14.15 illustrates two contrastive settings of a hypothetical vocal tract excited by regular laryngeal vibration with Fx = 125 Hz. In Figure 14.15a the vocal tract is adjusted for the production of the close front vowel [i]. Here, the volume of the oropharyngeal cavity is fairly big and the volume immediately between the lips and the point of maximum constriction is relatively small compared with other vowel settings. In general, it is not appropriate to refer to separate parts of the vocal tract as being totally responsible for particular resonances. However, when there is a very close constriction, then, to a first approximation, this representation of different cavities within the vocal tract as being associated with different resonances is acceptable. It is certainly convenient to think of cavity

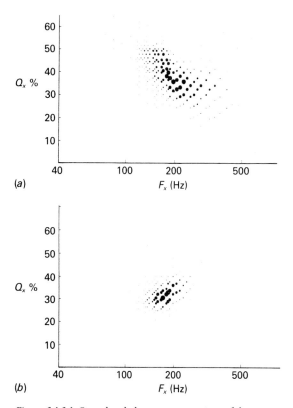

Figure 14.14 Qx – closed phase as a percentage of the period of vocal fold vibration versus frequency of phonation, Fx, for (*a*) a normal adult female speaker, (*b*) an adult female patient with Reinke's oedema. (From Singh and Soutar, 1993)

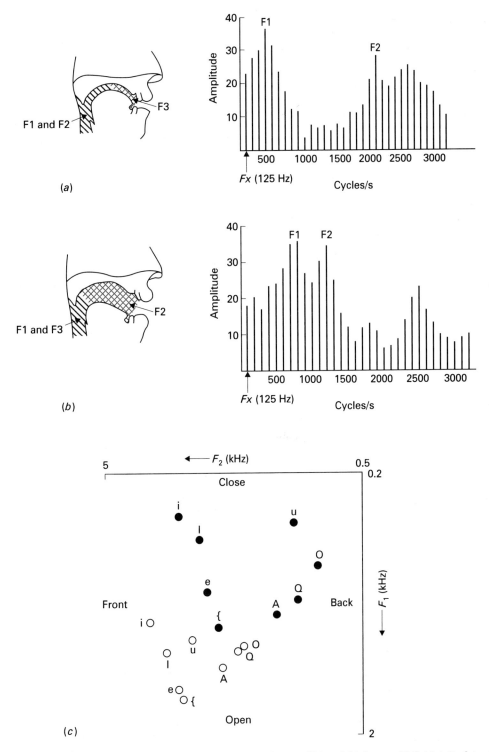

Figure 14.15 Shape of the vocal tract and sound spectrum for: (*a*) the vowel [i], and (*b*) the vowel [A]. (*c*) Articulatory and acoustic representations of English vowels. The formant frequencies for adult male speakers are shown by solid circles, the open circles representing frequencies for 4-year-old children

resonances in arriving at an understanding of the contribution of the vocal tract to the shaping of the speech spectrum of a sound. In the case of [i], the large back cavity produces a low frequency resonance.

In speech work the resonances of the vocal tract are referred to as formants and numbered in sequence going from low to high frequencies. This lowest resonance for [i] is, in consequence its first formant, F1. The back cavity is also responsible for the second formant, F2. The very small front cavity is responsible for the definition of F3, the third formant. The [i] vowel, as a consequence of this resonance shaping, tends to be characterized by a wide separation between the first and second formants. These resonances serve as frequency regions which are associated with the best transmission of energy from the laryngeal source and it is important to note the relatively close frequency spacing of F2 and F3, contributed to respectively by the back and front cavity resonances. Larynx excitation at intervening frequencies, between formant peaks, is not well transmitted simply because the impedance acoustically presented by the vocal tract to the laryngeal source, is greater at points on the overall frequency response which are distant from these resonances. The resonances are not appropriately described as sources of amplification, they are as it were 'windows' in the transmission of excitation through the vocal tract. Changing the shape of the vocal tract, by the adjustment of the articulators, alters the frequencies of the resonances and, correspondingly, the overall frequency response curve.

The relationship is highly complex in physical terms but there are simple acoustic pattern rules which may be learnt by the child in the first months and years of life. For the vowel [A], the oral cavity as a whole is very much larger than for the close front vowel [i] and the back cavity is smaller. The second formant is now essentially defined by the resonance of this front oral cavity, rather than being associated with the back cavity, and is lower in frequency. Ordinarily, it is supposed that the formants themselves provide the main auditory targets which the listener has to observe and the speaker has to strive to produce, in order to provide an adequate basis for communication. Sometimes spectacular formant movements take place, as for example in the diphthong [Ai], due to the swapping over of formant attributions with resonant cavities as the diphthongal evolution proceeds. For the first stages of speech acquisition, there is little conflict between formants and cavity affiliations. This is not the case later on and the pattern processing ability of the human auditory system might well be able to profit more from a representation of cavity to resonance affiliations than formant patterned changes by themselves. It is, however, the convention still that phonetically important contrastive systems, when represented in acoustic terms, are shown in relationship to the

formant frequencies rather than to the intrinsic vocal tract cavities with which they may be associated and by which they are in fact produced. The essential point, of course, is that the auditory system is primary in providing the guidelines relative to which productive success must be judged and it is the simplest auditory pattern criteria which decide the nature of phonetic contrasts, within the context of what it is possible to produce with the vocal tract.

In the lower part of Figure 14.15*c*, the relationships between F1 and F2 for an average young English man, producing a subset of the vowel tokens of Table 14.2, is given with the same representation of formant frequencies for the same vowels but now produced by 4-year-old children. Two important aspects of these different physical distributions of formant frequencies for the same phonetic entities should be noted. First, for the children, the formant values are higher, corresponding to their smaller vocal tracts. Second, the relative disposition of the formant frequencies for the children is largely similar to that of the adults. Two factors are at issue here. First, the children necessarily are employing a contrastive system, which corresponds to that of the models provided by the world around them and used by both siblings and adults. Second, the children are still at the stage of learning how best to produce these contrasts and, in consequence, their systems of contrasts are not as completely organized as they will be at a later stage of development. Auditorily, the normal listener is capable of making adjustments for both of these factors. First, it is possible to interpret widely different formant frequencies as being associated with the same phonetically definable vowel quality, by a process of inference which is called 'normalization'. Normalization is one of the pattern processing activities which make speech communication possible, by the inference and application of rules of pattern organization. Second, allowance is made for an inadequate system of contrasts produced by the immature speaker.

Rehabilitation and habilitation

Speech acquisition

In the progression from the first stages of speech receptive and productive ability to the development of mature competence, an increasing auditory ability to classify the sounds of speech goes hand in hand with the development and application of an increasing knowledge of the phonetically contrastive systems on which meaningful communication depends. One useful tool for the study of this development is provided by the availability of synthetic speech which, although artificially constructed, is so natural that it can be taken for a real human utterance. When this type of sound is used to test aspects of development, stimuli can be made which cover an acoustic continuum between two minimal pair extremes. Individual sounds can then be responded to with labels corresponding to the extreme target words.

Figure 14.16*a* illustrates this process in terms of labelling functions of response versus range. At the two ends of the range are two contrastive tokens which would be easily recognized by the mature adult. They could be two vowels, or they could be a minimal pair as in 'bee and pea' or 'date and gate'. In Figure 14.16*a* four possible types of response coming from a test of this sort are illustrated. The first, Figure 14.16*a*(i) is essentially random no matter whether a stimulus token is at one end of the range or at the other, the ability to categorize or label is indifferent. With exposure to the need for contrastive communication, the child develops the ability to categorize the extreme end-point stimuli (the mother

tends to use extreme exemplar forms in speaking with her infant in the first months of life). This type of labelling is shown in Figure 14.16*a*(ii), only the end-points are consistently labelled and in between there is uncertainty in label assignment. With increasing use of speech communication and developing ability, the situation shown in Figure 14.16*a*(iii) obtains. The 'progressive' labelling is associated with increased confidence at the extremes of the range and a progressive change in response for stimuli which lie in between the two extremes. Finally, in Figure 14.16*a*(iv) there are two well-defined categories in the perceptual labelling process. The stimuli, which are at points along a continuous physical range, are separated out into two classes, and they are confidently assigned to these two groups no matter in which order they are presented.

The results from an experiment performed with

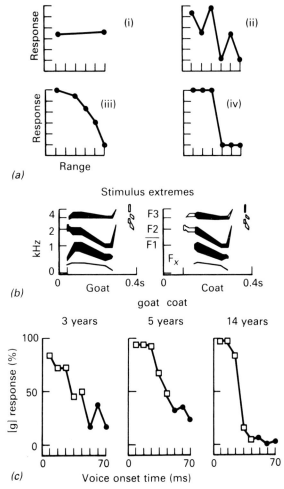

Figure 14.16 Normal developmental sequences. (*a*) (i–iv) Types of labelling in the progression through random, end-point, progressive, and finally complete categorical labelling; (*b*) end-point stimuli for the continuum from 'goat' to 'coat'; (*c*) averaged results of labelling responses along 'goat' versus 'coat' continuum for groups of normally hearing children. Note the development with age of end-point through progressive to the final establishment of categorical labelling

groups of children age grouped for every year between 3 and 14 years, with approximately 20 children in each group, produced the results which are shown in Figure 14.16c for the 3-year, 5-year and 14-year age groups. The formant patterning of the stimuli at the two extremes for the minimal pair items 'goat' and 'coat' are shown in Figure 14.16b. The labelling response for the 3-year-old children is similar to that shown in Figure 14.16a(ii), for moderately confident end-point categorization. At the age of 14 years, well defined categorical labelling is established which is identical with that obtained from adult listeners. The 5-year-old children give responses which are intermediate between these two extremes. The 5-year olds are obviously beginning to acquire greater confidence and are more truly producing progressive labelling with the beginning of categorization.

It is really important to distinguish between the categorical labelling results shown in Figure 14.15 and those which have been reported in work with neonates and children in the first 6 months of life, and indeed with animals. Phonetic targets cannot be used as the basis for the responses elicited from these very young children and animals, because no contrastive communication ability has been established. It is, however, possible to do work with children who are profoundly hearing-impaired and to go from the situation in which they are operating effectively randomly to one in which they are beginning to categorize. Their development of ability may be the result of training or the result of use of an appropriate hearing aid, together with associated communicative experience in the use of speech. Figure 14.17 shows a particular example taken from the responses of one member of a group of profoundly deaf children in which a range of intonation contours was used as the stimulus continuum (Figure 14.17a). An interactive speech pattern element display, working in real time, was used as the basis of training with both visual and auditory presentations being used (for 20 minutes a day over a 6-week period). Before training, typically only random responses were obtained from the children. They neither knew the targets nor heard effectively the real phonetic difference between the extreme tokens. After a period of 2 months' training, using the visual real-time intonation displays and combined acoustic presentations, the synthetic stimuli were labelled much more confidently for all of the children (excepting for one in the group of nine

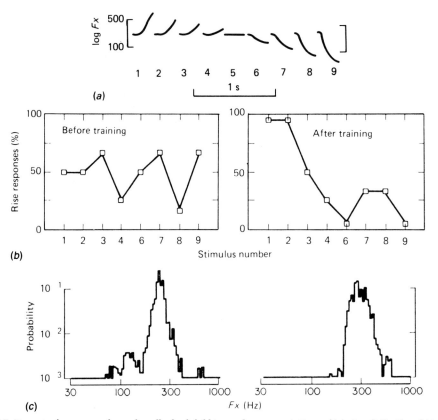

Figure 14.17 Perceptual response of a profoundly deaf child to random presentations of (a) stimuli (1–4) and (6–9) of stimulus range; (b) before and after training; (c) the change in voice characteristics

who had no effective hearing at all). In Figure 14.17*c* the larynx frequency distributions associated with the analysis of samples of the child's speech are shown. Both range and regularity have substantially improved, this was the case for all the children in the group.

A similar situation is shown in Figure 14.18 for the development of vowel contrastive ability, using synthetic stimuli once more for the definition of both the extremes and the intermediate values in a range, continuum, of synthetic vowel sounds. A profoundly deaf child has acquired the ability to label categorically at the end of a 7-month period. During this time the child has gone from being able to recognize the end-point sounds in progressive labelling to be confident in regard to the classification of the individual members of nearly all of the sounds presented in the continuum (different random presentations were used for each test and the sounds used were not otherwise heard). The process of acquisition has been based on speech communication in an ordinary oral environment in a school which is intensively dedicated towards the provision of speaking and hearing skills for the profoundly hearing-impaired child. No special training either in regard of displays or acoustic presentations has been used. New developments are now, however, at the point of making it feasible to assist this process of speech skill acquisition. These developments rely on the presentation of simplified acoustic stimuli which concentrate on the phonetic identity of the contrastive sound systems in a lan-

guage environment. They depend on the use of the techniques which are beginning to emerge in signal processing and spoken language engineering, structured for use in the classroom and home and applied also in the design of a new generation of phonetically appropriate hearing aids.

Signal and phonetically-based speech processing methods

The first really substantial advance in respect of speech presentation to the hearing-impaired took place in the 1950s when miniature body worn prostheses became generally available. These paved the way for the present day behind and in-the-ear hearing aids. Now, some 40 years later, further developments of basic consequence are in progress which are beginning to make use of the special characteristics of speech in order to enhance its intelligibility for different classes of user. In addition to processing at the purely acoustic level, a new generation of aids to hearing has come from the first work, also begun some 40 years ago, directed towards the electrical elicitation of a sensation of hearing in an otherwise totally deaf ear by the use of electrical stimulation of the cochlea. The following brief discussions are intended to link the summary of basic speech principles to some of the developments currently in progress in the field of hearing prostheses.

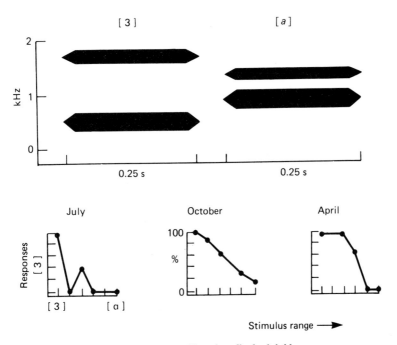

Figure 14.18 Vowel contrastive development in a 7-year-old profoundly deaf child

Speech stretching

This chapter has given special attention to the voice components of speech. This is a dominant physical characteristic of the speech of all languages. It is beginning to be employed as one means for the temporal simplification of speech signals for those whose receptive processing agility is not quite sufficient to cater for the normal rapidity and variability of the acoustic forms of spoken presentations. Even in continuous speech, approximately 50% of the time is occupied by silence because of the necessary intervals used for demarcation, for breathing and for the more detailed levels of speech organization involved in the production of consonantal contrasts. New methods of signal processing are beginning to be introduced which operate synchronously, so that the speed of the acoustic signal is effectively reduced without changing the fundamental pitch of the voice. This is achieved by the addition in synchrony with the original vibration of the speaker's vocal folds of additional speech waveform periods interpolated within the main stream of the speech signal. This process makes it feasible to take up some of the temporal slack in ordinary conversation or, for example, speech presentations on the radio, television or film and gives the listener greater time for receptive auditory processing. There is a necessary delay inherent in these types of processing at the segmental and word levels so that it is not readily feasible to avoid interference with lipreading.

Transition processing

At a more segmental level of processing, the relative imbalance of intensities between consonants and vowels can be redressed by the use of 'phonetically' sensitive dynamic changes in amplification of the speech signal. This minimizes the intrinsic limitations of the speaker's need to associate all consonantal productions with a degree of intensity reduction. It is a simple but, as yet, only laboratory based example of the way in which speech contrastive knowledge may be more effectively applied to overcome limitations inherent in the speech signal itself.

Speech pattern elements

A related approach involves a rather more analytic dissection of the speech signal into component parts, each one of which may be treated separately. This applies both in respect of the methods for its analysis and also the methods for its presentation to the impaired ear. In an obvious example, the voiced sounds may be separately processed from the voiceless fricatives.

The perception of voice in speech is a fundamental attribute which complements lipreading. An application of the discussions in the first part of this chapter would be to derive an acoustic method for ordinary speech analysis of the components which underlie its voiced excitation and which correspond to the laryngograph signal itself. In Figure 14.19 an example is given of the application of this type of technique to the extraction from noisy and reverberant speech of information relating to the epoch of excitation and duration of the closed phase. The uppermost figure is the acoustic speech signal taken from a complete speech sequence. The middle waveform is the corresponding larynx (Lx) waveform, while the lower signal is the output of the pattern processing, multi-level perception (mlp) algorithm. This algorithm gives a response to an input acoustic signal corresponding to the Lx waveform associated with that acoustic signal. The multilevel perception output has the epoch of excitation and a rough correspondence with the Lx closed phase associated with the shape of each one of its individual responses. It should be noted, however, that the multilevel perception system has been trained to detect epochs of excitation and closed phase but not to respond to amplitude variation and this is clearly evident in the particular example of Figure 14.19. Although the computer processing basic to this type of output is of some complexity, it is now quite feasible to have this facility provided in a wearable hearing aid. In conditions of noise and reverberation, the profoundly hearing-impaired user can be given an acoustic stimulation which is matched to the residual hearing. It gives a clear acoustic input devoid of noise and reverberation. The supplement to lipreading which is provided can be of very great help, not only in the enhancement of receptive communication but also in the improvement of the actual speech productive ability of the user. Indeed, when this type of hearing aid is employed, it is our experience that very often the comment of friends and family is not only that receptive ability has been assisted, but also that the user's speech has notably improved.

Figure 14.20 shows another aspect of this type of processing applied in the form of a visual presentation and also implemented in the form of a wearable hearing aid. The fundamental frequency curves corresponding to intonation are supplemented with a width modulation, which is associated with the intensity of the signal and linked to the visual association of bands of frication energy of the sort which are very evident in the complete spectrogram of the same utterance, shown in Figure 14.3. Here the transformation of the individual speech elements to quite different frequency ranges makes it possible to match the hearing ability of the deaf user. The purposes of visual display and interactive training are substantially assisted by these matching transformations, which make possible the cognitive linking of otherwise disparate physical components of speech. The real time analysis, basic to the visual displays and the acoustic presentations, are also available for work

file=temp.db speaker=ajf token=arl

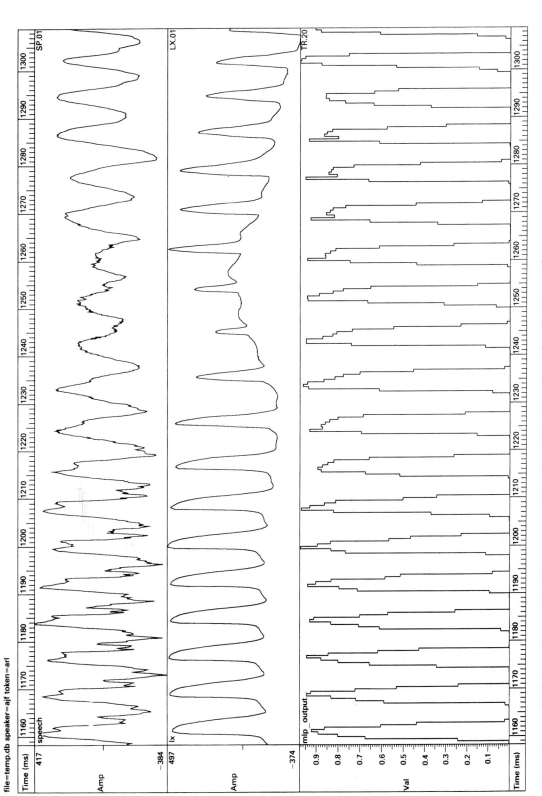

Figure 14.19 Vocal fold closure detection from the acoustic waveform of speech by a 'neural net' algorithm. Input at the top; laryngograph waveform used for training in the centre; computer output at the foot of the figure

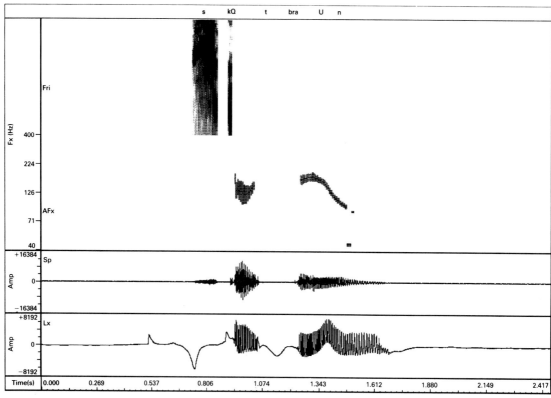

Figure 14.20 Pattern element spectrogram. At the top of the figure, the speech information contained in the standard spectrogram of Figure 14.3 is represented here with regard to the elements of frication, voice pitch and loudness as a function of time. These perceptually important components of speech have been derived physically by the use of the Sp, speech and Lx, laryngograph, waveforms shown below. The utterance is, as before, 'Scott-Brown'

in the speech pathology clinic as a means of interactive training and as a means of quantitative examination of the speaking skill of the client. Exactly the same type of approach can be used in respect of timbre processing in terms of formant, or resonance, pattern inference from the complete acoustic signal.

Future needs and possibilities
Recognition and synthesis

Spoken language engineering is especially concerned with the production of devices which are capable of giving phonetic segmental, or word response to, continuous speech inputs. This work is paralleled by the development of complementary techniques for the provision of synthetic speech outputs on the basis of either orthographic or phonetic segmental symbol inputs of the form of SAMPA. In principle, though not yet in practice, the combination of robust noise resistant speech recognition and real-time synthesis is of potential help to the hearing impaired and could be combined with speech pattern element auditory

matching. In speech pathology, the additional development of reliable normalization processing will be a key to the clinical use of recognition as an aid to computer-supervised interactive training.

Electrocochlear prostheses

A comprehensive overview of approaches to the electrical stimulation of the auditory system by means of electrocochlear hearing prostheses is given by Rosen in Chapter 15 of Volume 2 of this series.

Examples discussed in the present chapter may be found to be of some help in regard to the background support needed for a fuller understanding of the different prosthetic approaches discussed. The Vienna-House whole signal hearing aids are in effect waveform based devices making use of the speech pressure signal, but with appropriate amplitude compression and controlled in frequency range (even in the case of the House device this in fact is the final result of the output of more complex processing). The Ineraid approach simply uses bandpass filtering and it is only the energy which is contained in a small number (e.g. four to six) of contiguous frequency bands across the frequency spectrum of speech that is actually transmitted for use via the stimulating electrodes to the impaired auditory peripheral system. In earlier versions of the Nucleus electrocochlear device, the phonetic pattern element approach, discussed above, was basic to the signal processing system contained within the prosthesis. It is still not the case, however, that sufficiently robust processing is available to accomplish all of the operational criteria for this type of hearing aid and there has been a gradual change in the emphasis given to phonetically based signal processing, so that more technically motivated methods of signal presentation are employed. Continuously interleaved sampling has been used recently with the Ineraid devices. This simply avoids simultaneous connection to the stimulating electrodes, and consequent interaction between them. The Ineraid devices have been used because these have offered the best transparency in regard to complete control of the mode of signal presentation to the stimulating electrodes. Quite promising, even spectacular, improvements were derived from this approach compared with other methods of speech signal processing. The whole area is, however, in the very early stages of its evolution and given the extreme crudity of present techniques and the rapid parallel evolution of much more effective speech processing methods in other areas, substantial progress is to be expected. The percutaneous connector has the distinct advantage over transcutaneous techniques in respect of this intermediate phase of development because of the much greater control it affords in stimulation.

Reference

SINGH, W. and SOUTAR, D. S. (eds) (1993) *Functional Surgery of the Larynx and Pharynx*. Oxford: Butterworth-Heinemann

Further reading

ABBERTON, E. R. M., HOWARD, D. M. and FOURCIN, A. J. (1989) Laryngographic assessment of normal voice: a tutorial review. *Clinical Linguistics and Phonetics*, 3, 281–296
BAKEN, R.J. (1986) *Clinical Measurement of Speech and Voice*. London: Taylor and Francis
CODE, C. and BALL, M. (eds) (1995) *Experimental Clinical Phonetics*, 2nd edn. London: Whurr Publishers, vol. 30, no. 2, pp. 101–148
EUROPEAN SYMPOSIUM ON ELECTROLARYNGOGRAPHY and ELECTROPALATOGRAPHY (1995) *European Journal of Disorders of Communication*, 30,
HIRANO, M. and BLESS, D. (1993) *Videostroboscopic Examination of the Larynx*. London: Whurr Publishers
OWENS, F. J. (1993) *Signal Processing of Speech*. Basingstoke: Macmillan Press
PARSONS, T.W. (1987) *Voice and Speech Processing*. New York: McGraw-Hill
ROSEN, S. and HOWELL, P. (1991) *Signals and Systems for Speech and Hearing*. London: Academic Press
TITZE, I.R. (ed.) (1993) *Vocal Fold Physiology*. San Diego: Singular Publishing Group Inc

Acknowledgements

We are glad to acknowledge the help, data and advice that we have received from our colleagues: Evelyn Abberton, Darryl de Cunha, David Howells, Xinghei Hu, Angela King, David Miller, Ann Parker, Jianing Wei and Claude Simon.

15

Surgical anatomy of the skull base

C. M. Bailey

This chapter presents the surgical anatomy of the undersurface of the skull as it relates to the practice of otolaryngology; the intracranial aspect of the skull base is not discussed.

The description falls into two sections: first, a systematic topographical description of the anatomy of the skull base and structures beneath it; and second, an account of the anatomical basis of the lateral surgical approach to the skull base.

Overall topography of the skull base

The inferior aspect of the skull base is bounded in front by the upper incisor teeth, behind by the superior nuchal line of the occipital bone, and laterally by the remaining upper teeth, the zygomatic arch and its posterior root, and the mastoid process.

The region may be divided into posterior, central and anterior parts. The posterior part is separated from the central part by an arbitrary line drawn transversely through the anterior margin of the foramen magnum. The boundary between the central and anterior parts is the posterior border of the hard palate.

The *posterior skull base* comprises the occipital (muscular) area.

The *central skull base* can be subdivided into different bone areas that correspond to compartments underneath (van Huijzen, 1984) (Figure 15.1). It contains the pharyngeal, tubal, neurovascular, auditory and articular areas, and the infratemporal fossa.

The *anterior skull base*, on a lower level than the part behind, is formed by the hard palate and alveolar arches. It is part of the faciomaxillary structure, and will not be described further here (see Chapters 5 and 8).

Osteology of the skull base

Behind the faciomaxillary bones, the cranial base is made up of the occipital bone, temporal bones and part of the sphenoid bones.

Occipital bone

The occipital bone is convex posteriorly and encloses the foramen magnum, through which the cranial cavity communicates with the vertebral canal. The broad, curved plate behind and above the foramen magnum is termed the squamous part; the occipital condyle on each side of the foramen arises from the lateral part; and the thick, square piece in front of the foramen is the basiocciput.

The foramen magnum is oval in shape, with its long diameter lying anteroposteriorly. The fibrous dura mater is attached to the margins of the foramen; below, it is projected down the spinal canal as the spinal dura mater (theca); above, it sweeps up into the posterior cranial fossa. Within the dural sheath in the subarachnoid space, passing through the foramen, lie the lower medulla with the cervical roots of the spinal accessory nerves, the spinal arteries and veins, and the vertebral arteries.

The anterior margin of the foramen magnum gives attachment to a number of ligaments ascending from the axis: the membrana tectoria, vertical limb of the cruciform ligament, and the apical and pair of alar ligaments of the odontoid peg. The anterior atlanto-occipital membrane is attached to a ridge that joins the anterior poles of the occipital condyles; the posterior atlanto-occipital membrane is attached to the posterior edge of the foramen magnum.

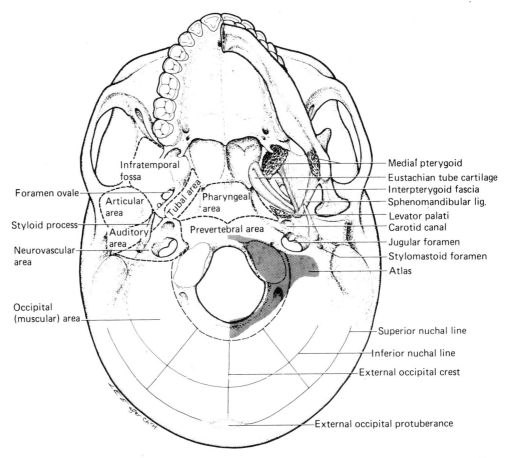

Figure 15.1 The skull base viewed from below. On the right half of the skull are indicated the regions of the central base; in the left half the mandible has been added in occlusion, with the interpterygoid fascia and eustachian tube in position. (From van Huijzen, 1984 with permission of the publishers, S. Karger)

The *squamous part* of the occipital bone gives attachment to the muscles of the back of the neck, and is described further in the section on the occipital (muscular) area of the skull base.

The *lateral part* gives rise to the occipital condyle on each side. Each condyle has a convex surface covered in hyaline cartilage which articulates with the concave surface of the atlas; these atlanto-occipital joints permit nodding only, rotation being the function of the atlanto-axial joints. Behind the condyle is a shallow fossa often perforated by the tiny posterior condylar canal, carrying a vein from the sigmoid sinus to the suboccipital venous plexus. In front of the condyle, just medial to the jugular foramen, lies the anterior condylar canal through which passes the XIIth nerve.

The *basiocciput* is an oblong block of bone which extends forward from the foramen magnum and fuses with the basisphenoid just behind the nose. The pharyngeal tubercle is a small protuberance in the midline, one-third of the way from the anterior margin of the foramen magnum to the posterior edge of the nasal septum. In front of the tubercle, the bone forms the roof of the nasopharynx and lies in the 'pharyngeal area' described in a following section. Behind it are attached the uppermost prevertebral muscles, with the longus capitis lying in front of the rectus capitis anterior. Separating the nasopharynx from the prevertebral region is the pharyngobasilar fascia with the prevertebral fascia just behind it.

Temporal bone

The temporal bone is made up of four parts which ossify separately and later fuse. The squamous part contributes the 'articular area' to the skull base, but most of it is in the temporal fossa on the side of the skull. The petromastoid part forms an important and complicated portion of the skull base lateral to the occipital bone. The tympanic plate, rolled like a tube open at the top, lies below the petrous and squamous parts, and just behind it the styloid process projects from the petrous bone.

The *squamous temporal bone* contains the hollow of the glenoid fossa with, in front, the convex eminentia articularis joined laterally to the zygomatic process. This area lies almost wholly within the temporomandibular joint, with only a small triangular part anterior to the joint forming part of the infratemporal surface of the skull.

The *petromastoid bone* projects forwards and medially at 45°, wedged between the basiocciput and the greater wing of the sphenoid; at the apex of the wedge the three bones do not quite meet, leaving a gap termed the 'foramen lacerum'. Although called a foramen, this is a canal almost 1 cm long through which no structure passes completely, although some do partially. The most important of these is the internal carotid artery which enters the posterior wall, together with its venous and sympathetic plexus, and traverses the superior part of the foramen.

More laterally, along the junction between the petrous bone and the greater wing of the sphenoid, lies the cartilaginous portion of the eustachian tube, running posterolaterally into the bony part of the tube where it is overhung by the spine of the sphenoid. Just posterior to this is the carotid foramen, separated by a ridge of bone from the jugular foramen behind.

Lateral to the carotid and jugular foramina lies the *tympanic bone*. Laterally, it forms the bony part of the external auditory canal, articulating with the squamous bone of the glenoid fossa in front (squamotympanic fissure) and the mastoid bone behind (tympanomastoid fissure). Medially, it forms the floor of the hypotympanum. The medial part of the squamotympanic fissure becomes divided by a thin flange of petrous bone (the projecting margin of the tegmen tympani), so creating a petrosquamous fissure in front and a petrotympanic fissure behind.

Lateral to the jugular foramen, and tucked in close behind the tympanic bone, projects the *styloid process*, which is of very variable length. Behind its base lies the stylomastoid foramen, and further posteriorly the mastoid bone is indented by the digastric notch, medial to which there is a groove for the occipital artery.

Sphenoid bone

The greater wing of the sphenoid, with the medial and lateral pterygoid plates, contributes to the base of the skull.

The *greater wing* articulates with the squamous temporal bone to form the roof of the infratemporal fossa. Anteriorly, this infratemporal surface ends in the inferior orbital fissure behind the maxilla. Medially, the greater wing is edge-to-edge with the petrous bone, perforated by the foramen ovale anteriorly and the foramen spinosum posteriorly; in front, it ends in the pterygoid plates, and behind, in the spine of the sphenoid which is an important surgical landmark. Occasionally two smaller foramina exist as well: the foramen of Vesalius (medial to the foramen ovale) and the innominate foramen (posterior to the foramen ovale).

The *medial pterygoid plate* projects back from the lateral margin of the choanal opening, where it articulates with the vertical plate of the palatine bone. Inferiorly, it ends in the pterygoid hamulus, superiorly in the pterygoid tubercle which projects back into the foramen lacerum. Halfway up the posterior edge is a spur, from which a ridge runs upwards and laterally towards the opening of the bony eustachian tube, enclosing the concave scaphoid fossa lateral to the pterygoid tubercle.

The *lateral pterygoid plate* extends back and laterally into the infratemporal fossa. Its only purpose is to give attachment to the pterygoid muscles.

Occipital (muscular) area

The superior nuchal line is a rather faint ridge that runs from the mastoid process to the external occipital protuberance, in a curve concentric with the foramen magnum (see Figure 15.1). Halfway between the superior nuchal line and the foramen magnum, and concentric with them, is another ill-defined ridge, the inferior nuchal line. The external occipital crest separates the two sides of the occipital area, running from the foramen magnum to the external occipital protuberance. Each half is then bisected by a very vague line radiating outwards from the foramen magnum to the superior nuchal line.

Thus each half of the occipital region is subdivided into four areas. The two alongside the foramen magnum receive the recti muscles. The medial area receives the rectus capitis posterior minor, which arises from the posterior arch of the atlas, is supplied by the posterior primary ramus of C1, and acts to extend the head. The lateral area receives the rectus capitis posterior major, which arises from the spinous process of the axis, is also supplied by C1, and acts to extend and rotate the head.

Between the superior and inferior nuchal lines, the medial area receives the semispinalis capitis, which arises from the transverse vertebral processes of C4–C7 and T1–T6, is supplied segmentally by posterior primary rami of the spinal nerves, and is the chief extensor of the head. The lateral area receives the superior oblique muscle, which arises from the lateral mass of the atlas, is supplied by C1, and acts primarily as a lateral flexor of the head; this muscle is covered laterally by the posterior parts of the insertions of splenius and sternomastoid into the superior nuchal line.

Pharyngeal area

Situated centrally in the skull base, this area forms the roof of the nasopharynx, and its boundaries are formed by the line of attachment of the pharyngeal wall. The pharyngeal constrictor muscles do not extend right up to the base of the skull but are attached to it by a rigid membrane, the pharyngobasilar fascia, and it is this which makes up the wall of the nasopharynx.

The *pharyngobasilar fascia* is attached to the skull base and medial pterygoid plates (that is to the back of the nose), and is thickened posteriorly into a pharyngeal ligament that continues inferiorly as the pharyngeal raphe. It is separated from the prevertebral muscles posteriorly by the prevertebral fascia. The origin of the pharyngobasilar fascia can be traced laterally from the pharyngeal tubercle across the basiocciput, to the petrous temporal bone just in front of the carotid foramen (see Figure 15.1). It then swings anteromedially, its attachment running along the cartilaginous eustachian tube to reach the sharp posterior edge of the medial pterygoid plate, to which it is attached all the way down to the hamulus. The lower edge of the pharyngobasilar fascia lies at the level of the hamuli and the hard plate, within the superior constrictor muscle.

It will be seen that the apex of the petrous bone (and the foramen lacerum) lies within a lateral recess of the nasopharynx, the fossa of Rosenmüller. The levator palati muscle arises here and is, therefore, intrapharyngeal, covered medially by mucous membrane. A postnasal carcinoma involving the fossa of Rosenmüller may invade upwards through the foramen lacerum, sometimes producing a lateral rectus palsy by compressing the VIth nerve where it crosses the apex of the petrous bone and enters the cavernous sinus.

Tubal area

The tubal area lies just lateral to the pharyngeal area, and simply comprises the region occupied by the eustachian tube (see Figure 15.1). Anteriorly, it includes the scaphoid fossa at the base of the medial pterygoid plate, from where it runs posterolaterally along the slit that lies between the petrous bone and the greater wing of the sphenoid until the bony eustachian tube is reached just in front of the carotid canal.

The bony part of the *eustachian tube* is about 1 cm long, and tapers down from the anterior wall of the middle ear to its junction with the cartilaginous part of the tube. This junction, the isthmus, is the narrowest part of the tube and lies just medial to the spine of the sphenoid. The cartilaginous part of the eustachian tube (2 cm long), runs forwards and medially at 45° and downwards at 30°, to open into the nasopharynx

by way of a trumpet-shaped orifice attached to the back of the medial pterygoid plate just above the pharyngobasilar fascia. The eustachian tube cartilage is an important landmark in base of skull anatomy. Along its lateral aspect, a straight line passes from the lateral pterygoid plate along the medial lip of the foramen ovale to the foramen spinosum and into the petrotympanic fissure (Bosley and Martinez, 1986).

The *salpingopharyngeus* muscle arises from the posterior margin of the tubal orifice and runs vertically down inside the pharynx to be inserted into the posterior border of the thyroid cartilage and the adjacent pharyngeal wall. It is innervated by the pharyngeal plexus from the pharyngeal branch of the vagus nerve and its contraction assists in opening the tube.

The pharyngobasilar fascia is attached to the undersurface of the eustachian tube, and the two 'paratubal' muscles arise one on each side of it. The levator palati arises medially (within the pharynx) and the tensor palati arises laterally (outside the pharynx). Both muscles are partly attached to the tube, and so open it during the act of swallowing. The paratubal muscles are fully described in the section on the parapharyngeal space.

Neurovascular area

Posterior to the tubal area lies the neurovascular area, containing the structures of the carotid sheath and styloid apparatus, as well as the facial nerve (see Figure 15.1).

Carotid sheath

The carotid sheath itself is not a membranous fascia, but a dense feltwork of areolar tissue that surrounds the internal carotid artery and vagus nerve; it is virtually absent over the internal jugular vein, which enables it to expand greatly during periods of increased blood flow. The carotid sheath is attached to the skull base around the carotid foramen and continues downwards as far as the aortic arch.

In the neck, the carotid sheath, together with the pretracheal fascia, is firmly attached anteriorly to the deep surface of sternomastoid. Posteriorly, it is not attached to the prevertebral fascia, but is free to slide over it. This means that pus tracking laterally from a parapharyngeal abscess passes behind the sheath and behind the sternomastoid, to a point in the posterior triangle.

The *internal carotid artery* passes vertically upwards from the carotid bifurcation in the neck to enter the carotid foramen (see Plate 1/15/I). It has no branches, but carries with it the carotid plexus of sympathetic nerves from the superior cervical ganglion.

The jugular foramen is divided by two transverse septa of fibrous dura (which may ossify) into three compartments. The anterior compartment is occupied by the IXth cranial nerve and the inferior petrosal sinus; the middle compartment is shared by the Xth and XIth nerves; and the posterior compartment is filled by the emerging internal jugular vein. The IXth and XIth nerves lie more laterally than the Xth in the foramen.

The *internal jugular vein* descends from the jugular bulb to lie behind the internal carotid artery on the lateral mass of the atlas (see Plate 1/15/II) just below the base of the skull, it receives the inferior petrosal sinus. As it descends, it passes across on to the lateral side of the internal carotid artery, receiving tributaries from the pharyngeal plexus of veins, and crossed on its lateral side by the accessory nerve. Also on the lateral side of the vein lie the deep cervical lymph nodes.

The *glossopharyngeal nerve* (IX) lies lateral to the inferior petrosal sinus as it emerges from the anterior part of the jugular foramen (see Plates 1/15/III and 1/15/IV). The nerve passes down on the lateral surface of the internal carotid artery and then gently curves forward around the lateral side of stylopharyngeus, medial to the external carotid artery towards the tongue.

The *vagus nerve* (X) emerges from its superior ganglion in the middle compartment of the jugular foramen and runs straight down in the back of the carotid sheath between the carotid artery and jugular vein (see Plates 1/15/III and 1/15/IV). Just below the skull base, it is dilated into its inferior ganglion, where it receives a connection from the accessory nerve carrying fibres from the nucleus ambiguus.

The *accessory nerve* (XI) is just lateral to the vagus in the middle compartment of the jugular foramen (see Plates 1/15/III and 1/15/IV). It immediately begins to curve away posteriorly across the lateral surface of the internal jugular vein, medial to the styloid process and posterior belly of the digastric, giving a branch to the sternomastoid before piercing the muscle to gain the posterior triangle.

The *hypoglossal nerve* (XII) emerges from the anterior condylar foramen, medial to the carotid sheath, and spirals in a lateral direction behind the vagus between the internal jugular vein and internal carotid artery (that is through the carotid sheath) (see Plates 1/15/III and 1/15/IV). It then swings forward lateral to the carotid arteries, deep to the styloid muscles and digastric, on its way to the tongue.

The *cervical sympathetic trunk* lies behind the carotid sheath in front of the prevertebral fascia, just medial to the vagus nerve. It ends superiorly at the superior cervical ganglion.

Styloid apparatus

From the tip of the styloid process, the stylohyoid ligament passes downwards and forwards to the lesser cornu of the hyoid bone. All these structures are derived from the second branchial arch cartilage. The stylomandibular ligament is not a distinct structure, but merely a condensation of the deep layer of the parotid fascia between the base of the styloid process and the angle of the mandible almost directly below it.

Three muscles diverge from the styloid process: the stylopharyngeus, the stylohyoid and the styloglossus (see Plate 1/15/V). All three have a different nerve supply, but all three participate in the mechanism of swallowing.

The *stylopharyngeus* arises from the deep aspect of the base of the styloid process, slopes down across the lateral aspect of the internal carotid artery, and is inserted into the thyroid cartilage and side wall of the pharynx. It is supplied by the IXth nerve, and elevates the larynx and the pharynx.

The *stylohyoid* arises from the back of the base of the styloid process, and slopes downwards and forwards to be inserted by two slips (which pass on either side of the intermediate tendon of the digastric) into the base of the greater cornu of the hyoid. It passes lateral to the external carotid artery. It is supplied by the VIIth nerve, and elevates and retracts the hyoid.

The *styloglossus* arises from the front of the styloid process and upper part of the stylohyoid ligament. It crosses lateral to the internal carotid artery and then swings forward medial to the lingual nerve to reach its insertion into the side of the tongue. It is supplied by the XIIth nerve, and retracts the tongue.

The external carotid artery is closely adjacent to the muscles of the styloid apparatus. It passes deep to the stylohyoid (and the digastric), but lies superficial to stylopharyngeus and styloglossus muscles, on its way to enter the parotid gland. The retromandibular vein, on the other hand, runs superficially to all elements of the styloid apparatus.

Facial nerve (VII)

The stylomastoid foramen transmits the facial nerve and the stylomastoid artery. As soon as it emerges from the foramen, the facial nerve gives off the posterior auricular nerve (supplying the occipital belly of occipitofrontalis) and a muscular branch (supplying posterior belly of digastric and stylohyoid). It then swings forward into the parotid gland, dividing as it does so into upper and lower divisions which then redivide to form the plexus of the pes anserinus within the substance of the gland.

Auditory area

This small area anterolateral to the neurovascular

area comprises the steeply sloping face of the tympanic bone, forming as it does the floor and anterior wall of the external auditory canal and middle ear.

At the anteromedial edge of the area lies the petrotympanic fissure of Glaser (already described in the section on the osteology of the temporal bone). This transmits the chorda tympani and anterior tympanic branch of the maxillary artery, and the corresponding veins which drain into the pterygoid plexus.

The *chorda tympani* emerges from the petrotympanic fissure and indents the spine of the sphenoid before joining the lingual nerve 2 cm below the skull base.

Articular area

This area, immediately in front of the auditory area, is the surface on which the head of the mandible articulates (by way of an intervening fibrocartilaginous disc). It is bordered by the attachment of the joint capsule, anteriorly just in front of the eminentia articularis, posteriorly to the squamotympanic fissure, and medially and laterally to the margins of the mandibular fossa.

Infratemporal fossa

The infratemporal fossa lies below the middle cranial

fossa, between the ramus of the mandible and the lateral wall of the pharynx (Figures 15.2, 15.3 and 15.4).

Its roof is the infratemporal area of the skull base, which is made up by the greater wing of the sphenoid with a small triangular contribution posteriorly from the squamous temporal bone. It has no anatomical floor and continues down into the neck. Anteriorly lies the posterior wall of the maxilla with the pterygomaxillary and inferior orbital fissures; posteriorly, it is bounded by the carotid sheath and styloid apparatus. The fossa is limited medially by the medial pterygoid muscle and interpterygoid fascia, and laterally by the mandible.

The contents of the fossa are the lateral and medial pterygoid muscles, the maxillary artery and its branches, the pterygoid venous plexus, the maxillary veins, and the branches of the mandibular nerve.

Lateral pterygoid muscle

This muscle arises from two heads: the upper head from the whole infratemporal surface of the skull, and the lower head from the outer surface of the lateral pterygoid plate. The heads converge posteriorly into a tendon which is inserted into the pterygoid pit at the medial end of the mandibular condyle (see Plate 1/15/VI). It is supplied by the Vth nerve (mandibular division); bilateral contraction opens the mouth and protrudes the chin by pulling the condyles

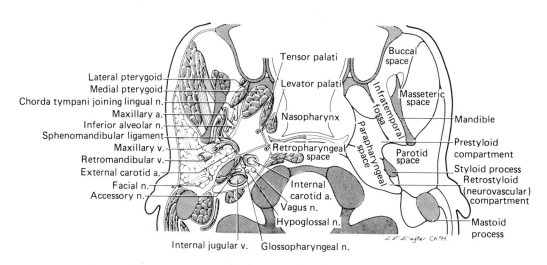

Figure 15.2 Central part of a horizontal section of the head passing through the foramen magnum, between the eustachian tube and the palate. In the left half all relevant structures have been drawn; on the right the different compartments are indicated as they appear at this level. (From van Huijzen, 1984 with permission of the publishers, S. Karger)

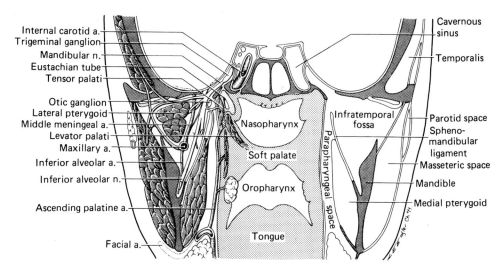

Figure 15.3 Coronal section of the head passing through the foramen ovale. On the left all relevant structures are illustrated; on the right the main compartments are shown. (From van Huijzen, 1984 with permission of the publishers, S. Karger)

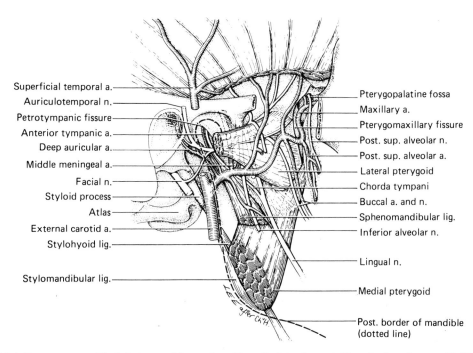

Figure 15.4 The structures of the infratemporal fossa, viewed from the lateral aspect. The veins have been omitted in order to permit a better view of the other structures. Part of the zygomatic arch has been removed. The posterior border of the mandible is indicated and the plane of attachment of both pterygoid muscles to the mandible can be seen. (From van Huijzen, 1984 with permission of the publishers, S. Karger)

forwards onto the eminentia articularis. Conversely their slow relaxation aids controlled jaw closure. Unilateral contraction swings the jaw to the opposite side.

Medial pterygoid muscle

The medial pterygoid arises from the medial surface of the lateral pterygoid plate and the fossa between the two plates; a small slip joins from the tuberosity of the maxilla and tubercle of the palatine bone. It passes outwards, downwards and backwards at 45° to its insertion into the angle of the mandible (see Plate 1/15/VI). It is supplied by the Vth nerve (mandibular division). Contraction aids closure of the jaw and in concert with the lateral pterygoids plays an important role in mastication.

Maxillary artery

The external carotid artery has two terminal branches, the superficial temporal and the maxillary (see Plate 1/15/I). The maxillary artery enters the infratemporal fossa between the sphenomandibular ligament and the neck of the mandible, and passes forward either lateral or medial to the lateral pterygoid muscle. If it takes the medial course, the artery then turns laterally again to emerge between the two heads of the muscle. It leaves the infratemporal fossa through the pterygomaxillary fissure to enter the pterygopalatine fossa.

The artery is traditionally described in three parts: before, on and beyond the lateral pterygoid muscle, with five branches coming from each part. From the first and third parts, the five branches all enter foramina in bones; from the second part, none of the branches go through bony foramina but supply the muscles of mastication (Last, 1973).

The *first part* gives off the inferior alveolar, middle meningeal, accessory meningeal, deep auricular and anterior tympanic arteries. The inferior alveolar artery passes down to join the inferior alveolar nerve and enter the mandibular foramen. The middle meningeal artery passes straight up through the foramen spinosum, while the accessory meningeal artery goes through the foramen ovale. The deep auricular artery passes superiorly to supply the external auditory canal and the anterior tympanic artery enters the petrotympanic fissure on its way to the middle ear (Davies, 1967).

The *second part* of the maxillary artery gives off five branches to the soft tissues: the lateral and medial pterygoid muscles, the temporalis muscle, the lingual and long buccal nerves.

The *third part* of the artery divides in the pterygopalatine fossa and will not be described further here.

The pterygoid plexus and maxillary veins

The pterygoid plexus of veins lies within and on the lateral surface of the lateral pterygoid muscle, and receives tributaries corresponding to the branches of the maxillary artery. The plexus drains into two short, large maxillary veins which pass horizontally backwards deep to the neck of the mandible to join the superficial temporal vein and form the retromandibular vein (see Plate 1/15/II).

The pterygoid plexus has three important communicating veins. The inferior ophthalmic veins pass to it through the inferior orbital fissure; a connecting vein passes vertically downwards from the cavernous sinus by way of the foramen ovale or, when present, the foramen of Vesalius; and the deep facial vein runs forwards beneath the zygoma to join the anterior facial vein. These connections can allow infection from the face to spread by way of the pterygoid plexus to the cavernous sinus and produce thrombosis.

The mandibular nerve

The mandibular nerve drops down through the foramen ovale and, after a short course just deep to the upper head of the lateral pterygoid muscle, the main trunk divides into anterior and posterior divisions (see Plate 1/15/III). Before it does so, the *main trunk* gives off the sensory nervus spinosus (which re-enters the middle fossa through the foramen spinosum), and the motor nerve to the medial pterygoid, which also supplies the tensor palati and tensor tympani.

The *anterior division* is entirely motor except for one branch, the long buccal nerve. The latter passes between the heads of the lateral pterygoid to swing forwards and downwards on the deep surface of the temporalis muscle, and then pierces the buccinator to supply the mucous membrane of the cheek. The motor branches supply the temporalis, masseter (by a branch which emerges through the mandibular notch) and the lateral pterygoid.

The *posterior division* is entirely sensory except for one branch, the mylohyoid nerve. The auriculotemporal nerve springs from two roots which pass either side of the middle meningeal artery, and passes backwards between the sphenomandibular ligament and neck of the mandible. The inferior alveolar nerve swings downwards on the surface of the medial pterygoid muscle, passes between the sphenomandibular ligament and neck of the mandible, and gives off the mylohoid nerve before entering the mandibular foramen. The lingual nerve is joined by the chorda tympani 2 cm below the base of the skull and passes downwards and forwards on the medial pterygoid, grooving the mandible before entering the mouth.

The *otic ganglion* lies close to the mandibular nerve just below the foramen ovale, between the nerve and the tensor palati muscle. It relays secretomotor fibres to the parotid gland, which it receives by way of the lesser superficial petrosal nerve and transmits to the auriculotemporal nerve. The lesser superficial petrosal nerve leaves the middle fossa through the foramen ovale, or sometimes through its own foramen, the foramen innominatum.

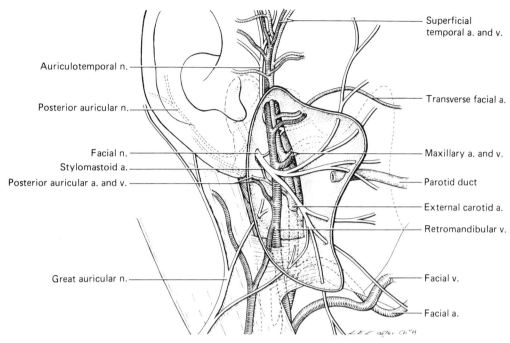

Figure 15.5 The structures of the parotid space viewed from the lateral aspect. The parotid gland has been removed from its capsule, leaving the vessels and nerves intact. (From van Huijzen, 1984, with permission of the publishers, S. Karger)

The sphenomandibular ligament

The sphenomandibular ligament is a fibrous band joining the spine of the sphenoid to the lingula of the mandibular foramen. It is derived from the first branchial arch (Meckel's) cartilage. Anteriorly, it blends into the interpterygoid fascia, which separates the lateral and medial pterygoid muscles, stretching forward as a sheet to be attached to the posterior edge of the lateral pterygoid plate.

Parotid space

The space enclosed within the capsule of the parotid gland lies partly superficial to the mandible, and extends through the retromandibular space behind the infratemporal fossa to abut against the parapharyngeal space (Figure 15.5 and see Figure 15.2). The parotid space is described in Chapter 9.

Parapharyngeal space
Prestyloid compartment

This compartment contains the two palati muscles and two arteries, the ascending palatine and ascending pharyngeal (Figure 15.6 and see Figures 15.2 and 15.3).

The *tensor palati muscle* arises from the skull base in a line from the scaphoid fossa along the edge of the greater wing to the spine of the sphenoid, and is also attached to the lateral side of the eustachian tube. It tapers down to a tendon which takes a right-angled turn around the hamulus to enter the pharynx, where it broadens into a flat aponeurosis; this triangular sheet blends with its counterpart on the opposite side and is attached to the posterior edge of the hard palate (the crest of the palatine bone). It is supplied by the Vth nerve by way of the nerve to the medial pterygoid. The action of this muscle is to tense the palate so that other muscles can raise and lower it.

The *levator palati muscle* arises from the petrous apex anterolateral to the carotid foramen and from the medial end of the tubal cartilage, and is inserted into the upper surface of the palatal aponeurosis. Supplied by the Xth nerve by way of the pharyngeal plexus, it acts to raise the soft palate and close off the nasopharynx.

The *ascending palatine artery*, a branch of the facial artery, ascends close to the pharyngeal wall to supply the soft palate and tonsil.

The *ascending pharyngeal artery*, a branch of the external carotid artery, ascends a little more posteriorly along the superior constrictor to supply the pharynx, the middle ear and the meninges. It is often a major feeding vessel to a glomus tumour.

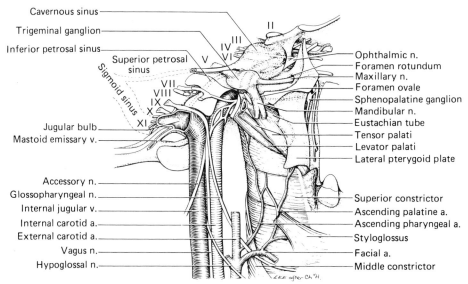

Cavernous sinus
Trigeminal ganglion
Inferior petrosal sinus
Superior petrosal sinus
Sigmoid sinus
Jugular bulb
Mastoid emissary v.
Accessory n.
Glossopharyngeal n.
Internal jugular v.
Internal carotid a.
External carotid a.
Vagus n.
Hypoglossal n.

Ophthalmic n.
Foramen rotundum
Maxillary n.
Foramen ovale
Sphenopalatine ganglion
Mandibular n.
Eustachian tube
Tensor palati
Levator palati
Lateral pterygoid plate
Superior constrictor
Ascending palatine a.
Ascending pharyngeal a.
Styloglossus
Facial a.
Middle constrictor

Figure 15.6 The structures of the parapharyngeal space and of the skull base above it, seen from the lateral aspect in a saggital section passing through the foramen ovale. (From van Huijzen, 1984 with permission of the publishers, S. Karger)

Retrostyloid compartment

This corresponds to the neurovascular space, and contains the carotid sheath (see previous section).

Structures within the skull base

The *internal carotid artery* curves forwards in the petrous bone from the carotid foramen, and then curves upwards into the upper part of the foramen lacerum in the middle fossa. It emerges at the apex of the petrous bone and immediately enters the cavernous sinus. It lies in front of the cochlea and middle ear cavity, separated from the middle ear and eustachian tube by a thin plate of bone which may be dehiscent. It gives off some small intrapetrous branches, including the caroticotympanic arteries, which may enlarge as feeding vessels for a glomus tumour.

The *jugular bulb* is the point at which the sigmoid sinus feeds into the upper end of the internal jugular vein. It usually lies below the posterior part of the floor of the middle ear, although its bony covering may be dehiscent, with only mucosa separating it from the middle ear cavity. However, its position is extremely variable and it may intrude right up into the middle ear ('high jugular bulb') (Graham, 1977). The inferior petrosal sinus joins the jugular bulb at the skull base; it emerges from the skull in the

anterior part of the jugular foramen and crosses either lateral or medial to the IXth, Xth and XIth nerves to enter the bulb. It is variable and may consist of three or more channels (Goldenberg, 1984).

The internal carotid artery diverges from the jugular bulb beneath the middle ear, leaving a wedge of bone between the two vessels (see Plate 1/15/IV) which is clearly shown on lateral hypocycloidal polytomography. Erosion of this 'keel' of bone is an early finding in patients with a glomus jugulare tumour.

The paths of the *IXth, Xth and XIth cranial nerves* in the jugular foramen, and of the XIIth cranial nerve at this level, have already been described (see subsection on the carotid sheath).

The *greater superficial petrosal nerve* enters the foramen lacerum from the middle fossa and is joined there by the deep petrosal nerve, which is a branch of the sympathetic carotid plexus. The two nerves unite to form the nerve of the pterygoid canal (Vidian nerve) which leaves the foramen lacerum in the pterygoid canal and runs forward to the pterygopalatine ganglion.

The *tympanic branch of the IXth nerve* (Jacobson's nerve) leaves the glossopharyngeal nerve at the petrous ganglion and passes through a canaliculus in the keel of petrous bone between the jugular and carotid foramina to supply the middle ear (tympanic plexus).

The *auricular branch of the Xth nerve* (Arnold's nerve) passes behind the internal jugular vein and enters the mastoid canaliculus on the lateral wall of the jugular foramen, from which it emerges by way of the tympanomastoid fissure to supply the skin of part of the external auditory meatus.

The anatomy of the ear within the petrous temporal bone is described in Chapter 1.

Muscles superficial to the lateral skull base

Four muscles which lie lateral, superficial to the base of the skull, are important in surgical exposure of the area (see Plate 1/15/VI).

The *masseter muscle* arises from the zygomatic arch and is inserted into a wide area on the lateral aspect of the mandible from the angle forwards along the lower border, and upwards over the lower part of the ascending ramus. It is supplied by the Vth nerve by way of the masseteric branch from the anterior division of the mandibular nerve, and its action is to close the jaws.

The *temporalis muscle* arises from the temporal fossa on the side of the skull, and from this large origin it converges in the shape of a fan to be inserted into the coronoid process of the mandible, mainly on its inner surface. It is supplied by the Vth nerve by way of the deep temporal branches of the anterior division of the mandibular nerve. Its contraction closes the jaws and its posterior fibres also retract the mandible.

The *sternomastoid muscle* arises from two heads: from the manubrium and clavicle. It is inserted into a curved line extending from the tip of the mastoid process to the superior nuchal line of the occiput. It is supplied by the XIth nerve together with branches of the IInd and IIIrd cranial nerves which may be sensory (proprioceptive). Its main action is to protract the head (moving it forwards while keeping it vertical with a horizontal gaze).

The *digastric muscle* arises from the digastric notch on the medial surface of the mastoid process and has as its name suggests, two bellies. The posterior belly narrows into an intermediate tendon which passes through a fibrous sling on the hyoid near the lesser cornu, and then expands into the anterior belly which runs beneath the mylohyoid to its insertion into the digastric fossa on the lower edge of the mandible. The posterior belly is supplied by the VIIth nerve (nerve to digastric) and the anterior belly by the Vth nerve (mylohyoid nerve). Its action is to depress and retract the chin.

Anatomical principles of the lateral surgical approach to the skull base

Many different surgical approaches have been employed to reach lesions in the rather inaccessible region of the skull base (Sasaki, McCabe and Kirchner, 1984; Samii and Draf, 1989; Jackson, 1991; Sekhar and Janecka, 1993). However, it is the lateral approach that has become established as the approach of choice for most otolaryngologists who work in this area (Goldenberg, 1984).

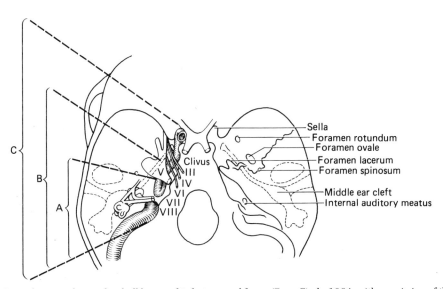

Figure 15.7 Lateral approaches to the skull base and infratemporal fossa. (From Fisch, 1984, with permission of the publishers, S. Karger)

The main difficulty in creating adequate exposure has been the long, tortuous course of the facial nerve, which prevents direct access. However, the technique of anterior transposition of the nerve demonstrated by Fisch (1977) has provided the access necessary for control of the internal carotid artery and internal jugular vein, and so has permitted satisfactory exploration of the lateral skull base. Fisch has developed four variants of this lateral approach,

which he loosely terms the 'infratemporal fossa approach' (Fisch, 1984) (Figures 15.7 and 15.8).

The type A approach provides access to the infralabyrinthine section of the temporal bone. The type B involves a more anterior approach and allows access to the petrous apex, the basiocciput and clivus. The type C approach takes the exposure even further forward, allowing the surgeon to remove lesions in the nasopharynx and parasellar regions, while the

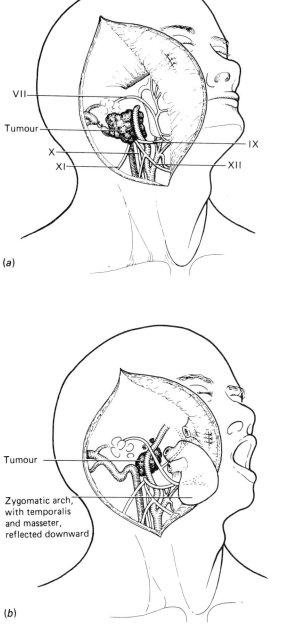

(a)

(b)

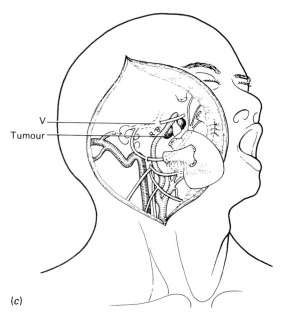

(c)

Figure 15.8 (*a*) Tumour exposure achieved by type A approach; (*b*) tumour exposure achieved by type B approach. The facial nerve is shown in anterior transposition (this is not necessary for lesions limited to the petrous apex); (*c*) tumour exposure achieved by type C approach. The superior division of the facial nerve with the frontal branch has been mobilized and transposed inferiorly. (From Fisch, Fagan and Valavanis, 1984, with permission of the publishers, W. B. Saunders)

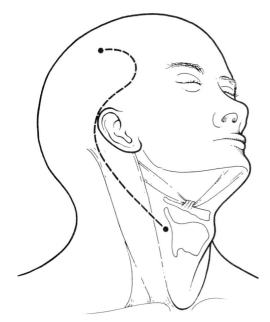

Figure 15.9 Skin incision for type A approach. (From Fisch, 1984, with permission of the publishers, S. Karger)

type D approaches are designed for access to the orbit and pterygopalatine fossa when control of the internal carotid artery is not critical.

Type A approach

This approach is employed primarily for the removal of glomus jugulare tumours and involves anterior transposition of the facial nerve.

A postauricular incision is extended down into the neck and up into the temporal region (Figure 15.9). An anteriorly based skin and periosteal flap is raised which transects the external auditory canal at the junction of its bony and cartilaginous parts. The external auditory meatus is closed as a blind sac, reinforced posteriorly by a musculoperiosteal flap. The remaining skin in the deep canal, together with the tympanic membrane, malleus and incus is completely removed.

Attention is then focused on the neck. The greater auricular nerve is identified and transected at a point where as much can be preserved as possible, in case it is needed as a graft later on. The facial nerve is exposed at the anterior border of the posterior belly of the digastric muscle, traced into the parotid gland and its main branches mobilized. The common, external and internal carotid arteries are then identified in the neck together with the hypoglossal, vagus and accessory nerves. Control tapes are passed around the external and internal carotid arteries and the carotid bifurcation is then elevated and dissected towards the jugular foramen.

The sternomastoid muscle is stripped from the mastoid tip and the digastric muscle transected in its mid-portion. This allows further dissection of the major vessels towards the skull base. A very thorough mastoidectomy is performed in which all the pneumatic spaces are exenterated and the fallopian canal skeletonized from the geniculate ganglion to the stylomastoid foramen. The remaining bone over the fallopian canal is then removed so that the facial nerve can be completely mobilized and transposed anteriorly into a groove cut in the tympanic bone (Figure 15.10). Following this, the sigmoid sinus is exposed from the sinodural angle down towards the jugular bulb. All overlying bone is removed and the sinus is clipped or ligated immediately below the mastoid emissary vein.

Attention is then directed to the anterior part of the dissection. The intratemporal part of the internal carotid artery is identified medial to the eustachian tube and the whole artery from its bifurcation in the neck to the horizontal segment in the temporal bone is exposed. The mucosa is stripped from the remaining eustachian tube, as far as the isthmus. The tube is then obliterated with muscle and bone wax so that CSF cannot track into the nasopharynx. Additional anterior exposure is obtained by removal of the styloid process and forward displacement of the ramus of the mandible. This gives complete control of the internal carotid artery and facilitates safe dissection of the anterior pole of the glomus tumour. Caroticotympanic arteries are encountered at this stage and need to be coagulated.

The superior and posterior tumour poles of the glomus tumour are dissected off the otic capsule and posterior fossa dura. Separation from the dura is achieved by opening the ligated sigmoid sinus and removing its lateral wall in continuity with the jugular bulb. Control of the inferior petrosal sinuses, which enter the medial wall of the jugular bulb, is achieved by packing each with haemostatic gauze. Finally, the inferior pole is removed in continuity with the rest of the tumour by separating it from the lower cranial nerves, IX, X, XI and XII, at the jugular foramen.

Large glomus jugulare tumours with intradural extension may demand a neurosurgical approach to remove the intradural portion of the tumour once the extradural part has been excised.

Type B approach

The type B approach is employed to expose the clivus in order to remove such lesions as chordomas, petrous apex cysts and cholesteatomas. The intitial stages of the operation are identical to those of the type A approach, but anterior facial nerve transposition is not usually necessary. However, in dissection of the intraparotid facial nerve, the frontal branch must be

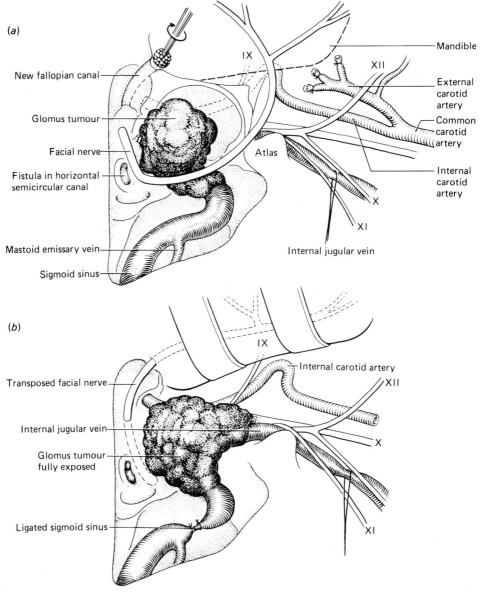

(a)

New fallopian canal

Glomus tumour

Facial nerve

Fistula in horizontal semicircular canal

Mastoid emissary vein

Sigmoid sinus

IX

XII

Mandible

External carotid artery

Common carotid artery

Atlas

Internal carotid artery

X

XI

Internal jugular vein

(b)

Transposed facial nerve

Internal jugular vein

Glomus tumour fully exposed

Ligated sigmoid sinus

IX

Internal carotid artery

XII

X

XI

Figure 15.10 (*a*) Exposure of glomus jugulare tumour by type A approach; (*b*) exposure of glomus jugulare tumour by type A approach after transposition of the facial nerve and ligation of the sigmoid sinus. (From Fisch, 1984, with permission of the publishers, S. Karger)

dissected free from the parotid as far forward as the lateral rim of the orbit, so that it can be displaced inferiorly without tension or stretching. The zygomatic arch is divided at its root and at the lateral aspect of the orbit following which the temporalis muscle together with the zygomatic arch and attached masseter muscle is reflected inferiorly, taking with them the mobilized frontal branch of the facial nerve.

The bone of the glenoid fossa is drilled away to

expose the temporomandibular joint and this allows the mandibular condyle to be removed or displaced inferiorly with a retractor. Further bone removal exposes the horizontal segment of the intratemporal portion of the internal carotid artery. With care, this can be completely mobilized and access gained to its entire medial surface as far as the foramen lacerum, together with the clivus. To achieve the maximum anterior exposure, the middle meningeal artery must be identified, coagulated and divided at the point where

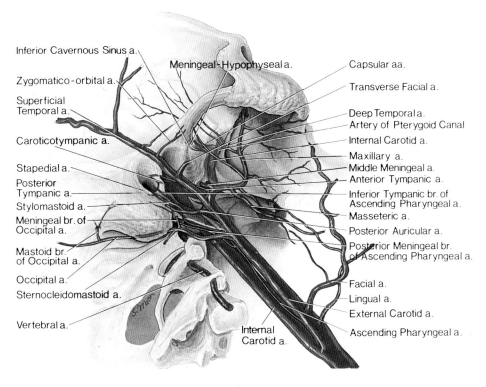

Plate 1/15/I The arteries of the central skull base.
(From Goldenberg, 1984, with permission of the author and publishers, *Laryngoscope*)

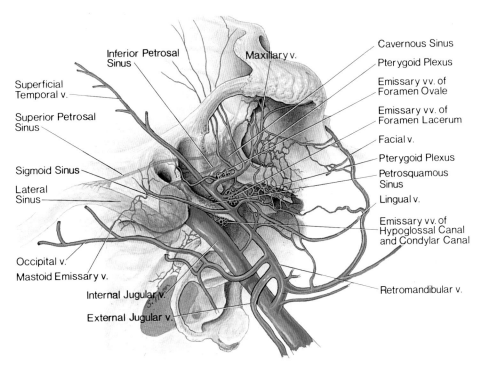

Plate 1/15/II The veins of the central skull base.
(From Goldenberg, 1984, with permission of the author and publishers, *Laryngoscope*)

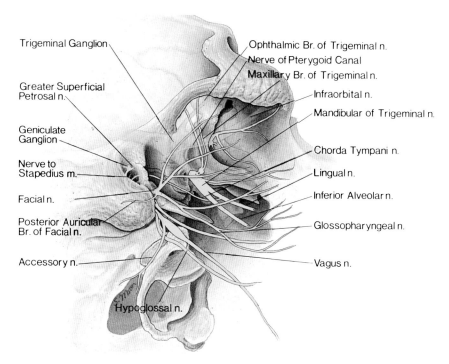

Trigeminal Ganglion

Ophthalmic Br. of Trigeminal n.

Nerve of Pterygoid Canal

Maxillary Br. of Trigeminal n.

Greater Superficial Petrosal n.

Infraorbital n.

Mandibular of Trigeminal n.

Geniculate Ganglion

Nerve to Stapedius m.

Chorda Tympani n.

Lingual n.

Facial n.

Inferior Alveolar n.

Posterior Auricular Br. of Facial n.

Glossopharyngeal n.

Accessory n.

Vagus n.

Hypoglossal n.

Plate 1/15/III The nerves of the central skull base.
(From Goldenberg, 1984, with permission of the author and publishers, *Laryngoscope*)

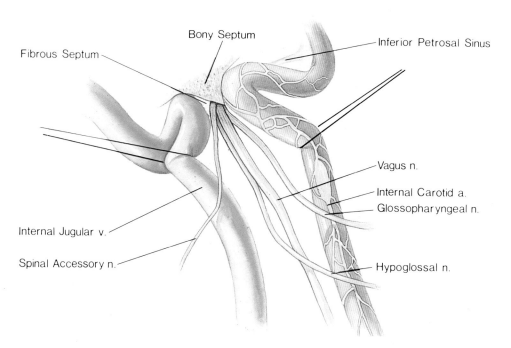

Fibrous Septum

Bony Septum

Inferior Petrosal Sinus

Vagus n.

Internal Carotid a.

Glossopharyngeal n.

Internal Jugular v.

Spinal Accessory n.

Hypoglossal n.

Plate 1/15/IV The structures in the jugular foramen.
(From Goldenberg, 1984, with permission of the author and publishers, *Laryngoscope*)

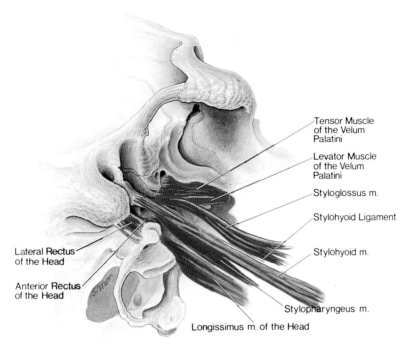

Tensor Muscle
of the Velum
Palatini

Levator Muscle
of the Velum
Palatini

Styloglossus m.

Stylohyoid Ligament

Stylohyoid m.

Lateral Rectus
of the Head

Anterior Rectus
of the Head

Stylopharyngeus m.

Longissimus m. of the Head

Plate 1/15/V The deep muscles of the central skull base.
(From Goldenberg, 1984, with permission of the author and publishers, *Laryngoscope*)

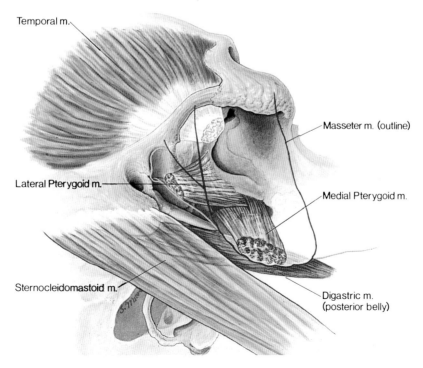

Temporal m.

Masseter m. (outline)

Lateral Pterygoid m.

Medial Pterygoid m.

Sternocleidomastoid m.

Digastric m.
(posterior belly)

Plate 1/15/VI The superficial muscles of the central skull base.
(From Goldenberg, 1984, with permission of the author and publishers, *Laryngoscope*)

it enters the foramen spinosum just anteromedial to the spine of the sphenoid. On rare occasions when even further anterior access is necessary, the mandibular nerve must be sectioned at the foramen ovale and it may also be necessary to remove the cochlea.

Type C approach

This approach can be employed for very anteriorly placed lesions in the nasopharyngeal, parasellar, retromaxillary and paratubal regions. A subtotal petrosectomy is carried out as for the type A and type B approaches, but anterior transposition of the facial nerve is not required.

The surgery is completed as for a type B approach, and then continues with detachment of the upper head of the lateral pterygoid muscle to expose the lateral pterygoid plate. Both pterygoid plates are removed and the maxillary nerve is sectioned at the foramen rotundum. The internal carotid artery can then be followed upwards as far as the cavernous sinus. Next, the pterygopalatine fossa is entered and, after division of the vidian nerve, the maxillary sinus, nasopharynx and sphenoid sinus may be exposed.

Type D approach

These recently described approaches are advocated for the resection of lesions in the orbit, the pterygopalatine fossa and posterior infratemporal fossa. Their use is restricted to the removal of tumours for which constant control of the infratemporal internal carotid artery is not necessary. As a result, these approaches offer the surgeon and the patient the potential benefit of maintaining hearing acuity on the affected side as the eustachian tube is neither opened nor removed.

A pre-auricular parotid incision is made, extended coronally as necessary to access the lateral orbital rim. A subtotal petrosectomy is not undertaken – in other words, the middle ear and its contents lie outside the operative field and remain intact. In the posterior variant of the type D approach, reflection of the zygomatic arch and subsequent removal of the temporomandibular joint and bone from the roof of

the infratemporal fossa is identical to that of the type C approach outlined above, but with the exception that the integrity of the eustachian tube is maintained and the internal carotid artery is not skeletonized. The anterior variant of the type D approach is the same but with osteotomies of the lateral orbital rim rather than the anterior zygomatic arch. This allows the entire lateral orbital complex, in continuity with the zygomatic arch, to be reflected inferiorly so that good access to the orbital can be achieved.

References

BOSLEY, J. H. and MARTINEZ, D. MCN. (1986) Practical surgical anatomy of the skull base. *Ear, Nose and Throat Journal*, **65**, 52–56

DAVIES D. V. (ed.) (1967) *Gray's Anatomy*, 34th edn. London: Longman. p. 794

FISCH, U. (1977) Infratemporal fossa approach for extensive tumors of the temporal bone and base of the skull. In: *Neurological Surgery of the Ear*, edited by H. Silverstein and N. Norrell. Birmingham: Aesculapius. pp. 34–53

FISCH, U. (1984) Infratemporal fossa approach for lesions in the temporal bone and base of the skull. *Advances in Oto-Rhino-Laryngology*, **34**, 254–266

FISCH, U., FAGAN, P. and VALAVANIS, A. (1984) The infratemporal fossa approach for the lateral skull base. *Otolaryngologic Clinics of North America*, **17**, 513–552

GOLDENBERG, R. A. (1984) Surgeon's view of the skull base from the lateral approach. *Laryngoscope*, **94** (Suppl. 36), 1–21

GRAHAM, M. D. (1977) The jugular bulb: its anatomic and clinical considerations in contemporary otology. *Laryngoscope*, **87**, 105–125

JACKSON, C. G. (ed.) (1991) *Surgery of Skull Base Tumors*. New York: Churchill Livingstone

LAST, R. J. (1973) *Anatomy, Regional and Applied*, 5th edn. London: Churchill Livingstone. p. 604

SAMII, M. and DRAF, W. (eds.) (1989) *Surgery of the Skull Base*. Berlin: Springer-Verlag

SASAKI, C. T., MCCABE, B. F. and KIRCHNER, J. A. (eds.) (1984) *Surgery of the Skull Base*. Philadelphia: Lippincott

SEKHAR, L. N. and JANECKA, I. P. (eds.) (1993) *Surgery of Cranial Base Tumors*. New York: Raven Press

VAN HUIJZEN, C. (1984) Anatomy of the skull base and the infratemporal fossa. *Advances in Oto-Rhino-Laryngology*, **34**, 242–253

16

Clinical neuroanatomy

John Philip Patten

Although this chapter is included in the basic sciences volume, the applied aspect is of such importance in differential diagnosis of diseases affecting neuro-otolaryngological function that some licence has been taken to indicate, whenever possible, the significance of both anatomy and physiology in disease states and differential diagnosis.

In some instances gross anatomy is of great importance and in others complex central connections require detailed elaboration to illustrate and explain clinical disorders. The following account is always biased in the direction of practical applications and information of limited or dubious clinical importance has been excluded.

The cranial nerves fall into three major groupings both in functional and gross anatomical similarities and share common anatomical relationships and pathology. Differing patterns of involvement within these groups allow very accurate differential diagnoses to be advanced, based on both the sequencing and ultimate extent of damage to nerves in these groups. The advent of computer assisted tomography and magnetic resonance imaging, has added remarkably to our ability to confirm or refute clinically-based diagnosis in this hitherto investigational no-man's-land. The ability to reconstruct slice scans in both sagittal and coronal planes has further transformed diagnostic accuracy. Interpretation still requires a very good grasp of gross anatomical relationships of the intracranial and extracranial courses of the cranial nerves and these anatomical features will form the bulk of this chapter.

The groupings are:

1 Cranial nerves I, II, III, IV and VI and the final distribution of the cervical sympathetic nerve
2 Cranial nerves V, VII and VIII

3 Cranial nerves IX, X, XI and XII and the cervical components of the sympathetic chain.

The influences of cerebellar, pyramidal, extra-pyramidal and corticobulbar dysfunction on these nerves and peripheral evidences of disordered brain-stem function will be detailed at the end of the chapter, or where appropriate.

Group one

In the first group the close relationship of the olfactory and optic nerves and the varying relationships of the three nerves supplying the extraocular muscles is considered. It is also necessary to note the relationships of the first division of the Vth nerve, which traverses the orbit, to these structures, although the detailed anatomy of this nerve is dealt with in group two.

The olfactory nerve (I)

Anatomy (Figure 16.1)

The olfactory epithelium lies in the olfactory cleft which occupies the upper 10 mm of the nasal septum, the roof of the nasal cavity and down the lateral wall towards the origin of the superior concha. In humans its total surface area is some 5 cm². It is a yellowish colour. In other species increasing pigmentation is associated with increased sensitivity to odours. The mucosa is bathed in a lipid-rich secretion from the epithelial Bowman's glands, indicating that lipid solubility may be a critical factor in odour detection. The olfactory receptor cells, some 5 million in all, lie on

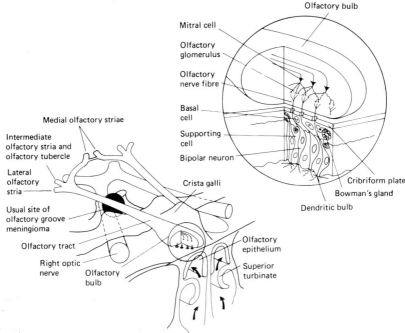

Figure 16.1 The olfactory pathways

the basal epithelium and extend vertically to the surface from which the terminal enlargement protrudes and gives rise to 8–20 olfactory cilia. Although these have the $9 + 2$ fibril arrangement of mobile cilia in other areas, they are thought to be non-motile and form a dense mat of fibrils lying on the surface of the epithelium. Pinocytic vacuoles have been demonstrated in the terminal enlargement of the receptor cells but their functional significance is uncertain (Fitzgerald, 1985).

The receptor cells are derived from ectoderm and are unique in being replaced from stem cells every 30–50 days. They also enter the CNS as very thin $(0.1–0.4\ \mu m)$ non-myelinated axons without synapse. These axons become grouped and ensheathed by Schwann cells forming some 20 fasciculi which, invested by pia and arachnoid mater, pass through the orifices of the cribriform plate to enter the olfactory bulbs, lying each side of the crista galli in the floor of the anterior cranial fossa. These axons synapse with dendrites of the large mitral cells in the olfactory glomeruli and each glomerulus receives axons from a wide area of the epithelium – there seems to be no functional grouping of axons. This allows a relatively small number of receptor cells to distinguish a large number of different odours. The axons of the mitral cells form the bulk of the olfactory tract but centrifugal axons of uncertain origin pass to the olfactory bulb and undoubtedly modify activity in the olfactory glomeruli, perhaps by both inhibitory and facilitatory action.

The olfactory tracts pass posteriorly and slightly laterally crossing the floor of the anterior cranial fossa, the optic nerves and immediately above the optic chiasm; just in front of the anterior perforated substance each divides into medial, intermediate and lateral olfactory striae.

The termination of the medial striae is uncertain. Many fibres decussate to the opposite medial striae and these may become the centrifugal fibres of the opposite olfactory tract having facilitatory and inhibitory effects on the opposite olfactory bulb. The intermediate striae terminate in the olfactory tubercle but its further functional anatomy is unknown. The lateral olfactory striae synapse with neurons in the lateral anterior perforated substance, the lateral olfactory gyrus, the pre-pyriform cortex and the medial group of amygdaloid nuclei – a group of tissues which in humans represents the primary olfactory cortex. These are the *only* sensory pathways in humans that do not relay in the thalamus. The distribution in the limbic system then contributes to both pleasurable and unpleasant consequences of odour detection at conscious level and the appropriate autonomic responses via the hypothalamus. This is related to activity in a secondary olfactory cortex in the entorhinal complex including the uncus and a tertiary olfactory cortex in the posterior orbitofrontal cortex. Descending pathways from these areas enter the pontine reticular formation in the brain stem, and mediate reflex activity such as salivation (Tanabe, Iino and Takagi, 1975).

Physiology

The receptor proteins lie in the olfactory cilia and it is likely that many different types of protein are involved. A smell must be volatile to enter the cavity, actively sucked into the area of the olfactory epithelium by sniffing, to create turbulant flow in the nasal passages, and lipid soluble to facilitate access to the fluid-bathed cilia.

Once stimulated, the activity in the neuron is difficult to study. Attempts at single fibre analysis are technically almost impossible and such studies as are available demonstrate no similarities in evoked potentials from similar groups of substances or stimuli. There is considerable evidence that some odours inhibit as well as excite and one must add to this an anatomical arrangement which allows not only local inhibition and excitation but crossed and possibly centrally-mediated control by both lateral and negative feedback mechanisms. This allows humans to identify some 3000 different odours. The central pathways clearly allow for further discrimination and perhaps clarification of odour recognition. In contrast is the remarkable process of adaptation that allows continuous exposure to an unpleasant smell to diminish perception so that the smell no longer registers.

Several theories to explain odour appreciation exist. One is based on receptor site configuration but it seems unlikely that sufficient variation in shape exists to explain the full range of odours. The lack of structural similarity between chemicals that smell the same makes this explanation unlikely as a sole mechanism (Amoore, 1963). A second theory, partially utilizing structural chemical considerations combined with molecular vibration, has been proposed and some support for this is found in that chemicals with similar frequency of vibration but different chemical structure, do have a similar smell (Wright, 1964). The most acceptable theory suggests that a dissolved molecule of specific size and shape is adsorbed onto and penetrates the receptor membrane leaving a temporary hole, which allows local depolarization of a size, rate and duration proportional to the molecule characteristics. Even this cannot explain all the features of olfaction and it is probable that a combination of all three possibilities is involved (Davies and Taylor, 1959).

Applied anatomy and physiology

Of immediate otolaryngological concern are simple mechanical factors interfering with access of the odour to the receptors, with simple airway obstruction, complicated by oedema or drying up of the mucosa as the most common causes of trouble. Mechanical destruction or blockage of the nasal passages by pathology ranging from allergic rhinitis to complex vascular diseases such as Wegener's granulomatosis

can occur. Simple polyps, nasal fractures and foreign bodies all have similar effects.

Many drugs and generalized medical conditions that can damage or interfere with a highly metabolically active tissue with a 30–50 day turnover rate, can also affect smell. These include generalized metabolic disorders such as renal failure, hepatic failure, endocrine disorders, including diabetes and influenza. Drugs affecting membrane moistness (antihistamines), cell turnover (antibiotics, antimetabolites) and cell function (anti-inflammatory agents, antithyroid drugs) may all affect both smell and taste (Schiffman, 1983).

Traumatic lesions of the olfactory fasciculi are caused by the shearing effect of brain movement when the head decelerates during a head injury. This complicates some 30% of serious head injuries particularly where immediate anteroposterior forces are applied to the head, so that a fall squarely onto the occiput is particularly likely to result in this complication. In such cases little or no recovery can be anticipated. Severe injury of this type may also tear the arachnoid cuffs and lead to CSF rhinorrhoea with a significant risk of subsequent meningitis.

There is circumstantial evidence that viral infections may gain access to the meninges via the same route in the absence of prior injury, herpes simplex encephalitis being a notable example. In the latter condition the initial localization of the infection to the anterior temporal lobes gives support to this theory of aetiology, the virus presumably gaining access along the olfactory tract, possibly by axonal transport (Johnson and Mims, 1978). This is not the whole answer as in 25% of cases the virus isolated from the serum is a different strain to that in the oropharyngeal mucosa.

Inside the skull, tumours of the olfactory groove, notably meningiomas will produce unilateral anosmia, usually unrecognized by the patient. Due to the local anatomy, progressive visual loss in the same eye follows – also often unrecognized by the patient. It is very important to test the sense of smell in any patient with sudden loss of vision in one eye.

At central level, disorders of smell appreciation are not recognized. Most patients who complain of a constant awful smell sensation or altered smell appreciation are suffering from a depressive or psychotic illness. The most readily identifiable centrally-based disorder is uncinate epilepsy, in which an epileptic event originating in the temporal lobe is ushered in by the hallucination of an unpleasant smell (and occasionally taste). These olfactory hallucinations are characterized by being both unpleasant and of extremely short duration, usually only a matter of seconds, often insufficient to enable the patient to identify the odour as other than unpleasant – burning rubber or rotting rubbish being the commonest description volunteered.

Considerable degeneration of the olfactory

glomeruli occurs with age and olfaction is the first sensory modality to be impaired by increasing age and is probably responsible for the decreasing appetite and loss of interest in food noted by the elderly (Schiffman, 1979).

The optic nerve (II)

The orbit is entirely surrounded by structures of otolaryngological significance, only the lateral border being relatively spared from possible infection or invasive pathology. The frontal, ethmoid and maxillary sinuses and the lateral wall of the nose bound the orbit superiorly, medially and inferiorly and are all prone to infection or malignant pathology.

The optic nerve enters the orbit through a tight canal, the optic foramen. The nerve is a direct extension of the brain and is invested with glial-derived tissue to the back of the globe, consisting of three membranes. The inner pial sheath invests the nerve and sends septae into the nerve itself dividing the nerve into a bundle of fascicles. The intermediate arachnoid sheath is very delicate with a potential subarachnoid space inside it and a subdural space outside. These are covered by a thick extension of the dura which merges with the sclera in the back of the globe. These membranes form a direct communication to the intracranial space and are responsible for the direct transmission of raised intracranial pressure to the optic disc causing papilloedema, although the exact mechanism of the disc swelling remains uncertain, venous compression almost certainly playing a role.

The myelinated fibres of the optic nerve are derived from the rods and cones of the retina. As these cell processes form the most superficial layer of the retina, they are normally non-myelinated until they enter

the disc. Occasional patches of myelination of these fibres as they cross the retina produce a characteristic white, fan-shaped lesion in the fundus and a field defect which is unrecognized by the patient, in the same way that one is unaware of the normal blind spot. The important papillomacular fibres conveying macular vision lie in the medial part of the nerve, only assuming their central position in the nerve at the optic foramen. In spite of this anatomy, extrinsic compression of the nerve in the orbit and the canal specifically affects these papillomacular fibres, producing a central scotoma rather than a defect spreading in from the periphery, as might be anticipated based purely on anatomical considerations (Figure 16.2).

There are 1.2 million fibres in each optic nerve, just over half of which decussate in the optic chiasm. The fibres which cross are those derived from the nasal retina, conveying the temporal half field, and enter the contralateral optic tract. The temporal half fibres (conveying the nasal field) pass straight into the ipsilateral optic tract.

Lesions within the orbit tend to produce mechanical displacement of the globe with consequent proptosis and diplopia. The optic nerve itself seems remarkably resistant to damage by pressure and displacement in the orbit, although an infective process may be more damaging by vascular mechanisms (Forrest, 1949; Font and Perry, 1976).

Lesions in the optic canal readily cause visual disturbance and a central scotoma is often the first evidence of a lesion at this site, followed by extraocular nerve palsies and very much later, proptosis. Meningiomas or neurofibromas of the optic nerve sheath are perhaps the most frequent tumours in the posterior orbit. Neoplastic infiltration from the paranasal sinuses and nasopharynx can occur and metastatic spread from remote sites such as the

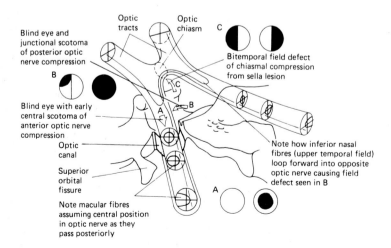

Figure 16.2 The visual pathways

prostate or suprarenal gland are well recognized. In general, the tempo of development of the signs and the presence or absence of pain will indicate the likely diagnosis (Takashi, 1956). The slow pain-less onset of symptoms usually indicates a benign lesion and rapidly evolving symptoms accompanied by pain indicate a metabolic or infective process in the area.

Involvement of the optic nerve immediately behind the optic foramen can produce bilateral visual prob-lems. The inferior nasal fibres of the opposite optic nerve not only cross in the chiasm but then sweep forwards into the optic nerve before turning sharply and then heading posteriorly into the chiasm and optic tract. They can be damaged by a lesion just *anterior* to the chiasm. A meningioma of the tubercu-lum sellae is the lesion most likely to be responsible. This can produce a blind eye, an upper temporal field defect in the contralateral eye (called a junctional scotoma) and, if large, can cause loss of smell on the same side as the blind eye and papilloedema in the *opposite* eye, disc swelling in the blind eye being prevented by the compressing lesion. This constitutes the famous but extremely rare Foster-Kennedy syndrome.

The optic chiasm itself lies more posteriorly than is generally appreciated – it lies above and behind the pituitary gland, not on the groove in front of the pitu-itary fossa seen on the skull. Pathological processes in the pituitary region include not only pituitary tumours but neoplasia arising in the ethmoid or sphenoid sinus, mucocoele of the sphenoid sinus and a variety of aneurysms arising from the circle of Willis or the great vessels themselves. The importance of excluding vascular anomalies or aneurysms *before* embarking on a transnasal approach to the pituitary fossa is perhaps even more important now than in the days of the subfrontal approach when unrecog-nized aneurysms were encountered with occasional fatal results. Lesions extending up from the pituitary region damage the underside of the chiasm anteri-orly. This produces a bitemporal hemianopia which spreads down from the upper temporal field (the lower fibres derived from lower retinal cells – there-fore upper field), although such a field defect is rarely appreciated by the patient at this stage or indeed occasionally even when complete. When testing the temporal fields particular attention should be paid to the upper temporal field to avoid missing a junctional scotoma (see previous section) or the earliest signs of a developing bitemporal hemianopia. In contrast, le-sions damaging the chiasm from above and behind, tend to affect the lower fields first – these include craniopharyngiomas, hypothalamic tumours and a dilated third ventricle. Field defects in this area are much more readily identified by the patient as they intrude into all activities especially reading and walk-ing down stairs.

Because there are many situations in which the visual fields are of help in otolaryngological diagnosis, it is worth describing simple field examination at the bedside. Carefully examined fields, using a red and white hatpin should be as accurate as screen testing and should only take a few minutes. The examiner should sit in front of the patient (in the traditional otolaryngological position) about 1 m from the pa-tient. The patient should cover one eye. A white 5 mm hatpin, preferably mounted on the handle of a tendon hammer, should be brought into the patient's field of vision on four arcs, upper and lower temporal and upper and lower nasal, respectively. If all are seen at the periphery, no field cut is likely. The pin should then be brought across from the temporal field on a horizontal meridian, the patient keeping the examiner's pupil in view. The blindspot should be detected readily and can be compared with that of the examiner, both parties losing the object in the same area. Following across into the nasal field any small scotoma will be indicated by the pin disappear-ing again. The size and shape of the scotoma can then be readily explored and even a small scotoma can be easily confirmed by this technique. At a more sophisticated level, the very earliest evidence of a field defect can be found with the red pin. Care has to be taken not to confuse the normal loss of brightness of a red object in the temporal half field as indicating an early field defect.

Differential diagnosis of the painful red eye (Sergott, 1983)

Otolaryngologists are often involved in cases where blurred vision and diplopia occur in the setting of an inflamed, proptosed eye and may well be the first doctors to see the patient. Diagnosis falls into four main groups of disorders – inflammatory, vascular, infective and neoplastic.

Inflammatory causes

Acute thyroid exophthalmos

The eye is often injected with chemosis. Lid lag is especially noticable on downward gaze. There may be diplopia due to globe displacement although paraly-sis of the superior and lateral rectus muscles is not uncommon. The condition is usually unilateral. Vision may be threatened and acute high dose ster-oids may be of value in treatment. A CT scan will show swelling of the extraocular muscles.

Pseudotumour of the orbit

This is an immunologically-based inflammatory disor-der affecting all tissues in the orbit. It can complicate sarcoid, systemic lupus erythematosus, tuberculosis, Wegener's granulomatosis, polyarteritis nodosa or the Tolosa-Hunt syndrome. Proptosis, pain and diplopia associated with a very high sedimentation rate, might all seem to indicate infection. As steroids are indicated, urgent exclusion of infective disease in the paranasal sinuses is vital. CT scans show normal extraocular muscles in the midst of oedematous orbital contents and will exclude coexistent sinus infection. The condition occurs in two main age groups – between 10 and 30 years and in the over 60s.

Vascular causes

Acute caroticocavernous fistula

This condition usually follows known trauma but occasionally an aneurysmal dilatation of the carotid may rupture into the cavernous sinus producing acute pulsating exophthalmus with marked arterial pulsation in the fundal veins. Carotid ligation or embolization is the procedure of choice.

Cavernous haemangioma

This produces a gradual exophthalmus with proptosis aggravated by bending or straining. There is usually no diplopia or field defect and little pain.

Infective causes

Local infections can readily spread into the orbit. Small boils on the nose, eyelids or face in the pre-antibiotic era had lethal potential. Paranasal sinus infection, especially of the ethmoids can easily extend directly into the orbit and frontal sinusitis, usually causes oedema of the eyelid and ptosis. In the diabetic patient all these infections carry even greater risk and additional specific problems such as mucormycosis and other rare fungal infections. The first vesicles of herpes zoster ophthalmicus usually erupt in the eyebrow after several days of severe pain and the acute red eye and oedematous lids may be mistaken for bacterial infection until the vesicles appear.

Neoplastic causes

Any primary or secondary neoplasm may involve the orbit, the latter by direct extension or from remote sites. Usually chemosis and injection are not marked. In the elderly, pseudotumour of the orbit can be a presenting symptom of lymphoma and, as always, the importance of a general physical examination must be emphasized.

Benign primary orbital tumours most often seen are lipomas, angiomas and haemangiomas. Less frequently, fibromas, myxomas and leiomyomas may be encountered.

Malignant primary orbital tumours are usually rhabdomyosarcomas which are locally invasive and usually occur in childhood. Rarely, fibrosarcoma, myxosarcoma, liposarcoma, chondrosarcoma, osteogenic sarcoma and haemangioendotheliomas may occur. Lacrimal gland tumours of variable malignancy occur and tend to be locally invasive through the roof of the orbit into the intracranial cavity.

Metastatic tumours in the orbit are due to carcinoma of the breast in 50% of cases. Tumours originating in the lung and kidney account for the rest. Malignant melanoma has been reported but is hard to distinguish from a primary melanoma of the ciliary body or retina. In children with neuroblastoma, orbital metastases occur in 20–50% of cases (Farnarier, Saracco and Blanc, 1972).

Pupillary abnormalities

As the main determinant of pupil size is the incident light, it is appropriate to discuss the major pupillary abnormalities at this stage.

In a blind eye, assuming that the cause of blindness has not simultaneously damaged the iris mechanism, the pupil will dilate or constrict in proportion to the light falling on the unaffected eye. The direct light reaction will be absent but the consensual light reflex from the opposite eye, intact. No consensual reflex in the normal eye will be seen when the affected eye is stimulated. This is quite a useful check for non-organic claimed loss of vision in one eye.

In acute retrobulbar neuritis the pupil reaction may be incomplete and the pupil may dilate in spite of a constant light source (pupillary escape phenomenon). In a patient with eye pain, aggravated by movement with blurred vision, this Marcus-Gunn pupil reaction is strongly indicative of demyelinating disease. The postulated mechanism is a decrease in fibres conveying light sensation.

In IIIrd nerve lesions, damage to the efferent pupilloconstrictor fibres will produce a fixed dilated pupil even though the patient perceives light normally. Incomplete lesions may merely cause a slightly dilated pupil with a sluggish reaction – an important stage in the evolution of a IIIrd nerve palsy in a patient who is deteriorating following a head injury. A useful clue in a conscious patient with a IIIrd nerve lesion is the almost invariable accompanying ptosis of varying degree followed by diplopia due to paralysis of the superior rectus muscle (see next main section). Argyll Robertson pupils due to meningovascular syphilis have become a great rarity. This is a small pupil, usually irregular, that does not react to light but does react to accommodation (Loewenfeld, 1969).

A sympathetic nerve lesion (Horner's syndrome) will be detected by only the most alert clinician. Due to loss of the less important pupillodilator fibres a slightly smaller pupil is found showing a normal light reaction because the light reflex pathway mechanisms are unaffected. A modest and variable degree of ptosis will occur which rarely goes lower than the edge of the pupil. As the cervical sympathetic pathway courses in and out of otolaryngological territory, a full understanding of the syndrome is essential to the otolaryngologist (see also section on cranial nerves IX, X, XI and XII) (Jaffe, 1950).

A Holmes-Adie (myotonic) pupil may present as eye pain because the affected pupil fails to constrict in bright light. The affected pupil may be variably larger or smaller than the other, depending on the incident light producing a slower constriction or dilatation of the affected pupil. The light reaction is very slow, definite constriction followed by slow dilatation may be demonstrated best by maintained forced convergence for about one minute. If the patient sits in a dark room, the pupil will stay very large but if they have just come into the clinic from a bright sunlit room, the affected pupil may be *smaller* than the normal pupil at first (Loewenfeld and Thompson, 1967).

The nerve supply to the extraocular muscles

The three nerves supplying the extraocular muscles and controlling eye movements have complex central control mechanisms and run peripheral courses that render them vulnerable both individually and as a group, to a wide range of surgical and medical disorders. They are of special interest to otolaryngologists because of their involvement in local neoplastic disease and in infective processes originating in the paranasal sinuses, nose and nasopharynx.

The oculomotor nerve (III) (Figures 16.3, 16.4 and 16.5a)

The IIIrd nerve exits from the brain stem in the interpeduncular fossa and runs forwards, laterally and slightly downwards in the subarachnoid space towards the roof of the cavernous sinus. In its distal subarachnoid course it runs parallel to the posterior communicating artery, hence its unique liability to damage by aneurysms which commonly arise at either end of this short vessel. It enters the roof and then the lateral wall of the cavernous sinus in between the two layers of dura dividing into two branches before it enters the superior orbital fissure. In the wall of the sinus it picks up sympathetic fibres from the plexus on the carotid artery, and additional parasympathetic fibres from the ophthalmic division of the Vth nerve.

The superior ramus supplies the levator palpebrae superioris and the superior rectus muscle. The inferior ramus supplies the medial and inferior recti, inferior oblique and carries the sympathetic and parasympathetic elements to the ciliary ganglion via the branch to the inferior oblique.

The anatomy of the pupillary fibres in the nerve itself is of great significance. The fibres lie dorsolaterally at first then medially and finally inferiorly but always in the periphery of the nerve. Their blood supply is derived from the pial plexus on the surface of the nerve, and the core of the nerve supplied by a vasa nervorum. If this latter vessel is occluded by vascular disease (diabetes, arteriosclerosis, arteritis) the pupillary fibres lying peripherally are spared. Conversely, if the nerve is damaged from without by a compressive surgical lesion (aneurysm, tumour,

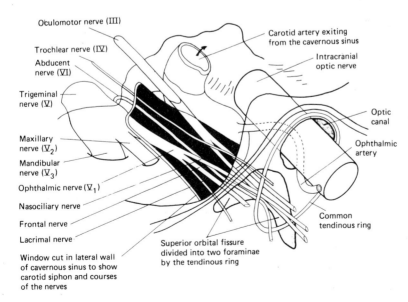

Figure 16.3 The cavernous sinus and orbital foramina

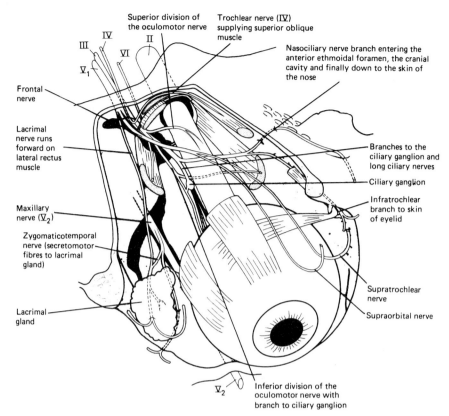

Figure 16.4 The orbital contents (right orbit from above and lateral)

abscess) the pupillary fibres are readily damaged. In IIIrd nerve lesions the involvement or otherwise of the pupil is a major diagnostic pointer. Pain tends to be a feature of surgical lesions so that a painful onset of a IIIrd nerve lesion with pupil involvement is almost certain to indicate a compressive lesion. No pain and a spared pupil is almost certain to indicate a medical cause (Wray, 1983). The major exception to these generalizations is a lesion due to diabetes which can be both painful and involve the pupil, mimicking a surgical lesion.

Central anatomy (see Figure 16.5*a*)

The detailed anatomical features of the oculomotor nucleus are beyond the scope of the present text. The nucleus is shaped like an inverted V, straddling the midline. The lateral nuclear columns supply the eyelid and the four extraocular muscles, the superior, medial and inferior rectus and the inferior oblique. The midline nuclei have mainly parasympathetic function especially the upper midline Edinger-Westphal nucleus, which is the main central control mechanism for pupil size. The fascicles of the IIIrd nerve fan out and traverse the red nucleus and

substantia nigra and then converge to form the main nerve trunk as it emerges just lateral to the midline in the interpeduncular fossa on the front of the midbrain.

The trochlear nerve (*IV*) (see Figure 16.3, 16.4 and 16.5*b*)

The fourth nerve is unique in several ways. It arises from the dorsal aspect of the brain stem at the level of the inferior colliculus. It then decussates in the superior medullary velum so that the right nucleus supplies the left superior oblique muscle and vice versa. It also has the longest intracranial course and is very slender, properties that possibly protect it from damage by external pressure around the brain stem and in the subarachnoid space. It enters the wall of the cavernous sinus beneath the IIIrd nerve but crosses it to reach a higher position as it enters the superior orbital fissure to supply the superior oblique muscle. The nerve is almost never damaged in isolation in cavernous sinus lesions, the IIIrd and VIth nerves being much more vulnerable. Vascular lesions of the nerve due to diabetes are probably the

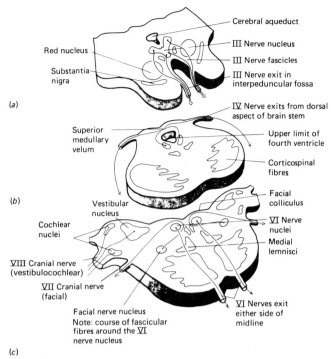

Figure 16.5 Brain stem connections of the extraocular nerves

commonest cause of pure IVth nerve lesions. Of particular importance to the otolaryngologist is the small fibrocartilaginous loop attached to the trochlear fossa in the upper medial orbit through which the muscle tendon passes. Accidental or surgical trauma may easily damage the tendon in this region and produce an apparent IVth nerve palsy (Burger, Kalvin and Smith, 1970).

The abducent nerve (VI) (see Figures 16.3, 16.4 and 16.5c)

The VIth nerve exits from the brain stem at the pontomedullary junction. It is the most medial of the three nerves arising from this groove, and ascends on the front of the pons and then angles forwards across the tip of the petrous bone to enter the bottom of the cavernous sinus in which it lies free, in close relationship to the intracavernous portion of the carotid artery. The long subarachnoid and meningeal course of the nerve renders it particularly liable to damage in acute and chronic meningitis and any other meningeal process, including remote or direct spread of malignancy. Its angulated entry into the cavernous sinus renders it vulnerable to stretch when the brain stem is pushed downwards by raised supratentorial pressure causing the classical false localizing VIth nerve palsy, which nearly always becomes bilateral.

The nerve may be involved in inflammation of the petrous bone secondary to otitis media. This is often combined with severe pain in the Vth nerve territory and loss of hearing. This constitutes Gradenigo's syndrome. Inflammatory disease of the cavernous sinus and aneurysmal dilatation of the carotid siphon within the cavernous sinus are particularly likely to involve the VIth nerve early, the IIIrd and IVth being involved later by the same process. Nerve trunk infarction by diabetes, arteritis and arteriosclerosis may also be seen exactly as for the IIIrd and IVth nerves as discussed above. Intracranially both cholesteatomas and acoustic neuromas may involve the nerve but such involvement is surprisingly rare. As it enters the orbit it passes laterally in order to reach its single muscle, the lateral rectus (see Figure 16.3). At this point it is particularly liable to damage by carcinoma infiltrating the orbit through the inferior orbital fissure from the nasopharynx (Rucker, 1966).

Central anatomy (see Figure 16.5c)

The nucleus of the VIth nerve lies in the floor of the IVth ventricle just lateral to the midline. The fibres of the facial nerve sweep round it. Although derived from the same nuclear column as the IIIrd and IVth nerve nuclei, it migrates during the massive developmental enlargement of the pons, but remains intimately linked to the other nuclei by the medial longitudinal bundle (discussed below). The fascicles of the VIth nerve have to traverse the whole depth of the pons to reach the point of emergence at the ponto-medullary junction. In its fascicular course it lies in close relationship to the ascending medial lemniscus and the descending corticospinal pathways.

Central mechanisms of nerves III, IV and VI (Figure 16.6)

The central control mechanisms for eye movement comprise a complex group of pathways which adjust eye position to movement and posture, mainly under the influence of vestibular and extrapyramidal pathways.

There are two forms of voluntarily controlled eye movements:

1 Visual pursuit where a specific target is fixed and followed, using parietal gaze centres closely integrated with the adjacent visual cortex
2 The ability to select a new target and relocate vision to suit, via frontal gaze centres utilizing direct pyramidal motor pathway mechanisms.

Damage in either of these areas causes conjugate gaze palsies and the range of movement of both eyes is identically affected so there is *no* diplopia.

At brain-stem level the need to integrate eye movements mediated by three different cranial nerve nuclei, widely spaced in the brain stem, requires complex and extremely rapidly conducting internuclear pathways. The most critical of these is the medial longitudinal fasciculus. Damage in this pathway causes internuclear ophthalmoplegias, with disconjugate gaze palsies. These will always cause diplopia. The cortical influences have final relays in the brain stem in the pons bilaterally – the lateral gaze centres. There are also four gaze centres in the midbrain, two on each side, one to look up and one to look down. Eye movements occur in saccades, a series of little jerk movements without over or under-shoot, until the new position is reached. This is achieved by rapid bursts at 1000 cycles/s by cells in the gaze centres. These bursts are initiated by voluntary information from the frontal eye fields via the anterior limb of the internal capsule. Automatic movements such as happen in reading are closely allied to visual information relayed via the optic tract without projection to the visual cortex. Feedback from stretch receptors in the ocular muscles is also of great importance in this type of movement. Tracking movements are controlled mainly by the superior colliculi, once the object to be followed has been located, using stereo-optic control. Vergence mechanisms require the voluntary frontal eye fields to work in conjunction with the parietal cortex with simultaneous inhibition of those brain-stem mechanisms which normally prevent convergence and divergence. Only animals with binocular stereoscopic vision have the need to converge to focus close objects.

Parietal lobe lesions

Poor object following or pursuit gaze problems are often difficult to demonstrate clinically as lesions in these areas also tend to cause a hemianopic field defect, so that the following movement ceases as the object moves into the blind half field. If however, the examiner is careful to keep the object in the patient's retained field of vision, a full range of pursuit movement should be achieved if there is no gaze palsy. A tendency to ignore objects on one side in the absence of a hemianopia (an attention field defect) may be related to the inability of the eye to scan peripherally due to lack of visual input.

Frontal lobe lesions

An irritative lesion such as a tumour or abscess in the frontal pole will drive the eyes away from the lesion. A right frontal tumour therefore may lead to focal fits with movement of the head and eyes to the left hand side before the patient loses consciousness. A destructive lesion such as surgical extirpation or a cerebrovascular accident will allow the eyes to gaze preferentially towards the side of the lesion due to unopposed push from the intact side. This phenomenon is readily seen in a drowsy, anaesthetized or unconscious patient.

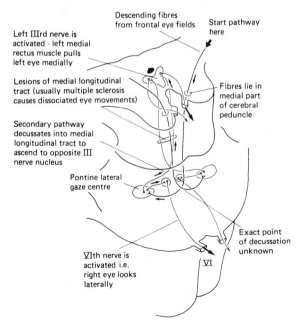

Left IIIrd nerve is activated - left medial rectus muscle pulls left eye medially

Descending fibres from frontal eye fields

Start pathway here

Lesions of medial longitudinal tract (usually multiple sclerosis causes dissociated eye movements)

Fibres lie in medial part of cerebral peduncle

Secondary pathway decussates into medial longitudinal tract to ascend to opposite III nerve nucleus

Pontine lateral gaze centre

Exact point of decussation unknown

VIth nerve is activated i.e. right eye looks laterally

VI

Figure 16.6 The internuclear pathways. (Pathway shown moves both eyes to the right side)

Midbrain lesions

Midbrain visual mechanisms are mainly concerned with up and down gaze. The classical lesion causing Parinaud's symdrome is a pineal tumour damaging the superior colliculus and the region of the posterior commissure. Such a lesion blocks the light reflex relays, producing fixed dilated pupils, impairs upward gaze and causes loss of convergence. Conversely, lesions of the inferior colliculus will only impair downward gaze. In some instances the ineffective movements of the extraocular muscles on attempting up or down gaze may pull the eyeball in and out of the socket, producing the very rare phenomenon known as retractory nystagmus.

Lesions affecting the thalamic nuclei, structural or pharmacological, may cause fixed deviations of up or down gaze. In patients with postencephalitic Parkinson's disease, oculogyric crisis was a classic feature. It can still be seen in some patients due to a sensitivity to phenothiazines. This is most common in young females. Divergence with one eye up and one eye down (skew deviation) with see-saw nystagmus on attempted lateral eye movement may be the result of lesions in the thalamus. A midline haemorrhage between the IIIrd nerve nuclei or multiple sclerosis can produce a divergent squint, with both eyes at the extremes of lateral gaze with intact up and down gaze limited only by mechanical factors at this extreme position.

Disorders affecting the midbrain

Anteriorly, aneurysms of the upper basilar artery or a tortuous basilar artery (basilar ectasia) may damage and distort the emergent IIIrd nerves. Posteriorly, pineal tumours or distortion and dilatation of the posterior end of the IIIrd ventricle due to aqueduct stenosis may cause Parinaud's syndrome. Infiltration of the superior medullary velum by direct spread of a medulloblastoma may cause bilateral IVth nerve lesions and impaired down gaze. Intrinsic lesions due to vascular occlusion, haemorrhage, demyelinating disease and tumour, may all cause anterior internuclear ophthalmoplegia, i.e. a divergent squint with loss of convergence but normal up and down gaze.

There are three named vascular syndromes of the midbrain due to combinations of IIIrd nerve lesions and local pathway damage:

1 *Nothnagel's syndrome*: a IIIrd nerve lesion with ipsilateral ataxia due to infarction of the superior cerebellar peduncle
2 *Benedikt's syndrome*: a IIIrd nerve lesion with contralateral cerebellar movement disorder due to a lesion of the red nucleus
3 *Weber's syndrome*: a IIIrd nerve lesion with contralateral hemiparesis due to a lesion of the basis pedunculi.

These syndromes have become extremely rare with the demise of meningovascular syphilis but are still occasionally seen in patients with small vessel disease (diabetes, cranial arteritis, lupus erythematosus, polyarteritis nodosa, polycythaemia rubra vera, etc.).

Pontine lesions

The pontine lateral gaze centres are often damaged by vascular lesions and demyelinating disease. This results in loss of gaze to the same side as the lesion, as their descending pathways have already decussated. In a drowsy or unconscious patient, this will result in the eyes deviating towards the good side.

Disorders affecting the pons

Anteriorly, the VIth nerves are often involved in bacterial, fungal or malignant meningitis due to their long meningeal course. Pontine tumours may involve the nerve nuclei or fascicular fibres and the posterior internuclear pathways. These tumours usually occur in children or adults with neurofibromatosis. Tumours blocking or infiltrating the IVth ventricle cause headache and vomiting due to CSF pathway block and VIth nerve palsies due to stretching of the nerves by raised intracranial pressure. If the VIth nerve palsy is due to direct tumour infiltration the VIIth nerve should also be involved as the fibres encircle the nucleus. These tumours include ependymoma, medulloblastoma, cerebellar astrocytoma or haemangioblastoma. Multiple sclerosis, haemorrhage and infarction, metabolic disorders (vitamin B deficiency), drug intoxication, fluid balance disturbance, viral infection and *Listeria monocytogenes* infection of the brain stem may cause a conjugate gaze palsy if damage is in the lateral pons or an internuclear ophthalmoplegia with nystagmus, if the lesion is in the central pons. Vascular occlusive lesions tend to cause unilateral internuclear ophthalmoplegia as the lesion extends only to the midline. There are numerous named vascular syndromes of the pons due to a variety of combinations of damage to the nuclei of nerves VI and VII and their fascicles and the sensory, motor and cerebellar pathways. There is no special advantage in learning these by heart, but the named syndromes include those of Millard Gubler, Foville, Grenet, Raymond-Cestan, Marie-Foix and Gasperini (Loeb, 1962). As a cautionary note, any hint of variability in diplopia should always raise the possibility of myasthenia gravis. If combined with variable dysarthria or intermittent swallowing difficulty a brainstem lesion may be incorrectly suspected. This is a very difficult diagnostic trap into which even experienced neurologists may fall.

Internuclear lesions (see Figure 16.6)

Internuclear lesions are caused by multiple sclerosis (bilateral) or vascular disease (strictly unilateral unless haemorrhagic). In these instances the lateral gaze centre is intact and abducts the ipsilateral eye normally – the relay to the opposite IIIrd nerve nucleus is blocked and the eye that should adduct in unison fails to move beyond the midline. With a bilateral lesion neither eye adducts while the abducting eye moves normally, and shows marked nystagmus at full abduction. This picture is almost diagnostic of multiple sclerosis. The integrity of the upper brain stem in such cases can be readily demonstrated by intact vertical gaze and convergence.

Nystagmus

Nystagmus is covered in detail in Chapter 4. From a simplistic neurological point of view, it is a less valuable physical sign than is often thought. The distinction into the different types, jerk, pendular, rotatory, etc., is often less easy to make than is suggested in most descriptions. Ultimately one is seeing a breakdown in the vestibular mechanisms as they affect the smoothness and stability of eye movements. Weak support from vestibular mechanisms will lead to poor maintenance of gaze (slow phase) and a quick restorative movement (the jerk phase) which is the feature used to define the direction of nystagmus. This is maximal when looking away from the side of a vestibular lesion, be it in the end organ, VIIIth nerve or vestibular nuclear connections. A controlling influence over vertical eye movements is also apparent in the phenomenon of vertical nystagmus which occurs with a structural or metabolic lesion of the brain stem. It is important to note that vertical nystagmus means vertical displacement of the eyes *not* side-to-side nystagmus which is seen when attempting upward and downward gaze. As defined, vertical nystagmus always indicates brain-stem damage. Another feature of brain-stem disease is jelly nystagmus, which is probably due to failure of inhibitory 'pause' neurons which normally stop the 'burst' neurons from producing visible little saccades. In this condition the eyes wobble with no clear-cut fast or slow component. Congenital nystagmus produces a similar type of nystagmus – the diagnostic feature being that the patient is quite unaware of it in spite of very dramatic nystagmus.

Cerebellar lesions, especially those affecting the flocculonodular lobes result in nystagmus due to the loss of the stabilizing effect of input from head posture receptors. In general the fast phase of cerebellar nystagmus is towards the side of a cerebellar lesion.

Group two

The second major grouping of cranial nerves consists of those lying in the cerebellopontine angle. The medial extent of the angle is defined by the VIth nerve, the upper extent by the Vth nerve and the lower extent by the IXth nerve. The VIIth and VIIIth nerves pass in close proximity across the subarachnoid space to enter the internal auditory canal at the start of their long intraosseous courses.

The trigeminal nerve (V)

The trigeminal nerve is the largest cranial nerve, and arises from the middle of the pons and passes forwards and laterally across the subarachnoid space. Its large ganglion lies over the tip of the petrous bone where the nerve divides into its three divisions.

The ophthalmic nerve (V_1) (see Figures 16.3 and 16.4)

The first division of the Vth nerve lies below the VIth nerve in the lateral wall of the cavernous sinus and is prone to damage by the same pathologies that cause extraocular nerve palsies (see above). Due to its extensive sensory distribution, severe pain in the forehead, nose and scalp, extending back as far as the vertex may result from such damage.

The nerve divides into three branches as it enters the superior orbital fissure:

1 The lacrimal nerve runs along the lateral rectus muscle to supply the lacrimal gland. It also supplies the skin over the lateral eyelid and brow. It picks up secretomotor fibres from the zygomaticotemporal nerve which it conveys to the lacrimal gland. In the skin it receives proprioceptive filaments from the facial nerve.
2 The frontal nerve divides into two, the supratrochlear and supraorbital nerves, which supply the skin of the forehead and scalp to the vertex. They are prone to damage by minor injuries over the brow and a causalgic syndrome may follow local trauma.
3 The nasociliary nerve has important autonomic and cutaneous functions:
  a The main trunk traverses the orbit and enters the anterior ethmoidal foramen into the intracranial cavity, runs across the cribriform plate and exits the skull through a slit in the crista galli to enter the nose. It supplies the mucosa of the nasal cavity and emerges at the lower end of the nasal bone to supply the skin over the tip of the nose, alar and vestibule.
  b In the orbit the nasociliary nerve gives off branches to the ciliary ganglion and two or three long ciliary nerves which carry the pupillo-dilator sympathetic fibres and convey sensation from the cornea. This is of cardinal importance for the protection of the very delicate cornea.
  c The infratrochlear branch is given off just behind the anterior ethmoidal foramen and lies on the

medial wall of the orbit and supplies the skin of the upper medial eyelid and upper side of the nose.

The corneal reflex

It is essential that otolaryngologists know how to elicit this reflex correctly. The afferent limb of the reflex is via the nasociliary nerve as above, and the efferent limb is via the facial nerve. A pointed wisp of cotton wool should be used. The examiner should ask the patient to look upwards, then resting the hand on the patient's cheek, the wisp should be applied to the lower cornea but taking care not to bring it into vision or a blink reflex will result. The patient will flinch, the eyeball will roll up and the eye will attempt to close. Even if the VIIth nerve is paralysed, the eyeball will roll up and the discomfort will be felt. The opposite eyelid will also close as this is a consensual reflex. Absence of the corneal reflex is often the first clinical evidence of Vth nerve damage and should be carefully tested in all patients with symptoms of vertigo, deafness or facial pain.

The maxillary nerve (V_2) (Figure 16.7)

The middle branch of the Vth nerve ganglion lies in the extreme lower lateral wall of the cavernous sinus and exits via the foramen rotundum, passes through the pterygopalatine fossa and enters the floor of the orbit via the inferior orbital fissure. At first it lies in a groove in the orbital floor and then enters the short canal and exits onto the face via the infraorbital foramen. It supplies the skin of the cheek, midlateral nose and lateral part of the alar, lower eyelid and the mucous membranes of the cheek and upper lip. In its course, it gives off the following branches:

1 Meningeal branches to the floor of the middle cranial fossa
2 Two branches to the sphenopalatine ganglion conveying the secretomotor fibres destined for the lacrimal gland
3 The zygomatic nerve which lies on the floor of the orbit, dividing into the zygomaticotemporal nerve (secretomotor to the lacrimal gland and carrying cutaneous sensation from the temporal area) and the zygomaticofacial nerve which, after penetrating the zygomatic bone, carries cutaneous sensation from the prominence of the cheek
4 The three alveolar nerves convey sensation from the teeth, gums and adjacent palate via the superior dental plexus. The anterior superior branch is the largest and supplies not only the incisor and canine teeth, but also the lateral nasal wall, nasal septum, the lower eyelid and the skin of the upper lip.

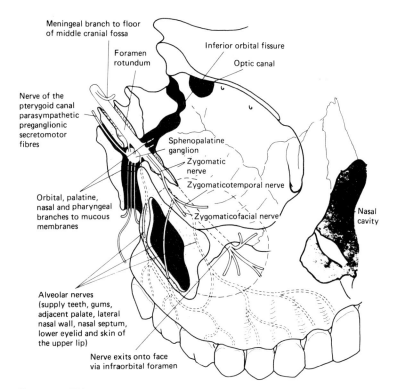

Figure 16.7 The maxillary nerve (V_2)

The pterygopalatine (sphenopalatine) ganglion

This very large ganglion is suspended from the maxillary division, deep in the pterygopalatine fossa. It receives its main connection from the nerve of the pterygoid canal. This carries preganglionic parasympathetic fibres derived from a pontine lacrimatory nucleus in the nervus intermedius (VIIth nerve) and sympathetic elements derived from the middle meningeal artery. Both groups of fibres are then relayed via their subsequent complex course to the lacrimal gland in the lacrimal branch of the nasociliary nerve. The main outflow, however is via the orbital, palatine, nasal and pharyngeal nerves to the mucous membranes of the orbit, nasal passages, pharynx, palate and upper gums.

The mandibular nerve (V₃) (Figure 16.8)

This is the largest branch of the Vth nerve and includes the motor component of the nerve. It exits from the skull via the foramen ovale, the main sensory trunk being joined by the much smaller motor root, in Meckel's cave, just outside the skull. A meningeal branch re-enters the skull with the middle meningeal artery through the foramen spinosum and supplies the lateral, middle and anterior cranial fossae. A small branch, the nerve to the medial pterygoid, supplies medial pterygoid, tensor tympani and tensor veli palatini.

The main nerve then divides into anterior and posterior trunks. The anterior trunk conveys the bulk of the motor root to supply masseter, temporalis and the lateral pterygoid muscles. The main branch of the anterior trunk is the buccal nerve which merges with the buccal branches of the facial nerve to convey sensation from the skin over the buccinator, the mucous membranes of the cheek and the posterior part of the buccal surface of the gum.

The posterior trunk is mainly sensory and divides into three main nerves:

1 The auriculotemporal nerve which passes behind the temporomandibular joint to join the facial nerve with which it is distributed to supply the skin over the tragus, helix, auditory meatus and tympanic membrane, and via superficial temporal branches, to the skin over temporalis. It also carries the secretomotor fibres to the parotid gland, and fibres derived from the tympanic branch of the glossopharyngeal nerve via the otic ganglion (see below).

2 The lingual nerve supplies sensation to the presul-

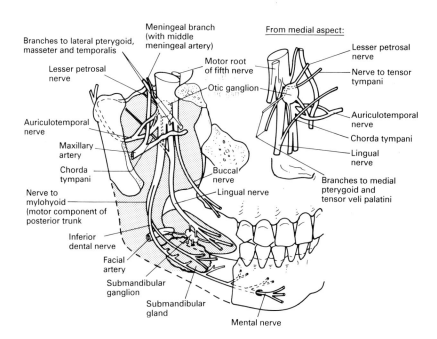

Figure 16.8 The mandibular nerve (V₃)

cal tongue, the floor of the mouth and lower gums. It carries the taste fibres of the chorda tympani from the mucous membranes of the tongue. It also conveys secretomotor fibres from the submandibular ganglion to the sublingual and anterior lingual glands. It communicates with the hypoglossal nerve.

3   The inferior alveolar (dental) nerve enters the mandibular canal running forwards in the mandible to re-emerge on the chin at the mental foramen dividing into the incisive and mental branches, supplying sensory fibres to the skin and mucous membrane of the lower lip, jaw, incisor and canine teeth. The motor component of the posterior trunk leaves the inferior alveolar nerve, just before it enters the mandibular canal, as the mylohyoid nerve supplying mylohyoid and the anterior belly of digastric.

Central mechanisms of the Vth nerve (Figure 16.9)

The central anatomy of the Vth nerve is very complicated. The small motor nucleus lies in a mid-position in the upper lateral pons opposite the nerve root. It receives bilateral supranuclear innervation from corticobulbar fibres which leave the main pyramidal pathways at the level of the nucleus. Direct connections from proprioceptive fibres in the adjacent main sensory nucleus allow a simple stretch reflex for mastica-

tion to operate. The jaw jerk tests the integrity of this pathway and if greatly enhanced, indicates a bilateral upper motor neuron lesion above midpontine level, the highest stretch reflex that can be elicited (McIntyre and Robinson, 1959).

The sensory nucleus is very extensive. The cell bodies of the sensory fibres lie in the gasserian ganglion at the petrous apex. At least 50% of the fibres do not enter the main sensory nucleus but are concerned with reflex activity. The other fibres form ascending and descending branches. The ascending fibres enter the mesencephalic nucleus of the Vth nerve. Their subsequent course and function is not understood. The descending fibres convey pain and temperature sensation and synapse in the nucleus of the descending tract of the Vth nerve which lies adjacent to the descending tract itself which extends as low as C2 cord level. The sensory fibres derived from the facial, glossopharyngeal and vagus nerves, all end in the same tract and are relayed in the same nucleus. The secondary ascending pathway fibres swing across the brain stem, ventral to the central canal to form the secondary ascending tract of the Vth nerve which is closely associated with the medial lemniscus, adding sensation derived from the face to that of the arm and leg in the same pathway. In the decussation these fibres are very vulnerable to damage by midline lesions, such as syringomyelia and syringobulbia, producing a sensory deficit typically extending forwards from the back of the head. This is the so-called 'onion peel' sensory deficit, which may leave sensation intact only over the nose and central face in the final stages of its development.

Clinical aspects of the Vth cranial nerve

Damage to the Vth cranial nerve is very important to the otolaryngologist. Branches of the nerve and its associated ganglia lie in areas often involved by otolaryngological disease, especially oropharyngeal and nasopharyngeal neoplasms.

Involvement of the motor root of the Vth nerve is quite rare as it seems to be resistant to pressure or distortion. If damaged, the wasting of the masseter is usually visible and easy to palpate on teeth clenching. The pterygoids are tested by attempted jaw opening against resistance, the jaw deviating towards the paralysed side.

Painless or painful loss of sensation over any part of the face, but particularly over V_2, is a very ominous finding and malignant disease in the antrum or nasopharynx is the most likely pathology. Repeated examination under general anaesthesia if necessary and biopsy of the nasopharynx are vital in such cases to attempt to establish the cause, even if CT or MRI scanning do not clearly indicate an abnormality. Involvement of V_1 is usually painful and nearly always accompanied by extraocular nerve palsies. It is most commonly caused by lesions in and around

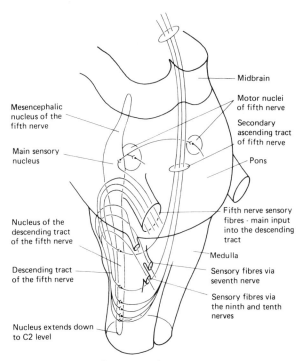

Mesencephalic nucleus of the fifth nerve

Main sensory nucleus

Nucleus of the descending tract of the fifth nerve

Descending tract of the fifth nerve

Nucleus extends down to C2 level

Midbrain

Motor nuclei of fifth nerve

Secondary ascending tract of fifth nerve

Pons

Fifth nerve sensory fibres - main input into the descending tract

Medulla

Sensory fibres via seventh nerve

Sensory fibres via the ninth and tenth nerves

Figure 16.9 Central sensory pathways

the cavernous sinus but may also be involved by malignant disease entering the orbit via the inferior orbital fissure.

Nasopharyngeal tumours most commonly arise in the fossa of Rosenmüller or near the orifice of the eustachian tube. They are usually squamous carcinomas. Tumours originating in the maxillary antrum or ethmoids are usually either squamous cell carcinomas or adenocarcinomas. Forty per cent of such tumours present as neurological problems. In 70% of cases the Vth nerve is involved, in 50% of cases the IIIrd, IVth and VIth nerves are involved. Visual pathways are affected in 8.5% of cases, and the lower cranial nerves in 10%. The favourite routes of entry into the skull are through the inferior orbital fissure or via the foramen lacerum with the carotid artery (Godtfredsen, 1944).

The maxillary division runs next to the mouth of the eustachian tube and the fossa of Rosenmüller, through the orbital floor just above the antrum and onto the face. Nasopharyngeal and antral carcinomas are particularly likely to damage this division and seem to cause loss of sensation more frequently than pain. The surface branches of both V_1 and V_2 are easily damaged by blunt trauma around the orbit and cheek, or divided by lacerations.

The mandibular division is involved in oropharyngeal, tonsillar and mandibular tumours and as noted above, painless numbness over the chin may be the presenting symptom, rather than pain. This remains a paradox when we consider that the common benign conditions cause exquisite facial pain and the most serious conditions are frequently quite painless.

Trigeminal sensory neuropathy is a very rare condition in which painless numbness develops over the Vth nerve territory, usually starting in the second division and eventually becoming bilateral. Only the passage of time and failure to demonstrate a responsible lesion allow this diagnosis to be made with certainty (Spillane and Wells, 1959).

The sensory root of the Vth nerve is very sensitive to distortion and pressure and loss of the corneal reflex is an important early sign of a lesion in the cerebellopontine angle. Rarely extensive loss of sensation over the face may be the presenting symptom of an acoustic neuroma, but again it is worth stressing the rarity of pain as the presenting symptom.

Trigeminal neuralgia

This is probably the most painful condition known, the cause of which seems to be minor ageing changes in the nerve or minor irritation by adjacent arteries. From a practical anatomical point of view, the very strict localization of the pain into Vth nerve territory is a vital diagnostic feature. There is no such thing as atypical trigeminal neuralgia and it is not acceptable to allow the pain to radiate behind the ear, onto the neck, or across the midline, and the anatomically precise distribution is the linchpin of diagnosis. The pain is

usually described in two characteristic distributions. The first runs from the lower canine tooth along the lower jaw to just in front of the ear and sometimes round into the upper jaw, i.e. it involves both V_3 and V_2. The second less frequent type runs from the upper incisor or canine, up the side or inside the nose and encircles the eye, involving both V_2 and V_1. It is probably this spread over two divisions that makes simple surgical section of the peripheral branch unsuccessful in managing the condition long term, although triggering is occasionally reduced. Although it is claimed that transient sensory deficit may follow a spasm of pain, any evidence of sensory loss, impaired corneal reflex or Vth motor weakness, should invalidate the diagnosis. Although trigeminal neuralgia may complicate multiple sclerosis it is very rare as a presenting symptom of this disease. The condition is dealt with in greater detail in Volume 4.

Herpes zoster ophthalmicus

Most patients with this condition develop severe pain in the distribution of V_1. The pain lasts 4–5 days. During this time the diagnosis of ruptured aneurysm, cranial arteritis or acute frontal sinusitis may all have to be seriously considered. The vesicles usually appear in the inner eyebrow. They then involve the entire distribution of the nerve branch. Severe chemosis of the eye and extraocular nerve palsies may further complicate the picture. Only the appearance of the vesicles will finally indicate the correct diagnosis.

Aneurysmal dilatation of the carotid artery

This is the other major condition in the elderly that can cause very severe pain in a V_1 distribution, with chemosis, extraocular nerve palsies and even blindness. This is usually of very sudden onset and typically develops in elderly females with long-standing hypertension.

The facial nerve (VII) (Figure 16.10)

The VIIth nerve is primarily motor to the muscles of facial expression. It also carries the important taste fibres from the tongue via the chorda tympani and taste from the palate via the nerve of the pterygoid canal. A small but clinically important cutaneous supply to the skin of the external ear is mediated in fibres carried from the nerve via the vagus. These sensory fibres are contained in a separate trunk, the nervus intermedius, which runs with the VIIIth nerve rather than the VIIth nerve in the subarachnoid space. The cell bodies of the sensory root lie in the geniculate ganglion. The nervus intermedius also carries preganglionic parasympathetic secretomotor fibres to the lacrimal, submandibular and sublingual salivary glands. These fibres originate in the lacrimatory nucleus and superior salivatory nucleus.

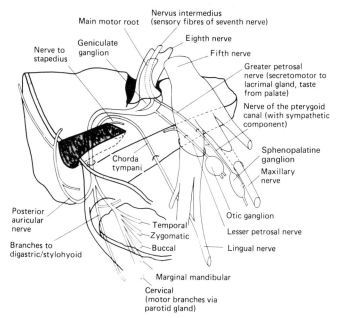

Figure 16.10 The facial nerve

Several important branches arise from the intra-petrous part of the nerve.

1 The greater petrosal nerve arises from the geniculate ganglion carrying taste fibres from the palate and conveying preganglionic parasympathetic fibres to the pterygopalatine ganglion, and via the zygomaticotemporal and lacrimal nerves to the lacrimal gland. It is joined by the deep petrosal nerve (derived from the sympathetic plexus on the carotid artery) to form the nerve of the pterygoid canal.
2 A branch from the ganglion joins the lesser petrosal nerve and is then carried to the otic ganglion. This conveys secretomotor fibres via the auriculotemporal nerve to the parotid gland. It also carries sympathetic fibres derived from the carotid artery to supply the blood vessels of the gland.
3 A small twig, the nerve to stapedius, arises 6 mm above the stylomastoid foramen.
4 The chorda tympani arises at the same level and runs forward across the middle ear and enters a canal in the petrotympanic fissure, grooves the spine of the sphenoid and joins the lingual branch of the Vth nerve with which it is distributed to the presulcal part of the tongue.
5 At the stylomastoid foramen twigs join both the vagus and glossopharyngeal nerve.
6 The posterior auricular nerve supplies the muscles of the ear and occipital belly of occipitofrontalis.
7 The branches to the muscles of facial expression are from above down, the temporal, zygomatic,

buccal, marginal and cervical; they pass through the substance of the parotid gland before emerging in the skin and are vulnerable to disease in the parotid gland and local surgical procedures.
8 Cutaneous fibres are distributed with the auricular branch of the vagus supplying the skin on both sides of the auricle and part of the external auditory canal and tympanic membrane.

The submandibular ganglion

The submandibular ganglion hangs from the lingual nerve. Its preganglionic fibres are derived from the superior salivatory nucleus, and reach it via the facial nerve, chorda tympani and lingual nerve. These fibres are secretomotor to the submandibular and sublingual glands. The sympathetic components are derived from the sympathetic plexus on the facial artery and pass uninterrupted through the ganglion to the blood vessels of the same glands.

The central connections of the facial nerve (see Figure 16.5)

The nucleus lies in a deep position in the central pons. The dorsal part of the nucleus receives bilateral supranuclear innervation whereas the lower part of the nucleus receives mainly contralateral supranuclear innervation. This has important consequences for the clinical varieties of VIIth nerve lesions. The nucleus is closely related to the Vth nerve and this proximity is vital for the important corneal reflex and its own reflex activity via the nucleus of the tractus solitarius. The fascicular course of the nerve is unusual in that the fibres course towards the floor of the IVth ventricle, wrap around the nucleus of the VIth nerve producing a visible enlargement on the floor of the IVth ventricle (the facial colliculus) and then retrace their course across the entire depth of the pons to exit at the pontomedullary junction. This complex arrangement is thought to be due to the embryological migration of the nucleus from its original position in the floor of the IVth ventricle to achieve its close relationship to the nucleus of the Vth nerve and the nucleus of the tractus solitarius.

Taste mechanisms (Figure 16.11)

Taste is mediated via taste buds; some 50 cells arranged in a pear-like cluster. These are found on the tongue, undersurface of the palate, palatoglossal folds, posterior wall of the pharynx, posterior surface of the epiglottis and the upper third of the oesophagus. They are most numerous on the lateral tongue and decrease in number with age by about 1% per annum. Each taste bud opens on the surface of the mucous membrane as a pore. The buds are found in the vallate, fungiform and foliate papillae. The lifespan of these cells, which are renewed from epithelial cells surrounding the bud, is about 10 days. They are therefore very vulnerable to factors inhibiting rapid cell turnover.

Two main receptor cells have been identified although they are possibly different types of the same cell. Some receptor cells have receptor sites for afferent neurons and small presynaptic vesicles, others contain larger vesicles and have more definite ciliary processes at their tip, just inside the pore. There is evidence of considerable cross-innervation of taste buds which may indicate inhibitory and facilitatory control similar to that seen in the smell receptors. It is thought that patterns of taste over a wide area of receptors is critical in perceiving different tastes

rather than that there are specific receptors for specific tastes. There is some evidence that sweet is more readily detected on the tip and medial dorsum of the tongue, salt and sour over the lateral tongue and bitter over the posterolateral tongue, where the circumvallate papillae are most numerous.

The neural connections of the taste receptor cells are the unipolar processes of cells in the geniculate ganglion of the VIIth nerve, the inferior ganglion of the IXth nerve and the inferior ganglion of the Xth nerve. The central processes of these cells form the tractus solitarius and they synapse in the adjacent nucleus of the tract. These fibres then ascend in the medial lemniscus to the opposite nucleus ventralis posterior medialis of the thalamus. The final pathway is via the internal capsule to the sensory cortex and insula. Some information from the pons relays direct to the hypothalamus for autonomic reflex purposes. The anatomy of the peripheral taste pathways is complex but for practical purposes, the supply to the anterior two-thirds of the tongue is mediated via the chorda tympani but finally distributed in the lingual branch of the mandibular division of the Vth nerve. The facial nerve also conveys sensation from the taste buds on the palate through the middle and posterior palatine nerves, via the greater petrosal nerve and the nerve of the pterygoid canal. Taste sensation from the vallate papillae, pharyngeal tongue and palatoglossal folds is conveyed by fibres carried in the IXth nerve. Taste sensation from the lowest part of the tongue, epiglottis and hypopharynx is carried by the vagus in fibres derived from its superior laryngeal branch.

Free nerve endings of the Vth nerve are also widespread, conveying somatic sensation from these same areas. They also undoubtedly contribute to the perception of extremely strong taste stimuli, such as curry powder, carbonated drinks and acid substances, and modifications of this pattern of gustatory and simple physical stimuli such as temperature, can alter taste sensation, heightening the unpleasant features of such highly flavoured compounds. It is clear that taste mechanisms are rather more complex than simple permutations of sweet, bitter, salt and sour. Parallel smell appreciation adds savour to taste. Patients with loss of smell describe all food as tasting like cardboard and only highly spiced or flavoured foods make any impact and often not necessarily a pleasant one. Adaptation again plays a role. The modification of fruit juice flavours by the previous use of mint toothpaste, is a universally appreciated phenomenon. Because of the vital role of smell in taste appreciation and the frequent simultaneous impairment of smell, it is difficult to isolate specific disorders of taste. For example, in Bell's palsy, patients identify tastes as having a metallic flavour in spite of the lesion being strictly unilateral and there being no impairment of the sense of smell. Chemicals and systemic diseases that modify taste and smell are listed in the section on smell above.

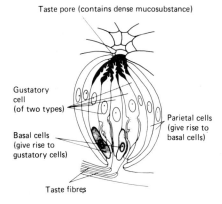

Taste pore (contains dense mucosubstance)

Gustatory cell (of two types)

Parietal cells (give rise to basal cells)

Basal cells (give rise to gustatory cells)

Taste fibres

Figure 16.11 The taste bud

Clinical disorders of the VIIth nerve

The VIIth nerve is frequently damaged by diseases of otolaryngological origin inside the skull, in the petrous bone and in the parotid gland (Tschiassny, 1953).

For reasons noted above, a cortical lesion affecting VIIth nerve function such as a vascular lesion or tumour in the motor strip, will cause weakness maximal in the lower face which is mainly contralaterally innervated. The upper face, in particular forehead movement and eye closure, is relatively spared, due to bilateral supranuclear innervation. This is an upper motor neuron facial weakness, and in many instances is more apparent on spontaneous smiling and speaking than during deliberate attempts to move the face to command.

Lesions affecting the whole facial nucleus or peripheral part of the nerve should cause total weakness. In some instances if weakness is more marked in the lower face, which may happen in the early or recovery phase of a simple Bell's palsy, an upper motor neuron lesion may be incorrectly suspected. Much less commonly, a very dense upper motor neuron lesion may mimic a lower motor neuron lesion affecting all facial movements. These difficulties are stressed as the distinction is of immense diagnostic importance and mistakes are easily made.

Lesions in the brain stem affecting the VIIth nerve usually also involve the VIth nerve because of the intimate anatomical relationship and long tract signs such as brisk reflexes or extensor plantar responses may also be detected on careful examination if the brain stem is distorted or infiltrated by the lesion.

The VIIth nerve lies in very close relationship with the VIIIth nerve as they cross the subarachnoid space to enter the internal auditory foramen. This is in the cerebellopontine angle and an acoustic neuroma is the most frequent lesion found at this site. Acoustic neuromas, although grossly distorting the VIIth nerve, very rarely present as a VIIth nerve palsy. If there is clinical evidence of a cerebellopontine angle lesion and if the VIIth nerve *is* involved, alternative pathology is more likely (Thomsen, 1976). Permanent damage to the VIIth nerve following surgical removal of an acoustic neuroma is unfortunately very common.

In the facial canal the nerve is liable to ischaemic damage and this is the probable mechanism of Bell's palsy where the nerve is thought to be damaged by compression caused by the inflammatory response to an antecedent viral infection. In nearly all cases very severe pain in the ear is experienced in the 24 hours before the onset of the Bell's palsy. It is particularly severe and persistent if herpes zoster is responsible (Ramsay Hunt syndrome). The pain and local swelling in the latter case may suggest bacterial infection until the vesicles appear 3–4 days later. The facial paralysis is usually complete on the second day and includes occipitofrontalis and platysma. Hearing distortion due to paralysis of stapedius and impaired taste due to simultaneous involvement of chorda tympani, do not always occur and in mild cases the lower half of the face may be more severely affected than the upper half mimicking an upper motor neuron lesion, as discussed above (Taverner, 1955).

Seventy-five per cent of patients make a good recovery over 3–6 weeks with or without treatment. Twenty per cent make an acceptable but slow recovery complicated by the development of facial synkinesis. This is due to nerve sprouting with subsequent loss of fine control which can turn a smile into a snarl and eye closure into a distorted grimace. Five per cent of cases make little or no recovery and may ultimately require plastic surgical repair. In some cases aberrant regeneration may lead to lacrimation instead of salivation on eating, so-called crocodile tears (Chorobski, 1951). It is most important that patients with Bell's palsy are not told that they have had a small stroke. Exclusion of underlying hypertension, diabetes, sarcoidosis and inflammatory arterial disease is important and more recently the recognition of Lyme disease in southern rural England requires blood tests for *Borrelia burgdorfii* to be added to the differential diagnostic list in appropriate areas, where there is a large deer population.

Middle ear infection carries a considerable risk of damaging the nerve by similar mechanisms. Fractures through the petrous bone are often complicated by facial nerve palsy. Those of immediate onset are usually due to nerve laceration. Those of delayed onset, usually 2–3 days after trauma are due to oedema and carry an excellent prognosis. Trauma to the nerve as it emerges from the stylomastoid foramen is a well recognized complication of forceps delivery.

Benign hemifacial spasm is seen in both sexes at any age but seems to be more common in elderly hypertensive females. Since the advent of scanning a surprising number of underlying lesions are found in this condition, such as cholesteatoma, acoustic neuromas, meningiomas, or aneurysms of the basilar artery. CT or MRI scanning should be regarded as a necessary investigation in all cases. The symptoms consist of a constant flickering and twitching of the facial muscles. This usually starts around the eye producing involuntary winking and later extends to involve the mouth. It is usually worse in company but continues 24 hours a day. It may respond to carbamazepine (Tegretol) but if the patient's age and condition allows, posterior fossa exploration to identify vascular irritation by a small vessel and exclude other lesions is indicated (Ehni and Woltman, 1945). Excellent control can be obtained using botulinum toxin injections in many cases. The need for repeat injection every 2–3 months and the expense at present limits the use of this valuable treatment.

Clinical testing of the VIIth nerve

A standard sequence of movements should be tested. Wrinkling the forehead, followed by forced eye closure will usually reveal weakness in the upper half of the face. The ability to flare the nostrils and wrinkle the nose should be tested, followed by the patient forcibly showing the teeth and attempting to blow out the cheeks. Eversion of the lower lip is difficult to achieve but tests the perioral muscles and produces striking contraction of platysma. It should only take about 30 seconds to perform these tests. Hearing should not be impaired to simple clinical testing although the patient may report distorted hearing. In the same way, formal testing of taste with standard test flavours may be performed but often the patient's own perception and description of altered taste will be adequate for diagnostic purposes.

Whenever the VIIth nerve is damaged it is important to exclude coexistent Vth nerve damage, in particular to confirm the presence of the corneal reflex. Not only will the absence of the corneal reflex exclude a simple Bell's palsy, but the considerable danger to an unprotected and anaesthetic cornea will be identified. Eye movements should be carefully tested to exclude a VIth nerve lesion, which could indicate a brain-stem lesion, and simple clinical tests of hearing should be performed, particularly if the corneal reflex is depressed, as simultaneous involvement of the Vth, VIIth and VIIIth nerves would strongly indicate a lesion in the cerebellopontine angle. It should be remembered that herpes zoster may affect several cranial nerves simultaneously and can cause severe pain which, when accompanied by multiple cranial nerve palsies, can present a very difficult diagnostic situation until the vesicles appear.

The vestibulocochlear nerve (VIII)

The anatomy and physiology of the specialized end organs of the VIIIth nerve are discussed in the first four chapters of this volume. Discussion here is therefore confined to the role of hearing impairment and balance disorders in the diagnosis of neurological disease.

Due to the anatomical proximity of the VIIth and VIIIth nerves, simultaneous involvement under many circumstances would seem likely. In reality such damage is quite unusual, with the exception of acute traumatic lesions of the petrous bone where both nerves are simultaneously lacerated. This peculiarity is of considerable clinical importance.

The cerebellopontine angle syndrome (Figure 16.12)

The most frequent tumour arising in the cerebellopontine angle is an acoustic neuroma (vestibular schwannoma). Although originating on the vestibular division of the nerve, the rate of growth is usually so insidious, that a purely vestibular presentation is extremely unusual. Gradual and often unrecognized

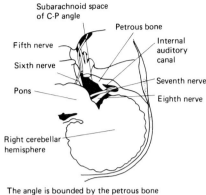

The angle is bounded by the petrous bone anteriorly, the pons medially, and the cerebellum posteriorly

Figure 16.12 The cerebellopontine angle

impairment of hearing is the rule. Similarly, the VIIth nerve may become grossly distorted but either benign facial hemispasm or weakness as a presenting symptom is similarly unusual. In contrast, minimal pressure on the Vth nerve root as the tumour extends upwards, or perhaps stretching of the Vth nerve root as the pons is displaced, commonly produces impairment of the corneal reflex. In spite of such distortion, frank pain or numbness of the face is also very unusual. Obviously a cerebellopontine angle tumour may present as facial hemispasm, facial weakness, facial numbness or a trigeminal neuralgia-like syndrome but, in all such instances, a cholesteatoma, or meningioma in the cerebellopontine angle becomes a more likely diagnosis. If the clinical picture has evolved extremely rapidly, both metastatic carcinoma or lymphoma could be responsible. Less frequently and usually in the 5–15 year age group, pontine glioma or cerebellar medulloblastoma can extend into the cerebellopontine angle to produce the typical combination of nerve lesions.

Balance disorders and vertigo

Unsteadiness is a very common symptom leading to referral to otolaryngological or neurological clinics. The most important historical feature to establish is what the patient means by the complaints of being 'off balance', 'giddy', or 'dizzy'. So often close questioning reveals that they mean 'light headed', 'floaty' or 'woozy', all non-specific symptoms more frequently due to anxiety. They do not describe the required illusion of movement of themselves or their surroundings, necessary to establish that they have true vertigo and therefore justify extensive and expensive otoneurological investigations to define the cause.

Disorders of balance, such as Menière's disease, vestibular neuronitis and benign positional vertigo,

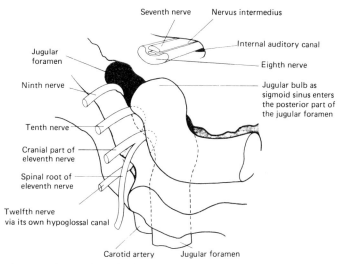

Figure 16.13 Schematic diagram of internal jugular foramen

will be discussed in detail elsewhere. The frequency with which vertigo is a symptom in migraine attacks also deserves mention. A feature of all these situations is that the attacks are episodic or provoked by change of position and in the case of migraine often accompanied by or associated with headache.

Disorders of balance due to structural organic disease in the CNS tend to produce continuing difficulty with balance and non-stop vertigo. The most frequent causes are multiple sclerosis and cerebrovascular accidents, affecting vestibular and cerebellar connections in the brain stem. Pure cerebellar lesions are less likely to produce vertigo unless they also distort the brain stem. They will usually also produce impaired coordination or a tendency to veer to one side while walking, rather than the drunken reeling in all directions, seen in association with vertigo in patients with brain-stem lesions.

For further discussion readers are referred to the first four chapters of this volume and later volumes in the series.

Group three

The final group of cranial nerves are not only anatomically bunched at their major exit, the jugular foramen, but share common nuclear origins. They also have peripheral cross connections for final distribution that make for poor physiological distinction of function as well as complex anatomy. Only the hypoglossal nerve, with its discrete nuclear origin and separate hypoglossal canal, can be discussed in isolation. Even then, its peripheral course brings it into close anatomical relationship with the other three nerves.

The glossopharyngeal nerve [IX] (Figures 16.13, 16.14 and 16.15)

The glossopharyngeal nerve has sensory, motor and autonomic components. The sensory ganglion cells lie in the superior and inferior ganglia of the nerve. The central processes pass to the nucleus of the tractus solitarius, conveying taste sensation, and to the nucleus of the spinal tract of the Vth nerve

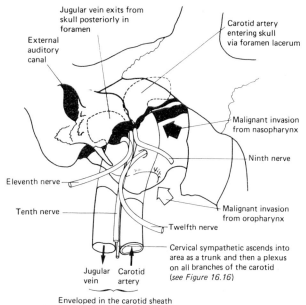

Figure 16.14 Schematic diagram of external jugular foramen

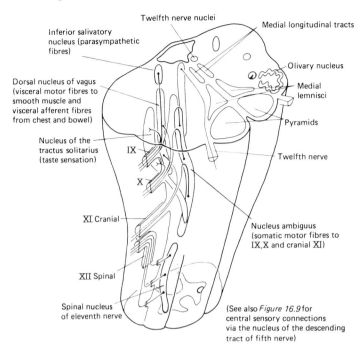

Figure 16.15 Central connections of nerves IX, X, XI and XII (viewed anterolaterally from the right side)

conveying somatic sensation. The motor nucleus lies in the upper part of the nucleus ambiguus which receives bilateral supranuclear innervation from corticobulbar fibres. This nucleus supplies the stylopharyngeus. The autonomic parasympathetic fibres arise in the inferior salivatory nucleus. These fibres are carried in the lesser petrosal nerve via the tympanic branch to the otic ganglion. The postganglionic fibres are distributed to the parotid gland via the auriculotemporal nerve.

The glossopharyngeal nerve emerges from the brain stem in line with the vagus and accessory nerves and exits from the skull via the jugular foramen. It descends between the jugular vein and carotid artery picking up sympathetic fibres from the carotid plexus as it loops forwards and medially to reach the soft tissues of the oropharynx, posterior tongue and palate. In its course it gives off the lesser petrosal nerve conveying the secretomotor fibres for the parotid gland to the otic ganglion. An important nerve, the carotid branch, innervates the carotid body and carotid sinus conveying respectively chemoceptor and stretch reflex information centrally for respiratory and circulatory reflex function. The final branches are the pharyngeal, tonsillar and lingual branches, conveying general sensation and taste sensation from the posterior third of the tongue and oropharynx.

The otic ganglion

The otic ganglion lies just below the foramen ovale,

attached to the mandibular nerve but functionally carries secretomotor fibres from the glossopharyngeal nerve. These parasympathetic fibres relay in it and supply the parotid gland via the auriculotemporal nerves originating from V_3. Sympathetic fibres derived from the middle meningeal artery pass through the ganglion and are also distributed to the blood vessels of the parotid gland by the auriculotemporal nerve.

Glossopharyngeal neuralgia

This is a rare condition which presents at about one tenth the frequency of trigeminal neuralgia. It consists of excruciatingly severe pain in the palate, throat and external auditory canal, locations demonstrating the somatic sensory distribution of the glossopharyngeal nerve. The pain has the typical burning, electric shock quality of neuralgia and is triggered mainly by swallowing. The incidence of underlying lesions inside the skull is thought to be very much higher than in trigeminal neuralgia. Both phenytoin and carbamazepine may control the pain. MRI scanning would seem a wise precaution in all instances, but small lesions may be missed and intracranial root exploration is necessary if medical treatment fails. Peripheral glossopharyngeal section has little to commend it, and can seriously interfere with normal swallowing mechanisms (Ekbom and Westerberg, 1966).

The vagus nerve (X) (see Figures 16.13, 16.14 and 16.15)

The vagus nerve (the wanderer) is the most widely distributed cranial nerve, hence only aspects essential to otolarynyologists will be detailed.

The central connections are similar to the IXth nerve.

1 The dorsal nucleus of the vagus contains motor and sensory components. The motor fibres are general visceral efferent to the smooth muscle of the bronchi, heart, oesophagus, stomach and intestine. The sensory fibres are general visceral afferent originating in the oesophagus and upper bowel with cell bodies in the superior and inferior vagal ganglia.
2 The nucleus ambiguus gives origin to those fibres controlling the striated muscle of the pharynx and intrinsic muscles of the larynx. It has a bilateral supranuclear innervation.
3 The nucleus of the tractus solitarius is shared with the glossopharyngeal nerve and receives fibres from the taste buds of the epiglottis and vallecula.
4 General somatic afferent fibres from the pharynx and larynx are found in the nerve and are believed to terminate in the spinal nucleus of the Vth nerve.

Because of these extensive nuclear connections multiple rootlets emerge from the brain stem and form a flat cord which enters the jugular foramen. The superior and inferior ganglia lie in the foramen and just below, an identical arrangement to the glossopharyngeal nerve. Both ganglia make connections with the accessory and hypoglossal nerves and the sympathetic plexus on the carotid artery. Below the inferior ganglion the cranial root of the accessory nerve merges with the vagus nerve which then distributes its fibres to the pharynx and larynx.

The vagal branches of practical importance are as follows:

1 A meningeal branch supplying the dura of the posterior fossa is given off in the jugular foramen.
2 The auricular branch arises from the superior ganglion, and is joined by a branch from the glossopharyngeal nerve and is distributed to the skin of the external ear with the branch of the facial nerve. These fibres eventually all enter the nucleus of the descending tract of the Vth nerve.
3 The pharyngeal branch arises just above the inferior ganglion and distributes the spinal accessory nerve components to the pharyngeal plexus, supplying the pharynx and palate.
4 The superior laryngeal nerve comes off the inferior ganglion and divides into two branches: the internal laryngeal nerve which supplies sensation to the mucous membrane of the larynx and conveys proprioceptive information from the neuromuscular spindles and stretch receptors of the larynx; and the external laryngeal nerve which supplies cricothyroid and contributes to the pharyngeal plexus, and is of considerable importance in speech mechanisms.
5 The recurrent laryngeal nerve has differing courses on each side. On the right it loops under the subclavian artery and on the left under the aortic arch. On both sides it then ascends on the side of the trachea. It supplies all the muscles of the larynx except cricothyroid and carries sensory fibres from the mucous membranes and stretch receptors of the larynx.

The spinal accessory nerve (XI) (see Figures 6.13, 16.14 and 16.15)

The cranial part of this nerve is a detached portion of the vagus and the spinal part is motor to the sternocleidomastoid and trapezius.

The cranial portion arises from the lower part of the nucleus ambiguus and a small component from the dorsal efferent nucleus of the vagus. The nerve rootlets emerge in line with the vagus, and are joined by the ascending spinal component and run laterally to enter the jugular foramen. The cranial portion merges with the vagus at the level of the inferior vagal ganglion and is then distributed with the pharyngeal and recurrent laryngeal branches of the vagus. These fibres probably supply the muscles of the soft palate.

The spinal root arises from ventral horn cells in the cord between C1 and C5. The fibres emerge from the cord laterally between the anterior and posterior spinal nerve roots to form a separate nerve trunk ascending into the skull through the foramen magnum. It then exits from the skull via the jugular foramen in the same dural sheath as the vagus. It runs posteriorly as soon as it emerges to supply the sternocleidomastoid and the upper part of trapezius and receives a major contribution from branches of the anterior roots of C3 and C4 to form a plexus which supplies the cervical musculature. Surgical evidence suggests that these additional root components make important contributions, as upper cervical root section is required to denervate completely the sternocleidomastoid and trapezius. The peripheral portion of the nerve is easily damaged in lymph node biopsy and other operations in the posterior triangle of the neck (Eisen and Bertrand, 1972).

The accessory nerve is unusual in that clinical evidence indicates that the supranuclear innervation of the motor cells supplying sternocleidomastoid is ipsilateral. In hemiparetic vascular lesions the weakness in sternocleidomastoid is on the *same side* as the lesion. In epileptic fits originating in the frontal pole, the head turns away from the side of the lesion, i.e. the *ipsilateral* sternocleidomastoid is contracting. Failure to recognize this distribution may seem to indicate that a patient with a left hemiparesis also has a right accessory nerve lesion, and hence a lower brain-stem lesion rather than a simple capsular cerebrovascular accident. This is an easy mistake to make unless this anatomical peculiarity is appreciated and the normality of the upper trapezius on the side of the weak sternocleidomastoid is also demonstrated.

The hypoglossal nerve (XII) (see Figures 16.13, 16.14 and 16.15)

The hypoglossal nerve arises from a nuclear column lying in the floor of the IVth ventricle and derived from the same cell group as the nuclei of nerves III, IV and VI. Like nerves III and VI, the fascicular fibres have to traverse the full sagittal diameter of the brain stem to exit from the ventral surface of the medulla between the pyramid and olive. The numerous rootlets combine and become two main roots with their own dural sleeves and exit via the hypoglossal canal just below the jugular foramen. The nerve therefore emerges deep to the other structures and has to course downwards and anteriorly to emerge between the jugular vein and carotid artery, cross the inferior vagal ganglion and then pass upwards and anteriorly on hyoglossus, distributing branches to all the muscles of the tongue. It receives sympathetic fibres from the superior cervical ganglion, some fibres from the vagus and the motor roots of C1 and C2 via the ansa cervicalis and numerous filaments connect to and are distributed with the lingual nerve.

Motor fibres derived from the hypoglossal nucleus itself supply styloglossus, hyoglossus, geniohyoid and genioglossus. The fibres derived from the C1 components are distributed to sternohyoid, sternothyroid, omohyoid, thyrohyoid and geniohyoid. Although a XIIth nerve lesion paralyses one side of the tongue as its most demonstrable feature, the larynx also pulls across to the opposite side on swallowing, because of failure of the hyoid to elevate on the paralysed side.

The supranuclear innervation of the hypoglossal nucleus is usually bilateral but can be mainly contralateral so that in some cerebrovascular accidents transient weakness of one side of the tongue may be found. The nerve is particularly vulnerable to surgical trauma in operations on the submandibular gland and ducts, and during carotid endarterectomy (Dehn and Taylor, 1983). Paralysis following central venous catheterization has also been reported (Whittet and Boscoe, 1984).

The cervical sympathetic nerve (Figure 16.16)

Horner's syndrome is due to damage to the cervical sympathetic nerve and is one of the most frequently

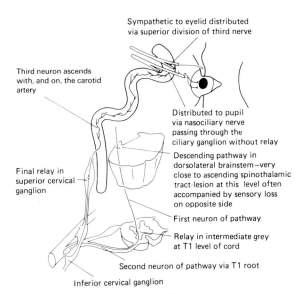

Figure 16.16 Schematic course of the cervical sympathetic nerve

missed physical signs in medicine. In the present context, its detection is of vital importance.

The cervical sympathetic nerve originates in the ipsilateral hypothalamus, runs through the entire dorsolateral brain stem to the central grey matter of the cervical spinal cord at T1 level. The sympathetic fibres leave the cord via the ventral root, join the sympathetic chain and ascend through the various ganglia to end as a plexus on the carotid artery, on which they re-enter the intracranial cavity. It ultimately supplies sympathetic fibres to *all* the cranial nerves innervating the pupil, glands and blood vessels of the head and neck.

The external evidences of Horner's syndrome are said to be fourfold:

1 Enophthalmos is rarely visible and of dubious authenticity

2 Loss of sweating over the face and forehead is rarely noted unless specifically tested by warming the patient

3 Ptosis of the eyelid may be very subtle and somewhat variable, as the nerve endings become sensitized to circulating adrenalin due to denervation hypersensitivity. The lid rarely drops lower than the edge of the pupil

4 Pupilloconstriction or more accurately the failure of pupillodilatation, leads to an entirely normally reactive pupil to light and accommodation but through a smaller range. At rest the affected pupil is small.

Horner's syndrome, may be congenital and this is associated with failure of pigmentation of the affected iris which remains blue.

Causes of Horner's syndrome

The causes of Horner's syndrome are as follows:

1 Lesions in the dorsolateral brain stem, especially vascular lesions in the medulla, multiple sclerosis at any level or pontine glioma
2 Lesions in the central cervical cord, syringomyelia, ependymoma, glioma or traumatic damage
3 Lesions of T1 roots, apical carcinoma of the lung, cervical rib, aortic aneurysm or avulsion of the lower brachial plexus
4 Lesions of the sympathetic chain in the neck, thyroid carcinoma, thyroid surgery, neoplastic lesions, local trauma, accidental surgical damage or surgical extirpation for various vascular syndromes of the arm
5 Lesions of the carotid plexus, carotid artery surgery, carotid artery thrombosis, migrainous spasm, local neoplastic destruction of the skull base or involvement by aneurysm or malignancy in the region of the carotid siphon or jugular foramen.

Clinical evaluation of the last four cranial nerves

Multiple involvement of these nerves is extremely common, so that the symptoms and signs of individual nerve lesions can be difficult to isolate, both from the history and on examination. Disorders of swallowing, speaking, coughing and pain syndromes are the usual presenting symptoms.

A glossopharyngeal nerve lesion will cause impaired taste sensation over the posterior third of the tongue but this is usually asymptomatic and impossible to test. The loss of somatic sensation over the palate and oropharynx will cause impaired swallowing reflexes as the initial stimulus to deglutition is the arrival of the bolus against the palate. This will lead to occasional choking on food and fluids. Pain in the throat and ear may develop with sensory fibre irritation and then true glossopharyngeal neuralgia may result. This characteristically will be triggered by swallowing.

Sensation over the palate should be tested by touching the palate with an orange stick and if sensation appears blunted, this can be confirmed using a long hatpin. A further check can be made by touching the posterior pharyngeal wall while the patient says 'Ah', to elevate the palate.

A vagal nerve lesion at brain stem or jugular foramen level, will affect the palate and vocal cords. Unilateral weakness of the palate causes nasal speech and a tendency for food to come back up the nose. Vocal cord paralysis will cause a hoarse, soft voice and prevent explosive coughing. The failure adequately to protect the airway, as swallowing is initiated, leads to spluttering of food and fluids, with secondary regurgitation through the nasal passages.

Pain in the ear may result from irritation of the sensory fibres in the nerve. In a peripheral recurrent laryngeal nerve lesion, the palate will not be affected, but the voice symptoms will be similar and also a tendency to choke on fluids. It has recently been recognized that the external laryngeal nerve and its supplied muscle, cricothyroid, has a greater effect on speech than previously realized. Damage causes more severe and lasting speech problems than results from a recurrent laryngeal nerve lesion (Kark *et al.*, 1984).

The integrity of the vagus can be assessed by the patient's voice, ability to cough, direct inspection of the palate and indirect laryngoscopy.

An accessory nerve lesion is really a spinal root lesion, as the cranial part of the nerve is distributed with the vagus. Weakness and wasting of sternocleidomastoid and the upper part of trapezius is readily demonstrable, provided it is carefully sought. Like Horner's syndrome, this is a physical finding that is easily missed.

A hypoglossal nerve lesion produces paralysis of the intrinsic musculature of the tongue on the same side. This causes surprisingly little disability and often is discovered accidentally by the patient or his dentist. Once recognized, some slight difficulty with chewing may be appreciated by the patient.

On examination at rest in an established lesion, the affected side of the tongue will be shrivelled and fasciculating. On attempted tongue protrusion, the tongue may deviate towards the affected side.

Clinical involvement of nerves IX, X, XI, XII and cervical sympathetic nerve (see Figures 16. 13 and 16.14)

As the last four cranial nerves lie in close proximity inside the skull and even closer outside the skull, multiple involvements are the rule and a variety of named syndromes have been reported. Of immediate practical importance are four major anatomical features (Svien, Baker and Rivers, 1963):

1 The proximity of the nucleus of nerves IX, X and XI in the brain stem to the spinothalamic tract and descending cervical sympathetic nerve produces a combination of multiple nerve involvement, sparing nerve XII and affecting spinothalamic sensation on the opposite side of the body and associated with an ipsilateral Horner's syndrome. This is seen in Wallenberg's syndrome (dorsolateral medullary infarction).
2 The XIIth nerve lies in a different brain stem vascular territory and the nerve emerges lateral to the pyramid. A vascular lesion of this area will produce a XIIth nerve lesion with contralateral hemiplegia and contralateral impairment of posture sense and touch. As the nerve exits through a separate foramen it is often spared by a lesion involving the jugular foramen structures from above.

3 Outside the skull all four nerves lie so close together that the XIIth nerve is less likely to be spared and is often the first structure affected by lesions infiltrating the area from the oropharynx. Any mass in this region is often palpable.
4 As the cervical sympathetic nerve has ascended into the region, its involvement (provided there is no evidence of a brain-stem lesion such as a spinothalamic sensory loss down the opposite side) is certain evidence of an external jugular foramen lesion.

The named syndromes

Eponymous syndromes have been applied to every conceivable permutation of nerve and tract involvement affecting the last four cranial nerves. Those terms in regular use are as follows:

Vernet's syndrome (of the internal jugular foramen) is characterized by involvement by nerves IX, X and XI only (an identical syndrome has been attributed to Schmidt).

Aveills's syndrome (of the brain stem) involves nerve X and the contralateral spinothalamic tract (loss of pain and temperature only).

Tapia's syndrome involves nerves X and XII. It is difficult to see how this syndrome arises at either brain stem or peripheral level for anatomical reasons above. Presumably this would be a chance association.

Jackson's syndrome is characterized by involvement of nerves X, XI and XII. Again it is difficult to see how this combination could develop on any logical basis; presumably as a consequence of a chance peripheral combination of lesions.

Collet-Sicard syndrome (of the posterior lacerocondylar space). This is basically an external jugular foramen syndrome involving nerves IX, X, XI and XII but sparing the cervical sympathetic nerve.

Villaret's syndrome (of the posterior retropharyngeal space). This is involvement of nerves IX, X, XI and XII *and* the cervical sympathetic nerve and is diagnostic of an external jugular foramen syndrome.

Wallenberg's syndrome (infarction of the dorsolateral medulla). This consists of lesions of nerves IX and X, the cervical sympathetic nerve, contralateral spinothalamic loss in the limbs, ipsilateral spinothalamic loss over the face and severe vertigo, vomiting and hiccoughs.

Causes (*excluding cerebrovascular accidents affecting brain stem*)

Intracranial lesions

Neurinomas of the XIIth nerve, less frequently nerves IX, X and XI, and rarely an acoustic neuroma may extend down into the internal jugular foramen.
Meningioma of the lateral recess.

Cholesteatoma (particularly likely to affect nerves VII and IX).
Meningitis (especially malignant or chronic fungal meningitis).
Fracture of skull base.

Extracranial lesions

Thrombosis of the jugular bulb.
Metastatic tumour in carotid sheath lymph nodes.
Retropharyngeal abscess or neoplasm.
Carotid body tumour (of the glomus jugulare), may start externally and erode in through the petrous bone, or start in the petrous bone and erode through the skull base, in either direction.

The presenting symptoms in these cases may be the following:

1 Persistent occipital headache often resembling migraine
2 Persistent otalgia, which may be worsened on swallowing
3 Hoarse voice, pain in the throat or persistent sore throat
4 Difficulty in swallowing, choking or nasal regurgitation.

CT and MRI scanning have revolutionized the investigation of these syndromes. Previously plain skull films, tomography, and carotid angiography were used and often failed to establish a diagnosis. CT scanning will reveal very early evidence of skull base erosion or infiltration by tumour, conversely MRI scanning, by not demonstrating the bony component, will often detect a small neuroma within the jugular foramen; impossible by any other technique.

Bulbar palsy

The differential diagnosis of lower cranial nerve lesions includes those conditions destroying motor nuclei in the brain stem. Poliomyelitis has fortunately become an historical condition, the commonest cause is now motor neuron disease. The presenting symptoms consist of a tendency to cough and splutter initially on fluids but then extending to include all consistencies of food. Nasal regurgitation and aspiration are common. Speech becomes progressively unintelligible and the patient typically arrives in the clinic clutching a handkerchief to the mouth, with a written list of complaints. In the early stages poor palatal movements, poor tongue movements and weakness of jaw closure and opening, may be found, but the symmetry of involvement may make it difficult to identify mild disability. Fasciculation may be seen in the tongue and facial muscles, or palpated in the masseter. Long tract signs are important and a brisk jaw jerk, increased reflexes and extensor plantars would provide strong supporting evidence for the diagnosis. Myasthenia gravis of the bulbar type is the most important differential diagnosis. Although variability ought to be the hallmark of this disorder, occasionally non-fatiguable and apparently progressive difficulty produces a confusing picture. This is further compounded by the typical occurrence of bulbar myasthenia gravis in the elderly, the same age group who tend to develop bulbar motor neuron disease.

Pseudobulbar palsy

In earlier discussion we have noted that certain motor cranial nerve nuclei have equal bilateral upper motor neuron innervation. Only the part of the facial nerve nucleus controlling the lower face shows a major difference in having mainly contralateral supranuclear innervation. Both the palate and tongue are occasionally visibly affected by upper motor neuron lesions suggesting a variable pattern of supranuclear innervation with mainly contralateral innervation in some cases. The accessory nerve is unique in having mainly ipsilateral supranuclear innervation. The significance of these variations is in the occurrence of pseudobulbar palsy. This is usually consequent upon vascular disease but is occasionally seen in motor neuron disease and the degenerative Steele-Richardson syndrome. These latter conditions produce symmetrical bilateral supranuclear degeneration. In vascular disease a unilateral lesion will usually cause little or no dysfunction of the lower cranial nerves (Willoughby and Anderson, 1984). In a patient with the usual upper motor neuron facial weakness, transient ipsilateral weakness of sternocleidomastoid and upper trapezius and a transient weakness of the palate and tongue may be detected on careful examination in the early hours following the incident. Some time later a stroke on the opposite side will deprive the lower cranial nerves of the residual 50% of their supranuclear innervation. This will result in acute inability to speak and swallow, and is often accompanied by severe emotional lability. In stroke-related disease, these problems will always be of acute onset. In degenerative disease such as Steele-Richardson syndrome or motor neuron disease of upper motor neuron type, the onset is insidious. In all instances pseudobulbar palsy is the end result.

Extrapyramidal disease

Fine control of articulation, swallowing and the facial movements associated with speech are achieved by extrapyramidal mechanisms.

Parkinson's disease

The loss of spontaneous facial expression and infrequent blinking, consitute two of the cardinal features of this disease. In the later stages, hypophonic, tachy-phemic speech is characteristic, the short, sharp whispered phrases being virtually unintelligible. Chewing food is extremely slowed and the patient may seem to lack the will to initiate swallowing. When one adds the slowness of cutting up and transporting food to the mouth, the often cachectic state of a patient with terminal Parkinson's disease is easy to understand. The apparent sialorrhoea of Parkinson's disease actually represents a decreased swallowing rate with a normal production of saliva; it is not due to excessive secretion.

Choreiform syndromes

Choreiform movements of the tongue, palate and mouth conspire to produce spluttering, slurred, explosive speech. This may be seen in Sydenham's chorea as a transient phenomenon but constitutes a severe and progressively disabling problem in Huntington's chorea.

Dyskinetic syndromes

The so-called buccal-lingual-masticatory syndrome is usually a complication of prolonged neuroleptic therapy but is also seen in mental subnormality and dementia. In these conditions the movements do not seem to interfere with speech or swallowing, as the movements subside while speaking and eating. They are mainly a feature at rest.

The oromandibular syndrome (Meige's syndrome) in which slow dystonic opening of the jaw and mouth, in association with tongue protrusion and blepharospasm, is usually seen without neuroleptic provocation. In this condition, any attempt to talk and eat aggravates the movements.

Another possibly related dystonic syndrome is spasmodic dysphonia, a disorder characterized by choking of the voice while speaking normally due to laryngeal spasm, especially on initial vowel sounds. The patient can usually whisper, hum and sing normally. During the choking phase, spasms in the face and neck muscles and blepharospasm may be observed (Bicknell, Greenhouse and Pesch, 1968). Treatment with botulinum toxin can be a successful form of treatment.

Cerebellar disorders

Dysarthria is a feature of generalized cerebellar disease. It typically consists of a slurred, spluttering type of dysarthria as breathing mechanisms are desynchronized with speech. There is also incoordination of tongue, palatal and facial movements. Inherited cerebellar degeneration and multiple sclerosis are the commonest causes, although in the latter condition the disability is compounded by coexistent spastic dysarthria, producing the typical scanning dysarthria of the disease. Cerebellar neoplasms rarely seem to produce definite speech disturbances.

Conclusion

Although much clinical material has been included in this chapter to emphasize the salient features of the anatomy and physiology of the cranial nerves in the clinical situation, the coverage is by no means comprehensive. It is hoped that the clinical physiology of cranial nerve function included here will enable the reader to perform a competent clinical examination of the cranial nerves in those otolaryngological situations that have a high likelihood of causing anatomical damage to these structures.

References

AMOORE, J. E. (1963) Stereochemical theory of olfaction. *Nature*, **198**, 271–272

BICKNELL, J. M., GREENHOUSE, A. H. and PESCH, R. N. (1968) Spastic dysphonia. *Journal of Neurology, Neurosurgery and Psychiatry*, **31**, 158–161

BURGER. L. J., KALVIN, N. H. and SMITH, J. L. (1970) Acquired lesions of the fourth cranial nerve. *Brain*, **93**, 567–574

CHOROBSKI. J. (1951) The syndrome of crocodile tears. *Archives of Neurology and Psychiatry*, **65**, 299–318

DAVIES, J. T. and TAYLOR. F. H. (1959) The role of adsorption and molecular morphology on olfaction. *Biology Bulletin of Maine Biology laboratory, Woods Hole*, **117**, 222–238

DEHN, T. C. H. and TAYLOR, G. W. (1983) Cranial and cervical nerve damage associated with carotid endarterectomy. *British Journal of Surgery*, **70**, 365–368

EHNI, C. and WOLTMAN, H. W. (1945) Hemifacial spasm – a review of 106 cases. *Archives of Neurology and Psychiatry*, **53**, 205–213

EISEN, A. and BERTRAND, G. (1972) Isolated accessory nerve palsy of spontaneous origin – a clinical and electromyographic study. *Archives of Neurology*, **27**, 496–502

EKBOM, K. A. and WESTERBERG, C. E. (1966) Carbamezipine in glossopharyngeal neuralgia. *Archives of Neurology*, **14**, 595–596

FARNARIER, G., SARACCO, J. B. and BLANC, P. (1972) L'action du traitement medical sur les carcinomes secondaires oculo-orbitaires. *Archives d'Ophthalmologie*, **32**, 29–40

FITZGERALD, M. J. T. (ed.) (1985) Smell and taste. In: *Neuroanatomy Basic and Applied*. London: Balliere-Tindall. pp. 190–193

FONT, R. L. and PERRY, A. P. (1976) Carcinoma metastatic to the eye and orbit. III: a clinical pathologic study of 28 cases metastatic to the orbit. *Cancer*, **38**, 1326–1335

FORREST, A. W. (1949) Intraorbital tumours. *Archives of Ophthalmology*, **41**, 198–232

GODTFREDSEN. E. (1944) Ophthalmologic and neurologic symptoms of malignant naso-pharyngeal tumours: a clinical study comprising 454 cases with special reference to histopathology and the possibility of early recognition. *Acta Psychiatrica et Neurologica*, Suppl. 34, 1–323

JAFFE, N. S. (1950) Localisation of lesions causing Horner's syndrome. *Archives of Ophthalmology*, **44**, 710–780

JOHNSON, R. T. and MIMS. C. A. (1978) Pathogenesis of virus infections of the nervous system. *New England Journal of Medicine*, **278**, 23–30, 84–92

KARK, A. E., KISSIN. M. W., AUERBACH, R. and MEIKLE, M. (1984) Voice changes after thyroidectomy: role of the external laryngeal nerve. *British Medical Journal*, **289**, 1412–1415

LOEB, C. (1962) *Strokes Due to Vertebrobasilar Disease*. Springfield: Charles C Thomas

LOEWENFELD. I. E. (1969) The Argyll Robertson pupil: a re-evaluation. *Survey of Ophthalmalogy*, **14**, 199–299

LOEWENFELD, I. E. and THOMPSON, H. S. (1967) The tonic pupil: a re-evaluation. *American Journal of Ophthalmalogy*, **63**, 46–89

MCINTYRE, A. K. and ROBINSON, R. F. (1959) Pathway for the jaw jerk in man. *Brain*, **82**, 468–471

RUCKER, C. W. (1966) The causes of paralysis of the third, fourth and sixth cranial nerves. *American Journal of Ophthalmology*, **62**, 1293–1298

SCHIFFMAN, S. S. (1979) Changes in taste and smell with age. In *Sensory Systems and Communication in the Elderly*, edited by J. M. Ordy and K. R. Brizzee. New York: Raven Press. pp. 227–246

SCHIFFMAN, S. S. (1983) Taste and smell in disease. *New England Journal of Medicine*, **308**, 1275–1279, 1337–1343

SERGOTT, R. C. (1983) Neuro-opthalmic evaluation of the red orbit syndrome. *Neurology Clinics*, **1**, 897–908

SPILLANE, J. D. and WELLS, C. E. C. (1959) Isolated trigeminal neuropathy. A report of 16 cases. *Brain*, **82**, 391–416

SVIEN, H. J., BAKER, H. L. and RIVERS, M. H. (1963) Jugular foramen syndrome and allied syndromes. *Neurology (Minneapolis)*, **13**, 797–809

TAKASHI, M. (1956) Carcinoma of the paranasal sinuses: its histogenesis and classification. *American Journal of Pathology*, **32**, 501–520

TANABE, T., IINO, M. and TAKAGI, S. F. (1975) Discrimination of odours in olfactory bulb, pyriform amygdaloid areas and orbito-frontal cortex of monkey. *Journal of Neurophysiology*, **38**, 1284–1296

TAVERNER, D. (1955) Bell's Palsy – a clinical and electromyographic study. *Brain*, **72**, 209–215

THOMSEN, J. (1976) Cerebellopontine angle tumours other than acoustic neuromas. Report of 34 cases. *Acta Otolaryngologica*, **82**, 106–111

TSCHIASSNY, U. (1953) Eight syndromes of facial paralysis and their significance in localising the lesion. *Annals of Otology and Laryngology*, **62**, 677–685

WHITTET, H. B. and BOSCOE, M. J. (1984) Isolated palsy of the hypoglossal nerve after central venous catheterisation. *British Medical Journal*, **288**, 1042–1043

WILLOUGHBY, E. W. and ANDERSON, N. E. (1984) Lower cranial nerve motor function in unilateral vascular lesions of the cerebral hemisphere. *British Medical Journal*, **289**, 791–794

WRAY. S. H. (1983) Neuro-ophthalmologic diseases. In: *The Clinical Neurosciences*, vol. 2, edited by R. N. Rosenberg. New York: Churchill Livingstone. pp. 797–840

WRIGHT, R. H. (1964) *The Science of Smell*. London: Allen and Unwin

17

Imaging and radiography

P. D. Phelps

Ever since their discovery around the turn of the century, X-rays have been used with variable success for the investigation of diseases of the ear, nose and throat. In the first half of the century, such imaging was limited to plain radiographic demonstration of bony structures of the petromastoid, sinuses and skull base, and to the assessment of normally air-filled structures in the upper aerodigestive tract. This was assisted by the administration of positive contrast agents, especially those containing barium, to show the pharynx and oesophagus. Air encephalography was the only means of demonstrating intracranial structures and lesions, but as vascular and intrathecal contrast agents became less toxic, angiography began to play a greater part.

Tomography, or sectional imaging, was a useful addition to these techniques, demonstrating specific anatomy and lesions without overlap of other bony structures. The highest refinement of this process was complex motion tomography using a spiral or hypocycloidal movement of the X-ray tube. In spite of many claims to the contrary, polytomography still gives a lower radiation dose to the eyes than any other craniofacial radiological technique if the examination is performed in the prone position or lead eye shields are used.

It is computerized tomography (CT) which has, in the last few years, made the most important contribution to radiology in otolaryngology. Initially, CT represented a great advance in soft tissue imaging because of its greatly improved density resolution. Recently, improved spatial resolution for structures of high inherent contrast, such as bone, has meant that high resolution CT using thin sections and a bone algorithm gives excellent bone detail in the petrous temporal bone and the paranasal sinuses. Clear demonstration of air/soft-tissue interfaces in conjunction with this bone detail makes high resolution CT a necessary

preoperative procedure for functional endoscopic sinus surgery.

Reconstruction of an image from a set of measurements, rather than a direct recording of the image on film, is now a feature of many imaging techniques, especially that of CT. Proton magnetic resonance imaging (MRI) is used to produce sectional images not unlike those of CT, and the reconstruction methods are virtually identical. However, MR differs from CT in not using any external source of ionizing radiation. MR images are derived from radio signals emitted by substances in the body in response to an alternating applied magnetic field. In essence it is the hydrogen nucleus consisting of a single proton that is examined primarily and thus MRI is concerned with the distribution and binding of water molecules. As water is present in all soft tissues almost all areas of the body can be examined by MRI except compact bone which nevertheless can be recognized as regions of signal void. The properties measured by MRI vary widely between different soft tissue types. The main advantage of MR over X-ray techniques is its superior soft tissue differentiation. A further advantage is the accessibility of any desired image plane without physical adjustment of either the imaging system or the patient. Initially it was thought that the greatly improved contrast resolution of soft tissues by MR would obviate the need for intravenous contrast enhancement, as used with CT. However, the paramagnetic contrast agent gadolinium DTPA has been found to be very effective for defining certain tumours of the head and neck and thus magnetic resonance with or without contrast enhancement is now replacing CT for the assessment of most neoplastic lesions. Finally the sensitivity of MR to flow is making possible the assessment of blood vessels by a non-invasive technique. Magnetic resonance angiography (MRA) has now developed to the point where it is replacing conventional catheter angiography and digital subtraction angiography in diagnostic assessment, leaving only the preoperative investigation of vascular tumours and therapeutic embolization as the remaining roles for conventional angiography.

Barium studies with fluoroscopic screening have for a long time been a standard means of investigation of the upper digestive tract and are particularly good at demonstrating lesions below the cricopharyngeus. It is believed by some that any complaint of a 'lump in the throat', as well as of true dysphagia, warrants a barium swallow (Figure 17.1), but it should never be forgotten that lesions of the oesophagus, hiatus hernia and even gastric neoplasms may present with unexpected symptoms. Lesions below the cricopharyngeus are more clearly demonstrated. Dynamic studies of swallowing using cine- or videoradiography have added a new dimension to the investigation of dysphagia and are further discussed in Volume 5, Chapter 2, but a barium swallow is of rather dubious value in the identification of ingested foreign bodies.

Imaging equipment and techniques
Plain radiography

It is possible to obtain good plain film views of the head and neck by using almost any basic radiographic unit; however, for maximum detail and contrast, a specialized skull unit, which keeps the film and incident X-ray beam central, is a distinct advantage. High energy X-ray tubes, with a fine focus and with small cones to limit the field size, also improve resolution. There are now advanced skull units available (Figure 17.2) which allow the X-ray tube to be adjusted to any point on the surface of a sphere. The X-ray film is located opposite and perpendicular to the central beam, and the part of the skull to be investigated is positioned in the centre of the sphere. With the skull immobilized in the supine position, accurate angulation in three reference planes is easily reproduced and there is constant magnification with no distortion of the radiographs. For a base view, however, the head has to be extended from the fixed supine position, and the advantages of the fixed reference planes are forfeited if a special table is not used or if the examination is not undertaken with the head supine. Mathematically, accurate positioning can be achieved using the reference planes, and a full description of the technique has been given by the Swedish authors, Radberg and Thibaut (1971).

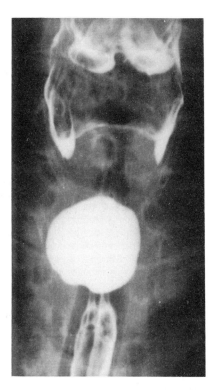

Figure 17.1 Routine barium swallow on a patient with vague dyspeptic symptoms. This anteroposterior projection shows a large unsuspected pharyngeal pouch. Above this, barium can be seen in the pyriform fossa and the valleculae

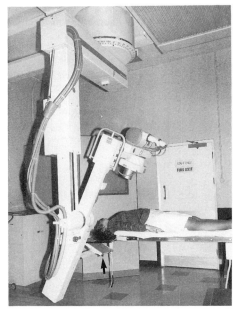

Figure 17.2 A modern isocentric skull unit. The patient is in position for a submentovertical view; this is the only projection for which the head needs to be moved from the fixed supine position. The arrow indicates the tray for the cassette

Lines and planes used in basic skull radiography (Figure 17.3) are as follows.

Radiographic baseline – orbitomeatal baseline

This is a line drawn from the outer canthus of the eye to the centre of the external auditory meatus. In the neutral position it is regarded as being always perpendicular to the film. It is raised by extending the head and lowered by flexing it. The base line is always kept at 90° to the film unless stated otherwise.

Infraorbital plane (also known as the Frankfurt plane)

This passes through the lower orbital margins and the roofs of the external auditory canals. An angle of 10° exists between the orbitomeatal baseline and the Frankfurt plane.

Auricular plane

This is at right angles to the infraorbital plane, and passes through the external auditory canals.

Median sagittal plane

A vertical plane running anteroposteriorly which bisects the skull into two equal halves. It must be aligned at right angles to the film for anteroposterior projections, and parallel to it for lateral projections. Rotation of the head around the vertical axis is referred to as rotation of the sagittal plane – the face being turned to whichever side is indicated.

Coronal plane

This is a vertical plane at right angles to the median sagittal plane, parallel to the film in anteroposterior projections. The meatal or auricular plane is a coronal plane passing through the external auditory meatus.

Tube angulation

This refers to the direction followed by the central ray emerging from the tube, which can be either 'cephalad', towards the head, or 'caudal', towards the feet. If fluid levels are being sought, a horizontal beam should be used, regardless of whether the patient is in a sitting or recumbent position.

Radiographic positions

These are named according to the direction of the central ray, with the part in contact with the film being positioned last; e.g. 20° occipitofrontal means the central ray is angled 20° caudally, and directed through the occiput to emerge through the frontal bone positioned against the film.

Immobilization

The head must always be carefully immobilized, with either head bands or special clamps, and respiration must be arrested during exposure to reduce lack of sharpness caused by movement.

Film quality

Film definition (a combination of detail and contrast) is improved if:

1 A Potter-Bucky diaphragm or grid is used, to reduce the amount of scattered radiation reaching the film
2 The beam is collimated to include only the structures under examination
3 The patient's head is immobilized to prevent movement during exposure
4 The smallest focal spot is used compatible with acceptable exposure times, optimum exposure factors, and tube focus loading
5 Suitable intensifying screens are used for optimum resolution consistent with the tube or generator output available. Rare earth screens may improve the diagnostic result if exposure factors are limited.

Conventional tomography

The basic radiograph is an image of the entire part being X-rayed with the result that structures of

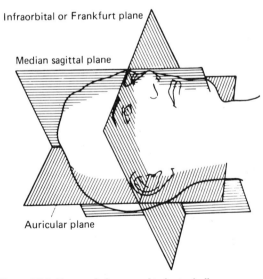

Figure 17.3 Lines and planes used in basic skull radiography. The orbitomeatal baseline (not shown) is close to the Frankfurt plane

varying density through that body area are super-imposed on each other. The tomograph consists of a radiograph visualizing just a horizontal slice of the area in question with the overlying and underlying structures blurred out by motion. This generally means that the tube and the film are the moving components while the patient remains still.

The simplest type of movement, which also has the shortest exposure time, is linear. It is, therefore, most suitable for the larynx and the tracheobronchial tree. Complex motion of the X-ray tube, either hypocycloidal or spiral, gives the most uniform blurring of structures outside the plane of section, as well as producing thinner sections of 1–2 mm thickness, although the investigation is now virtually obsolete.

Computerized tomography

Computerized tomography is the reconstruction by computer of a tomographic plane of an object (section or slice). It is developed from multiple absorption or attenuation measurements made around the periphery of the object (a scan). CT scanners use a highly collimated X-ray beam, but the radiographic film of conventional imaging has been replaced by a battery of ionization detectors which enable the required information to be obtained with maximum dose efficiency. The small volumes (voxels) of tissue, for which an attenuation value is derived, have a cross-sectional area normally less than 1 mm^2 and a depth equal to the thickness of the slice, which may be from 0.5 to 13 mm depending on the machine and the type of examination. The picture elements (pixels) are a two-dimensional reconstruction in the scan plane, displayed as a grey-scale picture on a television monitor. Computerized mathematical techniques are required to give accurate determination of the attenuation values at all points of the matrix within the section. These, as well as further considerations of how scanners function, are beyond the scope of this account. However, a brief consideration of image quality and limitation, as they affect radiology, would seem to be pertinent.

The success of CT can be attributed to its great sensitivity for very small changes in X-ray attenuation. This is known as contrast resolution. The quality of the CT image, however, depends on a complex relationship between radiation dose, spatial resolution, contrast resolution and noise. Noise is the mottling or granularity which affects the image when there is insufficient information from the detectors available for assessment. To some extent, therefore, there is a trade-off between optimum contrast resolution and optimum spatial resolution (raising the radiation dose to unacceptable levels still only partially overcomes this problem). In practice, most scanners have two options for image production, namely standard resolution for optimum density discrimination,

as when demonstrating brain tumours, and high resolution for fine detail discrimination, especially that of small bony structures in the sinuses and temporal bone. With the new rotate-only scanners, it is possible to obtain images in both soft tissue and bone resolution, using the same raw data but, inevitably, the reprocessing increases the length of the examination.

Twenty years ago, the demonstration of fine detail in the ear was considered the ultimate achievement of polytomography. In some respects the same is now true of high resolution CT, and a brief consideration of some of the limiting factors of this technique for examination of regions such as the middle ear seems desirable.

1 Partial volume averaging is a phenomenon that is seen with CT when the dimensions of the object being imaged are smaller than the slice thickness or the individual voxel. Non-representative attenuation values may be generated when all the densities within an individual voxel are averaged to produce a single attenuation coefficient. Bone or air in a voxel depicting soft tissue will significantly raise or lower the averaged attenuation reading of that voxel.
2 Soft tissue silhouetting is the outlining of small dense structures which may happen when soft tissue densities, such as normal adjacent brain, haemorrhage, tumour or fluid, are contiguous with a structure usually bordered by air. The difference in density between the structures and the background density may be insufficient for their visualization. This phenomenon is an even greater problem with the low contrast images of polytomography and is important in the evaluation of ossicular abnormalities in conjunction with soft tissue masses or small erosions. Some practical aspects of these two phenomena are demonstrated in Figure 17.4.

The standard axial or horizontal sections are used for almost all CT imaging in the ear, nose and throat, but further coronal views are often desirable, particularly for the sinuses and temporal bones. These may be obtained directly by elevating the patient's chin or by putting the head back (Figure 17.5), but it may be necessary to alter the algorithm if demonstration of soft tissue rather than bone is required (Figure 17.6). Direct CT imaging is not often used in other planes, but several projections for the temporal bones have been described in the literature (Zonneveld *et al.*, 1984). The alternative to direct imaging is reconstructed imaging from the raw data obtained from multiple axial sections. This can be done in any desired plane (Figure 17.7), but multiple axial images and, therefore, considerable extra irradiation are required. For the temporal bone, intervals of 1 mm are recommended. Even then, however, the quality of the 'reformatted' pictures will be inferior to direct

High resolution CT: partial volume averaging

Thin plate of bone at 2 different planes to the tomographic section

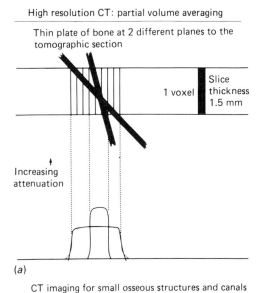

(a)

CT imaging for small osseous structures and canals

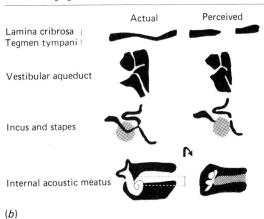

(b)

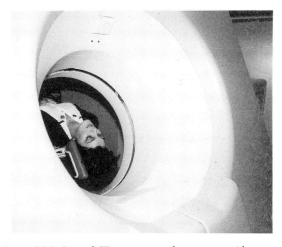

Figure 17.5 Coronal CT scan on a modern scanner with the patient in the 'head hanging' position and the scanner gantry tilted 20°

Figure 17.4 (*a*) The difficulties of imaging a thin plate of bone. At certain angles to the X-ray beam the plate will appear thicker than it should and averaging of attenuation values may mimic soft tissue. (*b*) Some practical aspects of problems with CT imaging in otolaryngology. Thin bony plates may not be demonstrated and may be thought to be eroded or dehiscent. Small canals may not be shown and may be considered to be obliterated. A soft tissue mass surrounding thin bony structures may obscure the bone detail, as in a cholesteatoma around the incudostapedial joint, and partial volume averaging may suggest a soft tissue mass within the internal auditory meatus at air meatography

imaging because of the interpolation process between adjacent slices and the problems of patient movement.

Administration of iodine-containing contrast agents, as used for many routine radiological investigations, such as excretion urography, was found in the earliest days to improve the demonstration of many intracranial pathological processes, especially that of tumours. 'Contrast enhancement', as it will henceforth be called, is still necessary for the demonstration of masses in the posterior cranial fossa. No CT brain scan investigation for suspected acoustic neuromas is complete without contrast enhancement. This enhancement is mainly a result of two factors:

1 Increased opacification of vessels
2 Extravasation into the extracellular spaces.

Outside the cranial cavity, the second phenomenon, in particular, is less apparent. Timing and degree of enhancement have been used in an attempt to differentiate tumours with little stroma, such as glomus tumours – which show instant enhancement in the vascular phase followed by rapid washout – from other vascular tumours such as meningioma, where there is no such rapid enhancement, but a more pronounced and persistent opacification beyond the initial vascular phase. Such rapid scans of the same slice, followed by a plot of time versus attenuation, are known as 'dynamic CT'. Because CT imaging involves computer assessment of X-ray attenuation, it is relatively easy to obtain attenuation values for any particular structure or discrete lesion, provided that partial volume averaging is avoided. Such densitometry studies are used for the assessment of otospongiosis (see Volume 3).

Radiotherapy planning

Computerized tomography images provide accurate information on the extent and location of tumours, which would be difficult or impossible to detect with conventional X-ray apparatus. Until recently, the information obtained had to be entered manually into the planning system with the inevitable losses in

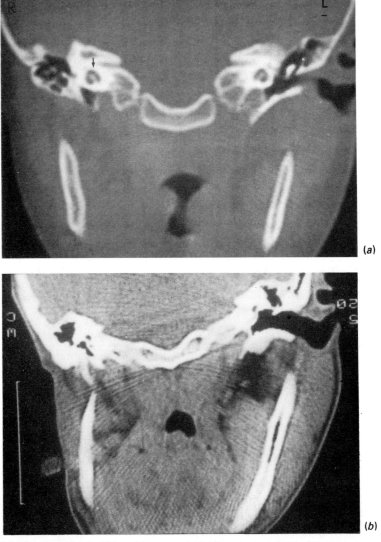

Figure 17.6 (*a*) Coronal CT scan at the level of the cochlea (arrow) in a case of right-sided hemifacial microsmia; this section on a high resolution setting and a window width of 4000 Hounsfield units also shows the deformed ossicles in the air-containing right middle ear, but does not adequately demonstrate the soft tissues below the temporal bones. (*b*) A similar coronal CT section in another case of right hemifacial microsmia showing the hypoplastic muscles; this picture on a narrow window setting has many artefacts because the high resolution mode for bone detail was used

time and accuracy. Various planning systems have been developed which enable CT slice data to be entered directly. A sophisticated dose calculation model provides three-dimensional dose distribution. This appears to be particularly useful in the area of the paranasal sinuses and nasopharynx where, in one series, 86% of patients had the planned field enlarged on the basis of CT planning scans (Adam *et al.*, 1984). However, unless therapy scans can be taken in the treatment plane, they have little advantage over diagnostic CT scans which can be used to reconstruct the tumour limits on a simulator film. If CT scans are to be used within a radiotherapy planning computer, it is important that the diagnostic images are taken with the same section orientation as will be used on the therapy equipment.

Magnetic resonance

Just as CT proved initially to be a valuable technique for imaging the brain, so MRI has shown its main

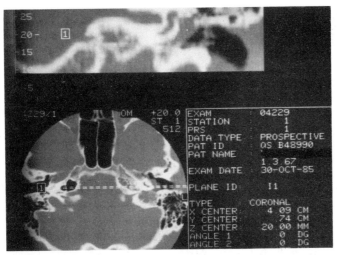

Figure 17.7 The left-sided glomus jugulare tumour has eroded the jugular fossa and extended into the middle ear cavity. A coronal reconstruction was done in the plane shown by the dotted line, and the resultant 'reformatted' coronal image shows the soft tissue mass in the lower part of the middle ear cavity below the lateral semicircular canal as well as air in the external auditory meatus and in the attic

value in the demonstration of neurological disease (Figure 17.8). A high level of contrast and an absence of artefacts characterize, in particular, the posterior cranial fossa, where MR is now superior to CT, especially as it makes possible direct coronal and sagittal imaging. Thus, CT is superior in imaging the temporal bone and sinuses because of its special ability to demonstrate soft tissue abnormalities together with fine bone detail. Magnetic resonance appears most useful for the infratemporal fossa and the

parapharyngeal regions, where tumours are well demonstrated. The relationship of masses to the various major blood vessels is better shown by MR than by contrast-enhanced CT (Figure 17.9). MR imaging relates almost exclusively to the behaviour of hydrogen protons. When the radiofrequency field which has disturbed a sample of protons is terminated, the

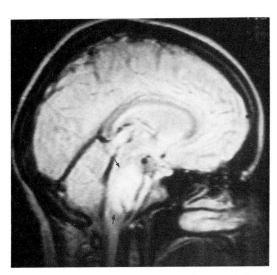

Figure 17.8 Magnetic resonance scan in the sagittal plane showing a brain stem glioma (arrows)

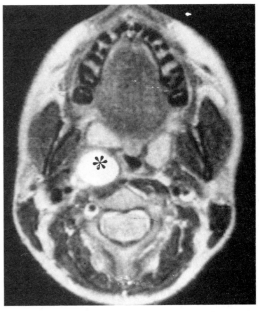

Figure 17.9 Axial T2-weighted MR scan showing high signal from a branchial cyst (asterisk)

protons return to their state of equilibrium and, in so doing, give a measurable MR signal. The magnitude of the signal is an indication of the number of protons affected and is referred to as the proton density. Only those hydrogen protons which are part of highly mobile molecules are affected; hence, at present, the technique is effectively limited to the display of water and mobile lipids. In most body tissues, it is the hydrogen of water which provides the biggest component of the MR signal. The other properties are the T1 or longitudinal relaxation time, and T2 or transverse relaxation time of these same protons.

Radiofrequency (RF) pulses applied at the correct frequency tip the magnetization away from the longitudinal direction towards the transverse plane. It takes some time for the magnetization to return to equilibrium or 'relax' to the original longitudinal orientation. This is the T1 time constant which varies for different tissues. Fat has a short T1 time and water a much longer time. After an isolated radiofrequency pulse that tips the longitudinal magnetization 90°, the magnetization resides in the transverse plane. It is mostly the decay of this transverse magnetization that gives rise to the MR signal. If a series of excitation pulses is applied with a time interval (TR) which is less than the T1 of a tissue the sequence is said to be T1 weighted. In practice such a sequence has a time interval of around 5 ms or less. It must be realized, however, that only transverse magnetization can be detected and most MR pulse sequences form an echo of the original free induction decay of the transverse magnetization which is the signal that is collected. Echo formation is achieved by following the initial 90°, radiofrequency pulse with a second 180° pulse. If T2 relaxation rates between tissues are to be accentuated, large time to echo (TE) must be used. This is called T2 weighting. In practice a second echo can be used to give more T2 weighting and this is known as 'double echo' protocol giving two sets of images; the first proton density and the second T2 weighted.

Formerly a standard investigation usually used T1- and T2-weighted protocols. The T1 images show better spatial resolution and give a high signal from fat. The fat in the alveolar tissue planes differentiates the soft tissue structures of the neck, and enables them to be seen clearly. The T2 images show poorer spatial resolution and take longer, but there is higher signal from water containing soft tissues. Thus cysts are particularly well shown (see Figure 17.9) but also tumours such as neoplasms usually have a higher than normal water content. Now, however, the T2 sequences are tending to be replaced by Gd-enhanced T1 protocols in the initial MR investigation.

A recent development has shown greatly improved spatial resolution for T2-weighted images. *Fast spin echo* (FSE) is a new fast scanning method that uses spin echoes and altered k-space filling, k-space being the amount of space which must be filled with information (raw data) to create an image. It is designed to provide more conventional spin-echo-type contrast in shorter time. In the fast spin echo pulse sequence the initial 90° pulse is followed by the acquisition of from 2 to 16 spin echoes. Each echo is acquired with a different phase-encode gradient, meaning that this information can be collected sixteen times faster than normal spin echo. The number of echoes selected is called the echo train length and the time between each echo is called the echo space. This not only shortens the examination time but enables a finer matrix to be used. Thinner sections (3 mm instead of 5 mm) can also be made and the greatly improved spatial resolution using four acquisitions means that it is possible to demonstrate the individual nerves in the internal auditory meatus. Although gadolinium-enhanced T1-weighted images have proved the gold standard for demonstrating all acoustic neuromas large and small, nevertheless this is not an entirely non-invasive procedure as an intravenous injection is necessary. The cost of the examination is also increased by the cost of the gadolinium and the presence of a radiologist is necessary. As the greatest MR workload in otolaryngology is the search for acoustic neuromas it would seem that a quick non-invasive protocol such as fast spin echo that can demonstrate the individual nerves in the internal auditory meatus, and thereby exclude an acoustic neuroma, is desirable (Figure 17.10).

Pulse sequences used in practice are:

1 *Spin echo*. This is the basic and most commonly used protocol. The initial 90° pulse is followed after an interval by a 180° pulse. The effect of the 180° pulse is to rephase the dephased protons, and neutralize external magnetic field inhomogeneities which results in a stronger signal which we call a spin-echo. The time between switching off the initial 90° pulse and the spin echo is called TE: the time to echo. Lengthening the time to echo increases the T2 weighting and the difference in signal intensity between different tissues, in particular muscle and fluid. Tumours contain increased fluid and so usually appear brighter than muscle on T2-weighted images. In practice a second 180° pulse can be applied and so two sets of images may be obtained in the same sequence, the so-called 'double-echo'. The first echo being neither T1 nor T2 weighted is known as the proton density scan: the second echo is mainly T2 weighted. A spin echo sequence with a time interval between 500 and 800 ms and a short time to echo of around 10 ms is used for the standard T1-weighted sequence. High field scanners tend to use longer time interval values than low field scanners, because T1 values are longer.

2 *Inversion recovery*. The protons are inverted by an initial 180° pulse prior to the 90° pulse resulting,

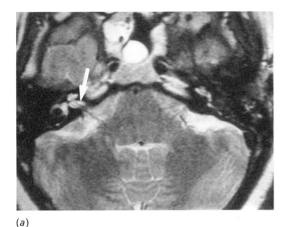

(a)

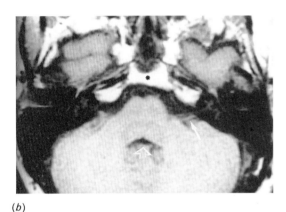

(b)

Figure 17.10 (a) Axial fast spin echo section through the internal auditory meatus showing the cranial nerves (arrow). (b) A standard T1-weighted MR section of the posterior cranial fossa. Note the high signal from marrow fat in the clivus (asterisk) and petrous apex. The cranial nerves in the cerebellopontine angle are shown (arrow) and the fourth ventricle (open arrow)

since they recover at different rates, in very heavily T1-weighted images.

3 *STIR.* The short tau inversion recovery sequence was introduced as a fat suppression sequence to demonstrate lesions in areas of high fat such as the orbit. The time to inversion is shorter than on the standard inversion recovery protocol and is set to null the signal from lipids. It does this by catching the fat protons just as they are recovering through a state of zero magnetization. The sequence works because fat has a shorter T1 than most tissues. In practice the STIR sequence shows increased signal intensity from most tumours and

has been found to be particularly useful in regions where there is much fat, such as the paranasopharyngeal spaces and around the parotid gland. Most tumours within the parotid gland are well demonstrated (Figure 17.11).

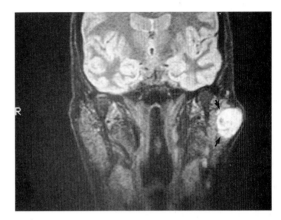

Figure 17.11 A large superficial pleomorphic adenoma of the parotid gland (arrows), which appears non-homogeneous on this coronal STIR section

4 *Enhanced scans with a paramagnetic agent.* Gadolinium (Gd) DTPA has been found to be very effective for showing neoplasms, not only intracranial tumours but those in other parts of the body. Gadolinium has the strongest magnetic moment of any paramagnetic element and has been incorporated into metal chelates to form dose effective highly stable and well tolerated proton relaxation agents. The mode of action of Gd appears to be similar to that of the iodine-containing compounds used in enhanced CT. There would seem to be two phases of enhancement: the vascular phase which occurs soon after injection, and later extravasation into the extracellular spaces. Both T1 and T2 relaxation times are reduced by Gd. The effect is most useful on T1-weighted sequences because it increases signal. On T2 sequences Gd reduces signal, which can be equivocal. T1 sequences also have the practical advantage that they give high resolution in a short scan time. Slow flowing blood gives a strong signal on T1-weighted protocols and this becomes even brighter when the blood contains Gd. Thus high signal after Gd comes from the nasal mucosa, especially over the turbinates, from the venous blood, the cavernous sinus and from inflammatory tissue. These tissues almost always enhance more than the tumour and so can be differentiated. The differentiation of tumour from oedema is also helped by Gd.

Angiography

Apart from the recently developed digital vascular imaging, almost all angiography of the head and neck is now achieved by catheterization of the femoral artery, followed by manipulation of the tip of the catheter into the appropriate vessel under fluoroscopic control. High resolution image intensification together with rapid automatic film changing and advances in catheter technology have led to selective and super-selective examination of the area of interest (Figure 17.12). The success of CT has superseded the diagnostic role of angiography in some conditions and modified it in others. Angiography is now used principally in cases of cerebral ischaemia and of intracranial haemorrhage, and in the diagnosis of aneurysms and angiomatous malformation. It still has an important role for vascular tumours, particularly glomus jugulare, and there has recently been an increased therapeutic application, particularly in the treatment of glomus tumours. The types of investigation may be listed as follows:

1 Arch aortography. This is used, although rarely now, for a demonstration of the major vessels of the neck.
2 Common carotid injection.
3 Internal carotid injection. This is used mainly for intracranial lesions.
4 External carotid injection. This is used principally for lesions of the face, and for demonstrating the blood supply of meningiomas (Figure 17.13). Super-selective demonstration of branches of the external carotid, particularly the ascending pharyngeal and the maxillary artery, is important for embolization techniques. Anastomoses with the internal carotid supply can also be demonstrated.
5 Vertebral angiography. This was formerly used for diagnosing lesions in the posterior cranial fossa. Although it is no longer used in the diagnosis of acoustic neuromas, this type of investigation is considered advisable by many surgeons for showing the vascular architecture preoperatively and, in some cases, to exclude vascular loops.
6 Retrograde jugulography. This was occasionally used to confirm the diagnosis of a glomus jugulare tumour and to show its lower limits. The sigmoid sinus and the jugular bulb can often be shown in the venous phase of a carotid angiogram, but such procedures have now been almost entirely supplanted by MRI and MRA.

Digital angiography

Digital subtraction angiography is a modified form of the subtraction technique used in vascular imaging. The essential difference between digital subtraction angiography and photographic subtraction lies in the digitalization of the video signals from an image intensifier/television system. This is followed by subtraction contrast enhancement and reconversion to analogue signals, which are subjected to further enhancement by windowing and grey-scale manipulation methods similar to those used for viewing CT images. In some systems, image enhancement is performed digitally and the resultant data are subsequently converted into analogue form for the television display.

It was hoped initially that intravenous digital

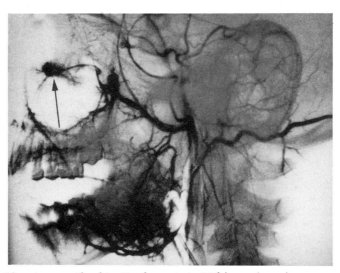

Figure 17.12 External carotid angiogram with subtraction demonstrates Little's area (arrow)

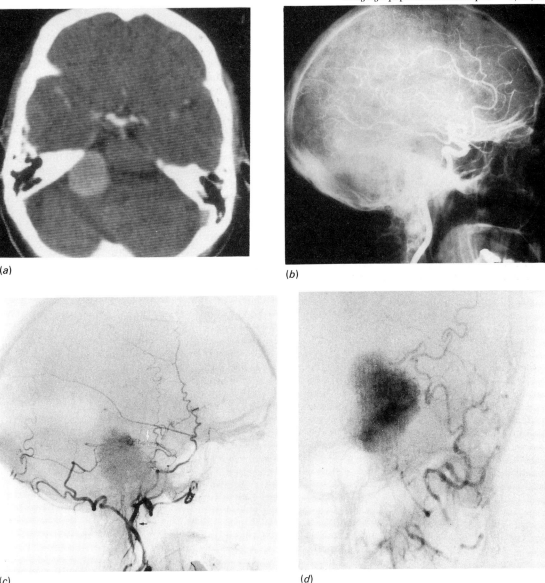

(a)

(b)

(c)

(d)

Figure 17.13 (*a*) Posterior fossa CT scan with contrast shows a dense homogeneously enhancing round mass in the posterior cranial fossa with the typical appearance of a meningioma. (*b*) The internal carotid angiogram shows no abnormality. (*c*) The external carotid angiogram with subtraction shows the pathological vessels of the tumour and its supply from the ascending pharyngeal artery (black arrow), and from the middle meningeal artery (white arrow). (*d*) Another view of the tumour showing blood supply from branches of the external carotid artery. (Courtesy of Dr Anthony D. Lloyd)

subtraction would completely replace intra-arterial procedures, but such techniques necessitate large doses of contrast agent, and movement by the patient is a problem. Movement downgrades the quality of the images recorded, but the problem can be partially overcome by what is called 're-registration' of the patient, whereby further views for the subtraction process are made during the examination.

The main applications of intravenous digital subtraction angiography are in the study of the extracranial arteries, of certain intracranial lesions, such as large aneurysms, and arteriovenous malformations, as well as in the diagnosis of cerebral venous sinus disease.

Intra-arterial digital subtraction angiography allows a low concentration of contrast medium and finer catheters to be used, reducing the risk of arterial damage. The rapid subtraction with real time display and the ability to study selected frames make this an ideal preliminary to interventional studies, although the inferior resolution for small vessels can be a problem. The efficacy of embolization and any alterations of flow which might take place can be immediately assessed (Figure 17.14).

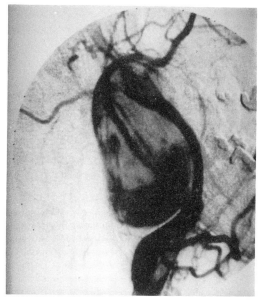

Figure 17.14 Arterial digital vascular imaging showing an aneurysm arising from the carotid system

Embolization techniques

Embolization is a technique of intravascular occlusion in which catheters are selectively manipulated into a pathological vascular territory for the purpose of injecting occlusive or embolic agents. Detachable balloons have been used to obliterate large vascular fistulae, and a great variety of embolic agents, such as Gelfoam, silicone spheres, tantalum powder and various chemical agents, have been used to obliterate feeding vessels of tumours, usually as a prelude to surgery. Super-selective catheterization is an essential preliminary. Occlusion of the nidus of the lesion, and not merely of the feeding pedicle, should be performed, and the distal migration of the emboli to the venous circulation, and beyond it, must be prevented. Such procedures should be carried out only in a few specialist neuroradiological centres.

Magnetic resonance angiography

Flowing blood has a variable appearance on MR images depending on the velocity and direction of flow. Rapidly flowing blood generally appears dark and the streaks of signal void were recognized at an early stage in the development of MR to delineate blood vessels. This is explained on the basis of protons leaving the selected section prior to emitting a spin echo. Attempts to speed the process of producing an MR image led to the development of the so-called gradient echo sequences in which the initial 90° pulse is not followed by a 180° refocussing pulse as in a spin echo protocol, but by a gradient reversal. With the reduction of time interval and time to echo characteristic of gradient echo sequences, flow related enhancement often happens, but unfortunately dephasing, rephasing and time of flight phenomena can all operate in the same image and may make it difficult to determine which appearances reflect flow artefacts and which appearances indicate signal from stationary tissue such as thrombus. Gradient echo imaging is therefore unsatisfactory for demonstrating all but the largest embolic 'strokes'. Nevertheless, recent successful attempts have been made to overcome some of these limitations by using limited flip angle gradient echo techniques in which the flowing blood has high signal intensity, because fully magnetized protons continuously enter the section being imaged and replace partially saturated spins resulting from a transverse vector which is less than 40°. There is then no spatially selective 180° pulse to discriminate against flowing spins as in a standard spin echo sequence. Other methods involve even echo rephasing and 'time of flight' (TOF) three-dimensional acquisitions which allow thinner sections and shorter times to echo. This consists of gradient echo three-dimensional imaging of multiple thin regions (slabs). Each slab consists of a small set of very thin sections. A time to echo of between 5 and 8 ms was used at a flip angle of 30°. Phase contrast MRA uses phase differences to produce angiographic images and may develop into a superior technique to time of flight for imaging complex tortuous vessels.

Despite these promising results, MRA is a complicated technique that is currently practical in only a few specialist centres. Perhaps the most useful application of MRA is the demonstration of sigmoid sinus thrombosis, an important complication of suppurative ear disease. MRA shows a signal void in the affected sinus (see Volume 3, Figure 2.16).

Limitations include patient movement and poor spatial resolution relative to standard angiography, which limits the ability to be specific about abnormalities that affect small vessels. The contrast between small vessel and background is flow dependent, and this limits the contrast to noise ratio and vessel visibility in pathological states that are characterized by slow flow. Catheter angiography will be irreplaceable for the demonstration of small blood vessels for the foreseeable future.

MRI with fat suppression

High signal from fat on T1-weighted sequences contrasting with adjacent soft tissues is the basis of much of the successful image formation by MR but, sometimes, in situations of high fat content such as the orbit or below the skull base this high signal can obscure relevant pathology. Consequently, a sequence to null the signal from lipids was produced. Fat has a shorter T1 than most tissues, and on the short tau inversion recovery (STIR) sequences the 90° pulse is timed to occur when the signal intensity of fat is zero. In practice the STIR sequence shows increased signal intensity from most tumours and has been found to be particularly useful in regions where there is much fat, such as the paranasopharyngeal spaces and around the parotid gland. Most tumours within the parotid gland are well demonstrated (see Figure 17.11). Unfortunately the STIR sequence cannot be used with Gd enhancement as signal from the enhanced tumour is suppressed along with the fat, and they are very susceptible to movement artefact.

The simplest way to show the presence of an enhancing tumour in an area containing much high signal fat is by photographic subtraction of the pre- and post-contrast images, and we have found this particularly useful for recurrent glomus jugulare tumours. However, good registration of the images is necessary in a completely immobile patient. Recently fat suppression techniques which do not affect the Gd enhanced tumours have been developed. This is known as chemical shift imaging and consists of a selective presaturation pulse technique which is centred on the resonant frequency of fat followed by a crusher gradient to disperse the fat signal (Barakos, Dillon and Chew, 1991). Unfortunately a uniform fat suppressed image is not achieved in all instances and susceptibility artefacts may occur at the periphery of the field in areas of changing body volume and at the interface of air and soft tissues to give asymmetric fat suppression. Nevertheless in situations of constant volume, chemical shift imaging can give a good demonstration of enhancing tumours. This enthusiasm for fat suppressed MR now includes all malignant tumours of the neck and below the skull base, and in one series optimal imaging to delineate squamous cell carcinomas both in the primary site and in nodal metastases was by T2-weighted fat suppressed images (Tien and Robbins, 1992). Post-contrast T1-weighted imaging with fat suppression was equally good and may improve delineation of the internal texture of lymph nodes.

Despite the undoubted improvements in soft tissue imaging brought about by MR, the ultimate goal of effective tissue characterization, the clear and distinctive demonstration of specific tumour tissue, remains as elusive as ever. This is especially true for the post-irradiation and post-surgical state where demonstra-tion of recurrent or continuant neoplasia and differentiation from chronic inflammatory tissue is extremely difficult. Specific isotope tracers like gallium have not been a success, but recently a new method has shown more promise.

Positron emission tomography (PET)

PET has been shown to be effective in detecting intracranial malignancies based on cerebral glucose metabolism. Measurement of regional tissue metabolic rates is made using radioisotopes with short half-lives. These decay with emission of positively charged particles. The positrons travel short distances in tissues before combining with a negatively charged electron, thus converting mass into energy emitted as gamma rays, which can be detected. The metabolism of glucose within cells is characterized following the administration of radiolabelled F-2-fluoro-deoxy-D-glucose (FDG). This technique has recently been applied in the detection of extracranial primary squamous cell carcinomas of the head and neck (Bailet *et al.*, 1992). In nine operative patients, PET was highly accurate in correlating tumour extent as seen on preoperative images, with the magnitude of tumour infiltration noted intraoperatively and in the surgical specimens. In one patient who received radiation therapy for a nasopharyngeal carcinoma, PET accurately delineated recurrent disease within the nasopharynx confirmed by intraoperative biopsies. Neither MRI nor CT were able to differentiate post-radiation changes from persistent tumour. These authors also found that PET appeared to be more accurate than CT or MR for demonstrating positive nodal malignancies, but like CT and MR was unable to differentiate reactive hyperplasia in some cases. PET with FDG has also been used to evaluate response to radiation and chemotherapy in patients with oro- and hypopharyngeal carcinomas. PET has been used for measuring activity-related changes in regional cerebral blood flow in response to single word processing at cortical level.

Imaging nodal metastatic disease

Although PET appears to promise a significant role in the future, the demonstration of nodal metastases is generally agreed to be slightly but significantly better by CT or MR than by clinical examination alone. At present both CT with contrast enhancement and MR are used for staging, neither having a definite advantage. CT is quicker and gives a good demonstration of 'ring enhancement', spread outside the node and other signs of neoplasia. The optimum protocols for MR have not been fully agreed and Gd enhancement tends to make the edge of the enhanced node indistinguishable from the surrounding fat. However, the fat suppression technique described above may well prove the most useful as post-contrast fat suppressed T1-weighted images can show clearly the thickened enhancing necrotic walls of metastatic nodes. An excellent review of current imaging practice for metastatic adenopathy is given by Som (1992).

Subsidiary imaging techniques

Radiological and other imaging investigations, which are sometimes used in otolaryngology but whose main application is in related specialties, will be described briefly.

Xeroradiography

A conventional source of X-rays is used for this technique; however, instead of recording on film, use is made of specially charged selenium plates to produce an image. Tomography can be used in the same way as with radiographic methods. Low contrast detail within the soft tissues is improved by the phenomenon of edge enhancement, providing a good demonstration of the air/soft-tissue interface in the pharynx and larynx (Figure 17.15).

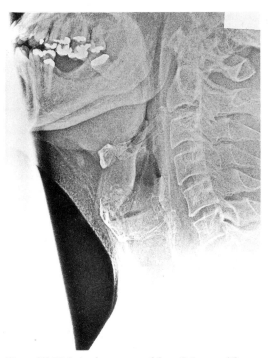

Figure 17.15 Lateral xerogram of the soft tissues of the neck showing the outlines of pharynx and larynx as well as the hyoid bone and laryngeal cartilages

The wide exposure latitude provides, in the same image, good detail of both soft tissue and bone. The disadvantages of xeroradiography are those of the increased radiation dose, which must be considered when examining children, the increased cost, and some loss of bone detail. Practical experience has shown that the improvement in soft tissue detail is useful in examining the pharynx and larynx, but there is little call for the technique in other areas, such as the sinuses, and therapy planning is now probably better done with CT and MR.

Panoramic radiography (orthopantomography)

Synchronous and reciprocal movement of the X-ray tube and film cassette around the lower part of the head of the patient constitutes the basic design of the panoramic X-ray machine. The curved focal plane is engineered to correspond to the size and shape of the average dental arch. It is possible to achieve, on one film, a complete demonstration of all bony structures in the upper and lower jaws, as well as of all teeth, both erupted and unerupted. These machines are now available, especially in dental clinics where their main use is for dental surveys; they are particularly useful to the orthodontist in the case of children with devel-opmental abnormalities, as a comparison between the two sides can easily be made. The patient is examined standing or sitting when using the commonest type of orthopantomograph. A bite block or jaw support automatically positions the jaws within the focal plane, but some repositioning may be necessary to obtain views of the antra and the temporomandibular joints. Spring loaded or movable head-clamps are normally used because of the long X-ray exposure times (between 15 and 22 s).

A quick and simple demonstration of the temporomandibular joints and parotid regions can be achieved (Figure 17.16), although the slightly oblique view of the temporomandibular joint demonstrates the neck and condyle of the mandible better than the articular fossa and eminence. A 'reversed orthopantomograph', an option available only on certain types of orthopantomograph, gives a rather better demonstration of the joint (Figure 17.17). However, the best demonstration of bone detail in the temporomandibular joint is by lateral complex motion tomography, but CT, MR or arthrography are necessary to show the state of the intra-articular disc.

The patient is examined in the supine position on a sophisticated and versatile, but more expensive, development of the basic panoramic X-ray machine. The panoramic image comes from a combination of linear and circular movements of the X-ray tube around the patient's head. The exposure is made throughout or during only certain segments of the

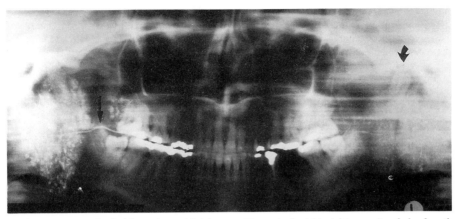

Figure 17.16 Orthopantomograph of a bilateral parotid sialogram. The main duct (straight arrow) and gland on the right are well demonstrated, but on the left the gland architecture has largely emptied of contrast. There is a punctate sialectasis. The curved arrow points to the temporomandibular joint on the left side

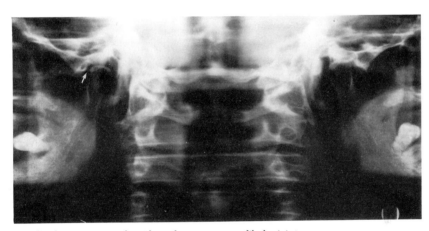

Figure 17.17 Reversed orthopantomograph to show the temporomandibular joints

tube movement and planned programmes for the middle third of face anatomy; temporomandibular joints (lateral view), cervical vertebrae, optic foramina and dentition are available. There is no need to turn or move the supine patient during the examination, and a good demonstration of facial anatomy makes this an excellent apparatus for assessing a badly injured patient. However, for dental surveys and demonstrations of the temporomandibular joints, this technique has no advantage over simpler panoramic X-ray machines. Other options available, such as views of the temporal bones, are, in the opinion of the author, of little value.

Attachments for cephalometric skull radiography are sometimes added to panoramic machines for use in dental clinics. Cephalometric radiographs are used primarily by orthodontists and oral and maxillofacial surgeons in the evaluation of facial growth and devel-

opment. The lateral and posteroanterior radiographs are made at a standard anode film distance of 152 cm (60 inches), the patient's head should be stabilized to produce a true lateral projection and the soft tissues of the face must be seen in addition to the skeletal structures. Such cephalometric methods have been used to estimate the size of the adenoid pad.

Ultrasonography

Although ultrasound has been used for the investigation of sinus disease, its practical value in otolaryngology is very limited and depends on its ability to identify fluid-filled cavities. Ultrasound may help, therefore, to confirm the cystic nature of masses in the neck – particularly in or around the thyroid gland – in the salivary glands and branchial cysts. A typical cystic lesion which proved to be vascular is shown in Figure 17.18. Recently, ultrasound has been used for the assessment of nodal metastases. Enlarged nodes are well shown but the examination is less specific than CT or MR.

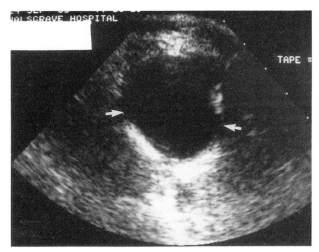

Figure 17.18 An ultrasound scan of a cystic mass in the neck which proved to be an aneurysm. In the neck, ultrasound is only of value in confirming the fluid-filled nature of the mass

Isotope scanning

The introduction of radioactive tracer materials, especially the technetium phosphate analogues, together with improved camera techniques and better diagnostic image resolution, have today resulted in the ready adaptation of bone scanning to the diagnosis of a variety of clinical problems. The major role of bone scanning in medicine generally remains that of the search for occult bony metastases in patients harbouring cancers known to have a predilection for the bony skeleton (that is breast, lung and prostate). Bone scans demonstrate areas of increased osteoblastic activity; however, this is a non-specific finding which may indicate a variety of disease processes including fracture, osteomyelitis, arthropathy, bone dysplasia, or primary or secondary tumour in bone. Carcinoma of the oral cavity, and particularly of the floor of the mouth, frequently invades the mandible subclinically before there is any evidence of bone destruction on plain films or orthopantomography. The extent of surgical resection depends greatly on whether or not there is bone involvement by the tumour; osteoblastic reaction on delayed bone scanning is often the earliest indication (Figure 17.19).

Formerly, radionuclide studies had an important role in neuroradiology where they were able to demonstrate approximately 80% of brain tumours. However,

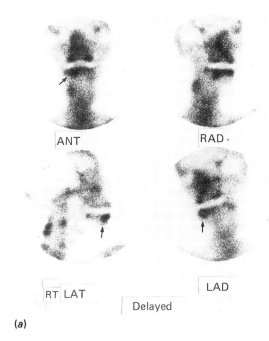

(a)

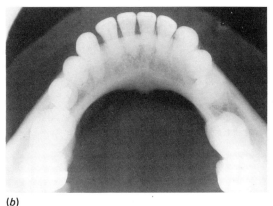

(b)

Figure 17.19 (a) A technetium-based isotope scan of the jaws showing an area of increased uptake in the anterior part of the mandible (arrow). The patient had a carcinoma of the floor of the mouth and the bone scan confirms that the mandible was involved. This was proved at surgery. (b) An intraoral view of the anterior part of the mandible shows no evidence of any involvement by this tumour. (Courtesy of Dr Arnold M. Noyek, Toronto)

these investigations have now been almost completely superseded by CT scanning and MRI. Dynamic and functional studies of the cerebrospinal fluid pathways, using labelled proteins or labelled inorganic chelating agents, still have a place; but CT, combined with cerebrospinal fluid water-soluble contrast agents, has the advantage of morphological display. Similarly, radionuclide cisternography has been used with variable success in the evaluation of cerebrospinal fluid leaks, particularly rhinorrhoea. This technique is even less satisfactory for demonstrating fistulae through the ear, and it is not required if a congenital deformity of the labyrinth is demonstrated by tomography or CT and the discharge of cerebrospinal fluid is confirmed by analysis of the fluid or the use of fluorescein or other tracers (see Volume 6, Chapter 2).

Temporomandibular joint disorders can be usefully assessed by bone scanning. Most discomfort and/or pain in or about the temporomandibular joint relates to altered muscle tension about the joint by the powerful muscles of mastication, probably on account of dental malocclusion which causes a change in bite dynamics. Isotope studies have also been used for the assessment of facial fractures and osteomyelitis or to predict the likely growth rate of osteomas. The salivary glands normally concentrate technetium-99m sodium pertechnetate. Originally, this was considered to be a nuisance on brain scans, but it is now used for the functional assessment of the gland parenchyma. Hyperfunction is seen in acute sialadenitis, granulomatous diseases, lymphoma and the sialoses; decreased activity with Sjögren's syndrome and most primary and metastatic tumours. Exceptions are Warthin's tumours and oncocytomas which intensely accumulate the radionuclide. The larynx is another organ which has been investigated with radioactive isotopes. Anterior extension of laryngeal cancer into the pre-epiglottic space is an important finding which may affect management of the disease. Extensive pre-epiglottic space involvement, sufficient to reach the hyoid bone, will incite a delayed osteoblastic response on the bone scan. For an account of this and other aspects of radionuclide scanning in otolaryngology, the reader is referred to the work of Noyek (1979).

Dacrocystography

Ultrafluid Lipiodol injected into the inferior canaliculus through a very fine catheter is used to demonstrate the patency of the canaliculi, lacrymal sac and the nasolacrimal duct. When disease is present, the site and degree of obstruction and the presence of fistulae, diverticula and concretions are shown. The exposure of the films is made during the actual injection of the contrast medium, and in normal patients will produce an image which is continuous throughout the duct system (Figure 17.20). Subtraction studies are particularly useful for demonstrating the common canaliculus. Common canaliculus blocks are characterized by the regurgitation of contrast medium through the upper punctum, and the outlining of both the upper and lower canaliculi on the radiographs, without filling of the lacrimal sac if the obstruction is complete. Complete or partial obstruction shows as a dilatation or 'mucocoele' of the lacrimal sac; it may be caused by congenital stenosis, inflammatory processes, trauma or neoplasms.

Sialography

Injection of radiopaque contrast medium into Stenson's or Wharton's duct to demonstrate the glandular ductal system is still the principal means of investigation into diseases of the parotid and submandibular salivary glands.

Before the contrast medium is introduced, plain films are obtained to demonstrate any radiopaque calculi or calcification within the gland. For the parotid gland, lateral and oblique views should be obtained in the open

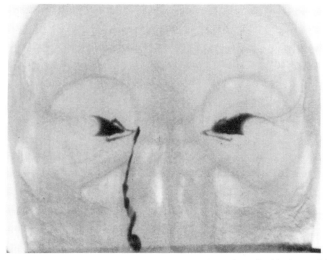

Figure 17.20 Bilateral dacrocystogram shows normal appearances on the right and a blockage of the common canaliculus on the left

mouth position. The lateral view for the submandibular gland should be taken with the floor of the mouth depressed by the patient's finger or a wooden spatula pressing the tongue downwards. An intraoral occlusal film is necessary to exclude a stone in Wharton's duct.

For the injection, either a water soluble or an oily contrast medium may be used. The present author uses ultrafluid Lipiodol, which allows good filling of the smallest calibre salivary ducts, and, being more viscid than the water-soluble agents, is easier to keep in the ductal system.

The opening of Stenson's duct of the parotid gland is opposite the second upper molar tooth. The orifice of Wharton's duct of the submandibular gland lies under the tip of the tongue on the sublingual papilla, and is smaller than that of Stenson's duct. In either case, the opening needs to be gently dilated with suitable dilators of the lacrimal type. Cannulation is by a catheter or sialographic cannula, and a hand injection technique is used. A sialogram can be considered in three phases – ductal filling, acinar filling, and evacuation. Acinar filling can be accomplished in most patients. The patient should be warned that discomfort will be felt in the region of the injected gland and should be told to signal when this occurs.

Conventional sialography is still the best examination for the duct architecture and for diseases of the duct system, such as sialectasis (Figure 17.21). It is less satisfactory for the demonstration of mass lesions, which appear as filling defects in the normal sialogram. Tumours within the parotid gland are better demonstrated and outlined by MRI. The parotid glands usually show lower CT attenuation than the adjacent muscles, and this feature also occurs with intraparotid tumours. Parotid sialography may give a better demonstration of the situation and extent of such a mass; however, with the improved resolution of the latest scanners, it is now less necessary than it was previously and in any case MRI is to be preferred.

Arthrography of the temporomandibular joint

The best demonstration of the bony components of the temporomandibular joint, i.e. condyle of the mandible and articular fossa and eminence, is obtained with lateral complex motion tomography. Plain film views and panoramic tomography are less satisfactory, especially for showing the articular fossa. However, none of these conventional techniques will show the thin fibrocartiliginous disc that divides this synovial joint into an upper and lower compartment. Recently, CT has been used to delineate the soft tissues of the temporomandibular joint, but positioning is difficult for direct sagittal sections and the definition of reformatted images is not really adequate. Magnetic resonance has also been used to show the disc.

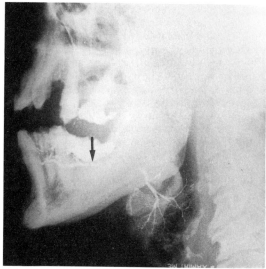

(a)

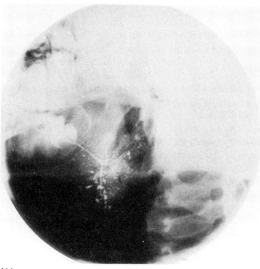

(b)

Figure 17.21 (*a*) Submandibular sialogram. The arrow points to the main duct. (*b*) Parotid sialogram with some degree of punctate sialectasis

In the meantime, arthrography, although not widely used, can be performed to provide evidence of disc displacement, disc perforation or both. The examination is most helpful diagnostically in those cases which have little or no bony abnormality shown on the tomograms, but in which the clinical features nevertheless suggest disc derangement. Either or both joint spaces may be injected, but usually just the lower compartment is opacified (Figure 17.22), although disc perforation will allow the upper compartment to fill as well. Further elaboration of the tech-

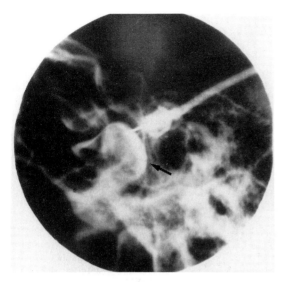

Figure 17.22 Temporomandibular joint arthrography.
Contrast is in the inferior compartment (arrow).
(Courtesy of Dr Ferraro)

nique can be achieved by use of tomography, double
contrast (using air as well as water-soluble contrast
agents), fluoroscopy and cineradiography.

Conclusions

The foregoing is an account of the imaging techniques which are, or can be, used in the practice of
otolaryngology for the demonstration of normal and
abnormal anatomy; for showing the situation and
extent of disease processes; and, in some instances,
for indicating the nature of the lesion. Few, if any,
should be considered routine examinations, and they
should be requested only after an adequate clinical
examination has been made. Most hospitals in the
UK have open access to radiographic facilities for
general practitioners, but whether such otolaryngological radiographic investigations should be ordered
by general practitioners is debatable. A barium swallow is perhaps the only satisfactory investigation that
may be undertaken without a prior otolaryngological
opinion. The most frequent examination requested is
that of plain film views of the sinuses in cases referred
from general practitioners, otolaryngologists and
other specialties, for a variety of symptoms, some of
which are quite non-specific. Clear sinus X-rays not
uncommonly exist in the presence of a nasopharyngeal carcinoma; which can result in a false sense of
security unless this is appreciated. The author believes that a radiological examination of the petrous
bone should be requested only by a specialist in this
field. Radiographs of the cervical spine in the case of
dizziness in an elderly patient serve no purpose.

The greatest change in the last 5 years has been
the development of computerized imaging, both CT
and MRI. Radiologists can now demonstrate not only
the bony changes that are produced by abnormalities
of the head and neck, but also the soft tissue changes.
The deep extent of a lesion can be shown and not
just the encroachment on the adjacent lumen. CT is
the optimum means of showing the soft tissue and
bone abnormalities in sinus disease and in the middle
ear. High resolution CT is now available at district
general hospital level, and the greatly improved demonstration of bone and soft tissue structures in the
head and neck gives an added impetus for radiologists
and otolaryngologists to become familiar with the
sectional anatomy displayed.

Three-dimensional imaging

It is now possible to obtain three dimensional (3-D)
reconstructions from a series of two-dimensional CT
scan slices by using a specific 3-D software computer
program. The scanning parameters in the 2-D plane
have a major influence on the quality of the resultant
3-D image, especially spatial resolution and contrast.
Important considerations when planning 3-D are the
slice thickness and bed increment of the original
study. Obviously the thinner the slice the greater the
resolution of the 3-D image but at the cost of a
possible increase in radiation dose to the patient as
the total number of scans in any one plane is increased. However, this may eliminate scanning in
both axial and coronal positions if other reconstructions are to be obtained. Patient movement is to be
avoided so good radiographic techniques must be
employed and scanning parameters such as zoom
factor must not be altered. For a typical 3-D reconstruction approximately 20 to 30 slices are required
in order to gain a good 3-D image. Depending on the
software, magnification plus rotation functions and
other manipulations such as 'cutting planes' can be
executed relatively easily providing further useful
information. It is also possible to undertake 3-D
images selecting differing tissue parameters such as
bone or soft tissue.

The full advantages of this imaging technique are
as yet not fully explored, but it has proved particularly useful for facial reconstructions in cases of congenital deformity or due to major trauma. The surgeon can be given a more complete appraisal of the
overall anatomy (Figure 17.23). However, 3-D imaging of the petrous temporal bone has failed to demonstrate fine bone detail such as the ossicles and dehiscences in the tegmen tympani and cannot be considered particularly advantageous at present (Astinet *et
al.*, 1992), although it has been suggested that a 3-D
study is helpful when exploration of a congenital
aural atresia is planned (Andrews *et al.*, 1992).

The subsidiary techniques listed previously have

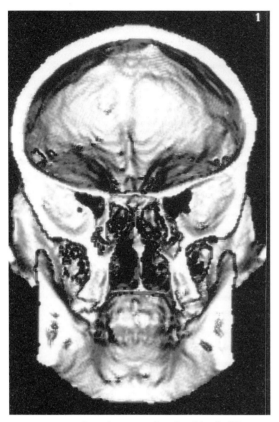

Figure 17.23 A three-dimensional study of the skull base

only occasional application in otolaryngology and, depending on availability, need to be used after discussion with a radiologist in the attempt to solve a specific problem. The latest computer-assisted methods can readily be used to measure certain properties of the normal and abnormal tissues being imaged, particularly X-ray attenuation by CT, and proton density and relaxation times by magnetic resonance. However, the attempts to chart a limited range of such values without overlap and to provide a means of 'tissue characterization' have so far proved largely unsuccessful.

What of the future of imaging in otolaryngology? The rapid advance of new technology during the last 5 years is indicative of certain trends. The limitations of plain radiographs, the cost of silver and the problems of storage of X-ray film probably mean that the traditional imaging methods will be used less. Tomographic methods will have increasing application. The demand for increasing the spatial resolution in CT means increasing the number of detectors and, simultaneously, the concomitant radiation exposure of the patient. A possible solution to this problem is provided by partial scanning. The mathematical reconstruction is made over a limited target volume or all detectors are directed towards a limited region of interest within the body, and only this region is scanned. The procedure reduces X-ray exposure, and all the detectors can be used to provide a high-resolution image of the scanned region. However, slice reconstruction does pose some problems. Another solution is to use imaging with non-ionizing radiation. The ionizing effect of X-rays restricts their usefulness in diagnostic imaging, in view of the need to limit the radiation exposure received by the patient. Hence all kinds of imaging with non-ionizing radiation are attractive alternatives, provided that acceptable image quality can be achieved. In this context, image quality mainly means spatial resolution, a process which, for magnetic resonance, is being rapidly improved although, generally speaking, the latter remains inferior to CT.

Digital radiography, the manipulation of digital data storage and the retrieval of pictorial information, will be increasingly used as a consequence of the availability of powerful small computers, very fast dedicated image processors and large storage capacity. The latest digital storage media could be the nucleus of an overall information system within a hospital. This could incorporate one year's image storage. The picture source can be any kind of imaging system, such as CT or ultrasound, and even conventional X-ray film can be converted into digital data, making basements full of 'old films' a thing of the past.

References

ADAM, J. C., BERRY, R. J., CLITHEROW, S. and BEDFORD, A. (1984) Evaluation of the role of computed tomography in radiotherapy treatment planning. *Clinical Radiology*, **35**, 147–150

ANDREWS, J. C., ANZAI, Y., MANKOVICH, N. J., FAVILLI, M., LUFKIN, R. B. and JABOUR, B. (1992) Three-dimensional CT scan reconstruction for the assessment of congenital aural atresia. *American Journal of Otology*, **13**, 236–402

ASTINET, F., LANGER, M., KESKE, U., ZWICKER, C., HIPPEL, K., FELIX, R. *et al.* (1990) High resolution computerized tomography of the petrous bone with two-dimensional and three-dimensional reconstruction. *Fortschritte auf dem Gebiete der Rontgenstrahlen und der neuen Bildgebenden Verfahren*, **153**, 14–21

BAILET, J. W., ABEMAYOR, E., JABOUR, B. A., HAWKINS, R. A., HO, C. and WARD, P. H. (1992) Positron emission tomography: a new, precise imaging modality for detection of primary head and neck tumours and assessment of cervical adenopathy. *Laryngoscope*, **102**, 281–288

BARAKOS, J. A., DILLON, W. P. and CHEW, W. M. (1991) Orbit, skull base and pharynx: contrast-enhanced fat suppression MR imaging. *Radiology*, **179**, 191–198

NOYEK, A. M. (1979) Bone scanning in otolaryngology. *Laryngoscope*, **89** (suppl. 18), 1–88

RADBURG, C. and THIBAUT, A. in collaboration with DELVAUD, G. (1971) *Supine Skull Radiography with Orbix*. Sölna, Sweden: Elema Schonander AB

SOM, P. (1992) Detection of metastasis in cervical lymph nodes: CT and MR criteria and differential diagnosis. *American Journal of Radiology*, **158**, 961–969

TIEN, R. D. and ROBBINS, K. T. (1992) Correlation of clinical, surgical, pathologic, and MR fat suppression results for head and neck cancer. *Head and Neck*, **14**, 278–284

ZONNEVELD, F. W., VAN WAES, P. F. G. M., DAMSMA, H., RABISCHONG, P. and VIGNAUD, J. (1984) Direct multiplanar CT of the petrous bone. *Head and Neck Imaging*, **16**, 754–778

18

Basic immunology

Lee S. Rayfield, Charles G. Kelly and Stephen J. Challacombe

Immunology is the study of the immune system and has its historical foundations in the way the body combats infectious disease. Long before the principles of microbiology and immunology were understood, it had been recognized that not all individuals became ill during an epidemic, and that those who recovered were resistant to future outbreaks. This state was termed 'immunity', meaning exemption.

In order effectively to resist an invading organism, whether virus, bacterium, fungus, protozoan or worm, the immune system has to be able to distinguish between the body's own constituents ('self') and those of the invader ('non-self'). Normally an individual fails to respond to (is tolerant of) self, but in autoimmune disease this tolerance breaks down. In immunodeficiency there is a partial or complete failure of some part of the immune system, which results in recurrent, and sometimes life-threatening, infections. In transplantation reactions, the graft, which is desirable to the body, is nevertheless rejected because it is foreign.

Damage to the surrounding tissues during the course of an immune response may sometimes exceed the potential benefits. Such exaggerated responses are termed 'hypersensitivity reactions'.

As immunological processes are involved in the majority of human diseases, including those of the ear, nose and throat, an understanding of the cellular and molecular basis of the immune system is essential. This chapter summarizes fundamental immunological mechanisms and their role in defence and disease states.

Immunity to infection

The means by which the body protects itself from invasion and infection can be broadly classified into two types. Those where prior exposure to the particular organism enhances a second immune response, namely specific, acquired or adaptive immunity, and those which are only minimally affected, namely nonspecific, innate or natural immunity. Innate immunity is the more primitive type and will be considered first.

Innate immunity

A variety of factors contributes to innate immunity. The most obvious obstacle to a potential invader is perhaps the physical barrier provided by the skin and mucous membranes. Although these surfaces are by no means impervious, the severe infections found in patients suffering from burns show how important this primary mechanical barrier is. Secretions which bathe mucosal surfaces cleanse and hamper colonization by microorganisms. The cilia of the lungs and the motility of the gastrointestinal tract contribute to expulsion. A number of inhibitory or microbicidal substances are present on the skin and in seromucous secretions, including lactic acid, saturated and unsaturated fatty acids and basic polypeptides.

In saliva and milk, lactoferrin inhibits bacterial growth by chelating the available iron. Lactoperoxidase, in the presence of hydrogen peroxide and thiocyanate ions, kills bacteria. Lysozyme is an enzyme which splits the mucopeptides of the bacterial cell wall by cleaving N-acetylmuramic acid from N-acetylglucosamine. It is found in tears, nasal secretions, saliva, blood and on the skin. Lysozyme is particularly toxic to Gram-positive bacteria, and it can also kill Gram-negative organisms if the cell wall is damaged to allow the enzyme access.

Non-pathogenic, commensal or symbiotic organisms constitute the normal mucosal flora. In addition to providing essential nutrients (e.g. vitamin K), they prevent colonization by virulent organisms through competition or by the production of microbicidal agents.

If a potentially pathogenic organism breaches the external barriers and enters the blood, two vital second lines of non-specific defence are provided by phagocytic cells and the complement system.

Phagocytic cells

Phagocytosis (literally 'cell-eating') involves the recognition, engulfment, killing and digestion of particulate matter. The latter may be whole cells or debris, and of foreign or host origin; phagocytes are thus not only defenders but also scavengers. The task is principally undertaken by two, morphologically distinct populations of bone-marrow derived leucocytes. Neutrophils are part of the granulocyte lineage and comprise between 45 and 70% of the adult leucocyte population. They are short-lived, lasting about 2 days, and have a high turnover rate in the bone marrow. The diameter is 12–14 μm and the cells have a characteristic multilobed nucleus. Within the cytoplasm there are many azurophilic granules (lysosomes), which hold a battery of proteolytic and hydrolytic enzymes (Figure 18.1*a*).

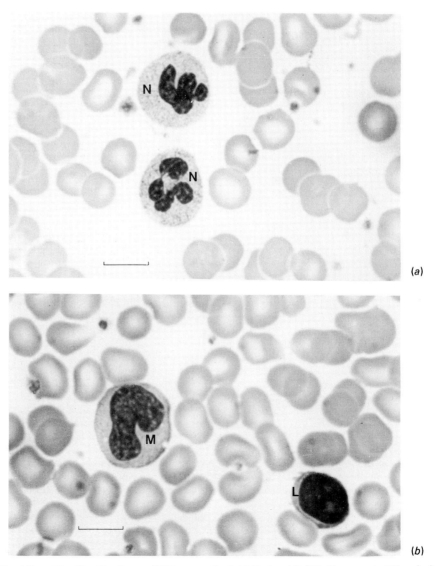

(a)

(b)

Figure 18.1 Blood films stained by May-Grunwald/Giemsa method. (*a*) Neutrophils (N); (*b*) monocyte (M) and a lymphocyte (L). Scale measures 10 μm. (Courtesy of Dr V. Sljivic)

In contrast to neutrophils, which are relatively uniform in appearance, the second group of phagocytes, monocytes and macrophages, form a heterogeneous collection of cell types. Both monocytes and macrophages derive from a common precursor, the promonocyte, but the macrophage is generally regarded as a terminally differentiated cell.

Fixed tissue macrophages comprise the mononuclear phagocyte system or reticuloendothelial system and function as an extremely effective filter. The Kupffer cells of the liver, alveolar and peritoneal macrophages, histiocytes of the skin, sinusoidal lining cells of the spleen, bone osteoclasts and, possibly, the microglia of the brain all belong to the mononuclear phagocyte system. Monocytes and macrophages are long-lived, having a lifespan of many weeks. They range in size from 15 to 40 μm and possess potent cytocidal and digestive substances within the small membranous lysosomes of the cytoplasm. Monocytes make up between 2 and 8% of normal peripheral blood leucocytes and are distinguished by their indented, horseshoe-shaped nucleus (Figure 18.1*b*).

Stages in phagocytosis

Phagocytosis can be divided into several distinct phases (Figure 18.2).

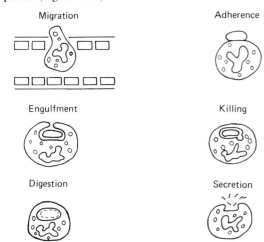

Migration

Adherence

Engulfment

Killing

Digestion

Secretion

Figure 18.2 Stages in phagocytosis by neutrophils, monocytes and macrophages

Migration

Blood-borne neutrophils and monocytes are attracted to sites of inflammation where the integrity of the tissues has been disturbed and a variety of pharmacological mediators have been activated, including chemotactic factors (see below). Vasoactive substances, such as histamine and serotonin (5-hydroxytryptamine), cause the blood vessels to become leaky and facilitate the adherence of phagocytes to the endothelium. The phagocytes form pseudopodia, which push between the endothelial cells and allow the cell to squeeze through the vessel wall.

Adherence

Contact between the particle to be engulfed and the phagocyte results in adherence to the cell membrane. This adherence may be greatly enhanced by the presence of opsonins, which coat the particle and bind to specific receptors on the phagocyte surface (see below). In the absence of opsonins, adherence most probably results from electrostatic interactions between particle and membrane. Whatever the nature of the binding, adherence triggers a metabolic or respiratory burst and the formation of a plethora of oxygen-dependent and highly microbicidal agents within the lysosomes.

Engulfment

Spreading of the initial site of attachment to the cell continues until the particle is completely surrounded by membrane. This is then pinched off to form an intracellular vacuole known as a phagosome.

Killing

The lysosomes fuse with the phagosome to form a phagolysosome, releasing toxic and digestive substances into the vacuole. Of the oxygen-dependent mechanisms activated during the respiratory burst, the generation of hydrogen peroxide (H_2O_2) and the formation of free oxygen radicals, such as superoxide anions (O_2^-), singlet oxygen ($^1O_2$) and hydroxyl groups (OH), are perhaps the most significant.

Digestion

Breakdown of phagocytosed particles may be brought about by the action of hydrogen peroxide and myeloperoxidase, and by proteolytic and hydrolytic enzymes.

Secretion

Following killing and digestion, the contents of the phagolysosome are expelled from the cell after fusion with the cell membrane. Macrophages, but not neutrophils, may retain some of the breakdown products on the cell membrane and present them to lymphocytes (this interaction will be dealt with more fully later). The secretion of active enzymes or radicals may cause damage to other microorganisms that have not been phagocytosed. However, local tissue damage may also result.

The complement system

The complement system consists of a series of glyco-proteins (Table 18.1) that circulate in the extracellular fluid compartment. They participate in a triggered enzyme cascade which comprises an initiation phase, amplification and the assembly of a membrane attack sequence. It involves a precise, sequential activation of inactive components, some of which are proenzymes. These, in turn, act enzymatically on components further along the pathway and cause the release of biologically active portions of the components (cleavage fragments). The process is one of amplification because an initial stimulus can cause the activation of millions of later components.

There are two major pathways of complement activation: the classical pathway, which was discovered first, and the alternative pathway, which is probably the more primitive phylogenetically. Both pathways lead to the formation of an enzyme (convertase) which splits the third complement component C3, the lynch-pin of the complement system. Both pathways also share a terminal sequence (or attack sequence) involving the components designated C5, C6, C7, C8 and C9. Biologically, the triggering of the complement cascade by either pathway leads to the activation of cells, opsonization and the lysis of complement-coated cells. A simplified representation of the cascade is shown in Figure 18.3.

Complement activation by the classical pathway

The components of complement that take part in the classical pathway are C1, C4, C2 and C3 (Figure 18.3a) – because the numbers were assigned to the components as they were discovered, the activation sequence does not follow the numerical order. Furthermore, C1 consists of three subunits: C1q, C1r and C1s. The major initiating stimulus for the classical pathway is the binding of C1q to an antigen–antibody complex. However, in the absence of antibody the pathway can be activated by lipid A – a constituent of the cell wall of certain bacteria – and by the envelope of oncornaviruses.

Table 18.1 Components of the complement system

Pathway	Component	Fragments	Molecular weight (kilodaltons)	Activity
Classical	C1q		410	Binds to C1r and C1q receptors on T and B cells
	C1r		170	Activates C1s
	C1s		85	With C1q and r cleaves C4 and C2
	C4		210	
		C4a	10	Anaphylatoxin
		C4b	200	Complexed with C2b splits C3, weak immune adherence via CR1
	C2		115	
		C2a	35	None
		C2b	80	Complexed with C4b splits C3
Alternative	Factor B		93	Binds to C3b
		Ba	30	? None
		Bb	63	Complexes with C3b to form convertase
	Factor D		25	Cleaves factor B
	Properdin		184	Stabilizes C3bBb complex
Terminal common pathway	C3		195	
		C3a	9	Anaphylatoxin
		C3b	186	Immune adherence via CR1 on phagocytes
	C5		205	
		C5a	11	Anaphylatoxin, chemotaxin
		C5b	195	
	C6		128	Binds to C5b
	C7		121	Binds to C5bC6, complex attaches to lipid membranes
	C8		155	Polymerizes C9
	C9		75	Forms channel in membrane
Regulation	C1 INH		100	Inhibits C1r and C1s
	Factor H		150	Competes with factor B
	Factor I (C3 INA)		100	Converts C3b to inactive C3bi

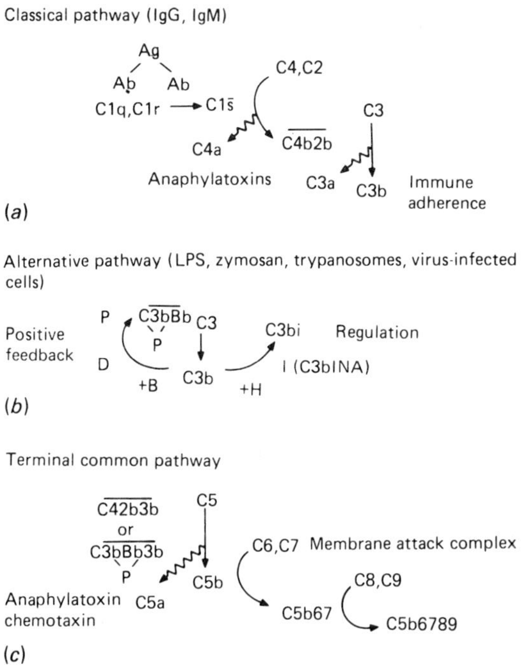

Classical pathway (IgG, IgM)

(a)

Alternative pathway (LPS, zymosan, trypanosomes, virus-infected cells)

(b)

Terminal common pathway

(c)

Figure 18.3 The activation of complement. A bar over a component, by convention, indicates an active enzyme. (Adapted from K. A. Joiner, E. J. Brown and M. Frank (1984) *Annual Review of Immunology*, Vol. 2, pp. 461–491)

Once activated, C1q converts C1r to an enzymatically active molecule capable of activating C1s. The C1qrs complex (also known as C1 esterase, C1s̄) binds and cleaves C4 into two: a large fragment C4b, which can covalently couple with the surface of a particle, and a smaller fragment C4a. C4b will bind C2 which is then cleaved by C1 esterase to produce a complex of C4b2b. It is this complex which acts as the C3 convertase.

C3, the most abundant of the complement components, is split into two fragments, C3a and C3b (see Table 18.1 and Figure 18.3a). The smaller fragment, C3a, is a peptide which causes the degranulation of mast cells and the consequent release of a variety of pharmacologically active substances. These include histamine, serotonin, a slow-reacting substance of anaphylaxis (SRS-A now renamed leukotriene C) and eosinophil chemotactic factor. C3a is termed an anaphylatoxin because of its effect on mast cells (see section on hypersensitivity). C3a causes smooth muscle contraction, both directly and through the substances released by mast cells, and the release of hydrolytic enzymes from neutrophils. It has been found that C4a also has anaphylatoxic properties.

Immune adherence

C3b, the larger cleavage fragment of C3, can covalently couple with cell surfaces around the site of complement activation. Such an interaction can lead to the cleavage of more C3 by the alternative pathway (see below). Bound C3b is the ligand for a receptor found on the surface of phagocytic cells – the C3b receptor (also known as CR1). Particles coated with C3b are readily phagocytosed by neutrophils and macrophages and are said to be opsonized (made ready for eating). Binding of C3b opsonized particles to the C3b receptor is called immune adherence.

The C4b2b complex is not very efficient in activating C3 but many hundreds of molecules are split by a single complex because of the abundance of C3 in plasma. However, only one C3b molecule combines directly with C4b2b to activate C5 and initiate the terminal sequence.

Complement activation by the alternative pathway

C3 spontaneously degrades to C3b in the plasma at a low level. In the presence of an initiator of the alternative pathway, the following events take place (see Figure 18.3b). C3b binds to factor B to produce a C3bB complex. This is susceptible to the action of another enzyme called factor D. Cleavage of factor B leaves a potent C3 convertase, C3bBb, capable of fixing additional C3b to the activating surface which leads subsequently to the formation of more C3bBb. As the formation of C3b by the alternative pathway produces more C3b, there is said to be positive feedback. The C3bBb complex is stabilized by another cofactor, properdin, which increases the half-life of the molecule from about 5 to 30 minutes.

Positive feedback by C3b to create more C3b would clearly exhaust C3, and later components of the pathway, if left unchecked. To prevent this happening there are a number of regulatory proteins (see Table 18.1). Factor H binds to C3b and inhibits its interaction with factor B; factor I (or C3b-INA) then rapidly cleaves the C3b to produce an inactive C3bi fragment. Although incapable of activating further C3, the C3bi is still bound to the activating surface and can interact with C3bi receptors (termed CR3), on the surface of the phagocytes. Further slow, proteolytic digestion eventually leads to a C3d fragment remaining on the surface.

The alternative pathway is initiated by cell wall polysaccharides of yeast (zymosan) and Gram-negative bacteria (lipopolysaccharide or endotoxin), bacterial dextrans and levans, parasites such as trypanosomes and schistosomes, and some virally transformed cells.

The terminal sequence of complement activation

Activation of the terminal complement components C5–C9 (see Figure 18.3c and Table 18.1) results in the formation of a membrane attack complex. This causes cell lysis when inserted in the lipid bilayer of cell membranes. The first step in this common pathway is the cleavage of C5 by the C4b2b3b (classical) convertase or the C3bBb properdin (alternative) convertase to generate C5b and C5a fragments (see Figure 18.3c). The smaller fragment, C5a, is a potent anaphylatoxin and has similar effects to C3a. In addition, C5a is itself chemotactic and attracts granulocytes and monocytes. The large fragment, C5b, associates with C6 to form a C5b6 complex which can non-covalently interact with biological membranes. C7 is then added to the complex.

It is possible for the C5b67 complex to become attached to membranes distinct from the activator surface where the complement system has been triggered. This can lead to the fixation of a membrane attack complex on bystander cells (reactive lysis). Membrane bound C5b67 binds one molecule of C8 and six of C9; although fixation of C8 can bring about some lysis, the addition of C9 vastly increases its efficiency. The final components (C8 and C9) result in the formation of a channel through the lipid bilayer and perturbation of osmotic stability.

The role of complement and phagocytic cells

Phagocytes have a central role in virtually all types of immune response, as will become clear below. Deficiencies in one or both classes of phagocytic cells lead to recurrent and life-threatening infections (see section on immunodeficiency). Nevertheless, in isolation, neutrophils and monocytes remove blood-borne parasites only poorly and certain microorganisms have developed antiphagocytic properties.

Many bacteria possess hydrophobic capsules which fail to adhere to the phagocyte cell membrane; often only the encapsulated variants of a bacterial species are virulent. These capsules may be polysaccharide in nature (e.g. pneumococci) or composed of polypeptides (e.g. *Bacillus anthracis*). The M-protein found on the surface of *β*-haemolytic streptococci (*Streptococcus pyogenes*) is antiphagocytic, and the production of

coagulase by *Staphylococcus aureus* (*Staph. pyogenes*) promotes the deposition of fibrin around the bacterium. Lipoprotein antigens of the plague bacillus *Yersinia pestis* and lipopolysaccharides in the cell wall of *Salmonella typhi* also inhibit adherence to the phagocyte membrane.

Activation of the alternative pathway of complement by cell wall constituents greatly enhances phagocytosis. The specific interactions between complement receptors, notably CR1, and opsonized particles are far more effective than electrostatic interactions. Furthermore, the release of inflammatory and chemotactic factors facilitate migration and intra-and extracellular killing.

Although phagocytic cells in combination with complement form a formidable barrier to invading organisms, they cannot deal with parasites which fail to activate complement or adhere to the phagocyte membrane; nor can they deal adequately with organisms which produce toxins or are resistant to the killing mechanisms of the phagocytes and take up residence within the cell, such as mycobacteria.

It is the adaptive or acquired immune system which meets this threat and provides a means by which any potential invader can be recognized and eliminated.

Acquired immunity

Acquired immune responses have the following characteristics:

1 They show memory – initial exposure to an infectious organism leads to a primary response; encountering the organism again produces an accelerated secondary response which persists (Figure 18.4)
2 They show specificity – the development of resistance following exposure to one organism does not confer resistance to unrelated organisms
3 They can be divided into responses which are

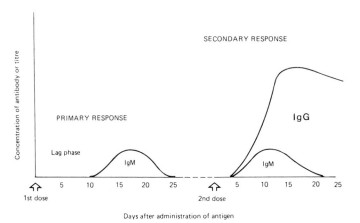

Figure 18.4 Production of immunoglobulins during primary and secondary immune responses

mediated by humoral factors (antibodies) and those mediated by specifically sensitized cells.

In practice, development of resistance generally involves both types of response, although the relative importance of antibody or cell-mediated immunity varies for individual organisms.

Antibody-mediated immunity

The structure of antibodies

Antibodies are proteins (immunoglobulins) found predominantly in the γ-globulin fraction of serum. There are five major classes of immunoglobulin (Ig): G, A, M, D and E. Although there are differences in molecular size, serum concentration, valency and function, the basic structure of these classes is similar, consisting of four chains: two identical heavy chains and two identical light chains (Figure 18.5). The heavy chain distinguishes the particular Ig classes and is denoted by a Greek letter (Table 18.2). The heavy (H) chains are composed of three (IgG, IgA, IgD) or four (IgM, IgE) constant domains (C_H) and a single variable domain (V_H). These domains comprise about 110 amino acid residues which adopt a conformation in which two β-sheets oppose each other stabilized by hydrophobic interactions. This conformation, termed the immunoglobulin domain, is further stabilized by a disulphide bond between the two β-sheets. As the name implies, constant domains are identical from one Ig molecule to another, provided that the molecules are of the same isotype.

Interchain disulphide bonds link heavy chains with one another and with light (L) chains; the precise number varies with different Ig classes. Light chains possess only two domains, one constant (C_L) and one variable (V_L); two kinds of L chain class exist, kappa (κ) and lambda (λ), and either one may associate with an H chain to form a functional Ig molecule.

Some Ig classes have subclasses (see Table 18.2) which contain slightly different amino acid sequences

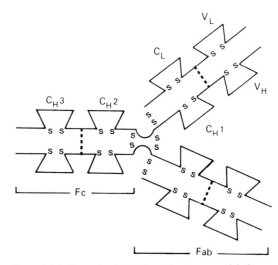

Figure 18.5 Generalized structure of an immunoglobulin molecule, based on human IgG1. The portion where the disulphide bonds hold the H chains together is the hinge region. The dotted lines mark the extent of the domains

within their C regions. Four subclasses of human IgG, two of IgA and two of IgM have been recognized. Another name given to Ig classes and subclasses is isotype.

Variable regions

Although antibodies of a single isotype are virtually identical in terms of protein structure, they are capable of binding to a wide range of different antigens – an antigen being defined here as any substance to which an antibody can bind. This discrimination is a function of the V regions, and variation between molecules of the same subclass is known as idiotypic variation.

It is the idiotype which determines the specificity for antigen. A comparison of the amino acid sequen-

Table 18.2 Immunoglobulin isotypes

Class	Heavy chain	Light chain	Molecular structure	Subclasses	Average molecular weight (daltons)	Concentration in serum (mg/ml)	Serum Ig (%)	Average half-life (days)
IgG	γ	κ or λ	H_2L_2	4	150 000	8–16	70–75	20–21 (7 for IgG3)
IgA	α	κ or λ	H_2L_2 $(H_2L_2)_2$ $(H_2L_2)_3$	2	160 000	1.5–4	15–20	6
IgM	μ	κ or λ	$(H_2L_2)_5$	2	900 000	0.5–2	10	10
IgD	δ	κ or λ	H_2L_2	1	160 000	0–0.4	1	3
IgE	ε	κ or λ	H_2L_2	1	170 000	< 0.0005	trace	2

ces of several different V regions highlights three defined regions which show considerable variation. These are termed hypervariable or complementarity determining regions and have been shown by X-ray crystallography to form the antigen binding site.

Fc and Fab fragments

Two proteases have been particularly informative in the analysis of IgG function. Papain splits the molecules into three: two antigen-binding fragments (Fab) which retain the capacity to recognize antigen, and a third crystallizable 'tail' fragment (Fc; see Figure 18.5). The Fab fragments are dimers of H and L chain constant and variable regions; Fc fragments are dimers of the second and third constant regions $C\gamma2$ and $C\gamma3$. Pepsin cleaves IgG to leave a $F(ab')_2$ fragment, two Fab fragments linked by the disulphide bridges at the hinge region; the rest of the molecule is degraded into small peptides.

Functions of immunoglobulins

These can be divided into Fab dependent and Fc dependent (or adjunctive) properties.

Binding of Fab portions of an Ig molecule to antigenic determinants (epitopes) on distinct particles leads to the formation of aggregates. If the epitopes are present on whole cells, this leads to agglutination; if the epitopes are on soluble elements, formation of large complexes leads to precipitation. Some bacteria, including the causative agents of diphtheria (*Corynebacterium diphtheriae*), tetanus (*Clostridium tetani*), cholera (*Vibrio cholerae*) and scarlet fever (*Strep. pyogenes*) produce toxins which cause local or systemic pathological changes. Immunoglobulins neutralize toxins by blocking the active site, either directly or by inducing a conformational change in the toxin molecule. Neutralization is also important in preventing infection, in this case the site of action is the receptor of the virus or bacterium for cell surface structures (e.g. influenza virus haemagglutinin). The adjunctive properties of Ig molecules depend upon an intact Fc region and vary with isotype (see below).

Complement fixation by way of the classical pathway is initiated, following antigen-binding, when two or more Fc regions are in close proximity. Receptors for the Fc portions facilitate phagocytosis (opsonize), allow cells to bind to antigen and release cytotoxic or inflammatory agents, and permit the passive transfer of antibody (IgG) from mother to fetus.

Role of different immunoglobulin isotypes

IgG is the principal Ig species found in blood and the extracellular spaces. Of the four human IgG subclasses, it is IgG1, IgG3 and, to a lesser extent, IgG2 which activate complement through the classical pathway and bind to the Fcγ receptor on phagocytic

cells; IgG can thus opsonize directly or through the generation of C3b. A population of leucocytes, defined functionally as K cells (for killer), can attach by way of Fcγ receptors to IgG-coated cells and, through the release of cytotoxins, bring about cell lysis. The phenomenon has been termed antibody-dependent cellular cytotoxicity, or ADCC for short. In addition to K cells, neutrophils and monocytes, eosinophils and platelets bear receptors for antigen-bound IgG and can cause damage to opsonized microorganisms by the release of cytotoxic agents, enzymes or mediators of inflammation. IgG is the only Ig class to be transferred across the placenta (see section on passive immunization) and is generally the major immunoglobulin synthesized during a secondary immune response (see Figure 18.4).

IgA is the second most abundant Ig in blood where it is found mainly as a monomer, although about 15% is present as dimers and trimers: two or three IgA molecules of identical antigen specificity are joined together at the Fc region by a J chain, a 15 kilodalton (kD) polypeptide. There are two subclasses of IgA. In blood, IgA1 represents about 80% of the total IgA, but in secretions. IgA2 is predominant (about 60%). The functions of serum IgA are unclear, but may be immunoregulatory as many IgC functions can be modulated by serum IgA.

IgA in secretions differs from that in serum and is called secretory IgA (SIgA). Those molecules in secretions are almost entirely dimeric and are independent of serum IgA. Sometimes referred to as mucosal paint, SIgA antibodies are found in the secretions covering mucosal surfaces, including gastric, bronchial and nasal secretions, colostrum, milk, tears and saliva. In viral infections of the middle ear, the concentration of specific IgA is two to six times higher than that of the IgC.

In addition to J chain, dimers of secretory IgA (Figure 18.6) are complexed with another protein, namely the 70 kD secretory component (SC or secretory piece). This is a polypeptide fragment derived from the polymeric immunoglobulin receptor which is

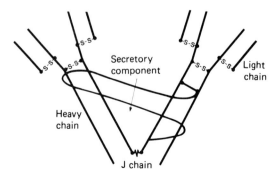

Figure 18.6 Schematic structure of a secretory IgA molecule showing the J chain and secretory component

synthesized by epithelial cells and acts as a vehicle for the transport of IgA from serum to mucosa (see section on the secretory immune system).

SIgA does not rely on opsonization or complement fixation for its biological activity; its main actions are neutralization of viruses, inhibition of adherence and growth of microorganisms on epithelial and other surfaces, neutralization of toxins, and antigen exclusion by preventing the access of antigen to the systemic immune system.

IgM exists in the blood as a pentamer and is the largest Ig species, sometimes known as macroglobulin, and diffuses only poorly into extravascular spaces. Its high valency for antigen and the proximity of five Fc portions make IgM antibodies very efficient agglutinins and activators of the classical complement pathway. During a primary response IgM is the major class of Ig synthesized (see Figure 18.4). The five monomers in IgM are joined by a single J chain. IgM can be complexed with secretory component and act as a secretory antibody.

IgD is a monomeric Ig found at a low concentration in the blood. Its principal role appears to be as a cell surface receptor on the antibody forming cell (see below).

IgE is normally found in only trace amounts (see Table 18.2), but in certain conditions, such as atopic allergy or during the course of infection with a parasitic worm, the level may be raised. Mast cells and basophils possess Fcε receptors which bind monomeric IgE molecules. This stabilization of the IgE increases its half-life from 2.5 days to around 12 weeks. Cross-linking, brought about by the simultaneous binding of antigen to adjacent IgE molecules, causes the rapid release of the contents of cytoplasmic granules into the surrounding medium. This is termed 'degranulation'. The vasoactive and inflammatory constituents include histamine, serotonin, eosinophil chemotactic factor, platelet aggregating factor and slow reacting substances of anaphylaxis (SRS-A) (see also section on hypersensitivity). Eosinophils also possess Fcε receptors and can bind to IgE-coated worms in the gut and contribute to parasite expulsion. IgE, like IgA, seems to play a major role in protecting external surfaces.

Some tests for antigen and antibody reactions

Precipitation of immune complexes forms the basis of some immunological tests for antibody or antigen, as outlined in Figure 18.7. If an antigen has two or more epitopes, antibody can cross-link antigen molecules. In gross antigen excess, each Fab binds to a separate antigen and causes formation of small complexes. As the concentration of antibody is increased, bigger, insoluble complexes form. At equivalence, all the antigen and antibody are complexed in a lattice structure. At antibody excess, the complexes tend to become smaller and more soluble because antibody

Double diffusion (Ouchterlony method)

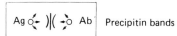

Precipitin bands

Single radial diffusion (Mancini method)

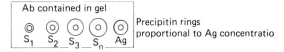

Precipitin rings proportional to Ag concentratio

Immunoelectrophoresis

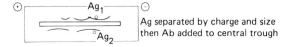

Ag separated by charge and size then Ab added to central trough

Rocket electrophoresis

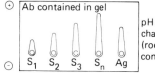

pH of gel adjusted to neutralize charge on Ab. Precipitin arcs (rockets) proportional to Ag concentration

Figure 18.7 Some tests for antigen and antibody reactions

fails to cross-link epitopes on different antigen molecules.

A rather different type of test for detecting antibody is the complement fixation test which is performed in two stages. In the first stage, the test serum is serially diluted and a constant amount of antigen is added, together with a source of complement. In the second stage, following incubation, antibody-coated red blood cells are added to indicate whether complement has been consumed in the first stage. If there is sufficient complement, these indicator cells will be lysed. If they are not, complement components must have been exhausted in the first stage by the formation of immune complexes. Hence antibody must have been present in the test serum. Radioimmunoassay and enzyme-linked immunosorbent assay (ELISA) techniques, which are extremely useful, are described in the section on diagnosis of autoimmune disease.

B lymphocytes and the synthesis of immunoglobulins

Antibodies are produced by plasma cells derived from B lymphocytes which differentiate, at least in mammals, in the bone marrow. The genes on only one of the two parental chromosomes are transcribed (allelic exclusion) and each B lymphocyte is committed to synthesizing immunoglobulin molecules with a single specificity. The immunoglobulin heavy chain gene locus is distinct from the two light chain gene loci. The heavy chain locus comprises many V gene segments (approximately 200, of which some are non-coding pseudogenes), each of which encodes most of the variable domain, as well as about 20 D (diversity) and 6 J (joining) gene segments. A functional exon which encodes an immunoglobulin variable domain is assembled by rearrangement of chromosomal DNA to bring together single V, D and J segments. The different possible combinations of V, D and J segments result in considerable diversity in antibody specificity. The diversity is further increased by mechanisms which introduce mutations at the joins between VD and DJ segments. The portion of the locus which comprises the V, D and J segments is followed by exons which encode the constant region of each immunoglobulin isotype. The two light chain gene loci are organized in a similar manner with multiple V gene segments (approximately 100 each) and a small number of J segments as well as exons encoding the constant region. There are no D segments.

Rearrangement of the heavy chain gene locus precedes that of the light chain loci. Some form of negative feedback prevents further gene rearrangement once a functional immunoglobulin molecule has been assembled.

Mature B lymphocytes, prior to exposure to antigen, express a surface bound form of monomeric IgM and, commonly, IgD which are the B-cell antigen receptors. Both have the same specificity for antigen. These receptors are associated with other heterodimeric signal transducing molecules.

During primary stimulation with antigen, mature B lymphocytes expand clonally to produce more cells capable of producing antibody. Some of the cells transform into plasma cells which are end cells and which secrete large quantities of immunoglobulin. There may be a switch in the class of Ig produced before the plasma cell is formed so that an isotype other than IgM is synthesized. During this expansion, a further mutational mechanism (somatic hypermutation) may operate on the immunoglobulin gene to increase antibody diversity further. A proportion of the B lymphocytes develop into memory cells which, on re-exposure to antigen, permit a more rapid response than unprimed cells (see Figure 18.4).

Monoclonal antibodies

The fusion of a B lymphocyte with a tumour derived from a plasma cell (plasmacytoma) has made it possible to create antibody secreting cells (hybridoma) which will divide indefinitely in culture and produce vast amounts of completely pure, monospecific antibody. These monoclonal antibodies have revolutionized diagnostic and research procedures because of their specificity, lack of batch-to-batch variation and ease of production.

The secretory or mucosal immune system

Many of the mucous membranes of the body are constantly exposed to microorganisms, and the secre-

tions which bathe epithelial surfaces play a major role in the local defence against such microorganisms (see previous section). The secretory immune system is a system of local immunity which protects mucosal surfaces and which can be stimulated independently of systemic immunity.

The system comprises the secretions which bathe the mucous membranes of the body and their associated glands. The organs involved include the eyes, middle ear, salivary glands, lungs, gastrointestinal tracts, genitourinary tract and the mammary glands. Specialized lymphoid tissue is associated with the secretory system in the gut (gut-associated lymphoid tissue or GALT) and in the lungs (bronchial-associated lymphoid tissue or BALT; see section on lymphoid tissues).

Stimulation of the secretory immune system

Antibodies can be induced in secretions by local immunization or, alternatively, by stimulation of gut-associated lymphoid tissue either by ingestion of antigen or by deposition in the small bowel. Antigen in the gut leads to the release of IgA precursor cells from Peyer's patches, which selectively migrate to (or are selectively retained in) mucosal tissues. These IgA plasma cell precursors are released into the local lymphatics where they migrate sequentially to the mesenteric lymph nodes, to the thoracic duct and into the blood stream, before migrating to the lamina propria of the gut and other secretory tissues, including the mammary glands. Local immunization leads to a proliferation of these cells, recruitment of others and an enhanced local SIgA response.

Synthesis and transport of SIgA

Plasma cells in the lamina propria (the connective tissue adjacent to the epithelium) secrete dimeric IgA, including one unit of J chain. This molecule has an affinity for the polymeric immunoglobulin receptor (pIgR) which is expressed on the surface of epithelial cells. The secretory component acts as a receptor for dimeric but not monomeric IgA. The whole complex is taken up into the cells within which partial proteolysis of the receptor takes place to give rise to the secretory component. The complex of dimeric IgA and secretory component is secreted into the lumen of the gland as SIgA (see section on secretory IgA). The secretory component confers a resistance to proteolysis on the IgA, which probably allows it to function in a hostile environment for longer periods.

Cell-mediated immunity

Although antibody provides an effective adaptive defence mechanism in the blood, in extracellular fluid and at the external surfaces, it is virtually ineffective once a microorganism has established intracellular residence. In the case of budding viruses, antibody may control the level of viraemia but it cannot eradicate the source. Macrophages and monocytes may provide a habitat for bacterial or protozoal parasites that are not killed during phagocytosis. The cell-mediated arm of the acquired immune system is suited to deal with intracellular parasites.

T lymphocytes and antigen recognition

The term 'cell-mediated' has been applied to immunity which is transferable with living cells, but not with serum from sensitized animals, and is mediated by lymphocytes that have differentiated under the influence of the thymus. These T lymphocytes, like B lymphocytes, are specific for a single antigen. Stimulation of T cells transforms them into activated T lymphocytes or lymphoblasts which have a much higher cytoplasm:nucleus ratio, a lower density and a greater diameter. Memory T cells are also generated during the course of clonal expansion.

In contrast to B lymphocytes, T lymphocytes neither recognize nor bind to antigen directly. They require the antigen to be taken up or produced by another cell, processed by a proteolytic degradation pathway and the resulting peptides to be presented on the cell surface in association with products of the major histocompatibility complex (MHC). This major histocompatibility complex restriction enables sensitized T lymphocytes to distinguish cells which bear foreign antigens from those which are free from infection. (A special case where T cells do not require the presence of self-histocompatibility markers is the recognition of tissue transplants, and this will be discussed later.)

The receptor for antigen is not Ig but a structurally related polypeptide dimer formed between non-identical α and β chains, each of 40–50 kD in size. Both chains comprise a constant region, shared between T cells of different specificities, and a variable region which determines antigen/major histocompatibility complex specificity. A third glycoprotein complex CD3, is required for insertion of the $\alpha\beta$ heterodimer into the cell membrane and is essential for signal transduction once antigen is bound.

T lymphocytes confer immunity through the production of cytokines and the generation of cytotoxic cells.

Cytokines, such as those of the interleukin series (IL-2, IL-4) recruit other cell types, modulate their action or lead to cell lysis (Table 18.3). Chemotactic factors attract monocytes and macrophages, and migration inhibition factors ensure that the recruited cells stay in the locality. Gamma interferon and macrophage-activating factor greatly enhance the capacity of macrophages to engulf and kill microorganisms; these cytokine-activated cells are called angry macrophages. Transmission of virus particles between cells is blocked by the action of interferon and the cytotoxic potential of natural killer cells (see below) is

increased. T cells themselves release lymphotoxins which kill some kinds of tumour cells.

T lymphocytes provide the main resistance to infections with obligate or facultative intracellular bacteria and protozoans, and to fungi. Organisms such as the tubercle and leprosy bacilli, *Brucella*, *Legionella* and *Toxoplasma* spp. are all susceptible to destruction by lymphokine-activated macrophages. In chronic infections, aggregates of macrophages form foci called granulomas.

Cytotoxic T lymphocytes are generated in response to viral infection or following the transplantation of histoincompatible tissue grafts. Cytotoxic T lymphocytes bind specifically to the infected or foreign cells and cause lysis.

The distinction between the two arms of the acquired immune response is useful in defining which protective mechanisms are most relevant in the case of particular infections. However, in the majority of infections, humoral and cell-mediated immunity both play a role in eliminating the organism (Figure 18.8), and this is most apparent when the regulatory interactions between T and B lymphocytes are examined. For this it is necessary to understand, in more detail, the role of the major histocompatibility complex.

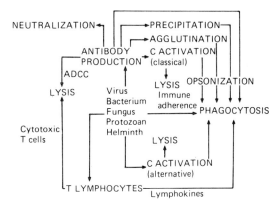

Figure 18.8 The interrelationship between various immune mechanisms

Cellular interactions between lymphocytes
The major histocompatibility complex

If skin grafts are transplanted between non-identical members of a species (allografts) or between members of different species (xenografts), there is an immunological reaction which results in destruction of the graft. Those antigens eliciting the strongest reactions are encoded by the major histocompatibility complex of a species, which in man is designated HLA, for human leucocyte antigen, and is located on the short arm of chromosome 6. The HLA is a complex because

Table 18.3 Characteristics of the main cytokines

Cytokine	Molecular weight (kD)	Cell source	Main cell target	Main actions
IFNγ	21–24	T cells, NK cells	Lymphocytes, monocytes, tissue cells	Immunoregulation, B cell differentiation, some antiviral action
IL-1α	33	Monocytes, dendritic cells, some B cells, fibroblasts, epithelial cells, endothelium, astrocytes, macrophages	Thymocytes, neutrophils, T and B cells, tissue cells	Immunoregulation, inflammation, fever
1L-1β	17			
IL-2	15	T cells	T cells, B cells, monocytes	Proliferation, activation, cytokine production
IL-3	20	T cells	Stem cells, progenitors	Panspecific colony stimulating factor
IL-4	20	T cells	B cells, T cells	Division and differentiation
IL-5	20 (dimer)	T cells	B cells, eosinophils	Differentiation
IL-6	26	Macrophages, T cells, fibroblasts, some B cells	T cells, B cells, thymocytes, hepatocytes	Differentiation, acute phase protein synthesis
IL-8 (family)	8	Macrophages, skin cells	Granulocytes, T cells	Chemotaxis
TNFα	50	Macrophages, lymphocytes	Fibroblasts, endothelium	Inflammation, catabolism (cachexia), fibrosis, production of other cytokines (IL-1, IL-6, GM-CSF) and adhesion molecules
TNFβ	50	Macrophages, lymphocytes	Fibroblasts, endothelium	Inflammation, catabolism (cachexia), fibrosis, production of other cytokines (IL-1, IL-6, GM-CSF) and adhesion molecules
IL-10	20 (dimer)	T cells	Monocytes, B cells	Inhibition, activation
IL-12	35–40 (dimer)	Macrophages	NK cells, T cells	Activation, differentiation

several genes or loci are clustered together over a relatively short distance (Figure 18.9). The complex can be divided into regions and subregions which encode functionally or biochemically distinguishable molecules.

Class I and class II histocompatibility molecules

The HLA-A, -B, and -C loci all code for class I histocompatibility molecules (see Figure 18.9). Structur-ally, they are composed of a 44-kD heavy α chain which associates with a light chain, β_2 microglobulin, encoded by a gene on chromosome 15. The three dimensional structure of a class I molecule has been determined. The α_3 region and β_2 microglobulin (see Figure 18.9) both form immunoglobulin-like domains supporting the membrane-distal α_1 and α_2 regions which together form a peptide binding domain. Class I molecules are found on almost all nucleated cells, but they are absent from human erythrocytes.

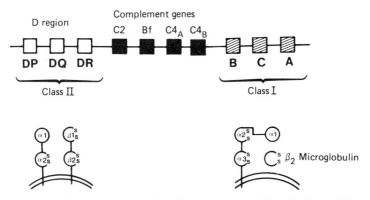

Figure 18.9 The HLA complex on chromosome 6 and the molecular structure of class I and class II histocompatibility antigens

The HLA-D region, containing DP, DQ and DR subregions, codes for class II histocompatibility molecules. These are integral, membrane-bound dimers formed between a 34-kD α chain and a 29-kD β chain. The three dimensional structure is very similar to that of the class I molecules with the α_2 and β_2 regions, both forming immunoglobulin-like domains. The α_1 and β_1 regions together form a single peptide binding domain (*see* Figure 18.9). DP, DQ and DR subregions contain genes for both α and β chains but the products only associate with complementary chains from the same subregion, e.g. DPα forms dimers with DPβ but not with DQβ or DRβ. Products of the subregions are codominantly expressed on selective cell types which are, in general, cells of the immune system – principally B lymphocytes, macrophages and other antigen presenting cells (see below) – and activated T cells. Gamma interferon induces class II expression on some cell types, such as thyrocytes. The class II histocompatibility molecules are sometimes referred to as I-region associated, Ia, antigens by analogy with the equivalent molecules in the mouse. The genes for classical and alternative complement components C2, C4 and factor B (Bf) are also found within the HLA complex and have been termed 'class III histocompatibility molecules'. They have no clear role in cellular recognition by T lymphocytes and are unrelated to the class I and class II molecules.

Detection of major histocompatibility antigens

Patients who have received deliberate or therapeutic blood transfusions develop antibodies to the histocompatibility antigens on leucocytes. Repeated pregnancies by the same father immunize mothers to paternal antigens carried by the fetus. By using such antisera, polymorphic forms of class I or II molecules can be serologically defined.

Class II antigens can also be detected by culturing lymphocytes from one individual with those of another, to form a mixed lymphocyte culture (MLC). If the cells express different class II antigens, the result will be a mixed lymphocyte reaction (MLR) and a clonal expansion of the reactive T cells. The reaction can be made one-way if the lymphocytes from one donor are pretreated so that they cannot proliferate. The magnitude of proliferation can be quantified by the addition of tritiated thymidine, which is taken up in dividing but not in static cells. Polymorphisms in class II antigens detected in this way are lymphocyte defined. The use of antibodies or lymphocytes or, increasingly, molecular biological techniques to detect histocompatibility antigens forms the basis of tissue typing (see section on transplantation).

Polymorphism

When there is more than one allele for a gene, the gene is said to be polymorphic. A minimum of 50 HLA-A, 97 HLA-B and 34 HLA-C specificities have so far been defined, indicating the remarkable degree of polymorphism within the HLA complex. Each allele is designated by a letter and a number, e.g. A1 and B7, and the combination of alleles expressed by an individual is known as a haplotype. Because HLA genes are inherited from both parents, a haplotype consists of up to six different class I alleles plus two D region specificities. There is a low frequency of recombination within HLA on account of the close genetic distance of the loci; thus haplotypes tend to be inherited *en bloc*.

Immune responses and their regulation

T-cell dependency of antibody responses

Although B lymphocytes are the only cells capable of synthesizing Ig, the antibody response to most antigens involves T lymphocytes. Congenital absence of the thymus impairs antibody production, particularly secondary responses, to many different types of antigen, and these have been termed 'thymus-dependent' (TD) antigens. A minority of antigens triggers B cells in the absence of T cells, and these are the so-called thymus-independent (TI) antigens. Two types of thymus-independent antigen have been described which, nevertheless, share a common feature in their both being large, polymeric molecules with a recurring structure. Often thymus-independent antigens stimulate polyclonal production of Ig, so that B lymphocytes other than those specific for the antigen are activated.

The cells which assist B lymphocytes to secrete Ig are helper or inducer T lymphocytes (T_H); they are specific for the same antigen as the B cell they help. The determinants to which T_H cells respond are termed 'carrier epitopes'. Cross-linking of Ig molecules on the surface of the B cell in the case of thymus-dependent antigens is a necessary but insufficient signal for antibody production. T_H cells provide a second activation signal, probably by way of direct cell-to-cell contact and the release of growth and differentiation promoting lymphokines (see Table 18.3). Antigen-specific and non-specific factors may be secreted. For optimal T–B-cell cooperation, the T_H and B lymphocytes must share HLA-D region polymorphism, so there is a major histocompatibility complex restriction through class II histocompatibility molecules.

Subsets of T lymphocyte

T lymphocytes are functionally heterogeneous, and several distinct T-cell subsets have been defined, including T_H (Table 18.4). T_H cells may be further divided into at least two subsets on the basis of the lymphokines they produce. Production of IL-2 and γ interferon but not IL-4 or IL-5 is characteristic of the T_H1 subset which generally promotes cell-mediated immune responses as well as IgM and IgG2 synthesis by B cells. Conversely, T_H2 cells are characterized by the production of IL-4 and IL-5 but not IL-2 or γ interferon, and stimulate increased production of IgG1 and IgE as well as increased numbers of eosinophils. Cytotoxic T lymphocytes (T_C), which kill virally infected cells, recognize viral antigens in the context of class I molecules. As for B lymphocytes, the precursors of T_C require specific T_H cells which recognize other viral determinants in association with class II molecules. Interleukin 2, a cytokine, is very important in the expansion of antigen-reactive T cells. The T lymphocytes responsible for delayed-type hypersensitivity (see below) represent another effector subset. Responses may also be suppressed by T cells.

Whether a distinct subset of suppressor T cells exists or whether suppression reflects different patterns of cytokine production by T cells is controversial. Suppression may be non-specific, i.e. affecting many different clones, or specific, thereby inhibiting only those that respond to the same antigen as suppressing T cells. Suppression can be effected both by soluble factors and cell-to-cell contact.

Antigen presentation

Because T lymphocytes do not recognize antigen without processing and presentation by compatible major histocompatibility complex molecules, there is a requirement for a cell to present antigen to the T cell. A number of cell types can perform this function, notably macrophages, dendritic cells and Langerhans cells. Antigens are endocytosed non-specifically and degraded (processed) into smaller fragments before association with major histocompatibility molecules. B lymphocytes can present antigen to T cells also, and in this case the uptake of antigen is specific as it occurs through the antigen-binding surface Ig.

Organization of lymphoid tissues

Lymphocytes in common with other blood cells are derived from the self-renewing pluripotent haemopoietic stem cells found in the fetal yolk sac and liver, and in the adult bone marrow. Lymphopoiesis, the generation of lymphocytes, takes place in the primary lymphoid organs: immature precursors multiply and produce more mature cells for release into the peripheral circulation and subsequent residence within secondary lymphoid organs.

Whether a precursor develops along the T- or B-lymphocyte lineage depends on the primary lymphoid organ to which it migrates, and this appears to be pre-programmed ('determined').

Primary lymphoid organs

Thymus

At about the sixth week of gestation, the thymus develops from the third and fourth pharyngeal pouches; it is seeded by lymphoid precursors, and lymphopoiesis begins around the eighth week. T lym-

Table 18.4 Functions of T-lymphocyte subsets

Subset	Function
T_H helper (inducer)	Enhance antibody production and cell-mediated immunity
T_C cytotoxic	Kill foreign or virally infected cells
T_D delayed-type hypersensitivity	Elicit delayed-type hypersensitivity reactions

phocytes are exported from the thymus from 12 weeks, but they are not yet fully functional. Within the thymus, T cells begin to express a variety of surface markers, some of which are unique to T cells, and characterize distinct subsets (Table 18.5). Anatomically, the thymus comprises two lobes which are subdivided into lobules; each has an outer cortex and an inner medulla. The more mature thymocytes probably migrate from the medulla.

Table 18.5 Some surface markers of human peripheral blood T lymphocytes

Marker	Expression on peripheral blood T lymphocytes
CD5	~ 100%; also on some B lymphocytes
CD3	~ 100%; non-covalently linked to T-cell antigen receptor
CD4	~ 65%; predominantly on T helper/inducer cells
CD8	~ 35%; predominantly on T cytotoxic cells
CD2	~ 100%; binds sheep erythrocytes and phytohaemagglutinin

Bone marrow

The fetal liver together with the bone marrow of both fetus and adult provide a lymphopoiesis-inducing microenvironment for B lymphocytes. Because birds have a specialized organ in which B cells differentiate, namely the bursa of Fabricius, the bone marrow and fetal liver of mammals are described as bursal equivalent tissues. Immature B lymphocytes, bearing surface IgM, can be found in the liver after 9 weeks of gestation. IgG and IgA are not normally produced until after birth. IgM synthesis begins shortly before birth to reach 10% of the adult value at birth, but it is dramatically increased if the fetus is congenitally infected (e.g. with Toxoplasma or rubella).

Secondary lymphoid organs

T and B lymphocytes are not fully mature when they leave the primary lymphoid organs and migrate to the secondary lymphoid organs, that is the lymph nodes, spleen and mucosal-associated lymphoid tissues (MALT). They home to particular areas of the organs and establish T-dependent and B-dependent regions.

Lymph nodes

The T-dependent paracortical zone lies within the B-dependent outer cortex (Figure 18.10). Lymphoid follicles contain B lymphocytes: primary follicles are unstimulated, while secondary follicles are larger with germinal centres and have been activated by antigen. The medullary region contains a mixture of

T and B lymphocytes, and plasma cells which secrete antibody lie along the chords. The lymph nodes draining the external ear are the superficial parotid nodes (tragus and anterior area), retroauricular nodes (posterior and cranial aspects) and superficial cervical nodes (lobule). The lymphatic vessels of tympanum and mastoid antrum drain into the parotid and upper deep cervical lymph nodes.

LYMPH NODE

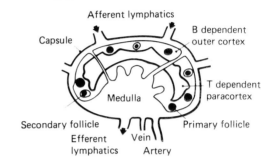

TONSIL

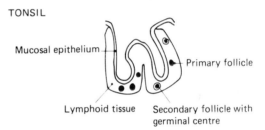

Figure 18.10 Schematic representation of lymph node and tonsil

Spleen

The leucocyte-rich white pulp is situated within an erythrocyte-rich red pulp. The T-dependent periarteriolar sheath surrounds the splenic arterioles, and outside this is a B-dependent marginal zone containing follicles and plasma cells.

Mucosal-associated lymphoid tissue

Mucosal-associated lymphoid tissue may be of the organized or diffuse type. Examples of mucosal-associated lymphoid tissue include the tonsils (see Figure 18.10), appendix, the Peyer's patches which lie along the gut, and the bronchial-associated lymphoid tissue. Unlike other secondary lymphoid organs, mucosal-associated lymphoid tissue is not encapsulated and has no afferent lymphatic vessels.

The primary and secondary lymphoid organs, with their connecting blood and lymphatic vessels, collectively make up the lymphon. A proportion of lymphocytes, after maturation in lymph node, spleen or mucosal-associated lymphoid tissue, recirculate through these organs. B- and T-lymphocyte responses take place within the secondary lymphoid organs; antigens may be carried on antigen presenting cells from local sites to the draining lymphoid tissue.

Immunization

The induction of immunity to particular infectious agents is known as immunization. This can be accomplished by the transfer of antibodies from one individual to another, called passive immunization, or by the administration of vaccines containing avirulent antigenic material to provoke an immune response, called active immunization.

Passive immunization

The transfer of immunoglobulins to fetus and neonate represents a natural form of passive immunization. In the former, antibodies of the IgG isotype are transported across the placenta by way of Fcγ receptors during the second and third trimesters. The process is selective; other Ig isotypes or proteins of similar molecular size to IgG do not cross the placenta. Up to about 6 months after birth, therefore, the fetus receives protection against a variety of potential pathogens that the mother has encountered. The protective effect is lost as a result of gradual catabolism. In some cases, transplacental passage of IgG can be harmful and cause autoimmune disease and rhesus haemolytic disease (see below).

The newborn infant receives additional protective antibodies from the mother in the colostrum and milk. In the first few days after birth this is very rich in SIgA, which coats the gut mucosa. Failure to provide secretory antibodies has been implicated in the development of food allergy.

Pooled γ-globulin fractions of normal human serum can be used to give temporary protection when needed, e.g. to protect premature infants who have failed to receive their full measure of maternal IgG or patients who are immunosuppressed for therapeutic reasons (such as transplant recipients), or individuals with immunodeficiency syndromes (see below). Preparations of γ-globulins are administered intramuscularly to avoid anaphylactic shock, as aggregated Ig could activate the complement cascade by way of the classical pathway.

Pooled γ-globulin fractions from other species (heterologous or xenogeneic γ-globulins) are used infrequently nowadays because of adverse reactions such as serum sickness (see below). Specific antibodies can be raised in animals (e.g. in horse) and given to non-immune individuals who have come into contact with the infective organism. If passive immunization with heterologous antibodies is necessary (e.g. as an antitoxin), it should always be accompanied by a schedule of active immunization. Protection afforded by passive immunization is rapid but transient because of normal catabolism of the Ig molecules.

Active immunization

Active immunization or vaccination involves the production of protective antibodies before natural infection and the provision of memory populations of T and B lymphocytes which will respond with second set kinetics when the appropriate organism is encountered. There are several different kinds of vaccine; generally the best are those which most closely mimic the natural infection.

Non-replicating vaccines

Killed organisms

For these vaccines to be successful the treatment employed to kill the microorganism – usually by means of heating and fixation with formalin or phenol – must preserve the antigenic structures necessary to establish immunity. Examples include the bacterial vaccines for whooping cough (*Bordetella pertussis*) and typhoid fever (*Salmonella, typhi, Salmonella paratyphi*), the rickettsial vaccine for typhus fever and the killed polio virus vaccine (Salk type).

Protective antigens derived from whole organisms

Toxoids are toxins that have been denatured and inactivated by treatment with formaldehyde. Some of the most successful vaccines, notably diphtheria and tetanus toxoids, have been produced by this means. These are particularly useful when the disease is caused by a toxin rather than by invasion of the organism.

Non-infectious subunits or components of the microorganism may be suitable vaccines; examples include the hepatitis B virus surface antigen and the pneumococcal polysaccharide vaccines. Although relatively safe and stable, the major disadvantage of non-replicative vaccines is that they have to be given in large doses by way of an unnatural (parenteral) route. They may be only weakly immunogenic and, as such, may require an adjuvant, a substance which boosts the immune response without necessarily inducing an antibody response to itself.

Live vaccines

Cross-protective organisms

A variant of the cowpox virus, vaccinia virus, is antigenically related to smallpox virus (variola) but, in the main, causes a mild local skin eruption in humans. Inoculation with vaccinia raises antibodies which cross-react with variola and confer immunity. The vaccine has been so effective that the smallpox virus, whose only reservoir is man, has been eradicated. Because vaccinia can occasionally produce complications, such as generalized vaccinia infection or encephalomyelitis, it is no longer ethical to vaccinate unless there is a clear risk of smallpox infection. Cross-protective vaccines are used for some animal diseases, e.g. human measles virus for canine distemper.

Attenuated organisms

Culture or treatment of infectious organisms, to render them avirulent yet able to induce protective immunity, is known as attenuation. There are numerous examples including the viral vaccines for German measles (rubella) and polio (Sabin type), and the bacillus of Calmette–Guérin (BCG), an attenuated strain of *Mycobacterium tuberculosis*. A novel approach to vaccine design – which is as yet at the research stage – is to construct attenuated viral vectors (such as vaccinia) which have been genetically engineered to contain important antigens of other viruses (e.g. hepatitis B, Epstein–Barr virus).

The great advantage of live vaccines is that they can be administered in small doses and can mimic natural infections to provide both local and systemic immunity. Indeed, cytotoxic T lymphocytes, which are crucial to the elimination of many viruses, are induced only by live viruses. Set against the advantages are the potential risks that organisms might re-acquire virulence, or that other viruses, possibly oncogenic, might contaminate the preparation. Even with attenuated organisms there may be a risk of disease if the inoculated individual is immunologically compromised.

Hypersensitivity reactions

An exaggerated or inappropriate immune response which damages host tissues is termed a 'hypersensitivity reaction'. Four main types of hypersensitivity, I–IV, have been classified by Coombs and Gell (1975): the first three cover hypersensitivity associated with antibodies, the fourth is mediated by T lymphocytes.

It is important to bear in mind that the mechanisms responsible for hypersensitivity are the same as those used in defence, the difference being that damage to the host outweighs the benefits.

Type I: immediate or reaginic hypersensitivity

The term 'immediate hypersensitivity' was originally applied because reactions occurred within minutes after exposure to a particular antigen. The principal mediators of immediate hypersensitivity or anaphylaxis are antibodies of the IgE isotype (so-called reaginic antibodies), and mast cells.

Local anaphylaxis

Atopic allergy, encompassing hay fever and some kinds of asthma and eczema, affects about 10% of the British population. By means of mechanisms that are poorly understood, repeated exposure of these individuals to an antigen (allergen) leads to the production of specific antibodies of IgE isotype. Common allergens include pollens and proteins of the house-dust mite. By way of receptors for Fcε, the antibodies bind to the surface of mast cells or basophils within the skin, and to mucosal membranes. Contact with the allergen leads to cross-linking of IgE molecules and explosive degranulation of the cell, with the release of the inflammatory mediators already alluded to in the section on the role of antibody. Vasodilatation, platelet aggregation, increased capillary permeability and the leakage of blood fluids (extravasation) produce an oedematous red wheal and flare reaction. Inflammation of the ducts draining the tears causes the eyes to run. In the lungs, slow-reacting substance of anaphylaxis brings about a gradual but long-lasting bronchoconstriction.

Systemic anaphylaxis

When an allergen is introduced directly into the bloodstream, degranulation can take place in any organ or tissue where there are sensitized mast cells. In man, the shock organs, which are most prone to anaphylactic responses, are the respiratory and circulatory systems. Anaphylactic shock is rare but very dangerous if not treated by injection of adrenalin; in extreme cases, an individual begins wheezing, and can collapse and die in a matter of minutes. Sensitivity to antibiotics or other drugs could lead to local or systemic anaphylaxis.

Type II: antibody dependent, cytotoxic hypersensitivity

The specific binding of antibody to the surface of a cell can lead to destruction by one of a number of different pathways: activation of complement, phagocytosis and targetting of cytotoxic macrophages, neutrophils, eosinophils or K cells.

Blood transfusion reactions

Human erythrocytes carry carbohydrate molecules which constitute the ABO blood group antigens. The alleles for these molecules are codominantly expressed, and phenotypically the red cells may be A,

B, AB, or O. Group A individuals have in their serum antibodies to group B and vice versa. These natural antibodies are found in the absence of previous transfusion; they are of the IgM class and are called isohaemagglutinins. (Similar antigens to the ABO substances have been found on bacteria and it is thought that sensitization by way of the gut induces antibodies which cross-react with human erythrocytes.)

Group O individuals possess only a backbone sugar molecule, substance H, and do not express A or B group antigens. For this reason, O blood is a universal donor because it can be given to any recipient. Conversely, AB individuals behave as universal recipients as they have antibodies to neither A nor B in their serum. If a blood transfusion is accidentally given to an incompatible recipient, an immediate and severe reaction ensues. The isohaemagglutinins agglutinate erythrocytes and fix complement. Symptoms include acute tubular necrosis of the kidneys, resulting from the sudden haemolysis, fever, hypotension, nausea and vomiting. Antigens other than those of the ABO system can elicit transfusion reactions, including those on leucocytes.

Rhesus haemolytic disease of the newborn

Erythrocytes also carry molecules encoded by the rhesus (Rh) system, of which the RhD antigen is the strongest and the only one of clinical significance. There are two alleles at the RhD locus, D and d; expression of D is dominant and about 85% of the British population are RhD$^+$. If a RhD$^-$ woman becomes pregnant by a RhD$^+$ father, the fetus may be RhD$^+$. At parturition, a significant leakage of fetal cells into the maternal circulation occurs, which immunizes the mother to RhD. In the course of a second pregnancy with a RhD$^+$ fetus, a small number of fetal erythrocytes leak across the placenta and induce a secondary response in the mother. IgG antibodies to RhD cross the placenta, giving rise to haemolysis and jaundice. In severe cases, exchange blood transfusion with RhD$^+$ blood is necessary *in utero* or following premature delivery.

To prevent sensitization of the mother, postpartum anti-RhD antibodies are given prophylactically. This has dramatically reduced the incidence of rhesus haemolytic disease in the newborn, presumably because the anti-RhD antibodies remove fetal cells before they sensitize the mother. The decreased chance of rhesus haemolytic disease when the mother and fetus are ABO incompatible can probably be explained in a similar fashion.

The mechanisms involved in type II hypersensitivity reactions may contribute to autoimmune diseases in which organ-specific autoantibodies are generated, e.g. pemphigus vulgaris and pernicious anaemia.

Type III: immune complex-mediated hypersensitivity

Immune complexes formed between antigen and antibody activate the complement cascade; type III hypersensitivity responses have immunopathological consequences.

Local, Arthus-type reactions

In 1903, Arthus and Breton found that the intradermal injection of horse serum into hyperimmunized rabbits induced a red oedematous lesion after about 6–8 hours. This Arthus reaction is brought about by the deposition of immune complexes in and around the local venules. Activation of complement produces chemotactic and anaphylatoxic factors. Neutrophils infiltrate the site and, unable to phagocytose trapped immune complexes, release their lysosomal enzymes, thereby causing damage and necrosis. Farmer's lung and pigeon fancier's disease are the result of type III hypersensitivity responses to inhaled antigen, with actinomycetes of mouldy hay being responsible for the former and serum proteins in the droppings of birds for the latter.

Systemic reactions

Following parenteral administration of a large dose of antigen to immune recipients, immune complexes may be deposited at many sites, notably the kidneys, heart, joints and skin. When passive immunization with horse γ-globulins was used in the treatment of diphtheria, formation of antibodies to the circulating heterologous proteins precipitated serum sickness. Small complexes, formed in conditions of antigen excess, are cleared only slowly by the mononuclear phagocyte system. Type III hypersensitivity reactions are mainly responsible for the pathology seen in non-organ-specific autoimmune disease (see below).

Type IV: delayed-type hypersensitivity

In 1890, Koch described a local erythematous indurated lesion in the skin of tuberculosis (TB) patients after the injection of tuberculin, an extract of *M. tuberculosis*. Because the reaction took between 24 and 72 hours to develop, he called it delayed. Delayed-type hypersensitivity reactions are mediated exclusively by T lymphocytes and are characterized by a mononuclear cell infiltration of lymphocytes (10–20%) and monocytes (80–90%); it is this dense cellular infiltration that gives the lesion a solid feel (induration). The release of lymphokines, and the recruitment and activation of monocytes, cause local tissue damage and vasodilatation.

The term 'delayed-type hypersensitivity reaction' is often used incorrectly to describe a protective immune response. Although the mechanisms involved in delayed hypersensitivity are part of the normal cell-mediated repertoire, a delayed-type hypersensitivity reaction does not necessarily indicate protective immunity. In some experimental models, immunity can be transferred with T lymphocytes independently of delayed-type hypersensitivity reactivity. Moreover, the immunopathology of diseases such as tuberculosis, and some kinds of leprosy, results from ineffective T-cell responses. In tuberculosis, the formation of granuloma in the lungs and other organs produces cavitation. In leprosy, the importance of T-lymphocyte responses in immunity to *M.leprae* is evident; weak T-cell reactivity is associated with many organisms (lepromatous type) and strong reactivity with a few (tuberculoid type). Borderline leprosy in the middle of the scale is associated with moderate T-cell reactivity, moderate *M.leprae* infection, but with severe granulomatous lesions.

A particular form of delayed-type hypersensitivity reaction, which has no apparent relevance to protective immunity, is that of contact sensitivity. Simple chemicals (haptens) that in isolation are non-immunogenic, can be absorbed through the skin to form immunogenic complexes with free or cell bound proteins. When the chemical is reapplied, a delayed-type hypersensitivity-like lesion develops. Nickel, constituents of rubber, clothing dyes and materials, and plant oils (e.g: poison ivy in the USA) can all elicit contact sensitivity.

Autoimmune disease

The immune system does not normally respond to the body's own antigens because there is normally an immunological tolerance to self-antigens. If this tolerance is broken, autoimmune responses against self-antigens can produce disease. Most autoimmune diseases are associated with the production of antibodies (autoantibodies), but autoreactive T lymphocytes may also be involved. A spectrum of autoimmune disease has been described, with organ-specific and non-organ-specific disorders at either ends of the spectrum.

In an archetypal organ-specific disease, autoantibodies are formed to antigens found on a single organ. Autoimmune diseases of the thyroid gland, such as Hashimoto's thyroiditis and thyrotoxicosis (Graves disease), would be cardinal examples (Table 18.6). Goodpasture's syndrome, in which autoantibodies react to a common antigen on glomerular and alveolar basement membranes, and myasthenia gravis (autoantibodies to the acetylcholine receptor at the neuromuscular junction of voluntary muscles), represent less absolute organ-specific diseases.

At the opposite end of the spectrum is systemic lupus erythematosus. The disease gets its name from the wolf (lupus)-like appearance of the facial rash. Systemic lupus erythematosus is associated with a plethora of autoantibodies (those to double-stranded DNA being of particular diagnostic value) and lesions in a variety of systems. Skin and joints are most commonly affected, but there may also be pulmonary, renal, cardiac, neurological and haematological involvement. Many of the non-organ-specific diseases are rheumatological, affecting joints and muscles.

Towards the middle of the spectrum are diseases where autoantibodies to an antigen present in many tissues nevertheless damage a rather specific target e.g. primary biliary cirrhosis, or where relatively specific autoantibodies cause systemic effects, e.g. autoimmune haemolytic anaemias.

Table 18.6 Some autoimmune diseases

Condition	Autoantibodies to	Target organ(s)	Effects
Hashimoto's thyroiditis	Thyroglobulin, thyroid microsomes	Thyroid	Hypothyroid (myxoedema)
Graves disease	TSH receptor	Thyroid	Thyrotoxicosis
Pernicious anaemia	Intrinsic factor	Gut	Malabsorption of vitamin B_{12}
Goodpasture's disease	Glomerular and alveolar basement membrane	Kidneys, lungs	Nephritis, alveolitis
Myasthenia gravis	Acetylcholine receptor	Voluntary muscles	Muscular weakness
Pemphigus vulgaris	Intercelluar substance	Skin	Bullous formation
Sympathetic ophthalmitis	Ocular proteins	Eye	Destruction of healthy eye
Primary biliary cirrhosis	Mitochondria	Small bile duct	Liver damage
Sjögren's disease	Salivary duct	Mouth, eyes, joints	Sicca complex, arthritis
Rheumatoid arthritis	IgG	Joints, skin, blood vessels, kidneys, heart	Arthritis, skin lesions, vasculitis, nephritis, etc.
Systemic lupus erythematosus	Double-stranded DNA, nuclear proteins, mitochondria, leucocytes	Skin, blood vessels, joints, kidneys, heart	Skin lesions, vasculitis, arthritis, nephritis, thrombocytopenia, etc.

Autoantigens and mechanisms of self-tolerance

Theoretically, any antigen can behave as an autoantigen, e.g. plasma proteins, cell-membrane components and receptors, extracellular antigens and intracellular constituents (see Table 18.6). In general, autoantibodies to antigens found at high concentrations throughout the body lead to non-organ-specific disease, while localized antigens are associated with organ-specific disorders. Autoantibodies are not confined to a single isotype. For example, in rheumatoid arthritis, IgG, IgA and IgM autoantibodies to IgG (rheumatoid factors) have all been described, although IgM is most common. The aetiology of the majority of autoimmune diseases remains unknown. In the normal state, self-tolerance is maintained by several mechanisms.

Lack of autoreactive cells

During lymphocyte development there is selection against cells which respond to self-antigens. Thus, potentially autoreactive T and B lymphocytes are functionally deleted from the immune system. It has been shown experimentally that the introduction of foreign antigens early in ontogeny induces long-lasting specific unresponsiveness to those antigens.

Lack of antigen presentation

Although self-reactive T and B lymphocytes may be present, they fail to respond because the antigen is sequestered and does not come into contact with lymphoid cells. This mode of tolerance operates for ocular proteins. Damage to one eye and the release of proteins into the circulation induce clones of self-reactive T and B lymphocytes which attack the other healthy eye and cause sympathetic ophthalmitis. The expression of class II histocompatibility molecules can allow cells to present self-antigens directly to self-reactive T lymphocytes. Such inappropriate class II expression has been implicated in autoimmune diseases of the thyroid.

Lack of T-lymphocyte help

In the case of T-dependent autoantigens, autoantibodies will not be produced if autoreactive T_H cells are absent. However, this requirement can be bypassed if the autoantigen is presented on an immunogenic carrier (the carrier determinants are those recognized by T cells). Drugs which chemically modify red cell or platelet antigens provide helper determinants in drug-induced autoimmune haemolytic anaemia and thrombocytopenia respectively. Agents which activate B cells polyclonally, such as the Epstein-Barr virus, could elicit autoantibody formation without T-cell cooperation.

Lack of suppression

A key question is whether autoreactive T and B lymphocytes are always present but not triggered, or whether new autoreactive clones are generated. It would seem that, for many self-antigens, autoreactive lymphocytes are present but are not activated. One of the reasons for the increased prevalence of autoimmune diseases with age may be a decreased efficiency of T cell-mediated suppression. Gross defects in suppression function have been implicated in the aetiology of systemic lupus erythematosus and may play a role in other autoimmune diseases.

Pathogenesis

Autoantibodies can damage cells by various hypersensitivity reactions; in autoimmune disease, the immune response is inappropriate because the antigens are self components. Organ-specific lesions involve antibody-dependent, cytotoxic mechanisms (type II hypersensitivity) while non-organ-specific lesions are mediated by immune complexes (type III hypersensitivity). The injection of many types of autoantibodies can be shown by experiment to induce organ-specific pathology. Although most of the damage in autoimmune diseases is mediated by antibody, it is likely that T-cell-mediated damage is also present in many organ-specific diseases, as autoreactive T lymphocytes have been able to transfer the disease in experimental models. Further, lymphocyte transformation *in vitro* to autoantigens in sympathetic ophthalmitis and pernicious anaemia, and the demonstration of autoreactive T lymphocytes in Graves disease, would suggest a role for type IV hypersensitivity in these diseases *in vitro*.

Stimulatory hypersensitivity

In autoimmune disease, a special form of antibody-mediated hypersensitivity, sometimes called type V or stimulatory hypersensitivity, has been described. Many patients with Graves disease have in their serum an antibody which mimics the action of the thyroid stimulating hormone (TSH) by binding to the TSH receptor on thyrocytes. Unlike TSH, the autoantibody, the long-acting thyroid stimulator, is not subject to negative feedback by way of the hypothalamus and thus causes excess production of thyroxine (thyrotoxicosis). In myasthenia gravis and a rare form of insulin-resistant diabetes (associated with acanthosis nigricans), antireceptor antibodies stimulate receptor turnover, leading to long-term depletion of the receptor.

Autoimmune diseases with head and neck manifestations

Sjögren's disease

Patients with primary Sjögren's disease usually present with sicca complex, a combination of dry mouth (xerostomia) and dry eyes (keratoconjunctivitis sicca). Autoantibodies to salivary duct antigens are present as well as a focal infiltrate of lymphocytes in the glands. An association between any non-organ-specific autoimmune disease, in particular rheumatoid arthritis, and sicca complex, is diagnostic of secondary Sjögren's syndrome.

Behçet's syndrome

This syndrome is a chronic, multisystem disease which involves the mouth, genital organs, skin, blood vessels, nerves, gut and joints. Oral ulceration is the most common presenting feature, and autoantibodies which bind to extracts of oral mucosa and other tissues are found in 70–80% of patients. Immune complexes are found in the serum of about 60%.

Pemphigus vulgaris

Pemphigus vulgaris is a serious blistering condition which had a mortality rate of about 50% before the advent of steroid therapy. Flaccid blisters, bullae, develop within the epidermis of mouth and scalp, rapidly disseminating over the body. Autoantibodies to the intercellular cement of the skin epithelium are present in serum.

Diagnosis of autoimmune disease

Autoantibodies present in serum may be detected by immunofluorescence, agglutination, radioimmuno-assays, enzyme-linked immunosorbent assays (ELISA) and complement fixation tests.

Immunofluorescence

After incubation with normal tissue specimens, auto-antibodies in serum are demonstrated by means of fluorochrome-conjugated antibody to human Ig. Auto-antibodies already fixed to the tissue can be detected in biopsy sections.

Agglutination

Autoantibodies to red blood cell antigens (e.g. rhesus D) which bind to but do not directly agglutinate the cells, can be shown by adding an anti-human Ig to the patient's red cells which then agglutinate (Coombs' test). Agglutination by antibodies of erythrocytes coated with antigen is known as passive haemagglutination. It forms the basis of the Rose-Waaler test for rheumatoid factor, although Latex beads coated with IgG may be used in place of red blood cells.

Radioimmunoassay

A radioactively-labelled antigen or secondary antibody (anti-human Ig) is used to detect autoantibodies to intrinsic factor, acetylcholine receptors, double-stranded DNA and glomerular basement membrane.

Enzyme-linked immunosorbent assay

In ELISA, serum from a patient is incubated with the relevant antigen, and any autoantibodies present are detected by means of an anti-human Ig conjugated to an enzyme. Addition of the appropriate enzyme substrate causes a colour change which is quantified by spectrophotometry and is proportional to the amount of autoantibody present.

Complement fixation

Complement fixation tests detect complement consumption by antigen–autoantibody complexes (see section on tests for antigen and antibody reactions).

Management of autoimmune disease

Treatment of autoimmune disease depends upon its clinical severity. Many organ-specific disorders can be treated by metabolic control, e.g. patients with Hashimoto's disease are given thyroxine, those with myasthenia receive anticholinesterase drugs, and patients with pernicious anaemia are supplemented with vitamin B_{12}. Immunosuppressive therapy is necessary in severe myasthenia gravis, pemphigus vulgaris, systemic lupus erythematosus and immune complex-mediated nephritis. Inflammation can be reduced in rheumatoid arthritis and related diseases by anti-inflammatory agents including indomethacin and salicylates. Plasma exchange (plasmapheresis) is helpful in life-threatening immune complex-mediated arteritis. Antimitotic agents, such as methotrexate, cyclophosphamide and azathioprine, have been used in the treatment of chronic active hepatitis, auto-immune haemolytic anaemia and systemic lupus erythematosus.

Immunodeficiency

Failure of one or more elements of the immune system causes immunodeficiency. Innate or acquired immune responses may be compromised and this may be either genetically determined, a primary immunodeficiency, or be secondary to another disease process. Recurrent infections with common pathogens or with opportunistic organisms which take advantage of the lowered defences typify immune deficiency and characterize the particular defect (Table 18.7).

Primary deficiencies of innate immunity

Phagocytic cells may show a reduced capacity to kill, e.g. chronic granulomatous disease, or may fail to migrate to chemotactic stimuli, e.g. lazy leucocyte syndrome. Natural killer (NK) cells are mononuclear, lymphocyte-like cells which are not readily characterized as either B or T lymphocytes and have been termed 'null cells'. They are cytotoxic for a variety of tumour cell lines *in vitro* but display no clear specificity or memory pattern and are, therefore, considered to be an innate immune mechanism. In patients with Chediak-Higashi disease, neutrophils, monocytes and natural killer cells possess abnormal giant lysosomes which inhibit locomotion and cytotoxic potential. These patients are particularly susceptible to bacterial infections and have a tendency to develop lymphomas. The latter observation supports the concept that natural killer cells play a role in surveillance against tumours.

Deficiencies in complement components can be broadly divided into those affecting the classical pathway, C3, or the terminal lytic sequence.

1 Deficiencies of C1, C2 or C4 are associated with increased risk of bacterial infection. More significantly, there is an increase in immune-complex-mediated hypersensitivity lesions, presumably as a result of decreased clearance of antigen–antibody complexes. A deficiency of C1 inactivator causes hereditary angioedema in which sudden oedema occurs in the deep dermis, subcutaneous or mucous membranes of skin, intestine or larynx.

2 C3 may be reduced directly or by defects in the C3 inactivator, with both cases being characterized by acute life-threatening infections.

3 Absence of a component of the terminal lytic sequence predisposes to infection with *Neisseria* species, *N. meningitidis* or *N. gonorrhoeae*. Lysis of *Neisseria* seems to be necessary for effective clearance of the organism.

Primary deficiencies of acquired immunity

Severe combined immunodeficiency

Failure of both antibody production and cell-mediated immunity results in severe combined immunodeficiency. Several subtypes have been classified (Table 18.8), most of which present with diarrhoea and failure to thrive in early infancy.

Deficiencies of T lymphocytes

Aberrant differentiation of the thymus results in the Di George syndrome. In the complete syndrome there is aplasia and involvement of heart and parathyroid glands. Partial Di George syndrome patients possess a hypoplastic thymus.

A defect in purine nucleoside phosphorylase, an enzyme of the purine salvage pathway, reduces cell-

Table 18.7 Infections associated with deficiencies in innate or acquired immunity

	Innate immunity		Acquired immunity	
	Complement defects	*Phagocyte defects*	*T-lymphocyte defects*	*B-lymphocyte defects*
Viruses			Polioviruses Echoviruses Vaccinia	
			Mumps Epstein-Barr virus Cytomegalovirus	
Bacteria	Staphylococci			
	Streptococci *Haemophilus influenzae* Neisseria	*Serratia* *Klebsiella* *Salmonella*	*Mycobacteria* *Legionella* *Listeria* *Nocardia asteroides*	Staphylococci Streptococcus (pneumococci, meningococci)
Protozoa			*Pneumocystis carinii* *Toxoplasma gondii* *Giardia lamblia*	
Fungi		*Candida*	Candida	

Table 18.8 Severe combined immunodeficiency (SCID) syndromes

Condition	Defect	Inheritance
SCID with leucopenia (reticular dysgenesis)	Absence of all leucocytes, erythrocytes and platelets present	Autosomal recessive
SCID ('Swiss type' agammaglobulinaemia)	Absence of T and B lymphocytes	Autosomal recessive or X-linked
SCID with adenosine deaminase deficiency	Enzyme lacking or inactive	Autosomal recessive (chromosome 20)
Cellular immunodeficiency with immunoglobulins (Nezelof's syndrome)	Normal B-lymphocyte numbers but low Ig levels	Autosomal recessive or X-linked
Bare lymphocyte syndrome	No HLA class I molecules on lymphocytes	Familial

mediated immunity; some T-cell subpopulations may be more susceptible to this deficiency than others, e.g. cytotoxic T cells. Other disorders which have a predominant effect on T lymphocytes are shown in Table 18.9. The distinction between deficiencies of cell-mediated immunity and antibody are somewhat blurred by the T-cell dependency of many antibody responses. For example, in late onset or common variable hypogammaglobulinaemia there is a profound decrease in Ig levels, and plasma cells are absent. Although the syndrome is heterogeneous, it is likely that the hypogammaglobulinaemia is a consequence of aberrant T-cell function, either increased suppressor or decreased helper activity.

Deficiencies of B lymphocytes

The first immunodeficiency syndrome was described by Bruton in 1952. In congenital or Bruton's agammaglobulinaemia, the concentration of all Ig isotypes is diminished, although it is most marked for IgM and IgA. Repeated infections with pyogenic bacteria and an opportunistic protozoan, *Pneumocystis carinii*, are observed from about 6 months postpartum when the protective effect of maternal IgG has waned. The lymphoid tissue is hypoplastic with no plasma cells and germinal centres, but T-cell reactivity is normal. Bruton's disease is X-linked and is treated by administration of whole plasma or γ-globulins.

There are a number of disorders with selective deficiencies in one or more Ig isotypes. The most common is selective IgA deficiency, with an incidence of about one in 800. It is associated with recurrent infections of the respiratory tract and paranasal sinuses. Allergic, type I hypersensitivity reactions may cause gastrointestinal damage if food antigens, normally neutralized by SIgA, trigger mast cell degranulation. The irritant effects of antigen in the lungs or gut may promote tumour growth or autoimmune disease. Autoantibodies to IgA are frequently present in selective IgA deficiency, but it is not clear whether they cause the disorder or whether they arise because tolerance, in the absence of IgA, is lost. The clinically observed effects of IgA deficiency might be expected

Table 18.9 Primary immunodeficiency predominantly affecting T lymphocytes

Condition	Defect	Inheritance
Di George syndrome complete partial	Thymic aplasia Thymic hypoplasia Cardiovascular abnormalities	Non-familial
Purine nucleoside phosphorylase deficiency	Enzyme lacking or inactive	Autosomal recessive (chromosome 14)
Wiskott–Aldrich syndrome	Slightly reduced T-cell numbers, T cells functionally abnormal, platelets and neutrophils decreased, elevated eosinophil levels	X-linked
Ataxia telangiectasia	Embryonic thymus, T-cell number reduced, loss of coordination, dilatation of capillaries in skin and eye, defective DNA repair	Autosomal recessive

from its role as a defender of mucosal surfaces. Nevertheless, a significant proportion of individuals are healthy and in many of these an increase in secretory IgM compensates for the loss of SIgA.

Secondary immunodeficiency

Most immunodeficiencies are secondary and result from immunosuppression, or increased loss or catabolism of Ig. There is a variety of causes, including protein or calorie malnutrition, lymphoproliferative diseases, radiotherapy or chemotherapy, and the use of immunosuppressive drugs.

Some organisms depress, rather than stimulate, the immune response. Perhaps the most extreme example is the virus responsible for the acquired immunodeficiency syndrome (AIDS). This virus, designated human immunodeficiency virus (HIV), is cytopathic for T lymphocytes bearing the CD4 surface marker, the majority of which are involved in inducing antibody or effector T-lymphocyte responses (see Table 18.5). In full-blown AIDS, the immunodeficiency mimics that of clinical immunosuppression and is so profound that rare opportunistic organisms, including *Pneumocystis carinii* and *Mycobacterium avium intracellulare*, can establish intractable infections. Infection with other viruses, including cytomegalovirus, rubella, Epstein-Barr virus and hepatitis B virus, can lead to immunosuppression.

Some tests for immunity and immunity deficiency

Grossly abnormal numbers of neutrophils, monocytes or lymphocytes can be detected by using routine haematological methods. Abnormalities in lymphocyte numbers can be investigated further by employing phenotypic markers of B and T cells (Table 18.10). All B lymphocytes express surface Ig (IgM for the majority of primary, blood-borne cells). Immunofluorescence with fluorochrome-conjugated anti-human Ig antibodies can be used to quantify the proportion.

T lymphocytes bear a variety of markers which can be detected with immunofluorescence, and these define functionally distinguishable T-cell populations (see Tables 18.5 and 18.10). In addition, human T lymphocytes spontaneously form rosettes with sheep erythrocytes by way of the CD2 surface glycoprotein, and this can be used to enumerate T-cell numbers microscopically.

Mitogens are substances which induce polyclonal expansion of lymphocytes, and they can be used to test the ability of lymphocytes to proliferate normally. Pokeweed mitogen (PWM) is mitogenic for T and B lymphocytes, and it elicits Ig secretion. Phytohaemagglutinin (PHA) and concanavalin A are T-lymphocyte mitogens.

Table 18.10 Some tests for immunity

Total leucocyte numbers
    proportion of surface Ig bearing cells
    proportion of T-lymphocyte subpopulations, e.g. CD4:CD8
Serum immunoglobulin levels
    different subclasses
    specific antibodies, e.g. isohaemagglutinins, anti-*Escherichia coli*
Lymphocyte transformation
    to mitogens, e.g. Con A, PHA
    to specific antigens, e.g. allogeneic cells (MLR, PPD)
In vivo tests
    to recall antigens, e.g. *Candida*, PPD (Mantoux, Heaf tests)
    to contact sensitizing agents
    of toxin neutralization, e.g. Schick test, Dick test

In vitro lymphocyte transformation to mitogens, allogeneic cells (MLR), or specific recall antigens to which the patient has previously been exposed, is evaluated by the incorporation of tritiated thymidine. Immunity to recall antigens can be assessed *in vivo* by the response to intradermal injection of antigen. A panel of common antigens is used, including PPD (a purified protein derivative of *M.tuberculosis*), streptokinase-streptodornase, *Candida albicans*, mumps virus and trichophyton. In children and infants, active induction of contact sensitivity by the application of dinitrochlorobenzene can be used to test for primary T-cell deficiency.

Clinical aspects of human leucocyte antigen (HLA)
Disease associations

A wide variety of diseases shows an association with particular HLA specificities or haplotypes. The most striking is that of ankylosing spondylitis with the HLA-B27 specificity. Approximately 90% of patients with the disease are positive for B27. This association does not mean that all B27 individuals will develop the disease, but that there is an increased risk of their doing so. An association between a disease and an allele may be very significant statistically yet carry little relative risk. Associations between HLA antigens and diseases related to infection (e.g. arthritis following *Salmonella* infection), autoimmune disease and even psychoses such as manic depression have been reported. A few of the disease associations are shown in Table 18.11.

It is not clear why there is such an association. One possibility is that the HLA product behaves as an immune response gene. According to this explanation, certain HLA specificities regulate whether there is a heightened or reduced response to a particular antigen. Therefore, an exaggerated response to an antigen might provoke an autoimmune disease or

Table 18.11 Associations between HLA and certain diseases

Condition	HLA	Frequency (%)		Relative risk
		Patients	Control	
Hodgkin's disease	A1	40	32.0	1.4
Behçet's disease	B5	41	10.1	6.3
Ankylosing spondylitis	B27	90	9.4	87.4
Reiter's disease	B27	79	9.4	37.0
Psoriasis vulgaris	Cw6	87	33.1	13.3
Multiple sclerosis	DR2	59	25.8	4.1
Goodpasture's syndrome	DR2	88	32.0	15.9
Dermatitis herpetiformis	DR3	85	26.3	15.4
Sicca syndrome	DR3	78	26.3	9.7
Graves disease	DR3	56	26.3	3.7
Myasthenia gravis	DR3	50	28.2	2.5
Systemic lupus erythematosus	DR3	70	28.2	5.8
Rheumatoid arthritis	DR4	50	19.4	4.2
Pemphigus (Jews)	DR4	87	32.1	14.4
Hashimoto's thyroiditis	DR5	19	6.9	3.2
Pernicious anaemia	DR5	25	5.8	5.4

Data updated from Svejgaard, A., Platx, P. and Ryder, L. P. (1983). *Immunological Reviews*, 70, 193–218.

hypersensitivity state, whereas a weak response to a pathogen will permit infection. It is also possible that the histocompatibility antigen acts as a receptor for an infective agent so that the disease is limited to certain specificities.

An alternative possibility is that the gene responsible for the disease is not HLA itself, but a gene in linkage disequilibrium with it. An allele is said to be in linkage disequilibrium with another if, at genetic equilibrium, the two alleles occur less or more frequently than would be expected from the frequencies of the individual alleles in the population. Linkage disequilibrium implies either a positive or negative selection for a combination of alleles, depending on whether there is a higher or lower frequency, respectively, than is to be expected. Where different HLA specificities are associated with the same disease in different populations, linkage disequilibrium is suspected as the cause of the association, e.g Grave's disease is associated with B8 in Caucasians but with Bw35 in Japanese.

Transplantation

Transplantation of tissue grafts between unrelated individuals results in rejection of the graft. In the special case of bone marrow transplantation, the graft itself contains immunologically reactive cells which may respond to the recipient's antigens and elicit a graft versus host disease. Although antigens coded for by the HLA on their own elicit strong transplantation reactions, a number of loci outside the HLA complex code for minor histocompatibility antigens which, in combination, induce rejection comparable to HLA disparity. Transplantation reactions are mediated by T lymphocytes, and T-deficient individuals or animals show impaired rejection responses. Indeed, athymic nude mice, the murine equivalent of Di George patients, accept skin xenografts. In the same way as for conventional antigens, re-exposure to histocompatibility antigens provokes accelerated or second-set rejection.

Antibody can play a role in hyperacute rejection, for instance of kidney allografts; high titres of antibody induced by multiple transplantation cause a type II hypersensitivity reaction and rapid necrosis of the transplant. Chronic rejection may also be brought about by antibodies.

The importance of the various HLA region products on the outcome of cadaver kidney transplants has been evaluated. At the HLA-A and -B loci, the recipient and graft may differ (mismatch) by up to four specificities; the greater the number of mismatches, the greater the incidence of rejection. More striking differences are seen with mismatches at the HLA-D locus, indicating a greater need for compatibility at this locus during transplantation.

Blood transfusion

Paradoxically, it has been found that the administration of a blood transfusion prior to kidney graft transplantation increases the chance of allograft acceptance and suppresses the reactivity of the recipient. In fact, the transfusion effect is so marked that it obviates the need for matching HLA-A and -B loci, although HLA-D matching is still beneficial.

Typing for HLA-D

Two methods have classically been used to type cells for HLA-D antigens, and both make use of one-way mixed lymphocyte reaction (see section on the HLA complex). The first involves the use of homozygous typing cells as the stimulator cell. A panel of cells homozygous for HLA-D specificities are cultured with the lymphocytes that are to be typed. If there is a positive reaction, the responder cells are not tolerant of the HLA-D antigens expressed by the homozygous stimulator cell and do not, therefore, possess that particular HLA-D polymorphism. If they fail to respond, it implies that they carry that HLA-D specificity.

The second test, primed lymphocyte typing, is more reliable because the presence of an HLA-D allele is demonstrated by a positive reaction. In primed lymphocyte typing, lymphocytes that have been primed to a particular HLA-D product are the responders, and the cells to be typed are the stimulators. If the stimulator cells bear the HLA-D antigen to which the responders are primed, the latter respond rapidly and strongly. The two typing techniques complement one another. HLA-D typing requires from 2 to 6 days to obtain a result and it is therefore not always practical to use it, for instance, in the case of cadaver organs. Typing for HLA-DR serological specificities is performed using antibody.

HLA-D, as well as some serologically defined HLA antigens, sometimes include the w designation, e.g. HLA-Dw6. This indicates that the final specificity is yet to be internationally agreed. Molecular biological techniques, such as the polymerase chain reaction, are currently transforming the typing of HLA specificities and may well form the basis of all tissue-typing in the future.

Immunology in otolaryngology

The contribution of the immune response to diseases of the ear, nose and throat has, in the case of some disorders such as diphtheria and allergic rhinitis, been recognized for many years. More recently, however, immunological mechanisms have been suspected in a number of other conditions. These include type I and type IV hypersensitivity reactions in otitis media with effusion and immune-complex deposition in hearing loss associated with Wegener's granulomatosis. Sensorineural hearing loss has been obtained in experimental animals following the induction of autoimmunity. Also immunomanipulation, by the administration of cytokines, has been used in the treatment of juvenile laryngeal papillomatosis. It seems likely that the interface between the disciplines of immunology and otolaryngology will lead to advances in our understanding of the aetiology of diseases of the ear, nose and throat, and will also facilitate the development of new therapies.

Reference

COOMBS, R. R. A. and GELL, P. G. H. (1975) Classification of allergic reactions responsible for clinical hypersensitivity and disease. In: *Clinical Aspects of Immunology*, 3rd edn, edited by P.G. Gell, R.R.A. Coombs and P.J. Lachmann. Oxford: Blackwell Scientific Publications. pp. 761–781

Further reading

BROSTOFF, J., SCADDING, G. K., MALE, D. K. and ROITT, I. H. (1992) *Clinical Immunology*. London: Gower Medical Publishing
CHAPEL, H. and HAENEY, M. (1993) *Essentials of Clinical Immunology*, 3rd edn. Oxford: Blackwell Scientific Publications
STITES, D. P., TERR, A.I. and PARSLOW, T. O. (1994) *Basic and Clinical Immunology*, 8th edn. Lauge: Prentice–Hall International Inc.

19

Microbiology

Alexander W. McCracken and Geoffrey A. Land

The evolution of modern medical microbiology

The age of scientific medical microbiology began in the middle of the 19th century with the pioneer discoveries of Louis Pasteur. By the end of the century, most of the major bacterial pathogens of man had been isolated, and the mechanisms by which bacteria cause diseases were being investigated. The concept of virulence had been introduced and the toxigenicity of bacteria had been applied to the development of active and passive immunization against diphtheria and tetanus. At the same time, advances were being made in understanding the reactions of human and animal hosts to infection, and there were inklings that the human immune system might consist of humoral and cellular arms. By the early 1900s, it was generally appreciated that the outcome of the interaction of microbes and man was predicated on the quantity and virulence of the microbe and the effectiveness of the local and systemic defence mechanisms of the human host. Beginning with the isolation of influenza virus in 1932, clinical virology advanced slowly until practical cell culture methods became available in the early 1950s. During the next 20 years, most of the viruses causing human disease had been isolated. About the same time, techniques such as immunofluorescence, followed later by enzyme immunoassays were applied to microbial identification and antibody detection. More recently, DNA probes and polymerase chain reactions have been used to detect microbial agents even in minute quantities.

The concept that safe drugs with specific antimicrobial action might be developed was the vision of Paul Erlich (1854–1915), who also foresaw the emergence of resistance to these drugs. The modern era of antimicrobial drugs began with prontosil in 1932, but the introduction of penicillin as a therapeutic agent truly revolutionized the management of infections and spawned an industry which continues to develop new antibiotics at an astonishing rate.

With the widespread use of immunosuppressive drugs, such as corticosteroids, antimitotic and anti-rejection agents, microorganisms which were previously rare or unknown as causes of human disease, have become increasingly common. Fungi, for example, have assumed a much greater role in human disease, and determining which microorganisms are pathogenic or non-pathogenic is no longer an easy task. Indeed, some argue that in the immunocompromised patient, almost any microorganism can cause disease.

Although the search for microbial causes of disease has been going on for nearly one and a half centuries, it is not yet over, as the discovery of the causes of Legionnaire's and Lyme diseases in recent years has shown. The most dramatic development in infectious diseases in many years has been the rapid spread across the world of the human immunodeficiency viruses. This has resulted in a very large population of people with acquired immunodeficiency syndrome (AIDS) who are highly susceptible to a wide range of opportunistic infections. Unfortunately at present, there are no antiviral drugs with effectiveness comparable to the antibiotics, and the epidemic of AIDS continues with little sign of abatement. In the USA, the recent recognition of hantavirus infections (Morbidity and Mortality Weekly Reports, 1993) and lethal outbreaks of *Escherichia coli* O 157: H7 food poisoning (Swerdlow *et al.*, 1991) are reminders that the microbial world is far from being conquered.

The interaction of the microbial world with man and his antimicrobial agents will continue to evolve. The most serious consequence of this is the development of bacterial drug resistance. As an example, strains of *Mycobacterium tuberculosis*, initially isolated from patients with AIDS in the USA, are often resistant to antituberculous drugs, and pose very serious challenges in clinical medicine and to public health.

In this chapter we attempt to present in concise form, the current state of clinical microbiology with special emphasis on those organisms which are associated with infections of the pharynx, larynx, paranasal sinuses, and the middle and external ear.

Using the clinical microbiology laboratory
Acquisition of specimens

In the world of data processing, the acronym *GIGO* stands for *garbage in, garbage out*. This evocative phrase is just as valid in clinical microbiology, where the quality of the final result is no better than that of the clinical specimen. Therefore, when specimens are submitted for microbiological investigation, the following should be kept in mind:

1 *Specimens should be representative samples of the pathological process.* As large a volume of pus, body fluid or tissue that can be safely removed should be sent to the laboratory. When a swab is used, it should hold as much exudate or as many superficial cells as possible.
2 *Specimens must be transported quickly to the laboratory.* If there are unavoidable delays, transport media should be obtained from the laboratory. If anaerobic organisms are suspected, specimens must be transported in containers from which oxygen has been excluded.
3 *Specimens must be accurately labelled for identification.* The patient's full name, and if possible a unique, identifying number should be on all specimens. Bar coding of specimens is emerging as a highly effective means of avoiding human error in specimen labelling and identification. Specimens should be accompanied by request forms, manually or computer-generated, which contain matching demographic information, the date, time and site of sampling, the procedures requested, and relevant clinical information, including antimicrobial treatment.
4 *Blood cultures should be drawn whenever there is evidence of systemic infection.* This is extremely important in immunosuppressed patients especially if their white blood cell count has fallen below $500/\mu l$, when there is a high risk of severe or fatal sepsis. Three blood cultures spaced about 30 minutes apart in any one day is recommended as the standard procedure in our institution.
5 *Specimens must be handled in a safe manner* to minimize the risk to anyone who may handle them from the bedside to the laboratory. Current national policy in the USA regards all clinical specimens, irrespective of their nature and source, as

dangerous. The greatest risks are from hepatitis B and C and human immunodeficiency viruses. All specimens must be handled under 'universal precautions', which include but are not limited to, wearing rubber gloves when collecting all patient samples, secure closure of specimen containers and the use of secondary containers such as sealable plastic bags. Similar precautions recommended by the Department of Health and Social Security are observed in the UK. All clinical microbiology laboratories should have clear, written criteria for the acquisition, identification and rejection of specimens.

Microbiological methods

Detailed descriptions of microbiological methods are beyond the scope of this text. However, it has long been evident that traditional manual methods for isolating bacteria in pure culture, identifying them by morphological, biochemical and serological properties and determining their antimicrobial susceptibilities, are slow. Specific antimicrobial treatment based on these methods can therefore be delayed as long as 3 or 4 days. Over the last 15–20 years, automated methods have been developed to a point at which, for faster growing bacteria, microbial identification and antimicrobial susceptibilities are available in 30–36 hours after receipt of the specimen. At some institutions, including our own, a data link between automated instruments in the laboratory and the hospital pharmacy enables a short list of antibiotics, based on susceptibility tests, to be recommended to the physician as soon as the results are available. This method has both clinical and economic advantages; the period when empirically selected antibiotics must be used is shortened by 24–48 hours, and very costly or toxic drugs can be avoided if equally effective, less toxic, and/or cheaper drugs are available.

Even more rapid bacterial identification can be achieved by methods in which techniques for antigen detection or nucleic acid probes are applied directly to clinical specimens, thus avoiding the long incubation periods required for isolating organisms in pure culture. Commercial kits for rapid diagnosis of such agents as group A streptococci have been widely used for several years; methods for the rapid identification of *Neisseria gonorrhoeae* and *Chlamydia trachomatis* based on chemiluminescent DNA probes are now available (Arnold *et al.*, 1989). Similar methods for detecting other organisms, including common viruses, are likely to become available in the near future. Ribotyping, in which ribosomal RNA is used as a probe for bacterial DNA (Stull, LiPuma and Edlind, 1988) may displace phage typing in the investigation of epidemics and nosocomial infections. Identification of *Mycobacterium* species, using this technique has already achieved considerable success (Good, 1991).

Whatever methods are used, it is imperative that microbiology laboratories process clinical specimens and report their results in a timely and efficient way. For instance, when a blood culture or an acid-fast stain is found to be positive, the patient's physician should be immediately notified. Many microbiology laboratories issue a preliminary report as soon as a presumptive microbial diagnosis is made. In those institutions which have laboratory information systems, urgent results can be automatically printed in the clinical unit as soon as the results are verified in the laboratory.

Methods specifically used for the laboratory diagnosis of certain microorganisms, such as anaerobes, chlamydia, fungi and viruses are discussed later in the text.

Antimicrobial susceptibility tests

Determining the antimicrobial susceptibility pattern of pathogenic bacteria is one of the main functions of the contemporary microbiology laboratory, since the susceptibilities of many bacteria cannot be predicted. The methods in common use are:

1 Disc diffusion tests
2 Broth or agar dilution tests
3 Automated procedures.

All of these methods, if standardized and quality controlled, can provide the necessary information for the successful management of serious infections. Disc diffusion and some semi-automated methods determine whether an organism is *susceptible, resistant* or *partially resistant* to a given antibiotic. This can be based on methods which relate the zone of bacterial inhibition to the minimal inhibitory concentration (MIC) of the organism (Bauer *et al.*, 1966) or by direct comparison of test and standard organisms grown under the same conditions in the presence of the antibiotic disc. Disc susceptibility tests may be unreliable for testing some fastidious bacteria, such as *Haemophilus influenzae* or *Neisseria gonorrhoeae* against penicillin. However, simple, rapid procedures are available which can directly detect beta-lactamase (penicillinase) production by these organisms, thus indicating their resistance to penicillin.

Dilution tests and most automated methods provide antimicrobial susceptibility results in the form of a minimal inhibitory concentration, which is the lowest concentration of the drug that will inhibit the growth of the test organism. Application of this method to treatment requires some knowledge of the pharmacokinetics and therapeutic blood levels of the antibiotic selected.

Many hospital laboratories issue antibiograms, based on the susceptibility patterns of bacteria isolated from patients in that institution, usually during the previous 6 months or year. Knowing the percentage likelihood that any organism will be susceptible to any antibiotic can be a useful, empirical guide to treatment while definitive susceptibility tests are being performed. When treatment is begun with potentially toxic antibiotics, in particular, the aminoglycosides, peak and trough serum levels should be measured to ensure adequate therapeutic blood levels without risking serious toxic effects.

Whatever drug or combination of drugs is selected for treatment of any infection, the response of the patient must be monitored. When a patient fails to respond clinically to adequate doses of an antibiotic, properly selected and administered, the laboratory data and the therapeutic choices must be critically reviewed. The presence of pus, however, is one of the most common causes of apparent failure of antibiotic treatment.

Indigenous microflora

The indigenous microflora (normal flora) of the nose, throat and external ear consists of a heterogeneous microbial population that is not well defined (Sommers, 1985). In addition, significant qualitative and quantitative differences can be found between the microflora of closely contiguous sites. For example, haemolytic streptococci are commonly isolated from the nasopharynx, but very infrequently from the nose: the opposite is true for *Staphylococcus aureus*. Determining the microbial species that normally colonize human body surfaces is subject to many variables, which include the age of the subject, hygiene, diet, and methods of sampling. For example, a diet rich in milk or other dairy products promotes growth of lactobacilli in the oropharynx, while dental disease appears to favour large numbers of Gram-positive cocci, fusiform bacteria and neisseria. Nevertheless, some knowledge of the 'normal' microflora in any site is essential before clinical significance can be assigned to any microbial isolate. The microorganisms which are generally accepted as making up the indigenous flora of the ear, nose and throat are listed in Table 19.1. Most of these organisms can also be isolated from the saliva (Russell and Melville, 1978). Included in Table 19.1 are a few known pathogens, such as *Staphylococcus aureus*, *Streptococcus pyogenes* and *Neisseria meningitidis*, which are sometimes present in the noses or throats of normal individuals. It is unclear why these potentially virulent organisms can be carried without ill effect on the host. However, it has been shown that the numbers of IgG- and IgA-coated bacteria in the nasopharynx increase with age suggesting that promotion of bacteriolysis and opsonization by IgG and prevention of epithelial attachment by IgA are important protective mechanisms against these potential pathogens (Stenfors and Raisanen, 1991).

The nasopharynx of the newborn infant is sterile,

Table 19.1 Indigenous microflora of the ear, nose/nasopharynx, mouth/oropharynx and skin

Site	Frequently and consistently isolated	Infrequently and inconsistently isolated
Ear	*Staphylococcus epidermidis* *Micrococcus* spp. Enterobacteriaceae Saprophytic mycobacteria	*Pseudomonas* spp. *Streptococcus pneumoniae*
Nose/nasopharynx	*Staphylococcus* spp. *Viridans streptococcus* *Propionibacterium* spp. Yeasts	*Staphylococcus aureus* *Streptococcus pyogenes* *Haemophilus* spp. *Neisseria* spp. *Streptococcus* spp.
Mouth/oropharynx	*Viridans streptococci* *Veillonella* spp. *Fusobacterium* spp. *Staphylococcus epidermidis*	*Neisseria* spp. inc. *meningitidis* *Haemophilus* spp. inc. *influenzae* *Staphylococcus aureus* *Bacteroides* spp. *Branhamella catarrhalis* *Lactobacillus* spp. *Actinomyces* spp. *Mycoplasma* spp. *Candida albicans*
Skin	*Staphylococcus epidermidis* *Corynebacterium* spp. *Propionibacterium acnes*	*Bacillus* spp. *Streptococcus* spp. *Peptococcus* spp.

but begins to be colonized by bacteria during the first 48 hours of life. Viridans streptococci, non-pathogenic neisseria and corynebacteria, are generally first to appear, followed by small numbers of *Streptococcus pneumoniae* and species of *Haemophilus*. Acquisition of these organisms appears to follow the start of breast-feeding and contact with maternal skin. Infants delivered in hospitals can rapidly acquire *Staphylococcus aureus* in their noses during the first few days of life. This organism can also be isolated from the anterior nares of about one-third of the adults in the general population, some of whom can carry the organism for months or years. *Streptococcus pyogenes* can be found in about 20% of throat cultures from children but only about 4% of adults harbour this organism in their throats. Some viridans streptococci found among the indigenous microflora can be shown to inhibit *Streptococcus pyogenes* and may be an effective natural defence against infection by this organism (Crow, Sanders and Longley, 1973). *Streptococcus salivarius*, for example, can prevent some individuals becoming colonized by *Streptococcus pyogenes* during an outbreak. Bacterial interference has also been used to displace virulent strains of *Staphylococcus aureus* causing outbreaks of neonatal sepsis. 'Avirulent' strains of *Staphylococcus aureus* (phage type 502A) instilled into infants' noses prevented colonization by virulent strains. However, enthusiasm for

this procedure should be tempered by reports of sepsis caused by the 'avirulent' staphylococcus (Drutz *et al.*, 1966). The mechanisms for these forms of bacterial interference are not known, although bacteriocines may be partly responsible.

Antimicrobial drugs can significantly alter the composition of the normal microflora in many sites in the body. With antibiotic treatment the normal bacterial population of Gram-positive and Gram-negative cocci and bacilli can be rapidly replaced with Gram-negative rods (Sprunt and Redman, 1968).

Bacteria affecting the ear, nose and throat

Staphylococcus

The genus *Staphylococcus* comprises 30 species (Table 19.2), many of which have only recently been defined or associated with human infection.

Morphology, culture and identification

Staphylococci are Gram-positive, spherical cocci, which divide in three dimensions and resemble a bunch of grapes. Except for one anaerobic subspecies (Table 19.2), they are aerobes and facultative anaerobes. They grow in high concentrations (9%) of

Table 19.2 Species of staphylococci which are indigenous microflora and/or pathogens

Coagulase-positive staphylococci	Coagulase-negative staphylococci
Staphylococcus aureus	Staphylococcus epidermidis
Staphylococcus aureus subspecies anaerobius	Staphylococcus saprophyticus
	Staphylococcus saccharolyticus
	Staphylococcus cohnii
	Staphylococcus capitis
	Staphylococcus haemolyticus
	Staphylococcus auricularis
	Staphylococcus lugdunensis
	Staphylococcus scheiferi
	Staphylococcus warneri
	Staphylococcus xylosis

sodium chloride and this together with the production of catalase distinguishes them from other genera of cocci such as *Streptococcus*, *Micrococcus* and *Enterococcus*. On blood agar, staphylococci grow as fairly large pigmented colonies, which range in colour from white through creamy yellow to lemon-yellow. For routine clinical purposes, a positive coagulase reaction is sufficient to identify an isolate as *Staphylococcus aureus*. Staphylococcal DNAase and phosphatase have the same significance as coagulase. Further identification of coagulase-negative staphylococci is by an array of biochemical reactions and susceptibility or resistance to novobiocin and polymyxin B.

Enzymes and toxins

Staphylococcus aureus produces many biologically active substances. *Exfolatin* is a complex staphylococcal toxin which causes separation of layers of the epidermis at the level of the stratum granulosum. The resulting 'scalded skin syndrome' (Ritter's disease) mainly affects young children. *Toxic shock syndrome toxin* (TSST-1) causes fever, hypotension, desquamative rashes and widespread organ dysfunction. *Staphylococcus aureus* produces four distinct *haemolysins* but their role in staphylococcal disease is not known. Some strains produce *enterotoxins* while the majority produce beta-lactamase which inactivates many of the penicillins.

Teichoic acid is an antigenic component of the staphylococcal cell wall. Demonstration of antibodies to teichoic acid has been used in the diagnosis of occult staphylococcal infections, including infective endocarditis.

Antimicrobial susceptibility

At Methodist Medical Center, Dallas, Texas, 97% of all strains of *Staphylococcus aureus* isolated are resist-

ant to penicillin. Similar figures are obtained in most tertiary care hospitals. These staphylococci are mainly beta-lactamase producers as most are susceptible to methicillin and the isoxazolyl penicillins. However, some strains are methicillin-resistant (MRSA) and by definition, have a minimal inhibitory concentration $> 8 \mu g/ml$. This form of resistance is due to induction in *Staphylococcus aureus* of a penicillin-binding protein PBP2a, which has a reduced affinity for methicillin and other antistaphylococcal penicillins. In our institution, 15% of all strains of *Staphylococcus aureus* are methicillin-resistant. In 1995, the incidence of methicillin-resistant *Staphylococcus aureus* in the USA continues to rise, while in Europe it is declining. Vancomycin is the drug of choice for treating these organisms. Penicillin tolerance is observed with some strains of *Staphylococcus aureus*. A minimal bactericidal concentration (MIC) of penicillin 32 times greater than the minimal inhibitory concentration (MIC) is necessary to kill these strains (normally the MBC = 4 × MIC). Many strains of staphylococci are susceptible to fusidic acid. While this drug has been used for many years in the UK, it has never been approved for use in the USA.

Clinical significance

Staphylococcus aureus is frequently found in the anterior nares of healthy individuals, and is the predominant staphylococcus that causes infections of the ear, nose and throat. These include some cases of localized otitis externa, otitis media, sinusitis and epiglottitis. Although most cases of toxic shock syndrome have been associated with tampon use, the disease has been reported in association with staphylococcal tracheitis (Solomon, Truman and Murray, 1985), pharyngitis (Hirsch *et al.*, 1984) and nasal packing (Hull *et al.*, 1983: Barbour, Shlaes and Guertin, 1984). Toxic shock syndrome has also been reported in males with staphylococcal infections of bone and soft tissues (Reingold, Margrett and Dan, 1982).

Coagulase-negative staphylococci

Staphylococcus epidermidis is a very common inhabitant of the skin, while *Staphylococcus capitis* and *Staphylococcus auricularis*, as their names indicate, are found as normal flora in the scalp and external ear. *Staphylococcus haemolyticus* and *Staphylococcus hominis* are found in areas of skin rich in apocrine glands. Among coagulase-negative staphylococci, *Staphylococcus epidermidis* is a frequent cause of opportunistic infections especially in association with percutaneous intravascular catheters and cardiovascular prostheses (Gill, Selepak and Williams, 1983) and has also been implicated as a rare cause of invasive ('malignant') otitis externa (Barrow and Levenson, 1992). However, all the coagulase-negative staphylococci listed in Table 19.2 have caused human infections (Pfaller and Herwaldt, 1988). The antimicrobial susceptibility pattern of *Staphylococcus epidermidis* and other coagulase-negative staphylococci is similar to that of methicillin-resistant *Staphylococcus aureus*; most isolates are susceptible to vancomycin and ciprofloxacin.

Streptococcus

Overview of the genus

The genus *Streptococcus* consists of Gram-positive cocci which form chains; it contains major pathogens and many of the indigenous bacterial flora of the ear, nose and throat. Recently, some of the organisms formerly included in the genus have been assigned to the genera *Enterococcus* and *Lactococcus* (Schliefer and Kilpper-Balz, 1984, 1987). The two most common pathogens of the genus are *Streptococcus pyogenes* and *Streptococcus pneumoniae*. Many streptococci are haemolytic and the type of haemolysis observed on blood agar plates separates them into three groups, i.e. those which cause (1) complete (β) haemolysis, (2) green (α) haemolysis or (3) lack haemolytic properties (γ haemolysis). Further distinction among the beta-haemolytic streptococci can be made by determining their polysaccharide cell wall (Lancefield) antigens.

Streptococcus pyogenes

Morphology, culture and identification

Streptococcus pyogenes (Lancefield group A streptococcus) is a Gram-positive, spherical coccus that forms chains of varying length. It grows on 2% blood agar as small transparent colonies surrounded by a zone of β-haemolysis. When many throat swabs have to be cultured, the organism is readily recognized when grown on sheep blood agar. However, if horse or rabbit blood agar is used, colonies of *Streptococcus pyogenes* cannot be distinguished from those of *Haemophilus haemolyticus*, a fairly common pharyngeal commensal.

Once isolated, β-haemolytic streptococci can be confirmed as *Streptococcus pyogenes* by serological grouping of the cell wall antigens (Lancefield grouping). Those reacting with group A antisera are *Streptococcus pyogenes*. Group A streptococci, with rare exceptions, are susceptible to low concentrations (0.04 units/ml) of bacitracin. Placing a bacitracin disc on the plate used for primary isolation allows simple rapid recognition of group A streptococci, whose growth is inhibited around the disc. Rapid grouping methods in which antibody-coated latex particles or protein A-rich staphylococci are agglutinated by streptococcal antigens are available for the determination of all the common Lancefield groups, especially A to G. Commercial kits which rapidly detect streptococcal antigen in throat swabs are likely to miss about 10% of group A streptococcal infections (Tenjarla, Kumar and Dyke, 1991).

Enzymes and toxins

Streptococcus pyogenes can produce many enzymes and toxins which have a role in the pathogenesis of streptococcal disease. Lysogenic strains can produce *erythrogenic toxin*. This substance causes fever, but its role in the typical rash of scarlet fever is debatable, since the rash may be the result of secondary hypersensitivity rather than a direct toxic effect on the microcirculation. Streptococcal oxygen-labile haemolysin (streptolysin O) is antigenic and antistreptolysin O (ASO) antibodies can be a useful laboratory aid to the diagnosis of non-suppurative post-streptococcal disease, particularly rheumatic fever. The M protein present on the surface of group A streptococci is a major determinant of virulence. This substance resists phagocytosis and the action of complement, and may have a role in the attachment of the organism to pharyngeal mucosa.

Antimicrobial susceptibility

Penicillin is still the drug of choice for the treatment of infections by *Streptococcus pyogenes*. Sulphonamides are effective for treating streptococcal carriers but not active infections. Erythromycin and the first generation cephalosporins are alternatives to penicillin.

Clinical significance

Streptococcus pyogenes frequently colonizes the throats of asymptomatic persons especially children. It accounts for up to 30% of all cases of acute pharyngitis in children between the ages of 5 and 10 years. Acute rheumatic fever and glomerulonephritis continue to be serious complications of streptococcal infection. In the last few years there has been a resurgence of rheumatic fever in parts of the USA (Veasy, Wiedmieir and Orsmond, 1987). A severe toxic shock-like syndrome attributable to *Streptococcus pyogenes* has also been described (Stevens *et al.*, 1989). Lancefield groups C and G are much less common causes of streptococcal pharyngitis, but rheumatic fever or glomerulonephritis can follow these infections.

Streptococcus pneumoniae

Morphology, culture and identification

Streptococcus pneumoniae is a Gram-positive, capsulated, lancet-shaped, diplococcus, which forms long chains in liquid culture. On blood agar, it forms small, draughtsman-like (checker-piece) colonies surrounded by a zone of alpha haemolysis. In culture

Streptococcus pneumoniae can be readily distinguished from other alpha haemolytic (viridans) streptococci by its susceptibility to a disc containing ethyl hydrocupreinate (optochin). The capsular polysaccharide can be typed serologically; 84 types are currently recognized.

Antimicrobial susceptibility

Most isolates of *Streptococcus pneumoniae* are susceptible to penicillin at a minimal inhibitory concentration of 0.06 µg/ml; a few more tolerant strains have a minimal inhibitory concentration between 0.12 µg/ml and 1.00 µg/ml. Penicillin resistant strains, first described from South Africa, are becoming increasingly common in the UK, the USA and other countries. Resistance is due to altered affinity of penicillin for penicillin-binding proteins (PBPs) (Handwerger and Thomasz, 1986). Penicillin-resistant strains are susceptible to vancomycin but resistant to tetracycline, erythromycin, clindamycin, rifampin and chloramphenicol.

Clinical significance

Streptococcus pneumoniae is fairly frequently isolated from throats of healthy individuals. Types 6, 9, and 23 are frequently isolated from healthy children, but, along with type 19, also account for about half of the paediatric cases of otitis media (Howie, Ploussard and Sloyer, 1975). The pneumococcus is also a common cause of sinusitis and a rare cause of mastoiditis. Pneumococcal sinusitis can be a severe complication of AIDS.

The mortality rate in systemic pneumococcal disease can range from 20% to 60%, despite antibiotics. Protective immunization with polyvalent pneumococcal vaccine is therefore recommended for elderly healthy adults, and patients with chronic lung, heart, liver or kidney disease, with sickle cell anaemia, or those who are immunosuppressed or have had a splenectomy.

Viridans streptococci

Viridans streptococci (i.e. alpha-haemolytic streptococci other than the pneumococcus) are commonly found among the indigenous flora of the oropharynx. However, they can cause infective endocarditis, and rarely soft tissue and visceral infections. The viridans streptococci are generally susceptible to penicillin.

Other streptococci

Streptococci which form tiny colonies on solid media have been given various specific names, for instance, *Streptococcus milleri*, *Streptococcus intermedius*, and *Streptococcus constellatus*. These streptococci are prob-

ably synonymous with *Streptococcus anginosus* (Coykendall, Wesbecher and Gustafson, 1987) and this name should perhaps take precedence. Small colony-forming streptococci may be α, β, or γ haemolytic and can possess Lancefield group A, C, F or G polysaccharides or, in some instances, may be ungroupable. *Streptococcus anginosus* (*Streptococcus milleri*) is found among the indigenous flora of the oro- and nasopharynx and can be isolated fairly frequently from clinical specimens (Ruoff, King and Ferraro, 1985). It has been implicated as a cause of pharyngitis (Cimolai *et al.*, 1988), buccal, dental and parotid abscesses. It can also cause abdominal abscesses, primary bacteraemias and infective endocarditis (Shlaes *et al.*, 1981). It is perhaps the most common facultative bacterium isolated from cerebral abscesses (De Louvois, Gortavai and Hurley, 1977; Shlaes *et al.*, 1981) and in many of these patients sinusitis or otitis are predisposing conditions (De Louvois, Gortavai and Hurley, 1977).

Enterococcus

Enterococcus faecalis and *Enterococcus faecium* (formerly enteric group D streptococci) are intestinal bacteria which are occasionally isolated from the nose and throat, especially from patients in hospitals. These organisms are noted for their high degree of resistance to most antibiotics, but they are often susceptible to penicillin when given with an aminoglycoside or vancomycin. Non-enteric group D streptococci such as *Streptococcus bovis* are susceptible to penicillin but the minimal inhibitory concentrations are higher than those for group A streptococci.

Corynebacteria

Overview of the genus

The genus *Corynebacterium* is now limited to those Gram-positive, aerobic, club-shaped rods, which have a cell wall containing, *meso*-diaminopimelic and arabinomycolic acids. *Corynebacterium diphtheriae* is the type species. Bacteria which morphologically resemble *Corynebacterium diphtheriae* and which are found among the normal microflora of the oropharynx and skin are often referred to as 'diphtheroids'. However, by present taxonomic criteria, some of these are likely to be placed in other genera. *Propionibacterium acnes* is an anaerobic organism commonly present on the skin, which closely resembles the corynebacteria, and is sometimes included among the 'diphtheroids'. There are currently 11 species of corynebacteria; but the organism long known as *Corynebacterium ulcerans* is not included (Collins and Cummings, 1986) and has yet to be accurately classified.

Corynebacterium diphtheriae

Morphology, culture and identification

As a result of incomplete cell division, *Corynebacterium diphtheriae* characteristically forms V, Y or Chinese letter shapes on Gram-stained preparations. When the organism is grown on Loeffler's medium and stained with methylene blue, typical metachromatic granules can be seen in the bacterial cell. The organism grows readily on blood agar, but forms more characteristic black colonies on media containing potassium tellurite. Identification of *gravis, intermedius* and *mitis* biotypes can be made on colonial morphology and patterns of carbohydrate fermentations. Rapid identification by immunofluorescence can be a useful method during epidemics (McCracken and Mauney, 1971). Demonstration of toxin production is essential to confirm the clinical diagnosis of diphtheria. Toxigenicity, which is dependent on the presence of a temperate phage carrying the *tox* gene, is demonstrable by immunodiffusion (Elek, 1949), by guinea-pig inoculation, or by cytotoxic effect in cell culture (Murphy, Bocha and Teng, 1978). Non-toxigenic strains are not infrequently isolated during epidemics.

Antimicrobial susceptibility

Penicillin and erythromycin are the drugs of choice for elimination of the organism in active cases of diphtheria and in carriers. Other effective drugs include cephalosporins, lincomycin, and clindamycin. The role of antibiotics, however, is secondary to antitoxin in the treatment of diphtheria.

Clinical significance

The diagnosis of diphtheria and its subsequent treatment with antitoxin must be made in the first instance on clinical findings. Treatment should not be delayed while waiting for bacteriological confirmation. Portions of the pseudomembrane from the throat, nose or larynx are preferable to swabs for bacterial isolation. A fairly common microbial 'red herring' is the simultaneous isolation of *Corynebacterium diphtheriae* and beta-haemolytic streptococci. When this happens, the diagnosis of diphtheria should not be overlooked and clearly must always take precedence for treatment.

Other Corynebacteria and Arcanobacterium haemolyticum

'*Corynebacterium ulcerans*' which can produce a diphtheria-like toxin is an uncommon cause of pharyngitis, which can be confused with diphtheria. *Corynebacterium pseudotuberculosis* is an animal pathogen which can occasionally cause granulomatous cervical adenitis, most cases of which have been reported from Australia and France (Lipsky *et al.*, 1982). This organism can produce a diphtheria-like toxin (Krech and Hollis, 1991), but isolates from human cases are non-toxigenic. *Corynebacterium xerosis*, *C. stratum* and *C. pseudodiphtheriticum* are sometimes found as indigenous flora of the skin and nasopharynx. They occasionally give rise to opportunistic infections in immunosuppressed patients.

Arcanobacterium (formerly *Corynebacterium*) *haemolyticum* can cause pharyngitis, scarlatiniform rashes, skin ulceration and septicaemia (Miller and Brancato, 1984; Clarridge, 1989). Unlike true corynebacteria, this organism is catalase negative. On Gram-stained smears, it can be easily confused with corynebacteria, haemolytic streptococci, actinomycetes or nocardia.

Haemophilus

Overview of the genus

The genus *Haemophilus* consists of species that, in the main are part of the normal respiratory flora. Members of this genus have a characteristic requirement for specific growth factors (X and/or V factors). X factor is haemin, a haemoglobin derivative, V factor is nicotinamide adenine dinucleotide (NAD). Recent taxonomic data indicate that *Haemophilus ducreyi*, the cause of chancroid, should be placed in some other genus. *Haemophilus influenzae* is by far the most common pathogen.

Haemophilus influenzae

Morphology, culture and identification

Haemophilus influenzae is a small, Gram-negative coccobacillus usually about 0.5 μm in length but occasionally forming long filaments. It requires both X and V factors for growth, both of which are provided by chocolate agar. In mixed cultures on blood agar (a source of X factor) with *Staphylococcus aureus*, *Haemophilus influenzae* grows as small satellite colonies around the staphylococci, a source of V factor. Colonies of *Haemophilus influenzae* are usually small, transparent discs, but some isolates are encapsulated and form much larger colonies. The organism can be typed serologically by its capsular antigens. Capsular type b causes the most serious human infections.

Antimicrobial susceptibility

Haemophilus influenzae is susceptible to several antibiotics used alone or in combination. Ampicillin or amoxycillin are satisfactory for the treatment of otitis media or sinusitis due to this organism, provided treatment is continued long enough. However, about 20% of type b strains produce beta-lactamase, and are therefore ampicillin-resistant. Suitable drugs for ampicillin-resistant infections include cefaclor, amoxycillin-clavulanate, and trimethoprim-sulphamethoxazole. For serious systemic infections, ampicillin given with chloramphenicol, cefuroxime or cefotaxime has been recommended.

Clinical significance

Haemophilus influenzae forms about 10% of the indigenous pharyngeal flora in adults. It is second only to the pneumococcus as a cause of otitis media (Feingold, Klein and Haslam, 1966), although many of these strains of *Haemophilus influenzae* are untypable. Non-capsulated strains are often isolated from patients with sinusitis. Most cases of acute epiglottitis in children and about 25% of adult cases are caused by type b (Mostoe and Strome, 1983). The most common and serious manifestation of *Haemophilus influenzae* type b is meningitis, especially among children 2 years of age and younger. The mortality rate is approximately 5% while between 25% and 30% have permanent neurological damage of varying degrees. These depressing consequences have resulted in the development of preventive vaccines. The first vaccine in the USA against type b was licensed in 1985 but although its efficacy was reported in Finnish studies to be 90% (Peltola *et al.*, 1984) it did not achieve a satisfactory level of protection when given to children in the USA (Osterholm *et al.*, 1988). The currently recommended vaccine in the USA is a polysaccharide vaccine conjugated with a diphtheria toxoid carrier (PRP-D vaccine) given at the age of 18–23 months with a second dose 2 months later (American Academy of Pediatrics: Committee on Infectious Diseases, 1988). Local reactions to the vaccine are found in 10% of vaccinees, while moderate to high fevers are reported in about 1%. Other more antigenic vaccines have been developed but are still not generally recommended. No vaccines have yet been developed against non-typable strains of *Haemophilus influenzae* that commonly cause otitis media. Such a prophylactic agent, based on bacterial somatic rather than capsular antigens could have considerable value in the prevention of this form of otitis media.

Other species of Haemophilus

Haemophilus parainfluenzae is the most common *Haemophilus* spp. in the normal oropharyngeal flora. Others are occasionally isolated from the mouth and from blood cultures (usually in infective endocarditis) including *Haemophilus haemolyticus*, *H. parahaemolyticus*, *H. aphrophilus*, *H. paraphrophilus*, and *H. segnis*. Ampicillin-resistant *Haemophilus aphrophilus* is a rare cause of acute epiglottitis (Jones, Slepak and Bigelow, 1976).

Bordetella

Bordetella pertussis

The genus *Bordetella* contains only one significant human pathogen, *Bordetella pertussis*, the cause of whooping cough. It is a small coccobacillus best isolated in cases of whooping cough from pernasal swabs plated on Bordet-Gengou medium, on which it forms colonies which resemble drops of aluminium paint. Rapid identification can be made from culture by immunofluorescence. Although *Bordetella pertussis* is susceptible *in vitro* to several antibiotics, only erythromycin is clinically effective.

Immunoprophylaxis of whooping cough

Pertussis vaccine, introduced around the 1950s, produced a dramatic fall in the incidence of whooping cough and reduced the morbidity in vaccinees who contracted the disease. Beginning in the 1970s, the use of this inactivated, whole-cell vaccine, usually given combined with tetanus and diphtheria toxoid (DTP), decreased in many countries because of its association with uncommon, though severe side effects. These included immediate hypersensitivity reactions, hyperpyrexia, shock with hypotonia, convulsions, and encephalopathy. As a result, the numbers of reported cases of whooping cough in England, Sweden and Japan increased significantly. It is probable that these serious reactions are not directly due to pertussis vaccine, but that the DTP vaccine accelerates the onset of latent neurological disorders, and there is little doubt, based on risk-benefit analysis that the benefits of pertussis immunization outweigh the risks (Cherry, 1988: Report of the Task Force on Pertussis and Pertussis Immunization, 1988). Acellular vaccines have been used successfully in Japan since 1981 (Tomodu, Ogura and Kirushige, 1991). The local and minor reactions to this form of pertussis vaccine appear to be less than with whole cell types, but whether serious neurological reactions are significantly reduced is uncertain partly because the vaccine is not given until 2 years of age, which is beyond the age when most serious adverse reactions occur. Meanwhile, the whole cell vaccine is still recommended in the USA, with the caveat that further vaccinations in the initial series are withheld if there are adverse systemic reactions.

Neisseria and Branhamella

Overview of the genera

At present the genus *Neisseria* consists of 10 species of which *Neisseria gonorrhoeae* and *Neisseria meningitidis* are major pathogens. *Neisseria catarrhalis* has now been reclassified as *Branhamella catarrhalis* (Doern, 1986), along with three other species which are found only in animals.

Neisseria gonorrhoeae and N. meningitidis

Morphology, culture and identification

Neisseria gonorrhoeae and *Neisseria meningitidis* are morphologically identical, Gram-negative, kidney-shaped diplococci. In inflammatory exudates they are seen typically within the cytoplasm of neutrophils. Both organisms, especially *Neisseria gonorrhoeae*, are vulnerable to adverse environmental conditions. Specially formulated transport media such as Thayer–Martin or Martin–Lewis media with a CO_2 atmosphere, are required when there is any likely delay in delivery of clinical specimens to the laboratory. Both species grow on chocolate agar in an atmosphere of 10% CO_2, as opaque, white discs, which give a positive oxidase reaction. Further identification of the species can be made by carbohydrate oxidation reactions or by immunofluorescence using monoclonal antisera. Meningococci can be further grouped serologically according to their capsular or outer protein membrane antigens. There are 13 groups of which groups A, B, C, Y and W135 are mostly frequently isolated.

Antimicrobial susceptibility

Penicillin-resistance due to beta-lactamase production is now found around the world in strains of *Neisseria gonorrhoeae*. In the UK 2% to 2.5% of strains are penicillin-resistant, and they are endemic in the major cities of the USA. Spectinomycin, ceftriaxone and enoxacin (Barry *et al.*, 1992) are active against penicillin-resistant strains. *Neisseria meningitidis* is generally susceptible to penicillin, but resistant strains are occasionally encountered. Elimination of nasopharyngeal carriage during outbreaks of *Neisseria meningitidis* can be achieved in a high percentage of carriers with a single dose of ciprofloxacin (Gauntt and Lambert, 1988) or ceftriaxone (Schwartz *et al.*, 1988).

Clinical significance

Neisseriae which colonize the naso- and oropharynx include *Neisseria cinerea*, *N. flavescens*, *N. lactamica*, *N. sicca* and *N. subflava*. Rare instances of systemic or central nervous system infection have been caused by these organisms. *Neisseria meningitidis* can be isolated from the nasopharynx of asymptomatic carriers during epidemics. The meningococcal groups isolated from nasopharyngeal carriers are usually but not exclusively those causing the epidemic. Group A causes most epidemics of meningococcal disease, while interepidemic cases are usually caused by groups B and C.

Severe exudative or ulcerative gonococcal pharyngitis, as a result of oral sexual transmission is well recognized, but many gonococcal pharyngeal infections can be asymptomatic (Weisner *et al.*, 1973).

Other Neisseria

Neisseria cinerea, *N. flavescens*, *N. lactamica*, *N. sicca* and *N. subflava* can be found among the indigenous microflora of the nasopharynx and throat. Rare instances of systemic or central nervous system infection have been caused by these organisms.

Branhamella catarrhalis

Branhamella catarrhalis is morphologically similar to the neisseriae but is distinguished by its production of deoxyribonuclease and lack of oxidative activity against carbohydrates. This organism was once thought to be a harmless inhabitant of the upper respiratory tract, but is now reported to be the third leading cause of otitis media, accounting for 10–15% of cases (Glebink, 1989). It is also regarded as a common cause of sinusitis (Brorson, Axelson and Holm, 1976) and of laryngitis in adults (Schalen *et al.*, 1980). Strains of *Branhamella catarrhalis* whose beta-lactamase inactivates both ampicillin and cefaclor are fairly common. These strains are susceptible to cephalosporins combined with clavulanic acid or sulbactam.

Enteric Gram-negative bacteria

The *Enterobacteriaceae* family consists of numerous genera and over a hundred species. However, only a few of these, notably *Escherichia coli*, *Klebsiella pneumoniae*, *Enterobacter aerogenes*, *Enterobacter cloacae* and *Serratia marcescens*, are occasional causes of otitis media and sinusitis. The *Enterobacteriaceae* are aerobic and facultative anaerobic, Gram-negative rods, which typically grow well in the presence of bile salts, e.g. on McConkey's medium. Numerous biochemical and serological reactions have been applied to the identification of these organisms and many identification schemes based on these tests have been devised. Rapid, automated methods of identification have been available for more than a decade (McCracken *et al.*, 1980; Smith, 1981) and have excellent correlation with standard manual methods. Antimicrobial susceptibilities of such a large, diverse group of organisms cannot be predicted with confidence, and susceptibility testing on all isolates of clinical significance is essential.

Klebsiella rhinoscleromatis and *K. ozoenae* are Gram-negative enteric bacteria, both of which are rare in the UK and the USA. *Klebsiella rhinoscleromatis* causes a chronic granulomatous infection of the upper respiratory tract mucosa (rhinoscleroma) which can progress to involve bone. There are areas of endemic rhinoscleroma in eastern Europe, parts of south America, central Africa, and southern Asia. Treatment is with tetracycline or trimethoprim-sulphamethoxazole given for several months. Whether *Kleb-*

siella ozoenae is the aetiological agent of chronic atrophic rhinitis is uncertain, although it can be isolated from some cases of the disease. It is generally susceptible to a wide range of antibiotics.

Pseudomonas

Characteristically, *Pseudomonas* spp. are motile, Gram-negative rods, which by contrast with the enteric bacteria, do not ferment carbohydrates, and are oxidase positive. Most of the 20 species currently recognized can cause human opportunistic infections (Von Graevenitz, 1985). *Pseudomonas aeruginosa* is by far the most common species causing sporadic infections and nosocomial outbreaks. It is the main cause of diffuse otitis externa, and has been isolated from 80% of patients with chronic otitis media (Brook and Finegold, 1979). Severe pseudomonas infections of the ear are uncommon but invasive ('malignant') otitis externa (Chandler, 1968; Rubin and Yu, 1988), mastoiditis and perichondritis of the auricle have been reported (Bassiouny, 1981). The antibiotics which are active against *Pseudomonas aeruginosa* include gentamicin, tobramycin, amikacin, ticarcillin and ciprofloxacin. Oral ciprofloxacin given alone (Lang *et al.*, 1990) and with rifampin for several weeks combined with surgical debridement (Rubin *et al.*, 1989) has been shown to be an effective alternative to systemic treatment for malignant otitis externa.

Borrelia and Treponema

Borrelia vincentii

Borrelia vincentii is a slender, irregularly curved, motile bacterium, about 10 μm to 20 μm in length. Microscopic examination of Giemsa or Wright stained smears from the mouth or pharynx is usually sufficient to establish a clinical diagnosis of Vincent's angina or acute necrotizing ulcerative gingivitis. In both conditions borreliae are accompanied by large numbers of fusobacteria, but the exact aetiological role of either organism in Vincent's infection or acute necrotizing ulcerative gingivitis is uncertain. Metronidazole is the drug of choice for fusospirochaetal infec-

tions, but the drug has not been officially approved for this purpose in the USA.

Treponema

Treponema pallidum, the cause of syphilis, is a regularly coiled, 6 μm to 10 μm, motile bacterium, which can be seen with the aid of darkground microscopy, immunofluorescence or silver-stained preparations. These techniques can be applied to material from primary or secondary lesions. Primary and secondary syphilis can involve the mouth with resulting enlargement of cervical lymph nodes, in which *Treponema pallidum* may be found using silver-stained histological sections. The diagnosis of all stages of the disease, especially late or latent syphilis is confirmed by serology. Current tests detect one of two distinct antibodies. First, antibody to cardiolipin antigen (Wassermann antibody) can be demonstrated by highly sensitive methods such as the Venereal Disease Reference Laboratory (VDRL) or rapid plasma reagin (RPR) tests. However, false positive reactions are fairly common in infectious mononucleosis, after viral vaccinations, in collagen-vascular diseases and even in pregnancy. Second, treponemal antibody can be detected by the fluorescent treponemal antibody–absorbed (FTA-ABS) or microhaemagglutination for *T. pallidum* (MHATP) tests, which are highly specific. Titres of Wassermann antibody roughly correlate with the *activity* of the disease, and most cases become nonreactive after successful treatment. Treponemal antibody persists permanently even after treatment. The application of serological tests to the diagnosis of syphilis is summarized in Table 19.3. Penicillin is the antibiotic of choice in all forms of syphilis. Alternative drugs include erythromycin, doxycycline and ceftriaxone.

Anaerobic and microaerophilic bacteria

The term *anaerobic bacteria* refers specifically to organisms which die in the presence of molecular oxygen even when it is in low concentrations. Microaerophilic bacteria can tolerate low concentrations of oxygen. There are many genera and species of

Table 19.3 Clinical interpretation of serological tests for syphilis

VDRL or RPR tests	MHATP or FTA-ABS tests	Usual clinical interpretation
Non-reactive	Non-reactive	No serological evidence of syphilis
Reactive	Reactive	Active syphilis
Non-reactive	Reactive	Treated syphilis
Reactive	Non-reactive	False positive

VDRL = Venereal Disease Reference Laboratory; RPR = rapid plasma reagin test; MHATP = microhaemagglutination test for *Treponema pallidum*; FTA-ABS = fluorescent *Treponema pallidum* (absorbed) test

anaerobes, among which Gram-positive and Gram-negative cocci and bacilli are all represented. Those commonly isolated from human infections are listed in Table 19.4. Whenever possible, if anaerobic infection is suspected, samples of pus or infected tissue should be obtained for culture; swabs should be avoided if at all possible, especially if the site being sampled has anaerobic normal microflora. Specimens should be collected into, and transported to the laboratory in containers that are free of oxygen such as those which can generate an inert atmosphere and/or contain prereduced media.

Table 19.4 Anaerobic and microaerophilic bacterial genera which can be isolated from the ear, nose and oropharynx

	Gram positive	Gram negative
Cocci	Peptococcus	Veillonella
	Peptostreptococcus	
Bacilli	Actinomyces	Bacteroides
	Arachnia	Fusobacterium
	Clostridium	
	Propionibacterium	

Methods of isolation include:

1 Inoculation of roll-tubes of media under a stream of nitrogen
2 Incubation of plated media in the anaerobic jar or disposable anaerobic pouches
3 Performing all microbiological procedures in an anaerobic chamber.

Identification is based on morphology and Gram reaction, biochemical tests and/or gas chromatography. Several commercial methods for rapid identification of anaerobes are available (Hussain *et al.*, 1987).

Most anaerobes are susceptible to chloramphenicol, clindamycin, metronidazole, and with the important exception of the *Bacteroides fragilis* group, to penicillin. Anaerobes form a large component of the normal microflora of the oropharynx. Anaerobes, either alone or in mixed culture, have been isolated from inflammatory and suppurative infections of the middle ear (Brook, 1987), nose and throat (Table 19.5). Anaerobes have been isolated from more than 50% of patients with chronic otitis media (Brook and Finegold, 1979).

Actinomyces and *Arachnia* spp. are microaerophilic oral flora which, as a result of local injury, as for example, during dental procedures, can gain access to soft tissues and establish infection, leading to cervicofacial actinomycosis. Despite their opportunistic characteristics, these bacteria rarely cause disease in patients with AIDS or other immunosuppressed conditions (Yeager *et al.*, 1986). Those associated with cervicofacial disease include *Actinomyces israelii*, *A. naeslundii*, *A. meyeri*, *A. odontolyticus*, and *Arachnia propionica*. It is not uncommon to find these organ-

Table 19.5 Recovery rates of anaerobes, alone and in mixed culture in inflammatory and suppurative diseases of the ear, nose and throat

Disease	No. cases studied	% Yielding anaerobes
Chronic sinusitis	83	53
Chronic otitis media	68	35
Perimandibular space infection	31	99
Peritonsillar abscess	21	76

Data extracted from Bartlett, J.G. (1990). Anaerobic bacteria: general concepts. In: *Principles and Practice of Infectious Diseases*, edited by G.L. Mandell, R.G. Douglas, and J.E. Bennett. New York: Churchill-Livingstone, p. 1834

isms in mixed cultures with other bacteria especially Gram-negative organisms, which may have a role in enhancing the low virulence of actinomycetes (Holm, 1950).

Specimens of pus from patients with actinomycosis often contain 'sulphur granules', which typically consist of masses of Gram-positive branching filaments. Growth of the actinomycetes in anaerobic culture is extremely slow and sometimes unsuccessful. The actinomycetes are susceptible to many antibiotics, but penicillin given in high doses over a prolonged period is generally successful. Alternative drugs include the cephalosporins, erythromycin, tetracycline and clindamycin.

Mycobacteria

Overview of the genus

The genus *Mycobacterium* consists of 25 species, which can be divided into *Mycobacterium tuberculosis* (which includes *Mycobacterium bovis*) and the 'non-tuberculosis mycobacteria'. The latter includes *Mycobacterium avium-intracellulare* (MAI) and *Mycobacterium kansasii* which commonly cause disseminated disease in patients with AIDS.

Morphology, culture and identification

Mycobacteria are characteristically acid- and alcohol-fast, aerobic, non-motile rods. A sensitive method for microscopic detection of mycobacteria is to stain smears with auramine-rhodamine and examine the slide by ultraviolet microscope. The bright orange fluorescent bacteria against a dark background are visually more easily detected than by conventional acid fast stains and light microscopy (Sommers, McClatchy and Monella, 1983). Lowenstein–Jensen, Petragnani, and semisynthetic media such as Middlebrook 7H-10 are usually used for isolation. Most clinically important species, including *Mycobacterium tuberculosis*, grow slowly, and cultures are maintained for 8 weeks before being discarded as negative. Final species identification is based on a wide array of biochemical tests and growth characteristics, including the effect of light and darkness on pigment production. Recently, nucleic acid probes for *Mycobacterium tuberculosis* and *Mycobacterium avium-intracellulare* have been developed (Gonzalez and Hanna, 1987) and may revolutionize the identification of mycobacterial infections, especially those which complicate AIDS.

Antimicrobial susceptibility

The first line drugs effective against *Mycobacterium tuberculosis* are isoniazid, rifampicin, pyrizinamide, ethambutol and streptomycin. Treatment with two or more drugs is the rule, to prevent the emergence of resistant strains. The recrudescence of tuberculosis and the rising incidence of *Mycobacterium avium-intracellulare* infections in patients with AIDS has been further complicated in the USA by the recent emergence of drug resistant strains of *Mycobacterium tuberculosis*.

Clinical significance

Tuberculous otitis media is a fairly rare manifestation of the disease, but should be suspected when 'sterile' cultures are obtained from a discharge from the middle ear. Laryngitis is also a fairly rare complication of tuberculosis (Bachman, Zizmor and Noyek, 1979). Otomastoiditis due to *Mycobacterium avium-intracellulare* has been described (Kinsella, Grossman and Black, 1986) while patients with cervical adenitis due to *Mycobacterium kansasii*, *M. scrofulaceum*, *M. avium-intra-cellulare* (Kinsella *et al.*, 1987) or *M. malmoense* have been reported, the last from northeast England (Connolly *et al.*, 1985).

Chlamydia

The Chlamydiae are tiny, Gram-negative, obligate intracellular bacteria that can cause of wide range of human infections. Characteristically, they form typical basophilic inclusion bodies, *in vivo* or *in vitro* as they replicate by binary fission in the cytoplasm of host cells. At present, three species are known: *Chlamydia psittaci*, the cause of psittacosis in man and ornithosis in birds, *Chlamydia trachomatis* which can cause ocular, genital or respiratory disease, and *Chlamydia pneumoniae* (formerly the TWAR agent) which can cause upper and lower respiratory infection (Grayston, Kuo and Wang, 1986). Although the evidence is inconclusive, *Chlamydia trachomatis* may cause some cases of nasopharyngitis and secretory otitis media (Harrison, 1986).

Identification of *Chlamydia* species is by inoculation of cycloheximide-treated cultures of McCoy cells, in which they form typical iodine-positive intracytoplasmic inclusions. Faster but less sensitive methods include detection of chlamydial lipopolysaccharide (LPS) antigens by enzyme immunoassay in nasopha-

ryngeal aspirates or swabs (Schachter, 1991). Most chlamydial infections are treated with tetracycline; erythromycin and sulphasoxazole are alternatives.

Mycoplasma

Mycoplasmas are highly pleomorphic bacteria as a result of having no cell wall. They can be grown in media enriched with serum and yeast, and with antibacterial substances such as thallium acetate, to inhibit competing bacteria. On solid media mycoplasmas grow as tiny colonies that often look like a fried egg. They can be further identified as to species by biochemical reactions and gaseous and pH requirements for growth. *Mycoplasma pneumoniae* is an established human pulmonary pathogen, but its role in infections of the upper respiratory tract remains uncertain. In experiments on human volunteers, some of those infected with *Mycoplasma pneumoniae* developed haemorrhagic bullous otitis (Rifkind, Chanock and Kravetz, 1962). Nevertheless, the organism, at best is a rare cause of naturally-occurring otitis media (Klein and Teele, 1976). Erythromycin and tetracycline are effective against *Mycoplasma pneumoniae* but clinical responses are often slow. *Mycoplasma orale* and *Mycoplasma salivarium* are part of the indigenous microflora of the oropharynx, but are not known to cause disease.

Fungi affecting the ear, nose and throat

Fungi are unique, eukaryotic organisms, which belong to the taxonomic kingdom, the *Myceteae*. They are characterized by a rigid cell wall composed of carbohydrate polymers, such as cellulose, chitin or glucan. They can reproduce sexually by spores or asexually by conidia, and the mechanisms by which they produce spores or conidia is used in their classification. Fungi exist as yeasts which are small unicellular forms, or molds which are composed of masses of multicellular filaments (hyphae). These may or may not have cross-walls, i.e. may be septate or non-septate. Some fungi, e.g. *Histoplasma capsulatum*, are dimorphic, and can form both yeasts and filaments, depending on the environmental conditions.

Until fairly recently, relatively few fungi caused human disease, but with the advent of antibiotics, cardiovascular catheters and prostheses, and immunosuppression either by disease, such as AIDS, or by therapeutic measures, scores of different fungi have been found to cause opportunistic infections (Land and McCracken, 1991). As exotic examples, the common mushroom *Schizophyllum commune* (Kern and Uecker, 1986) or the plant pathogen *Bipolaris* (Washburn *et al.*, 1988) have been isolated from patients with maxillary sinusitis. Most fungal infections in humans are acquired from the environment, animals, or from indigenous flora. With a few important exceptions, notably *Candida albicans*, person-to-person transmission does not take place.

Laboratory identification

In brief, the laboratory identification of fungi involves the following:

1 Microscopy

Slide preparations of clinical material are usually stained with methylene blue, Gram or periodic acid Schiff (PAS) stains. For fungi in tissue sections, methenamine silver (GMS) stain is the stain of choice.

2 Culture

Fungi will grow on blood or chocolate agar, but when fungi are suspected clinically, special media such as that of Sabouraud are essential; these usually contain antimicrobial agents, such as chloramphenicol and/or cycloheximide, to promote rapid, selective growth and aid in identification. Cultures are incubated at room temperature, 25° C and at 30° C for up to 6 weeks and beyond before being discarded as negative.

3 Identification

Identification of molds is based on colonial morphology and colour, and the microscopic structures seen in stained preparations of these colonies. Particular attention is paid to the structure of the hyphae and the type and arrangement of the spores or conidia. Yeasts can be identified by biochemical tests, such as determining their ability to assimilate or ferment various carbohydrates. Several rapid identification systems are now available which can identify yeasts in 4–24 hours (Land, McGinnis and Salkin, 1991).

4 Serological tests

Serology has limited value in mycology, although the serological detection of cryptococcal antigen in cerebrospinal fluid and in serum is a consistently valuable diagnostic procedure (Bloomfield, Gordon and Elmendorf, 1963).

Candida

Overview of the genus

With the inclusion of species previously classified in the genus *Torulopsis*, there are at least 150 species of *Candida*. Those which are of medical importance and are known to cause systemic disease are listed in Table 19.6.

Table 19.6 *Candida* species of medical importance

C. albicans
*C. glabrata**
C. guillermondii
C. krusei
C. lusitaniae
C. lipolytica
C. parapsilosis
*C. paratropicalis***
C. pseudotropicalis
C. tropicalis

Alternative names: **Torulopsis glabrata*; ***Sucrose-negative C. tropicalis*

Candida albicans

Morphology, culture and identification

Candida albicans is an ovoid, thin-walled yeast cell, about 4 μm × 6 μm, which grows at 25° C or 37° C. In inflammatory exudates or infected tissues, the presence of yeasts, pseudohyphae and/or true hyphae together with neutrophil polymorphs is good evidence of its pathogenicity. On mycological media and blood agar, the yeast forms smooth, creamy white colonies. Further distinction can be rapidly made from other *Candida* species by incubation of the organism in bovine serum, where it produces characteristic germ tubes. Definitive identification of *Candida* species is mainly by its morphology on special media, carbohydrate fermentation and assimilation reactions.

Antimicrobial susceptibility

Nystatin is effective against superficial candidal infections; amphotericin B is the drug of choice for systemic disease. About 50% of strains of *Candida albicans* are susceptible to 5-fluorocytosine (5FC), which can be given in combination with amphotericin to reduce the latter's toxicity. Susceptibility tests must be performed before 5-fluorocytosine is used to treat systemic candidal infection. The effectiveness of fluconazole in treating systemic candidosis is currently being evaluated.

Clinical significance

Candidal infections now account for 10–12% of all nosocomial infections in the USA. Their association with percutaneous, intravascular devices is well established. In clinical practice, careful attention should be paid to blood cultures that are positive for *Candida* species, since these are rarely the result of skin or laboratory contamination (Hurley, 1966). Acute candidal infections of the mouth are common in infants, but oral candidosis can also be an adverse effect of taking broad-spectrum antibiotics. Oropharyngeal candidosis is very common in patients with AIDS and is often one of the earliest signs of the severe immunosuppression. Chronic candidal pharyngitis and oesophagitis is typical of the syndrome of chronic mucocutaneous candidosis. Lawson, Bodey and Luna (1980) have described candida infections presenting as laryngitis.

Other pathogenic yeast forms

Histoplasma capsulatum, Blastomyces dermatitidis and *Paracoccidioides brasiliensis* are dimorphic fungi, but only their yeast phase is found in human tissue. The first two are fairly common pathogens in the USA but are rare in UK; the third is essentially confined to South America. All three fungi cause mucocutaneous infections which can affect the oropharynx and gingivae. In immunosuppressed patients with histoplasmosis, the disease may involve the larynx. Laryngeal infection in immunocompetent individuals can also be a feature of blastomycosis (Gwaltney, 1990).

Aspergillus

Overview of the genus

Aspergilli are ubiquitous molds which belong to the *Hyphomycetes* – the imperfect fungi. The genus *Aspergillus* contains numerous species, 20 of which can cause human infection. *Aspergillus fumigatus* is by far, the most common pathogenic species; *Aspergillus flavus* is an important cause of nasal and paranasal sinus infections, and along with *Aspergillus niger*, *Aspergillus terreus* and *Aspergillus nidulans* can cause systemic disease in immunodeficient patients.

Morphology, culture and identification

Microscopically, *Aspergillus* spp. have septate, dichotomously branching hyphae 2–4 μm in width, with a morphologically characteristic conidia-bearing aspergillum. These fungi are identified and distinguished from each other by colonial appearances, the structure of the aspergillum, and the arrangement of the conidial chains.

Antimicrobial susceptibility

The aspergilli are generally susceptible to amphotericin B, often combined with surgical treatment. The role of 5-fluorocytosine or rifampin in combination with amphotericin B remains uncertain. Itraconazole may possibly have a role in treating some cases of invasive aspergillosis (De Beule *et al.*, 1988).

Clinical aspects

Aspergilli can grow superficially in the external ear causing otomycosis, but occasionally, even in immunocompetent patients, the fungus can give rise to

necrotizing and invasive disease in this location (Cunningham *et al.*, 1988). In both immunocompetent and immunocompromised patients, infection of the nose and paranasal sinuses, usually by *Aspergillus flavus*, can be followed by fungal invasion of soft tissues and bone. Less aggressive forms of sinusitis, with fungus ball formation and granulomatous tissue reactions have also been associated with aspergillus infections (McGuirt and Harrill, 1979). Invasive ('malignant') otitis externa though frequently caused by *Pseudomonas aeruginosa* can also be caused by *Aspergillus* species. This form of otitis, caused by *Aspergillus fumigatus* has been described in patients with AIDS (Reiss *et al.*, 1991).

The term 'aspergillosis' is also used to describe infections by fungi which, in tissues, have very similar microscopic appearances but belong to different genera, such as *Penicillium*, *Fusarium*, *Acremonium* and *Scytallidium*. In tissues, all form dichotomously branched septate hyphae and culture is required for accurate identification.

The Mucorales

Overview of the order

The order *Mucorales* contains fungi which form broad, non-septate hyphae, on which they can produce a characteristic sexual propagating unit called a zygospore (hence the term zygomycosis, which is used synonymously with mucormycosis). The *Mucorales* comprise many genera including *Mucor*, *Rhizopus*, *Absidia*, *Rhizomucor*, *Saksenaea*, *Cunninghamella*, *Cokeromyces* and *Conidiobolus*. These fungi are widely distributed in soil, on foodstuffs, and some are readily isolated in hospitals, particularly from air-conditioning systems.

Morphology, culture and identification

On microscopic examination of PAS-stained tissues, these fungi have broad, ribbon-like non-septate hyphae, 10–25 μm in width, which typically branch at right angles. As a rule they form colonies in 24–48 hours at 30°C on enriched media containing no antimicrobial agents. Further identification is based on the morphology of the spore-bearing structures (sporangia) and the location of the rootlets (rhizoids).

Clinical significance

Mucormycosis (zygomycosis) affecting the nose, paranasal sinuses and sometimes extending to the brain, is exclusively a disease of those whose defence mechanisms are impaired. Once infection is established, it can be rapidly fatal. Neutropenic patients, or those whose neutrophil function is impaired, as for instance, in diabetic ketoacidosis, are particularly susceptible to these opportunistic fungi and the use of broad-spectrum antimicrobial drugs in these patients can increase the risk of mucormycosis. Fatal rhinocerebral mucormycosis in patients receiving haemodialysis has been associated with administration of the chelating agent desferrioxamine to control aluminium and iron toxicity (Goodill and Abuelo, 1987). Mucormycosis has been reported in patients receiving organ transplants (Morduchowicz *et al.*, 1986), but it is very uncommon in AIDS presumably because neutrophil function is not impaired. Treatment is with amphotericin B, usually combined with aggressive surgery.

In an attempt to reduce the toxicity of amphotericin B in treating mucormycosis and other serious fungal infections, two new forms of the drug have been introduced. In these preparations, amphotericin is incorporated into uni- or multilayered liposomes composed of dimyristoyl-phosphatidylcholine (DMPC) or dimyristoyl-phosphatidylglycerol (DMPG), or into particulate compounds with either of these two phospholipids. Early studies indicate that these compounds can offer considerable improvement over standard preparations of amphotericin B (Sculier *et al.*, 1988; Brajtburg *et al.*, 1990).

Entomorphthoramycosis is a painful, progressive infection of the nose and perinasal tissues caused by fungi of the genus *Conidiobolus*. It has been reported from Africa, Central and South America and from the USA (Dworzack *et al.*, 1978).

Phaeohyphomycosis

Phaeohyphomycosis is caused by the dematiaceous fungi, which are molds whose hyphae have darkly pigmented cell walls. Species of *Exserohilum* (Padhye *et al.*, 1986), *Curvularia* and *Bipolaris* can cause infection of the paranasal sinuses (Washburn *et al.*, 1988).

Sinus infection caused by the latter two species can progress to brain abscess. *Curvularia lanata* is also reported to cause allergic sinusitis (MacMillan *et al.*, 1987).

Rhinosporidium seeberi

Rhinosporidiosis is a chronic recurrent infection usually confined to the nasal turbinates, caused by *Rhinosporidium seeberi*. This organism has never been cultured but currently is thought to be a fungus. In a typical case, a friable polypoid mass forms in the nose, in which 10–200 μm cysts containing many spores can be seen. The disease is most common in the Indian subcontinent, but has been reported from many other countries. Treatment is surgical.

Viruses affecting the ear, nose and throat

Viruses which are of clinical interest to the otolaryngologist are first, those which cause upper respiratory infections, including pharyngitis and laryngitis (Table 19.7). It should be noted that many 'respiratory' viruses can cause a specific syndrome in some patients but a non-specific respiratory infection (a 'cold') in others; and that a coryzal illness can be the prodromal stage of a more serious illness such as measles. Second, congenital rubella and cytomegalovirus infections can have very serious effects on the central nervous system, including hearing loss. Third, the clinical effects of infections caused by the Herpesvirus family, quite often involve the ear, nose, throat and their adnexa. Fourth, hepatitis and human immunodeficiency viruses are of great importance in all fields of medicine.

Table 19.7 Virus groups and their usual serotypes that cause infections of the oropharynx and upper respiratory tract

Virus group	Usual serotypes	Disease or syndrome
Adenoviruses	1–8	Fever, coryza, pharyngitis
Coxsackievirus A	4, 5, 9, 10, 16	Hand foot and mouth disease
	1–6, 8, 10	Herpangina
	21	Common cold syndrome
Coxsackievirus B	2–5	Common cold syndrome
Coronavirus	1–2	Common cold syndrome
Epstein-Barr virus		Infectious mononucleosis
Herpesvirus hominis	1, 2	Gingivostomatitis
Influenza	A, B,	Influenza
	C	Common cold syndrome
Parainfluenza	1,2,3	Common cold syndrome (adults)
		Laryngotracheobronchitis (children)
Respiratory syncytial virus		Common cold syndrome (adults)
		Bronchiolitis (children)
Rhinovirus	100 + types	Common cold syndrome

General properties

Viruses are infective nucleoprotein; they are minute, obligate intracellular parasites, containing either DNA or RNA, which use the biosynthetic mechanisms of the host cell to replicate. For taxonomic purposes, they have been divided into families according to their size, type of nucleic acid, configuration (including the presence or absence of an envelope) and mode of replication. The nucleoprotein configuration of animal viruses is either helical or polyhedral.

Replication

Viral replication follows attachment of the virus particle to the surface of the host cell by specific receptor mechanisms. The virus enters the cell by fusion of its envelope with the cell membrane, or by pinocytosis, a process resembling phagocytosis. This is followed by dissociation of the nucleic acid from its protein capsid and synthesis of viral nucleic acid and protein at different sites in the cell at the expense of normal cellular biosynthetic mechanisms. Viral progeny are formed with assembly of new protein capsids and nucleic acid, and leave the cell either by causing its lysis or by budding from the cell membrane. In the latter event, the virus acquires an envelope and surface antigens from the host cell. A few viruses, notably the *Herpesviridae* family, can remain integrated with the host cell genome for long periods in a latent state, from which they can be reactivated to enter a replicative cycle that ends with release of new virus particles. After a period of replicative activity, the virus can return to the latent state.

Laboratory identification

In summary, the isolation and identification of viruses is by one or more of the following methods:

1 Microscopic examination

Microscopic examination of clinical specimens is sometimes complemented by fluorescence and/or electron microscopy. For example, smears from suspected herpetic or varicella-zoster lesions, stained by Geimsa, Papanicolaou or other suitable stains, can be useful for rapid confirmation of clinical impressions. Viral inclusion bodies in histological, cytological or fluorescent antibody preparations are perhaps the best microscopic indicators of viral infection.

2 Rapid detection of viral antigens

This can be carried out in clinical specimens by enzyme immunoassay for some viruses, including herpes simplex, using commercial kits. Third generation latex agglutination tests and haemagglutination tests for hepatitis B virus surface antigen, for example can be completed in about 1–2 hours.

3 Viral culture

This is generally limited to specialized reference laboratories, where inoculation of cell cultures is the method of choice. Virus replication is detected in infected cell cultures by morphological changes (cytopathic effect: CPE) such as cell death, giant cell or syncytium formation, or by demonstration of viral antigens in the cells or the cell culture fluids by immunological or serological methods.

4 Virus serology

Virus serology has a limited place in the management of patients with acute viral illnesses, since serological diagnosis based on fourfold or greater increases in antibody titres are frequently retrospective. Exceptions are serological tests which detect viral antigens or virus-specific IgM antibodies, which indicate current or very recent infection. Commercial methods are now available for IgM antibodies against cytomegalovirus, rubella, (Rubazyme; Abbott Laboratories, USA; Rubenz; Northumbria Biochemicals, UK) and hepatitis A and B (HAVAB-M and Corab-M respectively, both from Abbott Laboratories). Serological tests for human immunodeficiency, hepatitis B and Epstein–Barr viruses are widely used and valuable diagnostic procedures. Serological evaluation of patients' immunity to rubella or to hepatitis B is valuable when active or passive immunization is contemplated.

5 Clinical specimens

Air dried smears on glass slides, preferably transported in closed plastic containers, are adequate for microscopic diagnosis of superficial viral lesions, e.g. herpes simplex. For serological tests 5–10 ml of clotted blood in a sterile tube should be sent. For culture of most viruses that affect the upper respiratory tract, a throat swab taken with firm application to the mucosal surfaces to ensure an adequate sample of superficial cells, is satisfactory in most cases. Swabs should be placed in viral transport medium, sealed and transported to the laboratory in wet ice. Virus laboratories usually make available media and instructions for transportation of clinical specimens.

Adenoviruses

Adenoviruses are non-enveloped, double-stranded DNA viruses, measuring about 70 nm in diameter. Forty-seven types have been described so far. Most adenovirus respiratory infections are caused by types 1 to 8 and these can be isolated in HeLa and HEp2 cell cultures. The typical cytopathic effect consists of cells which round up and form clusters resembling a bunch of grapes. Identification of an isolate as an adenovirus can made by several methods including immunodiffusion, complement fixation or enzyme immunoassay (Meurman, Ruuskanen and Sarkinen, 1983), using infected cell culture fluid as antigen. Typing is a reference laboratory procedure. Adenoviruses are frequently the cause of epidemic or sporadic acute respiratory syndromes, which are often accompanied by conjunctivitis and preauricular node enlargement. In patients with AIDS or other immunosuppressed states, especially following bone marrow transplantation, adenoviruses can cause a wide range of clinical illnesses which include rash, upper respiratory illness, otitis media, pneumonitis, hepatitis, cystitis and central nervous system infection (Webb, Shields and Fife, 1987). These infections are often fatal.

Enteroviruses

Coxsackievirus A

Coxsackievirus A is small (25 nm), non-enveloped, polyhedral, contains RNA and belongs to the genus *Enterovirus*. Unlike most other enteroviruses, it does not replicate well in cell cultures, but is highly infective for newborn mice. There are 24 types of coxsackievirus A. Oropharyngeal syndromes associated with these viruses are:

1 Herpangina: a severe tonsillopharyngitis associated with fever and malaise and caused by types 1–6, 8 and 10.
2 Hand, foot and mouth disease: an epidemic infection that is characterized by sparse intraoral vesicles, with a similar eruption on the palms and soles, usually caused by type 16.

Coxsackievirus B

Coxsackievirus B is morphologically similar to but biologically distinct from coxsackievirus A. There are six serotypes. The virus is readily isolated in primary monkey kidney or human diploid cells in which it causes rapid cell death. Final identification requires neutralization of this cytopathic effect by type specific antisera. The isolation, identification and typing of the coxsackie and other enteroviruses is a labour-intensive, expensive process. The application of the polymerase chain reaction and nucleic acid hybridization methods to identification of enteroviruses may lead to much more rapid and economical diagnostic procedures (Chapman *et al.*, 1990). Coxsackievirus B, types 2–5, can cause acute coryzal illnesses; however, all six types are associated with more serious infections, especially myopericarditis, meningitis and epidemic myalgia.

Coronaviruses

Coronaviruses are large (80–120 nm) enveloped, single-stranded, RNA viruses. A unique feature of their morphology is the presence of petal-shaped projections on the viral envelope. There are four types of coronaviruses, which are extremely fastidious, and grow only in organ culture or some diploid fibroblast cultures. Laboratory isolation for diagnosis is not practical. Worldwide, coronaviruses account for about 15% of all human colds (Bradbourne, Bynoe and Tyrrell, 1967), but their clinical effects cannot be distinguished from those of other coryzal agents.

Herpesviruses

The *Herpesviridae* family are large (120 nm), enveloped, double-stranded DNA viruses, which have the common property of establishing latent infections of host cells *in vivo*. With the exception of Epstein–Barr virus, the herpesviruses that cause human infection characteristically produce eosinophilic intranuclear inclusion bodies and enlargement of infected cells both *in vitro* and *in vivo*.

Herpes simplex (Herpesvirus hominis: HSV)

There are two antigenically distinct forms of herpes simplex virus: type 1 is more likely to be isolated from facial or oropharyngeal lesions, while type 2 causes predominantly genital infection. However, either type can be isolated from either site. Scrapings taken from the base of recent active lesions, stained by Geimsa or haematoxylin and eosin stains are usually sufficient to confirm the clinical diagnosis. If culture is desired, material from a freshly opened vesicle inoculated speedily into susceptible cell culture can produce cytopathic effects in as little as 8 hours. Culture can be valuable in diagnosis when atypical herpetic lesions develop in patients with AIDS or other immunosuppressed states.

Primary gingivostomatitis, accompanied by fever and malaise is the most severe form of orolabial herpes. Recurrent 'cold sores' or 'fever blisters' are much more common, less severe and clinically characteristic. However, rare and atypical intraoral, palatal or pharyngeal lesions may require laboratory confirmation. Serological tests for herpes simplex virus, including those for anti-HSV-IgM are seldom helpful diagnostically. In herpetic infections IgM antibodies can be stimulated by recurrent as well as primary infections (Arvin and Prober, 1991). Acyclovir, although of benefit in primary genital herpes and serious recurring infections in immunocompromised patients, has yet to be shown to be effective in orofacial herpes.

Varicella-zoster virus

Varicella-zoster virus (VZV), the cause of both chicken-pox and shingles, has many biological similarities to herpes simplex virus but, in the laboratory, it requires cell cultures derived from human tissues for isolation and identification. Like herpes simplex virus, varicella-zoster virus typically causes enlargement of infected cells both *in vivo* and *in vitro* and forms prominent eosinophilic nuclear inclusions. These characteristics are readily observed in stained prepara-tions of scrapings made from fresh skin lesions in chickenpox and shingles.

The three clinical forms of varicella-zoster virus infection in humans are chickenpox, zoster (shingles), and atypical infections in immunocompromised pa-tients. Chickenpox is generally a fairly mild disease in children, typified by fever and crops of itching, vesicu-lar skin lesions. Oropharyngeal and lingual lesions are frequently present and are the most likely sources for the spread of the disease. Viral laryngitis and tracheitis can occasionally be seen in chickenpox. Varicella pneumonitis, which is usually a complica-tion of adult chickenpox, can be a life-threatening complication.

Zoster, which results from the reactivation of latent varicella-zoster virus can affect spinal or cranial nerves. Involvement of one of the three divisions of the trigeminal nerve is fairly common and results in painful eruptions in the areas of skin and mucous membrane supplied by that division of that nerve. In mandibular nerve zoster, for example, the tongue is characteristically affected on the same side as the skin lesions. Involvement of the geniculate ganglion of the VIIth cranial nerve causes severe facial paraly-sis, a vesicular eruption in the pharynx and external auditory canal (Ramsay–Hunt syndrome).

Zoster in immunodeficient individuals often presents in atypical forms. Local eruptions along the course of spinal or cranial nerves are often extensive, haemorrhagic and necrotic. Some patients present with generalized rashes that resemble chickenpox, while systemic infections resulting in fever, viral en-cephalitis, hepatitis, pancreatitis, small bowel infec-tion and pneumonitis are not uncommon (Simmons and Balfour, 1978). The treatment of choice of zoster, particularly in its more severe forms is acyclovir. Other agents active against varicella-zoster virus are vidarabine and α-interferon.

Cytomegalovirus (CMV)

Cytomegalovirus is a ubiquitious virus, morphologi-cally similar to herpes simplex virus. It can only replicate in human diploid cell cultures and grows at a much slower rate than herpes simplex virus. Its cytopathic effect in culture is the same as seen in infected tissues, (enlarged cells with prominent eosi-nophilic intranuclear inclusions). Cytomegalovirus

can be acquired in several ways. First, by congenital infection, which can be asymptomatic in both mother and infant, or in about 25% of cases, can result in serious, sometimes fatal disease in the infant. The ear is among many organs affected in congenital cytomegalovirus infection, and the virus has been demonstrated in the organ of Corti and the cochlea; 17% of congenitally infected infants develop hearing loss (Stagno *et al.*, 1977). Children with congenital cytomegalovirus infection can excrete the virus in the pharyngeal secretions and in the urine for years, and the virus can be isolated from either of these sources. Urine microscopy may show inclusion-bearing tubular cells, but although this method is virtually diagnostic, the sensitivity is low and urine culture is recommended for definitive diagnosis.

Second, primary cytomegalovirus infection in chil-dren and adults is very often asymptomatic, but cytomegalovirus mononucleosis can accompany pri-mary infection. This febrile illness resembles infectious mononucleosis in many respects, but pharyngitis and tonsillitis are rare. A similar syndrome can follow blood transfusion, or perfusion (post-perfusion syndrome).

Third, cytomegalovirus infection is a common com-plication of immunosuppressive treatment or diseases including AIDS. The lungs, alimentary tract, nervous and endocrine systems are the main target organs for infection.

Immunity to cytomegalovirus is complex and in its serological investigation, some tests are better than others. Complement-fixation tests should be avoided, as they lack sensitivity. Anticomplement immunofluores-cence tests are more sensitive and specific. Alternatives are enzyme immunoassay, indirect haemagglutination, and latex agglutination tests. For the rapid diagnosis of cytomegalovirus infections, tests for CMV-IgM antibod-ies can be used as an alternative to the conventional demonstration of seroconversion or significant in-creases in titre. This test, however, may not be a reliable indicator of acute infection, as both false negatives and false positives are fairly common. Treatment for severe cytomegalovirus infections, including the use of high doses of interferons and acyclovir, is still experimental.

Epstein–Barr virus

The structure of Epstein–Barr virus (EBV) is typical of the Herpesvirus family; it is a fairly large (120 nm) enveloped, double-stranded DNA virus. Like other herpesviruses, it can establish latent infection and has the unique property of transforming and immor-talizing human B lymphocytes. Epstein–Barr virus is now accepted as the cause of infectious mononucle-osis (Henle, Henle and Diehl, 1968), and may have an aetiological role in Burkitt's lymphoma and naso-pharyngeal carcinoma (Henle and Henle, 1974). Culture of the virus for diagnostic purposes is im-practical due to its complexity and duration.

The diagnosis of infectious mononucleosis is confirmed by serology. In addition to methods based on the time-honoured heterophile test of Paul and Bunnell, more specific methods which use various Epstein–Barr virus antigens are available. These antigens include viral capsid antigen (VCA), early antigen, diffuse component (EA/D), early antigen restricted component (EA/R) and EBV-induced nuclear antigen (EBNA). The presence of IgM antibodies to viral capsid antigen is good confirmatory evidence of acute Epstein–Barr virus infection. The significance of the various antibodies in Epstein–Barr virus infection is summarized in Table 19.8.

Influenza viruses

Influenza viruses belong to the *Myxoviridae* family, a name which reflects their affinity for mucoid substances. They are large (120 nm) enveloped, helical viruses with a segmented RNA core. Three groups, A, B, and C can be distinguished by their different complement-fixing antigens. Influenza C may eventually be placed in another genus as its biological activity differs sharply from influenza A and B; it causes a common cold syndrome, rather than influenza, and does not cause epidemics.

The surface envelope of influenza viruses has characteristic projections (peplomers), which allow attachment of the virus to the surface of host cells. There are two types: first a spike-like haemagglutinin (H), second, a mushroom-shaped neuraminidase (N). There are four antigenically distinct haemagglutinins (H0, H1, H2, H3) and two neuraminidases (N1, N2). One of eight possible combinations of H and N antigens is found on the surface of each influenza A virus, and major rearrangements of the H and N antigens take place about every 8–10 years ('antigenic drift'), usually resulting in large epidemics. Each strain of influenza A is identified by its place, and year of isolation, and its H and N antigens, e.g. influenza A/Scotland/74 (H3N2). The antigenic changes in influenza B are much less dramatic.

Influenza viruses can usually be isolated in primary monkey kidney cells within a week. They cause little or no cytopathic effect but can be detected by the haemagglutinating properties of the cell culture fluids. They can also be identified more rapidly, after 3 days' incubation, by application of fluorescent antibody or enzyme immunoassays to the cell cultures. The clinical diagnosis of 'classical' influenza during an epidemic is relatively easy, but sporadic influenza, especially in children may be more difficult to recognize. The severity of influenza A and B can range from asymptomatic infection, through a mild coryzal illness, to fatal influenzal pneumonia. Effective vaccines prepared against current strains of influenza A and B are recommended for patients with chronic diseases, especially of the heart, lungs and kidneys. Patients with AIDS, however, respond poorly to these vaccines, although this can be partly corrected by administration of zidovudine (Nelson *et al.*, 1988). Amantadine and rimantidine are equally effective in the chemoprophylaxis of influenza (Dolin, 1985).

Paramyxoviruses

The *Paramyxoviridae* family is comprised of three genera of human and animal viruses. Those causing human disease are listed in Table 19.9. The paramyxoviruses are very large (200–300 nm), enveloped, helical, RNA viruses. The parainfluenza viruses are the only members of the family which have neuraminidase on their envelopes. The paramyxoviruses replicate well in primary monkey kidney cells, in which syncytial giant cells are typically formed by measles, mumps and respiratory syncytial (RSV) viruses. Some paramyxoviruses do not produce cytopathic effects and can be detected in cell culture by immunofluorescence (IF), enzyme immunoassay (EIA), or haemagglutination (HA). For rapid diagnosis, immunofluorescence or enzyme immunoassay can be performed directly on clinical specimens.

Parainfluenza viruses types 1, 2 and 3 cause acute laryngotracheobronchitis in children and the common cold syndrome in children and adults. Type 3 may also cause bronchiolitis and pneumonia and is second only to respiratory syncytial virus in causing severe lower respiratory disease in young children. Mumps and measles are readily recognized clinically and seldom require laboratory confirmation. However, in patients who develop atypical measles, as a result of previous immunization with killed measles vaccine,

Table 19.8 The significance of various antibodies in Epstein–Barr infections

Antibody	Non-immune	Active primary	Recent primary	Past	Reactivated	NPC
VCA-IgM	− ve	+ ve	− ve	− ve	− ve	− ve
VCA-IgG	− ve	− ve	+ ve	+ ve	+ ve	+ ve
EA/D-IgG	− ve	+ ve	+ ve	− ve	+ / −	+ ve
anti-EBNA	− ve	− ve	+ / −	+ ve	+ ve	− ve

VCA = Viral capsid antigen; EA/D = early antigen, diffuse; EBNA = Epstein–Barr virus induced nuclear antigen; NPC = nasopharyngeal carcinoma

Table 19.9 The Paramyxoviridae family

Paramyxoviruses	*Morbillivirus*	*Pneumovirus*
Parainfluenza viruses 1–4 Mumps virus	Measles virus	Respiratory syncytial virus

laboratory diagnosis may be necessary. Virus culture or assay of measles IgM antibody are appropriate in these cases. Haemagglutination-inhibition or enzyme immunoassay tests can be used to determine a patient's immunity to measles and mumps, or to confirm the diagnosis by rising titres of antibodies to these viruses.

Rhinoviruses

The rhinoviruses are small, non-enveloped RNA viruses, of which over 100 types are known, and which cause about half of all cases of the common cold. They have also been implicated as primary causes of sinusitis and otitis media (Evans, Sydnor and Moore, 1975). The isolation of these viruses is not indicated for purely clinical purposes and no specific treatment or immunoprophylaxis is available.

Rubella virus

Rubella virus is an enveloped, (60 nm), helical, RNA virus. Its generic name is *Rubivirus* and it is in the *Togaviridae* family. Although the virus can be grown in African green monkey or rabbit kidney cells, the methods of isolation and identification are laborious and expensive. Except in infants with congenital rubella syndrome, in whom culture of nasopharyngeal secretions is usually positive, laboratory diagnosis is therefore almost exclusively by serological methods. Immunity or non-immunity can be determined by demonstrating rubella antibody by any one of several methods including passive haemagglutination (PHA), haemagglutination-inhibition (HI), solid-phase immunoassay (SPIA) and complement-fixation (CF) tests. Commercial kits are available for each of these. A positive antibody test is when the titre equals or exceeds a standard baseline titre or in the case of solid-phase immunoassay a baseline binding ratio or optical density.

Serology is particularly useful when a pregnant woman develops a rash after contact with another individual, usually a child, with rubella. Any of the above methods can be used. A fourfold or greater rise in titre or significant change in optical density in the solid-phase immunoassay test over 5–7 days is diag-

nostic. Rubella IgM antibody assayed by the solid-phase immunoassay method, can be performed between the third day and the end of the third week of the illness, and its presence confirms rubella infection. The serological diagnosis of congenital rubella can be confirmed by the presence of rubella IgM antibody in the infant's serum; sustained levels of rubella antibody in the first 6 months of life are also consistent with congenital rubella.

Permanent hearing loss and developmental abnormalities of the ear are frequent consequences of congenital rubella and can result from infection contracted up to the 20th week of gestation. The incidence of rubella has progressively decreased since the introduction of live vaccines. The vaccine widely used in Europe and exclusively in the USA is the RA 27/3 vaccine, which has excellent immunogenicity, due at least in part to its ability to stimulate both secretory as well as humoral IgA.

Hepatitis viruses

Many viruses can cause hepatitis, including cytomegalovirus and Epstein-Barr virus, but the term 'hepatitis viruses' is reserved for a heterogeneous group of five agents* – hepatitis viruses (HV) A, B, C, D, and E. Hepatitis viruses B, C and D can be parenterally transmitted, and can have serious sequelae. They are therefore of great concern to all medical practitioners and healthcare workers because blood and blood components are the main source of infection. The identity of the specific virus causing hepatitis must be made in the laboratory, as the acute illnesses caused by each of these viruses are for all practical purposes, identical. Laboratory diagnosis is exclusively by serological methods.

Hepatitis A virus

Hepatitis A virus (HAV) is a small RNA virus spread by the orofaecal route, has an incubation period of 4–7 weeks, and gives rise to outbreaks of hepatitis in which complications are rare. The diagnosis is made by demonstrating HAV-IgM in serum. This antibody appears about 3 weeks after exposure and persists for about 3 months. Exposed persons can be passively immunized with immune serum (gamma) globulin.

Hepatitis B virus

Hepatitis B virus (HBV) is an enveloped DNA virus, recently allocated to the *Hepadnavirus* family. Its antigenic components include a complex protein surface antigen (HBsAg), a nucleoprotein core antigen (HBcAg), and a protein antigen closely linked to the

---

* In 1995, three new hepatitis viruses belonging to the Flavivirus group were identified.

viral core (HBeAg). During the usual course of infection, antibodies to each of these antigens, HBsAb, HBcAb, and HBeAb respectively, are formed. Transmission of hepatitis B virus is mainly by parenteral infection by transfusion of blood or blood components, and by skin injury with sharp instruments contaminated with these substances. Some infections are acquired by splashing of mucous membranes with blood or blood products; others are transmitted sexually or acquired by sharing of contaminated needles among intravenous drug abusers. The incubation period is between 30 and 180 days.

The diagnosis is based on detection of various hepatitis B virus antigens and antibodies as follows:

1 Active hepatitis B infection, whether symptomatic or not, is accompanied by the presence of HBsAg in blood
2 In the usual (benign) course of the disease, recovery is accompanied by:
  a falling levels and finally disappearance of HBsAg
  b the appearance and rising serum levels of HBsAb
3 In 10–15% of all patients with hepatitis B virus infection, there is a period up to 4 weeks, when HBsAg and HBsAb are *both* undetectable. To prevent the serological diagnosis being missed, HBcAb-IgM can be performed. This antibody is *always* present from early in the illness until well into the convalescent phase, and indicates active hepatitis B virus infection.
4 In about 10% of hepatitis B virus infections, clinical recovery is incomplete and the patient develops persistent hepatitis. HBsAg remains positive and, for unknown reasons, HBsAb does not develop. HBeAg, which can be regarded as an indicator of high infectivity, may also be present. If it is absent, however, the patient is still infectious. The serological findings in asymptomatic carriers are similar to those found in patients with persistent hepatitis. Some individuals, even after long periods of being HBsAg positive, can eventually form HBsAb with simultaneous clearing of HBsAg from their blood, and resolution of hepatic abnormalities.
5 In all forms of symptomatic and asymptomatic

hepatitis B virus infection, antibodies to the viral core antigen (HBcAb) are found from the early stages of the illness. Therefore this antibody is evidence of past or present hepatitis B.

The serological diagnosis of hepatitis B is summarized in Table 19.10. The methods available for hepatitis B virus serology include, haemagglutination, latex agglutination, radio- and enzyme immunoassay. Weak positive reactions, e.g. in latex agglutination tests should be confirmed by more sensitive procedures such as radioimmunoassay.

Recombinant hepatitis B virus vaccines in current use are free of extraneous agents and protective immunity is achieved in about 90% of people vaccinated. When non-immune individuals are exposed to hepatitis B virus, passive immunization can be achieved with high titre hepatitis B immune globulin (HBIG) or if this is unavailable, with immune serum globulin (ISG). Hepatitis B virus vaccine can be given at the same time, if continued exposure to the virus is likely.

Hepatitis C virus

Hepatitis C virus (HCV) is an enveloped RNA virus, between 35 nm and 60 nm in diameter. At present it is thought to be either a togavirus (similar to rubella virus) or a flavivirus (similar to yellow fever virus). The disease has an incubation period of 2–20 weeks. In some countries, including the UK and the USA, hepatitis C virus causes most cases of post-transfusion hepatitis. In the USA serological tests for the detection of this agent have been in use for the screening of all blood donors since 1992. Hepatitis C virus can also cause some cases of sporadic hepatitis. Persistent infections, similar to those seen with hepatitis B virus, develop in about 25–50% of persons contracting hepatitis C virus and can progress to cirrhosis.

Hepatitis D virus

Hepatitis D (HDV, delta agent) is a small (30 nm) RNA virus, which has a hepatitis D virus nucleopro-

Table 19.10 Serological diagnosis of hepatitis B virus (HBV) infections

Test	Acute HBV infection	Past HBV infection	Chronic HBV infection
HBsAg	+ ve (but can be − ve)*	− ve	+ ve
HBsAb	− ve	+ ve	− ve
HBcAb-IgM	+ ve	− ve	− ve
HBcAb-IgG	+ ve	+ ve	+ ve
HBeAg	+ ve or − ve	− ve	+ ve or − ve

HBsAg = Hepatitis B surface antigen; HBsAb = hepatitis B surface antibody; HBcAb-IgM = hepatitis B core antibody, immunoglobulin M type; HBcAb-IgG = hepatitis B core antibody, immunoglobulin G type; HBeAg = hepatitis B e antigen
* See text

tein core, but is surrounded by an envelope containing HBsAg. It is a defective virus; coinfection with hepatitis B virus is necessary for hepatitis D virus to replicate in liver cells. Hepatitis D virus is particularly common in Italy and other Mediterranean countries. It can be associated with clinically severe hepatitis, acute hepatic necrosis, and exacerbations of hepatitis in hepatitis B virus carriers.

Hepatitis E virus

Hepatitis E is a small RNA calicivirus, which previously, together with hepatitis C and D comprised the 'non-A, non-B hepatitis agents'. It causes some cases of epidemic and sporadic enterically transmitted hepatitis.

Human immunodeficiency viruses

Human immunodeficiency viruses (HIV) are the cause of the acquired immunodeficiency syndrome (AIDS), first recognized in homosexual males in the USA, who developed pneumocystis pneumonia and/or Kaposi's sarcoma (Center for Disease Control, 1981). There are two known related but distinct viruses, HIV 1 and 2. HIV 1 is now distributed worldwide, while HIV 2 is found mainly in West Africa, but is being reported with increasing frequency from parts of Europe and Brazil.

HIV 1 is a single-stranded, RNA virus averaging 100 nm in diameter, with an envelope from which glycoprotein spikes protrude. The nucleic acid core contains reverse transcriptase, a unique enzyme mainly found in oncogenic viruses. The core protein (p24; sometimes referred to as p25) is present in relatively large amounts in infected cells, and is used as the antigen in some serological tests for HIV. HIV is readily inactivated by detergents including soap, and is rapidly eliminated by 0.5% sodium hypochlorite. It is inactivated by heating to 56°C for 30 minutes, by organic iodophores, ultraviolet and X-irradiation (Barnett and Levy, 1991).

Detection and isolation of HIV

Venous blood is generally the specimen used for isolation of HIV as well as serological detection of its antibodies. Blood for isolation must be either heparinized or in EDTA. The virus can also be isolated from cerebrospinal fluid, saliva, tears, milk, urine and genital secretions as well as from biopsies from infected tissues such as lymph nodes and the intestinal tract. Virus isolation can be achieved from both freshly collected specimens and specimens treated with dimethylsulphoxide and stored in liquid nitrogen. When collecting specimens, the use of gloves, the appropriate handling of needles and other sharp instruments and the safe transport of specimens to the laboratory are mandatory.

Heparinized blood is the preferred source for viral culture. Up to 30 ml of blood may be required to ensure sufficient virus-infected peripheral blood mononuclear cells are present. Cells from suspected cases are mixed with stimulated normal mononuclear cells and incubated for up to 5 weeks, during which time the cultures are monitored for virus replication. Replication is recognized by assay of reverse transcriptase, the p24 *gag* antigen, or by immunofluorescence. Isolation of HIV, however, is only available in a few specialized centres. The detection of HIV antigens can be achieved by several methods. These include immunoperoxidase and *in situ* hybridization techniques which are applicable to infected tissues and peripheral blood monocytes (Richman, McCutchan and Spector, 1987), and detection of HIV RNA or DNA by polymerase chain reactions. The Western blot technique which is widely used to detect antibodies to HIV can also be used to detect HIV proteins in infected-cell lysates. Many of these methods are at least as sensitive as culture, and may have important applications in diagnosis and in screening blood donors.

Virus serology

The enzyme-linked immunosorbent assay (ELISA) technique, which detects viral antigens is presently widely used as a screening procedure. Various antigens and antigen combinations have been used. Currently in the USA, antigens consisting of recombinant DNA-derived or synthetic HIV proteins or oligopeptides related to HIV glycoprotein gp41 are used (Ng *et al.*, 1989). The ELISA method which is primarily used to screen blood donors for HIV antibody is highly sensitive. 'Positive' tests are repeated in duplicate. If duplicate tests repeat as positive such results are probably best referred to as 'repeatedly reactive'. A repeatedly reactive test, which is generally taken to indicate active HIV infection must be confirmed by the immunoblot (Western blot) method. This technique can also distinguish between HIV 1 and HIV 2 infection. If the ELISA is negative in low risk individuals, a Western blot is generally not performed. In high-risk individuals, a negative ELISA test should be followed up by another ELISA test within 6 months.

Pathogenesis

The main target cell for HIV is the T4 lymphocyte, whose CD4 surface molecule provides a receptor for the HIV gp120 envelope antigen. HIV infection of the lymphocytes takes place, followed by their slow destruction leading to loss of their vital immune functions. This, in turn, leaves the host highly vulnerable to a great variety of opportunistic infections (Table 19.11). Currently, the diagnosis of AIDS is defined by a T4 lymphocyte count of $200/\mu l$ or less. Secondary

Table 19.11 Opportunistic pathogens associated with AIDS

Bacteria	Fungi
Mycobacterium avium-intracellulare	*Candida albicans*
Myobacterium tuberculosis	*Cryptococcus neoformans*
Legionella pneumophila	*Histoplasma capsulatum*
Nocardia asteroides	
Campylobacter jejuni	
Salmonella spp.	
Listeria monocytogenes	

Viruses	Protozoa
Herpes simplex	*Pneumocystis carinii*
Cytomegalovirus	*Isospora hominis*
Varicella-zoster	*Cryptosporidium* spp.
	Giardia lamblia
	Microsporidium spp.

viral infection of macrophages allows spread to the central nervous system, where in turn, neurons with CD4 receptors may be invaded. The combined effects of neuronal invasion and neurotoxic viral glyco-proteins account for the central nervous system syndromes that are common in advanced AIDS.

Clinical aspects

AIDS may present in several ways to the otolaryngologist. A heterophile-negative mononucleosis-like illness, with an exudative pharyngitis, and atypical lymphocytes in the peripheral blood, may follow soon after primary HIV infection (Cooper *et al.*, 1985). In the later stages of the disease, particularly when the T4 lymphocyte count is between $200/\mu l$ and $400/\mu l$, persistent lymph node enlargement is common. When T4 lymphocytes fall below $200/\mu l$, hairy leukoplakia of the tongue, and/or *Candida albicans* and/or cytomegalovirus infections of the pharynx and oesophagus are likely. Oral and pharyngeal lesions of Kaposi's sarcoma may also develop. Sinusitis due to *Streptococcus pneumoniae* is a serious bacterial complication of HIV infection. Malignant otitis externa due to one of several organisms has already been described.

Many antiviral drugs have undergone clinical trials for treatment of AIDS, but at present only zidovudine (AZT) is widely used. Unfortunately, it is neither completely suppressive nor free from serious side effects and its benefits in the management of AIDS appear to be limited. Small scale trials of experimental vaccines have begun in the USA, but it seems very unlikely that a vaccine for general use will be available in the near future.

References

AMERICAN ACADEMY OF PEDIATRICS (1998) *Haemophilus influenzae* infections. *Report on the Committee on Infectious Diseases*. Illinois: Elk Grove Village. 1988 pp. 204–210

ARNOLD, L. J. JR, HAMMOND, P. W., WEISE, W. A. and NELSON, N. C. (1989) Assay formats involving acridinium ester-labelled DNA probes. *Clinical Chemistry*, **35**, 1588–1594

ARVIN, A. M. and PROBER, C. G. (1991) Herpes simplex viruses. In: *Manual of Clinical Microbiology*, 5th edn, edited by A. Balows, W. J. Hausler, Jr, K. L. Hermann, H. D. Isenberg, and H. J. Shadomy. Washington, DC: American Society for Microbiology. p. 826

BACHMAN, A. L., ZIZMOR, J. and NOYEK, A. M. (1979) Tuberculosis of the larynx. *Seminars in Roentgenology*, **14**, 325–328

BARBOUR, S. D., SHLAES, D. M. and GUERTIN, S. R. (1984) Toxic shock syndrome associated with nasal packing: analogy to tampon-associated illness. *Pediatrics*, **73**, 163–165

BARNETT, S. W. and LEVY, J. A. (1991) Human immunodeficiency viruses. In: *Manual of Clinical Microbiology*, 5th edn, edited by A. Balows, W. J. Hausler, Jr, K. L. Hermann, H. D. Isenberg, and H. J. Shadomy, Washington, DC: American Society for Microbiology. p. 1011

BARROW, H. N. and LEVENSON, M. J. (1992) Necrotizing malignant otitis externa caused by *Staphylococcus epidermidis*. *Archives of Otolaryngology – Head and Neck Surgery*, **118**, 94–96

BARRY, A. L., COHN, M. A., SENSIE, J. C., FUCHS, P, C., WASHINGTON, J. A., MUNIEZ, P. R. *et al.* (1992) Interpretative criteria and quality control limits for testing susceptibility of *Neisseria gonorrhoeae* to enoxacin. *Journal of Clinical Microbiology*, **30**, 813–816

BASSIOUNY, A. (1981) Perichondritis of the auricle. *Laryngoscope*, **91**, 422–423

BAUER, A. W., KIRBY, W. M. M., SHERRIS, J. C. and TURCK, M. (1966) Antimicrobial susceptibility testing by a standardised single disc method. *American Journal of Clinical Pathology*, **45**, 493–496

BLOOMFIELD, N., GORDON, M. A. and ELMENDORF, D. F. JR (1963) Detection of *Cryptococcus neoformans* antigen in body fluids by latex particle agglutination. *Proceedings of the Society for Experimental Biology and Medicine*, **114**, 64–67

BRADBOURNE, A. I., BYNOE, M. L. and TYRRELL, D. A. J. (1967) Effects of the 'new' human respiratory viruses in human volunteers. *British Medical Journal*, **3**, 767–769

BRAJTBURG, J., POWDERLY, W. G., KOBAYASHI, G. S. and MEDOFF, G. (1990) Amphotericin B delivery systems. *Antimicrobial Agents and Chemotherapy*, **34**, 381–383

BROOK, I. (1987) The role of anaerobic bacteria in otitis media: microbiology, pathogenesis, and implications on therapy. *American Journal of Otolaryngology*, **8**, 109–117

BROOK, I. and FINEGOLD, S. M. (1979) Bacteriology of chronic otitis media. *Journal of the American Medical Association*, **241**, 487–488

BRORSON, J. E., AXELSON, A. and HOLM, S. E., (1976) Studies in *Branhamella catarrhalis* with special reference to maxillary sinusitis. *Scandanavian Journal of Infectious Diseases*, **8**, 151–156

CENTER FOR DISEASE CONTROL (1981) *Morbidity and Mortality Weekly Report*, **30**, 305

CHANDLER, J. R. (1968) Malignant external otitis. *Laryngoscope*, **78**, 1257–1294

CHAPMAN, N. M., TRACY, S., GAUNTT, C. J. and FORTMUELLER, V.

(1990) Molecular detection and identification of enteric viruses using enzymatic amplification and nucleic acid hybridization. *Journal of Clinical Microbiology*, **28**, 843–850

CHERRY, J. D. (1986) The controversy about pertussis vaccine. In: *Current Clinical Topics in Infectious Diseases*, edited by J. S. Remington and M. N. Swartz. New York: MCGraw-Hill. pp. 216–238

CIMOLAI, N., ELFORD, R. W., BRYAN, L. C., ANAND, C. and BERGER, P. (1988). Do the β-hemolytic, non-group A streptococci cause pharyngitis? *Review of Infectious Diseases*, **10**, 587–601

CLARRIDGE, J. E. (1989) The recognition and significance of *Arcanobacterium haemolyticum*. *Clinical Microbiology Newsletter*, **8**, 32–34

COLLINS, M. D. and CUMMINGS, C. S. (1986) The genus *Corynebacterium*. In: *Bergey's Manual of Systematic Bacteriology*, edited by M. E. Sharpe and J. G. Holt. Baltimore: Williams and Wilkins Company. pp. 1266–1276

CONNOLLY, M. J., MAGEE, J. G., HENDRICK, G. J. and JENKINS, P. A. (1985) *Mycobacterium malmoense* in the northeast of England. *Tubercle*, **66**, 211–217

COOPER D. A., GOLD, J., MCLEAN, P., DONOVAN, B., FINLAYSON, R., BARNES, T. G. *et al.* (1985) Acute AIDS infection. Definition of a clinical illness associated with seroconversion. *Lancet*, i, 537–540

COYKENDALL, A. L., WESBECHER, P. M. and GUSTAFSON, K. B. (1987) 'Streptococcus milleri', *Streptococcus constellatus*, and *Streptococcus intermedius* are later synonyms of *Streptococcus anginosus*. *International Journal of Sytematic Bacteriology*, **37**, 222–228

CROW, C. C., SANDERS, W. E. and LONGLEY, S. (1973) Bacterial interference, II: role of the normal flora in preventing colonization by group A streptococci. *Journal of Infectious Diseases*, **128**, 522–526

CUNNINGHAM, M., YU, V. L., TURNER, J. and CURTIN, H. (1988) Necrotizing otitis externa due to aspergillus in an immunocompetent host. *Archives of Otolaryngology – Head and Neck Surgery*, **114**, 554–556

DE BEULE, K., DE DONCHER, P., CAUWENBERGER, G., KOSTER, M., LEGENDRE, R., BLATCHFORD, N. *et al.* (1988) The treatment of aspergillosis and aspergilloma with itraconazole: clinical results of an open international trial. *Mykoses*, **31**, 476–485

DE LOUVOIS, J. D., GORTAVAI, P. and HURLEY, R. (1977) Bacteriology of abscesses of the central nervous system: a multicentre prospective study. *British Medical Journal*, **2**, 981–984

DOERN, G. V. (1986) *Branhamella catarrhalis*: an emerging human pathogen. *Diagnostic Microbiology and Infectious Disease*, **4**, 191–201

DOLIN, R. (1985) Antiviral chemotherapy and chemoprophylaxis. *Science*, **227**, 1296

DRUTZ, D. J., VAN WAY, J. H., SCHAFFNER, W. and KOENIG, G. (1966) Bacterial interference in the therapy of recurrent staphylococcal infections: multiple abscesses due to the implantation of the 502A strain of staphylococcus. *New England Journal of Medicine*, **275**, 1161–1165

DWORZACK, D. L., POLLOCK, A. S., HODGES, G. R., BARNES, W. G., AJELLO, L. and PADHYE, A. (1978) Zygomycosis of the maxillary sinus and palate caused by *Basidiobolus haptosporus*. *Archives of Internal Medicine*, **138**, 1274–1276

ELEK, S. D. (1949) The plate virulence test for diphtheria. *Journal of Clinical Pathology*, **2**, 250–258

EVANS, E. O., SYDNOR, J. B. and MOORE, W. E. C. (1975) Sinusitis of the maxillary antrum. *New England Journal of Medicine*, **293**, 735–739

FEINGOLD, M., KLEIN, K.O. and HASLAM, G. E. (1966) Acute otitis media in children. *American Journal of Diseases of Children*, **111**, 361–365

GAUNTT, P. N. and LAMBERT, B. E. (1988) Single dose ciprofloxacin for the eradication of pharyngeal carriers of *Neisseria meningitidis*. *Journal of Antimicrobial Chemotherapy*, **21**, 489–496

GILL, V. S., SELEPAK, S. T. I and WILLIAMS, E. C. (1983) Species identification and antimicrobial susceptibilities of coagulase-negative staphylococci isolated from clinical sources. *Journal of Clinical Microbiology*, **118**, 1314–1319

GLEBINK, G. S. (1989) The microbiology of otitis media. *Pediatric Infectious Diseases Journal*, **5**, 518–520

GONZALEZ, R. and HANNA, B. A. (1987) Evaluation of gene probe DNA hybridization systems for the identification of *Mycobacterium tuberculosis* and *Mycobacterium avium-intracellulare*. *Diagnostic Microbiology and Infectious Diseases*, **8**, 69–78

GOOD, R. C. (1991) Current methods for rapid detection and identification of Mycobacteria. In: *Rapid Methods and Automation in Microbiology and Immunology*, edited by A. Vaheri, R. C. Tilton and A. Balows. New York: Springer-Verlag. pp. 228–237

GOODILL, J. J. and ABUELO, J. G. (1987) Mucormycosis: a new risk in deferrioxamine therapy in dialysis patients with aluminum or iron overload. *New England Journal of Medicine*, **317**, 34–36

GRAYSTON, J. T., KUO, C-C. and WANG, S-P. (1986) A new *Chlamydia psittaci* strain TWAR isolated in acute respiratory infections. *New England Journal of Medicine*, **315**, 161–168

GWALTNEY, J. (1990) Acute laryngitis. In: *Principles and Practice of Infectious Diseases*, 2nd edn, edited by G. L. Mandell, R. G. Douglas, Jr and J. E. Bennett. New York: Churchill Livingstone. p. 499

HANDWERGER, S. and THOMASZ, A. (1986) Alteration in the kinetic properties of penicillin-binding proteins of penicillin-resistant *Streptococcus pneumoniae*. *Antimicrobial Agents and Chemotherapy*, **19**, 726–735

HARRISON, H. R. (1986) Chlamydial infections in neonates and children. In: *Neonates and Children in Chlamydial Infections*, edited by D. Oriel, G. Ridgway and J. Schachter. Cambridge: Cambridge University Press. pp. 283–292

HENLE, G., HENLE, W. and DIEHL, V. (1968) Relation of Burkitt's tumor-associated herpes type virus to infectious mononucleosis. *Proceedings of the National Academy of Sciences, USA*, **94**, 94–101

HENLE, W. and HENLE, G. (1974) Epstein-Barr virus and human malignancies. *Cancer*, **34**, 1368–1374

HIRSCH, B., STAIR, T., HOROWITZ, B. Z. and BROALUS, C. (1984) Toxic shock syndrome from staphylcoccal pharyngitis. *Ear, Nose and Throat Journal*, **63**, 494–497

HOLM, P. (1950) Studies in the aetiology of human actinomycosis and their importance. *Acta Pathologica et Microbiologica Scandinavica*, **27**, 736–751

HOWIE, V. M., PLOUSSARD, J. J. and SLOYER, J. L. JR (1975) The 'otitis-prone' condition. *American Journal of Diseases of Childhood*, **129**, 676–678

HULL, H. F., MANN, J. M., SANDS, C. J., GREGG, S. H. and KAUFMAN, P. W. (1983) Toxic shock syndrome related to nasal packing. *Archives of Otolaryngolgy – Head and Neck Surgery*, **109**, 624–626

HURLEY, R. (1966) Pathogenesis of the genus *Candida*. In:

Symposium on Candida Infection, edited by H.I. Winner and R. Henly. Edinburgh: Churchill Livingstone. pp. 13–14

HUSSAIN, Z., LANNIGAN, R., SCHICVEN, B. C., STOAKES, L., KELLY, T. and GROVES, D. (1987) Comparison of RapID-DNA and Minjtek with a conventional method for biochemical identification of anaerobes. *Diagnostic Microbiology and Infectious Diseases*, **6**, 69–72

JONES, R. N., SLEPAK, J. and BIGELOW, J. (1976) Ampicillin-resistant *Haemophilus paraphrophilus* laryngo-epiglottitis. *Journal of Clinical Microbiology*, **4**, 405–407

KERN, M. E. and UECKER, F. A. (1986) Maxillary sinus infection caused by the homobasidiomycetous fungus *Schizophyllum commune*. *Journal of Clinical Microbiology*, **23**, 1001–1005

KINSELLA, J. P., GROSSMAN, M. and BLACK, S. (1986) Otomastoiditis caused by *Mycobacterium avium-intracellulare*. *Pediatric Infectious Diseases*, **5**, 704–706

KINSELLA, J. P., CULVER, K., JEFFREY, R. B., KAPLAN, M. J. and GROSSMAN, M. (1987) Extensive cervical lymphadenitis due to *Mycobacterium avium-intracellulare*. *Pediatric Infectious Diseases*, **6**, 289–291

KLEIN, J. O. and TEELE, D. W. (1976) Isolation of mycoplasmas and viruses from middle ear effusions. A review. *Annals of Otorhinolaryngology*, **85**, 140–144

KRECH, T. and HOLLIS, D. G. (1991) *Corynebacterium* and related species. In: *Manual of Clinical Microbiology*, 5th edn, edited by A. Balows, W. J. Hausler, Jr, K. L. Hermann, H. D. Isenberg and H. J. Shadomy. Washington, DC: American Society for Microbiology. pp. 277–286

LAND, G. A. and MCCRACKEN, A. W. (1991) Fungal infections in the compromised host. In: *Handbook of Applied Mycology*, vol. 2, edited by D. K. Arora, L. Ajello and K. G. Mukerji, New York: Marcel Dekker, Inc. pp. 75–116

LAND, G. A., MCGINNIS, M. R. and SALKIN, A. (1991) Rapid diagnosis of mycoses: evaluation of commercial kits and systems. In: *Rapid Methods and Automation in Microbiology and Immunology*. New York: Springer–Verlag. pp. 353–366

LANG, K., GOSHEN, S., KITGES–COHEN R. and SADE J. (1990) Successful treatment of malignant otitis externa with oral ciprofloxacin. *Journal of Infectious Diseases*, **161**, 537–540

LAWSON, R, BODEY, G. and LUNA, M. (1980) Candida infection presenting as laryngitis. *American Journal of Medical Sciences*, **280**, 173–177

LIPSKY, B. A., GOLDBERGER, L. S., TOMPKINS, L. S. and PLORDE, J. J. (1982) Infections caused by non-diphtheria corynebacteria. *Review of Infectious Diseases*, **4**, 1220–1235

MCCRACKEN, A. W. and MAUNEY, C. U. (1971) Identification of *Corynebacterium diphtheriae* by immunofluorescence during a diphtheria epidemic. *Journal of Clinical Pathology*, **24**, 641–644

MCCRACKEN, A. W., MARTIN, W. J., MCCARTHY, L. J. and COOPER, B. H. (1980) Evaluation of the MS-2 system for the rapid identification of the Enterobacteriaceae. *Journal of Clinical Microbiology*, **12**, 730–734

MCGUIRT, W. E. and HARRILL, J. A. (1979) Paranasal sinus aspergillosis. *Laryngoscope*, **89**, 1563–1568

MCMILLAN, R. H. III, COOPER, P. H., BODY, B. A. and MILLS, A. S. (1987) Allergic fungal sinusitis due to *Curvularia lunata*. *Human Pathology*, **18**, 960–964

MEURMAN, O., RUUSKANEN, O. and SARKINEN, H. (1983) Immunoassay diagnosis of adenovirus infection in children. *Journal of Clinical Microbiology*, **18**, 1190–1195

MILLER, R. A. and BRANCATO, F. (1984) Peritonsillar abscess associated with *Corynebacterium haemolyticum*. *Western Medical Journal*, **141**, 449–451

MORBIDITY AND MORTALITY WEEKLY REVIEW (1993) Update on Hantavirus disease – United States, 1993. **42**, 612–614

MORDUCHOWICZ, G., SHMUELI, D., SHAPIRA, Z., COHEN, S. L., YUSSIM, A., BLOCK, C. S. *et al.* (1986) Rhinocerebral mucormycosis in renal transplant recipients. *Review of Infectious Diseases*, **8**, 441–446

MOSTOE, T. and STROME, M. (1983) Adult epiglottitis. *American Journal of Otolaryngology*, **4**, 393–399

MURPHY, J. R., BOCHA, P. and TENG, M. (1978) Determination of toxigenicity of *Corynebacterium diphtheriae* by a colorimetric tissue culture assay. *Journal of Clinical Microbiology*, **7**, 91–96

NELSON, K. E., CLEMENTS, H. L., MIOTTI, P., COHN, S. and POLK, B. F. (1988) The influence of human immunodeficiency virus (HIV) on antibody response to influenza vaccine. *Annals of Internal Medicine*, **109**, 333–338

NG, V. L., CHIANG, C. S., DEBOUCH, C., MCGRATH, M. S., GROVE, T. H. and MILLS, J. (1989) Reliable confirmation of antibodies to human immunodeficiency virus (HIV) with an enzyme-linked immunoassay using recombinant antigens derived from the HIV-1 *gag*, *pol* and *env* genes. *Journal of Clinical Microbiology*, **27**, 977–982

OSTERHOLM, M. T., RAMBECK, J. H., WHITE, T. E., JACOBS, J. L., PIERSON, L. M., NEATON, J. D. *et al.* (1988) Lack of efficiency of *Haemophilus influenzae* b polysaccharide vaccine in Minnesota. *Journal of the American Medical Association*, **260**, 1423–1428

PADHYE, A. A., AJELLO, L., WEIDER, M. A. and STEINBRONN, K. K. (1986) Phaeohyphomycosis of the nasal sinuses caused by a new species of *Exserohilum*. *Journal of Clinical Microbiology*, **24**, 245–249

PELTOLA, H., KAYHTY, H., VISTANEN, M. and MAKELA, P. H. (1984) Prevention of *Haemophilus influenzae* type b bacteremic infections with the capsular polysaccharide vaccine. *New England Journal of Medicine*, **310**, 1561–1566

PFALLER, M. A. and HERWALDT, L. A. (1988) Laboratory, clinical, and epidemiologic aspects of coagulase-negative staphylococci. *Clinical Microbiology Reviews*, **1**, 281–299

REINGOLD, A. L., MARGRETT, N. T. and DAN, B. B. (1982) Nonmenstrual toxic shock syndrome. A review of 130 cases. *American Journal of Medicine*, **96**, 871–874

REISS, P., HADDERINGH, R., SCHOT, L. J. and DANNER, S. A. (1991) Invasive otitis externa caused by *Aspergillus fumigatus* in two patients with AIDS. (Letter). *AIDS*, **5**, 605–606

REPORT OF THE TASKFORCE ON PERTUSSIS AND PERTUSSIS IMMUNIZATION (1988) *Pediatrics*, **81** (suppl.), 939–984

RICHMAN, D. D., MCCUTCHAN, J. A. and SPECTOR, C. A. (1987) Detecting human immunodeficiency virus RNA in peripheral blood mononuclear cells by nucleic acid hybridization. *Journal of Infectious Diseases*, **156**, 823–827

RIFKIND, D. R., CHANOCK, R. M. and KRAVETZ, H. (1962) Ear involvement (myringitis) and primary atypical pneumonia following inoculation of volunteers with Eaton agent. *American Review of Respiratory Disease*, **85**, 479–489

RUBIN, J. and YU, V. L. (1988) Malignant external otitis: insights into pathogenesis, clinical manifestations, diagnosis and therapy. *American Journal of Medicine*, **85**, 391–396

RUBIN, J., STOEHR, G., YU, V. L., MUDER, L. L., MATADOR, A. and KAMERER, D. B. (1989) Efficacy of ciprofloxacin plus rifampin for treatment malignant external otitis. *Archives of Otolaryngology – Head and Neck Surgery*, **115**, 1063–1069

RUOFF, K. L., KING, L. J. and FERRARO, M. J. (1985) Occurrence of *Streptococcus milleri* among α-hemolytic streptococci isolated from clinical specimens. *Journal of Clinical Microbiology*, **22**, 149–156

RUSSELL, C. and MELVILLE, T. H. (1978) A review. Bacteria in the human mouth. *Journal of Applied Microbiology*, **44**, 163–168

SCHACHTER, J. (1991) Chlamydiae. In: *Manual of Clinical Microbiology*, 5th edn, edited by A. Balows, W. J. Hausler, Jr, K. L. Hermann, H. D. Isenberg and H. J. Shadomy. Washington, DC: American Society for Microbiology. pp. 1045–1053

SCHALEN, L., CHRISTENSEN, P., KAMME, C., MIORNER, H. and PETERSEN, K. I. (1980) High isolation rate of *Branhamella catarrhalis* from the nasopharynx of adults with acute laryngitis. *Scandanavian Journal of Infectious Diseases*, **12**, 277–280

SCHLEIFER, K. H. and KILPPER–BALZ, R. B. (1984) Transfer of *Streptococcus faecalis* and *Streptococcus faecium* to the genus *Enterococcus*. *International Journal of Systematic Bacteriology*, **34**, 31–34

SCHLEIFER, K. H. and KILPPER–BALZ, R. B. (1987) Molecular and chemotaxonomic approaches to the classification of streptococci, enterococci, and lactococci. A review. *Systematic Applied Microbiology*, **10**, 1–19

SCHWARTZ, B., AL–TOBAQI, A., AL–RUWAIS, A., FONTAINE, R. E., A'ASHI, J., HIGHTOWER, A. W. *et al.* (1988) Comparative efficiency of ceftriaxone and rifampicin in eradicating pharyngeal carriage of group A *Neisseria meningitidis*. *Lancet*, i, 1239–1242

SCULIER, J. P., COUNE, A., MEURNIER, F., BRASSINE, C., LADURON, C., HOLLAERT, C. *et al.* (1988) Pilot study of amphotericin B entrapped in sonicated liposomes in cancer patients with fungal infections. *European Journal of Cancer and Clinical Oncology*, **24**, 527–538

SHLAES, D. M., LERNER, P., WOLINSKY, E. and GOPALAKRISHNA, K. V. (1981) Infections due to Lancefield group F and related streptococci. *Medicine*, **60**, 197–201

SIMMONS, R. L. and BALFOUR, H. H. JR (1978) Complications of disseminated varicella-zoster. *Surgery*, **83**, 486–490

SMITH, P. B. (1981) Systems approach to the identification of Enterobacteriaceae. In: *Rapid Methods and Automation in Microbiology*, edited by R. Tilton. Washington, DC: American Society for Microbiology. p. 207

SOLOMON, R., TRUMAN, T. and MURRAY, D. L. (1985). Toxic shock syndrome as a complication of bacterial tracheitis. *Pediatric Infectious Diseases*, **4**, 298–299

SOMMERS, H. M. (1985) The indigenous microbiota of the human host. In: *The Biologic and Clinical Basis of Infectious Diseases*, 3rd edn, edited by G. P. Youmans, P. Y. Paterson and H. M. Sommers. Philadelphia: W. B. Saunders. pp. 70–72

SOMMERS, H. M., MCCLATCHY, J. K. and MONELLA, J. A. (1983) The laboratory diagnosis of the mycobacterioses. In: *Cumitech 16*, edited by H. M. Sommers and J. K. McClatchy. Washington, DC: American Society for Microbiology. pp. 7–8

SPRUNT, K. and REDMAN, G. (1968) Evidence suggesting importance of role of interbacterial inhibition in maintaining a balance of normal flora. *Annals of Internal Medicine*, **68**, 579–590

STAGNO, S., REYNOLDS, D. W., AMOS, C. S., DAHLE, A. J., MCCOLLISTER, F. P., MOHINDRA, I. *et al.* (1977) Auditory and visual defects resulting from symptomatic and subclinical congenital cytomegalovirus infection. *Pediatrics*, **59**, 669–678

STENFORS, I.-E. and RAISANEN, S. (1991) Secretory IgA- and IgG-coated bacteria in the nasopharynx of children. *Acta Otolaryngologica*, **111**, 1139–1145

STEVENS, D. L., TANNER, M. H., WINSHIP, J., SWARTS, R., RIES, K. M., SCHLIEVERT, D. M. *et al.* (1989) Severe group A streptococcal infections associated with a toxic shock-like scarlet fever toxin A. *New England Journal of Medicine*, **321**, 1–7

STULL, T. L., LIPUMA, J. J. and EDLIND, T. D. (1988) A broad spectrum probe for molecular epidemiology of bacterial ribosomal RNA. *Journal of Infectious Diseases*, **157**, 280–286

SWERDLOW, D. L., WOODRUFF, B. A., BRADY, R. C., GRIFFIN, P. M., TIFFEN, S., DONNELL, H. D., JR, *et al.* (1991) A waterborne outbreak in Missouri of *Escherichia coli* O 175: H7 associated with bloody diarrhea and death. *Annals of Internal Medicine*, **117**, 812–819

TENJARLA, G., KUMAR, A. and DYKE, J. W. (1991) Testpack Strep A kit for rapid detection of group A streptococci in 11,088 throat swabs in a clinical pathology laboratory. *American Journal of Clinical Pathology*, **96**, 759–761

TOMODU, T., OGURA, H. and KIRUSHIGE, T. (1991) Immune responses to *Bordetella pertussis* infection and vaccination. *Journal of Infectious Diseases*, **163**, 359–364

VEASY, L. G., WIEDMIEIR, S. E. and ORSMOND, G. S. (1987) Resurgence of acute rheumatic fever in the intermountain region of the United States. *New England Journal of Medicine*, **316**, 412–414

VON GRAEVENITZ, A. (1985) Ecology, clinical significance and antimicrobial susceptibility of infrequently encountered glucose non-fermenting gram negative rods. In: *Non-fermentative Gram Negative Rods*, edited by G. L. Gilardi. New York: Marcel Dekker Inc. pp. 181–232

WASHBURN, R. G., KENNEDY, D. W., BEGLEY, N. D., HENDERSON, D. K. and BENNETT, J. E. (1988) Chronic fungal sinusitis in apparently normal hosts. *Medicine*, **67**, 231–247

WEBB, D. H., SHIELDS, A. F. and FIFE, K. H. (1987) Genomic variation of adenovirus type 5 from bone marrow transplant recipients. *Journal of Clinical Microbiology*, **25**, 305–308

WEISNER, P. J., TRONCA, E., BONIN, P., PEDERSEN, A. H. B. and HOLMES, K. K. (1973) Clinical spectrum of pharyngeal gonococcal infections. *New England Journal of Medicine*, **288**, 181–183

YEAGER, B. H., HOXIE, J., WEISMAN, R. A., GREENBERG, M. S. and BILANIJK, L. T. (1986) Actinomycosis in the acquired immunodeficiency-related complex. *Archives of Otolaryngology – Head and Neck Surgery*, **112**, 1293–1295

20

Cell biology

Wilson C. Mertens

Seasoned physicians and experienced basic scientists possess a deep understanding of various cancers in terms of the natural history and clinical implications of the disease, as well as the properties of malignant cells. However, even these experts find it difficult to define succinctly what 'cancer' is. Neoplasm, a term meaning 'new growth' is often used interchangeably with the term 'tumour' when describing cancer. Tumours are of two basic types: benign and malignant. The ability to distinguish between benign and malignant tumours, as well as normal tissue, is crucial in determining the appropriate treatment and prognosis of the patient. It is also important in determining what basic mechanisms underlie the development of these conditions. The following features characterize a malignant tumour, or cancer (Ruddon, 1987):

1 Cancers are made up of abnormal cells derived from a specific normal tissue.
2 Cancers consist of a greater number of abnormal cells than benign tumours.
3 Cancers invade and destroy adjacent normal tissue. Benign tumours grow by expansion, are usually encapsulated, and do not invade surrounding tissue.
4 Cancers may spread to distant sites (metastasize) through lymphatic channels, or blood vessels to regional lymph nodes or distant organs.

Surgeons, radiotherapists and oncologists are familiar with the progressive nature and potentially lethal consequence of these abnormal cell proliferations. Advanced forms of treatment, whether for an established malignancy or precancerous lesions, are resting more and more heavily on scientific discoveries surrounding the molecular mechanisms involved in neoplastic transformation, proliferation, invasion and metastasis. Although it is impossible in a chapter to give a comprehensive review of this vast topic, a working knowledge of current concepts useful to clinicians will be explored. This will be with particular reference to advances surrounding the most common malignancies otolaryngologists have to face, namely, squamous cell carcinomas of the head and neck.

Cancer: a genetic disease

There is now substantial evidence that changes in the genomes of cells (including transitions, inversions, deletions, chromosome rearrangements, gene amplification, and point mutations) can cause cancer (Squire and Phillips, 1992). Most carcinogens, whether chemical or physical, given chronically or administered for a short period, can induce a variety of mutations in cells (Pitot, 1993). Defects in the organism's ability to repair lesions in DNA are associated with an increased cancer risk (Thompson, 1989). Mutations, if they arise in an organism's germ line (and hence are present in all cells), may result in cancers which are inherited like other genetic traits, and indeed there are several examples of inherited human cancers (Squire and Phillips, 1992). In addition, most cancers appear to have a clonal origin, with each tumour developing from a single mutant cell (Wainscoat and Fey, 1990). Recent research has made progress in understanding how genetic abnormalities may contribute to the development of cancer. Describing these changes is complicated by the interrelated aspects of these observations. What were once separate fields of inquiry, now can best be understood as complementary research endeavours. The growing relevance of this topic to the clinical practice of oncology makes an understanding of it essential.

Chromosome abnormalities

The genetic information of an organism is encoded in the DNA contained in the genome of each cell. This DNA is carried along the length of chromosomes. Each somatic cell contains two copies of the genome, one from each parent, and each copy contains 50 000–100 000 genes (Seth and Papas, 1993). These genes are differentially expressed within cells to produce all genetic characteristics, including cellular functions. It appears likely that important cellular changes resulting in cancer may be related to chromosomal abnormalities. Much work has been performed on haematological malignancies, particularly leukaemia, primarily because of the ease with which these cells can be analysed. However, data are now accumulating on solid tumours (Mitelman, 1991). Initial reports concentrated on chromosomal abnormalities associated with particular malignancies (Rowley and Potter, 1976), but as will be seen below, molecular rearrangements associated with some chromosomal abnormalities have now been characterized, as have their cellular implications.

It appears that nearly all cancers have an abnormal chromosomal karyotype. Some of these appear to be random, but many chromosomal abnormalities have been identified which are non-random, or 'clonal'. This is defined as at least two cells with the same extra chromosome or chromosome structural rearrangement, or three cells with the same missing chromosome (Rowley and Mitelman, 1993). Chromosomal changes observed in cancers can be classified generally into three categories:

a Reciprocal translocation, with portions of two chromosomes exchanged, resulting in no net change in genetic content
b An increase in DNA from a specific chromosome region
c Non-reciprocal changes resulting in either deletion or addition of chromosome regions.

Reciprocal changes

Reciprocal changes may result in genes from one chromosome being placed abnormally close to other genes, altering the expression of these genes. It may also result in a change in gene structure at the site of the translocation. The first, and perhaps the best known clonal chromosomal abnormality is the Philadelphia chromosome (Ph[1]) commonly found in the leukaemic cells of patients suffering from chronic myeloid leukaemia (Rowley, 1973). The Ph[1] chromosome is the result of a reciprocal translocation between chromosomes 22 and 9, with a structural alteration of the *abl* oncogene (carried on chromosome 9) as a consequence (de Klein *et al.*, 1982). Virtually all patients suffering from acute promyelocytic leukaemia have a translocation involving chromosomes 15 and 17, with a translocation breakpoint (a chromosome location which appears 'weak' and allows alterations in the genome) on chromosome 17 near the gene encoding the retinoic acid receptor (Borrow *et al.*, 1990). The breakpoint in chromosome 15 is in a transcription gene. The translocation thus results in a chimeric product causing overproduction of a retinoic acid receptor (de The *et al.*, 1990). This may explain why this form of leukaemia appears to be sensitive to treatment with all-trans retinoic acid (Huang *et al.*, 1988).

Increased DNA in specific chromosomal regions

Increased genetic material in areas on chromosomes referred to as homogeneously staining regions (HSR) or abnormally banding regions (ABR) are associated with multiple gene copies resulting in amplification. Similar gene amplification is seen as multiple gene copies in an extra-chromosomal form called double minutes (DM). A number of these small chromosomal 'bits' may be present, and may represent the first stage in the assembly of homogeneously staining regions.

Cytogenetic studies in patients with squamous cell carcinomas of the head and neck are currently being reported. Although no basic defect has yet been found, in most patients with these carcinomas, non-random abnormalities have been seen. Kao-Shan *et al.* (1987) reported that subjects who smoked were more susceptible to damage at a specific breakpoint on the long arm of chromosome 11 (11q13) in otherwise normal cells. Jin and associates (1990) noted, in their cultured squamous cell carcinomas of the head and neck, a translocation between chromosome 9 and chromosome 11, with the breakpoint on chromosome 11 being 11q13. Other investigators have described deletions in chromosome 11 (especially deletions on the short arm of chromosome 11, at 11p13), and in chromosome 18 (18q) in long-term cultures (Sacks *et al.*, 1988; Carey *et al.*, 1989). Other breakpoints have been described in squamous cell carcinomas of the head and neck including breakpoints on chromosome 1 (1p36), chromosome 9 (9q32), and other areas of chromosome 11 (11q23, 11q14) (Owens *et al.*, 1992; Sen *et al.*, 1993). 11q13 is a chromosome locus for a number of oncogenes including *int*-2 (which encodes for a fibroblastic growth factor, FGF3), *hst*-1, *bcl*-1, and *prad*-1 (Lammie and Peters, 1991). Three known oncogenes, *L-myc*, *N-ras*, and *jun*, are located near 11p13. Some of these oncogenes have been found to be amplified in squamous cell carcinomas of the head and neck (see below).

In contrast to other reports, Owens and associates (1992) found cytogenetic abnormalities only in patients who had previously been treated with irradiation. This raises the question of the stability of these abnormalities throughout the duration of the disease as well as the effect of therapy. More extensive work with a larger bank of tumours will be required in order to assess this aspect.

Non-reciprocal changes

Non-reciprocal exchanges such as the very common deletion of the short arm of chromosome 3 (3p-) in small cell carcinoma of the lung and other broncho-genic carcinomas, suggest that loss of this chromosome material results in a loss of tumour suppression activity (Campbell *et al.*, 1989). Similar deletions are also present in renal carcinomas (Kovacs and Frisch, 1989). Recently, investigators have determined that similar deletions are found in squamous cell carcinomas of the head and neck (El-Naggar *et al.*, 1993). In one report of 18 carcinoma specimens, 75% had deletions at 3p21, and 33% at 3p24. In addition to determining that deletions at 3p are frequent abnormalities in these tumours, there appeared to be a correlation between poor histological differentiation, DNA aneuploidy, and such deletions; most poorly and moderately differentiated aneuploid carcinomas manifested a deletion at 3p. Latif *et al.* (1992) determined a significant deletion rate on the short arm of chromosome 3, with a commonly deleted region including several possible tumour suppressor genes involved in other malignancies. Hence, not only does the loss of chromosomal material at 3p appear to result in the loss of tumour suppressor activity, and may possibly be associated with aggressively malignant biological behaviour, but it also seems to be a common abnormality in squamous cell carcinomas of the head and neck. The genes associated with such changes remain to be determined.

Oncogenes and proto-oncogenes

In 1911, Rous described a sarcoma of chickens which could be transmitted to other chickens by either the injection of tumour cells or of a cell-free extract. It was ultimately determined that such tumours were caused by a retrovirus (known as the Rous sarcoma virus) carrying transforming genetic information into a normal cell, and resulting in the development of a cancerous cell (Stehelin *et al.*, 1989). Although animal tumour models have been the mainstay for such research, new techniques now allow human cancers to be evaluated. This is important as it appears that relatively few cancers have a viral association (see below). Inherited cancer syndromes such as Wilms' tumour, neurofibromatosis, and Li-Fraumeni syndrome have clarified the mechanisms of oncogenesis and have made this aspect of cell biology clinically relevant.

An oncogene is a distinct segment of DNA, or gene, which is involved in processes leading to the transformation of a normal cell to a malignant cell through its protein product. The initial oncogenes were described in studies employing retroviruses such as the Rous sarcoma virus. These RNA-containing viruses use their genome as a template for the synthesis of viral DNA through the action of RNA-directed DNA polymerase or reverse transcriptase (Benchimol, 1992). This newly formed viral DNA then becomes integrated into the host cell DNA as a provirus. The potential consequences of this integration into the host genome, in light of the earlier discussion on chromosomal abnormalities, is clear. If the provirus contains a gene with transforming activity (such as a viral oncogene, or v-*onc*: genes acquired by the retrovirus from the genome of a host cell), the expression of the gene's products may transform cells in culture after several days. These genes induce clinical tumours in infected animals quickly, as they are under the control of efficient retroviral promoters that are not normally regulated. The viral oncogene expression transforms every infected cell. These retroviruses have been intensively studied, and are termed acute transforming retroviruses (Perkins and Vande Woude, 1993). Although few human cancers are caused by this mechanism, v-*onc* sequences, compared with normal human genes of similar structure, have resulted in considerable insight into the makeup and function of human (or cellular) oncogenes. Another group of retroviruses has been described which induce cancers after a long latency period. These retroviruses, known as chronic tumour viruses or slow-acting retroviruses, do not contain viral oncogenes, but rather appear to transform infected cells through aberrant activation of normal host genes adjacent to the insertion of the provirus (Perkins and Vande Woude, 1993). The long latent period of disease may be the result of the low probability that the proviruses will integrate into the genome adjacent to the appropriate host cellular gene. Although the latter retroviruses have not been described as causing human cancer through insertional activation, many oncogenes have been described by the insertion of these proviruses into specific loci within the genome in experimental models.

Several oncogenes have been described, as well as their analogous normal genes, or proto-oncogenes (Cooper, 1990). The widespread belief that proto-oncogenes represent cancer-causing grenades waiting to explode, is unjustified. The DNA sequences of proto-oncogenes are highly conserved between species, and it is presumed that the functions of the proto-oncogene, expressed through its product, are vital to the normal development of multicellular organisms. The protein products normally appear to regulate cell growth and differentiation. Alteration or over-expression of these proteins, as a result of mutations, can result in cell proliferation.

The products of proto-oncogenes and oncogenes can be grouped according to their biochemical activity as well as location within the cell. These include (a) growth factors, (b) growth factor receptors with tyrosine kinase activity, (c) cytoplasmic tyrosine kinases, (d) guanine nucleotide-binding proteins, (e) cytoplasmic serine-threonine specific protein kinases and (f) nuclear proteins (Minden and Pawson, 1992) (Figure 20.1; Table 20.1).

Table 20.1 Selected oncogenes

Oncogene class	Oncogene	Proposed function
Growth factor	*int*-1	Matrix protein
	int-2 (FGF3)	Fibroblast growth factor related protein
Growth factor receptor	*erb*-B	Epidermal growth-factor-receptor
	fms	Colony-stimulating factor-1 receptor
Cytoplasmic kinases	*bcr-abl*	Tyrosine kinase
	src	Tyrosine kinase
	mos	Serine-threonine kinase
Guanine nucleotide binding proteins (*ras* family)	H-*ras*	GTPase
Nuclear proteins	L-*myc*	Transcription factor
	myc	Transcription factor
Others	*bcl*-1 (*prad*1)	Cyclin D

Growth factors

Growth factors are small proteins that bind to specific receptors at the cell surface. When binding takes place, a variety of effects may result. These include cell differentiation, cell proliferation, and mainten-

ance of the viability of the cell. For example, v-*sis* is homologous to the gene which encodes the β-chain of platelet-derived growth factor (PDGF) (Waterfield *et al.*, 1983). This growth factor acts by binding to its cell surface receptor, inducing tyrosine kinase activity. V-*sis* induces cellular transformation in culture when co-expressed with the receptor for PDGF. However, PDGF alone does not induce a malignant phenotype, presumably because of some form of receptor down-regulation after the binding of exogenous growth factor (Minden and Pawson, 1992).

Growth factor receptors with tyrosine kinase activity

Transmembrane receptors that possess protein kinase activity have an extracellular ligand-binding portion, a transmembrane section, and a cytoplasmic domain which contains a tyrosine kinase region (Hunter, 1987). Examples include epidermal growth-factor receptor (EGF-R), platelet-derived growth factor receptor (PDGF-R), as well as insulin receptor, insulin-like growth factor-1 receptor, and colony-stimulating factor-1 (CSF-1) receptor (Minden and Pawson, 1992). A growth factor's ability to express cellular characteristics appears to be dependent on the kinase activity of its specific receptor. In normal cells, activated growth factor receptors are rapidly internalized (that is, removed from the cell surface), and are also subject to structural modifications that inhibit their activity (Wells *et al.*, 1990). Down-regulation results in a growth factor having only a transient stimulating effect on the cell. Mutations producing structural alterations can result in the tyrosine kinase domain being continuously active, even in the absence of the growth factor (Roussel *et al.*, 1988). Cells expressing these variant growth factor receptors are subject to continuing proliferative signals that contribute to neoplastic transformation.

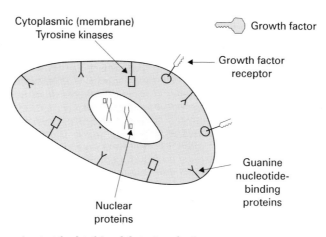

Figure 20.1 Oncogene classes (see text for details) and their sites of action

Cytoplasmic tyrosine kinase

Other tyrosine kinases are found entirely within the cytoplasm, often associated with the inside of the plasma membrane (Bishop, 1991). Several genes encoding for these kinases have been identified. It is uncertain what function the cytoplasmic tyrosine kinases play, but observations such as the activation of *src*, the product of which is a cytoplasmic kinase, by PDGF-R, suggests that the transmembrane tyrosine kinase may stimulate the cytoplasmic tyrosine kinase, possibly resulting in signal amplification (Cantley *et al.*, 1991). Other observations suggest that cytoplasmic tyrosine kinases may function in signal transduction and are an important adjunct in malignant transformation (Cross and Dexter, 1991; Hunter, 1991).

Guanine nucleotide-binding proteins

Guanine nucleotide-binding proteins such as the protein products of the *ras* gene family, possess guanosine triphosphatase (GTPase) activity (Gibbs *et al.*, 1984). Oncogenic activation of these genes appears to have several effects, such as DNA synthesis, cell proliferation, malignant transformation, and production of metastases (Sigal, 1988; Cooper, 1990; Chambers and Tuck, 1993). One mechanism of action is signal transduction (through its protein product, known as p21^{ras}) as an intermediate between the surface growth factor receptor and the nucleus (McCormick, 1989; Graziadei, Riabowol and Bar-sagi, 1990). Mutations in the *ras* gene family have been shown to play an important part in the development of several cancers. High levels of *ras* mutations have been found in pancreatic adenocarcinomas as well as cancers of the colon, thyroid and lung (Rodenhuis *et al.*, 1987; Almoguera *et al.*, 1988; Vogelstein *et al.*, 1988; Harris, 1991). K-*ras* mutations have been demonstrated in both precancerous colon polyps and in the adjacent adenocarcinomas, suggesting the development of genomic abnormalities in both cancer and precancerous lesions (Vogelstein *et al.*, 1988).

Cytoplasmic serine-threonine-specific protein kinases

Serine-threonine-specific protein kinases such as protein kinase C, and the product of the *raf* gene, seem to be stimulated by activated tyrosine kinases and *ras* proteins (Lee, Rapp and Blackshear, 1991; Troppmair *et al.*, 1992). Specific protein kinases may directly regulate the transcriptional and translational control of gene expression.

Nuclear proteins

Nuclear proteins encoded by oncogenes and proto-oncogenes are directly related to the regulation of gene expression (Lewin, 1991). These proteins bind to DNA in a site-specific manner and can activate or suppress transcription from adjacent transcription units. *Myc*-encoded proteins possess a structure (including a helix-loop-helix domain) indicative of DNA binding. They also contain a leucine zipper region which participates in dimerization. The products of the oncogenes *fos* and *jun* are components of the transcription complex AP-1. These two gene protein products combine into a heterodimer at the leucine zipper region, with a higher affinity for DNA than either protein alone (Lewin, 1991). These two oncogenes are examples of a number of transcription factors which can dimerize with one another. This results in many potential complexes, each of which may have distinct effects on gene expression, and consequently on cell biology.

Oncogenes and head and neck cancer

Several oncogenes have been studied in head and neck cancers, and attempts have been made to correlate these with pathological results and clinical outcome. Amplification of growth factors genes such as *int-2*, alone or coamplified with *hst-1* has been demonstrated (Tsutsumi *et al.*, 1988; Zhou, Casey and Line, 1988; Merritt *et al.*, 1990; Somers, Cartwright, and Schechter, 1990). These genes encode for members of the fibroblast growth factor family. Other investigators have found amplification of the *bcl-1* (or *prad-1*) gene alone or with *int-2*. The significance of this finding is uncertain (Berenson, Yang and Mickel, 1989), although *bcl-1* appears to encode a protein called cyclin (see cell proliferation, below) (Xiong *et al.*, 1991). All of the above oncogenes are closely related to chromosomal locus 11q13, which suggests that this breakpoint is important in the development of several cancers including squamous cell carcinomas of the head and neck (Lammie and Peters, 1991).

Tyrosine kinase type growth factor receptors and head and neck cancer

Tyrosine kinase type growth factor receptors are also important in squamous cell carcinomas of the head and neck. The epidermal growth factor receptor (EGF-R) is the normal protein product of the *erb*-B1 oncogene (Perkins and Vande Woude, 1993). Epidermal growth factor stimulates proliferation of cells by interacting with its receptor. Amplification of the receptor appears to be an inconsistent finding in these cancers (Field, 1992), but over-expression of the receptor gene (*erb*-B1) was found in 53% of squamous cell carcinomas of the head and neck in one study. In addition, four of the fifteen tumours studied had amplified *erb*-B1 gene, and this appeared to correlate with the level of differentiation of the tumours (Ishitoya *et al.*, 1989). The protein product of the *erb*-B2 oncogene, a transmembrane protein with considerable homology to EGF-R (Yamamoto *et al.*, 1986), has been found in the cytoplasm of many squamous cell carcinomas of the head and neck according to Field *et al.* (1992a). Although *erb*-B2 in breast cancer cells is associated with over-expression of the oncogene and a poorer prognosis, its implications in squamous cell carcinomas of the head and neck are unknown.

Geographical differences in *ras* gene alterations

An unusual geographical difference in the incidence of *ras* oncogene mutations appears to exist. H-*ras* mutations appeared in 20 of 57 (35%) samples evaluated from Indian oral cancers (Saranath *et al.*, 1991). Amplification of K-*ras* and N-*ras* was also seen in 33% of oral cancers in India, a result not seen in the West (Saranth *et al.*, 1989; Sakai *et al.*, 1992). Apart from reports from India, there is little evidence to suggest that alterations to the *ras* gene play a significant role in the development of squamous cell carcinomas of the head and neck (Sheng *et al.*, 1990; Field, 1992). The geographical differences in *ras* alterations remain unexplained, but may relate to the prevalence of betal chewing, and reverse smoking, which are thought to be carcinogenic and are habits which are not practised in the West. One group found that changes in the level of H-*ras* expression in squamous cell carcinomas of the head and neck were not due to genetic alteration of the gene. This suggests some other, as yet to be determined mechanism for the over-expression of this gene (Field, 1992).

The p21^{ras} and c-myc genes

Field *et al.* (1992b) demonstrated that patients with low levels of p21^{ras} protein had a poorer prognosis than those with positive staining for this oncogene. Three per cent of patients with negative p21^{ras} staining were alive at 60 months, compared with 54% of patients with positive staining ($P < 0.05$). It will remain to be seen whether other groups can reproduce this interesting finding.

Nuclear protein-producing oncogenes such as the *myc* gene family have also been extensively studied. Amplification or mutations of *myc* genes have been infrequently noted in the West (Merritt *et al.*, 1990; Field, 1992), but again in India, both c-*myc* and N-*myc* were amplified in up to 39% of cancers (Saranth *et al.*, 1989). Two groups found amplification of *int*-2 oncogene with the c-*myc* oncogene in a few squamous cell carcinomas of the head and neck (Merrit *et al.*, 1990; Leonard *et al.*, 1991), the implications of which remain unclear.

Over-expression of the c-*myc* gene has been seen without gene amplification in some cancers, including squamous cell carcinomas of the head and neck. Elevated c-*myc* protein product correlated with a poor prognosis in patients with squamous cell carcinomas of the head and neck (Field *et al.*, 1989), a finding found in other cancers as well. C-*myc* protein

product has been found in the nuclei of precancerous oral lesions, as well as some benign keratoses which did not exhibit any cytological atypia, suggesting that c-*myc* expression correlates with progressive cell transformation and oral cancer (Eversole and Sapp, 1993).

A multiplicity of chromosomal rearrangements, oncogene point mutations, amplifications, and over-expression are seen in squamous cell carcinomas of the head and neck. There tend to be more chromosomal abnormalities and oncogene activations as disease progresses, suggesting a complex process of carcinogenesis, including 'multiple hit' gene mutations as well as genomic instability with time. Furthermore, oncogenes may be simultaneously or sequentially activated in malignancy, and different carcinogens appear to activate different oncogenes.

Tumour suppressor genes or recessive oncogenes

Several cancers exhibit chromosomal deletions, suggesting that these tumours arise in part after the loss of tumour suppressor activity. These tumours include retinoblastoma, Wilms' tumour and the Li-Fraumeni (or cancer family) syndrome. These inherited cancers, or familial cancer syndromes, appear to result from the loss or mutation of one (recessive) tumour suppressor gene as one abnormal allele is already present in the germ line. Non-familial cancers would require that both alleles be affected in some way.

The first example of this type of process was described in retinoblastoma. A tumour suppressor gene known as RB1, located on chromosome 13, produces a nuclear phosphoprotein which is involved in the cell cycle regulation (Cooper and Whyte, 1989). Patients inheriting a germline mutation in RB1 are at high risk for developing retinoblastoma. In most families the penetration of the mutation is 90–95%, with about 80% of patients with a germline mutation developing bilateral disease. Hence this lesion is inherited as an autosomal dominant trait. In addition to retinoblastoma, individuals inheriting a germline mutation at RB1 are at high risk for developing other primary tumours.

Knudson (1971), employing a mathematical model, suggested that the transformation of normal cells into cancer cells requires two mutations. Mutation frequencies are low, and hence the non-hereditary form of retinoblastoma is an uncommon disease. However, when the first mutation takes places in the germline, every potential 'normal' cell has undergone the first mutation. As the numbers of cells at risk are large, it is almost a certainty that one or more cells will undergo a second mutation and develop into cancers.

Since then, other tumour suppressor genes have been described. Much recent work has involved a gene located on the short arm of chromosome 17 known as p53 (Levine, Momand and Finlay, 1991). Patients with the Li-Fraumeni, or cancer family syndrome, have germline mutations in one allele of the p53 gene, and develop tumours that possess mutations at both alleles (Malkin *et al.*, 1990). The protein product of this gene is usually localized to the nucleus where it is phosphorylated. However, some genetic mutations cause an abnormal p53 protein product to accumulate in the cytoplasm due to its longer half-life, hence providing a marker for gene abnormalities. Although cancer cells lacking a normal p53 gene can demonstrate lengthened cell doubling times or growth arrest when a normal p53 gene is introduced, it remains unclear how this gene regulates cell growth and cell cycling (Perkins and Vande Woude, 1993). Half of all adult cancers contain p53 mutations, and abnormal p53 gene expression is felt to be a very common genetic feature in a wide range of cancers (Levine, 1990). Over-expression of p53 protein product in squamous cell carcinomas of the head and neck has been evaluated by many investigators who have found a high proportion of tumours with abnormalities (Field *et al.*, 1991; Gusterson *et al.*, 1991; Brachman *et al.*, 1992; Langdon and Partridge, 1992; Sakai *et al.*, 1992; Sakai and Tsuchida, 1992; Watling, Gown, and Coltrera, 1992).

Increasing data are accumulating regarding the relationship between p53 gene and smoking. This gene has been found to be mutated and over-expressed in lung cancers associated with smoking (Iggo *et al.*, 1990). Field *et al.* (1991) also demonstrated that heavy smoking and increased p53 expression were correlated in squamous cell carcinomas of the head and neck. An association has also been found between heavy smoking and significant alcohol consumption in patients suffering from squamous cell carcinomas of the head and neck with elevated p53 expression (Field, Spandidos, and Stell, 1992).

Recent work has evaluated the expression of p53 in malignant and premalignant squamous epithelium in the aerodigestive tract. Positive staining for the p53 protein is seen in undifferentiated cancer cells. However, in non-adjacent mucosa demonstrating various stages of dysplasia, positive staining was also noted (Sozzi *et al.*, 1992). These results suggest that alteration of the p53 gene is an early event in the development of malignancy. Others have also evaluated primary squamous cell carcinomas of the head and neck and second primary tumours which often develop in these patients (Chung *et al.*, 1993). Within the same patient, primary tumour mutations are discordant with those of the second primary tumour, but the class of p53-base mutations (i.e. transitions from pyrimidine to pyrimidine or purine to purine) is the same in the majority of the cancers. These data support the concept of field carcinogenesis resulting from the exposure to a common carcinogen which initiates both primary cancers

and second primary tumours. It also suggests a practical use of abnormal p53 protein product (as well as other gene products, such as c-*myc*). Their presence within cells should refine the definition and identification of premalignant lesions, with implications for both therapy of established cancers as well as prevention of second malignancies (Lippman and Hong, 1993).

Oncogenic viruses

Although most human cancers do not appear to have a viral origin, there does appear to be a role for viruses in the development of some malignancies. This has been best described for the Epstein-Barr virus in nasopharyngeal carcinoma and Burkitt's lymphoma, and hepatitis B in hepatocellular carcinoma. Human papilloma virus (HPV) has been described in carcinomas of the cervix, vulva, and penis, as well as oesophagus and larynx (Howley, 1993). HPV has also been found to be associated with oral squamous cell carcinomas (Scully *et al.*, 1988). HPV-16 induces the production of transforming proteins E6 and E7 which form complexes with tumour suppressor gene products from p53 and RB1, respectively (Field, 1992). In the case of the p53 gene, the E6 proteins appear to promote degradation of the protein product, hence inactivating it. There also appears to be an interaction between HPV and the c-*myc* gene in cervical carcinoma; HPV DNA sequences have been demonstrated in the genome of genital squamous carcinomas in regions near the locus of c-*myc* and N-*myc* genes. In these cancers, the *myc* genes were structurally altered or over-expressed (Couturier *et al.*, 1991). Most squamous cell carcinomas of the anus with amplified c-*myc* oncogene are HPV positive (Crook *et al.*, 1991).

It also appears that tonsillar squamous cell carcinoma has a specific association with HPV. One group found HPV DNA in 10 cases of tonsillar carcinomas, compared with a rate of 30% HPV DNA detection in other aerodigestive tract carcinomas (Snijders *et al.* 1992). Brachman *et al.* (1992) evaluated 30 tumours, and determined that only 10% of these contained HPV DNA; interestingly, two of these three cases were tonsillar primaries, with only three tonsillar tumours included in the sample.

Cancer: a cellular disease

Tissues differ in their proliferation rates: some tissues are constantly being renewed, such as those in bone marrow and the gastrointestinal tract, others proliferate slowly, but may renew their population in the face of insult or injury (such as liver). Still others are static (e.g. nerve tissue). Most cancers arise in renewing or proliferating cell populations. If the tissue does not normally proliferate, then the development of cancer is often preceded by an insult which induces cell proliferation (such as hepatitis B infection or tobacco use).

Underlying all proliferating tissues is a small number of 'stem cells', which have a high capacity for cell proliferation as well as cell renewal. These cells generate other cells which expand and ultimately mature (differentiate) to develop into functioning tissue. This process of self-renewal, expansion and maturation is under tight control, probably by growth factors and hormones acting through tissue-specific receptors.

As noted above, human cancers are monoclonal, suggesting their origin from a single transformed cell. However, cancers also demonstrate considerable heterogeneity. Some of these differences may be related to the tendency of cancer cells to be genetically unstable, exhibiting a high rate of random mutation. This results in the development of subclones, some of which may develop greater autonomy and growth (Buick and Tannock, 1992). Other differences may relate to differentiation-related factors, as well as environmental differences within the cancer deposits, resulting from the abnormal vascularity of cancers (and most commonly manifested by central tumour necrosis), and sometimes the effect of treatment.

Growth factors

One of the more important mechanisms of cell growth regulation and differentiation results from the secretion of polypeptide growth factors. These growth factors are virtually undetectable in the blood stream, although platelets store platelet-derived growth factor (PDGF) as well as transforming growth factor-alpha and -beta (TGF-α and TGF-β). These factors presumably have roles in the stimulation of healing in the area of injury after their release from platelets (Deuel, 1987). Most of these growth factors exert their effects by binding to membrane receptors. When these receptors are activated, most of them exhibit tyrosine kinase activity (Hunter, 1987). Subsequent biochemical reactions can result in the activation of protein kinase C, a serine-threonine kinase, which is thought to result in further gene transcription regulation (Kikkawa, Kishimoto, and Nishizuka, 1989).

Alterations of growth factors, their receptors, or signalling pathways can lead to malignant transformation. Protein products of certain oncogenes may represent growth factors, growth factor receptors, or other proteins that participate in signal transduction anywhere from the level of receptor to the level of the chromosome (Mendelsohn and Lippman, 1993).

Epidermal growth factor receptors (EGF-R) appear to have increased expression in many cancers (Mendelsohn and Lippman, 1993) (see above). Transforming growth factor alpha (TGF-α) avidly binds to EGF-R, despite the fact that TGF-α and EGF have only 35% homology (Brachmann *et al.*, 1989). TGF-α is capable of inducing epithelial proliferation, and appears to be more active than EGF in stimulating angiogenesis (Schreiber, Winkler and Derynck, 1986). Many tumours which express EGF-R also produce TGF-α (Derynck *et al.*, 1987). This suggests that TGF-α and EGF-R function as a true autocrine pathway, providing a natural circuitry for cells to self-stimulate growth (Rosenthal *et al.*, 1986; Di Marco *et al.*, 1989; Wong, 1993).

Santini and colleagues (1991) evaluated EGF-R content in 70 squamous cell carcinomas of the head and neck as well as control tissue. High levels were seen in cancers, correlating with tumour size and stage of disease, but not with tumour differentiation. In contrast, Scambia *et al.* (1991) evaluated EGF-R by immunohistochemical techniques in 42 squamous cell carcinomas of the head and neck. Cancer tissue contained higher EGF-R levels than controls, with the only correlation between receptor levels being found with tumour differentiation (more poorly differentiated tumours were more likely to be positive).

As an example of possible future therapy based on growth factors and their receptors, Yoneda and colleagues (1991b), employing a murine model of a transplanted human squamous cell carcinoma from a patient exhibiting a paraneoplastic syndrome (hypercalcaemia, leucocytosis, and cachexia) evaluated both EGF and an anti-EGF-R antibody (Yoneda *et al.*, 1991a) on syndrome development and tumour growth. When epidermal growth factor was administered, the growth of tumours was accelerated, along with an increase in hypercalcaemia. A monoclonal antibody (mAb-108) which recognizes the extracellular domain of EGF-R was then administered by intraperitoneal injection. This therapy retarded tumour formation, and delayed the onset of hypercalcaemia and cachexia. Antibody injection into mice bearing heavier tumour burdens and demonstrating significant hypercalcaemia and cachexia resulted in reversal of both tumour growth as well as paraneoplastic symptoms. Baselga *et al.* (1993) have reported enhanced antitumour efficacy of the combination of an anti-EGF-R monoclonal antibody with the chemotherapy drug doxorubicin *in vitro* and in mouse xenografts of both an adenocarcinoma and a squamous cell carcinoma line. Although evaluation in clinical trials is required, manipulation of growth factors and their receptors may emerge as a therapeutic approach for patients with squamous cell carcinomas of the head and neck.

Recently, it was found that elevated levels of TGF-α and EGF-R may represent early markers of carcinogenesis in squamous cell carcinomas of the head and neck. In patients with squamous cell carcinomas of the head and neck, both TGF-α and EGF-R were increased in most samples of histologically normal mucosa, when compared with control patients (Grandis and Tweardy, 1993). Like the data presented above for the tumour suppressor gene p53 and *myc* oncogene, this finding confirms the molecular nature of the 'field cancerization' concept, and may serve as an important future marker in chemoprevention trials. It may also suggest a new use for growth factor-based therapies in the prevention as well as for the treatment of established cancer.

Cancer cell proliferation and the cell cycle

Proliferation rates vary considerably between cancers. Recent advances in the evaluation of cells by flow cytometry have resulted in the accumulation of considerable data with regard to cancer cell proliferation. However, evaluation of physical growth rates of treated human cancers is limited by the fact that many tumours are now aggressively treated and that accurate measurements can be made of such tumours only when evaluable by radiography or by clinical measurements such as palpation (Tannock, 1992). Another difficulty is the relatively short period in the tumour's natural history that this evaluation can be undertaken. Superficial or palpable tumours may be detected clinically usually only when they approach a diameter of 1 cm. Such cancers contain approximately 10^9 cells, and will have undergone around 30 doublings in volume before clinical detection. Ten further doublings in volume would result in a tumour that weighs approximately 1 kg (containing approximately 10^{12} cells), a size that is at the upper limit of cancer burden compatible with life. Preclinical estimates of growth rate for tumours can only be established indirectly. Experimental animal models employing injections of known numbers of cancer cells, as well as clinical studies of cancer recurrence in a local region after it is potentially cured by surgery, can be used to try to determine growth rates of cancers in their preclinical phase. For some cancers, the preclinical growth phase appears to be more rapid than the growth of tumours that are clinically obvious. Such growth cell deceleration is probably due to limitations of cell nutrition, as well as an increasing rate of cell death (Tannock, 1992).

The initial descriptions of the cell cycle were based on morphological criteria, with further evaluation by radio-labelled DNA precursors employing autoradiography. The cell cycle is divided by nuclear division, or mitosis, and nuclear replication, or DNA synthesis, which take place at different times (Figure 20.2). Hence the cycle is divided into M-phase, the period when mitosis happens, and the S-phase, when the cell is undergoing DNA synthesis. Most cells appear to pause between these two events, at stage G1 (between the M- and S-phase), and G2 (the gap between S-and the M- phase). Cells which are differentiated can go into a state of arrest following mitosis and before DNA synthesis. Such cells may be irrevers-

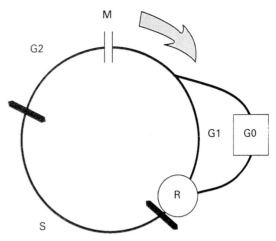

Figure 20.2 Schematic representation of the cell cycle (for explanations of abbreviations see text)

ibly out of cycle (due to final maturation), or may be reversibly out of cycle (due to poor nutrition or absence of growth factor support) but retain the capacity to proliferate if stimulated. The latter cells are termed G0. The 'intersection' of the G1 and G0 phase is the point where cells in G1 are committed to enter DNA synthesis and is known as the restriction point or 'R'. The distinction between G0 and G1 appears to be important, as the rate of increase of a population of cells is dependent on the fraction of cells that are in cycle, compared to those that are not in cycle (i.e. in G0).

A series of steps has been described by Pardee (1989) as being necessary to initiate DNA replication and hence proliferation. These steps include the binding of growth factor(s) to specific receptors, followed by transmission of growth factor-initiated signals to the nucleus and activation of genes, particularly those involved in the production of nuclear proteins such as *myc*. Binding of these nuclear proteins to DNA then alters the regulation of other genes, the products of which are important for the cell cycle to proceed. Many of these proteins are enzymes which increase in mid-to-late G1, and include thymidine kinase, DNA polymerase, thymidylate synthase, dihydrofolate reductase and ribonucleotide reductase.

Several investigators have demonstrated that cytoplasm from cells in metaphase (the time during mitosis or meiosis when doubled chromosomes line up along an equatorial plane between the spindle poles and begin to separate) can induce frog oocytes to enter meiosis (Masui and Markert, 1971; Smith and Ecker, 1970). This activity of the cytoplasm was termed maturation-promoting factor (MPF). Subsequent experiments in yeast have led to the identification of cell division cycle (*cdc*) genes which produce substances that control the transfer of cells through the cell cycle. Such genes have also been described in human cells, and one particular gene, *cdc*-2, has been studied in detail (Lee and Nurse, 1987). This gene encodes a protein which functions as a serine-threonine protein kinase (Draetta, 1990). This protein kinase (p34^{cdc-2}) becomes activated when dephosphorylated and bound to a regulatory protein (cyclin) which slowly accumulates during interphase to peak levels during mitosis. Cyclin is then quickly degraded, presumably by proteases (Kirschner, 1992). Loss of cyclin results in loss of kinase activity, and this loss of enzyme activity results in reduced protein synthesis and allows nuclei to exit mitosis. The loss of protein kinase activity also allows cyclin to accumulate again, permitting the cycle to repeat itself.

A family of cyclin proteins has been identified; so-called G1 cyclins appear before S-phase and permit the cell to enter S-phase when associated with p34^{cdc-2} (Perkins and VanDe Woude, 1993). Other cyclins function primarily during M-phase. A gene encoding for a G1 cyclin (*prad*-1 or *bcl*-1) has been found to be amplified in squamous cell carcinomas of the head and neck, and is near to the chromosomal breakpoint 11q13, a site of chromosomal abnormalities frequently described in squamous cell carcinomas of the head and neck.

This clock-like complex has potential implications for the treatment of squamous cell carcinomas of the head and neck. The p34^{cdc-2} kinase phosphorylates several substrate proteins. The p34^{cdc-2}-cyclin complex appears to be a kinase for the histone H1, a nuclear protein bound to DNA, which may be involved in chromosomal condensation at mitosis; cyclin may function to direct the complex to this area. Other potential substrates include the products of the tumour suppressor genes p53 and RB1. The retinoblastoma protein appears to exist in unphosphorylated form in phase G1 or G0, but in the S-phase and the G2/M-phases, it becomes heavily phosphorylated (Perkins and Vande Woude, 1993). This protein can be phosphorylated by p34^{cdc-2} *in vitro*. The p53 protein is phosphorylated by p34^{cdc-2}-cyclin complex in M-phase, and by the same kinase in complex with a different regulatory unit near the onset of the S-phase. It is therefore possible that phosphorylation of the inhibitory products of p53 and RB1 genes results in their inactivation, allowing progression of cells through the cell cycle. Inactivation of these genes has been associated with malignant transformation which, in part, results in impaired control of the cell cycle.

It is known that DNA damage results in an arrest of cells in the G2 phase of the cell cycle. This 'G2 block' induced by irradiation or the cytotoxic drug etoposide, may be mediated by the inhibition of p34^{cdc-2} kinase activity. Activation of p34^{cdc-2} kinase was demonstrated by one group to be inhibited in the PC-9 human lung cancer cell line by the chemotherapy agent cisplatin. Cyclin levels were not affected by the cisplatin, but the dephosphorylation kinase was blocked by the cytotoxic drug, suggesting that the cisplatin-induced cell cycle block in G2 could involve p34^{cdc-2} as a primary target (Nishio *et al.*, 1993).

Growth fraction and cell loss

Growth fraction has been defined as a proportion of cells in a tumour population that is proliferating. Assays employing tritiated thymidine incorporated into DNA, allows estimations of the duration of cell cycle phases, from which the proportion of proliferating cells can be calculated and expressed as the 'labelling index' (Tannock, 1992). More modern techniques such as evaluating the presence of specific enzymes or antigens by flow cytometry are now employed and described as the 'S-phase fraction'. The details of the methods for both techniques are beyond the scope of this chapter, but have been well described by Tannock (1992). Typical values for the labelling index, or for the S-phase cell proportion are in the range of 3–15% for most common cancers. This rate of cell proliferation is usually less than some normal renewing tissues such as intestinal mucosa (where the labelling index ranges from 12 to 18%), although higher rates of cell proliferation may be demonstrated for some rapidly growing cancers such as high grade lymphomas.

The potential doubling time of human cancers, assuming no cell loss, ranges from 4.5 to 20 days. However, the clinical volume doubling time for most human tumours tends to be about 2 months. It is therefore felt that the rate of cell loss in many human cancers is approximately 75–90%, based on data obtained from mathematical models (Tannock, 1992).

Although proliferating cells in human cancers may cycle quickly, relatively slow tumour growth seen clinically is the result of a relatively small proportion of proliferating cells combined with a high rate of cell death. It appears that squamous cell carcinoma of the head and neck is a relatively rapidly proliferating tumour. This is consistent with clinical data revealing median doubling times to be as low as 5 days and more aggressive behaviour than that of many other common cancers (Shackney, McCormack, and Cuchural, 1978; Molinari *et al.*, 1984; Wilson *et al.*, 1988). Molinari and associates (1984), reporting their data on proliferative activity, noted a trend toward higher proliferative activity in tumours with cervical lymph node metastases. The same group found a higher relapse rate after surgery for squamous cell carcinomas of the head and neck in those patients with high proliferation rates, a finding seen by others. A higher response rate to radiotherapy is seen in those patients with fast proliferating tumours, although no statistically significant correlation with clinical outcome was possible.

A considerable amount of effort has been applied to treatment of squamous cell carcinomas of the head and neck with chemotherapy agents that affect specific areas of the cell cycle. For example, the vinca alkaloids (including vincristine and vinblastine) are very cell-cycle specific, with major cytolytic effects on proliferating cells entering M-phase through the induction of mitotic arrest, as well as in non-proliferating cells in the G1 phase. Bleomycin appears to be most active during the premitotic or G2 phase. Antimetabolites such as methotrexate and 5-fluorouracil are most active against rapidly proliferating cells, particularly during the S-phase of the cell cycle. With longer drug exposure more cells enter the target portion part of the cycle and may become sensitive to cell cycle-specific agents. For this reason, increasing interest has been shown in continuous infusion of these agents, particularly 5-fluorouracil in combination with cisplatin (an agent with less cell-cycle specificity) in combination therapy of these diseases.

Cancer: invasion and metastasis

Although haematogenous metastases develop relatively late in squamous cell carcinomas of the head and neck, distant tumour deposits are a considerable clinical problem, with cervical lymphadenopathy being a frequent feature of these diseases, and one which results in difficulties for both surgeon and radiotherapist. They also have an effect on survival. Highly aggressive malignant cells, which are highly metastatic, appear early in the development of the primary tumour (Fidler and Hart, 1982). In breast carcinoma, perhaps the best studied solid tumour, it has been calculated that most metastases are initiated and disseminated when the primary tumour has attained a volume of < 0.125 cm^3 (Liotta, Kleinerman and Saidel, 1974; Liotta and Stetler-Stevenson, 1993). If this complex and multi-step process can be abrogated, it is likely that curative therapies will result, even though cells displaying a malignant phenotype already exist.

The process of invasion from the primary tumour into the surrounding stroma, intravasation into fluid-bearing vessels, and subsequent circulation of tumour cells followed by extravasation into distant tissues, producing metastases, is a step-wise selectional process which results in the survival of a fraction of the potentially metastatic cells that exist within the primary tumour. Work by Kerbel (1990) suggests that the cells with metastatic potential are actually predominant in the primary cancer early in its development. In accordance with this observation is the finding that certain molecular markers, such as amplified oncogenes measured in the primary tumour can be correlated with the propensity to develop metastases and impair survival in patients suffering from breast cancer (McGuire *et al.*, 1990).

The development of metastases is the result of a complicated and incompletely understood set of occurrences. As cancers progress to become locally invasive, new blood vessel formation (angiogenesis) develops. These newly formed blood vessels are often defective and easily invaded; however, cancer cells also invade pre-established vessels. It appears that in some rapidly growing cancers, even those of approximately 1 cm in size (representing the normal lower limit of clinical detection) millions of cancer cells can enter the circulation daily (Liotta, Kleinerman, and Saidel, 1974). Although only a small proportion of these cells (less than 0.01%) initiate viable metastatic tumours (Liotta and Stetler-Stevenson, 1993), metastatic disease in these cancers is a virtual certainty. Entrance of cancer cells into lymphatics ultimately results in most of these cells entering the venous drainage. It appears that, for many cancers, lymphatic and haematogenous dissemination take place in parallel, and that lymph nodes do not act as an effective barrier to further disease dissemination (Liotta and Stetler-Stevenson, 1993).

Cancer cells, either in clumps, or singly along with other structures such as leucocytes, fibrin or platelets, embolize into smaller blood vessels by mechanical impaction. They can also attach to blood vessel walls, induce retraction of capillary endothelium, attach and subsequently induce local dissolution of basement membrane, and extravasate into other tissues. Once a metastasis has formed, a new vascular supply is induced, and the process may then be repeated (a metastasis can then metastasize) (Liotta and Stetler-Steven son, 1993).

Cell surface proteins and glycoproteins

Several cell surface proteins and glycoproteins have been identified and may play a role in the development of metastases. These macromolecules borne on cancer cell surfaces appear to be different from those of normal cells, with (for example) increased chain branching, and reduced mannose content. Increased sialic acid content has also been described, and Yogeeswaran (1983) noted increasing metastatic potential in several cancer cell lines with higher sialic acid content. Lectins, proteins with binding sites that interact with sugars, such as those contained on glycoproteins and glycolipids on the cell surface, may result in agglutination. It has been noted that some cancer cells which bind a particular type of lectin (L-phytohaemagglutinin) have enhanced metastatic properties (Dennis, 1988). *In vitro* treatment of these cell populations with swainsonine (a drug which in other research appears to be both an immunomodulator as well as a chemoprotectant) alters the increased branching of oligosaccharides, resulting in a consequent loss of metastatic capability. How this form of investigation will translate into clinical terms remains to be seen.

Integrins, membrane glycoproteins which can interact both with the cytoskeleton of one cell, as well as a number of ligands on other cells (such as platelets and endothelial cells), may be important in metastasis development. Integrin expression appears to be modulated by growth and differentiation factors, including transforming growth factor-β. Integrin distribution is altered in malignant cells (Hynes, 1987). Recently, short synthetic peptides which contain the specific binding sequence which recognizes integrins have been found to prevent metastasis formation by tumour cells when injected simultaneously with the cells (Humphries, Olden, and Yamada, 1986), suggesting a possible new future therapy. Other surface antigens including those of the major histocompatibility complex (MHC) are also implicated in the process, but their role in the development of the metastatic phenotype remains uncertain.

Cadherins are cell surface glycoproteins which also participate in intercellular adhesion. Cadherins are important for epithelial calcium-dependent cell-to-cell adhesion (Schipper *et al.*, 1991). One type of cadherin molecule, E-cadherin, has been demonstrated to be important in the prevention of cancer cell invasion (Frixen *et al.*, 1991). Down-regulation of the E-cadherin gene has been associated with both invasion and metastasis, and hence may provide a method to assess the invasive potential of human cancers. Schipper *et al.* (1991) demonstrated E-cadherin in well- and moderately-differentiated squamous cell carcinomas of the head and neck, but could not detect this protein in poorly-differentiated cancers. In addition, most lymph node metastases were found to have lower levels of E-cadherin regardless of the differentiation of the primary cancer. Mattijssen *et al.* (1993) found a significant inverse correlation between expression of E-cadherin and differentiation grade in laryngeal tumours, but no correlation with the stage of the cancer. Although numbers were small, 2-year disease-free survival was poorer in patients with fewer than 25% of their cancer cells staining for E-cadherin (8/16), when compared with those patients with >25% of positive cancer cells (8/9). This suggested that E-cadherin expression may be related to prognosis in laryngeal carcinoma and that the E-cadherin gene may function as an antimetastasis gene. The gene encoding E-cadherin has been localized to chromosome 16 (16q22), and this locus may represent a new tumour suppressor gene in breast cancer as well as other tumours (Field, 1992). Chromosome translocations at 16q22 have been described in two squamous cell carcinomas of the head and neck (Owens *et al.*, 1992); correlation with E-cadherin expression will be an interesting subject for further study.

Oncogenes and metastasis genes

Oncogenes appear to play a central role in the development of the metastatic phenotype. Transfec-

tion studies employing *ras* genes, particularly the H-*ras* oncogene, can induce metastatic properties in some cells (Chambers and Tuck, 1993), with rising levels of the *ras* protein product (p21^{ras}) being correlated with metastatic capability. Expression of the *ras* oncogene can cause several changes in cells, including increased secretion of metalloproteinases (type IV collagenases) and cysteine proteinases (such as cathepsin L), and decreased expression of inhibitors of metalloproteinases and cysteine proteinases (tissue inhibitors of metalloproteinases, or TIMPs and cystatins, respectively). Several other genes, including the E-cadherin gene noted above, appear to be related to the prevention of metastases. The prototype of these antimetastasis genes is the *nm23* gene described by Steeg *et al.* (1988). Low expression of the gene product is associated with enhanced metastatic potential, suggesting that the *nm23* gene may be a metastasis suppressor gene. The protein product appears to function as a nucleoside disphosphate kinase that probably participates in signalling pathways within the cell (Liotta and Steeg, 1990). Recent data suggest that phosphorylation of the *nm23* protein, rather than its kinase activity, is correlated with the development of metastatic capability, and this may be important in the suppression of the anti-metastatic capabilities attributed to the *nm23* gene (MacDonald *et al.*, 1993). Recently, two squamous cell carcinomas of the head and neck tumour lines were evaluated for *nm23* gene mutations. In these two lines, it did not appear that *nm23* allelic deletion resulted in these tumour lines' biological behaviour (Chen, Shuler, and Milo, 1992).

One potential practical aspect of research into the development of metastases is the development of potential agents to interrupt the process. Carboxyamidotriazole (CAI,L651582) is a synthetic compound which inhibits calcium influx and certain calcium-regulated signal effector systems including receptor-associated tyrosine kinases (Kohn and Liotta, 1990). This agent has inhibited growth in colony formation in *in vitro* tumour lines. When administered to mice bearing human cancer xenografts, it reduced tumour incidence and retarded primary tumour growth and growth of established metastatic tumours as well as tumour cell motility and adhesion (Kohn, Sandeen, and Liotta, 1992). This agent is now undergoing phase I clinical trials, without producing undue toxicity thus far (Kohn *et al.*, 1993). Further clinical work will be required in order to determine whether this agent represents a useful adjunct in the treatment of metastatic and pre-metastatic human malignancies.

Conclusions

The subject of cancer biology is a varied, wide ranging, complex, highly interrelated topic. It is now proving to be an indispensable foundation upon which novel anticancer treatments are based. However, basic science data describing discoveries in squamous cell carcinomas of the head and neck are still coming slowly compared with many other cancer types: as well, sample sizes are often modest, requiring cautious interpretation of reports. Nevertheless, the basic science of oncology is becoming increasingly relevant to the practice of head and neck oncology, and further progress is likely to bear significant therapeutic fruit in the next decade.

References

ALMOGUERA, C., SHIBATA, D., FORRESTER, K., MARTIN, J., ARN-HEIM, N. and PERUCHO, M. (1988) Most human carcinomas of the exocrine pancreas contain mutant c-K-ras genes. *Cell*, **53**, 549–554

BASELGA, J., NORTON, L., MASUI, H., PANDIELLA, A., COPLAN, K., MILLER, W. H. JR *et al.* (1993) Antitumour effects of doxorubicin in combination with anti-epidermal growth factor receptor monoclonal antibodies. *Journal of the National Cancer Institute*, **85**, 1327–1333

BENCHIMOL, S. (1992) Viruses and Cancer. In: *The Basic Science of Oncology*, 2nd edn, edited by I. F. Tannock and R. P. Hill. New York: McGraw-Hill. pp. 88–101

BERENSON, J. R., YANG, J. and MICKEL, R. (1989) Frequent amplification of the bcl-1 locus in head and neck squamous cell carcinomas. *Oncogene*, **4**, 1111–1116

BISHOP, J. M. (1991) Molecular themes in oncogenesis. *Cell*, **64**, 235–248

BORROW, J., GODDARD, A. D., SHEER, D. and SOLOMON, E. (1990) Molecular analysis of acute promyelocytic leukemia breakpoint cluster region on chromosome 17. *Science*, **249**, 1577–1580

BRACHMAN, D. G., GRAVES, D., VOKES, E., BECKETT, M., HARAF, D., MONTAG, A. *et al.* (1992) Occurrence of *p53* gene deletions and human papilloma virus infection in human head and neck cancer. *Cancer Research*, **52**, 4832–4836

BRACHMANN, R., LINDQUIST, P. B., NAGASHIMA, M., KOHR, W., LIPARI, T. NAPIER, M. *et al.* (1989) Transmembrane TGF-α precursors activate EGF/TGF-α receptors. *Cell*, **56**, 691–700

BUICK, R. N. and TANNOCK, I. F. (1992) Properties of malignant cells. In: *The Basic Science of Oncology*, 2nd edn, edited by I. F. Tannock and R. P. Hill. New York: McGraw-Hill. pp. 139–153

CAMPBELL, L., BROWN, J., GARSON, O. M. and MORSTYN, G. (1989) Cytogenetic abnormalities in lung cancer. In: *Basic and Clinical Concepts of Lung Cancer*, edited by H. Hansen. Boston: Kluwer Academic Press. pp. 123–136

CANTLEY, L. C., AUGER, K. R., CARPENTER, C., DUCKWORTH, B., GRAZIANI, A., KAPELLER, R. *et al.* (1991) Oncogenes and signal transduction. *Cell*, **64**, 281–302

CAREY, T. E., VAN DYKE, D. L., WORSHAM, M. J., BRADFORD, C. R., BABU, V. R., SCHWARZ, D. R. *et al.* (1989) Characterization of human laryngeal primary and metastatic squamous cell carcinoma lines UM-SCC-17A and UM-SCC-17B. *Cancer Research*, **49**, 6098–6107

CHAMBERS, A. F. and TUCK, A. B. (1993) *Ras*-responsive genes and tumour metastasis. *Critical Reviews in Oncogenesis*, **4**, 95–114

CHEN, J. C., SHULER, C. F. and MILO, G. E. (1992) *NM23* in

human squamous cell carcinoma of the head and neck. *Proceedings of the American Association for Cancer Research*, **33**, A1079

CHUNG, K. Y., MUKHOPADHYAY, T., KIM, J., CASSON, A., RO, J. Y., GOEPFERT, H. *et al.* (1993) Discordant p53 gene mutations in primary head and neck cancers and corresponding second primary cancers of the upper aerodigestive tract. *Cancer Research*, **53**, 1676–1683

COOPER, G. M. (1990) *Oncogenes*. Boston: Jones and Bartlett

COOPER, J. A. and WHYTE, P. (1989) RBs and the cell cycle: entrance or exit? *Cell*, **58**, 1009–1011.

COUTURIER, J., SATRE GARAU, X., SCHEIDER MOUNOURY, S., LABIB, A. and ORTH, G. (1991) Integration of papilloma virus DNA near myc genes in genital carcinomas and its consequences for proto-oncogene expression. *Journal of Virology*, **65**, 4534–4538

CROOK, T., WREDE, D., TIDY, J., SCHOLEFIELD, J., CRAWFORD, L. and VOUSDEN, K. H. (1991) Status of c-myc p53 and retinoblastoma genes in human papilloma virus positive and negative squamous cell carcinomas of the anus. *Oncogene*, **6**, 1251–1257

CROSS, M. and DEXTER, T. M. (1991) Growth factors in development, transformation, and tumourigenesis. *Cell*, **64**, 271–280

DE KLEIN, A., VAN KESSEL, A. G., GROSVELD, G., BARTRAM, C. R., HAGEMEIER, A., BOOTSMA, D. *et al.* (1982) A cellular oncogene is translocated to the Philadelphia chromosome in chronic myelocytic leukemia. *Nature*, **300**, 765–767

DENNIS, J. W. (1988) Asn-linked oligosaccharide processing and malignant potential. *Cancer Surveys*, **7**, 573–595

DERYNCK, R., GOEDDEL, D. V., ULLRICH, A., GUTTERMAN, J. U., WILLIAMS, R. D., BRINGMAN, T. S. *et al.* (1987) Synthesis of messenger RNAs for transforming growth factors alpha and beta, and epidermal growth factor receptor by human tumours. *Cancer Research*, **47**, 707–712

DE THE, H., CHOMIENNE, C., LANOTTE, M., DEGOS, L. and DEJEAN, A. (1990) The t(15;17) translocation of acute promyelocytic leukemia fuses the retinoic acid receptor a gene to a novel transcribed locus. *Nature*, **347**, 558–561

DEUEL, T. F. (1987) Polypeptide growth factors: roles in normal and abnormal cell growth. *Annual Review of Cell Biology*, **3**, 443–492

DI MARCO, E., PIERCE, J. H., FLEMING, T. P., KRAUS, M. H., MOLLOY, C. J., AARONSON, S. A. *et al.* (1989) Autocrine interaction between TGF-α and EGF-receptor: quantitative requirements for induction of the malignant phenotype. *Oncogene*, **4**, 831–838

DRAETTA, G. (1990) Cell cycle control in eukaryotes: molecular mechanisms of *cdc2* activation. *Trends in Biochemical Science*, **15**, 378–383

EL-NAGGAR, A. K., LEE, M-S., WANG, G., LUNA, M. A., GOEPFERT, H. and BATSAKIS, J. G. (1993) Polymerase chain reaction-based restriction fragment link polymorphism analysis of the short arm of chromosome 3 in primary head and neck squamous carcinoma. *Cancer*, **72**, 881–886

EVERSOLE, L. R. and SAPP, J. P. (1993) C-myc oncoprotein expression in oral precancerous and early cancerous lesions. *Oral Oncology, European Journal of Cancer*, **29B**, 131–135

FIDLER, I. J. and HART, I. R. (1982) Biologic diversity in metastatic neoplasms – origins and implications. *Science*, **217**, 998–1001

FIELD, J. K. (1992) Oncogenes in tumour-suppressor genes in squamous cell carcinoma of the head and neck. *Oral Oncology, European Journal of Cancer*, **28B**, 67–76

FIELD, J. K., SPANDIDOS, D. A. and STELL, P. M. (1992) Overexpression of the p53 gene in head and neck cancer, linked with heavy smoking and drinking (letter). *Lancet*, i, 502–503

FIELD, J. K., SPANDIDOS, D. A., STELL, P. M., VAUGHAN, E. D., EVAN, G. I. and MOORE, J. P. (1989) Elevated expression of the c-*myc* oncoprotein correlates with poor prognosis in head and neck squamous cell carcinoma. *Oncogene*, 4, 1463–1468

FIELD, J. K., SPANDIDOS, D. A., MALLIRI, A., GOSNEY, J. R., YIAGNISIS, M. and STELL, P. M. (1991) Elevated p53 expression correlates with a history of heavy smoking and squamous cell carcinoma of the head and neck. *British Journal of Cancer*, 64, 573–577

FIELD, J. K., SPANDIDOS, D. A. YIAGNISIS, M., GOSNEY, J. R., PAPADIMIRIOU, K. and STELL, P. M. (1992a) C-erb-2 expression in squamous cell carcinoma of the head and neck. *Anticancer Research*, 12, 613–619

FIELD, J. K., YIAGNISIS, M. SPANDIDOS, D. A., GOSNEY, J. R., PAPADIMITRIOU, K., VAUGHAN, E. D. *et al.* (1992b) Low levels of rasp21 oncogene expression correlates with the clinical outcome in head and neck squamous cell carcinoma. *European Journal of Surgical Oncology*, 18, 168–176

FRIXEN, U., BEHRENS, J., SACHS, M., EBERLE, G., VOSS, B., WARDA, A. *et al.* (1991) E-cadherin-mediated cell-cell adhesion prevents invasiveness of human carcinoma cell. *Journal of Cell Biology*, 113, 173–185

GIBBS, J. B., SIGAL, I. S., POE, M. and SCOLNICK, E. M. (1984) Intrinsic GTPase activity distinguishes normal and oncogenic ras p21 molecules. *Proceedings of the National Academy of Sciences of the United States of America*, 81, 5704–5708

GRANDIS, J. R. and TWEARDY, D. J. (1993) Elevated levels of transforming growth factor alpha and epidermal growth factor receptor messenger RNA are early markers of carcinogenesis in head and neck cancer. *Cancer Research*, 53, 3579–3584

GRAZIADEI, L., RIABOWOL, K. and BAR-SAGI, D. (1990) Co-capping of *ras* proteins with surface immunoglobulins in B lymphocytes. *Nature*, 347, 396–400

GUSTERSON, B. A., ANBAZHAGAN, R., WARREN, W., MIDGELY, C., LANE, D. P., O'HARE, M. *et al.* (1991) Expression of p53 in premalignant and malignant squamous epithelium. *Oncogene*, 6, 1785–1789

HARRIS, C. C. (1991) Chemical and physical carcinogenesis: Advances and perspectives for the 1990's. *Cancer Research*, 51, 5023s–5044s

HOWLEY, P. M. (1993) Principles of carcinogenesis: viral. In: *Cancer: Principles and Practice of Oncology*, 4th edn, edited by V. T. DeVita Jr., S. Hellman and S. A. Rosenberg. Philadelphia: J. B. Lippincott. pp. 182–199

HUANG, M. E., YE, Y. C., CHEN, S. R., CHAI, J. R., LU, J. X., ZHOA, L. *et al.* (1988) Use of all-*trans* retinoic acid in the treatment of acute promyelocytic leukemia. *Blood*, 72, 567–572

HUMPHRIES, M. J., OLDEN, K. and YAMADA, K. M. (1986) A synthetic peptide from fibronectin inhibits experimental metastasis of murine melanoma cells. *Science*, 233, 467–470

HUNTER, T. (1987) A thousand and one protein kinases. *Cell*, 50, 823–829

HUNTER, T. (1991) Cooperation between oncogenes. *Cell*, 64, 249–270

HYNES, R. O. (1987) Integrins: a family of cell surface receptors. *Cell*, 48, 459–555

IGGO, R., GATTER, K., BARTEK, J., LANE, D. and HARRIS, A. L. (1990) Increased expression of mutant forms of p53 oncogene in primary lung cancer. *Lancet*, i, 675–679

ISHITOYA, J., TORIYAMA, M., OGUCHI, N., KITAMURA, K., OHSHIMA, M., ASANO, K. *et al.* (1989) Gene amplification and over-expression of the EGF receptor in squamous cell carcinomas of the head and neck. *British Journal of Cancer*, 59, 559–562

JIN, Y., HEIM, S., MANDAHL, N., BIORKLUND, A., WENNERBURG, J. and MITELMAN, F. (1990) Multiple clonal chromosome abberations in squamous cell carcinomas of the larynx. *Cancer Genetics and Cytogenetics*, 44, 209–216

KAO-SHAN, C. S., FINE, R. L., WHANG-PENG, J., LEE, E. C. and CHABNER, B. A. (1987) Increased fragile sites and sister chromatid exchanges in bone marrow and peripheral blood of young cigarette smokers. *Cancer Research*, 47, 6278–6282

KERBEL, R. S. (1990) Growth dominance of the metastatic cancer cell: cellular and molecular aspects. *Advances in Cancer Research*, 55, 87–131

KIKKAWA, U., KISHIMOTO, A. and NISHIZUKA, Y. (1989) The protein kinase C family: heterogeneity and its implications. *Annual Review of Biochemistry*, 58, 31–44

KIRSCHNER, M. W. (1992) The biochemical nature of the cell cycle. In: *Important Advances in Oncology 1992*, edited by V. T. DeVita Jr., S. Hellman and S. A. Rosenberg. Philadelphia: J. B. Lippincott. pp. 3–60

KNUDSON, A. G. (1971) Mutation and cancer: statistical study of retinoblastoma. *Proceedings of the National Academy of Sciences of the United States of America*, 68, 820–823

KOHN, E. C. and LIOTTA, L. A. (1990) L651582: A novel antiproliferative and metastasis agent. *Journal of the National Cancer Institute*, 82, 54–60

KOHN, E. C., SANDEEN, A. M. and LIOTTA. L. A. (1992) *In vivo* efficacy of a novel inhibitor of selected signal transduction pathways including calcium, arachidonate and inositol phosphates. *Cancer Research*, 52, 3208–3212

KOHN, E. C., FELDER, C., DAY, A., FREER, R. and LIOTTA, L. A. (1993) Signal transduction therapy of metastasis. *Proceedings of the American Association for Cancer Research*, 34, 570–571

KOVACS, G. and FRISCH, S. (1989) Clonal chromosome abnormalities in tumour cells from patients with sporadic renal cell carcinomas. *Cancer Research*, 49, 651–659

LAMMIE, G. A. and PETERS, G. (1991) Chromosome 11q13 abnormalities in human cancer. *Cancer Cells*, 3, 1–8

LANGDON, J. D. and PARTRIDGE, M. (1992) Expression of the tumour suppressor gene p53 in oral cancer. *British Journal of Oral and Maxillofacial Surgery*, 30, 214–220

LATIF, F., FIVASH, M., GLENN, G., TORY, K., ORCUTT, M. L., HAMPSCH, K. *et al.* (1992) Chromosome 3p deletions in head and neck carcinomas: statistical ascertainment of allelic loss. *Cancer Research*, 52, 1451–1456

LEE, M. G. and NURSE, P. (1987) Complementation used to clone a human homologue of the fission yeast cell cycle control gene cdc2. *Nature*, 327, 31–35

LEE, R-M., RAPP, U. R. and BLACKSHEAR, P. J. (1991) Evidence for one or more Raf-1 kinase(s) activated by insulin and polypeptide growth factors. *Journal of Biological Chemistry*, 266, 10351–10357

LEONARD, J. H., KEARSLEY, J. H., CHENEVIX-TRENCH, G. and HAYWARD, N. K. (1991) Analysis of gene amplification in head and neck squamous cell carcinomas. *International Journal of Cancer*, 48, 511–515

LEVINE, A. J. (1990) Tumour suppressor genes. *BioEssays*, 12, 60–66

LEVINE, A. J., MOMAND, J. and FINLAY, C. A. (1991) The p53 tumour suppressor gene. *Nature*, **351**, 453–456

LEWIN, B. (1991) Oncogenic conversion by regulatory changes in transcription factors. *Cell*, **64**, 303–312

LIOTTA, L., KLEINERMAN, J. and SAIDEL, G. (1974) Quantitative relationships of intravascular tumour cells, tumour vessels and pulmonary metastases following tumour implantation. *Cancer Research*, **34**, 997–1004

LIOTTA, L. A. and STEEG, P. S. (1990) Clues to the function of the *n23* and *awd* proteins in development, signal transduction and tumour metastasis. Provided by studies of *Dictyostelium* and *Discoideum*. *Journal of the National Cancer Institute*, **82**, 1170–1172

LIOTTA, L. A. and STETLER-STEVENSON, W. G. (1993) Principles of molecular cell biology of cancer: cancer metastases. In: *Cancer: Principles and Practice of Oncology*, 4th edn, edited by V. T. DeVita Jr., S. Hellman and S. A. Rosenberg. Philadelphia: J. B. Lippincott. pp. 134–149

LIPPMAN, S. M. and HONG, W. K. (1993) Not yet standard: retinoids versus second primary tumours. *Journal of Clinical Oncology*, **11**, 1204–1207

MCCORMICK, F. (1989) *Ras* GTPase activating protein: signal transmitter and signal terminator. *Cell*, **56**, 5–8

MACDONALD, N. J., DE LA ROSA, A., BENEDICT, M. A., PEREZ FREIJE, J. M. and STEEG, P. S. (1993) A novel phosphorylation of *nm23*, and not its NDPK activity correlates with metastatic potential. *Proceedings of the American Association for Cancer Research*, **34**, A393

MCGUIRE, W. L., TANDON, A. K., ALLRED, D. C., CHAMNESS, G. C. and CLARK, G. M. (1990) How to use prognostic factors in axillary node negative breast cancer patients. *Journal of the National Cancer Institute*, **82**, 1006–1015

MALKIN, D., LI, F. P., STRONG, L. C., FRAUMENI, J. F. JR., NELSON, C. E., KIM, D. H. *et al.* (1990) Germ line p53 mutations in a familial syndrome of breast cancer, sarcomas, and other neoplasms. *Science*, **250**, 1233–1238

MASUI, Y. and MARKERT, C. (1971) Cytoplasmic control of nuclear behaviour during meiotic maturation of frog oocytes. *Journal of Experimental Zoology*, **177**, 129–146

MATTIJSSEN, V., PETERS, H., SCHALKWIJK, L., MANNI, J. J., DE MULDER, P. H. and RUITER, D. J. (1993) E-cadherin expression in head and neck squamous cell carcinoma. *Proceedings of the American Association for Cancer Research*, **34**, 32

MENDELSOHN, J. and LIPPMAN, M. E. (1993) Principles in molecular cell biology of cancer: growth factors. In: *Cancer: Principles and Practice of Oncology*, 4th edn, edited by V. T. DeVita Jr., S. Hellman and S. A. Rosenberg. Philadelphia: J. B. Lippincott. pp. 114–133

MERRITT, W. D., WEISSLER, M. C., TURK, B. F. and GILMER, T. N. (1990) Oncogene amplification in squamous cell carcinoma of the head and neck. *Archives of Otolaryngology and Head and Neck Surgery*, **116**, 1394–1398

MINDEN, M. D. and PAWSON, A. J. (1992) Oncogenes. In: *The Basic Science of Oncology*, 2nd edn, edited by I. F. Tannock and R. P. Hill. New York: McGraw-Hill. pp. 61–87

MITELMAN, F. (1991) *Catalogue of Chromosome Aberrations in Cancer*, 4th edn. New York: Wiley-Liss

MOLINARI, R., COSTA, A., SILVESTRINI, R., MATTAVELLI, F., CANTU, G. and CHIESA, F. (1984) Cell kinetics in the study and treatment of head and neck cancer. In: *Head and Neck Oncology*, edited by G. T. Wolfe Boston: Martinus, Nijhoff. pp. 229–248

NISHIO, J., OHMORI, T., FUJIWARA, T. *et al.* (1993) Cis-diamminedichloroplatinum (II) inhibits dephosphorylation of the cdc2 kinase in human lung cancer cells. *Proceedings of the American Association for Cancer Research*, **34**, 398

OWENS, W., FIELD, J. K., HOWARD, P. J. and STELL, P. M. (1992) Multiple cytogenetic aberrations in squamous cell carcinomas of the head and neck. *Oral Oncology, European Journal of Cancer*, **28B**, 17–21

PARDEE, A. B. (1989) G_1 events and regulation of cell proliferation. *Science*, **246**, 603–608

PERKINS, A. S. and VANDE WOUDE, G. F. (1993) Principles of molecular cell biology of cancer: oncogenes. In: *Cancer: Principles and Practice of Oncology*, 4th edition, edited by V. T. DeVita, Jr., S. Hellmann and S. A. Rosenberg. Philadelphia: J. B. Lippincott. pp. 35–59

PITOT, H. C. (1993) The molecular biology of carcinogenesis. *Cancer*, **72**, 962–970

RODENHUIS, S., VAN DE WETERING, M. L., MOOI, W. J., EVERS, S. G., VAN ZANDWIJK, N. and BOS, J. L. (1987) Mutational activation of the K-RAS oncogene: a possible pathogenic factor in adenocarcinoma of the lung. *New England Journal of Medicine*, **317**, 929–937

ROSENTHAL, A., LINDQUIST, P. B., BRINGMAN, T. S., GOEDDEL, D. V. and DERYNCK, R. (1986) Expression in rat fibroblasts of a human transforming growth factor-alpha cDNA results in transformation. *Cell*, **46**, 301–309

ROUS, P. (1911) A sarcoma of fowl transmissible by an agent separable from the tumor cells. *Journal of Experimental Medicine*, **13**, 397–411

ROUSSEL, M. F., DOWNING, J. R., RETTENMIER, C. W. SHERR, C. J. (1988) A point mutation in the extracellular domain of the human CSF-1 receptor (C-fms proto-oncogene product) activates its transforming potential. *Cell*, **55**, 979–988

ROWLEY, J. D. (1973) A new consistent chromosomal abnormality in chronic myelogenous leukemia. *Nature*, **243**, 290–293

ROWLEY, J. D. and POTTER, D. (1976) Chromosomal banding patterns in acute non-lymphocytic leukemia. *Blood*, **47**, 705–721

ROWLEY, J. D. and MITELMAN, F. (1993) Principles of molecular biology of cancer: chromosome abnormalities in human cancer in leukemia. In: *Cancer: Principles and Practice of Oncology*, 4th edn, edited by V. T. DeVita, Jr., S. Hellman and S. A. Rosenberg. Philadelphia: J. B. Lippincott. pp. 67–91

RUDDON, R. W. (1987) *Cancer Biology*, 2nd edn. New York: Oxford University Press

SACKS, P. G., PARNES, S. M., GALLICK, G. E., MANSOURI, Z., LICHTNER, R., SATYA-PRAKASH, K. L. *et al.* (1988) Establishment and characterization of two new squamous cell carcinoma cell lines derived from tumours of the head and neck. *Cancer Research*, **48**, 2858–2866

SAKAI, E. and TSUCHIDA, N. (1992) Most human squamous cell carcinomas in the oral cavity contain mutated p53 tumour-suppressor genes. *Oncogene*, **7**, 929–933

SAKAI, E., RIKIMARU, K., UEDA, M., MATSUMOTO, Y., ISHII, N., ENOMOTO, S. *et al.* (1992) The p53 tumour-suppressor gene and *ras* oncogene mutations in oral squamous-cell carcinoma. *International Journal of Cancer*, **52**, 867–872

SANTINI, J., FORMENTO, J-L., FRANCOUAL, M., MILANO, G., SCHNEIDER, M., DASSONVILLE, O. *et al.* (1991) Characterization, quantification, and potential clinical value of the epidermal growth factor receptor in head and neck squamous cell carcinomas. *Head and Neck*, **13**, 132–139

SARANATH, D., PANCHAL, R. G., NAIR, R., MEHTA, A. R., SANGHAVI, V., SUMEGI, J. *et al.* (1989) Oncogene amplification in squamous cell carcinoma of the oral cavity. *Japanese Journal of Cancer Research*, **80**, 430–437

SARANATH, D., CHANG, S. E., BHOITE, L. T., PANCHAL, R. G., KERR, I. B., MEHTA, A. R. *et al.* (1991) High frequency mutations in codons 12 and 61 of H-ras oncogene in chewing tobacco-related human oral carcinoma in India. *British Journal of Cancer*, **63**, 573–578

SCAMBIA, G., PANICI, P. B., BATTAGLIA, F., FERRANDINA, G., ALMADORI, G., PALUDETTI, G. *et al.* (1991) Receptors for epidermal growth factor in steroid hormones in primary laryngeal tumours. *Cancer*, **67**, 1347–1351

SCHIPPER, J. J., FRIXEN, U. H., BEHRENS, J., UNGER, A., JAHNKE, K. and BIRCHMEIER, W. (1991) E-cadherin expression in squamous cell carcinomas of the head and neck: inverse correlation with tumour de-differentiation and lymph node metastasis. *Cancer Research*, **51**, 6328–6337

SCHREIBER, A. B., WINKLER, M. E. and DERYNCK, R. (1986) Transforming growth factor alpha: a more potent angiogenic mediator that epidermal growth factor. *Science*, **232**, 1250–1253

SCULLY, C., COX, M. F., PRIME, S. S. and MAITLAND, N. J. (1988) Papilloma viruses: the current status in relation to oral disease. *Oral Surgery, Oral Medicine and Oral Pathology*, **65**, 526–532

SEN, P., SRIVATSAN, E. S., TAYLOR, D. and GOEPFERT, H. (1993) Cytogenetic alterations and allele loss in chromosome 11q and 18q in squamous cell carcinoma of the head and neck (SCCHN). *Proceedings of the American Association for Cancer Research*, **34**, 129

SETH, A. and PAPAS, T. S. (1993) Principles of molecular cell biology of cancer: general aspects of gene regulation. In: *Cancer: Principles and Practice of Oncology*, 4th edn, edited by V. T. De Vita, Jr., S. Hellman and S. A. Rosenberg. Philadelphia: J. B. Lippincott. pp. 23–34

SHACKNEY, S. E., MCCORMACK, G. W., and CUCHURAL, G. J. JR (1978) Growth rate patterns of solid tumours and their relation to responsiveness to therapy: an analytic review. *Annals of Internal Medicine*, **78** 107–121

SHENG, Z. M., BARROIS, M., KLIJANIENKO, J., MICHEAU, C., RICHARD, J. M. and RIOU, G. (1990) Analysis of the c-Ha-ras-1 gene for deletion, mutation, amplification and expression in lymph node metastases of human head and neck carcinomas. *British Journal of Cancer*, **62**, 398–444

SIGAL, I. S. (1988) The ras oncogene-a structure and some function. *Nature*, **332**, 485–486

SMITH, L. D. and ECKER, R. E. (1970) Regulatory processes in the maturation and early cleavage of amphibian eggs. *Current Topics in Developmental Biology*, **5**, 1–38

SNIJDERS, P. F. J., CROMME, F. V., VAN DE BRULE, A. J. C., SCHRIJNEMAKERS, H. F., SNOW, G. B., MEIJER, C. J. *et al.* (1992) Prevalence of expression of human papillomavirus in tonsillar carcinomas indicates a possible viral etiology. *International Journal of Cancer*, **51**, 845–850

SOMERS, K. D., CARTWRIGHT, S. L. and SCHECHTER, G. L. (1990) Amplification of the int-2 gene in human head and neck squamous cell carcinomas. *Oncogene*, **5**, 915–920

SOZZI, G., MIOZZO, M., DONGHI, R., PILOTTI, S., CARIANI, C. T., PASTORINO, U. *et al.* (1992) Deletions of 17p and p53 mutations in preneoplastic lesions of the lung. *Cancer Research*, **52**, 6079–6082

SQUIRE, J. and PHILLIPS, R. A. (1992) Genetic basis of cancer. In: *The Basic Science of Oncology*, 2nd edn, edited by I. F. Tannock and R. P. Hill. New York: McGraw-Hill. pp. 41–60

STEEG, P. S., BEVLIACQUA, G., KOPPER, L., THORGEIRSSON, U. P.,

TALMADGE, J. E., LIOTTA, L. A. *et al.* (1988) Evidence for a novel gene associated with low tumour metastatic potential. *Journal of the National Cancer Institute*, **80**, 200–204

STEHELIN, D., VARMUS, H. E., BISHOP, J. M., and VOGT, P. K. (1989) DNA related to the transforming gene(s) of avian sarcoma viruses is present in normal avian DNA. *Nature*, **260**, 170–173

TANNOCK, I. F. (1992) Cell proliferation. In: *The Basic Science of Oncology*, edited by I. F. Tannock and R. P. Hill. New York: McGraw-Hill. pp. 154–177

THOMPSON, L. M. (1989) Somatic cell genetic approach to dissecting mammalian DNA repair. *Environmental and Molecular Mutagenesis*, **14**, 264–281

TROPPMAIR, J., BRUDER, J. T., APP, H., CAI, H., LIPTAK, L., SZEBERENYI, J. *et al.* (1992) RAS controls coupling of growth factor receptors in protein kinase C in the membrane to Raf-1 and B-Ras protein serine kinases in the cytosol. *Oncogene*, **7**, 1867–1873

TSUTSUMI, M., SAKAMOTO, H., YOSHIDA, T., KAKIZOE, T., KOISO, K., SUGIMURA, T. *et al.* (1988) Coamplification of the hst- 1 and int-2 genes in human cancers. *Japanese Journal of Cancer Research*, **79**, 428–432

VOGELSTEIN, B., FEARON, E. R., HAMILTON, S. R., KERN, S. E., PREISINGER, A. C., LEPPERT, M. *et al.* (1988) Genetic alternations during colorectal-tumour development. *New England Journal of Medicine*, **319**, 525–532

WAINSCOAT, J. S. and FEY, M. F. (1990) Assessment of clonality in human tumours: a review. *Cancer Research*, **50**, 1355–1360

WATERFIELD, M. D., SCRACE, G. T., WHITTLE, N., STROOBANT, P., JOHNSSON, A., WASTESON, A. *et al.* (1983) Platelet-derived growth factor is structurally related to putative transforming protein p28sis of simian sarcoma virus. *Nature*, **304**, 35–39

WATLING, D. L., GOWN, A. M. and COLTRERA, M. D. (1992) Over-expression of P53 in head and neck cancer. *Head and Neck*, **14**, 437–444

WELLS, A., WELSH, J. B., LAZAR, C. S., WILEY, H. S., GILL, G. N. and ROSENFIELD, M. G. (1990) Ligand-induced transformation by a non-internalizing epidermal growth factor receptor. *Science*, **247**, 962–964

WILSON, G. D., MCNALLY, N. J., DISCHE, E. S., SAUNDERS, M. I., DES ROCHERS, C., LEWIS, A. A. *et al.* (1988) Measurement of cell kinetics in human tumours *in vivo* using bromodeoxyuridine incorporation in flow cytometry. *British Journal of Cancer*, **58**, 423–431

WONG, D. T. W. (1993) GF$\beta\alpha$ and oral carcinogenesis. *Oral Oncology, European Journal of Cancer*, **29B**, 3–7

XIONG, Y., CONNOLLY, T., FUTCHER, B. and BEACH, D. (1991) Human D-type cyclin. *Cell*, **65**, 691–699

YAMAMOTO, T., IKAWA, S., AKIYAMA, T., SEMBA, K., NOMURA, N., MIYAJIMA, N. *et al.* (1986) Similarity of protein encoded by the human c-erb B-2 gene to epidermal growth factor receptor. *Nature*, **319**, 230–234

YOGEESWARAN, G. (1983) Cell surface glycolipids and glycoproteins in malignant transformation. *Advances in Cancer Research*, **38**, 289–350

YONEDA, T., ALSINA, M. M., WATATANI, K., BELLOT, F., SCHLESSINGER, J. and MUNDY, G. R. (1991a) Dependence of a human squamous cell carcinoma and associated paraneoplastic syndromes on the epidermal growth factor receptor pathway in nude mice. *Cancer Research*, **51**, 2438–2443

YONEDA, T., AUFDEMORTE, T. B., NISHIMURA, R., NISHIKAWA, N., SAKUDA, M., ALSINA, M. M. *et al.* (1991b) Occurrence of hypercalcemia and leukocytosis with cachexia in a human squamous cell carcinoma in maxilla in athymic nude mice: a novel experimental model of three concomitant paraneoplastic syndromes. *Journal of Clinical Oncology*, **9**, 468–477

ZHOU, D. J., CASEY, G. and LINE, M. J. (1988) Amplification of the *int*-2 in breast cancers and squamous carcinomas. *Oncogene*, **2**, 279–282

21

The principles of radiotherapy in head and neck cancer

Margaret F. Spittle

In an attempt to produce some improvement in survival and quality of life of patients, modern cancer management is multidisciplinary. It is particularly important in the head and neck region that those with a knowledge of surgery, radiotherapy, and chemotherapy should be intimately aware of the indications for other methods of treatment together with their potential advantages and disadvantages. It is by combining roles, not always in an intuitive manner, that small improvements may be seen in the management of such patients. The most important time for multidisciplinary review of management is when the patient first presents so that the sequencing, timing, and type of treatment which is most beneficial to the patient, can be optimal. As in most cancer treatments, it is the initial management programme for patients with head and neck malignancies that is the most likely to have a successful outcome. Subsequent attacks on recurrent disease are much less likely to be attended by success.

Patients with head and neck cancer should be seen in joint clinics where radiology and pathology can be demonstrated and reviewed, where the help of a dentist, speech therapist, dietitian, social worker, and counsellor is available. Fortunately combined clinics for head and neck cancer have been long-established and should be found in every large centre. Patients should be referred to these centres for advice and treatment. Only in this way is it possible to provide a concentrated range of expertise, a research base for improvement and development of cancer management where randomized control trials of treatment can be undertaken so that the outlook for patients with these diseases might be improved. Notwithstanding this, surgery, radiotherapy, and chemotherapy are taken to the limit of their toxicities in the management of patients with head and neck cancers. Knowledge of the management of combined toxicities, e.g.

avoiding toxicity of a less effective mode of therapy which prevents the full impact of a more effective treatment, is important expertise which only comes from multidisciplinary management.

Roentgen discovered X-rays in 1895 (Roentgen, 1931) and they were quickly brought into use for the treatment of cancer. Initially radiotherapy developed on an empirical basis but has subsequently benefited from developments in radiobiology, some of which were accelerated by military strategy in the world wars. Surgeons specializing and operating on patients with head and neck cancer must be completely conversant with the effects, both acute and chronic, of high dose radiotherapy and chemotherapy and be aware of the different forms of toxicity, tissue change and morbidity, associated with different treatment machines and field arrangements. In this chapter the types of radiation are discussed in the context of their particular application to specific areas of head and neck cancer management.

Types of radiation therapy

Orthovoltage

This is the most basic form of radiotherapy treatment and is rarely used now in the management of head and neck cancers. X-rays are produced when electrons are suddenly decelerated. Orthovoltage machines produce X-rays with energy below one million electron volts. As this form of radiation penetrates poorly, it is useful for superficial lesions, particularly skin tumours; but when used for other lesions, orthovoltage X-rays have the disadvantage that the maximum dose is on the surface of the skin. Skin tolerance is usually the limiting factor and may prevent adequate treatment of a lesion lying at a significant depth. The radiobiological efficiency of orthovoltage radiation is higher than that of supervoltage radiation. The unit of radiation is the Gray (Gy). One Gray of orthovoltage radiation produces the same biological effect as 1.15 Gy of supervoltage irradiation. However, because of photoelectric absorption there is a disproportionately increased absorption in bone and tissues of high density with low voltage radiation. The radiation energy is absorbed in proportion to the cube of the atomic number of the absorbing material. In the early days of radiation these machines were, by necessity, used for the treatment of advanced head and neck cancers and as a result bone and cartilage necrosis often developed. Radionecrosis of bone and cartilage is rarely seen today with modern supervoltage treatment.

Supervoltage

This type of radiation is most frequently used to treat head and neck cancers. The advantages are greater penetration, skin sparing and relatively homogeneous dose distribution (Meredith and Massey, 1968). All super voltage beams have a skin sparing effect due to forward scatter of their energy which allows the incident skin to receive a smaller dose than the maximum produced by that beam. Instead the dose rapidly builds up under the surface of the skin. The higher the energy of the linear accelerator, the more its skin-sparing effect, e.g. 5 MeV gives 1.25 cm of skin sparing and 8 MeV gives 2 cm. While this is an obvious advantage in areas where the skin tolerance would be the limiting factor in achieving a dose at depth, it is clearly important to allow for this when tumours are superficial or where there is skin involvement. If the maximum dose has to be on the surface of the skin, tissue equivalent build-up, or bolus, can be used. This is placed on the skin and absorbs the area of submaximal dose.

Long distance radioactive cobalt-60 machines produce a supervoltage quality beam of gamma rays. However, although the size of the isotope source is small, the beam does not arise from a point and there is therefore some penumbra at the edges of the beam. This lack of a sharp edge to the beam may be a disadvantage when treating close to areas of high radiation sensitivity such as the spinal cord and the lens.

By contrast, linear accelerators produce X-rays from a point source and have an extremely sharp fall-off at the edges of the field. The treatment volume produced by these machines can be close to radiosensitive structures and yet give little or no chance of damaging them. Beams of different energy have distinct depth characteristics and the machine manufacturers and physicists spend much time in ensuring sharp, flat isodoses and sharply cut-off beams. The absorption of supervoltage X-rays does not depend as heavily on the atomic number of the material it passes through as does an orthovoltage beam. The more homogeneous dose distribution through tissues of different density avoids damage to bone and cartilage. The photon beam can be modified by the use of filters. These are wedge-shaped pieces of brass which, when placed in the beam, absorb more of the dose at the thick end and less at the thin end. This has the effect of turning the main axis of the beam through an angle. Wedged fields are particularly useful when compensating for changes in the contour and shape of a patient or when used in combination to produce isodoses that homogeneously cover the tumour volume (Figure 21.1). When several planned fields are arranged around the tumour volume the dose to the tumour can be greater than the dose to the skin or surrounding tissue. To produce a penetrating beam of photons from a linear accelerator the electrons are accelerated along a radar wave. Linear accelerators between 4 MeV and 10 MeV are the appropriate energies for treating tumours in the head and neck region.

Electron beam

X-rays are produced when accelerated electrons bombard a target. It is possible to remove the target in a linear accelerator and treat the patient with the electrons instead. Electron beams have particular depth dose and absorption characteristics which make them different from the photons produced by an X-ray or gamma ray beam. A photon beam is absorbed exponentially, but electron energy is largely absorbed at a finite depth dependent on the energy of the electrons. There is a sharp fall off of dose at depth and therefore tissues lying under the maximum depth dose of the electrons will receive a very small relative dose. This property is exploited when treating over radiosensitive areas such as the spinal cord. An electron beam is employed for the final phase of radiotherapy treatment to the neck when the spinal cord has received maximum tolerable dose, but structures lateral to it must still be given further treatment to reach a tumoricidal dose. Electrons may therefore be introduced from fields placed laterally on each side of the neck. The depth of the spinal cord can be calculated and the electron energy chosen to deliver the dose homogeneously from just below the skin to just short of the cord.

Low energy electrons can be made into a relatively poorly penetrating beam. However, in contrast to orthovoltage radiation which is also poorly penetrating, the advantage of electrons lies in the fact that the beam is absorbed by a process which is not so dependent on the density of the material absorbing the radiation. Treatment can therefore be given to areas of bone and cartilage with a superficial beam of electrons without as great a risk of osteoradionecrosis and cartilage necrosis. A superficial electron beam is

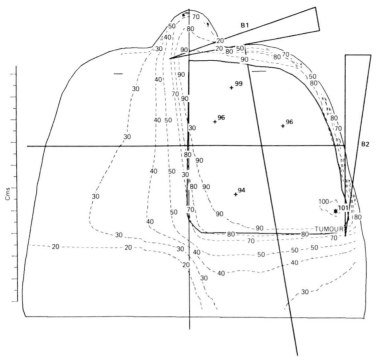

Figure 21.1 Treatment plan for a maxillary antrum carcinoma using two 45° wedges with beams angled in such a way to avoid the spinal cord and opposite eye

also useful in treating primary skin tumours round the cartilages of the nose or the pinna (Miller and Spittle, 1982). With this technique, high cure rates can be achieved often with a better cosmetic result than that of a wide surgical excision. Wedge resection of skin lesions of the ear, which was frequently performed because of the intolerance of the pinna to orthovoltage irradiation, is now rarely necessary and radiotherapy gives the patient a better cosmetic result.

In anteriorly placed tumours of the frontal sinus or the ethmoid sinus, a mixed treatment using electrons for the anterior field and supervoltage photons for the lateral fields, gives an excellent dose distribution. An electron beam can also be used to treat widespread superficial tumours of the scalp, such as angiosarcomas (Spittle, 1981). In this case a uniform dose distribution can be produced by arcing the electrons, treating the full thickness of the scalp to a radical dose and sparing the underlying brain tissue.

Neutrons

High energy machines can produce a beam of neutrons which are heavy uncharged particles and have several theoretical advantages for the irradiation of tumours. They produce a beam of high energy trans-fer with a low oxygen enhancement ratio. Radiobiologists have shown both *in vitro* and *in vivo* that cells are more sensitive to radiation if they are well oxygenated (Gray *et al.*, 1953). Cells that are well oxygenated are approximately three times more sensitive to irradiation with X-rays than poorly oxygenated cells (oxygen enhancement ratio of 3). However, only parts of tumours are well oxygenated. It is probable that the central areas of large tumours are necrotic and anoxic. Potentially viable cells on the rim of necrotic areas are relatively radioresistant to a photon beam because of anoxia. It may be these poorly oxygenated radioresistant cells which are responsible for the recurrences that develop after radical X-ray therapy. A neutron beam has the advantage that the oxygen enhancement ratio is low, approximately 1.5 and therefore cells, whether well oxygenated or anoxic, are relatively similarly affected by radiation. Neutrons were exploited for the management of tumours in 1926 by Stone (Stone, 1940) and, although the initial clinical response was good, an enhanced late damaging effect on normal tissues after irradiation caused considerable concern. Further enthusiasm for neutron therapy was expressed in the 1960s and results, particularly from the Hammersmith Hospital, London (Catterall and Bewley, 1973), showed some very good local control rates. However, late radiation damage was more severe than might have been predicted and led to complications, particularly when salvage surgery was attempted (Catterall, 1974). As the linear energy transfer of the neutrons is different from that of photons, the equivalent dose for the equivalent early effect had to be determined (Goldstein, Phillips and Fu, 1981). It may be that the late changes seen with neutrons are either due to the inherent severity of late effects or to the selection of non-equivalent doses. Comparative trials of neutrons and photons have not convincingly demonstrated a more favourable survival rate with neutrons and, as a result, it has been suggested that some early studies have used non-equivalent doses (Duncan, Arnott and Batterman, 1984).

In the UK, the use of neutrons is now reserved for the management of parotid gland tumours (Batterman and Breuer, 1981). Consistently more favourable results than those obtained with other forms of radiation have been shown for neutrons in several small international series of parotid gland tumour treatment (Griffin and Mortimer, 1989).

Protons

In a few selected centres worldwide, a heavy positively charged proton beam is available. Protons have the advantage that their depth/dose distribution characteristic gives an area of deposition of maximum energy at a depth in tissue called the Bragg peak. This is a small defined area of very much heightened effect which can be arranged to coincide with the tumour, thereby leaving a very much lower dose at the entry and exit point of the beam. Like neutrons, the proton beam does not rely on oxygenation of tissues for its effect and in some centres, in particular the Massachusetts General Hospital, excellent results have been obtained in the management of patients with traditionally radioresistant lesions such as chondrosarcomas of the base of skull and chordomas of the clivus (Austin-Seymour *et al.*, 1989). As yet, there are few of these machines and so it is imperative to identify specific indications for their use. In other words, diseases which would be more successfully treated entirely with protons or which would be helped by a boost or top-up treatment.

Hyperbaric oxygen

In an attempt to overcome the oxygen effect using conventional irradiation, treatment under hyperbaric oxygen has been investigated. This was initially pioneered by Van den Brenk and necessitated enclosing the patient in a cylinder at 3 atmospheres of oxygen (Van den Brenk, 1969). After allowing time for tissue oxygen equilibrium to take place it was considered that the whole tumour would have become well oxygenated and therefore uniformly radiosensitive.

The radiation was then given while the patient was in the tank. The apparatus used was unfortunately extremely heavy and there was a considerable fire risk with the regular use of high pressure oxygen in the radiotherapy department. The patient also became subject to barotrauma while pressurized and often needed grommets inserted in the ears. The cumbersome nature of the apparatus also meant that intricate radiotherapy fields were difficult to plan and treat while the patient was in the tank. The treatment plan was, therefore, less sophisticated. Since patients found the experience unpleasant it was considered inappropriate that the traditional 30 fractions of radiotherapy should be given in hyperbaric oxygen. An alteration in fractionation was made so that the patients could be treated with a once a week equivalent dose. It is possible that the altered fractionation which the hyperbaric oxygenation technique required altered the radiobiological response of the tumour in several ways and may have prejudiced the trial results. Two trials of the treatment of head and neck tumours under hyperbaric oxygen condition by Henk in Cardiff (Henk *et al.*, 1970; Henk and Smith, 1977) showed a slight advantage for the hyperbaric oxygen, more so in some sites than others, but in view of the many technical difficulties surrounding this form of treatment the benefits did not seem to outweigh its disadvantages.

Brachytherapy

Brachytherapy is short distance radiotherapy and usually entails either endocavitary or interstitial therapy. The advantage of brachytherapy is that it gives a very high dose to the target tissue with a rapid fall-off of isodoses at a distance. The disadvantage is that only a small volume may be raised to the target dose. Radioactive isotopes of iridium, caesium and cobalt have replaced the traditional radium brachytherapy. Endocavitary brachytherapy is employed when an additional top-up dose is needed to an organ or viscera which can be approached from the surface. Radioactive insertions have been part of the management of gynaecological cancers for many years and have the advantage that they supplement external beam therapy with high dose local treatment to the area of primary interest. Endocavitary irradiation may be used in the head and neck, for example, when a boost to the nasopharynx needs to be delivered to treat a carcinoma, either as part of the primary treatment or as part of re-treatment for recurrence. The advantage of using brachytherapy for recurrences is that the additional radiation does not have the same depth/dose distribution as external beam therapy and when used in an intracavitary manner does not add to skin toxicity. If used, it is frequently employed at the end of a course of external beam therapy as the main disadvantage of brachytherapy is that the depth of penetration of the beam is poor and, therefore, best used when the tumour is reduced to as small a size as possible (Goffinet *et al.,* 1980).

Interstitial treatment is frequently used in the management of tumours of the head and neck. Caesium needles and seeds are used to give an elegant radical treatment for small carcinomas of the anterior two-thirds of the tongue (Pierquin *et al.,* 1971). Following biopsy and staging, these lesions are assessed by a radiation physicist and a clinical oncologist to determine the volume that needs to be treated. A plan, using a one or two plane implant, is derived so that the distribution of radiation delivered to the tumour from the needles is homogeneous. The needles are then inserted according to that plan under general anaesthetic. After surgery, radiographs are taken in two planes so that a reconstruction of the actual distribution of radiation can be made by the physicist and the resultant treatment again discussed. Since it is virtually impossible to implant an area in a geometrically perfect manner, there will be hot or cold spots which must be identified. The dose to be achieved from the implant will then be agreed and the time at which the implant should be removed, calculated. It is usual to give approximately 70 Gy which may take between 5 and 7 days. During this time the patient is nursed in a protected room with lead screens in order to protect nursing staff and visitors who are only allowed to attend for a limited period of time. The needles are removed at the required time.

The advantage of a brachytherapy implant in the head and neck area is that the isodoses are packed closely together around the linear sources and, therefore, the radiation at a distance from the source is minimal. Also, the low dose rate of radiation may spare normal tissues from damage. For example, when using brachytherapy to treat carcinoma of the tongue, the target is to limit the volume needing radical dose to an area only 1 cm larger than the tumour itself. Localized mucositis and filming may be seen but the contralateral side of the mouth and parotid gland, in particular, is spared. This avoids oral dryness which often follows external beam treatment of the mouth. A moist mouth and a well-functioning flexible tongue are the major benefits of brachytherapy for early tongue carcinoma.

Interstitial therapy in the form of iridium wires can be used for implanting node areas and are particularly useful to achieve a concentrated dose in an area where the tumour has recurred following previous treatment (Syed, Feder and George, 1977). In any area where the ingenuity of the surgeon and the clinical oncologist can be harnessed to place iridium wires, an additional boost of treatment can be given (Neblett *et al.,* 1985). Gold grains are also sometimes used and can be placed with a gold grain gun into a tumour bed. The disadvantage of gold grains is that

the penetration of the beam is very poor and it is used to treat only very superficial disease.

Hyperfractionation

The difficulty of curing head and neck cancers has resulted in a constant effort to apply newer techniques of radiation to advanced disease. Traditionally, radiotherapy is given on a daily basis with breaks at weekends and the standard radical dose is 60–70 Gy in 6–7 weeks of daily treatment, treating all fields each day. This daily treatment enables the normal cells to repair following the radiation dose and this, in itself, may enhance the therapeutic index if the malignant cells repair less well between fractions. Since normal tissues takes 4–6 hours to repair, radiation treatment could be given in several fractions each day. The radiation dose limiting factor is the damage caused to late responding tissues. The tumour can be regarded as an acutely responding tissue and, by manipulating the dose/time relationship of the radiation, a gain in tumour response relative to tissue damage could be achieved (Williams, Denekamp and Fowler, 1985). If the dose per fraction is reduced it is possible to spare the late-reacting tissues. This is the basis of hyperfractionation. Either the same dose could be given, but be broken down into smaller fractions over the same period, hyperfractionation, or the treatment could be given in the standard number of treatments, but given over a shorter period, accelerated fractionation. The tumour may continue to proliferate during the time between fractions and, therefore, continuous hyperfractionation has been thought to be possibly useful in preventing repopulation of tumours.

From the above, it can be seen that hyperfractionation attempts to enhance the therapeutic difference between fast-responding tumour and slowly-responding normal tissues. It magnifies differences in repair capacity in effect of division cycle redistribution and increases the relative 'biological dose rate' to the tumour. Hyperfractionated radiotherapy for the treatment of head and neck cancers was initially used by Wang of Boston (Wang *et al.,* 1986) and the increased fractionation was an attempt to reduce the normal tissue injury and therefore toxicity which can be a dose limiting factor in the management of head and neck cancers by radiotherapy.

Clinical trials have consistently shown an advantage for hyperfractionation. The RTOG trial (Cox *et al.,* 1991) and the EORTC trial (Horiot *et al.,* 1992) showed an important improvement in local control and also some improvement in long-term survival with hyperfractionated schedules. At present the CHART trial (continuous hyperfractionated accelerated radiotherapy) is in progress in several centres in the UK (Dische and Saunders, 1990). This large trial hopes to explore whether repopulation of the tumour during the course of radiation treatment is an important feature of the radiobiology of failure to cure. CHART causes considerable disruption of standard hospital schedules by treating throughout the weekend and necessitates patients being housed near the hospital during their treatment. However, even if the results are the same as conventional standard fractionation there may be patients who would be happier to complete their treatment within 36 fractions over 12 days, rather than over the standard 6–7 weeks. The early results of this trial show no overall statistical difference in disease control or survival with CHART.

Hyperthermia

Hyperthermia is used with radiation in recognition that tumour cells are more sensitive to radiation if the ambient temperature is raised and also that anoxic cells seem to be preferentially sensitive to radiation when heated. Hyperthermia is being used with low dose interstitial brachytherapy (Aristobal and Oleson, 1984). This is a research tool at present and any application to the head and neck area is awaited with interest.

Combination therapy
Chemotherapy

In view of the mediocre responses to treatment of advanced head and neck cancers, the traditional combination of surgery and radiotherapy has been extended to include chemotherapy. But, in spite of a long history of combined management of head and neck tumours, the place of chemotherapy is, as yet, not established. Many trials have taken place over several years which have addressed the effect of radiotherapy and surgery in combination with, and without chemotherapy (Forastiere, 1991; Wolf, Lippman and Laramore, 1994). Chemotherapy has been given with various agents, and variously related to the other treatment options.

Cytotoxic drugs that have a good reputation in head and neck cancer may also produce mucositis as a side effect. This may limit the dose of radiotherapy which is able to be achieved if the drugs are given concomitantly. Enthusiasm has been shown for adjuvant chemotherapy which has the ability to downgrade the tumour and test its chemosensitivity. Indeed, it has recently been suggested that the most useful effect of chemotherapy is in highlighting those tumours which are responsive to non-surgical treatment and may therefore be successfully treated by radiotherapy and chemotherapy. The major advantage of this for the head and neck cancer patient is that it could lead to increased organ sparing. In 1985, the VA Cooperative Study Programme (Hong,

Wolf and Fisher, 1989) studied 332 patients with stage 3 or 4 laryngeal cancer. They were randomized into two groups which received either conventional laryngectomy and postoperative radiotherapy or had three cycles of induction chemotherapy. Those patients who responded after the third cycle of induction chemotherapy underwent a full course of radical radiotherapy; and those with residual disease after radiotherapy together with patients who did not respond to the chemotherapy completed their treatment with a total laryngectomy. Although no differences were seen in overall survival between the two groups, organ preservation was possible in 60% of those who had responded to induction chemotherapy. A biological basis for the use of chemotherapy as an indicator of successful radiotherapy treatment is unexplained, but is a recognized clinical phenomenon.

It is disappointing that the exact place of chemotherapy is not yet decided. Of course, not all forms of head and neck cancer are equally chemosensitive and certainly, in several series, carcinoma of the nasopharynx has shown itself to be particularly responsive to chemotherapy. Since head and neck cancer in some subsites is fortunately relatively rare, the problem of deciding on appropriate therapy depends upon the amalgamation of results of treatment of cancers at many sites in the head and neck. It may be, however, that the subsites act differently and respond differently to chemotherapeutic drugs and the generality of head and neck cancers include some very sensitive tumours and others which are resistant to all forms of treatment. It is increasingly important that both host and tumour factors should be taken into account when considering treatment and that management should be individually tailored for each patient depending on their genetic make-up, environmental factors, the biological characteristics and spread of their tumours.

Frequently, chemotherapy produces an increase in local control rate but no significant difference in survival. This is unfortunate, for agents effective against local disease should also be effective against distant micrometastases. In the UK, trials of methotrexate as an adjuvant to radiotherapy have shown an advantage (Gupta, Pointon and Wilkinson, 1987). The SECOG trial (Stell and Rawson, 1990) used a combination of bleomycin, cyclophosphamide and vincristine to show an advantage for chemotherapy. This group is currently exploring the question of concomitant or sequential treatment. The UKHAN trial compares various chemotherapy regimens given in different temporal relationships to radiotherapy.

There is considerable experience with cisplatin in the management of head and neck cancers and so it has been included in clinical trials, particularly in the USA. A combination of cisplatin and 5-fluorouracil is the regimen with the best general reputation in the treatment of head and neck cancer at present (Amrein, 1991). In the past, infusional chemotherapy using an intra-arterial catheter placed in the branch of the external carotid artery which supplied the tumour was advocated by some. This technique is hardly used nowadays as its effectiveness is matched by simple intravenous chemotherapy which does not have the same technical disadvantages and complications, e.g. partial tumour treatment, blockage of the arterial catheter and tissue infarction.

The toxicity of chemotherapy is often considerable and patients may complain of mucositis, nausea, vomiting, peripheral neuropathy, alopecia, weight loss and malaise. There has been no relevant evidence of a dose-response curve for chemotherapy. Although inadequate chemotherapy is not appropriate, high dose chemotherapy using growth factors to stimulate bone marrow stem cells or the use of autologous bone marrow transplants to reconstitute the bone marrow after high dose chemotherapy have not yet been shown to be efficacious. Management of patients who have residual or recurrent disease following radical therapy continues to be disappointing with chemotherapy. However, some palliation and improvement in the quality of their life may result from selected chemotherapy regimens in these difficult circumstances.

One of the problems which compounds the difficulties of achieving a complete cure for patients with head and neck cancer is that if prolonged local control is attained, an increased number of patients die of distant metastatic disease. Metastases have been shown by the RTOG to be present in approximately 20% of patients with head and neck malignancies and this number increases with time. This problem can realistically only be addressed by systemic therapy. A further factor which limits survival for patients with head and neck cancer is the increased tendency to develop tumours at other sites in the aerodigestive tract (Kogelnik, Fletcher and Jesse, 1975). These second primaries are usually related to a single aetiological factor – smoking. It is therefore possible to identify an at risk group for further aerodigestive cancers – those who have already suffered one squamous carcinoma in a smoking-related site. Young patients who develop head and neck cancer, especially if they have been non-smokers, also seem to have a genetic predisposition to development of further cancers in this area.

Retinoids have an anticarcinogenic effect with respect to squamous epithelium, possibly achieved by normalizing the effect of carcinogens. Hong *et al.* (1990), in a study of patients who had already suffered one head and neck malignancy, randomly compared a group of such patients who were given retinoids as prophylactic therapy, when considered *cured* of their primary disease, with a control *cured* group. This therapy neither increased the survival nor prevented recurrence from the primary cancer but, interestingly, there was a statistically significant decrease in the number of patients who developed a second primary in those who took the retinoids. At present, there is a

multicentre European study (Euroscan) of over 2000 patients which is comparing the use of retinol palmitate and N-acetylcysteine in patients who have previously been radically treated for head and neck cancer.

Chemotherapy and radiotherapy treatments are extremely taxing for patients with head and neck cancer. In many, there is a history of smoking and alcohol abuse. Poor general nutrition and low socioeconomic status also make it difficult for the patient to be adequately nourished during therapy. The skills of a dietitian, speech therapist, nurse counsellor and radiographer are all needed to ensure that the patients tolerate the radiotherapy as well as can be expected, that they understand the associated early toxicities and late complications, and that they complete their treatment in the best possible state. Patients should be weighed weekly, their oral hygiene checked regularly, and concomitant bacterial or fungal infections of the oropharynx treated early and effectively.

Treatment planning

The radiotherapy management of a patient with head and neck cancer will be described in detail. A patient with carcinoma of the maxillary antrum has been chosen as an example.

Initial assessment

The patient will have been seen in a joint clinic with surgical and clinical oncologists and have had the tumour biopsied. Once the characteristics of the disease have been documented and the patient has agreed to treatment, he will be referred to the planning department. It is important to review the patient's dental condition and have any carious teeth treated as radical irradiation alters the pH of saliva and dries the mouth and this may predispose to both periodontal and dental disease (Mossman, 1983). Teeth with a prognosis of less than 6 months are better extracted before irradiation as early dental trauma after treatment may predispose to osteoradionecrosis; radiation-induced endarteritis results in slower and less complete healing.

Definition of treatment volume

The clinical oncologist and senior radiographers will review and discuss the diagnostic MRI or CT scans with the radiologist and take these findings into consideration with those of the surgical oncologist, obtained at operation, to define the best treatment approach. When the maxillary antrum is involved with tumour, the aim of the clinical oncologist is to treat the whole of the maxillary antrum together with any obvious extension of disease. The treatment volume extends 1 cm across the midline to the contra-lateral side, to cover any extension of disease into other sinuses. Superiorly, the field is likely to extend so that it completely covers the ipsilateral frontal sinus. Inferiorly, the lower limit of the treatment volume will be the palate and posteriorly it will extend to the posterior margin of the maxillary antrum, which is approximately 1 cm anterior to the external auditory meatus. If there has been involve-ment of the inferior orbital margin then the ipsilateral orbital contents must be treated. If the bone is not breached, the ipsilateral eye can be protected from radiation by a lead block. Radiotherapy must be individualized for each patient, taking into full con-sideration the extent of the tumour and the general condition of the patient.

Preparation for treatment

In order to ensure that radiation is delivered accurately and reliably an immobilization shell is constructed. The patient is positioned supine so that the spinal cord is straight and horizontal. As the treatment field should not include the tissues below the palate, the mouth should be in a position of rest. If the treatment volume extends into the mouth, a gag is used to displace the lower jaw and tongue away from the treatment volume. Once in the appropriate position, a plaster shell is made of the patient's head and neck area. A plastic mask is then constructed from this by vacuum moulding and fitted to the patient to ensure reasonable comfort when it is fixed in the required treatment position. It is worth repeating that accurate immobilization is impor-tant in head and neck treatment where the linear accelerator field, with its sharp cut-off may be positioned close to the spinal cord or to the lens. Radical irradiation through the unprotected eye is sometimes necessary and causes conjunctivitis, keratitis, cataract formation and loss of vision. The dry eye which results needs intensive care with artificial tears and antibiotics.

The patient's mask is fitted to a headboard and a CT planning scan performed in the treatment posi-tion. This CT scan may not be identical in its display to that taken for diagnostic purposes and is not necessarily of diagnostic quality, but offers an ana-tomical registration of the patient's tumour in its treatment position. It is therefore important always to compare this scan with those performed prior to planning. The clinical oncologist is then able to out-line on each tomographic slice, through the area of interest, the volume of tissue which needs treatment to a radical dose. This volume will obviously include a margin for subclinical and microscopic spread of dis-ease and takes into account the histology of the disease, its rate of growth, and the general condition of the patient. The site of radiosensitive local structures such as the brain stem and the eye will be noted on the CT slices. The position of the contralateral eye which

becomes increasingly important if the eye on the ipsilateral side is to be sacrificed, is noted. The radiation physicist is then given enlarged CT slices with the treatment area marked on them. Using knowledge of the depth dose characteristics of the machinery avail-able in the department, the physicist is able to compute the optimum method in which the beam, or beams, may be placed to give maximum dose to the target volume while sparing adjacent normal structures. Such planning is computerized on the CT scan slice and is interactive with instant video display. Minimal dose to the surrounding tissues in the optimum field arrangement to treat a carcinoma of the maxillary antrum may be achieved with two wedged fields. As stated previously, the anterior field extends from the frontal sinus to the palate and from the medial canthus of the contralateral eye to cover the maxillary antrum and its most anterolateral area. The lateral field will be from just behind the external canthus of the ipsilateral eye anteriorly, to 1 cm in front of the external auditory meatus posteriorly. If these beams were to be placed at right angles, the anterior field would undoubt-edly exit through the contralateral eye giving a dose to that eye which would prejudice its vision. The field should, therefore, be angled backwards by approxi-mately 5° so that the beam exits behind the contra-lateral eye. The physicist normally produces several plans of different beam arrangements to discuss with the clinical oncologist, who then decides, in the light of all factors associated with the patient, which is the most appropriate treatment arrangement.

The tumour dose is quoted at the point of intersection of the radiation fields together with the maximum and minimum doses in the tumour volume. The dose that would be given to any radiosensitive structures such as the spinal cord or the lens is also calculated. When the treatment has been discussed with the radiogra-phers the patient returns for simulation. This involves being placed in the defined position in the mask on a treatment couch. The clinical oncologist, radiogra-phers, and physicist then ensure, by radiographic screening, that the set-up of the patient coincides with that of the plan. X-rays can be taken in this treatment position on the simulator or on the treating machine, and these give excellent verification of the arrangement of fields. A dose of 60–70 Gy to be given in 30–35 treatments over 6–7 weeks is traditionally prescribed.

Care during treatment

The clinical oncologist should see the patient regu-larly during the course of treatment. No systemic symptoms are expected but, during the second half of the treatment, skin erythema will develop together with a confluent area of mucositis on the soft palate as it is included in the treatment volume. Oral hy-giene is important throughout the treatment and a dental hygienist should also be available to the patient. Antifungal mouth washes are particularly useful as *Candida* infection is frequently acquired in an irradiated mouth. Every attempt should be made to avoid treating both parotid areas so that a dry mouth does not follow which is so unpleasant for the patient (Leslie and Dische, 1991). With the use of wedged fields for treatment of the maxillary antrum, only the ipsilateral parotid gland is included in the treatment volume or likely to receive radiation which would cause dryness of the mouth. In some, pilo-carpine in small doses may be enough to stimulate the parotid glands and help to overcome post-radia-tion mouth dryness, but it is clearly better to avoid it in the first place if this can be done without compro-mising the patient's chance of cure.

Every attempt must be made to deliver the required dose in the correct time as the dose/time relationship and its effect on the tumour and normal tissue is critical. Some studies have shown a reduction in local tumour control rates when there have been untoward interruptions in the treatment schedule, e.g. over bank holidays and as a result of machine breakdowns. Some compensation in dose can be made for a predictable break in treatment but, in general, every attempt should be made to counsel the patient that the treatment should go through as planned. Very occasionally the radiation reaction is so severe in some patients that treatment has to be delayed. At this stage a correction must be made so that the final treatment dose will be radiobiologically equivalent.

Additional treatment

In some tumours, such as supraglottic lesions, where there is a high potential for nodal involvement, the node areas of one or both sides of the neck can be prophylactically treated, adding little to the morbid-ity. At the end of treatment, a top-up dose may be given to coned-down fields, treating the site of bulk disease in the primary area to a higher dose. The patient must be advised that loss of hair may take place in both the areas of the incident and exit fields. When treating the maxillary antrum, the anterior field will exit through the back of the head and cause temporary alopecia, particularly distressing when unexpected.

Quality assurance is exceedingly important in radio-therapy as there are so many technical aspects of treatment. Machinery, the planning, the treatment aids, and the accuracy and reproducibility of treat-ment must be checked continually. If the patient is receiving concomitant chemotherapy while having radiotherapy, the radiation reaction is likely to appear sooner and to be more severe. If the radiation reaction appears to be approaching that which would cause the patient to stop the treatment, then the chemo-therapy should be suspended. Particular care must

also be taken when the patient is being irradiated at the nadir of the white blood count, 10 days post-chemotherapy, when infections are more common.

Clinical response to treatment

The response of a tumour to irradiation depends on the cell type and mitotic index. Lymphomas are more radiosensitive than carcinomas which in turn are more sensitive than sarcomas. Melanoma is generally radioresistant. Well differentiated lesions tend to be less radiosensitive yet more radiocurable than ana-plastic lesions. Cell death is normally manifest at cell division and since well-differentiated lesions normally have a longer cell cycle, radiation response may be slow. Although cure rate is highest in lesions that have disappeared at the end of a course of radiation therapy, the full impact of such treatment cannot be assessed until 4–8 weeks after completion of therapy. Thus assessing response midway through a planned radical treatment cannot predict eventual control (Rollo *et al.*, 1981).

Since complete surgical excision of a tumour does not mean that the disease will not recur locally, radiotherapy was usually employed postoperatively. When macroscopical residual disease was present postoperatively, the recurrence rate with postopera-tive radiotherapy was 55% and when microscopic disease was present local recurrence post radio-therapy was 31% (Mantravadi, Haas and Skolnick, 1983).

Combined modality treatment with radiotherapy and surgery has attracted much research and discus-sion to determine which modality should be employed first. Radiotherapy works best with a good blood supply and surgery is both easier and safer before radiotherapy. The treatment used first will have an undisturbed blood supply to favour its results. The advantages of pre- and postoperative radiotherapy are listed in Table 21.1.

An investigation was undertaken by the RTOG Group in the USA which evaluated 277 patients with various primary lesions of the oropharynx, oral cavity, supraglottis and hypopharynx. The patients were randomized and received either 50 Gy preopera-tively, followed by surgery 4–6 weeks later, or sur-gery followed by 60 Gy starting 2–4 weeks after completion of surgery (Kramer, 1985; Kramer *et al.*, 1987). Results showed that more of the patients who received radiotherapy postoperatively completed the therapy as planned (74% versus 56%). At 4 years the disease control was 65% in ·the group who received postoperative radiotherapy and 48% for the group who received preoperative radio-therapy. This was statistically significant (*P* = 0.04). Of those who completed the planned bi-modality pro-tocols, there was no difference in significant compli-cations from combined treatment. However, there

Table 21.1 Advantages and disadvantages of pre- and postoperative radiotherapy

Preoperative radiotherapy

Intact blood supply
Tissue planes not disturbed
Lymphatic drainage not disturbed
Clinical extent of disease obvious
Can irradiate skin which will be removed
Less delay in irradiation (contralateral neck)
Smaller fields, untreated grafts

Postoperative radiotherapy

Knowledge of extent of tumour
Knowledge of disease at margins
Less operative morbidity
No chance surgery will be refused
Safe use of high doses

was no significant difference in survival at 4 years, 33% in the preoperative arm and 38% in the postoperative arm ($P = 0.10$). There is therefore very little difference whether radiotherapy is given pre- or postoperatively although these results marginally favour postoperative therapy. It is not known what effect the addition of chemotherapy would have to these findings.

An enthusiastic head and neck surgeon who has understood the principles of radiotherapy as applied to malignancies of the head and neck, will give his patients the opportunity of a multidisciplinary approach to their disease. By using combined modality treatment, it is hoped that it may be possible not only to increase the cure rate of patients with head and neck malignancy but, perhaps more importantly, also to improve their quality of life.

References

AMREIN, P. (1991) Current chemotherapy of head and neck cancer. *Journal of Oral and Maxillofacial Surgery*, **49**, 864–870

ARISTOBAL, S. A. and OLESON, J. R. (1984) Combined interstitial irradiation and localized current field hyperthermia: results and conclusions from clinical studies. *Cancer Research*, **44**, 4457s–4760s

AUSTIN-SEYMOUR, M., MUNZENRIÐER, J. GOITEIN, M., VERHEY, L., URIE, M., GENTRY, R. et al. (1989) Fractionated proton radiation therapy of chordoma and low-grade chondrosarcoma of the base of the skull. *Journal of Neurosurgery*, **70**, 13–17

BATTERMAN, J. J. and BREUER, K. (1981) Results of fast neutron teletherapy for locally advanced head and neck tumors. *International Journal of Radiation Oncology, Biology and Physics*, **7**, 1045–1056

CATTERALL, M. (1974) The treatment of advanced cancer by fast neutrons from the Medical Research Council's cyclotron at Hammersmith Hospital, London. *European Journal of Cancer*, **10**, 343–449

CATTERALL, M. and BEWLEY, D. K. (1973) *Fast Neutrons in the Treatment of Cancer*. London: Academic Press. pp. 14–27

COX, J. D., PAJAKT, F., MARCIAL, V. A., COIA, L., MOHIUDDIN, M. and FU, K.K. (1991) Astroplenary: interfraction interval is a major determinant of late effects, with hyperfractionated radiation therapy of carcinomas of upper respiratory and digestive tracts: results from Radiation Therapy Oncology Group, protocol 83–13. *International Journal of Radiation Oncology, Biology and Physics*, **20**, 13–83

DISCHE, S. and SAUNDERS, M. I. (1990) The rationale for continuous hyperfractionated accelerated radiotherapy (CHART). *International Journal of Radiation Oncology, Biology and Physics*, **19**, 1339–1345

DUNCAN, W., ARNOTT, S. J. and BATERMAN, J. J. (1984) Fast neutrons in the treatment of advanced head and neck cancers: the results of a multi-centre randomly controlled trial. *Radiotherapy and Oncology*, **2**, 293–305

FORASTIERE A. A. (1991) Randomized trials of induction chemotherapy, a critical review. *Hematologic and Oncologic Clinics of North America*, **5**, 725–736

GOLDSTEIN, L. S., PHILLIPS, T. L. and FU, K. K. (1981) Biological effects of accelerated heavy ions. I. Single doses in normal tissues, tumors and cells in vitro. *Radiation Research*, **86**, 529–541

GRAY, L. H., CONGER, A. E., EBERT, M. et al. (1953) Concentration of oxygen dissolved in tissues at time of irradiation as factor in radiotherapy. *British Journal of Radiology*, **26**, 638–646

GRIFFIN, T. W. and MORTIMER, J. (1989) Overview of clinical trials and basis of future therapies, In: *Radiation Therapy of Head and Neck Cancer*, edited by G. Laramore. Springer-Verlag. pp. 219–234

GOFFINET, D. R., MARTINEZ, A., POOLER, D., PALOS, B. and COX, R. (1980) Brachytherapy renaissance. *Frontiers of Radiation Therapy*, **15**, 43–57

GUPTA, N. L., POINTON, R. C. S. and WILKINSON, P. M. (1987) A randomized clinical trial to contrast radiotherapy with radiotherapy and methotrexate given synchronously in head and neck cancer. *Clinical Radiology*, **38**, 575–581

HENK, J. M. and SMITH, C. W. (1977) Radiotherapy and hyperbaric oxygen in head and neck cancer. Interim report of 2nd clinical trial *Lancet*, ii, 104–105

HENK, J. M., KUNKLER, P. B., SHAH, N. K., SMITH, C.W., SUTHERLAND, W.H. and WASSIF, S.B. (1970) Hyperbaric oxygen in radiotherapy of head and neck carcinoma. *Clinical Radiology*, **21**, 223–231

HONG, W. K., WOLF, G. T. and FISHER, S. (1989) Laryngeal preservation with induction chemotherapy and radiotherapy in the treatment for advanced laryngeal cancer: interim survival data of VACSP 268. VA Laryngeal Cancer Study Group. *Proceedings of the American Society of Clinical Oncology*, **8**, 167 (abs 650)

HONG, W. K., LIPPMAN, S. M., ITRI, L. M., KARP, D.D., LEE, J.S., BYERS, R.M. et al. (1990) Prevention of second primary tumours with isotretinoin in squamous cell carcinoma of the head and neck. *New England Journal of Medicine*, **323**, 795–801

HORIOT, J. C., LE FUR, R., N'GUYEN, T., CHENAL, C., SCHIAUB, S., ALFONSI, S. et al. (1992) Hyperfractionation versus conventional fractionation in oropharyngeal carcinoma: final analysis of a randomized trial of the EORTC cooperative group of radiotherapy. *Journal of Radiotherapy and Oncology*, **25**, 231–241

KOGELNIK, H. D., FLETCHER, G. H. and JESSE, R. H. (1975) Clinical course of patients with squamous cell carcinoma of the upper respiratory and digestive tracts with no evidence of disease 5 years after initial treatment. *Radiology*, **115**, 423–427

KRAMER, S. (1985) Surgery and radiation therapy in the management of locally advanced head and neck squamous cell carcinoma. In: *Head and Neck Cancer*, edited by P. B. Chretein, M. E. Johns *et al*. Philadelphia: B. C. Decker. pp. 48–54

KRAMER, S. GELBER, R. D., SNOW, J. B., MARCIAL, V.A. LOWRY, L.D. and DAVIS, L.W. (1987) Combined radiation therapy and surgery in the management of advanced head and neck cancer: final report of the study 73–03 of the Radiation Therapy Oncology Group. *Head and Neck Surgery*, **10**, 19–30

LESLIE, M. D. and DISCHE, S. (1991) Parotid gland function following accelerated and conventionally fractionated radiotherapy. *Radiotherapy and Oncology*, **22**, 133–139

MANTRAVADI, R.U.P., HAAS, R. E. and SKOLNICK, E. M. (1983) Postoperative radiotherapy for persistent tumor at the surgical margin in head and neck cancer. *Laryngoscope*, **93**, 1337–1340

MEREDITH, W.J. and MASSEY, J. B. (1968) *Fundamental Physics of Radiology*. Bristol: John Wright & Sons Ltd

MILLER, R. A. and SPITTLE, M. F. (1982) Electron beam therapy for difficult cutaneous basal and squamous cell carcinoma. *British Journal of Dermatology*, **106**, 429

MOSSMAN, K. L. (1983) Quantitative radiation dose-response relationships for normal tissues in man II: response of the salivary glands during radiotherapy. *Radiation Research*, **95**, 392–398

NEBLETT, D. L., SYED, A.M.N., PUTHAWALA, A. A. and HARROP, R. (1985) An interstitial implant technique evaluated by contiguous volume analysis. *Endo/Hyperth/Oncol*, **1**, 213–222

PIERQUIN, B., CHASSAGNE, D., BAILLET, F. and CASTRO, J.R. (1971) The place of implantation in tongue and floor of mouth cancer. *Journal of the American Medical Association*, **215**, 961–963

ROENTGEN, W.C. (1931) On a new kind of rays 1895. *British Journal of Radiology*, **4**, 32

ROLLO, J., ROZENBOM, C. V., THAWLEY, S., KORBA, A., OGURA, J., PEREZ, C.A. *et al*. (1981) Squamous cell carcinoma of the base of the tongue: a clinicopathologic study of 81 cases. *Cancer*, **43**, 333–342

SPITTLE, M. F. (1981) Radiotherapy treatment of primary angiosarcoma of the skin. *International Journal of Radiation Oncology, Biology and Physics*, **7**, 1290 (abstract)

STELL P. M. and RAWSON, N.S.B (1990) Adjuvant chemotherapy in head and neck cancer. *British Journal of Cancer*, **62**, 779–787

STONE, R. S. (1940) Neutron therapy and specific ionization. *American Journal of Roentgenology*, **59**, 771–784

SYED, A.M.N., FEDER, B. H. and GEORGE, F. W. (1977) Persistent carcinoma of the oropharynx and oral cavity re-treated by after loading interstitial 192-Ir. *Cancer*, **39**, 2443–2450

VAN DEN BRENK, H.A.S. (1969) The oxygen effect in radiation therapy. *Current Topics in Radiation Research*, **5**, 197

WANG, C. C., SUIT, H. D., PHIL, D. and BLITZER, P.H. (1986) Twice-a-day radiation therapy for supraglottic carcinoma. *International Journal of Radiation Oncology, Biology and Physics*, **12**, 3–14

WILLIAMS, M. V., DENEKAMP, J. and FOWLER, J. F. (1985) A review of α/β ratios for experimental tumors: implications for clinic studies of altered fractionation. *International Journal of Radiation Oncology, Biology and Physics*, **11**, 87–95

WOLF, G., LIPPMAN, S. M., LARAMORE, G. *et al*. (1994) In: *Cancer Medicine*, edited by J. Holland and E. Frei. Baltimore: Lea and Febiger

The principles of chemotherapy

William J. Primrose

Squamous cell carcinomas constitute the majority of upper aerodigestive tract tumours and arise from the cellular unrest of a disturbed epithelium. Light microcopy only shows us one dimension of this complex, on going process to which we apply descriptive terms such as hyperplasia, dysplasia, metaplasia and anaplasia.

Many factors interplay in the phenomenon of carcinogenesis and this has been discussed in detail in Chapter 20. Hereditary factors, ageing, hormones, immune status and background radiation compound to varying degrees and remain largely beyond our control at present. They are inconsequential when compared to the role of environmental factors. Tobacco and alcohol are the most important risk factors in the Western world. They act synergistically (Cann, Fried and Rothman, 1985), both as tumour initiators and promoters, exerting their effects on the stem cells of the exposed epithelium. The cellular mechanisms involved (Table 22.1) are currently being unravelled, e.g. increased P53 expression correlates closely with heavy smoking and significant alcohol consumption (Field et al., 1991).

Millions of abnormal cells are produced on a daily basis, each one capable of forming a tumour if exposed to the right conditions. Epithelial growth, maturation and shedding dispose of many of these cells, others are recognized and destroyed by an intact immune system. Some clones of cells, with no territorial respect for their fellows, breach the basement membrane and establish a blood supply. These are the microinvasive cancers from which large tumours grow.

Cytokinetics

Cytokinetics, the study of the life cycle of cells at a cellular level, has developed rapidly since the

Table 22.1 Cellular mechanisms involved in carcinogenesis

Oncogenic virus transcription	e.g. Human papilloma virus in tonsil tumours, Epstein-Barr virus in nasopharyngeal carcinoma
Genotype changes	
Chromosome abnormalities	e.g. Reciprocal translocations, 3p deletions
Oncogenes	e.g. Growth factor Int/and Int 2, Growth factor receptor EGF-R, Nuclear proteins myc-L-myc, Cytoplasmic kinases, ras family
Recessive oncogenes Cyclin production	e.g. P53 expression
Phenotype changes Cytokeratins Envelope glycoproteins Blood antigens	

introduction of radioactively labelled substrates in the late 1940s. The development of tritiated thymidine, bromodeoxyuridine and flow cytometry have added further to the knowledge of the cell cycle and formed the backbone of early medical oncology research.

The cell cycle

Fundamental to the understanding of the growth and division of normal as well as cancerous cells is a dynamic process known as the cell cycle. This is defined as the interval between the midpoint of mitosis of one cell to the midpoint of subsequent mitosis of the daughter cells.

The non-dividing population of cells in any system is said to be in the G_0 phase; cells entering the cell cycle go through four phases as follows (Figure 22.1):

G_1 *phase (gap 1)*: the presynthetic/postmitotic phase. The majority of slow growing cell populations spend their time in this phase

S phase (synthetic): DNA transcription and replication as well as protein synthesis take place

G_2 *phase (gap 2)*: the postsynthetic/premitotic phase. RNA and protein synthesis continue

M phase (mitosis): Segregation of genetic material and cell division take place. During this phase the cell has divided into two, usually identical, daughter cells; the DNA content in each cell has been restored to the original, diploid amount. The cell may now mature and die, pass into the resting G_0 phase or replicate through the cycle again.

Tumour growth

Both normal tissue and tumours grow in volume by:

1 A net increase in cell numbers (most important)
2 A net increase in cell size (e.g. heart muscle hypertrophy)
3 A net increase in intercellular substance or products (e.g. colloid goitre)

At any one time tissue is composed of three distinct populations of cells:

Stem cells. These cells take an active part in the cell cycle and are therefore most sensitive to drugs or radiation. They have the capacity to proliferate, renew themselves, differentiate and be regulated (McCullough and Till, 1971). The last two features may be partly or totally lost in malignant tumours.

Dormant cells. These cells have left the cell cycle temporarily but may re-enter and proliferate when signalled to do so.

Differentiated cells. These cells have passed through several maturation stages after exiting from the cell cycle and, usually, have a finite function. They do not undergo further mitosis and ultimately die.

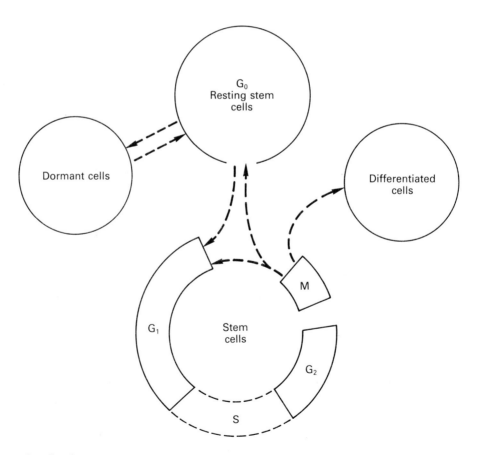

Figure 22.1 The cell cycle

The dynamics of any population of tumour cells is governed by the following three indices:

Cell cycle time. This varies as much between different normal tissues as it does between normal and malignant tissue. Normal bone marrow cells may cycle in 18 hours, whereas a basal cell carcinoma may cycle in 68 hours.

Growth fraction. This is the percentage of proliferating cells in a tumour, i.e. those actually passing through the cell cycle at a given point in time. It can be deduced mathematically from the tritiated thymidine labelling index or measured directly by a monoclonal antibody technique. It varies greatly from tumour to tumour and throughout the life-span of a particular tumour, being greatest in the early stages.

Cell loss. All tumours lose cells by various natural or induced means. Unsuccessful division, death, desquamation, metastasis and migration take their toll on the cell population. Cell loss may range from 30% in a lymphoma to 90% in a poorly differentiated bronchial carcinoma.

Doubling time is an observation which depends on all three of the above indices and shows a great variation between tumour classes. A bone sarcoma may take 20 days to double in volume compared to 100 days for a breast carcinoma. If it is assumed that a lung tumour is detected when it reaches 1 g (approximately 5×10^8 cells) then current mathematical models would suggest that it has been growing for several years before being clinically detected. The implications of this concept on the recurrence of tumours after treatment are self-evident.

Concepts in chemotherapy
Cell kill hypothesis

Basic concepts of drug-induced cell death were elucidated by Skipper, Schabel and Wilcox (1964) from experimental work on L1210 mouse leukaemia. It was recognized that a single inoculated leukaemia cell was capable of multiplying and eventually killing the host. Most cancers are now thought to have a clonal origin, each tumour developing from a single mutant cell.

Skipper, Schabel and Wilcox (1969) proved that cell destruction by drugs followed first order kinetics, i.e. a given dose of drug kills a constant fraction of cells, not a constant number, regardless of the number of tumour cells present at the time of treatment. Thus, a drug treatment which reduced a population of 10^6 cells to 10 should reduce a population of 10^5 cells to one cell.

Theoretically, if treatment is started early enough with large enough drug doses, repeated frequently enough, it is possible to reduce a tumour to a very small number of cells. Once a 'cure volume' is reached, anatomical and immunological factors may supervene to destroy the remaining tumour cells, as suggested by experiments on tumour transplantation (Fisher and Fisher, 1968). Immunological cell destruction is thought to follow zero order kinetics, that is all foreign cells up to a given number are killed.

Drug scheduling and dosage

Phenomenological models of tumour growth can be devised, with some complicated mathematics, to fit what is observed in reality. Most tumours exhibit exponential growth at some stage in their life-span; solid tumours in particular show a sigmoid-shaped growth curve called 'Gompertzian growth' (Norton and Simon, 1979) (Figure 22.2). This suggests that maximum growth and, by inference, maximum growth fraction, is achieved when the tumour reaches 37% of its expected volume.

Commencing treatment with cytotoxic agents on a tumour which is close to reaching its expected maximum volume will have little effect. It is not only the timing of the first treatment which is critical to a successful outcome, but also the timing of successive treatments. If a drug regimen is repeated too soon, the toxic effects on normal tissue will outweigh the benefits of the tumour cell kill, which will be reduced as it depends on a reasonable number of cells re-entering the cell cycle.

An optimal intertreatment interval exists (Figure 22.3) which maximizes cell kill while allowing bone

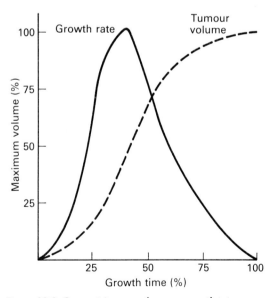

Figure 22.2 Gompertzian growth curve, growth rate superimposed. Growth rate is maximal at 37% of maximum tumour volume, but is very small at the extremes of tumour size

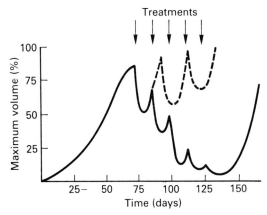

Figure 22.3 Gompertzian growth and theoretical regression induced by an intermittent chemotherapy schedule. The first three cycles have the maximum effect but all the tumour cells are never eradicated. Dotted line indicates progression of disease which occurs if intertreatment interval is too long

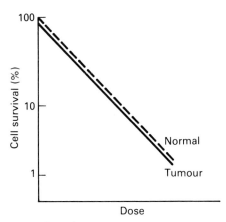

Figure 22.4 Class I drugs

marrow and other organs to recover. Retreatment delay in the case of a rapidly proliferating tumour may allow progression which may never be brought under control.

The treatment objective of every cytotoxic regimen is to achieve maximum tumour cell kill with minimum effect on normal stem cells. This narrows the therapeutic index of most drugs so that the drug dose and duration of action become important. Even if the tumour is susceptible to a drug, the drug will not work unless it reaches the tumour site and remains there long enough in sufficient tumoricidal concentrations. Hence, optimal concentration (C) and time of action (t) exist for every drug, but establishing this $C \times t$ ratio is not easy and falls into the complex field of pharmacokinetics. It is this area of risk/benefit that is most significant to our patients. Too little drug and the tumour progresses; too much and a toxic or even lethal dose is established.

Selective toxicity

It has been recognized for some time that most cytotoxic agents have a differential action on normal and malignant tissues. The full significance of this was not appreciated until a series of elegant experiments in the 1960s by Bruce, Meeker and Valeriote (1966). They studied bone marrow and lymphoma cells in the AKR strain of mouse and were able to develop a quantitative assay of the number of viable clonogenic cells which remained after treatment. Three classes of cytotoxic drug emerged with distinct differential actions.

Class I drugs (Figure 22.4) e.g. nitrogen mustard. These affect both the proliferating and resting cells

equally, affecting tumour and normal tissue in an equal dose-related manner. They are said to be 'non-specific'.

Class II drugs (Figure 22.5) e.g. methotrexate. These mainly kill proliferating cells during a specific part or parts of the cell cycle. These drugs are said to be 'phase specific'.

Class III drugs (Figure 22.6) e.g. cyclophosphamide. These kill both resting and cycling cells, but the latter are much more sensitive. These drugs are said to be 'cycle specific'.

All the major cytotoxic agents have now been studied extensively with regard to their specific sites of action in and out of the cell cycle. Some drugs act at more than one phase (Figure 22.7). The knowledge of this and other synergistic effects has become important in designing therapeutic regimens containing more than one drug.

Rationale for combination drug therapy

The combination of drugs in medicine to treat a single illness has been practised for many centuries.

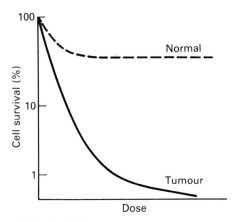

Figure 22.5 Class II drugs

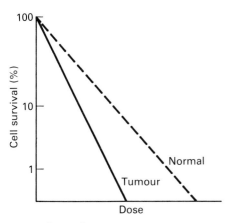

Figure 22.6 Class III drugs

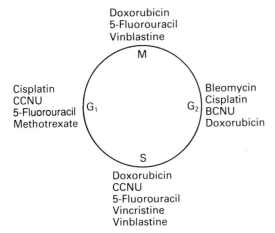

Figure 22.7 Cycle-specific drugs

Epilepsy, hypertension and life-threatening infections are a few modern day examples where drug combinations are used. The superiority of combination therapy to single agent therapy was first demonstrated conclusively in the case of childhood acute leukaemia by Frei *et al.* in 1961. This has now been confirmed in certain lymphomas, sarcomas and childhood tumours, to name but a few. The practical benefits of combining drugs may be explained, in part, by the following concepts.

Drug resistance

Drug resistant cell lines develop in most tumours, perhaps in part as a consequence of the mutagenic effects of the drug itself. If a drug which has an associated risk of resistance developing in one in a million cells (10^{-6}) is combined with an unrelated

drug with a similar risk then the cumulative risk is the product of both, that is 10^{-12}.

Biochemical blockade

Drug combinations can be designed with agents that produce breaks at multiple sites in the tumour cells' biosynthetic pathways. *Sequential blockade* develops when enzymes are blocked at various steps in the production of an essential metabolite. *Concurrent blockade* is said to be present when parallel pathways are affected. *Complementary inhibition* is achieved when a drug which blocks the biosynthesis of a macromolecule is combined with a drug which damages the macromolecule directly.

Cell cycle complementation

All tumours are composed of a heterogeneic population of cycling and non-cycling cells. The combination of alkylating agents and anthracyclines – which are effective against non-cycling cells – with 5-fluorouracil and methotrexate – which are cycle specific – possesses obvious theoretical synergism. Following treatment with non-cycle specific drugs, most tumours show a substantial increase in their growth fraction. This phenomenon is known as 'recruitment' and it may also happen in hormone dependent tumours in response to giving the appropriate hormone. Cycle-specific drugs show more effect after recruitment. *Synchronization* describes the phenomenon where cells are induced to pass simultaneously through the cell cycle. Cold shock, thymidine, vincristine and hydroxyurea are capable of producing synchronization *in vitro*. *Restriction point control* is another theoretical method described for preventing normal cells entering susceptible phases of the cell cycle.

Pharmacological considerations

Some cytotoxic agents may have their effects enhanced when used in combination with other inherently non-toxic agents by a series of unique interactions. Examples of these are:

1 Prolongation of action, e.g. probenicid
2 Facilitation of membrane transport, e.g. vitamin D
3 Reversal of toxic effects allowing greater cytotoxic dosage, e.g. folinic acid rescue after methotrexate.

The agents

In the last half century, nearly half a million substances have been screened world-wide for anticancer activity. One hundred or so of them have shown sufficient activity with tolerable toxicity to warrant human trials but only a handful have found their way into widespread clinical use.

Anticancer drugs can be classified according to their general characteristics (Table 22.2), although the specific mode of action of some substances is not fully known. Cytotoxic agents, by definition, are noxious substances with toxic side effects; they frequently produce unpleasant adverse reactions which are occasionally lethal. Hypersensitivity, idiosyncrasy and unexpected reactions can happen suddenly and contraindicate further use. A significant risk of teratogenicity and abortion precludes use of chemotherapeutic agents around the time of conception or during pregnancy.

Drugs and solutions should be carefully prepared and handled by experienced staff, with special regard to labelling and shelf life. Ideally, drugs should be prepared and reconstituted in a pharmacy setting by gowned, masked and gloved personnel using a vertical downflow laminar safety cabinet (Donner, 1978). Inexperienced persons or occasional users should familiarize themselves fully with the appropriate literature and data sheets. Information regarding shelf life, handling and contamination should be readily available (Table 22.3).

All doses and modes of delivery should be triple checked even by experienced personnel as severe, irreversible complications and even death have been reported. Intrathecal or intra-arterial injection increases the hazard of a miscalculated dose or mistaken drug. Patients should be closely monitored after the administration of the drug or drugs, regardless of whether they are given in an inpatient or outpatient setting.

The following is a brief pharmacopoeia of the common drugs likely to be encountered in the treatment of head and neck cancer.

Bleomycin sulphate

Bleomycin sulphate is a mixture of glycopeptide antibiotics first isolated in Japan from strains of *Streptomyces verticullus* (Umezawa, 1974). The precise mechanism of action is unknown, but it inhibits DNA, RNA and protein synthesis. The cycle-specific actions of this drug take place mainly in the G_2 and M phases. It concentrates in the skin and lungs but spares haemopoietic tissue. Plasma half-life is approximately 2 hours after intravenous administration, and 60–70% of the administered dose can be recovered in its active form in the urine.

Antitumour activity is seen in most squamous cell carcinomas, lymphomas and testicular tumours. When this drug is used as a single agent in head and neck cancer, 30% of patients show a response which is relatively short lived (Blum, Carter and Agre, 1973). Its major toxicities are directed to the lung and skin, with a 10% incidence of a non-specific pneumonitis, one in 10 cases of which progress to a fatal form of pulmonary fibrosis. Potentiation of lung damage may develop with oxygen administration,

Table 22.2 Classification of chemotherapeutic agents

Classification	Drug	Abbreviation
Alkylating agents	Busulphan	BUS
	Chlorambucil	CHL
	Carboplatin	CBDCA
	Cisplatin	DDP
	Cyclophosphamide	CYC
	Mechlorethamine	HN2
	Melphalan	MP2
	Thiotepa	THIO
Antibiotics	Actinomycin D	ACT
	Bleomycin	BLEO
	Daunorubicin	DNR
	Doxorubicin (Adriamycin)	ADR
	Mithramycin	MTH
	Mitomycin C	MTC
Antimetabolites	Cytosine arabinoside	ARA–C
	5-Fluorouracil	5–FU
	Ftorafur	FTOR
	Methotrexate	MTX
	6-Mercaptopurine	6–MP
	Thioguanine	6–TG
Enzymes	L-Asparaginase	L-ASP
Hormones	Adrenocorticoids	PRED
	Androgens	AND
	Oestrogens	ESTR
	Anti-oestrogens	Anti-ESTR
	Progestogens	PROG
Nitrosoureas	Carmustine	BCNU
	Lomustine	CCNU
	Semustine	MCCNU
	Streptozotocin	STZ
Plant alkaloids	Vinblastine	VBL
	Vincristine	VCR
	VM 16	VM 16
	VM 26	VM 26
Random synthetics	Dacarbazine	DTIC
	Dibromomannitol	DBM
	Hexamethylmelamine	HXM
	Hydroxyurea	HYD
	MethylGAG	MGAG
	Mitotane	o,p'DDD
	Procarbazine	PCB

e.g. during surgery. Regular chest X-rays and monitoring of pulmonary function are necessary. Dermatological toxicity can be troublesome, manifested by pigmentation, pruritus and dermatosclerosis. Fever, chills and vomiting are also quite common.

It is usually given as an intravenous or intramuscular bolus, typical dosages of 10–20 units/m² being

Table 22.3 Handling of anticancer drugs

Drug/route	Expiry time after reconstitution	Effect on skin, eyes and mucous membranes	Handling precautions	Action on contamination
Bleomycin sulphate i.m., i.v., i.a.	Use freshly prepared	Locally toxic, allergenic	Gloves and mask	Rinse thoroughly with water, then soap and water
Cisplatin i.v.	20 h at room temperature Refrigeration causes precipitation	Potentially allergenic	Gloves and mask necessary if spilt	Wash thoroughly with water
Cyclophosphamide i.v.	6 days at 4 °C	Skin irritation is rare	No special precautions	Wash thoroughly with water
Doxorubicin (Adriamycin) i.v.	2 days at 4 °C	Irritant	Gloves	Copious washing with soap and water
5-Fluorouracil i.v., infusion, i.a.	Dilute ampouled solution immediately before use	Minor local inflammation if skin is broken	Avoid contact with skin and mucous membrane	Flush affected parts with copious amounts of water
Methotrexate i.m., i.v., i.t., i.a.	2 weeks at room temperature	Irritant	Gloves	Wash with water. Apply bland cream. Calcium folinate cover if there is significant systemic absorption
Vinblastine i.v.	30 days at 4 °C	Irritant	Gloves	Thorough and immediate washing with large amount of water. Apply Heparin cream if accidentally injected into subcutaneous tissues

From D'Arcy 1986

prescribed on a weekly or twice weekly basis, up to a cumulative maximum of 400 units. It can also be administered as a 24-hour infusion.

Cisplatin (*cis*-diamminedichloroplatinum)

Cisplatin is a heavy metal complex containing a central platinum atom surrounded by two chloride and two ammonia molecules in the *cis* position. It was discovered in 1965 by Rosenberg, Van Camp and Krigas, who noted that platinum compounds produced around an electrode immersed in a culture medium have a bacteriostatic effect. This drug acts as a bifunctional alkylating agent, producing cross-linking of DNA strands, and was originally thought to be cell-cycle non-specific. It is now known that cisplatin blocks the dephosphorylation of serine-threonine protein kinase (P34^{cdc-2}) resulting in 'G$_2$ block' (Nishio *et al.*, 1993).

A single intravenous dose concentrates in the liver, kidneys and intestines but spares the central nervous system. It is protein bound in the plasma, demonstrating a bi-phasic plasma half-life with slow excretion over several days. Renal tubule damage is the major dose limiting adverse reaction encountered. Serum, urea and creatinine elevations are seen in approximately 30% of patients after a single intravenous dose of 50 mg/m². Repeated doses are cumulative but intravenous pre-hydration and man-

nitol diuresis can reduce nephrotoxicity. Anaphylactic-like reactions, CNS motor-toxicity, and myelosuppression are relatively common. In high doses it is almost 100% emetogenic but this can be controlled by 5-HT$_3$ antagonists such as ondansetron (Milne and Heel, 1991). Electrolyte disturbances and hyperuricaemia are secondary to renal tubule damage. Neurotoxicity takes the form of peripheral neuropathies and occasional seizures. Sudden death from cerebral herniation has been described and may indicate an occult brain metastasis (Walker, Cairncross and Posner, 1986). Extensive pre-treatment assessment to include blood and renal investigations, is necessary. Hearing impairment and platinum compound allergy contraindicate the use of this drug.

Antitumour activity is seen in germinal testicular tumours, ovarian cancer, sarcomas and advanced bladder tumours. When used as a single agent in squamous carcinomas of the head and neck, 30% of patients show a major response (Wittes, Cvitkovic and Strong, 1977). The addition of cycle-specific cytotoxic agents produces formidable major response rates approaching 90% in some series. It shows particular synergism with 5-fluorouracil, with response rates exceeding 50% in induction protocols (Kish *et al.*, 1984) (Table 22.4).

Typical dosages of 50–120 mg/m² are given intravenously over a 2–8 hour period while ensuring adequate hydration and urinary output. Subsequent

Table 22.4 Induction chemotherapy with cisplatin 5-fluorouracil (5-FU) response rates

No. evaluable patients	Regimen	Overall (%) response/ CR (%)
26	Cisplatin 100 mg/m² 5-FU 1 g/m²/d × 5 (2 cycles)	88/19
88	Cisplatin 100 mg/m² 5-FU 1 g/m²/d × 5 (3 cycles)	94/54
103	Cisplatin 100 mg/m² 5-FU 1 g/m²/d × 5 (3 cycles)	87/35
30	Cisplatin 100 mg/m² 5-FU 1 g/m²/d × 5 (3 cycles)	83/43
42	Cisplatin 100 mg/m² 5-FU 1 g/m²/d × 5 (3 cycles)	86/38
31	Cisplatin 80 mg/m² 5-FU 800 mg/m²/d × 5 (2–3 cycles)	84/23
53	Cisplatin 20 mg/m²/d × 6 5-FU 1 g/m²/d × 5 (2–4 cycles)	73/30

CR: complete response

doses should not be given for at least 3 weeks and until the serum creatinine has dropped below 114 μmol/l. Daily low dose cisplatinum, (6 mg/m²) per day for 30 days, given concurrently with radiotherapy has also been described (Tobias *et al.*, 1987).

Carboplatin (*cis*-diammine [11 cyclobutanedicarboxylato] platinum)

This close relative of cisplatin shows a similar range of activity against tumours as its parent compound. It demonstrates a shorter plasma half-life, 70% of a single intravenous dose can be recovered from the urine within 24 hours. It is less neurotoxic, ototoxic and nephrotoxic than cisplatin and can be given without prehydration even in patients with moderate renal impairment. Myelosuppression is the main dose limiting toxicity of carboplatin which usually precludes re-treatment within 30 days, but this may be overcome by the new generation of haematopoietic growth factors, e.g. Leucomax, Neupogen (Forastiere, 1992).

As a single agent it produces a slightly lower objective response rate in squamous cell carcinoma of the head and neck, but like cisplatin shows particular synergism when used in combination with 5-fluorouracil, producing response rates of around 55% (Decker *et al.*, 1983).

Typical dosages of 200–400 mg/m² are given intravenously over a 15–60 minute period. Leucopenia and thrombocytopenia may develop after 2–4 weeks and require regular monitoring.

Cyclophosphamide

Cyclophosphamide is a synthetic white crystalline powder with the molecular formula $C_7H_{15}Cl_2N_2O_2P$. H_2O and is related to the nitrogen mustards. It is activated by plasma and microsomal enzymes by way of intermediates to intracellular alkylating metabolites. It can be administered either orally or parenterally and distributes throughout most body tissues. Serum half-life after intravenous administration is 4–6 hours and most excretion takes place through the kidneys.

Antitumour activity is seen in a number of malignancies including lymphomas, multiple myelomas, leukaemias, neuroblastomas, retinoblastomas and carcinomas of the breast and ovary. This drug produces response rates of around 20% as a single agent in squamous cell carcinoma of the head and neck.

Serious adverse reactions include fatal haemorrhagic cystitis, cardiac toxicity and the development of secondary malignancies. Alopecia, leucopenia, nausea and vomiting are frequently reported. Potentiation of effects may develop with other cytotoxic agents and also with barbiturates. This drug is most frequently used in combination regimens. A typical intravenous loading dose of 40–50 mg/kg would be given over 2–5 days followed by oral maintenance therapy of 1–5 mg/kg. Total leucocyte counts of less than $3 \times 10^9/l$ may necessitate cessation of treatment.

Doxorubicin (Adriamycin)

Doxorubicin is a bright fluorescent red anthracycline antibiotic derived from *Streptomyces peucetius*. It binds between base-pairs of DNA, inhibiting DNA-dependent RNA synthesis and appears to be most effective during the G_2 phase of mitosis. Intravenous administration results in an initial plasma half-life of 30 minutes, with prolonged hepatic metabolism and excretion in bile and urine.

This drug has one of the widest antitumour spectra known, showing most activity in the acute leukaemias, lymphomas, sarcomas, paediatric malignancies, breast and lung carcinomas. When used as a single agent in head and neck cancer, response rates of around 20% have been described.

The major dose limiting toxicity is bone marrow suppression with nausea, vomiting, diarrhoea, mucositis and alopecia being frequently reported. Of special note is cardiac toxicity, manifest by ECG changes and congestive failure secondary to a diffuse cardiomyopathy. The risk of this developing increases very significantly if the total cumulative dose exceeds 550 mg/m². Synergism with cyclophosphamide may be apparent. Doxorubicin analogues, e.g. epirubicin and pyrarubicin are less toxic.

Typical dosages of 60–75 mg/m² can be given intravenously every 3 weeks. Extravasation at the site of infusion can produce cellulitis and massive tissue necrosis.

5-Fluorouracil

5-Fluorouracil is a fluorinated pyrimidine belonging to the antimetabolite group of cytotoxic agents originally discovered by Heidelberger, Chaudhuri and Weston in the 1950s. It is cell-cycle specific with maximum activity in the S-phase. It blocks DNA synthesis by inhibiting thymidylate synthetase, the enzyme responsible for thymidine formation. A single bolus intravenous dose leads to a short plasma half-life of 10–20 minutes because of rapid catabolism in the liver.

Antitumour activity is seen in a variety of carcinomas, including those arising in the gastrointestinal tract, breast, ovary and bladder.

When this drug has been used as a single agent in squamous cell carcinoma of the head and neck, response rates of 15–20% have been reported.

Side effects include anorexia, nausea, vomiting, mucocitis, leucopenia, alopecia and rarely cerebellar ataxia.

Typical dosages of 1000 mg/m² can be given daily by intravenous infusion for 4–5 days, repeated at 4-weekly intervals.

Methotrexate

Methotrexate, a sodium salt of 4-amino-10-methyl-folic acid, is an antimetabolite acting principally in the S phase of the cell cycle. It competitively inhibits dihydrofolate reductase, preventing the reduction of dihydrofolate to tetrahydrofolate, a necessary step in the process of DNA synthesis. However, this effect may be reversed by administering tetrahydrofolate (leucovorin) up to 24 hours later.

When this drug is parenterally administered, peak serum levels are seen in 30–60 minutes with a half-life of 2–10 hours, 40% being excreted unchanged in the urine. Daily doses result in sustained serum levels. To all intents and purposes it does not cross the blood-brain barrier and so has to be given intrathecally if necessary.

Initially introduced in 1940s for the management of acute leukaemias it shows antitumour activity in trophoblastic tumours, lymphomas and a variety of carcinomas. As a single agent used in the treatment of squamous cell carcinomas of the head neck, it demonstrates response rates of 40–50% (Wittes, 1980; Souhami and Tobias, 1986) which exceeds those observed with cisplatin. The major toxic effects of methotrexate are myelosuppression and gastrointestinal mucositis. Other adverse reactions include abdominal cramps, malaise, rashes, osteoporosis, renal and hepatic toxicity.

Typical dosages of 15 mg/m² daily for 3 days have prolonged survival in some recurrent cases, with few side effects. Dosages of 500–1000 mg/m² given intravenously on a weekly basis combined with leucovorin rescue are possible but do not necessarily improve survival (Browman *et al.*, 1990). Piritrexim, a lipo-philic analogue of methotrexate which is not subject to polyglutamation and therefore less toxic, has recently shown single agent activity in head and neck cancer (Uen *et al.*, 1992).

Vinblastine

Vinblastine is a plant alkaloid derived, along with vincristine, from the common garden periwinkle *Vinca rosea*. It inhibits both RNA synthesis and the formation of tubular structures found in the spindle fibres of mitotic metaphase. The exact mechanisms of tumour cell death induced by it are poorly understood. It is poorly absorbed from the gastrointestinal tract and has to be given intravenously. Vinblastine has a plasma half-life of 30 minutes, is metabolized in the liver and excreted in bile. Platelets may form a repository and so contribute to a sustained release.

This drug has a broad antitumour activity with the greatest response seen in rapidly dividing lymphomas and choriocarcinomas. When it is used as a single agent, response rates approaching 30% are seen in squamous cell carcinomas of the head and neck.

Vinblastine's toxic effects include nausea, vomiting, constipation, diarrhoea, granulocytopenia and peripheral neuritis. Typical dosages range from 4 to 20 mg/m² given intravenously on a weekly basis.

Definitions

Medical oncology has developed a jargon unique to itself. The terms used lead to misunderstanding by many and mistrust by a few, mainly surgeons. The author will attempt to define and expand some of the adjectives and phrases which are essential to the understanding of the subject and are frequently used.

Chemotherapy schedules

Adjunctive chemotherapy is the use of cytotoxic agents with intent to improve survival before, during or after standard local treatment by surgery, radiotherapy or both.

Induction chemotherapy (also known as neoadjunctive chemotherapy, up front or pre-emptive chemotherapy) is the use of cytotoxic agents with the intention of improving survival before progressing to standard local treatment.

Concurrent chemotherapy (concomitant chemotherapy) is the use of cytotoxic agents with the intention of improving survival during a course of radiotherapy. Synchronous chemotherapy/radiotherapy may precede or follow surgery, or be regarded as definitive treatment itself.

Adjuvant chemotherapy (maintenance chemotherapy) is the use of cytotoxic agents following definitive local treatment (surgery and/or radiotherapy) to improve survival.

Palliative chemotherapy is the use of cytotoxics, usually single agents, in an attempt to relieve symptoms in an incurable disease process. When administered to patients with advanced unresectable, recurrent or disseminated disease, prolonged life of reasonable quality has been reported in some cases.

Response

Cytotoxic agents should be given to consenting patients only on the basis of a reasonable expectation that a response will be produced. Although originally intended only as an end point in phase II trials, measurement, documentation and the correlation of a response seem to have assumed a much wider importance to medical oncologists.

Many parameters require consideration. Accurate tumour measurement, by various means, is necessary at the time of tumour staging. Response is usually measured 3–4 weeks after administration of induction chemotherapy which may consist of one or more cycles. More chemotherapy may be given if the response is favourable. Measurement of response in head and neck tumours is usually made on the basis of clinical parameters and occasionally by radiological assessment. Sometimes biopsies are taken at the tumour site to assess the 'pathological' response. Response at primary and nodal sites may vary, as may the duration of the response if not followed immediately by standard local treatment. Reassessment by the otolaryngologist who initially staged the patient is advisable. Responses are graded according to the following broadly accepted guidelines (Miller *et al.*, 1981).

Complete response (CR) indicates that there is total tumour regression, although a certain amount of tissue distortion or mucosal scarring may be allowed. A complete response should be maintained for at least 4 weeks.

Partial response (PR) indicates that there has been a 50% or greater reduction in the product of the two largest perpendicular diameters of *all* measurable lesions.

No response (NR) indicates no change in the size of the tumour, or a less than 50% reduction of *all* measurable lesions.

Progressive disease (PD) indicates a growth of measurable tumour of 25% or more, or the appearance of new lesions.

Major response implies complete or partial response.

Minor response implies less than 50% reduction in the bidimensional product.

Occasionally, responses are quoted after combined modality treatment, e.g. 'a partial response following chemotherapy and radiotherapy'. This can be misleading and older terms such as residual and recurrent disease are preferred after definitive treatment.

Survival

Traditionally, the term survival has taken the form of 3- or 5-year survival rates. In their crudest form, these figures record only whether the patient is alive or dead. The information can be made a little more sophisticated by stating if the patient is free of disease or not. Comparisons by simple non-parametric tests provide probability values from which significance may be deduced.

The last two decades have witnessed a blossoming of the use of survival curves, sometimes known as actuarial or Kaplan Meier plots (Kaplan and Meier, 1958), which are almost mandatory illustrations (Figure 22.8). These have the advantage that patients with different lengths of follow up may be included without fundamentally altering the shape of the curve, and 2- or 3-year survival rates may approximate to what will be observed at 5 years if numbers are large enough. Prognostic inferences may be made from complicated calculations based on the shape of the curves.

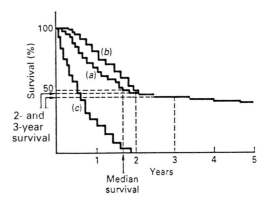

Figure 22.8 (*a*) Typical survival curve following standard treatment for stage III and IV head and neck squamous carcinoma. Most (95%) recurrences occur within 2 years, rendering this a valid approximation for 3- and 5-year survival. (*b*) Standard treatment followed by chemotherapy. (*c*) Control group (no treatment)

Median survival is frequently quoted – this is the time taken for 50% of the population being studied to die – and may be directly read from the curve or be calculated. Median survival values can vary greatly. In a large series of patients with recurrent intractable squamous cell carcinoma of the head and neck, median survival was reached in only 11 weeks (Stell and McCormick, 1986). Complete responders to chemotherapy, however, may not reach their median survival within 5 years of follow up. Similarly, patients with malignant salivary gland tumours (Conley and Dingman, 1974) may not reach their median survival in 5 years but, by contrast, display a completely different survival curve (Figure 22.9).

The timing of entry into a study is often overlooked

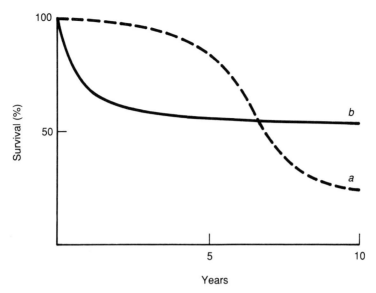

Figure 22.9 (*a*) Slow growing but malignant tumour. (*b*) Treatment initially very toxic but also therapeutic

but is a vitally important consideration. Entry at the commencement of treatment will produce a group of patients who do not complete their prescribed treatment and may not be worthy of comparison. Entry after completion of treatment may favourably skew the results in favour of the treatment by excluding early deaths from either disease or the therapy itself. It has been known in some studies for patients who failed to meet the stringent criteria for treatment on the study arm to be placed into the control arm, thus tipping the balance in favour of the former. Furthermore, if a large number of patients is lost to follow up, very close scrutiny of the claimed results is required before conclusions can be accepted.

Finally, reports of improved survival with any new treatment regimen over that which was experienced 10–20 years ago must be regarded with scepticism, even though numbers may be large and statistics convincing. The observed improvement may in fact be attributable to *stage migration*. This is best illustrated by the *Will Rogers* phenomenon. This famous American comedian proclaimed that 'when the Oakies moved from Oklahoma to California during the dust-bowl crisis, they raised the average IQ of both states'! Feinstein, Sosin and Wells (1985) produced disturbing evidence which suggested that contemporary improvements of survival rates in patients with lung cancer are a statistical artefact caused by a general drift of patients into higher clinical stages as a result of better diagnostic imaging techniques. Thus patients can move from stage I to stage IV on the basis of a CT or MRI scan, which was not available 20 years ago. This has the effect of improving the expected survival rates of both stage I and stage IV groups of patients.

Clinical trials

Most of the published literature about chemotherapy in head and neck cancer has been based on information obtained from properly conducted clinical trials. Anecdotal reports and retrospective reviews of casually applied but well intentioned treatment carry little credence. Many agents with proven efficacy for other tumours are still considered 'investigational' in head and neck cancer. All of the common drugs have been extensively investigated at phase I and phase II levels but useful phase III trial information is still scant.

The backbone of any drug trial is the protocol design. This needs to be 'watertight' with all possible eventualities anticipated before any patients are entered. Objectives need to be clearly defined and finite limits set on numbers and time. Contingency plans to deal with 'drop outs' and protocol violations are also necessary.

Eligibility criteria

Eligibility criteria are the set of rigid guidelines which have to be met before any particular patient can be entered into a trial. They are intended to ensure that all the patients in the trial fit into a well-defined population, and to screen against any conditions which may contraindicate chemotherapy. Thus the majority of patients entered into phase II and phase III trials have been carefully selected and do not necessarily reflect a typical sample of patients with advanced head and neck cancer. An example of typical selection criteria is given in Table 22.5. Common exclusions from entry into a trial include:

Table 22.5 Typical work up and eligibility criteria required

Full history and physical examination
Routine haematology and biochemistry
    White cell count (WCC) > $3 \times 10^9/l$
    Haemoglobin (Hb) > 12 g/100 ml
    Blood urea nitrogen (BUN) < 10 mmol/l
    Creatinine < 114 μmol/l
    Liver function tests normal
Radiology
    Chest X-ray
    Computerized tomographic/magnetic resonance scans
    Ultrasound liver
    Isotope scan liver/spleen/brain
Karnofsky performance status > 50%
Pulmonary function tests normal
Cardiac ejection fraction > 50%
Audiogram
    Pure-tone audiogram < 30 dB; s.d. > 80%
Dental opinion/clearance
Nutritional consultation
Immunobiological staging
    Delayed cutaneous hypersensitivity
    T-lymphocyte levels
    Lymphocyte function *in vitro*
    IgA and IgE determinations

1 Another synchronous primary tumour
2 Another recent primary tumour, e.g. within 3 years
3 Previous chemotherapy
4 Poor renal and lung function
5 Refusal to consent.

Phase I trials

Phase I trials are intended to be the initial evaluation of a new drug in humans. Ideally, the drug will have been previously evaluated in rodents, dogs and monkeys, and information should be available about its absorption, blood levels, distribution, excretion and toxicity. The object of the trial is to:

1 Establish antitumour activity
2 Establish toxicity
3 Establish the maximum tolerated dose
4 Gain information about uptake, metabolism, excretion and organ distribution.

These trials are often performed in patients with advanced disease refractory to other treatments. Interpretation of the results may be difficult and a false-negative result can potentially condemn a truly active drug to the shelf.

Phase II trials

Phase II trials are intended to identify the therapeutic efficacy of a single new drug or combination of drugs. Definitive answers about the ultimate value or precise role of each drug or combination of drugs are not expected. Ideally, the drug should be given at levels close to the maximum tolerated dose as determined by a phase I trial. Variation of the dose scheduling is permitted.

The object of a phase II trial is to assess response and measure the duration of response, if possible. Traditionally, new agents have been rejected for further study if the probability of response is less than 20%. If a phase II trial demonstrates no response in 14 patients, it is usually terminated because, by that stage, the true response rate in a larger trial would not exceed 20% ($P < 0.05$).

Broad trials may include a variety of *signal* tumours such as lymphomas, leukaemias and carcinomas of the breast, colon and lung. Head and neck cancer trials are much narrower disease orientated studies in which patient characteristics, site and stage are variables. Safeguards have to be taken to avoid making incorrect conclusions which take into account the possibility of false-negative results.

Phase III trials

Phase III trials are comprehensive studies of an active drug or drug combination. This usually involves a large randomized controlled clinical trial. Historical controls are virtually meaningless for this type of study as there is a great danger that two different populations might be compared. Patients should be matched, stratified and randomized into study and control arms before the treatment is begun.

The main object of a phase III trial is to measure and compare length of survival. Cross-overs should be avoided as they defeat the objectives of the trial and confuse the issues. Protocol design should include calculations of the necessary sample size, details of the statistical method of analysis and instructions on how to deal with excluded or *non-evaluable* patients. A multicentre trial may be required to obtain a sufficient number of patients within the time period allotted.

Few randomized trials have been performed which have been large enough to detect or exclude differences in survival which might be expected to be obtained from chemotherapy in head and neck cancer. Most trials have been reported to show no significant difference in outcome, but are too small to exclude differences that would be regarded as clinically important. Detection or exclusion of a 15% difference in absolute survival between the treatment and control arms usually requires about 250 patients, assuming a power of 0.9 and P value of 0.05. The two largest controlled trials, based on more than 1000 patients (Fazekas, Sommer and Kramer, 1980; Head and Neck Contracts Program, 1987), both showed no significant difference between the study and control arms. Small but clinically important differences may be exposed by meta-analysis. This statistical technique involves the pooling of results from all published (and if possible unpublished) properly conducted, randomized, controlled trials. If most of the trials reported show an improvement in the same direction, but none are significant in their own right, there may be an overall significant effect which can be revealed by meta-analysis. However, if about half the trials show improvement and the other half of equally sized and equally reliable trials show the opposite, meta-analysis is likely to show that such treatment is ineffective (Peto, 1987).

Ethical problems may arise in large trials when it becomes obvious that one arm is performing much better than the other. Happily, guidelines exist to deal with such a dilemma (Rubinstein and Gail, 1982).

Chemotherapy in practice

Between one-third and one-half of all head and neck cancer patients present with stage I or stage II disease and can expect a reasonable (70–90%) chance of cure with surgery or radiotherapy. Combined modality treatment is seldom necessary in this group. The remainder present with local or regionally advanced disease (stage III or stage IV), sometimes with established distant metastases (Table 22.6). Approximately one-third of these patients die from their disease, despite the efforts of surgeons, radiotherapists and oncologists.

For the past 30 years or so, the traditional role of chemotherapy in the management of head and neck cancer has been confined to the treatment of recurrence and/or metastatic disease (Clarke *et al.*, 1988; Pinto and Jacobs, 1991). The treatment goal is palliation, measured as prolongation of life or suppression of symptoms. However, since most major symptoms are due to the presence of tumour, effective palliation can only be achieved by reduction of tumour size

Table 22.6 Incidence of distant metastases in head and neck squamous cell carcinoma (by site)

Primary site	%
Oral cavity	8
Faucial arch	7
Oropharynx	15
Nasopharynx	28
Nasal cavity and sinuses	9
Supraglottic larynx	15
Vocal cord	3
Hypopharynx	24
Average	11

Adapted from Merino, Lindberg and Fletcher, 1977; an analysis of 5019 cases.

which, in turn, is likely to prolong survival. Although most of the drugs mentioned so far are thought to have activity in this setting, i.e. they produce partial response rates of up to 30% for periods of time, they do not necessarily prolong survival. Morton *et al.* (1985) reported their experience with cisplatin and bleomycin in a phase III randomized trial in advanced/recurrent disease. Cisplatin alone extended median survival by up to 63 days (Figure 22.10) compared with the control group whose survival curve was virtually identical to those patients receiving a combination of cisplatin and bleomycin. Those patients assigned to receive bleomycin alone had an even steeper survival curve and appeared to have been disadvantaged by the drug. Single agent methotrexate produces similar response rates to single agent cisplatin in advanced or recurrent disease. The Eastern Co-operative Oncology Group (ECOG) have compared methotrexate in combination with cisplatin and bleomycin in a large randomized trial (Vogl *et al.*, 1985). Improved response rates in the combination arm (48% versus 35%) failed to translate into improved survival.

The addition of 5-fluorouracil to cisplatin (the most potent combination in terms of response) in two large recent studies (Forastiere *et al.* (Southwest Oncology Group), 1992; Jacobs *et al.*, 1992) again failed to show a survival advantage. 5-Fluorouracil is generally given by continuous infusion over 4 days in hospital. This alone raised questions about the quality of life and cost effectiveness. Slow intravenous injections of methotrexate, 50 mg/m², given weekly on an outpatient basis remain a simple, well tried and practical regimen which does not require the strict supervision of an expert oncologist.

Induction chemotherapy

Rationale for induction chemotherapy

Impressive improvements in survival brought about by chemotherapy in leukaemias, lymphomas and some solid tumours, encouraged many oncologists to turn their attention to squamous cell carcinoma of the head and neck, where no improvements in survival had been seen for more than a generation (Stell and McCormick, 1986). The result of chemotherapy in cases of advanced recurrent disease were not impressive and so the treatment emphasis shifted to patients with early disease who had not yet undergone surgery or radiotherapy. The assumption of giving chemotherapy 'upfront' is to allow better assessment of a response, to enhance the later effects of radiotherapy and to eliminate the need for surgery in some patients. Other strong theoretical arguments for giving induction chemotherapy have been advanced for which a number of equally strong arguments against have emerged (Table 22.7).

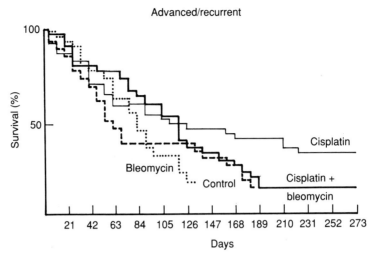

Figure 22.10 The results in a phase III trial

Table 22.7   Theoretical and practical arguments for and against induction chemotherapy

	Advantages	Disadvantages
1	Effective drug levels obtained because tumour vascularity unaffected by surgery or radiotherapy	Time spent giving chemotherapy delays surgery and radiotherapy which may be of more benefit
2	Better drug tolerance allows full effective courses to be given	Toxicity
3	Micrometastases eradicated	Immunosuppression promotes survival of micrometastases
4	Unresectable tumours rendered resectable	Tumour shrinkage confuses the surgical margin
5	Radiotherapy field and dose may be reduced, thus lowering morbidity	Potentiation of side effects of radiotherapy, e.g. mucositis, may compromise treatment
6	Chemotherapy predicts response to radiotherapy	Complete responders occasionally refuse further treatment until too late
7	Radiotherapy alone may be sufficient after a major response	Prolonged hospitalization

The significance of a complete response with induction therapy

Patients who have a good response to chemotherapy appear to have a better prognosis overall, regardless of treatment modality, than those who do not respond. This is especially true of patients who achieve a complete response after induction chemotherapy, followed by a standard treatment modality (Ensley *et al.*, 1984; Primrose *et al.*, 1985). Whether this benefit can be attributed, wholly or in part to the chemotherapy, is open to debate. Achieving a lesser response, as in other solid tumours, is much less predictive of ultimate cure. It is likely that complete responders have biologically favourable tumours which would do well with any established treatment modality. Radiotherapy alone, following a complete response, may be adequate treat-

ment (Primrose *et al.*, 1985) as the total tumour burden is obviously very small after chemotherapy.

Histological specimens of tumour sites following a complete response, are difficult to interpret. Increased differentiation, manifested by cellular enlargement, glycogen formation, desmosome activity and marked keratinization have been described (Michaels, Grey and Rowson, 1973). Up to 40% of complete responders have no detectable tumour in surgical specimens after resection of the previously involved area (Al-Kourainy *et al.*, 1987). However, most complete responders still have viable tumour cells present after chemotherapy, as evidenced by following a few patients who drop out from trials following a complete response to chemotherapy, and refuse all further treatment. Of the 100 patients reported by the present author in 1985, two such patients have been identified (complete remission after cisplatin and bleomycin) both of whom eventually died of disease at 5 and 6 years respectively. Four such patients were identified by Weaver *et al.* in 1982 (complete remission after cisplatin and 5-fluorouracil). Tumour recurrence was noted in three of these patients at 4, 6 and 7 months after chemotherapy; the fourth patient, with a base of tongue tumour, was said to be clinically and histologically disease free 18 months after chemotherapy.

Phase III trials of induction chemotherapy

The results of some of the larger randomized, control clinical trials that have evaluated the results of induction chemotherapy are summarized in Table 22.8. Many of these trials have been subsequently criticized for a number of reasons. The delivery of only one cycle of chemotherapy, or regimens which fail to include cisplatin, are considered by some as providing suboptimal treatment. Many of the trials have methodological limitations, such as exclusion of patients after randomization, and others have follow-up intervals which are too short to be definitive. Most are too small to detect clinically relevant differences in survival and therefore the vast majority report no significant difference in survival between the chemotherapy and control arms, although a trend is seen in some. One solution to these problems has been to pool the results and provide an overview which could be subject to meta-analysis.

Meta-analysis of induction chemotherapy

Stell and Rawson (1990) presented an overview of 23 randomized controlled trials of the management of head and neck cancer, two-thirds of which compared induction chemotherapy with standard treatment to a control group which received standard treatment alone. The remainder of the trials tested the effects of synchronous radiotherapy with chemotherapy compared to standard treatment. They looked at trial design, analysis of survival, response rates, site of failure, toxicity and cost. The minimal increase in survival that could be detected ranged from 11 to 51% with a median of 25%. No individual trial was big enough to detect the likely increase of survival, which they estimated at around 5%. The death rate of the 3398 patients who were randomized was 56.7% in the control arms and 56.2% in the treatment arms, i.e. an improvement of survival of 0.5% in the chemotherapy arms. This difference was not significant.

Subgroup analysis was carried out to compare the various agents used, whether singly or in combination, and when they were given. No single agent or combination of drugs produced a significant reduction of cancer deaths, although the combination of vincristine, bleomycin and methotrexate (VBM) significantly increased the number of deaths. Induction chemotherapy, synchronous chemotherapy and induction/maintenance chemotherapy did not affect

Table 22.8 Results of some of the larger randomized controlled clinical trials on induction chemotherapy

Authors and year	Patient numbers	Chemotherapy	Outcome
Archangeli *et al.*, 1983	142	Intra-arterial MTX	No significant difference in survival (favours chemotherapy arm)
Fazekas, Sommer and Kramer, 1980	638	MTX	No significant difference in survival
Head and Neck Contracts Program, 1987	462	DDP, BLEO	No significant difference in survival; distant metastases reduced with chemotherapy
Holoye, Grossman and Toohill, 1985	77	5FU	No significant difference in survival
Laramore *et al.* Intergroup study, 1992	442	DDP 5FU	No significant difference in survival; distant metastases reduced with chemotherapy
Jaulerry, Rodriguez and Brinin,* 1992	208	DDP 5FU VIN	No significant difference in survival
Knowlton *et al.*, 1975	96	MTX 5FU	No significant difference in survival
Kun, Toohill and Holoye, 1986	83	MTX 5FU BLEO	No significant difference in survival
Martin, Mazeron and Brun, 1988	107	MTX 5FU BLEO DDP	No significant difference in survival (favours control arm)
Schuller *et al.* (SWOG), 1988	158	MTX VINC BLEO DDP	No significant difference in survival; distant metastases reduced with chemotherapy
Stell *et al.*, 1983	86	MTX VINC BLEO 5FU	No significant difference in survival
Stolwijk *et al.*, 1983	68	MTX VINB BLEO 5FU CYC	No significant difference in survival
Taylor, Applebaum and Showell, 1985	82	MTX	No significant difference in survival
Toohill *et al.*,* 1987	143	MTX CYC MTX 5FU DDP	Significantly better survival in control arms

* Two studies combined. MTX = Methotrexate; BLEO = bleomycin; CYC = cyclophosphamide; VINB = vinblastine; DDP = cisplatin; 5FU = 5-fluorouracil; VINC = vincristine

cancer mortality, whereas synchronous/maintenance therapy significantly improved it. They also looked at the site of failure. Locoregional recurrence was 6.7% less in those patients who received chemotherapy, which was a highly significant finding. In contrast, distant metastases were 2% less common and this was not significant.

Similar results emerged from an overview of 43 prospective randomized studies of adjuvant and adjunctive chemotherapy in head and neck cancer carried out by the Winnipeg group (El-Sayed, 1992, personal communication). A small survival advantage with chemotherapy was apparent from the 5277 evaluable patients, at the expense of increased toxicity. Some patients with oral cavity lesions and those who received simultaneous and then maintenance chemotherapy appeared to be favourable subgroups, and confirmed Stell and Rawson's analysis.

More recently, Munro (1995) has undertaken an in depth overview of 54 randomized control trials using both the odds ratio method of Mantel-Haenszel (1990) and the rate difference method described by DerSimonian and Laird (1986). His pooled data suggested that chemotherapy increased absolute survival by 6.5% (95% confidence limits 3.1–9.9%). Subgroup analysis showed an even more striking survival benefit conferred by single agent chemotherapy given syncronously with radiotherapy, where overall absolute survival was increased by 12.1% (95% confidence limits 5–19%). A combination of platinum compounds and 5-fluorouracil was less effective (5.4% increase in survival) and induction chemotherapy even less beneficial (3.7% overall improvement in survival).

The conclusions are highly significant and appear relatively insensitive to publication bias, no single study being unduly influential. It would require a very large unreported trial with highly negative results to overturn the conclusions.

Although meta-analysis of potentially 'flawed' trials has been criticized by one or two eminent oncologists, it is now generally accepted that induction chemotherapy, even with the most active combinations of drugs, is unlikely to improve survival significantly, and should either be restricted to investigational settings or abandoned completely.

Reasons for failure

Not only has induction chemotherapy failed to show a survival advantage over standard local treatment, it has also been implicated in adversely affecting prognosis in a number of trials (Stell and Rawson, 1990). Toohill *et al.* (1987) documented the delay in progressing to standard local treatment caused by the administration of induction chemotherapy which averaged 66 days in their first study and 95 days in their second study. They cited this as the major factor responsible for their negative findings. There may

also be a biological explanation for the limitation of induction chemotherapy, based on the following hypotheses (Tannock, 1994):

1 *Inadequate cell kill.* Even pathologically confirmed complete responses may still contain a large number of viable tumour cells scattered through the original tumour location. These cells retain the capacity to proliferate and overwhelm the host again (Figure 22.11)

2 *Reduction in surgical margins or radiation fields.* A dramatic reduction in tumour volume with induction chemotherapy has rendered a number of hitherto unresectable tumours to be removed surgically. This *confusion* of the limits of the tumour has led to microscopically positive margins and ultimate tumour recurrence in a number of cases. Similar reductions in radiation fields and doses have happened after chemotherapy, and produced a similar effect on outcome

3 *Reduction in radiosensitivity after chemotherapy.* A number of mechanisms has been postulated to account for this phenomenon including reduced tumour cell oxygenation and induction into the cell cycle. Prior exposure to chemotherapy has been reported by some investigators to cause a decrease in the intrinsic radiosensitivity (Louie *et al.*, 1985). This effect has been described after treatment with alkylating agents such as cisplatin and doxorubicin, but varies with the cell lines that have been studied. One possible mechanism may

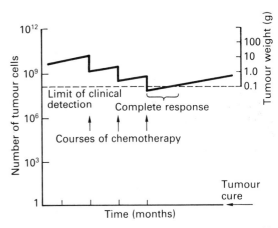

Figure 22.11 A hypothetical tumour containing 10^{10} viable cells (about 10 g) is treated with three courses of chemotherapy, each of which kills 90% of the cells. There is some repopulation between treatments. After three courses, the number of viable tumour cells is less than 10^8 (about 0.1 g) and the patient is judged to be in complete clinical and radiological remission. This is a small step toward tumour cure. Also, additional chemotherapy may not be helpful if drug-resistant cells have been selected after three courses of chemotherapy. (Reproduced with permission from Million and Cassisi, 1994, J. B. Lippincott Co.)

be drug-induced stimulation of glutathione synthesis, or induction of the enzymes glutathione-S-transferase and glutathione reductase which were involved in the inactivation of radicals produced by ionizing radiation and some anticancer drugs (Clarke, 1986).

Synchronous chemotherapy/radiotherapy

A number of interactions between radiotherapy and chemotherapy has been extensively studied in the laboratory setting and are summarized in Table 22.9. It is postulated that cells with intrinsic or acquired resistance to radiation should be sensitive to radiation in the presence of chemotherapy.

Two types of schedules of concomitant chemotherapy and radiotherapy have been subject to clinical trial. The first added a single agent at a low or moderate dose to the standard radiation treatment. A number of randomized trials have investigated this approach, all reported increased toxicity with synchronous treatment but also an increase in local control and disease-free survival (Shanta and Krisnamurthi, 1980; Fu *et al.*, 1987; Gupta, Pointon and Wilkinson, 1987; Bachaud *et al.*, 1991) and one, which used fluorouracil, reported that overall survival was improved for oral cavity lesions (Lo *et al.*, 1976).

A second approach to synchronous chemotherapy and radiation treatment attempted to optimize the chemotherapy component. Multiple agents were given at higher doses and in more intensive schedules which required regularly scheduled interruptions of radiation treatment. It is known that an interruption in the administration of radiation treatment, as a single treatment modality, results in lower rates of control (Pajak *et al.*, 1991). The risk inherent with these regimens, therefore, is the suboptimal delivery of the standard treatment (radiation) in order

Table 22.9 Interaction between chemotherapy and radiotherapy

Drug and radiation active against different tumour cell subpopulations
Decreased tumour cell repopulation following fractionated radiation
Increased tumour cell recruitment from G_0 into therapy-responsive cell cycle phase
Cell cycle synchronization
Improved drug delivery with shrinkage of tumour
Early eradication of tumour cells preventing drug and/or radiation resistance
Eradication of cells resistant to one treatment modality by the other
Inhibition of repair of radiation damage

Adapted from Vokes and Weichselbaum 1990

to optimize the administration of the experimental drug combination. Despite these reservations, a number of promising trials have reported encouraging rates of local or regional control and survival (Taylor *et al.*, 1989; Vokes *et al.*, 1989; Adelstein *et al.*, 1990a, b). Most of these have used infusional fluorouracil with one or more additional drugs and have uniformly reported mucositis as a dose limiting toxic effect. Combination chemotherapy with synchronous radiotherapy has been compared with induction chemotherapy (using the same drugs) followed by radiation in three trials. All indicated superior disease free or overall survival for the synchronous treatment groups (SECOG, 1986; Adelstein, 1990a, b; Merlano *et al.*, 1991). In addition one recent randomized trial, comparing rapidly alternating combination chemotherapy and radiation therapy with radiation alone, indicated superior survival for the group that received the combination drugs (Merlano *et al.*, 1992). Any beneficial effects of synchronous chemotherapy and radiation therapy may be due to the added toxic effects of the two modalities, with less than additive effects against dose limiting normal tissues. One mechanism may involve inhibition of cell proliferation, which may be stimulated in the tumour as shrinkage is accompanied by improved vascularity.

Similar effects on cell kill however could be obtained by using radiation treatment alone by hyperfractionation. Very promising initial results have been shown in a number of studies. The question remains whether synchronous chemotherapy and radiotherapy should be compared to hyperfractionated radiotherapy in a large controlled trial.

UKHAN I

UKHAN I is the largest multicentre UK-based trial in progress at the moment. It addresses both single agent methotrexate and combination VBMF (vincristine, bleomycin, methotrexate, 5-fluorouracil) synchronous chemotherapy with the possibility of adjuvant treatment in some patients. All head and neck cancer patients are eligible, including a postsurgical arm, apart from those with T1N0 and metastatic disease. Enthusiasm for the flexible protocol has come mainly from the encouraging results produced by the Christie Hospital in Manchester using single agent methotrexate (Gupta, Pointon and Wilkinson, 1987) and the SECOG participants from in and around London who prefer a VBMF regimen (SECOG, 1986).

Accrual began in January 1990, using an unbalanced randomization of four arms (Table 22.10) allowing a 2×2 factorial analysis. Six centres participated in the first year, this has now increased to 25 centres, which include three from overseas. Thirteen of these have opted for the methotrexate only regimen, the remainder for VBMF. The original intention to accrue 1000 patients by the end of 1994 has fallen behind schedule, but with 590 randomized

Table 22.10 UKHAN I trial design

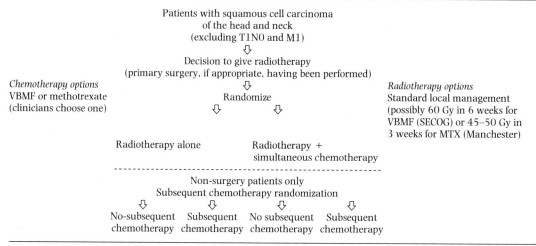

Patients with squamous cell carcinoma
of the head and neck
(excluding T1N0 and M1)
⇩

Decision to give radiotherapy
(primary surgery, if appropriate, having been performed)

Chemotherapy options	⇩	*Radiotherapy options*
VBMF or methotrexate	Randomize	Standard local management
(clinicians choose one)	⇩ ⇩	(possibly 60 Gy in 6 weeks for
		VBMF (SECOG) or 45–50 Gy in
		3 weeks for MTX (Manchester))

Radiotherapy alone   Radiotherapy +
simultaneous chemotherapy

- -

Non-surgery patients only
Subsequent chemotherapy randomization
⇩   ⇩   ⇩   ⇩
No-subsequent   Subsequent   No subsequent   Subsequent
chemotherapy   chemotherapy   chemotherapy   chemotherapy

MTX: methotrexate; VBMF: vincristine, bleomycin, methotrexate, 5-fluorouracil

patients at the end of 1993 this promises to be one of the largest phase III trials in the world, allowing a high probability of detecting a small (5–10%) difference in survival and other endpoints.

Organ preservation

The removal of the thyroid gland or major salivary glands can be accomplished with minimal disfigurement in the majority of patients, unlike the removal of the tongue, mandible or larynx. The larynx is the commonest organ to be affected by squamous cell carcinoma in the head and neck region (either as primary disease or direct spread from the hypopharynx) and consequently, for many years, surgeons have developed and refined conservation techniques to compete stage by stage with results obtained by primary radiotherapy.

It has been postulated for some time that chemotherapy can be substituted for surgery in advanced head and neck cancer patients who achieve a complete response (Jacobs *et al.*, 1987). Larynx preservation using induction chemotherapy followed by radiotherapy has slowly gained momentum as a treatment strategy (Karp *et al.*, 1991). The cooperative studies programme of the Department of Veterans Affairs began a multicentre trial in 1985 comparing total laryngectomy with induction chemotherapy/radiotherapy to test this concept. One hundred and sixty-six patients were recruited into each arm and assessed after 2 years, the 4% difference in survival (65% versus 61%) in favour of the laryngectomy group was not found to be significant. The difference in disease-free survival (Figure 22.12) is even more striking, though is not significant at 2 years (Depart-

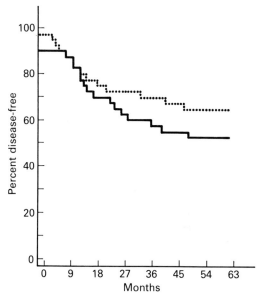

Figure 22.12 Disease-free interval for 332 patients randomly assigned to induction chemotherapy and radiation therapy (solid line) or conventional laryngectomy and postoperative radiation (dotted line). The disease-free interval survival was shorter in the chemotherapy group, but the difference was not statistically significant (*P* = 0.1195). (From Wolf *et al.*, 1991, reprinted by permission of *The New England Journal of Medicine*, **324**, 1688, 1991)

ment of Veterans Affairs Laryngeal Cancer Study Group, 1991). The authors brushed aside the highly significant finding that only 2% of the laryngectomy arm recurred locally compared to 12% of the chemotherapy arm and proclaimed that the major finding of the study was that 64% of patients randomly assigned to induction chemotherapy could retain their larynx.

This study has attracted criticism for not including a radiation only treatment arm which may have proven as effective as the induction chemotherapy arm. Hence, its conclusions are both fundamentally flawed and also prone to reporting bias. Despite these interpretations, organ preservation using chemotherapy at other sites in the head and neck is very much in vogue. All we can do is wait to see if similar trends in local recurrence and disease-free survival emerge.

Cost

The cost of chemotherapy cannot be overlooked in these days of audit, cost effectiveness and financial restraint. Stell and Rawson (1990) calculated the cost of induction and maintenance regimens based on the length of stay in an English teaching hospital (plus 3 days for assessment and recovery). Length of stay ranged from 3 to 50 days with a median of 22 and cost £3361. They dismissed the cost of drugs as relatively small, but clearly this can no longer by ignored with a single 450 mg vial of carboplatin costing £205 (MIMS, January 1994).

Typical 1989 costs for four cycles of outpatient cisplatin and bleomycin in the USA are estimated at $7360, with 5 days hospitalization for leucopenia adding another $5925 (Million and Sigal, 1994).

Chemoprevention

Chemoprevention is the administration of drugs to suppress carcinogenesis and prevent the development of invasive cancer. This is now recognized as an important treatment strategy, especially in the head and neck, where despite successful treatment of primary disease, second primary cancers develop at an annual rate of 3–7%. The commonest premalignant lesion in the head and neck is leucoplakia, easily recognized as white patches in the mouth, tongue or larynx caused by increased keratin production. The ability of synthetic natural retinoids to reverse leucoplakia has been studied extensively, with rates of response ranging from 50 to 100%. 13-*Cis*-retinoic acid has been evaluated in a number of randomized placebo controlled trials. When administered for 3 months at high doses, 67% of the lesions responded to isoretinoin compared with 10% of the lesions treated with placebo (Hong *et al.*, 1986), however, a number of the lesions which responded, progressed within 3 months after cessation of therapy and a significant number of side effects were reported including cheilitis, dermatitis, conjunctivitis and hypertriglyceridaemia.

In a subsequent trial, patients were treated for 3 months with high dose isoretinoin and then randomly assigned to receive maintenance therapy with either low dose isoretinoin or betacarotene (Lipman *et al.*, 1993). This trial again confirmed the activity and toxicity of high dose isoretinoin, which was more effective in low dose maintenance than the betacarotene, both of which were equally well tolerated. The use of high dose isoretinoin has also been investigated as adjuvant therapy after surgery and radiation treatment. It produces a significant overall reduction in second primary tumours (Hong *et al.*, 1990).

New dimensions and new directions

The search for effective new drugs and drug combinations continues with Taxol (paclitaxel) receiving much attention. This drug, which is derived from the bark of the Yew tree has already shown substantial activity in heavily pretreated and platinum refractory patients with advanced progressive ovarian cancer. In this setting it is infused over a 3-hour period at a dose of 175 mg/m²/every 3 weeks and produces significant responses in over 20% of patients. Adverse reactions include type 1 anaphylactic hypersensitivity, myelosuppression and peripheral neuropathy. It is not yet licensed for general head and neck use in the UK.

Interest is also growing in the biochemical modulation of 5-fluorouracil by folinic acid or interferon, where increased response rates have been seen in colorectal, gastric and oesophageal cancer (Wilke *et al.*, 1992). Both folinic acid and interferon inhibit the enzyme thymidylate synthetase by increasing the levels of 5-Fd VMP and Fd VMP respectively, thus preventing DNA synthesis.

Modulation of P glycoprotein (responsible for drug transport into tumour cells) can also be affected by a number of other non-cytotoxic drugs including nifedipine, verapamil, quinine, chloraquin, progestogens, tamoxifen, cyclosporin A, reserpine and tricyclic antidepressants.

In general terms, however, the use of chemotherapy in head and neck cancer has not shown the dramatic improvements of survival seen in other tumours and has not been adopted as part of our standard treatment. Some medical oncologists have expressed reservations about the use of chemotherapy outside the investigational setting of a clinical trial (Vokes and Weichselbaum, 1990; Tobias, 1992).

The most recent and largest overview of randomized trials performed by Munro (1995) now shows a robust and highly significant improvement of absolute survival of 6.5% conferred by the addition of chemotherapy; even more impressive is the 12.1% increase survival rate conferred by synchronously administered single agent drugs.

Perhaps at this stage more oncology centres should adopt the use of synchronous chemotherapy/radiotherapy as part of standard treament, as well as participate in large multcentred trials such as UKHAN I. It would also seem prudent at this stage to abandon the use of induction chemotherapy as it confers little, if any, benefit to the patient.

The continued use of platinum-based chemotherapy in selected patients with metastatic or recurrent disease should continue with the emphasis on particular subgroups of patients such as those with anaplastic tumours of the nasopharynx who have shown particular promise with maintenance treatment (Boussen *et al.*, 1991; Tannock, 1994).

References

ADELSTEIN, D.J., SHARAN, V.M., EARLE, A.S., SHAH, A.C., VLASTOU, C., HARIA, C.D. *et al.* (1990a) Long term results after chemotherapy for locally confined squamous cell head and neck cancer. *American Journal of Clinical Oncology*, **13**, 440–447

ADELSTEIN, D.J., SHARAN, V.M., EARLE, A.S., SHAH, A.C., VLASTOU, C., HARIA, C.D. *et al.* (1990b) Simultaneous versus sequential combined technique therapy for squamous cell head and neck cancer. *Cancer*, **65**, 1685–1691

AL-KOURAINY, K., KISH, J., ENSLEY, J., TAPAZOGLOU, E., JACOBS, J., WEAVER, A. *et al.* (1987) Achievement of superior survival for histologically negative versus histologically positive clinically complete responders to cisplatin combinations in patients with locally advanced head and neck cancer. *Cancer*, **59**, 233–238

ARCHANGELI, G., NERVI, C., RINGHINI, R., CRETON, G., MIRRI, M.A.M. and GUERRA, A. (1983) Combined radiation and drugs: the effect of intra-arterial chemotherapy followed by radiotherapy in head and neck cancer. *Radiotherapy and Oncology*, **1**, 101–107

BACHAUD, J.M., DAVID, J.M., BOUSSIN, G. and DALY, N. (1991) Combined post operative radiotherapy and weekly cisplatin infusion for locally advanced squamous cell carcinoma of the head and neck: preliminary report of a randomised trial. *International Journal of Radiation, Oncology, Biology and Physics*, **20**, 263–296

BLUM, R.H., CARTER, S.K. and AGRE, N. (1973) A clinical review of bleomycin – a new antineoplastic agent. *Cancer*, **31**, 903–914

BOUSSEN, H., CVITKOVIC, E., WENDTING, J.L., AZLI, N., BACHOUCHI, M., MAHJOUBI, R. *et al.* (1991) Chemotherapy of metastatic and/or recurrent undifferentiated nasopharyngeal carcinoma with cisplatin, bleomycin and fluorouracil. *Journal of Clinical Oncology*, **9**, 1675–1681

BROWMAN, G.P., GOODYEAR, M.D.E., LEVINE, M.N., RUSSEL, R.I., ARCHIBALD, S.D., YOUNG, J.E.M. *et al.* (1990) Modulation of the antitumour effect of methotrexate by low-dose bueovorin in squamous cell head and neck cancer: a randomised placebo-controlled clinical trial. *Journal of Clinical Oncology*, **8**, 203–208

BRUCE, W., MEEKER, B. and VALERIOTE, F. (1966) Comparison of the sensitivity of normal haematopoietic and transplanted lymphoma colony-forming cells to chemotherapeutic agents administered in vitro. *Journal of the National Cancer Institute*, **37**, 233–245

CANN, C., FRIED, M. and ROTHMAN, K. (1985) Epidemiology of squamous cancer of the head and neck. *Otolaryngologic Clinics of North America*, **18**, 367–388

CLARKE, E.P. (1986) Thiol-induced biochemical modification of chemo- and radio-responses. *International Journal of Radiation, Oncology, Biology and Physics*, **12**, 1121–1126

CLARKE, J.R., FALLON, B.G., DREYFUSS, A.I., HOSCHNER, J., KINZIE, J., LOH, J.J. *et al.* (1988) Chemotherapeutic strategies in the multidisciplinary treatment of head and neck cancer. *Seminars in Oncology*, **15**, 35–44

CONLEY, J. and DINGMAN, D.L. (1974) Adenoid cystic carcinoma of the head and neck. *Archives of Otolaryngology*, **100**, 81–90

D'ARCY, P.F. (1986) Handling anticancer drugs. In: *Iatrogenic Diseases Update*, 2nd edn. Oxford: Oxford University Press. pp. 224–230

DECKER, D.A., DRELICHMAN, A., JACOBS, J., HOSCHER, J., KINZIE, J., LOH, J.J. *et al.* (1983) Adjuvant chemotherapy with cis-diaminodichloroplatinum II and 120 hour infusion 5-fluorouracil in stage III and IV squamous cell carcinoma of the head and neck. *Cancer*, **51**, 1353–1355

DEPARTMENT OF VETERANS AFFAIRS LARYNGEAL CANCER STUDY GROUP (1991) Induction chemotherapy plus radiation compared with surgery plus radiation in patients with advanced laryngeal cancer. *New England Journal of Medicine*, **324**, 1685–1690

DERSIMONIAN, R. and LAIRD, N. (1986) Meta-analysis in clinical trials. *Controlled Clinical Trials*, **7**, 177–188

DONNER, A.L. (1978) Possible risks of working with antineoplastic drugs in horizontal laminar flow hoods. *American Journal of Hospital Pharmacy*, **10**, 127–130

ENSLEY, J., KISH, J., JACOBS, A., WEAVER, J., CRISSMAN, J., KINGIE, M. *et al.* (1984) Superior survival in complete responders achieved with chemotherapy alone compared to those requiring chemotherapy in patients with advanced squamous cell carcinoma of the head and neck. *ASIO Abstracts*, p. 181

FAZEKAS, J.T., SOMMER, C. and KRAMER, S. (1980) Adjuvant intravenous methotrexate or definitive radiotherapy alone for advanced squamous cancers of the oral cavity, oropharynx, supraglottic larynx or hypopharynx: concluding report of the RTOG randomized trial on 638 patients. *International Journal of Radiation, Oncology, Biology and Physics*, **6**, 533–541

FEINSTEIN, A., SOSIN, D. and WELLS, C. (1985) The Will Rogers phenomenon. Stage migration and new diagnostic techniques as a source of misleading statistics for survival in cancer. *New England Journal of Medicine*, **312**, 1604–1608

FIELD, J.K., SPANDIDOS, D.A. MALLIRI, A., GOSNEY, J.R., YIAGNISIS, M. and STELL, P.M. (1991) Elevated p53 expression correlates with a history of heavy smoking and squamous cell carcinoma of the head and neck. *British Journal of Cancer*, **64**, 573–577

FISHER, B. and FISHER, E.R. (1968) The proliferation and spready of neoplastic cells. *21st Annual Symposium on Fundamental Cancer Research MD Anderson Hospital and Tumor Institute*. Baltimore: Williams & Wilkins. pp. 552–582

FORASTIERE, A.A. (1992) Chemotherapy of head and neck cancer. *Annals of Oncology*, **3**, 511–514

FORASTIERE A.A., METCH, B., SCHULLER, D.E., ENSLEY, J.F., HUTCHINS, L.F., TRIOZZI, P. *et al.* (1992) Randomised comparison of cisplatin plus fluorouracil and carboplatin plus fluorouracil versus methotrexate in advanced squamous cell carcinoma of the head and neck: a Southwest Oncology Group study. *Journal of Clinical Oncology*, **10**, 1245–1251

FREI, E., FREIREICH E., GEHAN, E. and RINKEL, D. (1961) Studies of sequential and combination antimetabolite therapy in acute leukaemia: 6 mercaptopurine and methotrexate acute leukaemia group B. *Blood*, **18**, 431–454

FU, K.K., PHILIPS, T.L., SILVERBERG, I.J., JACOBS, C., GOFFINET, D.R., CHUN, C. *et al.* (1987) Combined radiotherapy and chemotherapy with bleomycin and methotrexate for advanced inoperable head and neck cancer: update of a Northern California Oncology Group randomised trial. *Journal of Clinical Oncology*, **5**, 1410–1418

GUPTA, N.K., POINTON, R.C.S. and WILKINSON, P.M. (1987) A randomized clinical trial to contrast radiotherapy with radiotherapy and methotrexate given synchronously in head and neck cancer. *Clinical Radiology*, **38**, 575–581

HEAD AND NECK CONTRACTS PROGRAM (1987) Adjuvant chemotherapy for advanced head and neck squamous carcinoma. *Cancer*, **60**, 301–311

HEIDELBERGER, C., CHAUDHURI, N. and WESTON, E. (1958) The metabolism of 5-fluorouracil -2-C¹⁴ in humans. *Proceedings of the American Association of Medicine*, **73**, 897–900

HOLOYE, P.Y., GROSSMAN, T.W. and TOOHILL, R.J. (1985) Randomized study of adjuvant chemotherapy for head and neck cancer. *Otolaryngology, Head and Neck Surgery*, **93**, 712–717

HONG, W.K., ENDICOTT, J., ITRI, L.M., DOOS, W., BATSAKIS, J.G., BELL, R. *et al.* (1986) 13-cis-retinoic acid in the treatment of oral leukoplakia. *New England Journal of Medicine*, **315**, 1501–1505

HONG, W.K., LIPPMAN, S.M., ITRI, L.M., KARP, D.D., LEES, J.S., BYERS, R.M. *et al.* (1990) Prevention of second primary tumours with isoretinoin in squamous cell carcinoma of the head and neck. *New England Journal of Medicine*, **323**, 795–801

JACOBS, C., GOFFINET, D.R., GOFFINET, L., KOHLER, M. and FEE, W.E. (1987) Chemotherapy as a substitute for surgery in the treatment of advanced resectable head and neck cancer: a report from the Northern California Oncology Group. *Cancer*, **60**, 1178–1183

JACOBS, C., LYMAN, G., VELEZ-GARCIA, E., SRIDHAR, K.S., KNIGHT, W., HOCHSTER, H. *et al.* (1992) A phase III randomised study comparing cisplatin and fluorouracil as single agents and in combination for advanced squamous cell carcinoma of the head and neck. *Journal of Clinical Oncology*, **10**, 257–263

JAULERRY, C., RODRIGUEZ, J. and BRININ, F. (1992) Induction chemotherapy in advanced head and neck tumours: results of two randomised trials. *International Journal of Radiation, Oncology, Biology and Physics*, **23**, 483–489

KAPLAN, E.L. and MEIER, P. (1958) Non parametric estimation from incomplete observations. *Journal of the American Statistical Association*, **53**, 57–81

KARP, D.D., VAUGHAN, C.N., CARTER, R., WILLETT, B., HEEREN, T., CALARESE, P. *et al.* (1991) Larynx preservation using induction chemotherapy plus radiation therapy as an alternative to laryngectomy in advanced head and neck cancer. *American Journal of Clinical Oncology*, **14**, 273–279

KISH, J.A., ENSLEY, J., WEINER, A., JACOBS, J.R., KINZIE, J., CUMMINGS, G. *et al.* (1984) Improvement of complete response rate to induction adjuvant chemotherapy for advanced squamous carcinoma of the head and neck. *Adjuvant Therapy of Cancer IV*, pp. 107–115

KNOWLTON, A.H., PERCAPIO, B., BOBROW, S. and FISCHER, J.J.

(1975) Methotrexate and radiation therapy in the treatment of advanced head and neck tumours. *Radiology*, **116**, 709–712

KUN, L.E., TOOHILL, R.J. and HOLOYE, P.Y. (1986) A randomised study of adjuvant chemotherapy for cancer of the upper aerodigestive tract. *International Journal of Radiation, Oncology, Biology and Physics*, **12**, 173–178

LARAMORE, G.E., SCOTT, C.B., AL-SARRAF, M., HASELOW, R.E., ERVIN, T.J., WHEELER, R. *et al.* (1992) Adjuvant chemotherapy for resectable squamous cell carcinoma of the head and neck: report on Intergroup Study 0034. *International Journal of Radiation, Oncology, Biology and Physics*, **23**, 705–713

LIPMAN, S.M., BATSAKIS, J.G., TOTH, B.B., WEBER, R.S., LEE, J.J., MARTIN, J.W. *et al.* (1993) Comparison of low dose isoretinoin with beta carotene to prevent oral carcinogenesis. *New England Journal of Medicine*, **328**, 15–20

LO, T.C.M., WILEY, A.L., ANSFIELD, F.J., BRANDENBERG, J.H., DAVIS, H.L., GOLLIN, F.F. *et al.* (1976) Combined radiation therapy and 5-fluorouracil for advanced squamous cell carcinoma of the oral cavity and oropharynx: a randomised study. *American Journal of Roentgenology*, **126**, 229–235

LOUIE, K.G., BEHRENS, B.C., KINSELLA, T.J., HAMILTON, T.C., GROTZINGER, K.R., MCKOY, W.M. *et al.* (1985) Radiation survival parameters of antineoplastic drug-sensitive and resistant human ovarian cancer cell lines and their modification by buthionine sulfoximine. *Cancer Research*, **45**, 2110–2115

MCCULLOUGH. E.A. and TILL, J.E. (1971) Regulatory mechanism acting on haematopoietic stem cells. *American Journal of Pathology*, **65**, 601–614

MANTEL HAENSZEL (1990) *Early Breast Cancer Trialists' Collaborative Group Treatment of Early Breast Cancer, volume 1 Worldwide Evidence 1985–1990*. Oxford: Oxford University Press

MARTIN, M., MAZERON, J.J. and BRUN, B. (1988) Neo-adjuvant polychemotherapy of head and neck cancer: results of a randomized study (abstract). *Proceedings of the American Society of Clinical Oncology*, **7**, 152

MERINO, O.R., LINDBERG, R.D. and FLETCHER, G.H. (1977) An analysis of distant metastases from squamous cell carcinoma of the upper respiratory and digestive tracts. *Cancer*, **40**, 145–151

MERLANO, M., CORVO, R., MERGARINA, G., BENASSO, M., ROSSO, R., SERTOLI, M.R. *et al.* (1991) Combined chemotherapy and radiation therapy in advanced inoperable squamous cell carcinoma of the head and neck: the final report of a randomized trial. *Cancer*, **67**, 915–921

MERLANO, M., VITALE, V., ROSSO, R., BENASSO, M., CORVO, R., CAVALLARI, M. *et al.* (1992) Treatment of advanced squamous cell carcinoma of the head and neck with alternating chemotherapy and radiotherapy. *New England Journal of Medicine*, **327**, 1115–1121

MICHAELS, L., GREY, P.A. and ROWSON, K.E.K. (1973) Effects of bleomycin on human and experimental squamous carcinoma. *Journal of Pathology*, **109**, 315–321

MILLER, A.B., HOOGSTATEN, B., STAQUET, M. and WINKLER, A. (1981) Reporting results of cancer treatment. *Cancer*, **47**, 207–214

MILLION, R.R. and CASSISI, N.J. (1994) *Management of Head and Neck Cancer, a Multidisciplinary Approach*, 2nd edn. Philadelphia: J. B., Lippincott Company

MILLION, R.R. and SIGAL, M.C. (1994) Cost of management of head and neck cancer. In: *Management of Head and*

Neck Cancer, a Multidisciplinary Approach, 2nd edn, edited by R. R. Million and N. J. Cassisi. Philadelphia: J. B. Lippincott Company. pp. 879–882

MILNE, R.J. and HEEL, R.C. (1991) Ondansetron, therapeutic use as an anti-emetic. *Drugs*, 41, 574–595

MIMS (1994) *Monthly Index of Medical Specialities*. London: Haymarket Medical Ltd, January 1994

MORTON, R.P., RUGMAN, F., DORMAN, E.B., STONEY, P.J., WILSON, J.A., MCCORMICK, M. *et al.* (1985) Cisplatinum and bleomycin for advanced or recurrent squamous cell carcinoma of the head and neck: a randomized factorial phase III controlled trial. *Cancer Chemotherapy and Pharmacology*, 15, 283–289

MUNRO, A.J. (1995) An overview of randomised controlled trials of adjuvant chemotherapy in head and neck cancer. *British Journal of Cancer*, 71, 83–91

NISHIO, J., OHMORI, T., FUJIWARA, Y., TAKEDA, Y. and SAIJO, N. (1993) Cis-diaminedichloraplatinum (II) inhibits disphophorylation of the cdc2 hinase in human lung cancer cells. *Proceedings of the American Association for Cancer Research*, 34, 399

NORTON, L. and SIMON, R. (1979) New thoughts on the relationship of tumour growth and characteristics to sensitivity to treatment. In: *Methods of Cancer Research vol XVII, Cancer Drug Development, Part B*, edited by V. T. DeVita Jr and H. Busch. New York: Academic Press. pp. 53–90

PAJAK, T.F., LARAMORE, G.E., MARCIAL, V.A., FAZEKAS, J.T., COOPER, J., RUBIN, P. *et al.* (1991) Elapsed treatment days – a critical item for radiotherapy quality control review in head and neck trials: RTOG report. *International Journal of Radiation, Oncology, Biology and Physics*, 20, 13–20

PETO, R. (1987) Why do we need systematic overviews of randomized trials? *Statistical Medicine*, 6, 233

PINTO, H.A. and JACOBS, C. (1991) Chemotherapy for recurrent and metastatic head and neck cancer. *Haematology/Oncology Clinics of North America*, 5, 667–686

PRIMROSE, W.J., VAUGHAN, C., HONG, W., KARP, D., WILLETT, B. and STRONG, M. (1985) Three year survival rates in advanced head and neck cancer after induction chemotherapy; significance of initial response. *New Dimensions in Otolaryngology – Head and Neck Surgery*, edited by E. N. Myers, vol II. Amsterdam: Excerpta Medica. pp. 1077–1078

ROSENBERG, B., VAN CAMP, L. and KRIGAS, T. (1965) Inhibition of cell division in *Escherichia coli* by electrolysis products from a platinum electrode. *Nature*, 205, 698–699

RUBINSTEIN, L.N. and GAIL, M.H. (1982) Monitoring rules for stopping accrual in comparative survival studies. *Controlled Clinical Trials*, 3, 325–343

SCHULLER, D.E., METCH, B., STEIN, D.W., MATTOX, D. and MCCRACKEN, J.D. (1988) Pre-operative chemotherapy in advanced resectable head and neck cancer: final report of the Southwest Oncology Group. *Laryngoscope*, 98, 1205–1211

SECOG (1986) A randomised trial of combined multidrug chemotherapy and radiotherapy in advanced squamous cell carcinoma of the head and neck: an interim report from the SECOG participants (1986). *European Journal of Surgery and Oncology*, 12, 289–295

SHANTA, V. and KRISNAMURTHI, S. (1980) Combined bleomycin and radiotherapy in oral cancer. *Clinical Radiology*, 31, 617–620

SKIPPER, H., SCHABEL, F. and WILCOX, W. (1964) Experimental evaluation of potential anti-cancer agents. *Cancer Chemotherapy Reports*, 35, 1–111

SOUHAMI, R.L. and TOBIAS, J.S. (1986) *Cancer and its Management*. Oxford: Blackwell Scientific

STELL, P.M. and MCCORMICK, M.S. (1986) Cancer of the head and neck: are we doing any better? *European Journal of Surgery and Oncology*, 12, 94–99

STELL, P.M. and RAWSON, N.S.B. (1990) Adjuvant chemotherapy in head and neck cancer. *British Journal of Cancer*, 61, 779–787

STELL, P.M., DALBY, J.E., STRICKLAND, P., FRAZER, J.G., BRADLEY, P.J. and FLOOD, L.M. (1983) Sequented chemotherapy and radiotherapy in advanced head and neck cancer. *Clinical Radiology*, 34, 463–467

STOLWIJK, C., WAGENER, D.J., VAN DEN BROEK, P., LEVENDAG, P. C., KAZEMI, I. and BRUASET, I. (1983) Ramdomised adjuvant chemotherapy trial for advanced head and neck cancer. *Netherlands Journal of Medicine*, 28, 347–351

TANNOCK, I.F. (1994) Chemotherapy. In: *Management of Head and Neck Cancer; A Multidisciplinary Approach*, 2nd edn, edited by R.R. Million and N. J. Cassisi. Philadelphia: J B Lippincott Company. pp. 143–156

TAYLOR, S.G., APPLEBAUM, E. and SHOWELL, J.L. (1985) A randomised trial of adjuvant chemotherapy in head and neck cancer. *Journal of Clinical Oncology*, 3, 672–679

TAYLOR, S.G., MURTHY, A.K., CALDARELLI, D.D., SHOWELL, J.C., KIEL, K., GRIEM, K.L. *et al.* (1989) Combined simultaneous cisplatin/fluorouracil chemotherapy and split course radiation in head and neck cancer. *Journal of Clinical Oncology*, 7, 846–856

TOBIAS, J.S. (1992) Current role of chemotherapy in head and neck cancer. *Drugs*, 43, 333–344

TOBIAS, J.S., SMITH, B.J., BLACKMAN, G. and FINN, G. (1987) Concurrent daily cisplatin and radiotherapy in locally advanced squamous carcinoma of the head and neck and bronchus. *Radiotherapy and Oncology*, 9, 263–268

TOOHILL, R.J., DUNCANVAGE, J.A., GROSSMAN, T.W., DUNCANVAGE, J. and MOLIN, T. (1987) The effects of delay in standard treatment due to induction chemotherapy in two randomised prospective studies. *Laryngoscope*, 97, 407–412

UEN, W.C., HUANG, A.T., MENNEL, R., JONES, S.E., SPAULDING, M.P. and KILLION, K. (1992) A phase II study of piritrexim in patients with advanced squamous head and neck cancer. *Cancer*, 69, 1008–1011

UMEZAWA, H. (1974) Chemistry and mechanism of action of bleomycin. *Federation Proceedings: Federation of American Societies for Experimental Biology*, 33, 2296–2302

VOGL, S.E., SCHOENFELD, D.A., KAPLAN, B.H., LERNER, H.J., ENGSTROM, P.F. and HORTON, J. (1985) A randomised prospective comparison of methotrexate with a combination of methotrexate, bleomycin and cisplatin in head and neck cancer. *Cancer*, 56, 432–442

VOKES, E.E. and WEICHSELBAUM, R.R. (1990) Concomitant chemotherapy: rationale and clinical experience in patients with solid tumours. *Journal of Clinical Oncology*, 8, 911–934

VOKES, E.E., PANJE, W.R., SCHILSKY, R.L., MICK, R., AWAN, A. M. and MORAN, W.J. (1989) Hydroxyurea, fluorouracil and concomitant radiotherapy in poor prognosis head and neck cancer: a phase I–II study. *Journal of Clinical Oncology*, 7, 761–768

WALKER, R., CAIRNCROSS, J. and POSNER, J. (1986) Acute neurological deterioration after cisplatin therapy for primary and metastatic brain tumours. *ASCO Abstracts*, 5, 135

WEAVER, A., FLEMING, S., KISH, J., VANDENBURG, H., JACOB, J., CRISSMAN, J. *et al.* (1982) Cisplatinum and 5-fluorouracil as induction therapy for advanced head and neck cancer. *American Journal of Surgery*, **144**, 445–448

WILKE, H., STAHL, M., SCHMOLL, H.J., PREUSSER, P., FINK, U. and MEYER, H.J. (1992) Biochemical modulation of 5-fluorouracil by folinic acid of alpha-interferon with or without cytostatic drugs in gastric, esophageal and pancreatic cancer. *Seminars in Oncology*, **19** (suppl. 3), 215–219

WITTES, R.E. (1980) Chemotherapy of head and neck cancer. *Otolaryngology Clinics of North America*, **13**, 515–520

WITTES, R., CVITKOVIC, E. and STRONG, E. (1977) The role of cisplatinum in the treatment of head and neck cancer. *Journal of Clinical Haematology and Oncology*, **7**, 711–716

WOLF, G.T., HONG, W.K., FISHER, S.G., ENDICOTT, J.W., CLOSE, L., FISHER, S.R. *et al.* (1991) Induction chemotherapy plus radiation compared with surgery plus radiation in patient with advanced laryngeal cancer. *New England Journal of Medicine*, **324**, 1685–1690

Principles and use of nuclear medicine

J. Watkinson

The principles and practice of otolaryngology are primarily concerned with the diagnosis and treatment of diseases which affect the mucosal structures of the upper aerodigestive tract, adnexal organs such as the thyroid gland, salivary glands and cervical lymph nodes as well as the cartilaginous and bony structures of the larynx and skull. Conditions affecting these structures can often be diagnosed with ease using traditional methods of history and examination combined with conventional radiography. Recent advances in imaging techniques (computerized tomography, ultrasound and magnetic resonance imaging) increase diagnostic sensitivity and specificity but suffer from distinct disadvantages since they usually provide only anatomical information. The use of nuclear medicine can add a physiological dimension to diagnostic imaging within the head and neck. By using a variety of radiopharmaceuticals, the metabolic functions of a number of head and neck organs and tissues affected by a variety of disease processes can be imaged.

This chapter describes the fundamental principles of nuclear medicine and then outlines the role of current techniques used for both diagnosis and treatment within the field of otolaryngology.

Fundamental principles

These may be conveniently divided under the following headings and are discussed in turn.

1 Structure of the atom
2 Radioactive decay
3 Interaction of radiation with matter
4 Production of radionuclides
5 Radionuclide generators
6 Radiopharmaceuticals
7 Radiolabelling of compounds
8 Radiopharmacy
9 Instrumentation
10 Radiation dosimetry: protection and regulations.

Structure of the atom

The atom consists of a positively charged nucleus which is composed of two types of bodies. These are neutrons and protons and are known collectively as nucleons. Around the nucleus are one or more negatively charged particles of smaller mass called electrons. The electronic structure of the atom determines its chemical properties, while the nuclear structure is responsible for its stability and radioactive decay properties. While the accepted model of atomic and molecular structure has arisen from the wave mechanical treatment of Schroedinger, it is convenient to employ an earlier model (of Bohr) in order to explain simple atomic electrical phenomena. Atoms may contain any number of electrons from one to more than 100. The electron is a high velocity particle that moves in an orbit around the nucleus. The electron possesses a known mass which is constant for all atoms. Two properties differentiate the electron from other particles in the atom: mass and electrical charge.

Electrons are negatively charged and exhibit forces of attraction or repulsion to other charged particles. Electrons exist in a series of energy shells, or orbits, around the nucleus (Figure 23.1), and each shell is subdivided into subshells or orbitals. These shells and subshells represent a hierarchy of energy levels, the shell nearest to the nucleus containing the electrons at the least 'energized' level. An electron can be excited to a higher orbit, and subsequently emits energy as electromagnetic radiation as it falls back to

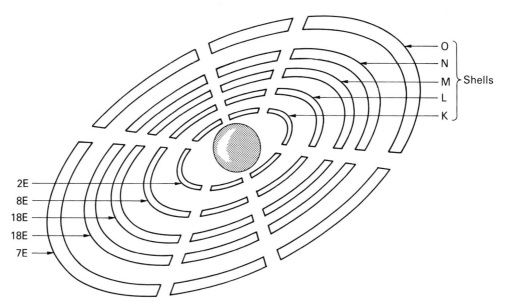

Figure 23.1 Electronic configuration in orbital shells. An atom of ^{123}I has 53 electrons. E = Electrons

a lower orbit. Electrons falling back to one of the outer orbits give rise to visible or ultraviolet light. Electrons falling back to one of the inner orbits give X- and γ-rays.

With regard to nuclear structure, the nucleus contributes almost all of the mass of an atom. The two particles which are significant in nuclear medicine are the proton and the neutron. The proton (p) has a known mass which remains constant and is 1836 times that of an electron. It has a positive charge. The neutron (n) also has constant mass (1840 times the electron) and has no electrical charge. It can neither attract nor repel charged particles. The mass number, A, is the total number of nucleons while N denotes the number of neutrons. There is a convention for expressing the nuclear composition of an element X (when Z, the atomic number, represents the number of protons) thus:

$$A_Z X_N$$
$$N = A - Z$$

where X = chemical symbol, A = mass number, Z = atomic number, N = neutron number.

For example, iodine (I) with 53 protons and 70 neutrons is represented as ^{123}I. All iodine atoms have the same atomic number which can therefore be omitted. An abbreviated way of denoting this atom would be ^{123}I or I-123. Nuclei with even numbers of protons and neutrons are more stable than those with odd numbers.

When a nucleus is specifically described by its mass number, atomic number and arrangement of nucleons, it is called a nuclide. Nuclides of the same atomic number are called isotopes and have the same chemical properties. Nuclides with the same numbers of protons and neutrons but different energy states and spins are called isomers. ^{99}Tc and ^{99m}Tc are isomers of the same technetium nuclide. When a nuclide is unstable it decays by spontaneous fission or the emission of alpha (α) particles, beta (β) particles or gamma (γ) ray emission. It is then called a radionuclide.

Radioactive decay

Soon after radioactivity was discovered it was found that the radiations emitted by radioactive substances could be classified into three categories. The distinguishing characteristics were the range of the radiation in matter and their deflection in electrostatic and magnetic fields. Alpha particles, as the most easily absorbed rays were called, were identified as helium nuclei. Beta particles had a radiation intensity of an intermediate range and were more easily deflected by magnetic fields than alpha particles. They were negatively charged and were recognized to be electrons. Gamma rays were the most penetrating radiations but were unaffected by magnetic or electrical fields.

Most of the 1800 known nuclides are unstable and decay or change their nuclear structure in such a way that they achieve greater stability. Radionuclides decay to obtain a neutron to proton ratio of the nearest possible stable nuclide. During the decay process the unstable nuclide may lose mass by emission of an alpha particle.

If the nucleus has too many neutrons or protons, stability may be achieved by changing the neutron to proton ratio. This is achieved by the emission of a β^- particle from the nucleus if it has an excess of neutrons, by emission of a β^+ particle (positron) or by capture of an electron if it is neutron deficient.

The nuclides formed by the decay processes above may be in an excited state having excess energy which can be lost by further decay in the emission of gamma rays.

Alpha decay

Heavy nuclei such as radon and uranium decay by emitting alpha particles. An alpha particle is a helium nucleus containing two protons and two neutrons. When a nuclide decays by this route the atomic number reduces by two and the mass number by four. Alpha particles play no routine role in nuclear medicine and will not be discussed further.

Beta decay

When a nuclide has more neutrons than the stable nucleus of that element it will decay by emitting a β^- particle. If the daughter nuclide is in an excited state, a gamma ray emission may ensue. The β^- particle (which is essentially an electron) may be decelerated by the Coulomb field of atomic nuclei in the surrounding medium to result in the production of X-rays. This is known as *Bremsstrahlung* (German for braking or slowing down). β particles have a short path length and are useful for therapy (e.g. ^{131}I and thyroid carcinoma). The additional gamma rays from ^{131}I may be also used for imaging purposes.

Positron or β^+ decay

Nuclei with an excess of protons decay by emission of positrons (e.g. ^{11}carbon, ^{13}nitrogen, ^{15}oxygen, ^{18}fluorine). These are important clinically because they are the only radioisotopes of these biologically important elements that can be used for imaging. Essentially, positron decay amounts to transformation of a proton into a neutron. Positrons have a short range in matter. They eventually combine with electrons and are thus annihilated with the production of two gamma photons, each with an energy of 0.51 MeV and travelling in exactly opposite directions (Figure 23.2). If these photons are detected simultaneously then their origin will lie on the line joining two detectors. By taking a number of views a series of intersecting lines is obtained which identifies the point of origin in three dimensions. This forms the basis of positron emission tomography (PET).

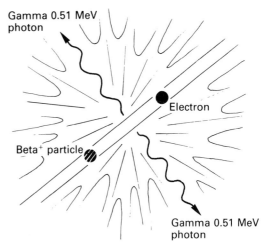

Figure 23.2 Annihilation reaction. A positron is attracted to an electron, both particles are annihilated and converted to energy (two gamma rays)

Electron capture

A proton-rich or neutron-deficient nucleus may, as an alternative to β^+ decay, follow the electron capture process in which an electron is taken from one of the atom's electron shells thereby transforming a proton into a neutron. The difference in electron energy appears as an X-ray. The probability of this reaction increases with increasing atomic number because in these atoms the electron shells come closer to the nucleus.

Isomeric transition

After radioactive decay, the daughter nuclide may be in an excited state and emit gamma rays in order to reach the ground state. This usually takes place in a fraction of a second but with some nuclides the excited state can exist for minutes or hours. These excited or isomeric states are called metastable states and are denoted by 'm'. Metastable isotopes are very useful in nuclear medicine. There is no β particle emission so the radiation dose per unit of radioactivity administered to the patient is low. They are also often readily available, e.g. technetium-99m (^{99m}Tc, half-life ($T_{\frac{1}{2}}$) = 6.03 hours).

Internal conversion

This process happens when an emitted gamma ray knocks an electron from the K-shell of its own atom. The vacancy in the K shell is filled by the transition of an electron from the L shell and a characteristic K X-ray is emitted. The effect is to prevent the gamma rays from leaving the atom. Various examples of decay schemes are shown in Figure 23.3.

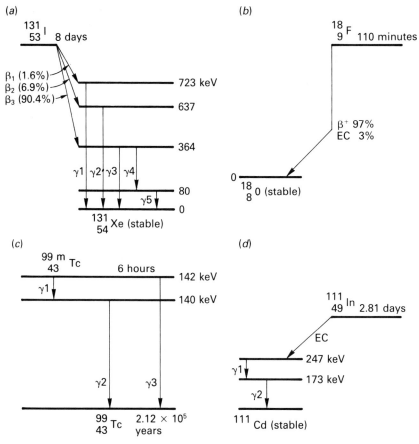

Figure 23.3 Some examples of decay schemes. (*a*) ^{131}I: main-transitions and energy levels, β- and γ-ray emissions; (*b*) ^{18}F: showing β^+ emissions; (*c*) ^{99m}Tc: isometric transition; (*d*) ^{111}In: electron capture and γ-ray emission

Radioactive decay equations

The rate at which a radionuclide decays is a characteristic of that nuclide and cannot be affected by temperature, pressure or light. The probability that any nucleus will disintegrate per unit time is a constant λ, the decay constant. The disintegration rate, $-dN/dt$, also termed the activity, A, is the product of the decay constant and the number, N, of atoms present.

$$-dN/dt = \lambda N$$

integrating this equation, $N_t = N_0 e^{-\lambda t}$
where N_0 and N_t are the numbers of atoms present at time $t = 0$ and $t = t$.

In terms of activity, therefore, $A_t = A_0 e^{-\lambda t}$.

The half-life, $T_{\frac{1}{2}}$ is the time required to reduce the initial disintegration rate, or activity, by half, and is characteristic of every radionuclide. The decay constant, λ, is related to the half-life by $\lambda = 0.693/T_{\frac{1}{2}}$.

Transient equilibrium

If the $T_{\frac{1}{2}}$ of the daughter radionuclide is small compared to the $T_{\frac{1}{2}}$ of the parent, then a relationship of transient equilibrium can occur between them (Figure 23.4). The difference in $T_{\frac{1}{2}}$ between parent and daughter is a factor of about 10–50 and is exemplified by the system molybdenum-99 ($T_{\frac{1}{2}} = 67$ hours) decaying to technetium-99m ($T_{\frac{1}{2}} = 6$ hours). This system is used extensively in nuclear medicine to produce ^{99m}Tc using a generator (see later).

Secular equilibrium

If the $T_{\frac{1}{2}}$ of the parent radionuclide is very much larger than the $T_{\frac{1}{2}}$ of the daughter radionuclide (i.e. 100 or more), then both radionuclides decay with the $T_{\frac{1}{2}}$ of the parent.

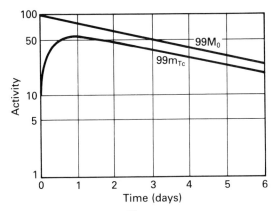

Figure 23.4 Transient equilibrium

Units of radioactivity

Radioactivity is now expressed in the SI unit, the becquerel (Bq) and is equal to one disintegration per second. Until recently, the unit activity was the curie, Ci, which was equal to 3.7×10^{10} disintegrations per second. The curie and the becquerel are related by $1\ Bq = 2.7 \times 10^{-11}\ Ci$ and $1\ Ci = 3.7 \times 10^{10}\ Bq$. For clinical use the megabecquerel, MBq, is a convenient multiple.

Interaction of radiation with matter

When a charged particle, such as an alpha or beta particle, passes close to an atom, electrostatic forces operate between it and the orbital electrons of the atom. If the particle is sufficiently close, one of the orbital electrons may acquire enough energy to escape from the atom. This is called 'ionization' and leaves the atom with a positive charge. The particle loses energy and an ion pair is formed. Gamma rays, being uncharged, do not cause ionization directly.

Alpha particles

An alpha particle has a relatively large mass and a low velocity. There is a high probability of interaction between an orbital electron and a passing alpha particle. Its range in a medium is short so that a sheet of paper will stop most particles. Its penetration in tissue is only a few cells so that all its energy is given up within this distance resulting in a high local radiation dose. Nowadays they are *not* used in nuclear medicine where external detection of radioactivity is required.

Beta particles

A beta particle has a mass 7000 times smaller than an alpha particle and leaves the nucleus at up to the speed of light. The particle is deflected from its path as it passes near the orbital electrons and the probability of reaction with them is high. The penetration of a beta particle in water and tissue is up to several millimetres, with all its energy being dissipated within this distance. Radiation dose to the cell is fairly high resulting in damage to the cell contents and, for this reason, beta-emitting radionuclides are often used in radiotherapy, i.e. ^{131}I and differentiated thyroid cancer.

Gamma rays

Gamma rays have well-defined energies. The penetration through tissue is high with a low probability of interaction with orbital electrons. The probability that it will dissipate its energy as it passes through a thickness of tissue is less than with alpha and beta particles. The higher the gamma ray energy, the lower the probability of interaction and the greater the penetration of tissue. This results in an increased likelihood of reaching an external detector, i.e. the gamma camera. For this reason, gamma-emitting radionuclides are used for imaging purposes, e.g. technetium-99m. Gamma rays may interact with matter in one of three different ways: the photoelectric effect, compton scatter, and pair production.

Photoelectric effect

In the photoelectric effect, a low energy gamma ray strikes an inner orbital electron which is ejected from the atom with the energy of the gamma ray. The gamma ray is completely stopped. Ejection of the orbital electron results in a vacancy in the inner orbit and this is filled by other orbital electrons with a subsequent emission of characteristic X-rays.

Compton scatter

Compton scatter happens when a gamma ray of medium energy strikes an outer orbital electron which is then ejected from its orbit. Some of the energy of the incident gamma ray is transferred to the electron. A gamma ray of reduced energy emerges from the atom with a change of direction.

Pair production

In pair-production, a high energy gamma ray interacts near the nucleus to produce two particles, a β^- particle and a positron. The ejected positron almost invariably collides with an electron resulting in annihilation of both particles and the emission of two gamma rays each of 0.51 MeV.

Production of radionuclides

All elements found in nature with atomic numbers higher than 83 are radioactive, i.e. they undergo spontaneous decay. Radioactivity can also be produced artificially by bombarding appropriate substances with high speed subatomic particles so that more than 1500 artificial radionuclides have now been produced. There are three main types of 'production factory' for radionuclides. These are the cyclotron, the nuclear reactor and the radionuclide generator.

The cyclotron

A cyclotron is an instrument in which charged particles such as protons and deuterons are accelerated in circular paths and in a vacuum, by means of a magnetic field. They can be passed around and around the circuit so that they achieve very high velocities and energies up to millions of electron volts. When a target of an appropriate stable element is placed in the path of the accelerated particles, the particles strike the target nuclei and some of their energy is transferred to these nuclei. This energy is dissipated by the emission of nucleons – neutrons and protons. This may be followed by emission of gamma rays. The greater the energy of the accelerated particles, the higher the number of emitted nucleons. An example of a cyclotron-produced reaction is:

$$^{111}\text{Cd (p,n)}^{111}\text{In}$$
$$\text{Cd = cadmium, In = indium.}$$

^{111}Cd is the target, p represents the irradiating particle (a proton), n (a neutron) is the emitted particle and ^{111}In is the radionuclide product. Depending on the nature and energy of the irradiating particle, the target nucleus may emit a proton, a neutron, one of each or more. Therefore in order to produce a specified radionuclide, an appropriate particle must be used at a calculated energy level. The target must be pure, and preferably mono-isotopic, to avoid unwanted reactions. Even then, a number of radionuclides may be produced.

Iodine-123 (^{123}I) is an important medical radionuclide. When it is produced directly by bombarding the stable nuclide, other isotopes such as ^{124}I and ^{125}I may result. This may be avoided by using an indirect method: a nuclear reaction is chosen in which xenon-123 (^{123}Xe) is produced. This then decays to produce ^{123}I. Recently, medical imaging techniques have been developed which utilize positron emission. These require radionuclides which have a very short life and emit positrons. They include ^{11}C, ^{13}N, ^{15}O and ^{18}F, all of which decay by positron emission. Because of their ultrashort lives they must be produced on site, either by a conventional cyclotron or by a medical cyclotron (smaller version) producing intermediate energy particles at high intensity.

The nuclear reactor

The nuclear reactor consists of fuel rods made of fissile material such as uranium-235 (^{235}U). These undergo spontaneous fission, in which a heavy nucleus breaks up into two fragments with the emission of two neutrons and the release of 200 MeV energy. This is removed by heat exchangers and is used to produce electricity. The emitted neutrons can cause fission of other nuclei in the fuel rod and a chain reaction can ensue – a nuclear explosion. This is prevented by the design of the reactor, choice of fuel rod material, etc. Neutrons emitted into the spaces between the fuel rod may interact with other nuclei and produce various radionuclides, particularly if they are moving slowly. In order to slow down neutrons which are too energetic the spaces between the rods are filled with substances such as heavy water, beryllium and graphite. A target element may be introduced into the reactor core and the low neutrons will interact with the target nuclei to produce radionuclides. Two types of reaction are particularly important for producing radionuclides in a reactor: fission of heavy elements and neutron capture.

Fission reaction: (n,f)

When a target of heavy elements such as ^{235}U is introduced into the reactor core, neutron bombardment breaks up the nuclei into two particles of approximately equal mass:

$$^{235}\text{U} + \text{n} \rightarrow {}^{236}\text{U} \rightarrow {}^{131}\text{I} + {}^{102}\text{Y} + 3\text{n}$$
$$\text{Y = yttrium.}$$

The resultant isotopes are separated by chemical procedures (precipitation, solvent extraction, etc). These fission products are usually neutron-rich and decay by β^- particle emission.

Neutron capture (n, γ)

In this reaction, the target nucleus captures one thermal (i.e. slow) neutron and emits gamma rays to produce an isotope of the same element. No particles are emitted. The specific activity of the radionuclide so produced is low. Since the target and product nuclei belong to the same element, chemical separation is not necessary. Among the useful radionuclides produced by neutron capture are tellurium-131 (^{131}Te) which decays to ^{131}I. Another example is ^{98}Mo (n, γ) ^{99}Mo which decays to ^{99m}Tc (see below).

Radionuclide generators

The cyclotron is a very expensive piece of machinery and the nuclear reactor even more so. This production of radionuclides in the above ways can take place only at a small number of institutions, which

sell radionuclides to distant establishments such as hospitals. However, very short-lived radionuclides, widely used in medicine, cannot be produced in this way because they decay too rapidly. The *radionuclide generator* is the answer to this problem, and its development has made possible the widespread use of short-lived radionuclides. Table 23.1 shows some radionuclides currently used in nuclear medicine and otolaryngology.

Table 23.1 Radionuclides currently used in nuclear medicine and otolaryngology

Nuclide	$T_{1/2}$	Mode of decay
^{18}F	110 minutes	$B^+ \rightarrow 2\gamma$
^{67}Ga	3.2 days	$\gamma:EC$
^{99m}Tc	6.0 hours	$\gamma:IT$
^{111}In	2.8 days	$\gamma:EC$
^{123}I	13 hours	$\gamma:EC$
^{125}I	60 days	$\gamma:EC$
^{131}I	8 days	β^-, γ
^{201}Tl	3.1 days	$\gamma:EC$

Radionuclides with short physical half-lives ($T_{\frac{1}{2}}$) are now widely used in nuclear medicine imaging procedures for the following reasons. First, because large quantities (up to 740 MBq) of radioactivity can be administered to a patient to provide good quality diagnostic images in a short imaging time and, second, because the rapid decay of these fairly large amounts of radioactivity ensures that the radiation burden to the patient is kept to a minimum acceptable level. However, a number of problems are associated with the use of short-lived radionuclides. These include a supply problem to the user who would lose a proportion of radioactivity during transportation and this loss would depend on the distance of the user from the source. These problems can be solved by the use of portable radionuclide generators located within the nuclear medicine department providing a ready supply of short-lived radionuclides.

Generator principles

Radionuclide generators are constructed on the principle of the decay-growth relationship between a 'parent' radionuclide and its daughter.

Parent $T_{\frac{1}{2}}p \rightarrow$ Daughter $T_{\frac{1}{2}}d \rightarrow$ Grandaughter $T_{\frac{1}{2}}q \rightarrow$ Stable isotope

where $T_{\frac{1}{2}}p$ = half life of 'parent' radionuclide
$T_{\frac{1}{2}}d$ = half life of 'daughter' radionuclide
$T_{\frac{1}{2}}q$ = half life of 'grandaughter' radionuclide.

An ideal radionuclide generator should be simple to use and easy to handle, allow for rapid elution

providing a high yield and be properly shielded to minimize radiation exposure. The daughter eluate must be free from parent radionuclide and absorbent material and there should be no other radioactive contaminants in the eluate. The daughter should decay to a stable or very long-lived radionuclide so that radiation dose to the patient is minimal. The daughter radionuclide should be in a form ready for administration to a patient, or readily converted to a suitable radiopharmaceutical and the maximum activity should be obtainable from the generator for early morning preparation.

A typical generator system is shown in Figure 23.5 together with some commonly used generator systems applicable to otolaryngology. These generators make use of the principle of the decay-growth relationship between a long-lived parent radionuclide and its short-lived daughter. The daughter radionuclide is chemically different from the parent and can thus be separated. The generator consists of a glass or plastic column containing a support material onto which the parent radionuclide is absorbed. The daughter radionuclide can be separated from the parent and removed from the generator in a carrier-free state by elution with a suitable eluant and leaving the parent on the column. After elution, the daughter radioactivity starts to grow again until an equilibrium is reached. The generator must be sterile, pyrogen free, ^{99}Mo and aluminium breakthrough must be controlled, and both the pH and radiochemical purity of the eluate must be assured.

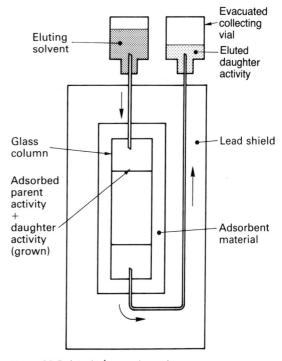

Figure 23.5 A typical generator system

Radiopharmaceuticals

A radiopharmaceutical consists of a radioactive component which provides a signal for detection outside the body, and is usually bound to a chemical moiety which directs the radionuclide to the target organ or system of interest. Some radionuclides localize in their target organ due to the natural biodistribution of that element. Radiopharmaceuticals for imaging studies are administered to patients, usually by the intravenous route, and then carried around the body in the circulation. By positioning a suitable detector (see instrumentation) over the surface of the body, target organs can be visualized as active areas against a non-radioactive or low activity background. Thus it is possible to study internal organs by a non-invasive technique.

In the design of the ideal radiopharmaceutical a number of factors requires consideration to achieve the best possible result with the minimum radiation dose to the patient. The factors are tabulated in Table 23.2 and some of the radiopharmaceuticals used in modern otolaryngological practice are listed in Table 23.3.

Table 23.2 Characteristics of an ideal radiopharmaceutical for organ imaging

Radionuclide	
Radiations	Pure γ emitter
	No particulate emissions (α or β)
	γ-ray energy of 100–300 KeV
$T_{1/2}$	Similar to length of investigation
	Facilitates waste disposal
Chemistry	Versatile
	Stable radiolabelling
Toxicity	Non-toxic to body organs and systems
Availability	Readily available at all times
Cost	Reactor produced radionuclides cost less than those produced by cyclotron

Radiopharmaceuticals
High target to background ratio
No adverse reactions
No unwanted pharmacological responses
Stable for *in-vitro* and *in-vivo* studies
Resident time in target organ should be long enough to complete the study
Cheap and easy to produce
Quality easily assayed by simple techniques

Dosage forms and administration

The dose of a radiopharmaceutical may be defined as that dose of radioactivity necessary to provide the maximum diagnostic information with the minimum radiation dose to the patient. Because the result of the test is dependent on the visual appearance of the scintigram, the dosage may sometimes depend on the sensitivity of the detection equipment. Modern gamma cameras (see instrumentation) tend to be more sensitive than their predecessors and dosage may be reduced accordingly. Most radiopharmaceutical preparations are given as injections and many nuclear medicine departments prepare multidose amounts in a 'stock container' usually with a preprepared kit.

Radiolabelling of compounds

The radiolabelling of a compound can be achieved either by the substitution of atoms or groups of atoms of the molecule by radioactive atoms, or by the chelation or complexing of radioactive atoms or groups by molecules of the compound. The majority of radiopharmaceuticals used for diagnostic purposes in nuclear medicine in otolaryngology are prepared by the second method.

Isotope exchange reactions

This method of radiolabelling usually involves the introduction of a radionuclide into a molecule by replacing an atom already present within the molecule. The atoms are replaced by isotopes of the same element having different mass numbers. The technique is generally used to prepare radioactive compounds which have *in-vitro* applications or to prepare radiopharmaceuticals labelled with iodine or with β-emitting isotopes for therapy.

Example

^{125}I-labelled triiodothyronine (T3) and ^{125}I-thyroxine for *in-vitro* radioimmunoassay work.

Introduction of a foreign radioactive element or group

In this technique of radiolabelling, the radionuclide is conjugated to the molecule to produce a radioactive compound with a desired biological distribution. The radioactive element or group is foreign to the molecule, an essential difference between this and the previous technique.

Examples

^{99m}Tc-methylene diphosphonate (MDP) for bone imaging
^{99m}Tc-(v)-dimercaptosuccinic acid (DMSA) for medullary thyroid cancer imaging
^{111}In – antibodies for tumour localization.

Radiopharmacy

Radiopharmacy may be defined as the science, practice and provision of radiopharmaceuticals. The

Table 23.3 Some radiopharmaceuticals used in current otolaryngological practice

Example	Clinical use
^{99m}Tc-methylene diphosphonate	Bone scanning
^{99m}Tc-pertechnetate	Thyroid, salivary gland imaging
^{99m}Tc-DTPA	CSF leaks
^{99m}Tc-red blood cells	Blood flow
^{99m}Tc-(v)-dimercaptosuccinic acid (pentavalent DMSA)	Medullary thyroid cancer
Iodine	
^{125}I	Radioimmunoassay
^{123}I	Thyroid imaging
^{131}I	Therapy for differentiated thyroid cancer
^{18}F-deoxyglucose (FDG)	Tumour imaging
^{67}Ga-citrate	Infection, tumour imaging
^{111}In-Wbc	Infection
^{123}I/^{131}I-MIBG	Imaging and therapy for medullary thyroid cancer
^{111}In-somatostatin (octreoscan)	Neuroendocrine tumours

radiopharmacy is the laboratory where radiopharmaceuticals are prepared. It must be suitable for the storage and handling of radioactive materials and should be designed in such a way that radiopharmaceuticals can be prepared under pharmaceutical conditions. Some functions of the radiopharmacy are shown in Table 23.4 and some commonly used radiopharmaceutical dispensing procedures are listed in Table 23.5.

Table 23.4 Some functions of a hospital radiopharmacy

Receiving radioactive packages
Preparation of radiopharmaceuticals
Dispensing
Quality control
Storage
Waste disposal
Documentation

Table 23.5 Some commonly used radiopharmaceutical dispensing procedures

Generator eluates
Kits
In-house preparation
Predispensed products
Products requiring dilution or subdivision
Oral products
Oral products requiring admixture with food
Labelled blood cells
Radioactive gases
Radioactive aerosols

Instrumentation

Almost all the detectors used in nuclear medicine are scintillation detectors. 'Scintillators' are substances which absorb energy from ionizing radiations and emit a weak flash of light. The intensity of the light flash, or scintillation, is proportional to the total energy absorbed within the scintillator. The main components of scintillation detectors are:

1 The scintillator
2 The photomultiplier tube
3 Pulse height analyser
4 Scaler/timer.

The scintillator

Radiation, usually in the form of gamma rays emitted from the patient, enters the scintillator which, in the gamma camera is usually a sodium iodide crystal containing small quantities of thallium. Secondary electrons are produced which deposit energy in the crystal and cause it to emit a flash of light. The size of the light flash depends on the energy absorbed in the crystal. Sodium iodide is a good scintillator since first, it has a relatively high atomic number and is, therefore, also an efficient absorber of radiation. Second, it has good light yield. Third, it is transparent to the light produced which can then escape from the crystal and, fourth, it is available as large single crystals suitable for use in gamma cameras.

The photomultiplier tube

The light flash emitted from the crystal is detected by a photomultiplier tube, a device which converts light into electrons and amplifies the pulse. When the light flash hits the photocathode of the photomultiplier tube, the energy of the light is absorbed and a few electrons are emitted from the photocathode. A series of dynodes attract the negatively charged electrons due to their applied positive potentials. As each electron reaches the first dynode it stimulates the emission of several further electrons. At each dynode this process is repeated for up to 13 dynodes. The final cascade of electrons produced by the process is connected at an anode resulting in a pulse of electrical charge.

Pulse height analyser

For a given gamma ray energy, a range of electrical pulses of different sizes is produced in the photomultiplier tube. Any particular radionuclide will produce a spectrum of pulses which depends largely on the gamma energies emitted, but also on the geometry of the source and detector, and on the amount of scatter present. The pulse height analyser detects differences in pulse size and enables the system to be adjusted so that only pulses corresponding to the radionuclide of interest are detected.

The scaler/timer

The scaler/timer counts the number of pulses in the 'window' set by the pulse height analyser in a given time interval.

The gamma camera

The block diagram of a gamma camera is shown in Figure 23.6. Gamma rays emitted from the patient interact with the sodium iodide crystal producing pulses in some of the photomultiplier tubes. The sum of all the pulses represents the total energy deposited in the crystal. The position computer determines the position of events in the crystal due to the relative sizes of the pulses. In this way, the image of the patient's organ can be built up. The image can be recorded on X-ray film or in a computer for further analysis.

The purpose of the collimator is to prevent scattered photons reaching the crystal. Only those photons travelling in the right direction will pass through one of the very many holes in the thick lead sheet of the collimator and reach the crystal. Collimators can be designed with variations in hole diameter to govern resolution of the image, and hole dimensions and number of holes to govern sensitivity.

Single photon emission computerized tomography (SPECT)

In SPECT, the same gamma emitters as in planar scintigraphy are used. Transaxial devices (Figure 23.7) allow the detector to rotate around the patient and collect information in a single slice through the body.

Positron emission tomography (PET)

In PET, two rotating gamma ray detectors are placed on opposite sides of an object containing a positron emitter. The simultaneous detection of the two annihilation photons places the original position of the annihilation (encounter of a β^+ particle with an electron) in the space between the two detectors. This technique allows a very accurate measurement of the concentration of the isotope and is, therefore, well adapted to quantitative functional studies.

Radiation dosimetry: protection and regulations

Ionizing radiations cannot be detected by the human senses but can be detected and measured by various techniques such as autoradiography, Geiger counters and scintillation detectors. It is not possible to measure directly the radiation dose absorbed by the body, or a part of the body, using these instruments when the radionuclide is localized in an internal body organ. However, if the activity is known, it is possible to calculate the dosage absorbed by the organ.

Units

Absorbed dose is the quantity of energy imparted by ionizing radiation to a unit mass of matter. The unit of absorbed dose is the *gray* (gy) and is equal to one joule per kilogram. *Dose equivalent* is equal to the absorbed dose multiplied by a factor that takes into account the way in which particular radiation distributes energy in the tissues. This influences the degree of radiation damage. The unit of dose equivalent is the *sievert* (Sv). *Effective dose equivalent* is the dose equivalent to various tissues and organs multiplied by a risk weighting factor for each tissue and organ and summing the products. The unit of effective dose equivalent is again the sievert.

Dosimetry

The radiation dose to a patient resulting from the administration of a radiopharmaceutical depends on the amount of energy deposited by the radiation in the patient. This dose can be calculated based on information derived from the pharmacokinetics and biodistribution of the radiopharmaceutical, the equilibrium dose constant for each radiation emitted by the radionuclide and geometry of the organs allowing calculation of the absorbed fraction. Details of such calculations are outside the scope of this chapter.

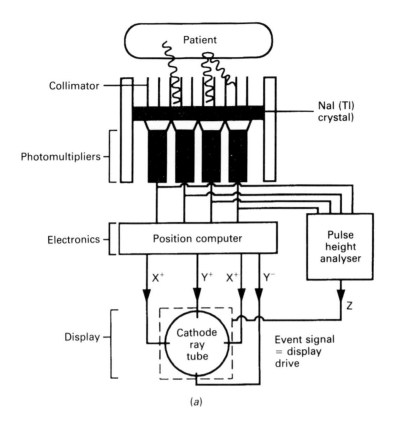

(a)

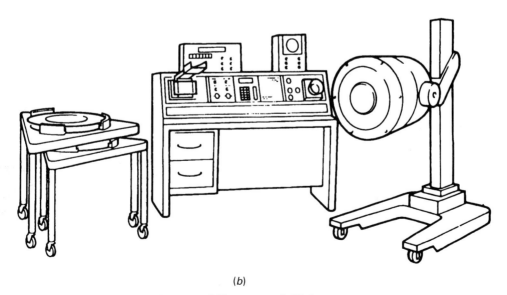

(b)

Figure 23.6 (*a*) A gamma camera block diagram and (*b*) a gamma scintillation camera

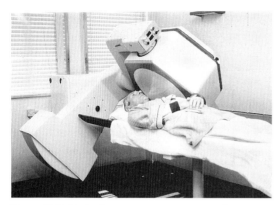

Figure 23.7 Single photon emission computerized tomography (SPECT). Transaxial devices allow the detector to rotate around the patient

Radiation protection

It is essential that people who handle radioactivity are protected from its hazards. It must also be borne in mind that patients who have received a dose of radiopharmaceutical are 'radioactive sources' and their urine or sputum etc., may also be radioactive. There are two main hazards to workers with radioactivity. These are external irradiation from gamma rays and internal irradiation resulting from ingestion, inhalation or absorption. External irradiation can be minimized by adhering to the rules of limiting time exposure, distance from source and using shielding. Methods to avoid internal irradiation are obvious.

Radiation regulations

There are regulations regarding the handling and use of radioactivity in the UK. These are outside the scope of this chapter but are available in the literature.

Fundamental techniques
Diagnostic

Diagnostic nuclear medicine tests can be classified into *in-vitro* and *in-vivo* investigations. *In-vitro* procedures play a small but important role in current otolaryngological practice and some of the substances which can be measured using radioimmunoassay are

Table 23.6 Substances measured by radioimmunoassay

T4, T3, thyroid stimulating hormone
Thyroglobulin
Parathormone
Calcitonin
Human growth hormone
Vasopressin
Hepatitis B antigen
Human immunodeficiency virus antibody

listed in Table 23.6. However, the majority of nuclear medicine tests now available to the otolaryngologist are *in-vivo* investigations and the organs and tissues which can be imaged are discussed below.

Thyroid

Diseases of the thyroid are common. Laboratory investigations are essential to confirm or exclude a clinical suspicion of either hyperthyroidism or hypothyroidism and a number of 'flow channels' exist depending which condition is suspected (IAEA, 1988). Further *in-vivo* investigations may be necessary to establish the clinical cause of hyperthyroidism and one of the most useful investigations for any goitre is a radionuclide thyroid scan with quantitative uptake using either technetium-99m-pertechnetate ($^{99m}TcO_4^-$) or iodine-123 (^{123}I-iodide).

The otolaryngologist is usually involved with the investigation of the solitary thyroid nodule and the preoperative diagnosis of malignancy, together with the postoperative assessment of residual thyroid tissue and the detection of residual or recurrent tumour. There are many clinical situations when the possibility of thyroid cancer arises but by far the commonest mode of presentation is as a palpable solitary nodule when the incidence of malignancy is 5–10% (Perlmutter and Slater, 1956).

The choice of agents for imaging differentiated (follicular and papillary) thyroid cancer has been reviewed elsewhere (Goulden, Glass and Silvester, 1968). With either $^{99m}TcO_4^-$ or ^{123}I, the majority of nodules greater than 0.5 cm in diameter can be identified and accuracy increased by using oblique views. Smaller lesions in the isthmus may contribute to false negative results but since they are often easier to palpate they do not constitute a significant problem. The function of all preoperative thyroid imaging is to increase the possibility of a diagnosis of malignancy by improving the predictive accuracy without any loss in sensitivity.

When a clinically solitary thyroid nodule is investigated, a ^{99m}Tc or ^{123}I scan may show a solitary nonfunctioning or hypofunctioning area (i.e. a 'cold' nodule), a functioning area (i.e. a 'hot' nodule) or a multinodular goitre, with or without retrosternal extension. The possibility of retrosternal extension should be investigated further using ^{131}I since its high gamma photon energy makes it preferable for visualizing a retrosternal thyroid. The probability of malignancy is increased if the scan demonstrates a solitary 'cold' nodule (Figure 23.8), but decreased to less than 1% if it shows a 'hot' nodule or a multinodular goitre. All solitary 'cold' nodules should be investigated further by fine needle aspiration biopsy and/or ultrasound which, in expert hands, increases the diagnostic sensitivity to at least 90%. Current practice dictates that uncomplicated solitary thyroid nodules are best evaluated initially by fine needle aspiration

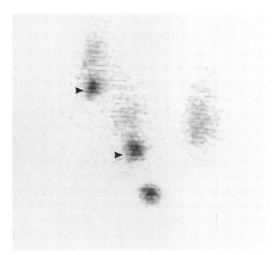

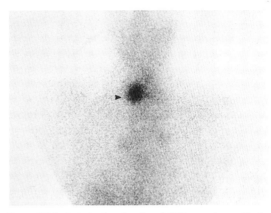

Figure 23.8 Anterior ^{99m}Tc pertechnetate thyroid scan showing a solitary cold nodule in the right lobe of the thyroid. Two markers (arrowed) have been placed on the upper and lower limits of the nodule and there is a lower marker on the suprasternal notch. Histology confirmed papillary carcinoma

Figure 23.9 Anterior head and neck ⁶⁷Ga scan in a patient with Hashimoto's disease who developed a solitary thyroid nodule. Avid uptake of ⁶⁷Ga is seen within the nodule (arrowed) and subsequent histology revealed lymphoma

cytology, but individual patterns of assessment will vary from unit to unit. In the future, nodules which are classed as 'indeterminate' on fine needle aspiration should probably be assessed further by scintigraphy before advising surgery.

There are some nodules which take up tracer on the ^{99m}Tc scan but not on an iodine scan. These discrepancies probably reflect an ability to trap but not organify iodine and such problems can usually be resolved by performing ¹²³I scans on any hot nodule which concentrates pertechnetate followed by a perchlorate discharge test which assesses the ability of a nodule to trap and organify iodine.

Many other radionuclides have been used to investigate the solitary thyroid nodule. Phosphorus-32, caesium-131, gallium-67 (⁶⁷Ga) citrate, ^{99m}Tc-bleomycin and thallium-201 (²⁰¹Tl) chloride have all been evaluated (Watkinson, 1990) in an attempt to increase diagnostic specificity without any loss in sensitivity. All these agents exhibit variable uptake in malignant lesions but at the present time, for malignancy, the false-negative rate is unacceptably high for them to have a place in the routine investigation of thyroid nodules. However, patients with long-standing Hashimoto's disease sometimes develop a solitary thyroid nodule. This is usually a lymphoma and, as such, accumulates ⁶⁷Ga (Figure 23.9).

In the postoperative assessment of differentiated thyroid cancer, radionuclide imaging techniques aim to establish the completeness of initial surgical treatment and to detect residual, recurrent or metastatic tumour. At present, the most widely used and accepted method of follow up is regular whole-body imaging using ¹³¹I combined with sequential serum thyroglobulin measurements (Ng Tang Fui *et al.*, 1979). Recent trends in conservative thyroid surgery have shown that total thyroidectomy is not always indicated, so that follow up will be clinical and biochemical (with thyroglobulin) since whole body imaging is not possible when normal functioning thyroid tissue remains in the neck. Differentiated thyroid malignancy exhibits minimal or no iodine uptake in the presence of normal thyroid tissue but thyroid ablation results in high serum thyroid stimulating hormone (TSH) levels and, subsequently, ¹³¹I will localize in residual, recurrent or metastatic tumour which can then be demonstrated as hot lesions on a whole-body scan. This method permits the detection of residual and recurrent tumour in the neck together with local or distant metastases and assesses the potential for radioiodine treatment.

The use of whole-body ¹³¹I scans to detect thyroid metastases in thyroidectomized patients has distinct disadvantages. Patients have to be rendered hypothyroid by curtailing thyroxine therapy and not all differentiated thyroid cancer continues to take up ¹³¹I. Recent attempts to combat these problems have involved the use not only of ¹²³I-anti-human thyroglobulin monoclonal antibody but also ²⁰¹Tl-chloride which has been used to detect residual and recurrent disease (Figure 23.10), and which, in combination with ¹³¹I, has an increased sensitivity for the overall detection of metastatic disease (Hoefnagel *et al.*, 1986).

Patients with medullary carcinoma of the thyroid can be imaged using a number of radiopharmaceuticals. Primary tumours appear as cold areas on ^{99m}Tc or ¹²³I scans with the classical pattern of bilateral symmetrical non-functioning nodules developing in the familial type. Unlike follicular carcinoma and papillary carcinoma with follicular elements, medullary carcinoma does not trap iodine which, therefore, plays no role in either imaging or therapy. Recently,

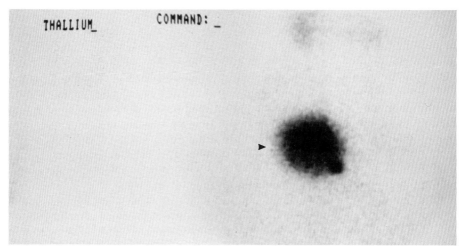

Figure 23.10 Anterior head and neck ^{201}Tl scan in a patient with recurrent papillary carcinoma of the thyroid. Uptake is seen at the site of known disease (arrowed) within the neck and upper mediastinum

two new radiopharmaceuticals have been developed which localize in medullary tumours. ^{131}I-metaiodobenzylguanidine (MIBG) was developed for imaging phaeochromocytoma and has subsequently been shown to be taken up by other neuroectodermally-derived tumours, including medullary carcinoma (Endo *et al.*, 1984) and paragangliomas (Khafagi *et al.*, 1987). Pentavalent ^{99m}Tc (v)- dimercaptosuccinic acid (DMSA) has been developed and its uptake has been described in medullary carcinoma of the thyroid (Ohta *et al.*, 1984). Reports have confirmed the uptake of both ^{131}I-MIBG and ^{99m}Tc (v)-DMSA in primary and recurrent medullary carcinoma but have shown ^{99m}Tc (v)-DMSA to have distinct advantages over ^{131}I-MIBG (Clarke *et al.*, 1988). At present, the main role of pentavalent DMSA is in the investigation of primary, recurrent and metastatic medullary carcinoma (Figure 23.11) and ^{131}I-MIBG scanning is reserved for use in any one individual to assess uptake and then, if positive, to use a therapeutic dose if indicated.

Parathyroid

Primary hyperparathyroidism is the commonest cause of hypercalcaemia and the introduction of the multichannel analyser for biochemical measurements has resulted in more patients being identified with elevated serum calcium levels. The accurate diagnosis of primary hyperparathyroidism is usually straightforward with precise measurements of parathormone now possible. Preoperative localization of parathyroid adenomas is now feasible using ^{99m}TcO$_4^-$/^{201}Tl subtraction scanning (Ferlin *et al.*, 1983) (Figure 23.12). ^{99m}Tc pertechnetate localizes in the thyroid gland, whereas ^{201}Tl localizes in both the thyroid and parathyroid glands. By subtracting the ^{99m}Tc image from

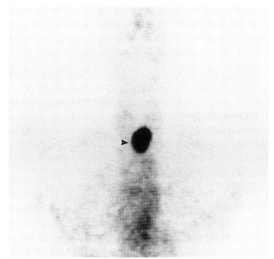

Figure 23.11 Anterior head and neck ^{99m}Tc (v)-DMSA scan in a patient with a solitary thyroid nodule due to medullary carcinoma of the thyroid. Positive uptake (arrowed) is seen at the site of known disease

the ^{201}Tl image it is possible to identify enlarged parathyroids within the neck and mediastinum. The technique has an overall sensitivity of 92% for detecting parathyroid adenomas (Ferlin *et al.*, 1983) and is particularly useful in the assessment of abnormally situated glands or in those patients having 'second-look' procedures. Sensitivity is related to number, size and position and is greatest for singly involved lower pole glands which exceed 1.5 cm in size. In general, the sensitivity is poor for those patients with diffuse parathyroid hyperplasia. The uptake of ^{201}Tl is non-specific and false positives can be seen with thyroid neoplasia, multinodular goitres, Hashimoto's disease, lymphoma, sarcoidosis and parathyroid carcinoma.

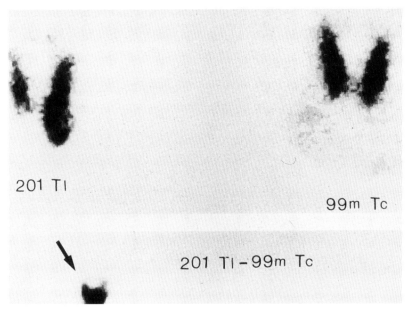

Figure 23.12 Anterior ^{99m}Tc/^{201}Tl subtraction scan in a patient with primary hyperparathyroidism. A parathyroid adenoma (arrowed) has been identified at the lower pole of the left thyroid lobe which measured approximately 2 cm in size

Carcinoma of the parathyroid is rare and the majority of patients present with severe hyperparathyroidism and markedly elevated serum calcium and parathormone levels (Shane and Bilezikian, 1982). Approximately 50% of patients have a palpable neck mass (Fujimoto and Obara, 1987) and non-invasive preoperative localization may be facilitated by a positive ^{67}Ga-citrate scan (Iwase *et al.*, 1986), although the diagnosis is usually made at operation. Persistently elevated serum calcium and parathormone levels should alert the surgeon to the possibility of recurrent disease, when localization should begin with cervical examination since approximately 50% of recurrences are palpable (Fujimoto and Obara, 1987). Recurrent tumour within the neck and mediastinum has been successfully located using ^{99m}Tc/^{201}Tl subtraction scanning (Iwase *et al.*, 1986). However, the thyroid lobe is usually totally excised along with the parathyroid carcinoma at operation, so local recurrence can be demonstrated using ^{201}Tl chloride alone. Suspected localization should be confirmed by CT scanning (Fujimoto and Obara, 1987).

Salivary glands

CT, MRI and ultrasound all demonstrate the soft tissue structure of the salivary glands and, therefore, provide an anatomical but not a physiological assessment of the gland. Contrast sialography, with or without CT, requires cannulation of one or more salivary ducts which may be difficult and require dilation or incision of the duct orifice. This can be uncomfortable for the patient and there is often an inflammatory response consequent upon the use of contrast material.

Salivary gland scanning using ^{99m}Tc-pertechnetate provides physiological images of the glands and assesses both function and drainage (Greyson and Noyek, 1982). The metabolism of pertechnetate is analogous to iodine. It is trapped but not organified by the thyroid, secreted by salivary duct epithelium and excreted in saliva.

Following i.v. injection of ^{99m}Tc-pertechnetate, rapid dynamic sequential images are obtained to demonstrate salivary gland blood flow. Serial planar images are then taken every 3 minutes to show the progressive symmetrical accumulation of tracer within the parotid and submandibular glands. After 15 minutes the patient is given a sialogogue orally which causes prompt salivation with drainage if the glands are innervated or the salivary ducts are patent. This test can be useful in the evaluation of ductal obstruction with intermittent pain or gland enlargement (Figure 23.13) and assesses innervation of the submandibular glands in patients with facial palsy.

The excretory function of each salivary gland as well as its relative blood flow can be assessed either visually or by using a nuclear medicine computer. Palpable lesions can be divided into vascular or non-vascular and functioning or non-functioning masses. Functioning salivary gland tumours tend to be benign with large numbers of oncocytes such as Warthin's tumours. Although malignant neoplasms are generally vascular but non-functioning on the scan, so are mixed tumours, lymphomas and abscesses. Since the

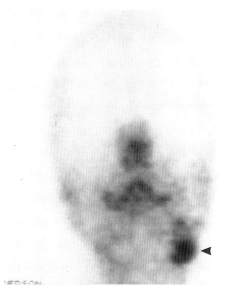

Figure 23.13 Anterior 15-minute [99mTc]-pertechnetate salivary gland scan in a patient with intermittent pain and swelling of the left submandibular gland. Following administration of an oral sialogogue, there has been prompt drainage of all the salivary glands except the left submandibular gland where retention of tracer is clearly seen (arrowed). Obstruction was due to a stone in Wharton's duct

[99m]Tc scan cannot differentiate between benign and malignant salivary swellings, it is of limited use in their investigation, although it may be of value in individual cases.

Overall salivary gland function can be useful in assessing xerostomia in patients with Sjögren's syndrome. Gallium-67 localizes faintly in normal salivary tissue but specific focal accumulation can develop in an abscess or malignancy. Non-specific uptake in both salivary and lacrimal glands is seen in sarcoidosis and can be used both for diagnosis and to monitor therapy and disease progression.

Lacrimal glands

Obstruction to tear duct drainage with clinical symptoms of epiphora may be due to tumours, infection and trauma of the paranasal sinuses affecting the nasolacrimal duct. Conventional imaging with contrast dacrocystography involves intubation of the canaliculi and injection to demonstrate the tear ducts. Manipulation may be difficult or contraindicated when gross anatomical distortion or infection are present.

When ^{99m}Tc-pertechnetate is instilled into the inferior recess of the eye, tracer spreads to label the tears and to demonstrate the drainage pathways. Sequential images using a gamma camera fitted with a pinhole collimator produce high-resolution images of the canal-

iculi, lacrimal sac and nasolacrimal duct. Under normal conditions, drainage into the nose is seen within one minute. Delayed drainage with stasis is easily recognized and may persist for up to 20 minutes. The level of obstruction can be defined as being proximal or distal to the nasolacrimal sac (Carlton, Trueblood and Rossomondo, 1973). Since this procedure is rapid and atraumatic, it provides a simple screening test for those patients requiring dacrocystography and is of particular value for preoperative and postoperative assessment.

Bone

Bone scanning of the head and neck provides images of altered bone physiology. Any lesion which produces an osteoblastic reaction, increased or decreased blood flow, or an increase in calcium turnover will result in altered biodistribution of the bone scanning agent, ^{99m}Tc-methylene diphosphonate (MDP). Although anatomical resolution is poor when compared with conventional radiography, early physiological changes can be detected which may be sufficient to confirm or refute pathological bony involvement.

Following an i.v. injection of ^{99m}Tc-MDP, static 4-h anterior, posterior, lateral and oblique projections are obtained as appropriate. Standard radiographic views (Waters' and Townes') may be of value. Improved resolution is possible using either converging or pinhole collimators for small structures and current research suggests that diagnostic sensitivity can be increased by digitizing nuclear medicine images with conventional X-rays. In addition to the static views, rapid sequential images (anterior, Waters' or Townes') taken at 3-s intervals following injection provide a low resolution angiogram and the activity on the scan relates to local blood flow. A 5-minute picture provides a 'blood pool' image and the intensity of activity on the scan indicates the size of the vascular compartment of the lesion. Static views show the extent of any osteoblastic bone reaction but the addition of dynamic pictures can increase diagnostic sensitivity and specificity (Noyek, 1979). Table 23.7 summarizes the findings of three-phase bone scanning in head and neck lesions.

When evaluating head and neck bone images, familiarity with normal scan appearances is essential. Increased areas of uptake in the mandible and the maxillary alveolar ridges may be seen in patients with periodontal and periapical inflammation, recent dental extractions, multiple cementomas and malfitting dentures (Matteson *et al.*, 1980). Although bone scanning is extremely sensitive and will demonstrate lesions before they are visible on plain radiographs, the findings are often non-specific and uptake is seen in malignancy, benign bone cysts, osteoid osteomas, osteomyelitis, trauma, and in metabolic disorders such as Paget's disease, fibrous dysplasia and hyperparathyroidism. Increased focal uptake of ^{99m}Tc-MDP

Table 23.7 Three-phase bone scanning of the head and neck

Lesion	Perfusion and blood pool	Static scan
Tumour (primary and secondary)	+	+
Acute sinusitis	+	+
Acute osteomyelitis	+	+
Chronic osteomyelitis	−	+
Recent fracture	+	+
Old fracture	−	+
Vascularized bone graft (early)	+	+
Free bone graft (early)	−	−
Free bone graft (late)	−	+
Paget's disease	+	+

is seen in the majority of primary head and neck bony tumours. However, these lesions are much better evaluated by other imaging modalities such as CT.

The clinical use of bone scanning using ^{99m}Tc-MDP in head and neck malignancy has been reported to be of value in the pretreatment evaluation of bony involvement from primary carcinoma, in the diagnosis of residual and recurrent disease, and to detect bony metastases to, and from, the head and neck (Noyek, 1979). However, since bone scanning is poorly specific (see Table 23.7), bony extension within the mandible cannot be reliably distinguished from benign dental disease (Matteson *et al.*, 1980). Distant bony metastases from head and neck carcinoma (excluding the thyroid) are uncommon and, consequently, bone scanning plays no part in either diagnosis or staging. However, metastases to the facial bones and calvarium frequently arise with carcinoma of the breast and lung and anterior and lateral skull views are recommended to exclude these lesions.

Bone scanning within the head and neck is of value in the evaluation of facial trauma and can demonstrate fractures undetected by conventional radiography (Noyek, 1979). It is also useful in the diagnosis and management of acute and chronic sinusitis with osteomyelitis and, using ^{67}Ga-citrate, it is possible to demonstrate an active focus within chronic osteomyelitis and distinguish chronic sinusitis from carcinoma. Paget's disease of the temporal bone producing auditory symptoms and pulsatile tinnitus can be detected with a ^{99m}Tc-MDP bone scan and photon-deficient areas further investigated with ^{67}Ga, when positive uptake will suggest an osteogenic sarcoma.

Single photon emission computerized tomography (SPECT) demonstrates anatomy and physiology in three dimensions and can increase diagnostic sensitivity for the detection of tumours and sepsis and is also of value in the evaluation of temporomandibular joint dysfunction (O'Mara, 1985). Combined ^{67}Ga-citrate and ^{99m}Tc-MDP scanning is more sensitive than either radiographs or CT for the early detection and follow up of malignant otitis externa and localization is improved using SPECT. Both planar and SPECT ^{99m}Tc-MDP bone scans may be of value in predicting the fate of free and pedicled bone grafts (Noyek, 1979; O'Mara, 1985).

Squamous cell carcinoma

In the management of head and neck squamous carcinoma, the most important prognostic factor at the time of initial presentation is the presence or absence, level and size of metastatic cervical lymphadenopathy (Stell, Morton and Singh, 1983; Grandi *et al.*, 1985). There is a large observer error when palpating the neck (Sako *et al.*, 1964), and although CT and MRI scanning have added a new dimension to the evaluation of metastatic neck disease, they are non-specific. In addition, nodes less than 1.0 cm in size are usually regarded as clinically non-significant and groupings of three or more 8–10 mm contiguous nodes contribute to false-positive results (Mancuso *et al.*, 1981; Watkinson, 1993).

The accumulation of mercury-197 chlormerodrin at sites of known head and neck squamous carcinoma was first reported in 1965 (Johnson, Larson and McCurdy, 1965). Since then, physicians and surgeons have employed a variety of radiopharmaceuticals to investigate head and neck tumours in an attempt to identify primary and occult tumour with cervical metastases together with residual or recurrent disease following surgery and irradiation. ^{67}Ga-citrate, cobalt-57 (^{57}Co)-bleomycin, indium-111 (^{111}In)-bleomycin, ^{99m}Tc-bleomycin, ^{99m}TcO$_4^-$ and some of the radiolanthanides have all been tried with some success (Kashima *et al.*, 1974; Cummings *et al.*, 1981; Watkinson, 1990). However, they suffer from low sensitivity and specificity, considerable cost, and prolonged blood clearance which may delay the scanning time for up to 48 hours.

One of the criticisms of using ^{67}Ga-citrate or ^{57}Co-bleomycin to image cervical lymphadenopathy was the inability to detect lesions less than 2 cm in size, by which time nodes were usually clinically palpable (Cummings *et al.*, 1981).

^{99m}Tc-sulphur colloid lymphoscintigraphy (Blakeslee *et al.*, 1985) and ^{111}In-labelled monoclonal antibody against the epidermal growth factor receptor (Soo *et al.*, 1987) have been used to image cervical lymph nodes. However, they have proved similarly unsuccessful due to an inability to detect nodes less than 2 cm in size and an unacceptable false-negative rate.

Recent reports have described the accumulation of ^{99m}Tc (v)-DMSA at known sites of primary and meta-

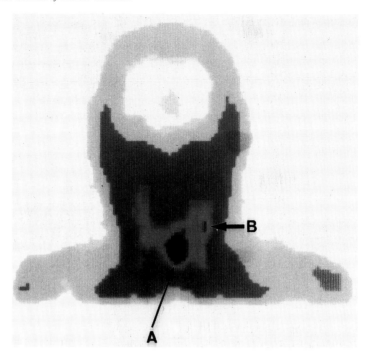

Figure 23.14 Coronal SPECT ^{99m}Tc (v)-DMSA scan in a patient with a clinically T3N0 transglottic squamous cell carcinoma of the left vocal cord (A). CT scan confirmed the extent of the primary tumour and showed no neck nodes. The patient underwent total laryngectomy and left modified radical neck dissection. The neck dissection specimen contained one positive node in level 3 (B)

static squamous carcinoma (Figure 23.14). It is as sensitive but more specific than ^{67}Ga-citrate, and the use of SPECT improves the sensitivity so that it is now possible to detect cervical nodes less than 2 cm in size which were neither palpable nor visible on CT (Watkinson *et al.*, 1991).

The advent of PET has added a new dimension to head and neck tumour imaging. Using ^{18}F-deoxyglucose (FDG), it is now possible to identify not only primary tumours but also metastatic neck disease (Baillet *et al.*, 1992). The problem with all neck imaging is that, as with CT and MRI, the sensitivity of the investigation decreases with the size of the lesion and what is required is an imaging study which can accurately identify microscopic disease in occult nodes measuring 1 cm or less. Whether PET can do this remains to be seen, so at present, elective neck surgery is probably better than elective neck investigation. The most likely role for PET in the future lies in the detection of the occult primary, residual and recurrent disease (Figure 23.15) following surgery and irradiation (to include anatomical/physiological interposition as dual coregistration with either CT or MRI) and to facilitate further research in neuro-otology, such as the evaluation of cochlear implantation and the investigation of non-organic hearing loss.

Lymph nodes

In 1969, Edwards and Hayes evaluted the potential of ^{67}Ga-citrate as a bone scanning agent and reported its concentration in the cervical lymph nodes of a patient with Hodgkin's disease. ^{67}Ga was subsequently described as a new 'tumour seeking' agent, not only for head and neck malignancy, but for tumours in general (Andrews and Edwards, 1975). Its current role in imaging head and neck cancer is now largely confined to the evaluation of lymphoma. ^{67}Ga can be used to assess patients before positive histology is obtained and during initial staging. However, it can be of particular value in the assessment and restaging of residual and recurrent disease following surgery and irradiation (Turner *et al.*, 1978). However, the clinician should be aware that bilateral symmetrical accumulation of the tracer can occur within the salivary glands following irradiation and that this normal phenomenon (Beckerman and Hoffer, 1976) may cause some confusion when interpreting images.

Cerebrospinal fluid

CSF leaks can be demonstrated using ^{111}Indiethylenetriaminepenta-acetic acid (DTPA). Sequential,

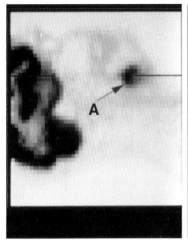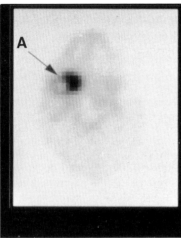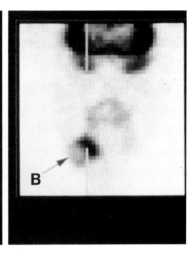

Figure 23.15 Sagittal, axial and coronal ¹⁸FDG-PET scans in a patient with radiorecurrent squamous cell carcinoma of the anterior tongue (left side). Marked uptake is clearly seen at the site of recurrent primary disease (A) and a tumour positive submandibular node (B). (By courtesy of Miss Elfy Chevretton)

anterior, posterior, lateral and vertex views are taken at 2, 4, 24 and 48 hours following a lumbar injection of ¹¹¹In-DTPA. In patients with CSF rhinorrhoea, radioactivity can be demonstrated in the nose, nasopharynx or paranasal sinuses. The location of the leak can be identified by counting the radioactivity in nasal packs placed in the anterior, middle and posterior aspects of the roof of the nose by an otolaryngologist. False positives secondary to cross-contamination and radioactivity are seen and should be related to blood levels. In those patients with otorrhoea, radioactivity can be dectected in the nasopharynx following passage of the tracer down the eustachian tube or on a cotton ball placed in the ear canal (Gilday, 1983).

Miscellaneous

Primary and metastatic melanomas have been demonstrated using ¹¹¹In and ¹³¹I-monoclonal antibodies (Buraggi *et al.*, 1985). ¹¹¹In-somatostatin (octreoscan) is a new radiopharmaceutical with exciting potential offering the ability to visualize neuroendocrine and pituitary tumours together with apudomas, and the uptake of ¹²³I/¹³¹I-MIBG in thymoma and malignant paragangliomas (Figure 23.16) has recently been described which may have diagnostic and therapeutic implications (Watkinson, 1990).

Therapeutic

The most commonly used radionuclide for therapy within the field of nuclear medicine in otolaryngology is iodine-131 (Table 23.8). This is because differentiated thyroid cancer (follicular, papillary, follicular mixed) retains properties allied to its tissue of origin

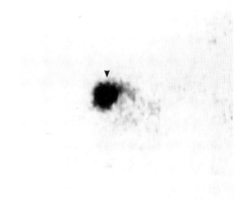

Figure 23.16 Left lateral 24 hour ¹³¹I-MIBG scan in a patient with a large glomus jugulare tumour. Marked uptake is seen (arrowed) at the site of known disease. The patient was subsequently treated with a therapeutic dose of ¹³¹I-MIBG

Table 23.8 Commonly used radiopharmaceuticals for radiotherapy within nuclear medicine and otolaryngology

Radiopharmaceutical	Target organ
Iodine-131	Differentiated thyroid cancer (follicular and follicular/papillary mixed)
¹³¹I-MIBG	Neuroendocrine tumours, e.g. glomus jugulare, carcinoid, medullary thyroid cancer
Rhenium-186-DMSA	Medullary thyroid cancer

and can therefore concentrate iodine against a gradient by using the iodine pump. This is always the case for follicular carcinoma but patients with papillary carcinoma may also concentrate radioiodine, since many of these tumours also contain follicular elements. Although there is now a move in some cases, towards more conservative thyroid surgery (lobectomy only), the standard conventional treatment for most differentiated thyroid carcinoma has been total thyroidectomy followed by radioiodine therapy with iodine-131.

It is virtually impossible for a surgeon to perform a 'total' thyroidectomy. Postoperative scanning will frequently show residual activity within the neck, irrespective of the presence or absence of differentiated tumour. As a consequence, all patients should receive postoperative ^{131}I radioablation in order to eradicate any residual normal thyroid tissue and then proceed through a carefully designed managment programme (Figure 23.17). Hence following definitive surgery or

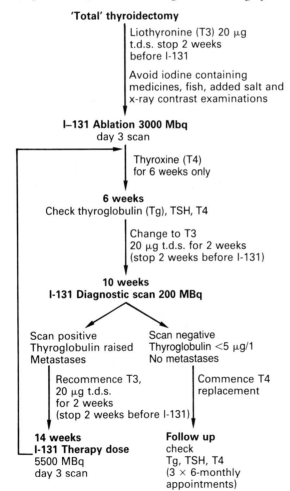

'Total' thyroidectomy

Liothyronine (T3) 20 μg t.d.s. stop 2 weeks before I-131

Avoid iodine containing medicines, fish, added salt and x-ray contrast examinations

I–131 Ablation 3000 Mbq
day 3 scan

Thyroxine (T4) for 6 weeks only

6 weeks
Check thyroglobulin (Tg), TSH, T4

Change to T3 20 μg t.d.s. for 2 weeks (stop 2 weeks before I-131)

10 weeks
I-131 Diagnostic scan 200 MBq

Scan positive Thyroglobulin raised Metastases

Scan negative Thyroglobulin <5 μg/1 No metastases

Recommence T3, 20 μg t.d.s. for 2 weeks (stop 2 weeks before I-131)

Commence T4 replacement

14 weeks
I-131 Therapy dose
5500 MBq
day 3 scan

Follow up
check
Tg, TSH, T4
(3 × 6-monthly appointments)

Figure 23.17 Treatment of differentiated thyroid carcinoma, Birmingham Oncology Centre protocol

cessation of T3/T4 (2 weeks for T3; 4 weeks for T4), the TSH rises and stimulates both the uptake of iodine and the growth of residual normal functioning thyroid tissue and residual differentiated tumour including differentiated metastases. During this period patients should be advised to avoid iodine-containing medicines, fish, added salt and X-ray contrast examinations. Commonly an empirical ablation dose of 3000 MBq ^{131}I is then given, recommencing thyroxine after 6 days (Figure 23.17).

Compulsory isolation of the patient in a purpose-built unsealed source radionuclide therapy room is mandatory until the radioactivity of the patient has decreased to an accepted safe limit, usually within a period of approximately 5 days. Radioiodine is eliminated in body fluids, including urine, faeces, sweat and saliva. The latter may be a problem if the patient has a tracheostomy. Therefore the fashioning of either a temporary or permanent alternative airway should be avoided if possible.

Patients are commenced on full thyroxine (T4) replacement which, after 6 weeks, should reliably suppress TSH. At this point a thyroglobulin (Tg) level is measured which has been shown to be a reliable marker of disease activity providing the TSH is fully suppressed (Black *et al.*, 1981). Hormone replacement is recommended with liothyronine (T3), for 2 weeks only, followed by an [131]I 200 MBq diagnostic scan at 4 weeks.

Those patients with an abnormal scan, whose thyroglobulin is raised or who are known to have metastatic disease are recommenced on liothyronine (T3) for a further 2 weeks only, followed by inpatient radioiodine therapy at 4 weeks, when a dose of [131]I (5500 MBq) is usually given. The interval between the initial ablation dose of 3000 MBq and the therapy dose of 5500 MBq is therefore approximately 14 weeks.

The patient is recommenced on full thyroxine replacement and the process is repeated until there is no evidence of abnormal ^{131}I uptake and the thyroglobulin level is undetectable. Subsequent follow up relies upon clinical and, where indicated, radiological examination together with thyroglobulin and TSH measurements. External beam radiotherapy is usually reserved for patients who have macroscopic residual disease which is resistant to, or fails to accumulate, radioiodine (Phillips *et al.*, 1993).

A move towards conservative surgery obviously leaves a significant amount of normal functioning thyroid tissue within the neck. This will produce thyroglobulin and concentrate radioiodine within the neck, thereby possibly preventing the detection of local distant micrometastases, unless the TSH is fully suppressed with exogenous thyroxine (T4). In this situation, follow up is clinical and biochemical (with thyroglobulin) in the first instance. In such patients, imaging with ^{201}Tl has proved helpful since this technique is independent of normal functioning thyroid tissue. It can also be used in patients who request not to be scanned with ^{131}I or where stopping T3/T4 is considered unnecessary or detrimental to the patient, particularly in elderly patients or in those with aggressive tumours since some cancers can grow rapidly during the period of T3/T4 cessation.

Neuroendocrine tumours of the head and neck concentrate metaiodobenzylguanidine (MIBG) and therefore it is possible to treat lesions such as glomus jugulare, carcinoid and medullary thyroid cancer using ^{131}I-MIBG. Treatment can be given primarily (Rockall *et al.*, 1990) or as an adjunct to surgery or external beam radiotherapy. Following extirpative surgery, it is possible also to administer interstitial brachytherapy at the time of the operation using ^{125}I seeds to treat any residual tumour.

Recent advances in radiopharmacy have utilized the uptake of [99m]Tc (v)-DMSA in medullary carcinoma of the thyroid and current research suggests that it may be possible to use the β^- emitter rhenium-186 to treat medullary carcinoma of the thyroid with rhenium-186-DMSA. Early results are encouraging (Allen *et al.*, 1990).

References

ALLEN, S. J., BLAKE, G. M., MCKEENEY, D. B., LAZARUS, C. R., BLOWER, P. J., SINGH, J. *et al.* (1990) A new radiopharmaceutical, [186]Re-V-DMSA, for therapy of medullary carcinoma of the thyroid (abstract). *European Journal of Nuclear Medicine*, **16**, 432

ANDREWS, G. A. and EDWARDS, C. L. (1975) Tumour scanning with gallium 67. *Journal of the American Medical Association*, **223**, 1100–1103

BAILLET, J. W., ABEMAYOR, E., JABOUR, B. A., HAWKINS, R. A., HO, C. and WARD, P. H. (1992) Positron emmission tomography: a new, precise imaging modality for detection of primary head and neck tumours and assessment of cervical adenopathy. *Laryngoscope*, **102**, 281–288

BECKERMAN, C. and HOFFER, P. B. (1976) Salivary gland uptake of ^{67}Ga-citrate following radiation therapy. *Journal of Nuclear Medicine*, **17**, 685–687

BLACK, E. G., CASSONI, A., GIMLETTE, T. M. D., HARMER, C. L., MAISEY, M. N. and OATES, G. D. (1981) Serum thyroglobulin in thyroid cancer. *Lancet*, ii, 443–445

BLAKESLEE, D. B., BECKER, D. G., SIMPSON, G. T., PATTEN, D. H. and SPRENGELMEYER, J. (1985) Lymphoscintigraphy of the neck. *Otolaryngology, Head and Neck Surgery*, **93**, 361–365

BURAGGI, G. L., CALLEGARO, L., MARIANI, G., TURRIN, A., CASCINELLI, N., ATTILI, A. *et al.* (1985) Imaging with ^{131}I-labelled monoclonal antibodies to a high molecular-weight melanoma-associated antigen in patients with melanoma: efficacy of whole immunoglobulin and its F(ab)$_2$ fragments. *Cancer Research*, **45**, 3378–3387

CARLTON, W. H., TRUEBLOOD, J. H. and ROSSOMONDO, R. M. (1973) Clinical evaluation of microscintigraphy of the lacrimal drainage apparatus. *Journal of Nuclear Medicine*, **14**, 89–92

CLARKE, S. E. M., LAZARUS, C. R., WRAIGHT, P., SAMPSON, C. and MAISEY, M. N. (1988) Pentavalent ^{99m}Tc DMSA, ^{131}I MIBG

and ^{99m}Tc MDP – an evaluation of three imaging techniques in patients with medullary carcinoma of the thyroid. *Journal of Nuclear Medicine*, **29**, 33–38

CUMMINGS, C. N., LARSON, S. M., DOBIE, R. A., WEYMULLER, E. A., RUDD, T. G. and MERELLO, A. (1981) Assessment of cobalt-57 tagged bleomycin as a clinical aid in staging of head and neck carcinoma. *Laryngoscope*, **91**, 529–537

EDWARDS, C. L. and HAYES, R. L. (1969) Tumour scanning with ^{67}Ga-citrate. *Journal of Nuclear Medicine*, **10**, 103–105

ENDO, K., SHIOMI, K., KASAGI, K., KONISHI, J., TORIZUKA, K., WAKAO, K. *et al.* (1984) Imaging of medullary thyroid cancer with ^{131}I-MIBG. *Lancet*, ii, 23

FERLIN, G., BORSATO, N., CAMERANI, N., CONTE, N. and ZOTTI, D. (1983) New perspectives in localising enlarged parathyroids by technetium-thallium subtraction scan. *Journal of Nuclear Medicine*, **24**, 438–441

FUJIMOTO, Y. and OBARA, T. (1987) How to recognize and treat parathyroid carcinoma. *Surgery Clinics of North America*, **67**, 343–357

GILDAY, D.'L. (1983) Special clinical problems in paediatrics. In: *Clinical Nuclear Medicine*, edited by M. N. Maisey, K. E. Britton and D. L. Gilday. London: Chapman and Hall. pp. 331–364

GOULDEN, A. W. G., GLASS, H. I. and SILVESTER, D. J. (1968) The choice of a radioactive isotope for the investigation of thyroid disorders. *British Journal of Radiology*, **41**, 20–25

GRANDI, C., ALLOISIO, M., MOGLIA, D., PODRECCA, S., SALA, L., SALVATORI, P. *et al.* (1985) Prognostic significance of lymphatic spread in head and neck carcinomas: therapeutic implications. *Head and Neck Surgery*, **8**, 67–73

GREYSON, N. D. and NOYEK, A. M. (1982) Radionuclide salivary scanning. *Journal of Otolaryngology*, **11** (suppl. 10), 1–47

HOEFNAGEL, C. A., DELPRAT, C. C., MARCUSE, H. R. and DE VIJLDER, J. J. (1986) Role of thallium-201 total body scintigraphy in follow-up of thyroid carcinoma. *Journal of Nuclear Medicine*, **27**, 1854–1857

IAEA (1988) Optimization of nuclear medicine procedures for the diagnosis and management of thyroid disorders. *Nuclear Medicine Communications*, **9**, 131–139

IWASE, M., SHIMIZU, Y., KITAHARA, H., TOKIOKA, N. and TAKATSUKI, K. (1986) Parathyroid carcinoma visualised by gallium-67 citrate scintigraphy. *Journal of Nuclear Medicine*, **27**, 63–65

JOHNSON, G. S., LARSON, A. L. and MCCURDY, H. W. (1965) Tumour localisation in the nasopharynx using radiomercury labelled chlormerodrin. *Journal of Nuclear Medicine*, **6**, 549–554

KASHIMA, H. K., MCKUSICK, K. A., MALMUD, L. S. and WAGNER, H. N. (1974) Gallium-67 scanning in patients with head and neck cancer. *Laryngoscope*, **84**, 1078–1089

KHAFAGI, F., EGERTON-VERNON, J., VAN DOORN, T., FOSTER, W., MCPHEE, I. B. and ALLISON, R. W. G. (1987) Localisation and treatment of familial malignant non-functional paraganglioma with iodine-131 MIBG: report of two cases. *Journal of Nuclear Medicine*, **28**, 528–531

MANCUSO, A. A., MACERI, D., RICE, D. and HANAFEE, W. (1981) CT of cervical node cancer. *American Journal of Roentgenology*, **136**, 381–385

MATTESON, S. R., STAAB, E. V., FINE, J. T. and HILL, C. (1980) Bone-scan appearance of benign oral pathologic conditions. *Journal of Oral Surgery*, **38**, 759–763

NG TANG FUI, S. C., HOFFENBERG, R., BLACK, E. G. and MAISEY,

M. N. (1979) Serum thyroglobulin concentration and whole-body radioiodine scan in the follow-up of differentiated thyroid cancer after thyroid ablation. *British Medical Journal*, **2**, 298–300

NOYEK, A. M. (1979) Bone scanning on otolaryngology. *Laryngoscope*, 89 (suppl. 18), 1–87

OHTA, H., YAMAMOTO, K., ENDO, K., MORI, T., HAMANAKA, D., SHIMAZU A. *et al.* (1984) A new imaging agent for medullary carcinoma of the thyroid. *Journal of Nuclear Medicine*, **25**, 323–325

O'MARA, R. E. (1985) Role of bone scanning in dental and maxillofacial disorders. *Nuclear Medicine Annual*, 265–284

PERLMUTTER, M. and SLATER, S. L. (1956) Which nodular goitres should be removed? *New England Journal of Medicine*, **255**, 65–71

PHILIPS, P., HANZEN, C., ANDRY, G., VAN HOUTTE, P. and PANA FRUULING, J. (1993) Postoperative irradiation for thyroid cancer. *European Journal of Surgical Oncology*, **19**, 399–404

ROCKALL, T., WATKINSON, J. C., DOUEK, E. and CLARKE, S. E. M. (1990) The scintigraphic evaluation of glomus tumours. A case report with a literature review. *Journal of Laryngology and Otology*, **164**, 33–36

SAKO, K., PRADIER, R. N., MARCHETTA, F. C. and PICKREN, J. W. (1964) Fallibility of palpation in diagnosis of metastases to nodes. *Surgery, Gynecology and Obstetrics*, **118**, 989–990

SHANE, E. and BILEZIKIAN, J. P. (1982) Parathyroid carcinoma: a review of 62 patients. *Endocrine Review*, **3**, 218–226

SOO, K. C., WARD, M., ROBERTS, K. R., KEELING, F., CARTER, R. L., MCCREADY, V. R. *et al.* (1987) Radioimmunoscintigraphy of squamous carcinomas of the head and neck. *Head and Neck Surgery*, **9**, 349–352

STELL, P. M., MORTON, R. P. and SINGH, S. D. (1983) Cervical lymph node metastases: the significance of the level of the lymph node. *Clinical Oncology*, **9**, 101–107

TURNER, D. A., FORDHAM, E. N., ALI, A. and SLAYTON, R. E. (1978) Gallium-67 imaging in the management of Hodgkins' disease and other malignant lymphomas. *Seminars in Nuclear Medicine*, **8**, 205–218

WATKINSON, J. C. (1990) Nuclear medicine in otolaryngology. Editorial. *Clinical Otolaryngology*, **15**, 457–469

WATKINSON, J. C. (1993) The clinically N0 neck: investigation and treatment. Editorial. *Clinical Otolaryngology*, **18**, 443–445

WATKINSON, J. C., LAZARUS, C. R., TODD, C., MAISEY, M. N. and CLARKE, S. E. M. (1991) Metastatic squamous carcinoma in the neck: an anatomical and physiological study using CT and SPECT Tc99m (v) DMSA. *British Journal of Radiology*, **64**, 909–914

24

Wound healing

S. R. Young and M. Dyson

In an age of cost-guided medical care in which the term 'clinical audit' has become standard practice (Department of Health, 1989), it is vital that the time a patient is under treatment is cut to the absolute minimum. We need to have quantitative and sensitive procedures for accurate wound diagnosis and strict protocols for prescribing the most appropriate therapies. An effective diagnostic procedure allows the clinician to follow the healing process once treatment has begun and also alerts him to any problems which develop so that an appropriate change of management can be effected as quickly as possible. To save even a few days by using the most effective therapy could, nationally, account for an enormous saving in health care costs. The government white paper (Department of Health, 1989) defines audit as: 'The systematic critical analysis of the quality of care, including the procedures used for diagnosis and treatment, the use of resources and the resulting outcome and quality of life for the patient'. As an example of how current resources are being stretched, consider the cost of pressure sore care in the UK. Estimates of the prevalence of pressure sores in hospitals and nursing homes are about 10% of all patients (Allman, 1989; Goode, Burns and Walker, 1992). The hospital population in the UK was approximately 300 000 in 1992 (HMSO, 1994). Therefore, 10% of this population equates to the 30 000 patients who suffer from pressure sores. In the UK there are almost 225 000 nursing home beds. Based on these figures, the total number of patients with pressure sores in the nursing home community is in the order of 22 500 (David, 1983; Potter, 1994). This makes the total number of patients suffering from pressure sores in hospitals and nursing homes 52 500. In terms of cost of treatment of pressure sores, the most frequently quoted figure is £150 million per year (Scales *et al.*, 1982; Hibbs, 1989; Livesey and Simpson, 1989;

Watson, 1989; Collier, 1990; Young, 1990; Morison, 1992). One estimate of the cost of treatment for a single patient with a pressure sore was £25 905 (Hibbs, 1988), which represented a 12-week period of treatment in hospital. It can be seen that the cost for just one particular type of wound is enormous. If the cost of all the other wounds is added, e.g. venous leg ulcers, diabetic ulcers, acute surgical wounds etc., the total is quite astronomical.

The aim of this chapter is to provide a detailed source of reference about wound healing from the basic cellular and chemical processes to the more applied clinical level. Ways in which wound healing can be affected, some positive, some negative, will also be examined. There is no general agreement in clinical and laboratory research literature as how best to treat each individual type of injury. Many clinicians, like all good chefs, have their own ideas how best to tackle the job presented to them. Also, no two injuries are identical and, for example, what may work for one venous leg ulcer may not for another. It is vital that the clinician has as much knowledge as possible about the biology of wound healing and how various therapies interact with it. Armed with this knowledge, the clinician is in a strong position to work out why a particular wound does not respond to therapy and how best to alter the treatment regimen to provide the much needed repair stimulus. It must be understood that some wounds may not repair because of the presence of some underlying deficiency in the wound environment which renders therapy ineffective.

Bearing this in mind, one of the first steps to be taken by clinicians before embarking on a course of therapy is to make sure that they have a full patient history so that any underlying complications are known, e.g. diabetes mellitus, venous insufficiency etc. These complications should be addressed before any course of therapy is undertaken. Failure to do this results in waste of time, money, and most important there is a likelihood of compounding the problem and placing the patient at further risk. Once therapy has begun, it is important to have sensitive, quantitative, easy to use and interpret, diagnostic techniques by which changes in a wound's response to therapy can be assessed. The more sensitive the technique the earlier the clinician can detect whether the therapy used is effective. A number of techniques will be discussed.

Wound healing

Wound healing may be defined as the restoration of tissue continuity after injury. Although tissues generally tend to heal without any need for further intervention, the healing process is not always as rapid as it could be. Also the end product both cosmetically and mechanically can be poor. It is interesting that in postnatal mammals, function is restored to the injured tissue by a process of repair which results in the formation of a scar. However, in the early fetus, form and function are restored completely to the injured tissue by a process of regeneration. To improve the quality of healing in postnatal mammals it is important that we fully understand the cellular and molecular events which take place during the repair process. In this way we may discover what mechanisms are responsible for the switch between the two types of healing that are apparent after birth – healing by first and second intention.

Healing by first intention

This type of healing is found in clean, incised, surgical wounds. In these there is a minimum of tissue destruction, the edges of the wound are closely opposed, and healing takes place without complication.

Healing begins with haematoma formation and an acute inflammatory reaction alongside the damaged tissue. Epithelial proliferation ensues rapidly (within 24 hours) sealing the wound at the basal cell layer of the epidermis. Granulation tissue develops by the third day. Fibroblasts both secrete and contract the immature connective tissue matrix. The end result is an intact epithelium (regeneration) and a small fibrous scar (repair) (Tighe and Davies, 1990). The preconditions for this process are that the wound edges should be smooth, have a good blood supply and be almost completely free from infection.

Healing by second intention

This type of healing is seen in traumatic wounds, where tissue is lost, the wound margins are not opposed, or when complications such as infection intervene.

In these types of wounds, the haematoma is larger and there is more inflammation due to the greater tissue destruction. Epithelial proliferation begins at an early stage, but union of the epithelium across the wound is delayed, as it has to grow down and spread progressively across the wound at the junction of viable and non-viable tissue. More granulation tissue is produced, an important factor in healing by secondary intention for the contraction of the wound by myofibroblasts, which reduce the size of the wound and hence, the degree of scarring. The end result is an intact epithelium (regeneration), but more tissue distortion and a large scar (repair) (Tighe and Davies, 1990).

The cellular and chemical response to injury

Following injury, a number of cellular and chemical events take place in soft tissues. The major cellular components of the repair process include platelets, mast cells, polymorphonuclear leucocytes, macrophages, lymphocytes, fibroblasts, pericytes and endothelial cells. These cells migrate as a module into the injury site in a well-defined sequence which is controlled by numerous soluble growth factors. These growth factors originate from a number of sources such as blood cells (e.g. platelets, macrophages and polymorphonuclear leucocytes), inflammatory cascade systems (e.g. coagulation and complement), or from the products of damaged tissue breakdown.

The whole repair process can, for convenience, be divided into three phases (Clark, 1990), although these phases overlap considerably lacking any distinct border between each other. The three phases are:

1 Inflammation
2 Proliferation/granulation tissue formation
3 Remodelling.

There is now overwhelming evidence which shows that the effectiveness of certain therapies is dependent upon the phase of repair in which they are employed. This will be discussed in more detail later in this chapter.

Inflammation

This early dynamic phase of repair is characterized initially by clot formation. The blood platelet is a major constituent of the blood clot and, in addition to its activities associated with clotting, platelets also contain numerous biologically active substances including prostaglandins, serotonin, platelet derived growth factor (PDGF), etc. These substances have a profound effect upon the local environment of the wound and its subsequent repair (Clark, 1990). Mast cells provide another source of biologically active substances and growth factors which help orchestrate the early repair sequences.

Neutrophils are the first polymorphonuclear leucocytes to enter the wound bed, attracted by an array of wound mediators present at the wound site. The neutrophils' function is to clear the wound site of foreign particles such as bacteria and damaged tissue debris.

Macrophages enter the wound bed, closely behind the neutrophils, where they phagocytose bacteria and wound tissue debris. They also produce wound mediators, including growth factors which direct granulation tissue formation (Leibovich and Ross, 1975).

Evidence will be presented later in this chapter which shows that, when used at the right time, during wound repair, certain therapies can influence the release of these wound mediators from the cells in and around the wound bed.

Proliferation and granulation tissue formation

During normal acute injury repair the inflammatory phase is followed within a few days by granulation tissue formation. This stage is often referred to as the proliferative phase. During this phase the wound void is filled with cells (mainly macrophages and fibroblasts), numerous blood vessels (angiogenesis), and a connective tissue matrix (containing fibronectin, hyaluronic acid and collagen types I and III).

A new epidermis forms during this phase of repair. The new epidermal cells migrate from the edge of the wound and from around hair follicles, sweat ducts and glands within the injury site (in the case of partial thickness wounds) towards the centre of the wound.

Wound contraction takes place during this phase of repair and can be defined as the process by which the size of a wound decreases by the centripetal movement of the whole thickness of surrounding skin (Peacock, 1984). In man, most of the skin is relatively immobile due to its attachment to underlying structures. In some instances where wounds have been sustained over joints, wound contraction may lead to immobilization as a result of tension developed through attachment of the skin to underlying structures. Excessive contraction is often seen as a serious complication to healing (Figure 24.1).

The stimuli controlling all these events come from numerous sources, the macrophage being the main one. Release of active factors from macrophages is thought to be controlled, in part, by the relatively hypoxic environment of the wound (Knighton *et al.*, 1983). The effect of various therapies on the macrophage will be discussed in detail later.

Remodelling

Remodelling may continue for many months or years after the proliferative phase of repair. During remodelling, granulation tissue is usually gradually replaced by a scar which is a relatively acellular and avascular tissue. The composition of extracellular matrix changes as the wound matures. Initially, the extracellular matrix is composed mainly of hyaluronic acid, fibronectin, collagens types I, III and V. During remodelling the ratio of collagen type I to III changes until type I is the dominant form. Scar tissue is a poor substitute for unwounded dermis. The rate at which a wound gains tensile strength is slow (Levenson *et al.*, 1965), gaining only 20–25 % of its maximum strength by the third week after injury. Increase in wound strength depends upon two main factors. First, the rate of collagen deposition. Second, it depends on collagen remodelling, its alignment and formation of larger collagen bundles (Kischer and Shetlar, 1974) and an alteration of intermolecular cross-links (Bailey *et al.*, 1975). It will be shown later that if used at the correct time after injury, certain therapies can improve both the cosmetic appearance and the mechanical properties of the resulting scar tissue.

A diagrammatic representation of the normal response of skin to wounding is summarized in Figure 24.2. This figure shows the main changes in relative cell numbers during the inflammatory, proliferative and remodelling phases of repair following skin incision.

Factors affecting wound healing
Infection

Bacterial contamination of a wound delays healing. Bacteria use the nutrients and oxygen supplied to a wound and this may lead to tissue anoxia and starvation. They cause tissue damage by producing lactic acid and secreting endotoxins and exotoxins which result in cell lysis and extracellular matrix digestion. The bacterial contamination also prolongs the inflammatory response which causes further tissue damage from protease release.

Infection tends to happen when the immune system is overwhelmed. Patients with complement deficiency states (e.g. those with poor nutrition, or those exposed to trauma or surgery) and those with opsonization defects (e.g. those with viral disease, anaemia, previous bacterial invasion), are particularly susceptible to bacterial infection. The susceptibility of a wound to infection is also increased by the presence of necrotic tissue, foreign particles and haematoma in the wound.

Bacterial killing by phagocytosis requires a high oxygen level. Oxygen deficiency favours the growth of anaerobic bacteria. Infected wounds have decreases in both bursting strength (Bucknall, 1980) and skin graft acceptability. The proliferation of fibroblasts is also reduced (Shulman, Petro and Hallgen, 1979). Apart from causing wound complications, bacteria may spread into the bloodstream causing bacteraemia and septicaemia which may be fatal.

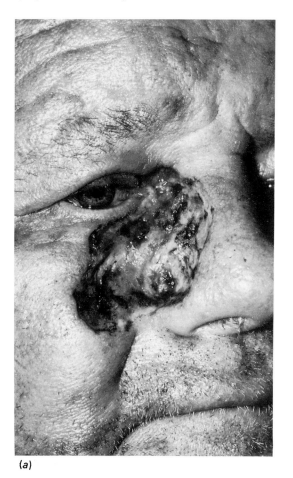

(a)

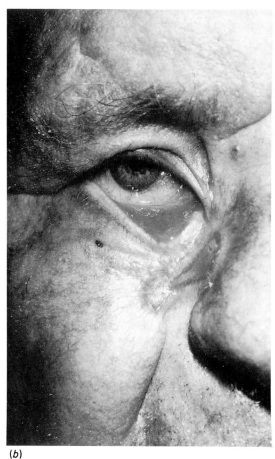

(b)

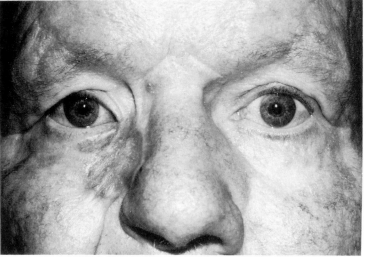

(c)

Figure 24.1 (*a*) Patient has had a skin cancer (basal cell carcinoma) removed from the side of his nose and cheek. The wound was allowed to heal by secondary intention. (*b*) Appearance of wound 4 weeks later. Note how the natural forces of wound contraction have produced a severe distortion of the eyelid (ectropion). (*c*) To repair the ectropion, scar was removed and a full thickness skin graft was applied to the area. Appearance 1 month following skin grafting. (Courtesy of William Panje)

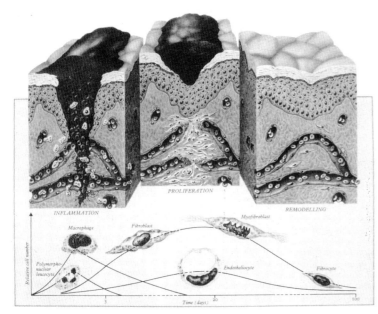

Figure 24.2 Schematic diagram summarizing the changes in relative cell numbers in an incised skin lesion during the inflammatory, proliferative and remodelling phases of repair (from *Gray's Anatomy*, 37th edn, courtesy of Churchill Livingstone)

Foreign bodies

Foreign bodies that have entered a wound, such as splinters of wood and fragments of glass or metal, lower the wound's oxygen tension. They also cause prolonged inflammation, further tissue destruction and increase the risk of bacterial infection (Hohn, 1980), and hence inhibit tissue repair.

Oxygen

The oxygen level in tissue has been shown to affect the rate of healing. Oxygen is required for both phagocytosis of bacteria and during collagen synthesis for the hydroxylation of proline and lysine.

Low tissue oxygen tension at the advancing edge of proliferation creates an oxygen gradient which stimulates macrophages to produce angiogenic factors. These attract blood vessels into the wound and raise the oxygen tension which facilitates collagen synthesis and epithelialization (Knighton *et al.*, 1983).

Many conditions are associated with the production of local tissue hypoxia; these include tissue trauma, inadequate haemostasis, atherosclerosis, diabetes mellitus, venous insufficiency and oedema. Tissue hypoxia reduces proliferation, bacterial resistance, and hence, delays healing. It can be resolved by applying hyperbaric oxygen to the wound and this has been shown to promote healing of leg ulcers (Heng, 1983).

Smoking

Smoking reduces the oxygen tension of blood and, hence, of wounds. Furthermore, nicotine-induced vaso-constriction causes local hypoxia and poor healing. Smokers also have an increased risk of tissue flap necrosis and peripheral ulcers and are often deficient in vitamin C, which is an essential co-factor in wound healing.

Wound tension

A wound which is closed too tightly with sutures may become ischaemic and necrotic.

Blood supply

An adequate blood supply is required to provide the wound with inflammatory cells, oxygen, nutrients, and to remove waste materials. Oxygen is required for the intensified metabolic processes which take place in a wound, for the oxidative degradation of foreign particles by phagocytic cells and for collagen synthesis.

Blood supply to a wound and the rate of healing is variable and depends on the position of the wound, e.g. facial wounds heal faster than those in the lower leg due to their better blood supply. The rate of healing also depends on the type of tissue damaged; tendons and fascia heal more slowly than muscle as their blood supply is less favourable. In a hypoxic wound, musculocutaneous flaps can be used to increase blood supply to the area.

Irradiation, which is frequently used to treat head and neck cancer, causes irreparable damage to the skin's microvasculature. As a consequence of reduced blood supply, resulting from irradiation, wounds heal poorly and are much more susceptible to infection than are non-irradiated tissue beds (Figure 24.3).

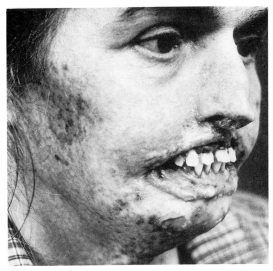

Figure 24.3 Patient had radiation treatment for acne 25 years previous to this photograph. Her lips are now infiltrated with invasive cancer. Note the extensive scarring resulting from the previous radiation. (Courtesy of William Panje)

Temperature

Hypothermia reduces the tensile strength of wounds and slows healing (Lofstrom and Zederfeldt, 1957). This may be due to altered haemodynamics and sludging of blood. Decreased environmental temperature, particularly, affects superficial cutaneous wounds.

Nutritional status

Healing requires adequate supplies of protein, vitamins and trace elements. Problems develop if supplies are inadequate due to poor intake (starvation and malnutrition), abnormal absorption (gastrointestinal tract disease or surgery), or greatly increased demand (burns). Patients with chronic wounds may need nutritional supplements to satisfy their increased metabolic demand. Wound healing is delayed in patients with cachexia as seen in cancer patients and those with immune deficiency. Obesity can also cause wound healing problems.

Protein and carbohydrates

Healing tissue requires amino acids for protein synthesis and as an energy source for gluconeogenesis. Amino acids are needed for cell growth and proliferation, the production of collagen and other matrix components, and the production of enzymes and antibodies. Severe protein deficiency inhibits all the basic phases of wound healing (Haydock and Hill, 1986), but particularly collagen synthesis.

Carbohydrates are necessary as a supply of energy for the wound healing process. They are particularly important in cell proliferation and phagocytosis.

Vitamin deficiencies

Vitamin A

Vitamin A is required for the maintenance of a normal epidermis, for the synthesis of the glycoproteins and proteoglycans which are necessary for re-epithelialization and for the cross-linking of collagen fibres. It is also vital for the inflammatory process, particularly for enhancing macrophage availability, and for the destabilization of lysosomal membranes, thereby enabling the release of their enzymes. Vitamin A can be used to counteract the effects of corticosteroids.

Vitamin C

Vitamin C is required for hydroxylation of proline and lysine during collagen formation. In vitamin C deficiency, collagen is underhydroxylated and hence subject to degradation. Wound dehiscence is much more common in patients with vitamin C deficiency. Vitamin C deficiency also causes capillary fragility, as it is required for the formation of the vascular basement membrane. Furthermore, deficiency affects glycosaminoglycan metabolism, the synthesis of complement factors and gamma globulins. Inflammation and resistance to infection are also compromised as macrophage and neutrophil function is impaired by vitamin C deficiency (Beisel *et al.*, 1981). Vitamin C deficiency is seen particularly in chronically ill patients.

Vitamin K

This is required for the synthesis of clotting factors VII, IX, and X (Nossel, 1983). Deficiency of this vitamin results in bleeding disorders, inadequate haemostasis and hence promotion of bacterial growth.

Vitamin B

Vitamin B deficiency causes a reduction of type III collagen secretion which results in decreased wound strength (Alvarez and Gilbreath, 1982). It is also responsible for decreased antibody production.

Vitamin E

This is an antioxidant which removes free-radical intermediates, many of which are produced by neutrophils, from the wound. A deficiency results in an increased availability of potentially toxic free radicals.

Minerals

Zinc, copper and iron are the most important minerals for wound healing. Zinc is required for epidermal cell proliferation. Zinc metalloenzymes degrade potentially damaging free oxygen radicals, and facilitate cell migration and proliferation (Nelder, 1983). It is also required for basement membrane synthesis and function (Bettger and O'Dell, 1981). Zinc deficiency causes a delay in wound healing, reduces cell mitosis, collagen and other protein synthesis and lysyl oxidase activity. Excess zinc also impairs wound healing by reducing chemotaxis and phagocytosis (Chandra, 1984). Copper and iron are important co-factors in collagen cross-linking.

Ageing

Ageing affects all stages of wound healing. Inflammation is delayed and lasts longer while wound contraction, cell proliferation and cell metabolism are all decreased. The rate of capillary growth into the wound and mast cell numbers decline with age. The diminished blood flow causes decreased clearance of metabolites and foreign materials, and tissue hypoxia which delays wound healing.

Wound remodelling also differs in the aged person. Fibroblast activity decreases and hence, collagen synthesis and degradation decrease. There is also a reduction in the amount of collagen organization and cross-linkage which results in decreased tensile strength.

Re-epithelialization is also slowed by ageing; keratinocytes from older patients proliferate less than those from younger patients (Gilchrest, 1983). The effects of ageing on wound healing are often compounded by malnutrition, vascular insufficiency or systemic disease.

Underlying disease

Diseases that cause tissue hypoxia, such as diabetes, arteriosclerosis and chronic venous insufficiency, all retard wound healing. In diabetics, vitamin C transport is impaired by the increased blood sugar level and this disturbs collagen synthesis. The chemotactic and phagocytic functions of leucocytes are also impeded, which increases the risk of infection.

Small vessel disease that accompanies diabetes, manifested by endothelial proliferation in small arterioles and by basement membrane capillary thickening, reduces oxygen availability for hydroxylation, prevents normal collagen synthesis and delays wound healing.

Drugs

Anti-inflammatory drugs

Glucocorticoids depress the inflammatory response by decreasing neutrophil and monocyte recruitment and by suppressing macrophage phagocytosis. They also suppress the release of enzymes from lysosomes by stabilizing the membranes of these vesicles. As a consequence there is delayed wound debridement

and bacterial elimination. Steroids also inhibit fibroblast proliferation and hence, collagen synthesis and granulation tissue formation (Salmela, 1981), which results in the production of a thin abnormal dermal matrix. Keratinocyte proliferation is also decreased, causing thinning of the epidermis.

The non-steroidal anti-inflammatory drugs have been reported to counteract inflammation by inhibiting prostaglandin synthesis (Moore and Hoult, 1980), which results in tissue hypoxia and delayed wound healing. However, more recent work (Cackett, Young and Dyson, 1995) has shown experimentally that non-steroidal anti-inflammatory drugs, specifically acetylsalicylic acid (aspirin) and 6-methoxy-α-methyl-2-naphthalenacetic acid (naproxen) do not inhibit wound closure. These compounds only reduce those inflammatory responses which if excessive are detrimental to the healing process, i.e. neutrophil accumulation (Weiss, 1989).

Cytotoxics

Cytotoxic drugs interfere with wound healing by inhibiting cell division, altering the nitrogen balance of the wound, inhibiting fibrosis, reducing collagen deposition and suppressing angiogenesis. They particularly affect the proliferative phase of wound healing by interfering with protein synthesis. Cytotoxic drugs also reduce resistance to infection.

Anticoagulants

These are substances which inhibit coagulation, e.g. warfarin and heparin. Warfarin displaces vitamin K, which acts as a coenzyme in prothrombin synthesis. Heparin binds to antithrombin III and enhances the inactivation of thrombin and prevents fibrin formation.

Immunosuppressives

These suppress the immune system and increase the risk of wound infection. Immunosuppressives inhibit DNA synthesis and by this mechanism interfere with cell proliferation and differentiation, consequently they retard wound healing.

Penicillamine

This inhibits the metalloenzyme lysyl oxidase by copper depletion and prevents cross-linking of collagen fibrils. This results in reduced collagen stability and wound strength (Nimni and Bavetta, 1965).

Wound dressings

The function of a 'modern' wound dressing is not merely to protect it from further physical trauma or prevent infection, but also to create the optimum environment within which the wound can heal rapidly and gain the best cosmetic and mechanical end result. These 'modern' dressings, which maintain a moist environment over the wound, first appeared on the market in the early 1960s and since that time the wealth of literature on the benefits of moist healing has been overwhelming. Yet there are still many clinicians who will not change a lifetime's habit of drying wounds out. It has been demonstrated both experimentally and clinically that wounds re-epithelialize more rapidly under moist conditions than under dry (Winter, 1962; Hinman, Maibach and Winter, 1963; Rovee, Kurowsky and Labun, 1972; Rovee, Linsky and Bothwell, 1975; Linsky, Rovee and Dow, 1981). Moist conditions also increase the rate of dermal repair (Dyson *et al.*, 1989). Angiogenesis, the development of new blood vessels has been shown to accelerate under moist conditions (Dyson *et al.*, 1992). Increased wound contraction has also been reported in wounds maintained in a moist environment (Rovee, Linsky and Bothwell, 1975; Linsky and Rovee, 1975).

Quantitative studies monitoring the relative changes in cell populations in moist and dry wound environments showed that the numbers of inflammatory cells (neutrophils and macrophages) decreased more rapidly under moist conditions (Dyson *et al.*, 1989). There was also a more rapid increase in the number of proliferative phase cells (fibroblasts and endothelial cells) in moist wounds. This work demonstrated a clear acceleration in the inflammatory and proliferative phases of repair. It should be added that when the wound has re-epithelialized completely, there is no further need to use an occlusive or semi-occlusive dressing as the new epidermis will act as the body's own natural semi-occlusive dressing. This will also ensure that maceration of the tissue does not happen at this time. The study showed clearly that one of the main reasons why a dry wound does not re-epithelialize as rapidly as a moist wound is because the hard eschar can act as a barrier preventing the epidermis finding a clear route across the wound surface (Figure 24.4). Another major problem with wounds covered with dry gauze dressings is that the dressing adheres to the wound surface and when removed takes a proportion of the new granulation tissue with it causing re-injury (Figure 24.5).

Dressings which can provide the correct environment are numerous and the choice depends very much upon the nature of the wound in question. A wound dressing protocol booklet compiled by Miller and Dyson (1994) provides a concise, logical guide to wound dressing choice. Figure 24.6 shows an example of how the booklet addresses one particular wound type. The style is that of an algorithm by which the final choice of dressing is based upon the clinician's answers to structured questions. Sloughy, granulating, infected, non-healing, sinus, malodorous wounds etc., are also dealt with in this booklet.

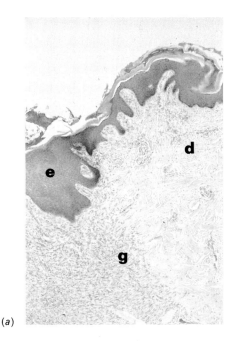

(*a*)

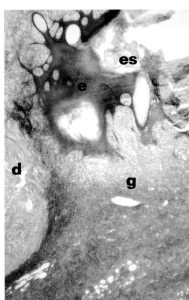

(*b*)

Figure 24.4 Photomicrographs of a section through the wound bed 7 days post surgery of: (*a*) a moist wound; (*b*) a dry wound. Note the irregularity of the advancing epidermis. e: epidermis; es: eschar; d: dermis of adjacent uninjured skin; g: granulation tissue; (magnification × 25)

Electrotherapy

Electrotherapy, the treatment of wounds by electrical means, can accelerate tissue repair. Electrical energy

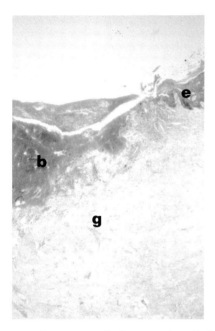

Figure 24.5 Photomicrograph of a section through the wound bed 14 days post surgery. Note the reinjury at the wound surface of this gauze dressed wound. b: blood; e: epidermis; g: granulation tissue; (magnification × 25)

is often transduced into some other form of energy, e.g. ultrasound or light. Both these forms of alternative therapy are now widely used to stimulate tissue repair and relieve pain, often for the same conditions. Ultrasound and light are very different forms of energy, one mechanical, the other electromagnetic, yet they both produce similar effects on tissues, accelerating the inflammatory phase of repair, so that the proliferative phase is entered more rapidly.

Ultrasound therapy

To say that ultrasound is a frequently used therapeutic modality in physiotherapy practice is a gross understatement. The results of a survey carried out in the UK in 1985 (ter Haar, Dyson and Oakley, 1985) showed that 20% of all physiotherapy treatments in NHS departments and 54% of all private treatments involved therapeutic ultrasound. It is obvious that if a modality is used so widely then it is vital that we understand fully its biological effects and mechanisms of action so that it can be used effectively and, more important, safely.

Physical effects of ultrasound

When ultrasound enters the body it exerts an effect on the cells and tissues by either, or a combination of, thermal or non-thermal mechanisms.

Thermal effects

When ultrasound travels through tissues a percentage of it is absorbed which leads to the generation of heat within that tissue. The amount of absorption depends upon the nature of the tissue, its degree of vascularization and the frequency of the ultrasound. Tissues with a high protein content absorb ultrasound more readily than those with a higher fat content. The higher the ultrasound frequency the greater the absorption. A biologically significant thermal effect can be achieved if the temperature of the tissue is raised to 40–45°C for at least 5 minutes. Controlled heating can produce desirable effects (Lehmann and DeLateur, 1982) which include pain relief, decrease in joint stiffness, increased blood flow, etc.

The advantage of using ultrasound to deliver this heating effect is that the therapist has control over the depth at which the heating develops. For example, by using high frequencies (e.g. 3 MHz) the heating is more superficial than when lower frequencies are used (e.g. 0.75 MHz). Structures which will be heated preferentially include periosteum, superficial cortical bone, joint menisci, fibrotic muscle, tendon sheaths and major nerve roots (Lehmann and Guy, 1972), and intermuscular interfaces (ter Haar and Hopewell, 1982). It is important that the clinician has knowledge of the structures which lie between the ultrasound source and the injured tissue, and also beyond it.

Once delivered, the heat is then dissipated by both thermal diffusion and local blood flow, which can present a problem when treating injuries where the blood supply has been restricted by either the nature of the injury or the relatively avascular nature of the tissue itself (e.g. tendon). Another complication can happen when the ultrasound beam hits bone or a metal prosthesis. Because of the great acoustic impedance difference between these structures and the surrounding soft tissues, up to 30% of the incident energy is reflected back through the soft tissue. This means that more energy is absorbed as heat during the beam's return journey and the temperature of the soft tissues increases, especially that immediately adjacent to the reflector.

Non-thermal effects

There are many situations where ultrasound produces bioeffects and yet a clinically significant increase in temperature cannot be detected. Evidence exists which suggests that non-thermal mechanisms play a primary role in producing a therapeutically significant effect: stimulation of tissue regeneration (Dyson *et al.*, 1968), soft tissue repair (Paul *et al.*, 1960; Dyson, Franks and Suckling, 1976), blood flow in chronically ischaemic tissues (Hogan, Burke and Franklin, 1982), protein synthesis (Webster *et al.*, 1978), bone repair (Dyson and Brookes, 1983).

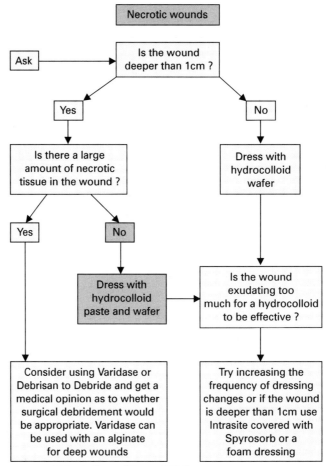

Figure 24.6 Wound dressing protocol (after Miller and Dyson, 1996)

The effect of ultrasound on the inflammatory phase of repair

As indicated previously the inflammatory phase is extremely dynamic. During this phase, numerous cell types enter and leave the wound site, e.g. platelets, mast cells, macrophages, neutrophils, etc. There is evidence to show that therapeutic ultrasound can interact with the above cells to influence their activity which can lead to the acceleration of repair.

Ultrasound has been shown to produce changes in platelet membrane permeability leading to the release of serotonin (Williams, 1974; Williams, Sykes and O'Brien, 1976). In addition to serotonin, platelets contain growth factors essential for successful repair (Ginsberg, 1981). If ultrasound can stimulate the release of serotonin it may also influence the release of these other factors (Hart, 1993).

Histamine is one of the major chemicals which modifies the wound environment. The mast cell is the major source of this factor and normally releases

it by a process known as degranulation, in which the membrane of the cell, in response to increased levels of intracellular calcium (Yurt, 1981), ruptures releasing histamine and other products into the wound site. It has been shown that a single treatment of therapeutic ultrasound if given soon after injury, i.e. during the early inflammatory phase, can stimulate mast cells to degranulate releasing histamine into the surrounding tissues (Fyfe and Chahl, 1982; Hashish, 1986). It is possible that ultrasound stimulates the mast cell to degranulate by increasing its permeability to calcium. Increased calcium ion permeability has been demonstrated by a number of researchers and it is known that calcium ions can act as intracellular messengers. When the distribution and concentration of calcium ions changes in response to environmental modifications of the plasma membrane they act as an intracellular signal for the appropriate metabolic response. There is much evidence that ultrasound can produce membrane changes in a number of cell types. These range from gross destructive changes to more subtle reversible changes. Gross changes can be achieved if levels of ultrasound are high enough. Even when using therapeutic levels of ultrasound it is possible to achieve the necessary conditions for destruction of tissue if a standing wave is allowed to form due to bad clinical practice in failing to keep the applicator head moving. Dyson *et al.* (1974) demonstrated that if this phenomenon happened in the region of fine blood vessels that it was possible to damage the endothelial cells lining the luminal side of the vessels.

Reversible membrane permeability changes to calcium have been demonstrated using therapeutic levels of ultrasound (Mummery, 1978; Mortimer and Dyson, 1988; Dinno *et al.*, 1989). The fact that this effect can be suppressed by irradiation under pressure suggests that cavitation is the physical mechanism responsible. Changes in permeability to other ions such as potassium have also been demonstrated (Chapman, Macnally and Tucker, 1979). Work by Dinno *et al.* (1989) demonstrated, in a frog skin model, that ultrasound can modify the electrophysiological properties of the tissue. The work reported an ultrasound-induced reduction in the sodium-potassium ATPase pump activity. Such a decrease in pump activity, if it developed in neuronal plasma membranes, might inhibit the transduction of noxious stimuli and subsequent neural transmission, which may account, in part, for the pain relief which is often experienced following clinical exposure to therapeutic ultrasound. It should be noted, however, that the mechanism of pain relief is still not fully understood and much of it can be attributed to placebo effects.

As discussed above, the evidence is clear that therapeutic ultrasound can alter membrane permeability to various ions. The ability to affect calcium transport through cell membranes is of considerable clinical significance as calcium, in its role as intracellular or second messenger, can have a profound effect on cell activity, e.g. increased synthesis and secretion of wound factors by cells involved in the healing process. This has been shown to take place in the macrophage in response to therapeutic levels of ultrasound (Young and Dyson, 1990a) which, as discussed earlier, is one of the key cells in the wound healing system, being a source of numerous growth factors. This *in vitro* study demonstrated that the ultrasound-induced change in growth factor secretion is frequency dependent. Ultrasound at an intensity of 0.5 W/cm^2 spatial and temporal average (SATA) and a frequency of 0.75 MHz appeared to be most effective in encouraging the immediate release of factors already present in the cell cytoplasm. A higher frequency (3.0 MHz) appeared to be most effective in stimulating the production of new factors, which were then released some time later by the cells' normal secretory processes. There appeared to be a delayed effect when treating with the higher frequency and the resulting liberated factors, when

tested, were more potent in their stimulating effect on the fibroblast population growth in comparison to those liberated using 0.75 MHz. One possible reason why these two frequencies induce different effects is the physical mechanisms involved. At the higher frequency, heating is the most dominant mechanism, whereas with the lower frequency non-thermal mechanisms predominate. Therefore, the differing proportions of non-thermal to thermal mechanisms present in each of the two treatments may explain the difference seen in the resulting biological effects. Hart (1993) also found that following the *in vitro* exposure of macrophages to ultrasound a growth factor was released into the surrounding medium which was mitogenic for fibroblasts.

It was often thought that ultrasound was an anti-inflammatory agent (Reid, 1981; Snow and Johnson, 1988). When viewed from a clinical standpoint, i.e. rapid resolution of oedema (El Hag *et al.*, 1985), this conclusion is understandable. However, research has shown that ultrasound is not anti-inflammatory in its action (Goddard *et al.*, 1983), rather it encourages oedema formation to develop more rapidly (Hustler, Zarod and Williams, 1978; Fyfe and Chahl, 1985) but then subside more rapidly than in control sham-irradiated groups, so accelerating the whole event, driving the wound more rapidly into the proliferative phase of repair.

Further confirmation of this has been shown experimentally in acute surgical wounds (Young and Dyson, 1990b). In this study, full-thickness excised skin lesions in rats were exposed to therapeutic ultrasound (0.1 W/cm^2 SATA, 0.75 MHz or 3.0 MHz) daily for 7 days (5 minutes per day per wound). By 5 days after injury the ultrasound-treated groups had significantly less inflammatory cells in the wound bed and more extensive granulation tissue than the sham-irradiated controls. Also, the alignment of fibroblasts, parallel to the wound surface, in the wound beds of the ultrasound-treated groups was indicative of a more advanced healing than the random alignment of fibroblasts seen in the sham-irradiated control wounds. The results obtained suggested that there had been an acceleration of wound healing through the inflammatory phase of repair in response to ultrasound therapy. It was also noted that there were no abnormalities such as hypertrophy of the wound tissue seen in response to ultrasound therapy. Therefore, ultrasound therapy appears to accelerate the process without the risk of interfering with the control mechanisms which limit the development of granulation tissue.

The effect of ultrasound on the proliferative phase of repair

The main events taking place during this phase of repair include cell infiltration into the wound bed, angiogenesis, matrix deposition, wound contraction and re-epithelialization. Cells such as fibroblasts and endothelial cells are recruited to the wound site by a combination of migration and proliferation. Mummery (1978) showed *in vitro* that fibroblast motility could be increased when they were exposed to therapeutic levels of ultrasound. With regard to cell proliferation, there is little evidence in the literature to suggest that ultrasound has a direct stimulatory effect on fibroblast proliferation. Most of the *in vitro* studies report either no effect or even an inhibitory effect on cell proliferation when exposed to therapeutic levels of ultrasound (Loch, Fisher and Kuwert, 1971; Kaufman *et al.*, 1977). However, the literature shows that when tissues are exposed to ultrasound *in vivo* a marked increase in wound bed cell number can be demonstrated (Dyson *et al.*, 1970; Young and Dyson, 1990b). This anomaly may be explained if we examine the cellular interactions which take place during healing. It was illustrated earlier that during wound repair much of the stimulus which controls the cellular events is derived from the macrophage. Therefore, it is highly likely that any increase in, for example fibroblast proliferation may be due, in part, to an indirect effect of ultrasound via the macrophage. Work by Young and Dyson (1990a) showed that if macrophages are exposed to therapeutic levels of ultrasound, *in vitro*, then removed and the culture medium placed on fibroblast cultures that there is a large stimulatory effect on the proliferation of the fibroblasts. It appears that the macrophage is sensitive to ultrasound and in response to therapeutic levels (0.5 W/cm^2 spatial average pulse average (SAPA)) releases a factor or factors which stimulate fibroblasts to proliferate.

Ultrasound can also effect the rate of angiogenesis. Hogan, Burke and Franklin (1982) showed that capillaries develop more rapidly when chronically ischaemic muscle was exposed to ultrasound. Other work has shown that the exposure of skin lesions to ultrasound can stimulate the growth of blood capillaries into the wound site as shown in Figure 24.7 (Hossein-pour, 1988; Young and Dyson, 1990c).

When fibroblasts are exposed to ultrasound *in vitro* a marked stimulation in collagen secretion can be detected (Harvey *et al.*, 1975). The degree of response was intensity dependent. When the fibroblasts were exposed to continuous ultrasound (0.5 W/cm^2 SA) a 20% increase in collagen secretion was recorded, however, when the ultrasound was pulsed (0.5 W/cm^2 SATA) a 30% increase was recorded. Webster *et al.* (1978) also demonstrated an increase in protein synthesis when fibroblasts were exposed to ultrasound.

Wound contraction can be accelerated by ultrasound. Work by Dyson and Smalley (1983) showed that pulsed ultrasound (3 MHz, 0.5 W/cm^2 SATA) could stimulate the contraction of cryosurgical lesions. More recently, Hart (1993) showed that exposure of full-thickness excised skin lesions to low levels of pulsed ultrasound stimulated contraction leading

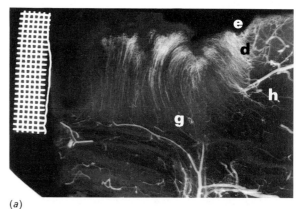

(*a*)

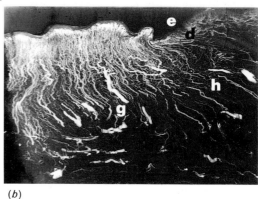

(*b*)

Figure 24.7 Microfocal radiographs showing the developing blood supply to the wound bed 7 days post surgery in: (*a*) a control sham-irradiated wound; (*b*) an ultrasound-treated wound. e: epidermis of adjacent uninjured skin; d: dermis of adjacent uninjured skin; g: granulation tissue containing the developing blood vessels; h: hypodermis (magnification × 2)

to a significantly smaller scar. Interestingly he found that the degree of contraction induced using an intensity of 0.5 W/cm^2 (SATA) could also be achieved using a much lower intensity of 0.1 W/cm^2 (SATA). This is a significant finding which implies that clinicians can reduce their ultrasound treatment intensities by a significant degree and still achieve the desired results, via non-thermal effects. It is vital that when treating tissues which have a compromised vasculature and hence no effective mechanism of dispersing excess heat that the lowest effective ultrasound intensity is used.

In humans, wound closure is achieved by granulation tissue formation and re-epithelialization, whereas in many other mammals (e.g. rats and mice), where the skin is more loosely connected to the underlying tissues, wound closure is due mainly to contraction. Dyson, Franks and Suckling (1976) found that ultrasonic therapy (3 MHz, pulsed, 0.2 W/cm² SATA), significantly accelerated the reduction in varicose ulcer area. Similar findings were reported by Roche and West (1984).

Callam *et al.* (1987) studied the effect of weekly ultrasound therapy (1 MHz, pulsed, 0.5 W/cm² SAPA) on the healing of chronic leg ulcers. They found that there was a 20% increase in the healing rate of the ultrasound-treated ulcers.

Accelerated wound closure has also been recorded in other chronic wounds such as pressure sores (Paul *et al.*, 1960; McDiarmid *et al.*, 1985). McDiarmid *et al.* also reported an interesting finding that microbially-infected sores were more responsive to ultrasound therapy than uninfected sores. It is likely that the low grade infection had in some way primed or upregulated the healing system by, for example, recruiting more macrophages to the area, which in turn would produce an amplified signal to herald an early start to the other phases of repair.

The effect of ultrasound on the remodelling phase of repair

During remodelling the wound becomes relatively acellular and avascular, collagen content increases, and the tensile strength of the wound increases. The remodelling phase can last from months to years depending upon the tissue involved and the nature of the injury. The mechanical properties of the scar are related to both the amount of collagen present and also the arrangement or alignment of the collagen fibres within the wound bed.

The effect of ultrasound on the properties of the scar depends very much upon the time at which the therapy was first instigated. By far the most effective regimens are those which are started soon after injury, i.e. during the inflammatory phase of repair. Webster (1980) found that when wounds were treated three times per week for 2 weeks after injury (0.1 W/cm² SATA) the resulting tensile strength and elasticity of the scar were significantly higher than those of the control group. Other groups have also demonstrated an increase in tensile strength and collagen content in incised lesions whose treatment was commenced during the inflammatory phase (Byl *et al.*, 1992). They also compared two different ultrasound intensities and found that the lower intensity (1 MHz, pulsed, 0.5 W/cm² SATA) was the most effective. Treatment with ultrasound during the inflammatory phase of repair not only increases the amount of collagen deposited in the wound but also encourages the deposition of that collagen in a pattern whose three-dimensional architecture resembled that of uninjured skin more than the untreated controls (Dyson, 1981). Jackson, Schwane and Starcher (1991) showed that the mechanical properties of injured tendon can be improved with ultrasound if treatment starts early enough, however, the levels

used were relatively high at 1.5 W/cm². Enwemaka, Rodriguez and Mendosa (1990) reported that increased tensile strength and elasticity can be achieved in injured tendons using much lower intensities (0.5 W/cm² SA).

Ultrasound application

Acute wounds

The weight of the evidence with regards to the effectiveness of ultrasound therapy indicates that the earlier it is used after injury, the more effective it is, i.e. during the early inflammatory phase of repair (Oakley, 1978; Patrick, 1978). During the inflammatory phase of repair macrophages and mast cells occupy the wound site and it has been shown that these cells are responsive to therapeutic ultrasound (Fyfe and Chahl, 1985; Young and Dyson, 1990a). This action of therapeutic ultrasound accelerates the inflammatory phase of repair resulting in a more rapid entry into the proliferative phase (Dyson, 1990). During the inflammatory phase of repair, treatments should be once a day for approximately a week, or until swelling and pain have subsided. Treatments through the subsequent proliferative phase of repair can then be reduced to three times per week (McDiarmid and Burns, 1987). This should be maintained until the condition is resolved.

Chronic wounds

The literature with regard to the treatment of chronic wounds is sparse and also mixed in respect to the efficacy of ultrasound treatments and also about the treatment intervals. In the case of venous leg ulcers the positive reviews state a treatment regimen of once per week (Callam *et al.*, 1987), and three times per week (Dyson, Franks and Suckling, 1976).

It is advisable to maintain treatment of chronic wounds beyond the inflammatory phase of repair into the proliferative phase as it has been shown that ultrasound can effect many of the processes that take place during that time, e.g. angiogenesis (Young and Dyson, 1990c), fibroblast activity (Webster, 1980; Dyson, 1987), and wound contraction (Hart, 1993). These effects have been achieved using low intensity ultrasound (maximum of 0.5 W/cm² SAPA) which utilizes primarily non-thermal mechanisms.

The duration of treatment depends upon the area of the injury. Typically the area should be divided into zones which are approximately 1.5 times the area of the ultrasound treatment head, and then treated for 1 or 2 minutes per zone (Oakley, 1978). Subsequent treatment times should then be increased by 30 seconds per zone up to a maximum of 3 minutes (Oakley, 1978). Hoogland (1986) recommended a total maximal treatment time of 15 minutes and that at least 1 minute should be spent in treating an area of 1 cm².

Potential hazards

Ultrasound can be an effective therapy or a potential hazard depending upon how it is applied. There exists a number of extensive lists of contraindications and precautions (Reid, 1981; Hoogland, 1986; Dyson, 1988). These include irradiation of:

- Uterus during pregnancy
- Gonads
- Malignancies and precancerous lesions
- Tissues previously treated by deep X-ray or other radiation
- Vascular abnormalities, e.g. deep vein thrombosis, emboli, severe atherosclerosis
- Acute infections
- Cardiac area in advanced heart disease
- Eye
- Stellate ganglion
- Haemophiliacs not covered by factor replacement
- Areas over subcutaneous bony prominences
- Epiphyseal plates
- Spinal cord after laminectomy
- Subcutaneous major nerves
- Cranium
- Anaesthetic areas

Many of these contraindications have been included in the list even though they are not based on any hard scientific evidence. However, even if there is a remote chance that damage may be sustained then ultrasound should not be used.

Laser therapy

There has been much interest in the biological effects of low level laser radiation since the pioneering work of Mester in the early 1970s (Mester, Mester and Mester, 1985). However, despite the rapid expansion in the number of investigations into this modality, doubts still exist with regards to its efficacy. There are a number of reasons for this (Basford, 1986; King, 1989). The main reasons appear to be the anecdotal nature of the many reports on the clinical use of laser where trials have been performed without adequate control groups and also with low numbers of patients. The reports often do not give adequate information with regard to the physical parameters of the laser used which precludes attempts by other research groups to repeat the work.

One characteristic of laser radiation is that it is coherent; however, it has been shown that significant biological effects can be achieved by exposure to non-coherent light (Karu, 1988; Young *et al.*, 1988). Even with a question mark hanging over the efficacy of light therapy, laser and light therapy machines can now be found in many physiotherapy departments and are being used routinely for pain relief and to accelerate tissue repair. The following section examines some of the clinical and laboratory evidence showing areas where light therapy may be effective.

Work on the effect of light on tissue repair was initiated by Mester (Mester, Mester and Mester, 1985) who showed that exposure of partial-thickness skin wounds to a ruby laser increased the rate of epithelial growth. More recently Dyson and Young (1986) showed that full-thickness excised lesions could be stimulated to repair more rapidly when exposed to a combined pulsed infrared and continuous helium neon laser. Laser irradiated wounds were shown to contract more than control wounds when the infrared was delivered at a frequency of 700 Hz. However, when the infrared was pulsed at 1200 Hz, wound contraction was inhibited. Differential cell counts carried out on the wound tissue showed that there were significantly more fibroblasts in the wounds treated with 700 Hz than in the other wounds, and also that their orientation was very specific, i.e. aligned parallel to each other at right-angles to the direction of blood vessel growth (Figure 24.8). This orientation is very indicative of a wound undergoing active contraction. The lack of orientation of the fibroblasts in the 1200 Hz treated wounds suggests that they were not yet fully cooperating with each other in inducing contraction, and this was probably why less contraction was seen in these wounds.

As with ultrasound, it appears that light therapy is particularly effective when used during the inflammatory phase of repair, therefore it is possible that its mode of action on the wound healing process is similar, i.e. the light interacts with the macrophages, encouraging them to release wound mediators which in turn stimulate the onset of the later stages of repair. Work was carried out to test this hypothesis (Young *et al.*, 1988). U937 cells (Sundstrom and Nilsson, 1976) were either sham-irradiated (control group) or exposed *in vitro* to one of a range of wavelengths of light. Some of the light sources were coherent, others were non-coherent. The average power output of all the sources was 15 mW, the energy density 2.4 J/cm^2 and the wavelengths were 660, 820, 870 and 880 nm. After irradiation the macrophages were placed in an incubator for 12 h to allow the synthesis and secretion of wound mediators into the surrounding medium. The medium was then removed and placed on fibroblast cultures and their proliferation assessed over 132 h. It was found that the following wavelengths, 660, 820 and 870 nm, encouraged the release of wound mediators which stimulated fibroblast proliferation, whereas 880 nm had the opposite effect. It was also noticed, that so far as the response was concerned, the light did not need to be coherent.

El Sayed and Dyson (1990) showed that another important inflammatory cell, the mast cell, can also be stimulated by light therapy. Wavelengths which appeared to be the most effective in causing an in-

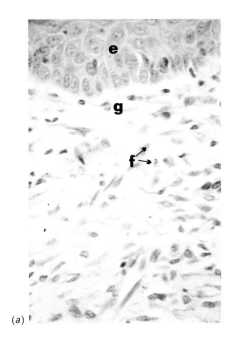

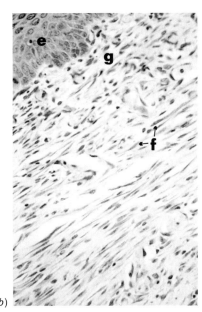

Figure 24.8 Photomicrographs of a section through the wound bed of: (*a*) a control sham-irradiated wound; (*b*) a laser-irradiated wound. Note the parallel alignment of fibroblasts. e: epidermis; g: granulation tissue; f: fibroblast; (magnification × 250)

crease in mast cell number and degranulation were 660, 820, 940 and 950 nm.

Many investigators have tried to produce hypotheses which explain how light can stimulate cells. First, light has to be absorbed to cause an effect. It

has been proposed (Karu, 1988) that the photoabsorbers in mammalian cells are the respiratory pigments or cytochromes which are found in the mitochondria of all cells. The hypothesis is that visible light is absorbed by these photoacceptors (infrared being absorbed at the cell membrane level) causing short-term respiratory chain activation and oxidation of the electron acceptor NAD (nicotinamide adenine dinucleotide). This leads to changes in the redox status of both mitochondria and cytoplasm. As a result, there is an increase in the ATP pool and cytoplasmic H^+ concentration. The change in cytoplasmic pH can lead to cell permeability changes to a variety of ions such as calcium which in turn can modify cell activity. Work has shown that light therapy can modify calcium uptake in macrophages (Young, Dyson and Bolton, 1990). The effect was shown to be wavelength, energy density and frequency dependent.

In summary, evidence suggests that both ultrasound and light may be useful therapeutic modalities. Although, physically, they are very different in their nature, the effects that they produce in injured tissues are very similar. They can both interact with cells such as macrophages and mast cells, stimulating the production of wound mediators. However, there is a need for more carefully controlled clinical trials (in particular in the field of light therapy) to assess the clinical value of these forms of electrotherapy.

Wound assessment

It is vital to have objective and sensitive techniques by which wound healing can be assessed. Chronic wounds present additional problems with regard to wound assessment. Because these wounds heal so slowly it is often difficult to obtain an early indication if they are healing, remaining static or deteriorating. Often much time is wasted using ineffective therapeutic modalities.

There are numerous methods for evaluating wound repair, which can be divided into two main groups: invasive and non-invasive techniques.

Invasive methods

These techniques provide quantitative information about the wound and its stage in healing. These methods include:

Biopsy

Histological evaluation of excised tissue to identify and measure the number of cell types present during the healing process (Young, 1988).

Biochemical analysis

Biochemical analysis of wound tissue biopsies and fluid to measure the various components involved in wound repair, e.g. collagen synthesis and deposition, mRNA synthesis, extracellular factors, etc. (Saperia, Glassberg and Lyons, 1986).

Tensile strength estimation

Tensile strength may be analysed by its tissue breaking point or its wound rupture stress (Charles *et al.*, 1992).

Angiography

Angiogenesis may be monitored by angiography (Young and Dyson, 1990c).

Although these methods are able to yield quantitative data regarding wound healing, they are invasive involving biopsy which results in the destruction of the tissue under investigation, thereby delaying the wound healing process. In addition, many patients find this procedure, at best, uncomfortable.

Non-invasive methods

These techniques tend to be less quantitative than the invasive methods, however, they are more acceptable to patients. Non-invasive methods include:

Transparency tracings

A double layer of sterile acetate or polythene film is placed over the wound, and the outline is traced using a permanent marker pen. By using a double layer film, the side which has been in contact with the wound, can be discarded preventing contact infection. The surface area of the wound can then be measured by either placing the acetate tracing onto graph paper and counting the squares, or evaluated using a computer, which scans and digitizes the traced outline and calculates the surface area automatically. The disadvantages of using the tracing method is that it is very hard to define the edges of the wound and so operator error can be high.

Photographic recording

Wounds can be photographed instead of traced. The operator must place a ruler or some other object of known size next to the wound to provide a scale against which measurements can be made. The wound surface area can then be calculated from photographs using computerized image analysis. Although accuracy is increased using photographic rather than tracing methods, errors can still arise for example due to varying ambient light conditions leading to variations in exposure from film to film.

Also, distortions of the vertical and horizontal axes arise if the wound is on a curved surface.

Depth gauges

A device known as the Kundin gauge (Kundin, 1989), has been developed which is able to measure the length, width and depth of a wound, and from which area and volume are calculated. This method is more accurate when used to measure circular and elliptically shaped wounds. When used for irregular wounds in which there are tracking and underlying cavities, the method often underestimates area and volume; this is the main disadvantage of this method. However, the method is easy to use, disposable, objective and inexpensive.

Volume

The volume of wounds can be measured by making moulds of the wound, using a variety of substances, including hydrocolloid gel, silicone rubber, silastic foam, and alginates (Covington *et al.*, 1989). The mould in then placed in water, and the displacement is the volume of the wound. The use of this method is restricted; it cannot be used over shallow wounds, or those which are circumferential around a limb, or for wounds with undermining and sinus formation. The orifice of the wound has to be sufficiently large to remove the material.

Another method to measure volume, is the use of saline (Berg *et al.*, 1990). The wound is covered by a film, and saline is injected into it. This is a simple and reproducible technique, but is not satisfactory for superficial sores.

Stereoscopic photography

This is used to overcome projection errors from the curved skin surface to a flat screen. This method uses two cameras so that a photograph is produced from which depth measurements can be recorded (Bulstrode, Goode and Scott, 1986). The area and volume of the wound can be calculated by a computer. The method is accurate, reproducible and non-invasive. Measurements of irregular defects in the wound, in three dimensions, can be made. However, the amount of specialized equipment and time involved restricts this method in its application in clinical practice.

Thermal imaging

This method detects infrared radiation emitted from the skin. The emissivity of the wound is variable and depends upon whether it has been exposed without a dressing, and if so for how long, and whether it is infected. It can be used to record temperature at the edges of a wound, to monitor blood perfusion, and it could also be useful for monitoring the effect of antibiotic therapy in an infected wound.

Video image analysis

Video cameras can be used to record lesions from different angles to optimize information, and to reduce the measurement problems caused by skin curvature (Smith, Bhat and Bulgrin, 1992). This method uses a video camera with a macro-lens, linked to an image processing computer, which produces high precision measurements of area, colour density and volume.

High frequency diagnostic ultrasound

One major drawback with all non-invasive techniques is that they only produce data which describe the outer surface of the wound and surrounding uninjured skin. None of the techniques gives any indication as to the quality of the underlying reparative tissue. However, there now exists a non-invasive method which allows the clinician to look deep into the wound bed with a high degree of resolution in order to assess the quality of the reparative tissue (Whiston, Melhuish and Harding, 1993; Whiston *et al.*, 1993; Young *et al.*, 1993; Karim *et al.*, 1994). This technique involves the use of high frequency ultrasound (Quality Medical Imaging Ltd, UMDS, Guy's Hospital, London).

This is a simple procedure which is able to produce a high resolution image of the dermis. The scan can be carried out through certain wound dressings, e.g. Geliperm, when a coupling gel is applied onto it, thereby avoiding risks of infection and also offering protection to the delicate wound surface during the scanning procedure. An axial resolution of 65 μm and a lateral resolution of approximately 200 μm can be obtained. Using image analysis, it is possible to monitor small changes in a wound, even before they become clinically evident, and recognize whether the wound is deteriorating or improving. This early detection can lead to large savings in treatment times. Wound depth can be calculated with this technique, e.g. in burn injuries. It is a rapid, sensitive and repeatable way of quantifying wound healing. The scanner can also look at other tissues below the skin providing they are within 2 cm of the skin surface, e.g. tendons (Figure 24.9). This is useful as clinicians currently do not have any precise non-invasive method for examining tendons after surgery. Using this technique, the clinician is able to monitor the healing tendon and know exactly when the time is right to begin light exercise.

Summary

Tissue repair consists of a number of overlapping phases, of which the inflammatory phase is particularly important, in that it determines the rate of onset of the proliferative phase, and hence the rate of the whole process. It is apparent from clinical observations that the rate and quality of the repair process can vary tremendously with excessive scarring at one extreme and delayed healing at the other. The possible causes of delayed healing are numerous and may include lack of reparative cells, inappropriate local conditions, poor nutritional status, underlying chronic disease, etc. Ideally, attempts to accelerate the healing process should address each of these individually. Finally, to optimize our therapies we should employ accurate, sensitive and preferably non-invasive wound assessment methods.

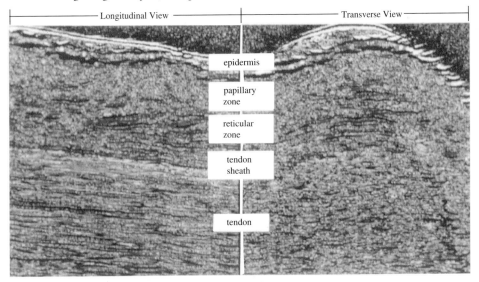

Figure 24.9 High frequency diagnostic ultrasound images showing the skin and underlying achilles tendon in traditional grey scale

References

ALLMAN, R. M. (1989) Epidemiology of pressure sores in different populations. *Decubitus*, **2**, 30–33

ALVAREZ, O. M. and GILBREATH, R. L. (1982) Thiamine influence on collagen during the granulation of skin wounds. *Journal of Surgical Research*, **32**, 24–31

BAILEY, A. J., BAZIN, S., SIMS, T. J., LELEUS M., NICHOLETIS, C. and DELAUNAY, A. (1975) Characterisation of the collagen of human hypertrophic and normal scars. *Aeta Biochemica et Biophysica Acta*, **405**, 412–421

BASFORD, J. K. (1986) Low-energy treatment of pain and wounds: hype, hope or hokum? *Mayo Clinic Proceedings*, **61**, 671–675

BEISEL, W. R., EDELMAN, R., NAUSS, K. and SUSKIND, R. M. (1981) Single-nutrient effects on immunologic function. *Journal of the American Medical Association*, **245**, 53–58

BERG, W., TRANEROTH, C., GUNNARSSON, A. and LOSSING, C. (1990) A method for measuring pressure sores. *Lancet*, i, 1445–1446

BETTGER, W. J. and O'DELL, B. L. (1981) A critical physiological role of zinc in the structure and function of biomembranes. *Life Science*, **28**, 1425–1438

BUCKNALL, T. E. (1980) The effect of local infection on wound healing: an experimental study. *British Journal of Surgery*, **67**, 851–855

BULSTRODE, C. J. K., GOODE, J. W. and SCOTT, P. J. (1986) Stereophotogrammetry for measuring rates of cutaneous healing: a conventional technique. *Clinical Science*, **71**, 437–443

BYL, N. N., MCKENZIE, A. L., WEST, J. M., WHITNEY, J. D., HUNT, T. K. and SCHEUENSTUHL, H. A. (1992) Low-dose ultrasound effects on wound healing: a controlled study with Yucatan pigs. *Archives of Physical and Medical Rehabilitation*, **73**, 656–664

CACKETT, P., YOUNG, S. R. and DYSON, M. (1995) The effects of nonsteroidal anti-inflammatory drugs on wound healing. *BSc Thesis*, University of London

CALLAM, M. J., HARPER, D. R., DALE, J. J., RUCKLEY, C. V. and PRESCOTT, R. J. (1987) A controlled trial of weekly ultrasound therapy in chronic leg ulceration. *Lancet*, ii, 204–206

CHANDRA, R. K. (1984) Excessive intake of zinc impairs immune response. *Journal of the American Medical Association*, **252**, 1443–1446

CHAPMAN, I. V., MACNALLY, N. A. and TUCKER, S. (1979) Ultrasound induced changes in the rates of influx and efflux of potassium ions in rat thymocytes *in vitro*. *British Journal of Radiology*, **47**, 411–415

CHARLES, D., WILLIAMS, K. III, PERRY, L. C., FISHER, J. and REES, R. S. (1992) An improved method of *in vivo* wound disruption and measurement. *Journal of Surgical Research*, **52**, 214–218

CLARK, R. A. F. (1990) Cutaneous wound repair. In: *Biochemistry and Physiology of the Skin*, edited by L. E. Goldsmith. Oxford: Oxford University Press. pp. 576–601

COLLIER, M. (1990) A sore point. *Community Outlook*, October, 29–30

COVINGTON, J. S., GRIFFIN, J. W., MENDIUS, R. K., TOOMS, R. E. and CLIFFT, J. K. (1989) Measurement of pressure ulcer volume using dental impression materials. *Physical Therapy*, **69**, 68–72

DAVID, J. A. (1983) *An Investigation of the Current Methods used in Nursing for the Care of Patients with Pressure Sores.* Guildford: Nursing Practice Research Unit University of Surrey

DEPARTMENT OF HEALTH (1989) *Working for Patients*. Medical Audit Working Paper 6. London: HMSO

DINNO M. A., DYSON, M., YOUNG, S. R., MORTIMER, A. J., HART, J. and CRUM, L. A. (1989) The significance of membrane changes in the safe and effective use of therapeutic and diagnostic ultrasound. *Physics in Medicine and Biology*, **34**, 1543–1552

DYSON, M. (1981) The effect of ultrasound on the rate of wound healing and the quality of scar tissue. In: *Proceedings of the International Symposium on Therapeutic Ultrasound*, Manitoba, 1981, edited by A. J. Mortimer and N. Lee. Winnipeg: Canadian Physiotherapy Association. pp. 110–123

DYSON, M. (1987) Mechanisms involved in therapeutic ultrasound. *Physiotherapy*, **73**, 116–120

DYSON, M. (1988) The use of ultrasound in sports physiotherapy. In: *International Perspectives in Physical Therapy, Sports Injuries*, edited by V. Grisogono. Edinburgh: Churchill Livingstone. pp. 213–232

DYSON, M. (1990) Role of ultrasound in wound healing. In: *Wound Healing: Alternatives in Management*, edited by L. C. Kloth, J. M. McCulloch and J. A. Feedar. Philadelphia: F. A. Davis. pp. 259–285

DYSON, M. and BROOKES, M. (1983) Stimulation of bone repair by ultrasound. In: *Ultrasound 82, Proceedings 3rd Meeting World Federation of Ultrasound in Medicine and Biology*, edited by R. A. Lerski and P. Morley. Oxford: Pergamon Press. pp. 61–66

DYSON, M. and SMALLEY, D. S. (1983) Effects of ultrasound on wound contraction. In: *Ultrasound Interactions in Biology and Medicine*, edited by R. Miller, E. Rosenfeld and U. Cobet. New York: Plenum Publishing Corporation. pp. 151–158

DYSON, M. and YOUNG, S. R. (1986) Effect of laser therapy on wound contraction and cellularity in mice. *Lasers in Medical Science*, **1**, 125–130

DYSON, M., FRANKS, C. and SUCKLING, J. (1976) Stimulation of healing varicose ulcers by ultrasound. *Ultrasonics*, **14**, 232–236

DYSON, M., POND, J. B., JOSEPH, J. and WARWICK, R. (1968) Stimulation of tissue repair by pulsed wave ultrasound. *IEEE Transactions on Sonics and Ultrasonics*, SU-17, 133–140

DYSON, M., POND, J. B., JOSEPH, J. and WARWICK, R. (1970) The stimulation of tissue regeneration by means of ultrasound. *Clinical Science*, **35**, 273–285

DYSON M., POND J., WOODWARD, J. and BROADBENT, J. (1974) The production of blood cell stasis and endothelial cell damage in the blood vessels of chick embryos treated with ultrasound in a stationary wave field. *Ultrasound in Medicine and Biology*, **1**, 133–148

DYSON, M., YOUNG, S.R., PENDLE, L., WEBSTER, D.F. and LANG, S. (1989) Comparison of the effects of moist and dry conditions on dermal repair. *Journal of Investigative Dermatology*, **91**, 434–439

DYSON, M., YOUNG, S.R., HART, J., LYNCH, J.A. and LANG, S. (1992) Comparison of the effects of moist and dry conditions on the process of angiogenesis during dermal repair. *Journal of Investigative Dermatology*, **99**, 729–733

EL HAG, M., COGHLAN, K., CHRISTMAS, P., HARVEY, W. and HARRIS, M. (1985) The anti-inflammatory effects of dexamethasone and therapeutic ultrasound in oral surgery. *British Journal of Oral and Maxillofacial Surgery*, **23**, 17–23

EL SAYED, S.O. and DYSON, M. (1990) Comparison of the effect of multiwavelength light produced by a cluster of semiconductor diodes and of each individual diode on mast cell number and degranulation in intact and injured skin. *Lasers in Surgery and Medicine*, **10**, 559–568

ENWEMAKA, C. S., RODRIGUEZ, O. and MENDOSA, S. (1990) The biomechanical effects of low-intensity ultrasound on healing tendons. *Ultrasound in Medicine and Biology*, **16**, 801–807

FYFE, M. C. and CHAHL, L. A. (1982) Mast cell degranulation: a possible mechanism of action of therapeutic ultrasound. *Ultrasound in Medicine and Biology*, **8** (suppl. 1), 62

FYFE, M. C. and CHAHL, L.A. (1985) The effect of single or repeated applications of 'therapeutic' ultrasound on plasma extravasation during silver nitrate induced inflammation of the rat hindpaw ankle joint *in vivo*. *Ultrasound in Medicine and Biology*, **11**, 273–283

GILCHREST, B. A. (1983) In vitro assessment of keratinocyte ageing. *Journal of Investigative Dermatology*, **81**, 184–189

GINSBERG, M. (1981) Role of platelets in inflammation and rheumatic disease. *Advances in Inflammation Research*, **2**, 53

GODDARD, D. H., REVELL, P. A., CASON, J., GALLAGHER, S. and CURREY, H. L. F. (1983) Ultrasound has no anti-inflammatory effect. *Annals of the Rheumatic Diseases*, **42**, 582–584

GOODE, F. G., BURNS, E. and WALKER, B. E. (1992) Vitamin C depletion and pressure sores in elderly patients with femoral neck fracture. *British Medical Journal*, **305**, 925–927

HART, J. (1993) The effect of therapeutic ultrasound on dermal repair with emphasis on fibroblast activity. *PhD Thesis*, University of London

HARVEY, W., DYSON M., POND, J. B. and GRAHAME, R. (1975) The stimulation of protein synthesis in human fibroblasts by therapeutic ultrasound. *Rheumatism and Rehabilitation*, **14**, 237

HASHISH, I. (1986) The effects of ultrasound therapy on post operative inflammation. *PhD Thesis*, University of London

HAYDOCK, D. A. and HILL, G. L. (1986) Impaired wound healing in patients with varying degrees of malnutrition. *Journal of Parenteral and Enteral Nutrition*, **10**, 550–554

HENG, M. C. (1983) Local hyperbaric oxygen administration for leg ulcers. *British Journal of Dermatology*, **109**, 232–234

HIBBS, P. (1988) *Pressure Area Care for the City and Hackney Health Authority*. London: St Bartholomew's Hospital

HIBBS, P. (1989) The economics of pressure sores. *Care of the Critically Ill*, **5**, 247–250

HINMAN, C. D., MAIBACH, H. I. and WINTER, G. D. (1963) Effect of air exposure and occlusion on experimental human skin wounds. *Nature*, **200**, 377–379

HMSO (1994) *Annual Abstract of Statistics no. 194*. London: HMSO

HOGAN, R. D. B., BURKE, K. M. and FRANKLIN, T. D. (1982) The effect of ultrasound on the microvascular hemodynamics in skeletal muscle: effects during ischemia. *Microvascular Research*, **23**, 370–379

HOHN, D. C. (1980) Host resistance to infections: established and emerging concepts. In: *Wound Healing and Wound Infection*, edited by T. K. Hunt. New York: Appleton-Century-Crofts. pp. 264–279

HOOGLAND, R. (1986) *Ultrasound Therapy*. Delft: Enraf Nonius

HOSSEINPOUR, A. R. (1988) The effects of ultrasound on angiogenesis and wound healing. *BSc Thesis*. University of London

HUSTLER, J. E., ZAROD, A. P. and WILLIAMS, A. R. (1978) Ultrasonic modification of experimental bruising in the guinea pig pinna. *Ultrasonics*, **16**, 223–228

JACKSON, B. A., SCHWANE, J. A. and STARCHER, B. C. (1991) Effect of ultrasound therapy on the repair of achilles tendon injuries in rats. *Medicine, Science. Sports, Exercise*, **23**, 171–176

KARIM, A., YOUNG, S. R., LYNCH, J. A. and DYSON, M. (1994) A novel method of assessing skin ultrasound scans. *Wounds*, **6**, 9–15

KARU, I. (1988) Molecular mechanisms of the therapeutic effect of low intensity laser irradiation. *Lasers in Life Sciences*, **2**, 53–74

KAUFMAN, G. E., MILLER, M. W., GRIFFITHS, T. D., CIARAVINO, V. and CARSTENSON, E. L. (1977) Lysis and viability of cultured mammalian cells exposed to 1 MHz ultrasound. *Ultrasound in Medicine and Biology*, **3**, 21–25

KING, P. R. (1989) Low level laser therapy. A review. *Lasers in Medical Science*, **4**, 141–150

KISCHER, C. W. and SHETLAR, M. R. (1974) Collagen and mucopolysaccharides in the hypertrophic scar. *Connective Tissue Research*, **2**, 205–213

KNIGHTON, D. R., HUNT, T. K., SCHEUENSTUHL, H. and HALLIDAY, B. J. (1983) Oxygen tension regulates the expression of angiogenesis factor by macrophages. *Science*, **221**, 1283–1285

KUNDIN, J. I. (1989) A new way to size up a wound. *American Journal of Nursing*, **89**, 206–207

LEHMANN, J. F. and GUY, A. W. (1972) Ultrasound therapy. In: *Interaction of Ultrasound and Biological Tissues*, edited by J. Reid and M. Sikov. DHEW Publication, (FDA) 73–8008, USA. Washington, DC: Government Printing Office. pp. 141–152

LEHMANN, J. F. and DELATEUR, B. J. (1982) Therapeutic heat. In: *Therapeutic Heat and Cold*, 3rd edn, edited by J. F. Lehmann. Baltimore: Williams and Wilkins, p. 404

LEIBOVICH, S. J. and ROSS, R. (1975) The role of the macrophage in wound repair. *American Journal of Pathology*, **78**, 71–92

LEVENSON, S. M., GEEVER, E. G., CROWLEY, L. V., OATES, J. F., BERARD, C. W. and ROSEN, H. (1965) The healing of rat skin wounds. *Annals of Surgery*, **161**, 293–308

LINSKY, C. B. and ROVEE, D. T. (1975) Influence of the local environment on the course of wound healing in the guinea pig. In: *Wound Healing*, edited by T. Gibson. Montreaux: Foundation for International Cooperation in Medical Science. p. 211

LINSKY, C. B., ROVEE, D. T. and DOW, T. (1981) Effects of dressing on wound inflammation and scar tissue. In: *The Surgical Wound*, edited by P. Dineen and G. Hildick-Smith. Philadelphia: Lea and Febiger. pp. 191–205

LIVESEY, B. and SIMPSON, G. (1989) The hard cost of soft sores. *Health Service Journal*, **99**, 231

LOCH, E. G., FISCHER, A. B. and KUWERT, E. (1971) Effect of diagnostic and therapeutic intensities of ultrasonics on normal and malignant human cells *in vitro*. *American Journal of Obstetrics and Gynecology*, **110**, 457–460

LOFSTROM, B. and ZEDERFELDT, B. (1957) Effects of induced hypothermia on wound healing: a study in the rabbit. *Acta Chirurgica Scandinavica*, **112**, 152

MCDIARMID, T. and BURNS, P. N. (1987) Clinical applications of therapeutic ultrasound. *Physiotherapy*, **73**, 155

MCDIARMID, T., BURNS, P. N., LEWITH, G. T. and MACHIN, D. (1985) Ultrasound and the treatment of pressure sores. *Physiotherapy*, **71**, 66–70

MESTER, E., MESTER, A. F. and MESTER, A. (1985) The biomedical effects of laser application. *Lasers in Surgery and Medicine*, **5**, 31–39

MILLER, M. and DYSON, M. (1996) *Principles of Wound Care*. London: Macmillan

MOORE, P. K. and HOULT, J. R. S. (1980) Anti-inflammatory steroids induce tissue prostaglandin synthetase activity and enhance prostaglandin breakdown. *Nature*, **288**, 269–270

MORISON, M. J. (1992) *A Colour Guide to the Nursing Management of Wounds*. London: Wolfe

MORTIMER, A. J. and DYSON, M. (1988) The effect of therapeutic ultrasound on calcium uptake in fibroblasts. *Ultrasound in Medicine and Biology*, **14**, 499–506

MUMMERY, C. L. (1978) The effect of ultrasound on fibroblasts *in vitro*. *PhD Thesis*, University of London

NELDER, K. (1983) The biochemistry and physiology of zinc metalloenzymes. In: *Biochemistry and Physiology of the Skin*, edited by L. Goldsmith. New York: Oxford University Press. pp. 1082–1101

NIMNI, M. E. and BAVETTA, L. A. (1965) Collagen defect induced by penicillamine. *Science*, **150**, 905–906

NOSSEL, H. L. (1983) Disorders of blood coagulation factors. In: *Harrisons Principles of Internal Medicine*, edited by R. G. Petersdorf, R. D. Adams and E. Braunwald. New York: McGraw-Hill Book Co. pp. 1900–1909

OAKLEY, E. M. (1978) Applications of continuous beam ultrasound at therapeutic levels. *Physiotherapy*, **64**, 169–172

PATRICK, M. K. (1978) Applications of therapeutic pulsed ultrasound. *Physiotherapy*, **64**, 103–104

PAUL, B. J., LAFRATTA, C. W., DAWSON, A. R., BAABE, E. and BULLOCK, F. (1960) Use of ultrasound in the treatment of pressure sores in patients with spinal cord injuries. *Archives of Physical and Medical Rehabilitation*, **41**, 438–440

PEACOCK, E. E. (ed.) (1984) Contraction. In: *Wound Repair*, 3rd edn. Philadelphia: W. B. Saunders and Company. pp. 39–55

POTTER, M. S. (1994) Incidence of pressure sores in nursing home patients. *Journal of Wound Care*, **3**, 37–42

REID, D. C. (1981) Possible contraindications and precautions associated with ultrasound therapy. In: *Proceedings of the International Symposium on Therapeutic Ultrasound*, edited by A. J. Mortimer and N. Lee. Winnipeg: Canadian Physiotherapy Association. p. 274

ROCHE, C. and WEST, J. (1984) A controlled trial investigating the effect of ultrasound on venous ulcers referred from general practitioners. *Physiotherapy*, **70**, 475–477

ROVEE, D. T., KUROWSKY, C. A. and LABUN, J. (1972) Effect of local wound environment on epidermal healing. In: *Epidermal Wound Healing*, edited by H. I. Maibach and D. T. Rovee. Chicago: Year Book Medical Publishers. pp. 159–181

ROVEE, D. T., LINSKY, C. B. and BOTHWELL, J. W. (1975) Experimental models for the evaluation of wound repair. In: *Animal Models in Dermatology*, edited by H. I. Maibach. New York: Churchill Livingstone Inc. pp.253–266

SALMELA, K. (1981) Comparison of the effects of methylprednisolone and hydrocortisone on granulation tissue. *Scandinavian Journal of Plastic and Reconstructive Surgery*, **15**, 87–91

SAPERIA, D., GLASSBERG, E. and LYONS, R. F. (1986) Demonstration of elevated type I and II pro-collagen mRNA levels in cutaneous wounds treated with helium-neon laser. *Bio-

chemical and Biophysical Research Communications*, **136**, 1123–1128

SCALES, J. T., LOWTHIAN, P. T., POOLE, A. G. and LUDMAN, W. R. (1982) 'Vaperm' patient support system: a new general purpose hospital mattress. *Lancet*, ii, 1150–1152

SHULMAN, G., PETRO, J. A. and HALLGEN, E. M. (1979) Quantitative bacteriology in wound care. *Annals of Surgery*, **45**, 374–377

SMITH, D. J., BHAT, S. and BULGRIN, J. P. (1992) Video image analysis of wound repair. *Wounds*, **4**, 6–15

SNOW, C. J. and JOHNSON, K. J. (1988) Effect of therapeutic ultrasound on acute inflammation. *Physiotherapy Canada*, **40**, 162–167

SUNDSTROM, C. and NILSSON, K. (1976) Establishment and characterisation of a human histiocytic lymphoma cell line. *International Journal of Cancer*, **17**, 565–577

TER HAAR, G. and HOPEWELL, J. W. (1982) Ultrasonic heating of mammalian tissue *in vivo*. *British Journal of Cancer*, **45**, (suppl. V), 65–67

TER HAAR, G., DYSON, M. and OAKLEY, E. M. (1985) The use of ultrasound by physiotherapists in Britain, 1985. *Ultrasound in Medicine and Biology*, **13**, 659–663

TIGHE J. R. and DAVIES, D. R. (1990) *Pathology*, 4th edn. London: Bailliere Tindall

WATSON, R. (1989) Pressure sores: a rational approach to treatment. *Nursing Standard*, **39**, 23–24

WEBSTER, D. F. (1980) The effect of ultrasound on wound healing. *PhD Thesis*, University of London

WEBSTER D. F., POND J. B., DYSON, M. and HARVEY, W. (1978) The role of cavitation in the *in vitro* stimulation of protein synthesis in human fibroblasts by ultrasound. *Ultrasound in Medicine and Biology*, **4**, 343–351

WEISS, S. J. (1989) Tissue destruction by neutrophils. *New England Journal of Medicine*, **320**, 365–376

WHISTON, R. J., MELHUISH, J. and HARDING, K. G. (1993) High resolution ultrasound imaging. *Wound Healing*, **5**, 116–121

WHISTON, R. J., YOUNG S. R., LYNCH J. A., HARDING K. G. and DYSON, M. (1993) Application of high frequency ultrasound to the objective assessment of healing wounds. In: *The 6th Annual Symposium on Advanced Wound Care*, edited by K. Harding. London: Macmillan Press. pp. 26–29

WILLIAMS, A. R. (1974) Release of serotonin from platelets by acoustic streaming. *Journal of the Acoustic Society of America*, **56**, 1640

WILLIAMS, A. R., SYKES, S. M. and O'BRIEN, W. D. (1976) Ultrasonic exposure modifies platelet morphology and function *in vitro*. *Ultrasound in Medicine and Biology*, **2**, 311–317

WINTER, G. D. (1962) Formation of the scab and the rate of epithelialisation of superficial wounds in the skin of the young domestic pig. *Nature*, **193**, 293–294

YOUNG, J. B. (1990) Aids to prevention of pressure sores. *British Medical Journal*, **300**, 1002–1004

YOUNG, S. R. (1988) The effect of therapeutic ultrasound on the biological mechanisms involved in dermal repair. *PhD Thesis*, University of London. pp. 169–174

YOUNG, S. R. and DYSON, M. (1990a) Macrophage responsiveness to therapeutic ultrasound. *Ultrasound in Medicine and Biology*, **16**, 809–816

YOUNG, S. R. and DYSON, M. (1990b) The effect of therapeutic ultrasound on the healing of full-thickness excised skin lesions. *Ultrasonics*, **28**, 175–180

YOUNG, S. R. and DYSON, M. (1990c) The effect of therapeutic ultrasound on angiogenesis. *Ultrasound in Medicine and Biology*, **16**, 261–269

YOUNG, S. R., DYSON, M. and BOLTON, P. A. (1990) Effect of light on calcium uptake in macrophages. *Laser Therapy*, **2**, 53–57

YOUNG, S. R., LYNCH, J. A., LEIPINS, P. J. and DYSON, M. (1993) Non-invasive method of wound assessment using high-frequency ultrasound imaging. In: *The 6th Annual Sympo-sium on Advanced Wound Care*, edited by K. Harding. London: Macmillan Press. pp. 29–31.

YOUNG, S. R., BOLTON, P. A., DYSON, M., HARVEY, W. and DIAMANTOPOULOS, C. (1988) Macrophage responsiveness to light therapy. *Lasers in Surgery and Medicine*, **9**, 497–505

YURT, R. W. (1981) Role of the mast cell in trauma. In: *The Surgical Wound*, edited by P. Dineen and G. Hildick-Smith. Philadelphia: Lea and Febiger. pp. 37–62

25

The principles of laser surgery

J. A. S. Carruth

It has been said that when the time in which we live is finally named, it will not be known as the atomic or space age but the laser age. At present, we are still only at the dawning of this age. The first laser was not produced until 1960, but since then a large number of lasers has been developed with a vast range of scientific, industrial and military uses. With these lasers astronomers have measured the distance to the moon to an accuracy of centimetres, huge numbers of telephone calls can be transmitted by flexible glass fibres and physicists have probed plasmas hotter than the sun.

These diverse uses of the laser (light amplification by stimulated emission of radiation) are all dependent on the basic characteristics of the laser beam: an intense beam of pure, monochromatic light which does not diverge and in which all the light waves are of the same length, travel in the same direction and are in phase, rising and falling together. The beam can be focused to a fine point to produce very high energy levels.

The development of lasers

The concept of stimulated emission of radiation was initially proposed by Albert Einstein in 1916 (van der Waerden, 1967). Until that time, physicists believed that there could be only two interactions between matter and light, absorption and emission. An atom is normally in a low energy or ground state but may be excited by the absorption of a photon (a quantum of radiant energy) of precisely the correct frequency and energy level. Conversely, an atom in the excited state can emit a photon spontaneously and drop to its ground state.

Einstein suggested the third possibility, stimulated emission, which forms the basis of the laser. He stated that under certain circumstances a photon could stimulate an excited atom or molecule to emit another photon with the same energy travelling in exactly the same direction. This could only happen if the stimulating photon had exactly the same energy as that which would normally be emitted spontaneously. Stimulated emission is unlikely when matter is in thermodynamic equilibrium as in this situation there is a greater population of atoms and molecules in the lower energy or ground state than in the excited state; and a photon is much more likely to be absorbed by a low energy atom or molecule than to stimulate emission from one in the excited state. With this concept it was possible to imagine that, in a population of excited atoms, a series of collisions would result in the release of an increasing number of photons – a beam of laser light.

In the 1930s, stimulated emission was referred to as *negative absorption*. Scientists did not proceed to the production of *net negative absorption* as they were obsessed with the principle of thermodynamic equilibrium, which was thought to be the normal condition of matter throughout the universe. This view was reiterated by Fabrikant (1940) who said that a population inversion was necessary for *molecular amplification*, the process that we call stimulated emission. He added, 'such a situation has not yet been observed in a discharge even though such a ratio of population is, in principle, obtainable. Under such conditions we would obtain a radiation output greater than the incident radiation and we could speak of a direct experimental demonstration of the existence of *negative absorption*'.

Schawlow and Townes (1953) are credited with the first published detailed proposal for the production of a laser which they called an *optical maser*. After further development, Townes, Basov and Prokhorov were awarded the Nobel Prize in 1964 for the *maser* (microwave amplification by stimulated emission of radiation) and the publication of their work stimulated intense laser research. Maiman (1960), while working at the Hughes Research Laboratory in California, made the first ruby laser despite a widely held belief that the ruby was unsuitable for a laser. In 1961, the first gas and continuous wave laser, the helium neon laser, and the neodymium laser were produced (Javan, Bennett and Herriott, 1961; Johnson and Nassau, 1961). In the latter, neodymium was present in a calcium tungstate host and this device demonstrated that a solid state laser could be operated at room temperature. The neodymium YAG, carbon dioxide, diode, ion, chemical, dye and metal vapour lasers were produced shortly afterwards (Geusic, Marcos and van Vitert, 1964; Patel, 1965). More recently, the excimer laser has been developed, an example of which is the argon fluoride laser. In these lasers, the medium is composed of two atoms which are only stable in the excited state.

Lasers in surgery and medicine

At about the same time, the xenon-arc photocoagulater was introduced into ophthalmology by Meyer–Schwickerath (1956) to treat threatened retinal detachment and certain other disorders. It was rapidly apparent that there were inherent problems with this system largely due to its lack of power. Ophthalmologists rapidly evaluated the more powerful pulsed ruby laser and concluded that it was superior for retinal photocoagulation (Kapany *et al.*, 1963; Flocks and Zweng, 1964). Encouraging results for the ruby laser's ability to destroy malignant tumours in animals and superficial malignancies in humans (McDuff *et al.*, 1965) were later countered by research which demonstrated that viable cancer cells were present in the debris which was ejected explosively during pulsed irradiation (Minton *et al.*, 1965; Ketcham, Hoye and Riggle, 1967). Theoretically, these cells could be forced into surrounding normal tissues, adjacent blood vessels and lymphatics and so disseminate the malignancy.

In 1965, Patel produced the carbon dioxide (CO_2) laser and first experiments showed that the focused beam could be used to divide a wide range of animal tissues in a precise and bloodless manner (Yahr and Strully, 1966). Further studies failed to reveal any viable cells in the plume emitted during vaporization of tissue using the CO_2 laser (Mihashi *et al.*, 1976). These findings have recently been challenged and it has been suggested that there may be viable, viral particles in the vapour produced by the destruction of tissue with this type of laser (Walker, Mathews and Newson, 1986).

Breidemeier (1969) developed an endoscopic coupler for the CO_2 laser which enabled the first *in vivo* studies to be carried out on the canine larynx. Dis-

crete lesions of a clinically desirable size could be produced on the vocal cords, in a bloodless field, using powers of 5–30 watts, with a spot size of 2 mm and an exposure time of 0.1–0.5 s. Healing of these lesions was excellent. This laser was then coupled to a Zeiss operating microscope and used in laryngeal microsurgery for vocal cord keratosis, carcinoma *in situ*, vocal cord nodules, polyps and papillomas (Strong and Jako, 1972).

At the same time that the CO_2 laser was being evaluated, ophthalmologists were experimenting with the continuous wave argon laser. It was found that the blue/green light produced by this laser was readily absorbed by vascular tissue and was thought to be of considerable value for the treatment of diabetic retinopathy (Zweng, 1971).

Although the pulsed, neodymium-glass laser was not found to have significant applications in medicine and surgery, the continuous wave neodymium YAG laser did. It could be transmitted by fibreoptics and in this form was used for the control of bleeding in the gastrointestinal tract (Nath, Gorisch and Kiefhaber, 1973).

Development of photodynamic therapy

The concept of photosensitization is far from new. Raab described the killing of *Paramecium* sensitized with acridine dye and exposed to light in 1900. Just five years later, Jesionek and Tappenier (1905) used topical eosin and white light to treat skin tumours. Although a wide range of photosensitizers has been and is being investigated, the majority of research work has focused on the porphyrins. In 1924, Policard demonstrated that a number of human and animal tumours exhibited a red fluorescence and attributed this to an accumulation of endogenous porphyrins from secondary bacterial infection.

More recently, haematoporphyrin derivative (HPD), a mixture of porphyrins, was used to demonstrate fluorescence in malignant tissues and to treat a breast tumour in combination with filtered light (Lipson, Baldes and Olsen, 1961, 1964). The chemistry of HPD has been extensively investigated as has its distribution within the body tissues. HPD is selectively retained within malignant tissues and also in the liver, spleen, kidneys and skin but the exact mechanism for this retention remains uncertain. The wavelength of light which best activates HPD and also penetrates most deeply into the tissues has been determined. Light with a wavelength of 630 nm appears to be optimal and is best produced by an argon-pumped dye laser, using a rhodamine dye and transmitted by flexible fibre. When HPD is activated by light, singlet oxygen is created by energy transfer from the excited porphyrin molecule (Weishaupt, Gomer and Dougherty, 1976). This is cytotoxic, probably acting at several sites by the oxidation of sensitive bonds.

The ability of photodynamic therapy to destroy tumours has been investigated in a large number of cultured, transplanted and naturally acquired animal tumours. Clinical studies have been undertaken to establish both the diagnostic and therapeutic potential in the management of human tumours. It has been shown that HPD-bearing tumour fluoresces when exposed to blue light. Under these conditions, a high level of diagnostic accuracy can be achieved at endoscopy when viewing lung and bladder tumours. Clinical therapeutic trials have been carried out on metastatic breast tumours, lung carcinomas, bladder tumours, head and neck cancer, brain gliomas and ocular tumours, all of which show that photodynamic therapy can eradicate tumours. However, many of the tumours treated to date are those which have failed all other treatment modalities and are exceedingly extensive. Despite this, considerable tumour responses with useful palliation have been achieved in some and encouraging results are being reported for small tumours treated for cure.

The laser
Production of coherent laser light

The lasing medium is contained within the laser tube which has a fully reflective mirror at one end and a partially reflective mirror at the other to allow access to the laser beam (Figure 25.1). The lasing medium is pumped and excited either electrically or by a high energy light source in order to create a population inversion of atoms in a high laser energy state. The high laser level must have a long lifetime compared to the low level if a population inversion is to be achieved (Figure 25.2). Stimulated emission then takes place as atoms spontaneously emit photons which, on collision with other excited atoms, stimulate these to emit identical photons travelling in the same direction as the original stimulating photons (Figure 25.3). These photons are released in all directions but, from time to time, photons are released in exactly the same axis as that of the laser tube. These photons are reflected back into the lasing medium by the mirrors to collide with other excited atoms which subsequently release their photons in the axis of the tube. By this means, there is a rapid build-up of light energy in the laser tube – the cascade effect – and the beam is emitted through the partially reflective mirror (Figure 25.4).

Beam characteristics

The laser beam is an intense, collimated (parallel) beam of pure, monochromatic, single wavelength light. All the light waves are the same length and travel both in phase and in the same direction. The beam can be focused by a lens or concave mirror to produce a small spot of light with extremely high energy.

Beam transmission

The coherent light from visible and low infrared lasers can be transmitted by fine, flexible fibres to appropriate delivery devices. As yet, no flexible fibre has been found which will transmit the far infrared CO_2 laser energy efficiently. The early CO_2 laser tubes were mounted directly onto the operating microscope and the beam was aimed at the target by a concave mirror controlled by a micromanipulator. These systems were inherently unstable and cumbersome. Today, the laser tube is mounted in a separate console and the beam transmitted to the microscope, handpiece or bronchoscope by means of a self-supporting, articulated arm which is hollow and contains mirrors at its articulations. The length of the arm, number of articulations and range of movements vary from machine to machine (Figure 25.5).

Beam aiming

The laser beam must be aimed accurately at the target before it is activated. With lasers operating in

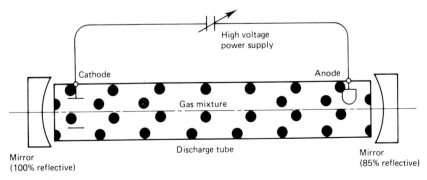

Figure 25.1 Gas laser configuration

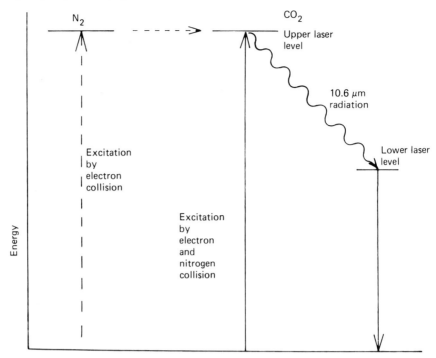

Figure 25.2 Laser energy diagram

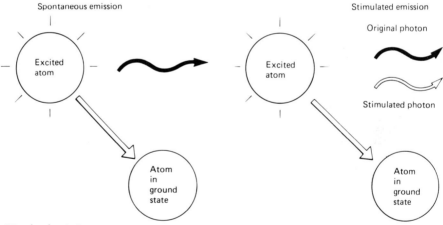

Figure 25.3 Stimulated emission

the visible wavelengths, an attenuated beam is used to define the beam path and target area; but with the invisible near and far infrared lasers, a coaxial low-powered visible helium neon laser is used for aiming. Either a concave mirror or zinc selenide lens focuses the beam, the latter system being able to transmit both the infrared and red wavelengths.

The focal point of the beam is adjusted to the focal length of the microscope lens, which for most microlaryngeal surgery is 400 mm, although shorter work-

ing distances have been used in oral surgery. Anderson (1981), when working on the cervix, recommended the use of a laser focused at 400 mm with a 250 mm focal length lens as this arrangement produced a wide, defocused beam of 2 mm in diameter.

The laser/microscope assemblies incorporate a micromanipulator which moves the final focusing mirror and enables the aiming beams to be positioned with great accuracy (Figure 25.6). Laser broncho-scopes have the working beam either 'fixed' in the

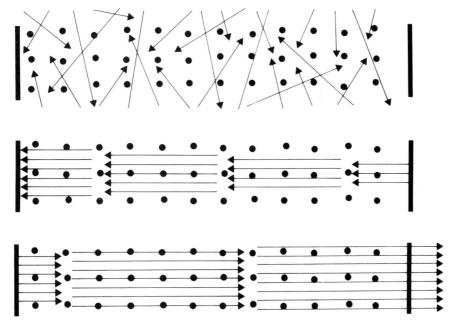

Figure 25.4 Production of the laser beam: the cascade effect

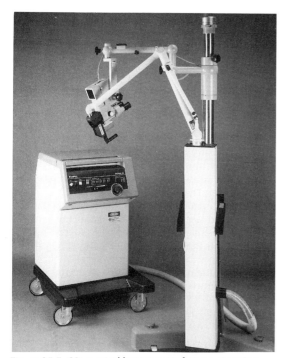

Figure 25.5 CO_2 surgical laser mounted on an operating microscope

centre of lumen without the facility of an aiming beam or have a small micromanipulator on the bronchoscope coupler.

The argon laser beam can be transmitted to a slit lamp, operating microscope, handpiece or endoscope by a flexible fibre. The Nd-YAG laser may also be used with an endoscope or hand piece. Design of the end of an endoscopic delivery fibre appears to be critical. The laser fibre has to be surrounded by a metal-tipped Teflon sheath down which compressed air is blown to keep the tip free from debris and secretions. If these adhere to the tip, they absorb energy and cause thermal damage to the fibre, which then has to be removed for cleaning and possibly also recutting during a long treatment session. The metal tip may even become so hot that the Teflon sheath swells to such an extent that it is impossible to remove it from the biopsy channel of the endoscope.

Laser beam parameters

Beam power

Power levels vary from laser to laser; milliwatts of power for low level laser therapy to 100 watts in high-powered CO_2 or Nd-YAG surgical lasers.

Power density

It is essential to know both the power and power density (irradiance) for all medical and surgical laser applications. The laser energy has a greater effect if delivered to a small spot rather than spread over a large area. Power density is measured in watts or milliwatts per square centimetre and is calculated by dividing the power by the area of the laser imprint.

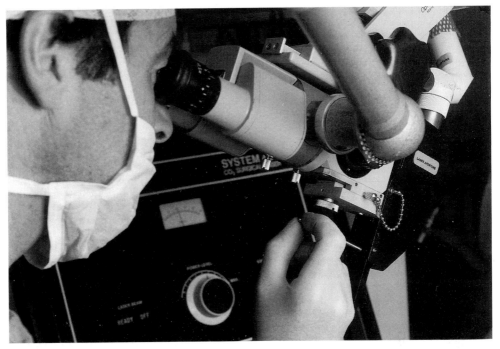

Figure 25.6 Micromanipulator

Energy distribution within the beam

In spite of the parallel nature of the laser beam, there may be profound differences in the energy distribution within the beam resulting from differences in the optical cavity, such as the radii of the mirrors and their spacing. There is a number of different transverse electromagnetic modes (TEM) of which the commonest is the fundamental mode (TEM_{00}). In this mode the distribution is circular but the power level does not have a sharp cut-off and the spot size is measured between points at which the power has fallen to 14% of the central level. This implies that there will be effects on the tissue outside the boundaries of the quoted spot size. The power distribution is doughnut shaped in TEM_{01} and with other modes the energy may be distributed to a number of points with the TEM number indicating the number of modes or points of zero energy.

Total energy delivered

This is measured in joules (watts/seconds) and is calculated from the output power and exposure time.

Laser/tissue interaction

The pattern of absorption of the laser is determined by its wavelength and the effect on tissue depends on

the intensity of the irradiation, total energy delivered and rate of delivery of the energy.

Biostimulation

Very low levels of laser energy are thought to be biostimulative. As laser energy levels increase inhibition develops until at high levels a thermal injury is inflicted (Mester, Mester and Mester, 1988). Low level therapy has been used to improve wound healing and to relieve the pain of sports injuries and arthropathies. Dyson and Young (1986) have shown that both wound contracture and cellularity are affected by mid-laser treatment. The results of carefully constructed studies are awaited with interest but the present status has been well outlined by King (1989). Different types of laser have been used for these purposes, ranging from low-powered, red helium neon and infrared gallium arsenide lasers to the CO_2, argon and Nd-YAG lasers which are used at very low subtherapeutic power levels.

Thermal effects

The temperature of tissues increase as they absorb energy. No change in tissue structure is evident between 37°C and 60°C, but above that temperature tissues begin to coagulate. Protein in collagen fibres denatures and this results in contraction of the tissue. It is this induced contraction that imparts haemostatic properties when the laser is applied to blood vessels. When the temperature of soft tissues is raised to 100°C, intercellular water is boiled and converted into steam. A thousand-fold increase in volume results in almost instantaneous vaporization. Once the water has been removed from the tissues, residual cellular debris is burnt at a temperature of 400–500°C. Burning does not cause significant damage to the surrounding tissues as there is poor thermal contact between the debris and adjacent normal tissues.

Non-thermal effects

Non-thermal effects may be photomechanical or photochemical. An example of the mechanical effects is the use of the pulsed Nd-YAG laser for destruction of opaque bodies within the eye. Nanosecond 10^{-9} pulses create minute balls of plasma in which the temperature can be higher than that of the sun and it is the shock waves from these that destroy the lesions. Longer pulses from this laser are being used to destroy renal and gallstones.

Direct interaction between laser photons and molecules is responsible for photochemical effects. Examples of this type of action are the photoactivation of haematoporphyrin derivative within malignant tumours, or the ultraviolet laser tissue interaction using the excimer lasers to reshape the cornea or in removal of atheroma from arteries.

Surgical lasers

The name of each laser is derived from its lasing medium. This also determines the wavelength of coherent light produced by that laser and, as stated previously, defines the pattern of tissue absorption and the clinical role of each. In clinical practice there is considerable overlap in the roles of the three most commonly used lasers (Table 25.1).

The CO_2 laser is used as a high precision, bloodless, light scalpel with an ability to seal blood vessels up to 0.5 mm in diameter. The argon laser is used mainly to coagulate blood vessels but may also be used at higher power levels to destroy tissues, albeit slowly and imprecisely. Thermal tissue destruction with the

Table 25.1 The most common roles of lasers

Laser	Tissue destruction	Vessel coagulation
Carbon dioxide	+ + +	+
Argon	+	+ + +
Neodymium-YAG	+ +	+ +

Nd-YAG laser is relatively imprecise and may be time-consuming, but superior to the CO_2 for haemostasis.

The carbon dioxide laser

The CO_2 laser produces continuous wave, far infrared, coherent light at a wavelength of 10 600 nm which is absorbed by water and by soft tissues as these contain 70–90% water. Although the cell contents are carbonized by the laser beam, falling as soot around the wound, it has been shown in several studies that there are no viable cells or cell components in the debris released by cell vaporization. Mihashi *et al.* (1976) studied the debris following vaporization of the tongues of dogs and found that, although some epithelial cells were recognizable, they had lost their *functional vitality*. Oosterhuis *et al.* (1982) vaporized Cloudman mouse melanomas and failed to find viable tumour cells by *in vitro* or *in vivo* culture, whereas controls of cells mixed with debris and smoke remained viable. As stated previously, it has recently been suggested that there may be viable viral particles in the vapour produced by the CO_2 laser ablation of viral lesions (Walker, Mathews and Newson, 1986). This finding has recently been challenged by Abrahamson, Di Lorenzo and Steinberg (1990) who were unable to find any viral particles in the plume during laser destruction of viral laryngeal papillomas.

There is no shock impact when the CO_2 laser beam strikes the tissues and, therefore, no tendency to force cells into adjacent normal tissues. As cell vaporization takes place at the relatively low temperature of 100°C (the boiling point of water) and tissues conduct heat poorly, there is a very thin layer of damaged cells adjacent to the laser wound. This margin of cells may be as narrow as 50 μm. Kiefhaber, Nath and Moritz (1977) demonstrated that 90% of the CO_2 laser's energy was absorbed in a depth of 100 μm. This laser sequentially removes layers of cells by vaporization to expose subjacent layers which are then vaporized, so deepening the wound in a precise controlled fashion.

Two techniques can be employed to remove lesions. First, after a representative biopsy has been taken, the laser is used to vaporize the whole lesion and adjacent normal tissues until a tumour free defect to appropriate margins has been achieved. The major disadvantage of this method is that it destroys the greater part of the lesion which is then unavailable for histological examination. The second technique is to use the laser beam, where possible, as a scalpel and excise the lesion with appropriate margins. The anterior border is first cut to an appropriate depth and then the lesion is undercut. The specimen must be kept under tension to prevent heat contracture. With this technique the final defect is no larger, is more precisely cut and the whole specimen is available for histological study.

Advantages of CO_2 laser surgery

Immediate tissue destruction

Tissue destruction by instantaneous vaporization is an obvious advantage over cryotherapy, in which a period of many days is needed to allow the tissue destroyed by freezing to separate. This period is frequently accompanied by pain, oedema and slough which are minimal or absent after CO_2 laser surgery.

Bloodless dissection

The focused CO_2 laser beam will seal blood vessels up to 0.5 mm in diameter. Larger vessels can be controlled by a defocused beam with lower power density. By necessity, a compromise power setting has to be used that provides both rapid cutting and good haemostasis. Surgery within the larynx is essentially bloodless, but if extended endoscopic resections are performed, some vessels will be encountered which will require diathermy coagulation. Some diathermy and ligatures are inevitably required with major resections of lesions in the oral cavity.

The laser beam also seals lymphatics and it has been suggested that this may reduce the spread of malignant cells by this route. Oosterhuis (1978) studied the lymphatic spread of labelled Cloudman 591 melanoma cells after scalpel and laser incisions and found significantly higher spread after a scalpel incision. The spread after laser incision was no higher than in controls which had not been cut. Holzer and Ascher (1979) studied severed peripheral nerves and found that their ends were smooth. The endoneurium had been sealed and amputation neuromas did not develop.

Minimal instrumentation

No instruments are needed to deliver the beam to the tissues when used with the operating microscope. An efficient sucker is required at the point of surgery to remove steam to prevent thermal injury and to provide a clear view of the target tissue. Minimal instrumentation is vitally important when access is limited, as in paediatric laryngology.

Unfortunately, the CO_2 laser beam cannot be transmitted by a fine flexible fibre and so the target area must be accessible to a rigid, straight endoscope. Stainless steel mirrors equipped with suction are available to reflect the laser beam so that lesions in inaccessible areas can be treated, e.g. the undersurface of the vocal cords, the laryngeal surface of the epiglottis or nasopharynx.

Precise dissection

In otolaryngology, almost all work is undertaken with an operating microscope, although some resections in the anterior part of the mouth are treated more easily with a hand piece. The microscope provides a well-illuminated, magnified operative field in which the bright-red helium neon aiming beam spot is positioned with great accuracy using the micromanipulator on the laser/microscope attachment. In modern machines, the spot size can be varied; a small spot size is suitable for laryngeal work whereas a wider beam would be appropriate for intraoral resections to facilitate the acquisition of adequate margins. Power levels are selected so that an energy density is delivered that provides the combination of rapid dissection and adequate haemostasis. Most modern machines offer *super pulsing* of the beam with a high peak power and exposure times measured in milliseconds. Both the theoretical evidence provided by McKenzie (1983) and early clinical results indicate that the use of a super pulsed beam with a 'short, sharp' dissection technique may reduce damage to adjacent normal tissues and reduce charring.

Most surgeons use an intermittent pulse of 0.1–0.2 seconds for work in the larynx rather than continuous exposure and have the machine in super pulsed mode to minimize laryngeal tissue damage. Intraoral resections are usually performed with a continuous beam, controlled by foot switch, with an energy level selected to provide an acceptable rate of tissue removal with satisfactory haemostasis.

Minimal damage to adjacent normal tissues

As stated previously, there is an extremely thin layer of damaged cells, only a few microns in width, between the laser wound and adjacent normal tissues. As a result, minimal postoperative oedema develops. Healing of CO_2 laser wounds in the larynx is associated with minimal inflammation, relatively few myofibroblasts and, therefore, only small amounts of collagen formation in wounds. Scarring or deformation of tissues is most unusual (Tranter, Frame and Brown, 1985). Similar results have been reported for laser wounds of the oral mucosa (Fisher *et al.*, 1983).

Healing of skin incisions cut by CO_2 would appear to be slower, with a reduced tensile strength after 7 days, compared with an incision cut by scalpel, although the final strength is the same (Cochrane *et al.*, 1980). This suggests that there is little to be gained from making skin incisions with CO_2 laser except in patients with a haemorrhagic tendency for whom better haemostasis can be achieved. The CO_2 laser is essentially a tool for cutting mucosa. It is of immense value in gynaecology, otolaryngology and also in neurosurgery when precise, atraumatic *no touch* surgery is required.

The argon laser

The argon laser produces coherent light which can be transmitted by way of a flexible fibre. The laser light consists of a number of discrete wavelengths, but most of its energy is at 488 and 514 nm. Coherent light at these wavelengths will pass through water and clear colourless structures without absorption and without causing thermal damage. The light is selectively absorbed by tissues which are red, its complementary colour.

The beam is scattered in skin and absorbed by chromophores, such as blood. It has an absorption depth of about 230 μm in skin whereas in blood it is 170 μm. The selective absorption pattern of argon laser energy makes it ideally suitable for the coagulation of both normal and abnormal blood vessels. Jain (1983) compared its use for blood vessel coagulation in neurosurgery with the bipolar coagulator and commented that the laser could perform photocoagulation precisely without spread of energy to adjacent tissues or contact with the vessel. The laser offered considerable advantages in comparison to bipolar coagulation. For example, there was no risk of clot dislodgement by instrumentation and the delivery of energy was precise with little risk of diffuse vessel wall damage or of electrical current leakage. The only advantages of the traditional bipolar system were that it remained relatively inexpensive and was less complex.

The argon laser was first used for photocoagulation of retinal lesions. The laser beam was delivered through a slit lamp and avascular areas of the retina in patients with diabetic retinopathy were photocoagulated in an attempt to reduce new vessel formation. This treatment could be carried out through, and without damage to, the clear anterior parts of the eye. It is still widely used in this field today with the krypton laser. It has also been used to treat port wine stains by photocoagulation of the abnormal capillaries in the outer dermis. Again, it can achieve this without damaging the clear overlying normal epidermis. Its selectivity in absorption offers unique advantages, for example, it could be used to coagulate small vessels lying on vital structures such as the vasa nervorum (Di Bartolomeo, 1981).

The absorption pattern of the argon laser results in slow and relatively imprecise thermal tissue destruction. Some early work on the photodestruction of bronchial tumours was performed with this laser by Hetzel *et al.* (1983). It has largely been replaced by the Nd-YAG laser for this purpose, although it is still occasionally used for tumours adjacent to vital structures or those which are inaccessible to the CO_2 laser.

Early machines were relatively immobile as they needed a continuous flow of water to cool the laser tube and three-phase electricity. Recently, air-cooled machines have been introduced which are easily movable and some are even portable. The majority of machines produce about 5 watts of power but 20 watt lasers are now available and are used to control haemorrhage from upper gastrointestinal ulcers and also for tumour ablation.

The beam is transmitted by a single flexible fibre, 100 μm in diameter, embedded in a protective sheath. The diverging beam is refocused by a lens at the distal end. With a slit lamp or microscope, spot sizes of 50–100 μm are generated, controlled by a micromanipulator and aimed with the help of an attenuated beam. Spot sizes of about 1 mm diameter are used with a handpiece. The operator could be at significant personal risk of retinal damage with lasers of visible wavelength. As a consequence, both slit lamps and microscopes incorporate a shutter which closes when the main beam is activated. This mechanism is fail safe in that the beam cannot be activated unless the shutter is closed.

The Nd-YAG laser

The Nd-YAG laser is the only one of the three commonly used lasers which does not have a gas as its lasing medium. Instead, it has a crystal rod made of yttrium aluminium garnet with dopant neodymium ions embedded in its lattice. The rod measures 100 mm long and is about 6 mm wide. The exciting energy is provided by a powerful light source which is usually a krypton arc lamp focused on the crystal rod. This is the most powerful surgical laser in current use, as more neodymium ions can be contained in a given volume of crystal than a gas and so power levels of up to 100 watts can be achieved.

The Nd-YAG laser produces near infrared, coherent light at a wavelength of 1060 nm. It can be transmitted by a flexible fibre and is aimed by a visible low-powered helium neon laser. The laser beam is absorbed by tissues to a considerable depth without colour or tissue specificity. Early work suggested that the absorption length of this wavelength could be as much as 90 mm and there was obvious concern that damage could be sustained by tissues beyond the organ being treated. More recently, work by Keifhaber, Nath and Moritz (1977) proved that this was not the case and that the beam was absorbed within a few millimetres. The Nd-YAG laser beam is scattered and diffused by tissue inhomogeneities. So great is the scattering/absorption ratio that a near infrared photon may be scattered many times before it is absorbed. This pattern of absorption means that the beam affects a far larger volume than the CO_2 laser and that for a given power the temperature rise is less (Figure 25.7).

At high power levels, the Nd-YAG laser is used to destroy tissue. In this respect it is relatively slow but does so with better haemostatic control than is possible with the CO_2 laser. The Nd-YAG laser can control vessels of up to 1.5 mm in diameter compared with 1.1 mm with the argon laser and 0.5 mm with the focused CO_2 beam (Kelly *et al.*, 1983).

Three distinct layers have been recognized in tissue that has been destroyed by the Nd-YAG laser. First,

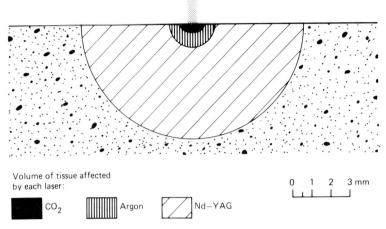

Figure 25.7 Depth of tissue affected by different lasers

there is a layer that has been vaporized; second, one which has been coagulated and will subsequently slough; and third, one in which cells have died and will be replaced by fibrous tissue without loss of physical integrity. There is, therefore, only a small risk of perforation when treating a tumour which involves the whole wall of the oesophagus or trachea.

Tissue removal with this laser lacks the precision which is possible with the CO_2 laser, but recently the Nd-YAG laser has been coupled to a synthetic sapphire *blade* so that it can be used like a scalpel. A wide range of general surgical procedures has been performed using this system. Wounds heal well and the overall morbidity has been low. Results from controlled clinical trials with this laser scalpel are awaited with interest.

Potassium titanyl phosphate (KTP) laser

This device is based on the standard Nd-YAG laser which generates infrared light at 1064 nm. The beam is passed through a crystal of KTP which doubles the frequency of the beam to produce green coherent light at a wavelength of 532 nm. This wavelength can be transmitted by a standard flexible fibreoptic cable and can be attached to an operating microscope. Like other devices, an attenuated beam can be used to aim the laser which is guided into the operative field by a micromanipulator. The delivery fibre may also be attached to a wide range of hand-pieces which facilitate its application in the ear, larynx and oral cavity.

The absorption characteristics of this laser beam are similar to those of the argon laser. More energy is

available with the KTP laser than with the majority of argon lasers. It is undergoing extensive evaluation for a wide range of otolaryngological procedures. At present, it appears to be less precise and operates at higher temperatures than the CO_2 laser but achieves superior haemostasis.

The dye laser

Dye lasers are used in two main clinical areas:

1 Photoactivation of intratumour haematoporphyrin derivative in the management of malignant tumours by photodynamic therapy
2 Selective destruction of blood vessels within the skin by continuous and pulsed wave lasers.

The dye laser uses an organic rhodamine dye as the lasing medium. The dye is continuously circulated to avoid heating and is excited either by a flash lamp or by an argon or copper vapour laser. As each dye molecule is composed of many atoms, it gives rise to a spectrum of laser lines and each dye can be used to lase over a range of about 50 nm. By changing the dye, coherent light in almost all parts of the visible spectrum can be obtained. The required laser line is selected from the available spectrum by the insertion of a birefringent filter which allows only one wavelength of light to pass through it depending on its angle in the beam. This ability to tune a dye laser is a very important feature. It offers the possibility to photoactivate future tumour sensitizers which may become operative at different wavelengths. Seemingly the only disadvantage is that the power available is, at best, only one-quarter of the exciting laser.

Light from the dye laser can be transmitted by

flexible fibres. A number of fibre tips for surface irradiation of tumours is available which include a cylinder for implantation into the centre of tumour tissue and a diffusing bulb tip for the irradiation of the inside of a viscus, for example, the bladder.

Metal vapour lasers

A wavelength of approximately 630 nm is required to photoactivate intratumour haematoporphyrin derivative. An alternative light source for this is the gold vapour laser. This machine can produce much higher power levels and is more stable, easier to use than many dye laser systems and more suited to clinical practice (Carruth and Mckenzie, 1986). This laser produces red light at a fixed wavelength of 628 nm and pulsed at rate of 10 kHz which, for practical purposes, is akin to a continuous beam. When other tumour photosensitizers become available, excited at different wavelengths, the metal could be changed to copper, which in turn could drive a tunable dye laser.

Excimer laser

These lasers have as their lasing medium substances which only combine in the excited state, e.g. argon fluoride. The majority produce coherent light in the violet/ultraviolet range and tissue removal is thought to result from molecular disruption rather than thermal processes. Some work has been undertaken using this type of laser for precise microlaryngeal procedures. The capacity for haemostasis is very limited with these lasers and there is already evidence that some of these laser wavelengths may be mutagenic. These factors together with their high cost limits their use in otolaryngology.

Erbium and holmium YAG

These lasers produce coherent light at wavelengths between 2 and 3 μm. There is now significant experimental evidence that they can be used to cut both soft and hard tissues with great precision and with little thermal damage to adjacent normal tissues. Soft tissues are probably better removed with the erbium YAG laser. Although ultraprecise tissue removal can be achieved with these lasers, haemostasis may be inferior to others and this could ultimately limit their clinical use.

Safety

The lasers used in medicine and surgery are much less powerful than many of their industrial counter-

parts. All therapeutic lasers are in the highest power class (class 4) and 'their use requires extreme caution'.

A wide range of national and international safety codes exist. In the UK the relevant codes are British Standards Code BS4803, *Radiation and Safety of Laser Products and Systems* 1983 and BS5724, *Electrical Safety of Laser Equipment*. A further document, *Guidance on the Safe Use of Lasers in Medical Practice*, has been published by the Department of Health and Social Security (DHSS). The European Community has funded a concerted action programme on medical laser development and a definitive code of safe practice has been produced which harmonizes all the codes of safe practice which are in existence in countries throughout the Community. In addition to the safety measures detailed below, it identifies certain required training standards for all doctors working with lasers. It is to be hoped that this code will shortly be ratified and will come into operation throughout the European Community.

Safety administration

The local health authority has overall responsibility for the implementation of health and safety advice. It is stated by the codes of safe practice that a laser safety officer should be appointed who will advise on all aspects of this problem and produce a code of safe practice for each laser in each clinical situation.

The safety officer is usually a medical physicist with a wide experience of lasers. He may be responsible for several hospitals within a district or region. A local laser protection supervisor should be appointed who may be either a doctor or a member of the operating theatre staff. He will be responsible for the implementation of the safety codes when lasers are being used clinically. A list of *nominated users* should be drawn up and access to the machine, by key control, should be limited to doctors on this list.

The machine

The machine must comply with the British Standard codes for electrical and laser safety and a number of specific features have been recommended in the DHSS guide.

Key control

All class 3A, 3B and 4 lasers must incorporate a master key control.

Emission warning

A visible or audible warning should be provided when the laser is switched on and operating.

Remote interlock

This should be available so that the operating theatre doors can be automatically locked when the laser is operational.

Aiming beam

An aiming beam must be fitted and it must not be possible to operate the laser in the event that this beam fails.

Emergency shut-off switch

An instant switch must be fitted.

Beam transmission system

The fibre or articulated arm should be securely fitted and a tool required for detachment.

Warning labels

Appropriate labels must be fitted.

Environmental

The room in which the laser is operated must be designated a *laser controlled area*. Access to this area must be strictly limited to those either essential to the procedure or specific visitors. Warning signs must be displayed outside and, ideally, these should be illuminated when the laser is switched on.

The eye hazard

The part of the eye that could be damaged by laser radiation is determined by the laser wavelength. Far infrared light produced by the CO_2 laser would be absorbed by the cornea and a retinal injury would not be sustained unless the beam had penetrated the whole globe. However, the near infrared laser light produced by the Nd-YAG laser and visible wavelengths would be focused on the retina, resulting in an increase in power to the area equal to 10^5 times the energy incident on the cornea.

The maximum permissible exposure has been calculated. For wavelengths transmitted to the retina, a factor of 10 times less than the level of exposure at which there is a 50% chance of producing a retinal injury is allowed. The maximum permissible exposure tables are available in *The British Standards Code*. The DHSS Code states that these levels should be used as a guide on the control of exposure and should not be regarded as precisely defined lines between safe and dangerous levels.

Eye protection

Adequate eye protection must be provided for both the patient and all the staff in the laser controlled area (Figure 25.8). It is obviously extremely unlikely that a member of staff would be exposed directly to the laser beam, but it is possible that they could be hit indirectly by reflection from an instrument or retractor. The design of, and specifications for, laser proof eye wear which should be provided are clearly defined in the safety codes. The eye wear must be marked to indicate the wavelengths against which protection is provided and the absorbence of the filter at these wavelengths. The glasses must attenuate the laser beam to below the maximum permissible exposure in the event of a direct hit and must not shatter or puncture if exposed directly to the maxiumum power of the laser.

Different eye wear will be required for use with each laser and glasses which conform to these specifications must be provided. The eyes of the patient should also be protected by glasses or carefully fixed pads which, in the case of the CO_2 laser, must be soaked in water to absorb the energy should the beam miss the target (Coleman and Conway, 1985) (Figure 25.9). Argon laser goggles or eye shields are also available. If work is to be performed close to the patient's eyes, stainless steel contact lenses are available and must be used.

When using the operating microscope, the surgeon will have the optics to protect his eyes against the

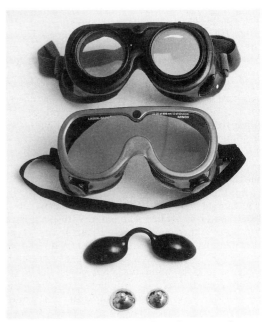

Figure 25.8 Eye protection from above down – CO_2 laser goggles, argon laser goggles, eye shields and contact lenses for use with the argon laser

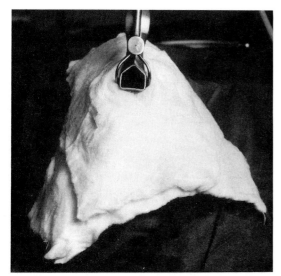

Figure 25.9 Head of patient draped with thick, wet swabs for CO_2 laser surgery to the larynx

CO_2 laser radiation. When the microscope or slit lamp is used with the argon laser, shutters which operate when the laser is activated are used for protection. With the Nd-YAG laser, filters on the endoscope are necessary to protect the eyes of the surgeon and goggles or pads must be provided for the patient. For all other usage, particularly with hand pieces, the surgeon must wear appropriate laser-proof glasses.

Skin injury

Skin injury is unlikely unless there is accidental exposure to the direct beam. The energy of a reflected beam is usually insignificant and protective clothing is not thought to be necessary for operating theatre personnel.

The plume

It must be stressed that the vapour produced during the removal of tissue with the CO_2 laser must be removed at source by powerful suction. There has always been concern about the possibility of there being viable viral particles within this vapour and the case at present remains 'not proven'. There is certainly no evidence, to date, that viable malignant particles have ever been implanted into the patient when any laser technique has been used. However, the CO_2 laser is often used to vaporize viral lesions or lesions in patients who have generalized viral diseases including AIDS. In the absence of positive evidence

to prove that there are no viral particles in the plume, suction must be meticulous. It would seem advisable for the surgeon and members of the staff to wear special viral filter masks to prevent inhalation of vapour.

Anaesthetic safety

Anaesthetic tube combustion is a hazard unique to laryngology when the CO_2 laser is used. A number of endotracheal fires have been recorded with some fatalities. An endotracheal tube, made of combustible material, will ignite if it is struck by the CO_2 laser beam. A number of *laser-resistant* tubes have been developed and several will not ignite if surrounded by a gas mixture with low oxygen and nitrous oxide content, or if used with a flow of carbon dioxide or nitrogen around the upper part of the tube above the cuff. All the tubes tested to date will ignite if surrounded by oxygen and the use of nitrous oxide does not ameliorate the situation as this gas supports combustion as well as oxygen.

In spite of the lack of a totally laser-proof, disposable, soft, flexible, anaesthetic tube, a number of *laser-safe* anaesthetic techniques have been developed, either without an endotracheal tube or involving the use of protected plastic or metal tubes. It is essential for the laryngologist to work as a team with an anaesthetist who is fully conversant with this hazard and the techniques to overcome it.

Anaesthetic techniques for microlaryngeal laser surgery
(See Figure 25.10)

Jet ventilation with no endotracheal tube

The Venturi ventilation principle has been known since the 18th century. In this technique, the patient is anaesthetized routinely and a fine endotracheal tube is inserted. When the patient has been positioned on the operating table, a laryngoscope is inserted and appropriately fixed. The endotracheal tube is then removed and a jet ventilation attachment is fastened to the laryngoscope which allows the paralysed patient to be oxygenated by intermittent jet ventilation of oxygen.

There are several disadvantages to this technique which is totally laser safe, as there is no combustible material in the airway. First, some patients are not suitable for the technique, particularly those who are grossly obese or who have severe chronic obstructive airway disease. Second, the cords abduct and vibrate on each injection of gas so that surgery has to take place between injections. Despite this, the surgeon soon learns the rhythm of injection and surgery can be carried out easily. Third, the subglottis cannot be protected with a wet swab although, it has to be

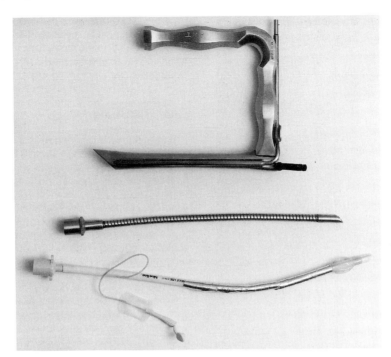

Figure 25.10 Anaesthetic equipment from above down – jet injector attached to laryngoscope, metal tube, Portex tube wrapped with aluminium foil

said, there have been no reports of problems from injuries to the subglottis from the defocused laser beam. Fourth, it has been suggested that jet ventilation may blow viable particles of papillomas into the lower airways with the risk of seeding, albeit theoretical.

Other jet ventilation techniques employ metallic catheters inserted into the trachea, but it is considered by some that the risk of causing a pneumothorax with these catheters, particularly in children, is significant.

Spontaneous respiration

In this technique, a nasopharyngeal airway is introduced, care being taken to ensure that it does protrude from behind the soft palate or appear in the operative field. There must be a constant high flow of gas down the airway so that aspiration of incandescent carbon fragments into the plastic airway during the expiratory phase cannot happen, otherwise there would be a risk of combustion. With the technique decribed by Spargo, Nielson and Carruth (1986), anaesthesia was maintained by the inhalation of anaesthetic gases. They considered that this technique was particularly appropriate for children with any degree of respiratory obstruction. Topical local anaesthetic should be applied to the vocal cords before surgery. More recently the use of the intra-

venous anaesthesia agent, propofol, in combination with an oxygen enriched air mixture delivered through a nasopharyngeal airway has been advocated (Rhys-Williams *et al.*, 1993). Other intravenous anaesthetic agents would be perfectly acceptable and be more appropriate for children, where the use of propofol is not universally accepted.

Protected endotracheal tube

It is easier to control and maintain adequate ventilation in difficult patients if an endotracheal tube is in place. While the subglottic structures can be protected with wet swabs, the tube itself must be protected by wrapping it with metal foil. The foil has to be relatively thick as it will absorb some of the laser energy if hit. Narrow 0.5–1 inch (1.3–2.6 cm) adhesive aluminium tape is wound up the tube from the proximal edge of the cuff to a point where the tube is well outside the operative field. The wrapping must start distally to avoid spaces appearing in the wrapping when the tube is flexed, as these might allow passage of the laser beam to strike the tube and cause ignition. The cuff cannot be wrapped and must be protected with a wet swab in the subglottis. This wrapping makes the tube rough and rigid. If great care is not taken, it can cause soft tissue damage to the larynx and pharynx. It certainly cannot be passed through the nose. Some have suggested that tubes can be protected merely with wet gauze, but in the author's opinion this is both difficult and dangerous.

Metal tube

Norton and de Vos (1978) have developed a flexible metal tube which is totally laser proof (Figure 25.10). It is somewhat rough and a little traumatic for the patient. A cuff must be attached to seal the airway and even though filled with saline, it must be protected. The internal diameter of these tubes is small in relation to their external diameter especially when compared with similar sized plastic tubes. Some anaesthetists use these metal tubes with some form of jet ventilation. A disposable metal tube is now commercially available which has a cuff attached but they are expensive and their cuffs also need to be protected.

Other techniques

A number of other techniques are currently being evaluated. They include high frequency positive pressure ventilation administered through transoral metal cannulae and by metal cricothyrotomy tubes. It seems likely that in the near future a soft, flexible disposable, endotracheal tube will be developed which will not ignite in any gas mixture and will be totally laser and foolproof.

Clinical use of lasers in otolaryngology

A laser should only be used when it offers significant advantages over established, conventional techniques. Applications have been found in the following aspects of otolaryngology.

Laryngeal surgery

The CO_2 laser in combination with a rigid laryngoscope, appropriately supported, is ideally suited to microlaryngeal work. Instruments have been designed to facilitate laser laryngeal microsurgery (Figures 25.11 and 25.12). Microlaryngeal suction forceps with a fine suction catheter built into an angled cupped forceps is useful, as is a malleable adjustable suction tube which can be clamped into the laryngoscope to provide adequate distal suction without encroaching significantly into the lumen of the laryngoscope. A number of other retractors and metal *paddles* is available with built-in suction, both to retract tissues in the exposure of lesions and to prevent damage by the beam or steam.

Lesions should not be completely vaporized if at all possible. The laser should be used as a scalpel so that the whole lesion can be submitted for histopathological examination. This of particular importance in the management of *leukoplakia*, where a solitary biopsy may be unrepresentative of the whole. Despite some early evidence to the contrary, it has been shown that it is not possible to remove mucosa from the anterior ends of both vocal cords without significant risk of webbing.

Traumatic *vocal cord nodules* have been resected using a microspot CO_2 laser and relatively low power settings of 1.0–3.0 watts with pulses of 0.1 second. These nodules are gradually *shaved* off the edge of the normal cord using a protected endotracheal tube together with wet gauze in the subglottis. *Vocal cord polyps* are usually drawn medially with microsuction forceps so that the pedicle can be divided by the laser. Stripping of the vocal cords for *Reinke's oedema* can be carried out with precision and without damage to the underlying cord. Yates and Dedo (1984) described a technique in which they used the CO_2 laser to incise the mucosa on the dorsum of the cord, retracted it medially, vaporized the submucosal oedematous tissue and then returned the mucosa to the surface of the cord. In a refinement of this technique, the residual mucosa can be fixed to the underlying cord with intermittent pulses of laser energy.

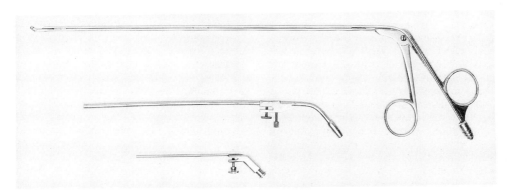

Figure 25.11 Microlaryngeal instruments: suction forceps, malleable adjustable suction tube and attachment for jet ventilation

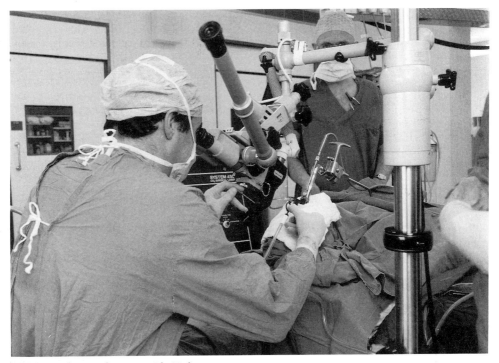

Figure 25.12 Microlaryngeal surgery with CO_2 laser

Attractive as it may seem, it was not in the above areas of laryngeal microsurgery that advances or improvements were required. At the outset it was hoped that laser therapy might offer more hope for conditions where conventional therapy largely failed, e.g. laryngeal stenosis and vocal cord webs.

Congenital or acquired subglottic stenosis in children has traditionally been managed by a tracheostomy with a fenestrated tube and speaking valve. This allowed the child to breathe out through the larynx, to speak and did not interfere with laryngeal growth. Although seemingly safe, this method of management had not been without complication. In a series of 25 children reported by Fearon and Cotton (1974), six (25%) died of causes related to their tracheostomy. A similar series of 85 children who required a tracheostomy described by Hollinger *et al.* (1976) was less alarming, but still 10 children died of whom five succumbed from causes related to their tracheostomy. Other forms of surgical treatment have been developed, e.g. laryngotracheoplasty (Evans and Todd 1974), but all are associated with a significant morbidity.

Kaufman, Thompson and Kohut (1981) described a series of 13 childeren with subglottic stenosis largely secondary to intubation. Eleven of these children were less than 3 years of age and eight had a tracheostomy at presentation. They were managed by injections of steroids into the lesion before laser vaporization. Stents were also used in three children but did not appear to be of benefit. In this series, three children could be decannulated and two had normal airways subsequently but were not decannulated for various reasons. Two other patients needed tracheostomies during the course of treatment. Ultimately, a satisfactory airway was achieved in 10 of the 11 children. In conclusion, Kaufman, Thompson and Kohut suggested that circumferential removal of the subglottic mucosa should not be performed as it encouraged scar formation and interrupted the mucociliary pathway. They considered that laser therapy in combination with dilatation, antibiotics and steroids, given systemically or by injection into the lesion, had an important part to play in the management of these cases.

Hollinger (1982) expressed similar enthusiasm in a preliminary report of the management of six children with severe subglottic stenosis who would have needed a tracheostomy but could be managed without one. The children required one to 11 endoscopic resections (average 6.5) but a successful outcome was achieved in all cases. He concluded that an infant with subglottic stenosis who, while needing a tracheostomy, was able to breathe spontaneously and undergo a general anaesthetic, was a suitable candidate for management with the laser.

However, in his paper there was mention of a further five children with the same problem who, for logistic or timing reasons, could not be treated with the laser. There was also another child who needed an urgent tracheostomy for very severe obstruction.

Without belittling either Hollinger's or Kaufman's achievements, it would seem that these reports have to be read with care before letting them influence the management of a child. Ten years after Hollinger's report the role of the laser in this field remains uncertain. Indications for the use of the laser may be minimal in cases of established stenosis and it may only have value in the immediate removal of granulation tissue following prolonged endotracheal intubation. Whatever, it is imperative that the child should be assessed or treated in a centre where there is a paediatric laryngologist with experience in the use of the laser.

Post-traumatic stenosis has posed significant management problems in adults as well. Endoscopic procedures are followed by a disappointingly high rate of recurrence and open surgical procedures are associated with significant morbidity. In 1980, Lyons *et al.* reported the use of the CO_2 laser in the management of six patients, five of whom had had previous treatment. After a relatively short period of follow up, the tracheostomies in four could be occluded and two patients had been decannulated. Shugar, Som and Biller (1982) described the management of 16 patients with the laser. Seven of their patients merely had redundant supraglottic soft tissues following hemilaryngectomy. This redundant tissue could be easily removed by the laser and, as a result, none required a permanent tracheostomy. Only two of the other cases could be decannulated; one had a web which was excised and a keel inserted for 2 weeks, the other had post-radiotherapy scarring which recurred 9 months after decannulation following laser excision of the stenosis. In a comprehensive paper Simpson *et al.* (1982) described the management of 60 patients with a wide range of stenotic lesions of the larynx and upper trachea. Soft silastic stents were used in 39. Success was defined as an adequate voice and airway without a tracheostomy and was achieved in 41 patients. It is somewhat difficult to compare exact results for laser surgery alone with the results for laser surgery followed by stenting. Simpson *et al.* concluded that features indicating a poor prognosis were circumferential scarring, stenosis longer than 1 cm, posterior inlet scarring with arytenoid fixation and bacterial infection of the tracheostomy.

Duncavage, Ossoff and Toohill (1985) reported a successful outcome in 11 out of 20 patients treated with the CO_2 laser. Seventeen were managed by laser excision of the stenosis alone while in the remainder *supplemental treatment* was given. This consisted of dilatation, intralesion steroids, grafts and, in three patients, the use of a stent. They concluded that success could be anticipated with small thin scars and redundant soft tissues and concurred with Simpson *et al.* (1982) about poor prognostic features.

A further technical modification for the management of stenosis in the posterior glottis and trachea, the micro-trapdoor flap, was described by Dedo and Sooy (1984). They made an incision on the superior, subglottic surface of the scar following which the submucosal tissue was removed with the laser. Incisions with a knife or microscissors were then made on either side of the trapdoor enabling it to be laid on the raw area. Suturing was not necessary as the mucosa readily adhered to the denuded area. They achieved success in eight out of nine patients with this technique.

The successful treatments of patients with total tracheal stenosis has recently been described (Shapsay, Beamis and Dumon, 1989). They opened the stenotic area with either the Nd-YAG or CO_2 laser and then inserted a T-tube which was retained for a period of 2–14 months.

In conclusion, it would appear that the treatment of upper airway stenoses with the laser alone may be unsuccessful in a significant number of cases. More patients can achieve a successful outcome if the laser resection is combined with endoscopic stenting, antibiotics, steroid injection and dilatation. Clinical experience to date suggests that a group of patients can be defined in which this form of therapy is unlikely to succeed.

Vocal cord webs are extremely easy to divide with a laser but many subsequently recur. Often the recurrent web is smaller than the orignal and, in many cases, one or two laser procedures will reduce the web to insignificant proportions. Several techniques have been described to overcome the problem of recurrence. The first is to open only the anterior end of the web, leaving a bridge at the posterior edge, which is divided when the anterior opening has epithelialized. The second technique is to remove the fibrin from the healing cords endoscopically at regular intervals to prevent reformation of the adhesions. The third technique is to provide cover for one cord using either an absorbable gelatin sponge or fibrin glue. Many surgeons use an endoscopically inserted keel of silastic sheeting which is fixed to the anterior commissure and secured with either a heavy nylon or stainless steel suture. This suture is passed percutaneously and secured over buttons. The keel is usually removed after 3–6 weeks and the procedure is normally accomplished without the need for a temporary tracheostomy.

A number of laser techniques has been described for the management of *bilateral vocal cord paralysis*. All involve some degree of cordectomy together with either partial or complete removal of the arytenoid. At first, a wide resection of the true cord was advocated (Croft, 1984), but it soon became apparent that a less destructive procedure was adequate. Removal of the posterior third of one cord was found to be satisfactory for some patients and the airway could be further improved by laser arytenoidectomy (Shaheen, 1984; Prasad, 1985; Dennis and Kashima, 1989). Some even found arytenoidectomy alone adequate (Ossoff *et al.*, 1984). Excellent results have been claimed by all and it would seem that the CO_2 laser is now the preferred treatment modality for this problem.

Recurrent respiratory papillomatosis is the one laryngeal condition for which the CO_2 laser has revolutionized treatment. Previous surgical techniques for their eradication have been accompanied by troublesome bleeding at the time of surgery. More importantly, those involving diathermy have been associated with significant thermal damage to normal tissues, postoperative oedema and late scarring with contraction and loss of function. Complete removal of all visible disease can be performed with the CO_2 laser without troublesome bleeding and with minimal damage to the underlying normal laryngeal tissues. It should now be possible to avoid a tracheostomy in this condition by routinely using the laser. Tracheostomy has a significant morbidity in small children and has sometimes been followed by the development of papillomas in the trachea and around the tracheostome. In 109 patients treated by a combination of laser and podophyllum, Dedo and Jackler (1982) reduced the need for a tracheostomy from 25% to 1.8% and the mortality from 7% to 0.

When removing papillomas from the mucosa it is important not to damage the subepithelial tissues or Reinke's space, otherwise scarring and contracture is inevitable. Debulking procedures rather than a total extirpation of disease at the anterior and posterior glottis minimize the risk of subsequent webbing and scarring (Crockett, McCabe and Shive, 1987).

Two management protocols for this condition have been derived. The first involves regular debulking procedures in the anticipation of a prolonged remission, while the second comprises on demand surgery, in other words laser microlaryngoscopy when the airway has become compromised. This latter management plan requires that the child has alert and sensible parents, easy access to the hospital and an ever ready surgical team. The main advantages of this latter approach are that, in practice, emergency procedures are extremely rare and the child has the least number of operative procedures.

Photodynamic therapy may have an important part to play in the treatment of recurrent respiratory papillomatosis. Abrahamson *et al.* (1992) reported a series of 30 patients who were treated with di-haematoporphyrin ether and red light from an argon pumped dye laser. In their series, 50% of the patients showed a reduction in the growth rate of the papillomas and three became free from the disease. There were some problems with skin photosensitization and there was

histological evidence of latent virus in the laryngeal tissues even after treatment.

The CO_2 laser is an ideal tool for the removal of *intubation granulomas*. However, its use does not seem to reduce recurrence rates (Benjamin and Croxson, 1985). It has also been found useful on the rare occasion that the larynx has been affected by *malignant granulomas*. In this rare condition, the ease of laser surgery, activity of the disease and the rate of recurrence seem to be related. In poorly controlled, active disease, surgery is usually accompanied by significant haemorrhage and the granuloma recurs rapidly; while on the other hand, in relatively inactive disease, surgery is usually bloodless and recurrence delayed.

Early *squamous cell carcinoma* of the larynx has also been treated by the laser. Strong (1975) introduced the idea of treating early vocal cord carcinoma with laser excision and the experience of the Boston group was updated by Blakeslee *et al.* (1984). In Strong's first series of 11 patients three had failed radiotherapy, all had tumour free margins and no patient had a recurrence. Strong commented that if margins were found to be involved by tumour, other treatment by radiotherapy or surgery would be necessary and that the voice was 'as good as the remainder of the larynx would allow'.

By 1984, a total of 113 non-irradiated patients had been treated in essentially the same way and their results had been published (Blakeslee *et al.*, 1984, Ossoff, Sisson and Shapsay, 1985). Both groups had excised the lesions with appropriate margins and taken biopsies for frozen section from the edge of the defect. The removal of tumour was continued until either the margins of the defect were shown to be tumour free or the thyroid cartilage was reached, in which case it was considered that further resection was inappropriate and radiotherapy should be given. For these workers the advantages of laser excision biopsy were clear. They were impressed by the ability to establish the diagnosis, stage and to provide adequate treatment for T1 lesions in one procedure. The technique was appropriate for radiotherapy-resistant tumours and for recurrent lesions after unsuccessful radiotherapy. Their patients were spared the short- and long-term problems that can develop with radiotherapy and, unlike radiotherapy, could have their treatment repeated as often as was either necessary or wise. The only disadvantage was that their patients' voices were not as good as those who had been given successful radiotherapy. Their patients' voices were serviceable after the removal of small lesions, and breathy or distinctly rough when larger tumours had been resected.

There is now a number of series reported in the literature in which the value of primary endoscopic excision of laryngeal malignant disease using the CO_2 laser has been proved. Two large series deserve further discussion (Motta, 1990; Steiner, 1993). Motta reported 93 cases of T1 glottic carcinoma in which a cure rate of 90% was achieved using the CO_2 laser alone and 95% after additional surgery for recurrent disease. An analysis of T1b tumours treated by CO_2 laser resection gave a cure rate by laser alone of 75% rising to 90% when recurrent lesions were treated by more extensive surgery. This series suggested that cure of anterior commissure lesions may be successfully achieved with this form of treatment in contrast to the finding of Krespi and Meltzer (1989) who, in a small series of tumours involving the anterior commissure had failed to control a single patient. Motta also treated 46 patients with T2a or T2b tumours and achieved control rates of 63% with the laser alone and 85% when further treatment was carried out for recurrent disease.

Steiner (1993) reported a series of 240 patients who received laser therapy as the primary mode of treatment for their laryngeal neoplasm. He divided the series into two groups. The first group (159 patients) consisted of 29 patients with carcinoma *in situ*, 96 patients with T1 tumours and 34 with T2 carcinomas. There were only six patients with recurrent disease in this cohort and only one patient subsequently required a total laryngectomy. In the second group (81 patients), 58 patients had T2, 17 T3 and six T4 tumours. There were 30 supraglottic carcinomas in this group and 38 glottic carcinomas classified as T2 lesions but with impaired vocal cord mobility; 22% of this group recurred locally and six patients required total laryngectomy.

It is claimed that the laser offers three further potential advantages in the management of advanced tumours. Laser debulking of the tumour at the time of the biopsy is said to enable more accurate staging of the tumour. It presents the radiotherapist with a reduced tumour bulk to treat and avoids either immediate laryngectomy or primary tracheostomy with its risk of tumour seeding around the stoma. It has to be said that none of these potential advantages has been proven by clinical trial to translate into a clinically significant effect.

Oral surgery

In the *oral cavity* and for surgery of the *tongue*, lasers offer significant benefits in terms of bloodless surgery, postoperative morbidity and the length of stay of the patient in hospital (Strong *et al.*, 1979a, b). A variety of hand pieces has been designed for use, but it is generally thought that these are only appropriate for the anterior part of the mouth. Much of the work in the mouth is still carried out using the operating microscope which provides a well illuminated magnified view of the operative field. The system is slightly rigid and so it is essential that lines of resection are clearly marked with laser impacts. These lines must be clearly visible at the beginning of the procedure or

must become evident during the course of the operation. As the laser beam cuts in a straight line, it is vitally important for the surgeon to confirm the lines of resection regularly throughout the procedures.

There is now considerable experience with use of the contact Nd-YAG and KTP lasers in the oral cavity and oropharynx (Strunk and Nichols, 1990). With one exception, there is no conclusive evidence to suggest that these offer significant advantages over conventional techniques or the CO_2 laser (Frame *et al.*, 1984; Rhys–Evans, Frame and Brandrick, 1986; Carenfelt, 1991). The exception to this statement is the recent technique of laser palatoplasty described by Ellis, Flowcs Williams and Shneerson (1993). In this, a 2-cm wide portion of palatal mucosa extending from the hard palate to the uvula is vaporized using the Nd-Yag laser down to the muscle. The deep penetration of this laser burn causes sufficient fibrosis of the underlying tissues to stiffen the palate. This results in a reduction of palatal flutter which is one of the causes of snoring.

The healing of wounds in the oral mucosa has been widely studied (Fischer *et al.*, 1983). When laser and scalpel wounds of the oral mucosa were compared, there was less damage adjacent to the laser wound, a reduced inflammatory reaction and minimal contracture. The submandibular duct can be cut without any fear of subsequent occlusion or stenosis. Despite all these features of improved wound healing, the same problem of osteoradionecrosis develops if the mandible is exposed in a previously irradiated patient.

There is a widely held opinion that postoperative pain is reduced following the resection of tongue lesions using the CO_2 laser, but this has never been proven fully by controlled clinical trials. In the author's series of 100 major tongue procedures carried out with the CO_2 laser, 45% of the patients required no analgesics whatsoever and a further 32% could be controlled with oral medication alone. In this series 85% of patients were discharged on the first or second postoperative day (Carruth, 1985).

Hypopharyngeal surgery

Endoscopic laser surgery has been performed in the hypopharynx. Overbeek, Hoeksma and Edens (1984) reported a series of 377 patients who had undergone endoscopic treatment for *pharyngeal pouch*. They adopted the technique first described by Dohlman (1949) but in 69 of their patients excised the party wall between the pouch and the oesophagus with a laser. Three patients developed mediastinitis in the laser group compared to five in the conventionally treated group. Overbeek considered that this was acceptable and that the final results were better in the laser group as they did not develop stenosis which was found on occasions in those treated by electrocoagulation.

Otological surgery

The argon, KTP and CO_2 lasers have been used in otology to perform a wide range of microsurgical procedures and some significant advantages over conventional techniques are claimed. At first there was concern that the laser energy might damage the delicate membranous structure of the inner ear. In 1972, Stahle, Hogberg and Engström focused an argon laser directly on the cochlea of guinea pigs and, although the beam parameters used did not penetrate the otic capsule, found histological evidence of damage to the adjacent stria vascularis. The effects of laser energy on the footplate of the stapes were first assessed by Sataloff (1976) who applied the Nd-YAG laser to both normal and otosclerotic footplates. He was only able to produce discrete lesions in the underlying membranes when the footplate had been painted with copper sulphate to improve laser energy absorption. Since then there has been a variety of reports concerning the potential structural and functional effects on the inner ear of footplate perforation by the laser. Perkins (1980) used the argon laser on post-mortem temporal bones to determine the parameters needed to vaporize small holes in the footplate. The utriculus and sacculus appeared unaffected but formal histological examination was not undertaken. A similar study was carried out by Di Bartolomeo and Ellis (1980) and similar results were obtained. Histological studies following penetration of the footplate with the argon laser were published by Gantz *et al.* (1982) in which three of eight ears sustained perforations of the sacculus. In addition to a rise in temperature within the inner ear, it has been suggested that laser irradiation produced fluctuations in endocochlear pressure which might cause functional damage (Thoma, Unger and Kastenbauer, 1981). Ricci and Mazzoni (1985) challenged this finding and demonstrated that following perforation of the footplate there was only a small rise in the perilymph pressure which they considered harmless. In a later publication Thoma, Mrowinski and Kastenbauer (1986) showed that when the CO_2 laser was used to perforate the footplate there was a very large rise in perilymph pressure which was of sufficient magnitude to damage the inner ear. These rather contradictory experimental findings have been largely superseded by the results of clinical applications which are summarized below.

Although it is possible to remove lesions from the pinna using the CO_2 laser, there would seem to be few advantages over conventional techniques. Similarly, it is extremely easy to open out a meatus stenosed by soft tissue, but this does not dispense with the need for an indwelling stent or pack to prevent a recurrence of the stenosis. It is hard to believe that in the performance of a simple *myringotomy* a laser could prove to be advantageous, but it has been suggested that if made with the CO_2 laser it

will remain open for a period of weeks. During this time the middle ear mucosa may return to normal and consequently a grommet may not be required. Goode (1982) found that he could produce 2 mm perforations with a single 0.1 second pulse of the CO_2 laser and recorded that the majority took up to 6 weeks to heal. In two patients the perforations failed to close. The first had been made intentionally larger (4 mm) so that permanent ventilation could be achieved, while the second had been made in a monomeric drum. A larger but uncontrolled series was reported by Lipman *et al.* (1987) in which 100 patients had their myringotomies performed by CO_2 laser. These remained patent for 2–4 weeks and only 40% developed recurrent effusions.

The argon and KTP lasers have been used to remove granulation tissue from the ossicular chain in *tympanoplasty*. Escudero *et al.* (1979) used the argon laser to spot weld a patch of temporalis fascia onto the eardrums and Di Bartolomeo and Ellis (1980) reported a similar technique but suggested that the laser impacts might cause shrinkage of the graft and, therefore, suggested that the graft should be made substantially larger than the perforation.

The argon laser has found use in *stapedectomy* to divide both the stapedius tendon and crura of the stapes and then to perforate the footplate. The first series of 11 cases was reported by Perkins (1980) who obtained satisfactory results in the short term. McGee (1983) reported a much larger series which compared the results of patients who had laser stapedectomy with a group who had small fenestrae created by conventional techniques. His conclusions were that laser stapedectomy caused very little trauma and a minimum of physiological disturbances. The initial results were good but not significantly better than those obtained by conventional techniques.

Rauch and Bartley (1992) compared argon laser stapedectomy to stapedectomy by traditional methods and found it to be superior. The incidence of footplate fracture or avulsion was five times greater with traditional techniques and sensorineural hearing loss four times more common in revision procedures. Perkins and Curton (1992) considered the choice of prosthesis to be an important factor. The results in their laser stapedectomies were significantly affected by the choice of prosthesis and material used to seal the fenestra. In a review of the use of lasers for otosclerosis, Lesinski (1990) considered that the argon and KTP lasers had the ideal beam profile for otological surgery but the wrong absorption characteristics, whereas the CO_2 laser had the correct absorption but a less than perfect beam profile.

The argon and CO_2 lasers have been used to remove *acoustic neuromas* and other cerebellopontine angle tumours (Glasscock, Jackson and Whitaker, 1981). The tumours are exposed conventionally and then exenterated using a power of 3–3.5 watts.

Tumour removal can be slow at these power levels but the laser is relatively atraumatic and has proved to be of some value in the removal of relatively inaccessible lesions (Powers *et al.*, 1984; Gardiner, Robertson and Clark, 1983).

Nasal surgery

Rhinophyma can be treated by precise dermabrasion with the CO_2 laser (Shapsay *et al.*, 1980). Other skin lesions on the nose can be removed by excision using the CO_2 laser as a scalpel, but with minimal advantages over conventional techniques. Some excellent results have been reported for the argon and pulsed dye lasers when used to treat *cutaneous vascular malformations*, e.g. port wine stains, telangiectases and the unsightly vessels that sometimes develop after rhinoplasty. This presents a true advance as these conditions were relatively untreatable before the development of laser techniques.

The application of this technology to intranasal telangiectases (*Osler's disease*) has not been particularly sucessful as new telangiectases develop in untreated areas. Healey *et al.* (1978) treated *choanal atresia* by using the CO_2 laser transnasally to remove the obstructing partition, but a clear advantage over conventional techniques has not been conclusively shown. Simpson, Shapsay and Vaughan (1983) reported a series of cases in which the CO_2 laser was used to remove a wide range of lesions from the nasal cavity including *papillomas*, *granulomas*, nasal *polyps* and *adhesions*, but again these may all be readily removed by conventional instruments and clear advantages for the use of the laser have not been shown.

The argon, KTP and CO_2 lasers have been used for the *reduction of the turbinates*, but although some advantages are claimed it would be very difficult to justify the cost of a laser for the performance of this type of surgery.

Photodynamic therapy

This technique represents a new and exciting approach to the management of many forms of localized malignant disease. The only tumour sensitizer which has been developed and subjected to clinical trials is the haematoporphyrin derivative (HPD). This sensitizer is activated by red light at a wavelength of 630 nm produced by either a tunable dye or gold vapour laser. A new group of sensitizers, based on the phthalocyanines shows great promise as they seem to incorporated into malignant tumours better than previous substances.

All clinical studies of photodynamic therapy have used the same technique. On the first day, the patient is given haematoporphyrin derivative or dihaemato-

porphyrin ether by intravenous injection. No significant side effects have been reported from the injection of sensitizer, but all patients develop severe but reversible skin photosensitization which lasts for 6–8 weeks. After 72 hours, the tumour is photoirradiated using a laser and delivery fibre. Subcutaneous disease is treated to a dose of 25 joules/cm^2 which destroys the tumour without damaging the overlying skin. Ulcerated lesions are treated by surface irradiation to a total dose of 100–200 joules/cm^2 which causes maximal tumour necrosis to a depth of 1 cm. Treatment can be repeated as often as necessary, both to remove further layers of thick tumour or to treat other lesions.

It has been estimated that more than 10 000 patients have now been treated by this technique and much of the work has been carried out on primary and secondary skin tumours. Local control can be achieved in 60–80% of patients with multinodular metastatic disease of the chest wall from breast carcinoma. Basal cell carcinomas which have failed other modalities can readily be treated with excellent results. Some head and neck tumours would appear ideal for this form of therapy as they are relatively small, remain localized and are easily accessible. More importantly, surgery for these conditions is usually mutilating in terms of the patient's appearance, ability to talk or swallow and photodyamic therapy might change this radically.

Wile *et al.* (1982, 1984) treated 114 tumour sites in 39 patients with photodynamic therapy. Complete tumour response was obtained in 28 sites and several remained tumour free for more than one year. A partial response was obtained in 42 sites but others were either not measurable or showed no response. They found that patients with persistent or recurrent disease in the primary site benefited substantially from treatment and that tumours of the tongue appeared to be particularly sensitive to this form of therapy. Others have reported the effect of photodynamic therapy on locally advanced disease and have demonstrated that it is possible to produce significant tumour necrosis with resultant palliation and local control in some (Carruth and McKenzie, 1985; Keller, Doiron and Fisher, 1985; Schuller, McCaughan and Rock, 1985).

It will surely not be long before this treatment gains universal acceptance. It could offer significant advantages to a multitude of patients with malignant disease. For example, it could aid palliation and local control for those with late stage head and neck carcinomas. Photodynamic therapy might prove to be curative for very early or localized lesions and could be used to sterilize wounds in which tumour cells may be spilt. Multicentric or cosmetically unacceptable malignant disease of the skin is another obvious potential application. This form of laser treatment offers much. Hopefully, future clinical trials will realize its full potential.

References

ABRAHAMSON, A. L., DI LORENZO, T. P. and STEINBERG, B. M. (1990) Is papilloma virus detectable in the plume of laser treated laryngeal papillomas. *Archives of Otolaryngology – Head and Neck Surgery*, **116**, 604–607

ABRAHAMSON, A. L., SHIKWITZ, M. I., MULLOOLY, V., STEINBERG, B. M., AMELACA, C.T. and ROTHSTEIN, H. R. (1992) Clinical effects of PDT in recurrent laryngeal papillomas. *Archives of Otolaryngology – Head and Neck Surgery*, **118**, 25–29

ANDERSON, M. C. (1981) Treatment of cervical intraepithelial neoplasia with the carbon dioxide laser: report of 543 patients. *Obstetrics and Gynecology*, **59**, 720–725

BENJAMIN, B. and CROXSON, G. (1985) Vocal cord granulomas. *Annals of Otology, Rhinology and Laryngology*, **94**, 538–541

BLAKESLEE, D., VAUGHAN, C. W., SHAPSAY, S. M., SIMPSON, G. T. and STRONG, M. S. (1984) Excisional biopsy in the selective management of T_1 glottic cancer: 3-year follow-up study. *Laryngoscope*, **94**, 488–494

BREIDEMEIER, H. C. (1969) *Laser Accessory for Surgical Applications*. U.S. patent, 3, 659, 613, issued 1972

CARENFELT, C. (1991) Laser uvulopalatoplasty in the treatment of habitual snoring. *Annals of Otology, Rhinology and Laryngology*, **100**, 451–454

CARRUTH, J. A. S. (1985) Resection of the tongue with the carbon dioxide laser: 100 cases. *Journal of Laryngology and Otology*, **99**, 887–889

CARRUTH, J. A. S. and MCKENZIE, A. L. (1985) Preliminary report of a pilot study of photoradiation therapy for the treatment of superficial malignancies of the skin, head and neck. *European Journal of Surgical Oncology*, **11**, 47–50

CARRUTH, J. A. S. and MCKENZIE, A. L. (1986) New concepts in cancer therapy: photoradiation therapy. In: *Head and Neck Oncology*, edited by H. J. Bloom. New York: Raven Press. pp. 315–318

COCHRANE, J. P. S., BEACON, J. P., CREASEY, G. H. and RUSSELL, R. C. G. (1980) Wound healing after laser surgery: an experimental study. *British Journal of Surgery*, **67**, 740–743

COLEMAN, M. F. and CONWAY, M. (1985) Prevention of facial burns during laser laryngoscopy. *Laryngoscope*, **95**, 349–350

CROCKET, D. M., MCCABE, C. B. F. and SHIVE, C. J. (1987) Complications of laser surgery for recurrent respiratory papillomatosis. *Annals of Otology, Rhinology and Laryngology*, **96**, 639–644

CROFT, C. B. (1984) The use of the carbon dioxide laser in the treatment of bilateral abductor paralysis of the vocal cords. *Proceedings of the Third Annual Conference of the British Medical Laser Association*

DEDO, H. H. and JACKLER, K. (1982) Laryngeal papilloma: results of treatment with the CO_2 laser and podophyllum. *Annals of Otology, Rhinology and Laryngology*, **91**, 425–430

DEDO, H. H. and SOOY, C. D. (1984) Endoscopic laser repair of posterior glottic, subglottic and tracheal stenosis by division and micro trapdoor flap. *Laryngoscope*, **94**, 445–450

DENNIS, D. P. and KASHIMA, H. (1989) Laser posterior cordectomy for treatment of bilateral vocal cord paralysis. *American Journal of Otolaryngology*, **98**, 930–934

DI BARTOLOMEO, J. R. (1981) The argon and CO_2 lasers in otolaryngology: which one, when and why? *Laryngoscope*, Suppl. **26**, 1–16

DI BARTOLOMEO, J. R. and ELLIS, M. (1980) The argon laser in otology. *Laryngoscope*, **90**, 1786–1796

DOHLMAN, G. (1949) Endoscopic operations for hypopharyngeal diverticula. *Proceedings of the 4th International Congress of Otolaryngology*. London. pp. 715–717

DUNCAVAGE, J. A., OSSOFF, R. H. and TOOHILL, R. J. (1985) Carbon dioxide laser management of laryngeal stenosis. *Annals of Otology, Rhinology and Laryngology*, **94**, 565–569

DYSON, M. and YOUNG, S. (1986) Effect of laser therapy on wound contraction and cellularity in mice. *Lasers in Medical Science*, **1**, 125–130

ELLIS, P. D. M., FLOWCS WILLIAMS, J. E. and SHNEERSON, J. M. (1993) Surgical relief of snoring due to palatal flutter: a preliminary report. *Annals of the Royal College of Surgeons*, **75**, 286–290

ESCUDERO, L. H., CASTRO, A. O., DRUMMOND, M., PORTO, S. P. S., BOZINIS, D. G., PENNA, A. F. S. *et al.* (1979) Argon laser in human tympanoplasty. *Archives of Otolaryngology*, **105**, 252–253

EVANS, J. N. G. and TODD, G. B. (1974) Laryngotracheoplasty. *Journal of Laryngology and Otology*, **88**, 589–597

FABRIKANT, V. A. (1940) Thesis. Quoted in Bertolotti, M. (1983) *Masers and Lasers: a Historical Approach*. Bristol: Adam Hilger Publishers

FEARON, B. and COTTON, R. J. (1974) Surgical correction of subglottic stenosis of the larynx in infants and children: progress report. *Annals of Otology, Rhinology and Laryngology*, **83**, 428–431

FISHER, S. E., FRAME, J. W., BROWNE, R. M. and TRANTER, R. M. D. (1983) A comparative histological study of wound healing following CO_2 laser and conventional surgical excision of canine buccal mucosa. *Archives of Oral Biology*, **28**, 287–291

FLOCKS, M. and ZWENG, H. C. (1964) Laser coagulation of ocular tissues. *Archives of Ophthalmology*, **72**, 604–611

FRAME, J. W., DAS GUPTA, A. R., DALTON, G. A. and RHYS EVANS, P. H. (1984) Use of the carbon dioxide laser in the management of pre-malignant lesions of the oral mucosa. *Journal of Laryngology and Otology*, **98**, 1251–1260

GANTZ, B., JENKINS, H. A., KISHIMOTO, S. and FISCH, U. (1982) Argon laser stapedectomy. *Annals of Otology, Rhinology and Laryngology*, **91**, 25–26

GARDINER, G., ROBERTSON, J. H. and CLARK, W. C. (1983) 105 patients operated upon for cerebello-pontine angle tumours – experience using combined approach and CO_2 laser. *Laryngoscope*, **93**, 1049–1055

GEUSIC, J. E., MARCOS, H. M. and VAN UITERT, L. G. (1964) Laser oscillation in Nd doped yttrium aluminium, yttrium gallium and gadolinium garnet. *Applied Physics*, **41**, 182–184

GLASSCOCK, M. E., JACKSON, C. E. and WHITAKER, S. R. (1981) Argon laser in acoustic tumour surgery. *Laryngoscope*, **91**, 1404–1416

GOODE, R. L. (1982) Carbon dioxide laser myringotomy. *Laryngoscope*, **92**, 420–423

HEALEY, G. B., MCGILLM, T., JAKO, G. J., STRONG, M. S. and VAUGHAN, C. W. (1978) Management of choanal atresia with the carbon dioxide laser. *Annals of Otology, Rhinology and Laryngology*, **87**, 658–662

HETZEL, A. R., MILLARD, F. J. C., AYESH, R., BRIDGES, C., NANSON, A. and SWAIN, C. B. (1983) Laser treatment of carcinoma of the bronchus. *British Medical Journal*, **286**, 12–16

HOLLINGER, L. D. (1982) Treatment of severe subglottic stenosis without tracheostomy: preliminary report. *Annals of Otology, Rhinology and Laryngology*, **91**, 407–412

HOLLINGER P. H., KUTNICK, S. L., SCHILD, J. and HOLLINGER, L. D. (1976) Subglottic stenosis in infants and children. *Annals of Otology, Rhinology and Laryngology*, **85**, 591–599

HOLZER, P. and ASCHER, P. W. (1979) Laser surgery of peripheral nerves. In: *Laser Surgery*, edited by I. Kaplan and P. W. Ascher, vol. 3, part 2. Jerusalem: Academic. p. 149

JAIN, K. K. (1983) Lasers in neurosurgery: a review. *Lasers in Medicine and Surgery*, **2**, 217–230

JAVAN, A., BENNETT, W. R. and HERRIOTT, D. R. (1961) Population inversion and continuous optical maser oscillation in a gas discharge containing a helium neon mixture. *Physical Review*, **6**, 106

JESIONEK, A. and TAPPENIER, H. VON (1905) Zur Behandlung der Hautcarcinome mit fluorescierenden Stoffen. *Archivs für Klinische Medizin*, **82**, 233–237

JOHNSON, L. F. and NASSAU, K. (1961) Infrared fluorescence and stimulated emission of Nd^{+3} Ca. *Proceedings of the Institute of Radio Engineers*, **49**, 1704–1706

KAPANY, N. S., PEPPERS, N. A., ZWENG, H. C. and FLOCKS, M. (1963) Retinal photocoagulation by lasers. *Nature*, **199**, 146–149

KAUFMAN, J. A., THOMPSON, J. N. and KOHUT, R. I. (1981) Endoscopic management of subglottic stenosis with the CO_2 surgical laser. *Otolaryngology Head and Neck Surgery*, **89**, 215

KELLER, G. S., DOIRON, D. R. and FISHER, G. U. (1985) Photodynamic therapy in otolaryngology – head and neck surgery. *Archives of Otolaryngology – Head and Neck Surgery*, **111**, 758–761

KELLY, D. F., BOWN, S. G., CALCER, B. M., PEARSON, H., WEAVER, B. M. Q., SWAIN, C. P. *et al.* (1983) Histological changes following Nd–YAG laser photocoagulation of canine gastric mucosa. *Gut*, **24**, 914–920

KETCHAM, A. S., HOYE, R. C. and RIGGLE, G. C. (1967) A surgeon's appraisal of the laser. *Surgery Clinics of North America*, **47**, 1249–1263

KIEFHABER, P., NATH, G. and MORITZ, K. (1977) Endoscopical control of massive gastrointestinal hemorrhage by irradiation with a high power Nd–YAG laser. *Progress in Surgery*, **151**, 140–155

KING, P. R. (1989) Low level laser therapy: a review. *Lasers in Medical Science*, **4**, 141–150

KRESPI, Y. P. and MELTZER, C. J. (1989) Laser surgery for vocal cord carcinoma involving the anterior commissure. *Annals of Otology, Rhinology and Laryngology*, **98**, 105–109

LESINSKI, S. G. (1990) Lasers for otosclerosis – which one if any and why? *Lasers in Surgery and Medicine*, **10**, 448–457

LIPMAN, S., ZIMM, E., MALONEY, R., GUELCHER, R. and ANON, J. (1987) Carbon dioxide laser myringotomy. *Lasers in Surgery and Medicine*, **7**, 99

LIPSON, R. L., BALDES, E. J. and OLSEN, A. M. (1961) Hematoporphyrin derivative: a new aid of endoscopic detection of malignant disease. *Journal of Thoracic and Cardiovascular Surgery*, **42**, 623–629

LIPSON, R. L., BALDES, E. J. and OLSEN, A. M. (1964) A further evaluation of the use of hematoporphyrin derivative as a new aid for the endoscopic detection of malignant disease. *Diseases of the Chest*, **46**, 676–679

LYONS, G. D., OWENS, R., LOUSTEAU, R. J. and TRAIL, M. L. (1980) Carbon dioxide laser treatment of laryngeal stenosis. *Archives of Otolaryngology*, **106**, 255–256

MCDUFF, P. E., DETERLING, R. A., GOTTLIEB, L. S., FAHIMI, H. D., BUSHNELL, D. and ROEBER, F. (1965) Laser surgery of malignant tumours. *Diseases of the Chest*, **48**, 130–139

MCGEE, T. M. (1983) The argon laser in surgery for chronic ear disease and otosclerosis. *Laryngoscope*, **93**, 1177–1182

MCKENZIE, A. L. (1983) How far does thermal damage extend below the surface of CO_2 laser incisions. *Physics in Medicine and Biology*, **28**, 914–920

MAIMAN, T. H. (1960) Stimulated optical radiation in ruby. *Nature*, **187**, 493–494

MESTER, E., MESTER, A. and MESTER, A. (1985) The biochemical effects of laser application. *Lasers in Surgery and Medicine*, **5**, 31–39

MEYER–SCHWICKERATH, G. (1956) Erfahrungen mit der Licht. Koagulation der Netzhaut und der Iris. *Documenta Ophthalmologica*, **10**, 91–131

MIHASHI, S., JAKO, G. J., INCZE, J., STRONG, E. W. and VAUGHAN, C. W. (1976) Laser surgery in otolaryngology – interaction of CO_2 laser and soft tissue. *Annals of the New York Academy of Science*, **267**, 263–294

MINTON, J. P., CARLTON, D. M., DEARMAN, J. R., MCKNIGHT, W. B. and KETCHMAN, A. S. (1965) An evaluation of the physical response of malignant tumour implants to pulsed laser radiation. *Surgery, Gynecology and Obstetrics*, **121**, 538–544

MOTTA, G. (1990) The treatment of laryngeal carcinoma by direct microlaryngoscopy using the CO_2 laser. *Lasers in Medical Science*, **5**, 143–148

NATH, G., GORISCH, W. and KIEFHABER, P. (1973) First laser endoscopy via a fibreoptic transmission system. *Endoscopy*, **5**, 208–213

NORTON, M. L. and DE VOS, P. (1978) A new endotracheal tube for laser surgery of the larynx. *Annals of Otology, Rhinology and Laryngology*, **87**, 554–558

OOSTERHUIS, J. W. (1978) Lymphocytic migration after laser surgery. *Lancet*, i, 446–447

OOSTERHUIS, J. W., VERSCHUEREN, R. C. J., EIBERGEN, R. and OLDHOFF, J. (1982) The viability of cells in the waste products of CO_2 laser evaporation of the Cloudman mouse melanoma. *Cancer*, **49**, 61–67

OSSOFF, R. H., SISSON, G. A., DUCAVAGE, J. A., MOSELLE, H. I., ANDREWS, P. E. and MCMILLAN, W. G. (1984) Endoscopic laser arytenoidectomy for treatment of bilateral vocal cord paralysis. *Laryngoscope*, **94**, 1293–1297

OSSOFF, R. H., SISSON, G. A. and SHAPSAY, S. M. (1985) Endoscopic management of selected early vocal cord carcinoma. *Annals of Otology, Rhinology and Laryngology*, **94**, 560–564

OVERBEEK, J. J. M. VAN, HOEKSEMA, P.E. and EDENS, E. TH. (1984) Microscopic surgery of the hypopharyngeal diverticulum using electrocoagulation or carbon dioxide laser. *Annals of Otology, Rhinology and Laryngology*, **93**, 34–36

PATEL, C. K. N. (1965) CW high power N_2-CO_2 laser. *Applied Physics*, **7**, 15–17

PERKINS, R. C. (1980) Laser stapedectomy for otosclerosis. *Laryngoscope*, **90**, 228–240

PERKINS, R. and CURTON, F. S. (1992) Laser stapedectomy: a comparative study of prosthesis and seal. *Laryngoscope*, **102**, 1321–1327

POLICARD, A. (1924) Etudes sur les aspects offerts par les fumeurs experimentales examinées à la lumière de woods. *CR Societe de Biologie*, **91**, 1423–1425

POWERS, S. K., EDWARDS, M. S. B., BOGGAN, J. E., PITTS, L. H., GUTIN, T. H. and HOSOIBUCHI, Y. (1984) Use of the argon surgical laser in neurosurgery. *Journal of Neurosurgery*, 60, 523–530

PRASAD, U. (1985) CO_2 surgical laser in the management of bilateral vocal cord paralysis. *Journal of Laryngology and Otology*, 99, 891–894

RAAB, O. (1900) Uher die Wirkung fluoreszirenden stoffe auf injusoria. *Zeitschrift für Biologie*, 439, 524

RAUCH, S. D. and BARTLEY, D. Y. M. L. (1992) Argon laser stapedectomy: comparison and traditional fenestration techniques. *American Journal of Otology*, 13, 556

RHYS EVANS, P. H., FRAME, J. W. and BRANDRICK, J. (1986) A review of carbon dioxide laser surgery in the oral cavity and pharynx. *Journal of Laryngology and Otology*, 100, 69–77

RHYS-WILLIAMS, S., VAN HASSELT, C. A., AUN, C. S. T., TONG, M. C. F. and CARRUTH, J. A. S. (1993) Tubeless anaesthetic technique for optimal carbon dioxide laser surgery of the larynx. *Americal Journal of Otolaryngology*, 14, 271–274

RICCI, T. and MAZZONI, M. (1985) Experimental investigation of temperature gradients in the inner ear following argon laser exposure. *Journal of Laryngology and Otology*, 99, 359–362

SATALOFF, J. (1967) Experimental use of the laser in otosclerotic stapes. *Archives of Otolaryngology*, 85, 614–616

SCHAWLOW, A. L. and TOWNES, C. H. (1953) Infrared and optical masers. *Physics Review*, 112, 1940–1949

SCHULLER, D. E., MCCAUGHAN, J. S. and ROCK, R. P. (1985) Photodynamic therapy in head and neck cancer. *Archives of Otolaryngology – Head and Neck Surgery*, 111, 351–355

SHAHEEN, O. H. (1984) The carbon dioxide laser in the treatment of bilateral vocal cord paralysis. In: *Problems in Head and Neck Surgery*. London: Baillière Tindall. p. 9

SHAPSAY, S. M., STRONG, M. S., ANASTASI, G. W. and VAUGHAN, C. W. (1980) Removal of rhinophyma with the carbon dioxide laser: a preliminary report. *Archives of Otolaryngology*, 106, 257–259

SHAPSAY, S. M., BEAMIS, J. F. and DUMON, J. F. (1989) Total cervical tracheal stenosis: treatment by laser, dilation and stenting. *Annals of Otology, Rhinology and Laryngology*, 98, 890–895

SHUGAR, J. M. A., SOM, P. M. and BILLER, H. F. (1982) An evaluation of the carbon dioxide laser in the treatment of traumatic laryngeal stenosis. *Laryngoscope*, 92, 23–26

SIMPSON, G. T., STRONG, M. S., HEALEY, G. D., SHAPSAY, S. M. and VAUGHAN, C. W. (1982) Predictive factors of success or failure in the endoscopic management of laryngeal and tracheal stenosis. *Annals of Otology, Rhinology and Laryngology*, 92, 384–388

SIMPSON, G. T., SHAPSAY, S. M. and VAUGHAN, C. W. (1983) Rhinological laser surgery. *Otolaryngology Clinics of North America*, 16, 837–839

SPARGO, P. M., NIELSON, M. S. and CARRUTH, J. A. S. (1986) Use of a carbon dioxide laser for the treatment of recurrent laryngeal papillomatosis in small children: experience with an anaesthetic technique. *Lasers in Medical Science*, 1, 211–216

STAHLE, J., HOGBERG, L. and ENGSTRÖM, B. (1972) The laser as a tool in inner ear surgery. *Acta Otolaryngologica*, 73, 27–37

STEINER, W. (1993) Results of curative laser microsurgery of laryngeal carcinomas. *American Journal of Otolaryngology, Head and Neck Medicine and Surgery*, 14, 116

STRONG, M. S. (1975) Laser excision of carcinoma of the larynx. *Laryngoscope*, 85, 1286–1289

STRONG, M. S. and JAKO, G. J. (1972) Laser surgery in the larynx. *Annals of Otology, Rhinology and Laryngology*, 811 791–798

STRONG, M. S., VAUGHAN, C. W., HEALEY, G. B., SHAPSAY, S. M. and JAKO, G. J. (1979a) Transoral management of localised carcinoma of the oral cavity using CO_2 laser. *Laryngoscope*, 89, 897–905

STRONG, M. S., VAUGHAN, C. W., JAKO, G. J. and POLANYI, T. (1979b) Transoral resection of cancer of the oral cavity: the role of the CO_2 laser. *Otolaryngology Clinics of North America*, 12, 207–218

STRUNK, C. L. and NICHOLS, M. L. (1990) A comparison of the KTP/532-laser tonsillectomy vs. traditional dissection/snare tonsillectomy. *Otolaryngology – Head and Neck Surgery*, 103, 966–971

THOMA, J., UNGER, V. and KASTENBAUER, E. (1981) Temperatur und Druckmessungen in Innenohr bei der Anwendung der Argon Lasers. *Laryngology Rhinology Otology [Stutts]*, 60, 587–590

THOMA, J., MROWINSKI, D. and KASTENBAUER, E. R. (1986) Experimental investigations on the suitability of the carbon dioxide laser for stapedectomy. *Annals of Otology Rhinology and Laryngology*, 95, 126–131

TRANTER, R. M. D., FRAME, J. W. and BROWNE, R. M. (1985) The healing of CO_2 laser wounds of the larynx. *Journal of Laryngology and Otology*, 99, 895–999

VAN DER WAERDEN (ed.) (1967) English translation in *Sources of Quantum Mechanics*. Amsterdam: North Holland Publishers

WALKER, N. P. J., MATHEWS, J. and NEWSON, S. W. B. (1986) Possible hazards from irradiation with the carbon dioxide laser. *Lasers in Surgery and Medicine*, 6, 84–86

WEISHAUPT, K. R., GOMER, C. J. and DOUGHERTY, T. J. (1976) Identification of singlet oxygen as the cytotoxic agent in photo-inactivation of a murine tumour. *Cancer Research*, 36, 2326–2329

WILE, A. G., DAHLMAN, A., BURNS, R. G. and BERNS, M. W. (1982) Laser photoradiation therapy of cancer following hematoporphyrin sensitization. *Lasers in Surgery and Medicine*, 21, 163–168

WILE, A. G., COFFEY, J., NAHOBEDION, M. Y., BAGHDESSARIAN, R., MASON, G. R. and BERNS, M. W. (1984) Laser photoradiation therapy of cancer: an update of the experience at the University of California, Irvine. *Lasers in Surgery and Medicine*, 4, 5–12

YAHR, W. Z. and STRULLY, K. L. (1966) Blood vessel anastomosis by laser and other biomedical applications. *Journal of the Association of Advanced Medical Instrumentation*, 1, 28–31

YATES, A. and DEDO, H. H. (1984) CO_2 laser enucleation of polypoid vocal cords. *Laryngoscope*, 94, 731–736

ZWENG, H. C. (1971) Lasers in ophthalmology. In: *Laser Applications in Medicine and Biology*, vol. I, edited by M. L. Wolbarsht. New York: Plenum. p. 239

26

Intensive and high dependency care

Gavin Lavery and Adrian Pearce

An intensive therapy unit (ITU) is a geographically defined area in the hospital which utilizes specialized personnel and equipment to provide care for the critically ill. Critical illness may be defined as an unstable condition with impaired vital organ function. Patients may also be admitted to ITU if they have a risk of developing serious and preventable complications. Patients with no chance of survival or whose survival will result in an unacceptably poor quality of life should not, in general, be admitted to the intensive care unit (European Society of Intensive Care Medicine Task Force, 1994).

In essence, ITU should offer the facilities for the early diagnosis, prevention and/or treatment of multiple organ failure. This role of organ support is most clearly seen in respiratory failure. Although ITUs developed as places where mechanical ventilatory support of respiratory function could be provided, it is now inappropriate to view the intensive care unit solely as a place where patients receive mechanical ventilation. The ITU should possess the means to support all the major organ systems, i.e. circulatory support, haemodialysis and other forms of renal support, nutritional support and the ability to treat coagulation disorders, severe infection and metabolic derangement (European Society of Intensive Care Medicine Task Force, 1994).

ITU should gather in one area, equipment, technical expertise and a high concentration of appropriately trained nursing staff which cannot be duplicated elsewhere in the hospital. Although ITU is always one of the most expensive areas for patient treatment in any hospital (£1000–1500+ per day in 1995), every acute hospital requires this capability and concentrating resources in one area is the most cost effective way to do this.

Patient management in ITU requires a team approach. Major elements of the team include medical, nursing, technical, physiotherapy and dietetic staff in addition to the input of radiology, bacteriology and other laboratory-based personnel. To weld this group together, ITU requires a medical director who has specific training and an on-going interest in ITU and who should spend the bulk (if not all) of his time in ITU (Knaus et al., 1986).

Medical responsibility for the patients in ITU varies from unit to unit and between medical systems. At one extreme, treatment is dictated by the referring service at all times. This seems most inappropriate since the people most influencing treatment only assess the patients intermittently and it is difficult for them to see all the pieces in the jigsaw. At the other extreme, all clinical decisions are taken by the ITU medical staff without any reference to the referring service. This seems also to be cavalier and unwise. Most well run units steer a middle path either using a formal written constitution or by informal arrangements between clinicians.

An ITU must function 24 hours every day. For this reason it should be large enough to ensure that it is never empty since this would result in the staff being deployed elsewhere and the unit being unable to respond quickly to clinical needs. Thus an ITU should probably have a *minimum* of six bed spaces. They should have a high nurse: patient ratio (1 : 1 is viewed as appropriate in the UK). To achieve this, each bedspace requires approximately 6.5–7.0 nurses to cover shifts, weekends, holidays, sick and study leave. In addition, each unit needs 24-hour resident medical cover, i.e. a doctor, who has no other clinical commitments, present physically in the unit at all times. Likewise, there must be 24 hour technical back-up available rapidly. Most units also have their own 'in house' laboratory which provides blood gas analysis (at least) and measurement of blood/plasma electrolytes, glucose, lactate, osmolarity and some drug levels.

A significant problem may develop when ITU patients are in the recovery phase of their illness. Often they reach a level of function which makes further ITU management unnecessary but which is still too unstable for care in a general ward. Such patients require admission to a 'step-down' unit providing a level of care which is intermediate between ITU and general ward care. Such units are often called high dependency units (HDUs) and are still relatively uncommon in the UK. The existence of HDUs is essential for the modern approach of progressive patient care in which patients are grouped together depending on their need for care. To confuse the issue further, some units, officially designated ITUs devote a significant or even the majority of their activity to the care of HDU-type patients.

A HDU may be defined as an area for patients requiring more intensive observation, treatment and/or nursing care than can normally be provided on a general ward (Association of Anaesthetists of Great Britain and Ireland, 1991). Such units would not normally accept patients requiring mechanical ventilation beyond a few hours. Costs and staffing of such units are significantly less than that of ITU and the usual nurse:patient ratio is 1 : 2 or 1 : 3.

This chapter outlines the current ITU/HDU management of critical illness in the major organ systems.

Airway and ventilation

The major reason for admission of otolaryngology patients to ITU is a respiratory problem. Although this is usually synonymous with airway obstruction caused by infections, tumours and surgery, there are, in addition, many other indications for the intensive care of our patients which can be follows:

Airway obstruction caused by infection, tumours or surgical intervention.

Lung substance problems e.g. cardiogenic pulmonary oedema, non-cardiogenic pulmonary oedema, aspiration with infection, mucus plugging with atelectasis, trauma to chest wall or lung substance, disease processes, e.g Wegener's granulomas, rheumatoid arthritis.

Pulmonary blood flow deficiency secondary to primary pulmonary hypertension, pulmonary emboli or right heart failure.

Central depression of respiratory centre as a result of drugs, e.g. opioids, benzodiazepines, CNS infections, trauma, epilepsy, cerebral venous or arterial pathology, electrolyte abnormality e.g. hyponatraemia.

Respiratory muscle weakness, phrenic nerve damage, diffuse muscle disease.

In health, a minute volume of ventilation 4–5 l/min and inspired O_2 of 21% will provide normal arterial tensions of CO_2 (5.1 kPa) and O_2 (13 kPa). The work of breathing is only 1–2% of the total oxygen consumption. With respiratory disease, minute volumes of 20 l/min and 100% inspired oxygen may not provide normal arterial gas tensions and the work of breathing may increase 10-fold to the point of cardiac failure. Increased work of breathing cannot be measured scientifically but is suggested by elevated respiratory and heart rates, use of accessory muscles and sweating. Adequacy of gas exchange is gauged by the estimation or measurement of blood gas tensions and pH. Arterial oxygen saturations below 85% will usually cause overt cyanosis. More accurate determinations of oxygen saturation can be made with pulse oximetry and arterial blood gas analysis.

Following assessment of a patient with respiratory difficulties, the following treatment plan, listed in ascending order of intervention, is usually suitable:

1 Raised inspired oxygen by means of nasal cannulae or facemask, with pulse oximetry monitoring. This may be carried out on the ward. A patient with oxygen saturations below 90% with 40% inspired oxygen needs high dependency care. With an appreciably raised work of breathing or saturations less than 85% with inspired oxygen concentrations of 60%, transfer to the ITU is indicated.
2 Continuous positive airway pressure, applied by tightly fitting facemask and suitable circuit with oxygen enriched air.
3 Tracheal intubation via the oro- or nasal route, with maintenance of spontaneous respiration, with or without continuous positive airway pressure.
4 Tracheal intubation and mechanical ventilatory support.

The indications for intubation are:

1 To provide intermittent positive pressure ventilation
2 To protect the airway from blood/secretions/CSF in a compromised patient
3 To maintain patency of the airway in cases of airway narrowing
4 To facilitate suctioning of airway secretions.

In general, it is acceptable to leave *in situ* an oro- or nasotracheal tube for 7–10 days. Beyond this time, in an adult, the laryngeal complications of prolonged intubation become more prominent and it is wise to insert a tracheostomy if intubation is, or will be, required beyond this time. Tracheostomy by percutaneous dilatational techniques in the intensive care unit has become well established (Hazard, 1994) and has substantially reduced the number of requests to the otolaryngological department for this procedure. It is not without problems and a learning curve can clearly be identified. The routine use of a fibrescope (Winkler *et al.*, 1994) to view the wires and dilators clearly entering the trachea may well become standard.

The indications for institution of mechanical ventilation in a patient breathing spontaneously are generally:

1 P_aO_2 < 6 kPa on 60% inspired oxygen
2 P_aCO_2 > 8 kPa with pH < 7.2
3 Patient fatigue
4 Cardiovascular decompensation
5 To stabilize the respiratory system
   a elective postoperatively
   b multisystem failure.

Modes of ventilation

Developments in ventilator design and understanding of respiratory physiology have increased the methods available to the intensivist (Downs, Räsänen and Smith, 1991; Tobin, 1994). Modern ITU ventilators can usually offer the following functions:

Controlled mandatory ventilation

A rigid programme where a set tidal volume and respiratory rate are delivered. Typically the ratio of time allowed for inspiration and expiration (I : E ratio) is 1 : 2 or 1 : 3, i.e. expiration takes longer. In some patients more effective ventilation may be achieved with inverse ratio ventilation of 2 : 1 or 3 : 1.

Intermittent mandatory ventilation

A set tidal volume and respiratory rate are delivered but, in-between machine breaths, the patient may breathe freely through the circuit.

Synchronized intermittent mandatory ventilation

This is a development of the above in which the timing of mandatory inspiratory breaths can be altered slightly to coordinate or synchronize with patient spontaneous breaths.

Pressure support

Pressure support has become a popular mode of ventilatory support. This mode depends on patient effort for initiation of ventilatory support. The ventilator senses the small negative pressure generated in the breathing circuit by the patient at the beginning of inspiration. The ventilator then delivers gas flow to the patient to reach a variable, but clinician adjusted, pressure. This mode of ventilatory assistance matches as closely as possible machine respiratory support with patient respiratory pattern. It cannot be used in patients who are paralysed or heavily sedated, who are then unable to initiate a spontaneous breath. Pressure support may be used to augment spontaneous patient breaths in intermittent mandatory ventilation mode.

In addition to the support provided above, it is possible to provide positive pressure during the expiratory phase. By convention, positive end-expiratory pressure applies to mechanical breaths and continuous positive airway pressure to spontaneous respiration. Clinically useful levels of positive end-expiratory pressure and continuous positive airway pressure are 5–20 cmH$_2$O.

In general, current practice aims to ventilate with the lowest inflation pressure possible, preferably not exceeding 30 cmH$_2$O. Higher pressures are thought to cause further lung damage or at least impair lung healing in adult respiratory distress syndrome. Pressure controlled ventilation with inverse ratio (Shanholtz and Brower, 1994) is in vogue, although there are few formal studies which demonstrate any definite benefit over traditional volume controlled ventilation with positive end-expiratory pressure. Limiting inspiratory pressures may reduce the minute volume delivered, resulting in an elevation of arterial CO$_2$ concentrations. This 'permissive hypercapnia' (Tuxen, 1994) does not seem to be disadvantageous. The inspired oxygen concentration should be at the lowest value that reliably maintains oxygen saturations above 90%. Often the addition of positive end-expiratory pressure or continuous positive airway pressure causes an increase in arterial oxygen saturations for a given inspired oxygen concentration. However, positive end-expiratory pressure may reduce cardiac output and oxygen flux (see later) may be reduced despite an increased saturation. Invasive monitoring of cardiac output may be necessary to select the 'best' positive end-expiratory pressure.

Weaning from ventilatory support

Weaning describes the process of reducing mechanical ventilation until the patient's own spontaneous respiration is sufficient to maintain gaseous homeostasis. Generally, a patient's spontaneous breathing activity is encouraged in order to prevent loss of respiratory muscle bulk from disuse. Ventilatory support is added to augment, rather than replace, spontaneous respiratory activity.

The rapidity of transfer from mechanical ventilation to full spontaneous respiration depends on the purpose and length of ventilation. Overnight elective postoperative ventilation may not require formal weaning before extubation. In those patients who have been on mechanical ventilatory assistance for more than 48 hours, the following manouevres (Beale, 1994) are common, depending on the mode of mechanical ventilation employed:

1 Allowing the patient to breathe spontaneously for short, but daily increasing, periods by disconnection from the ventilator. Often, continuous positive airway pressure is initiated during the periods of

spontaneous respiration. It is important that the patient is reconnected before exhaustion ensues.

2 Steadily decreasing the number of intermittent mandatory ventilation breaths from the ventilator, e.g. by one to two breaths per day. Once only four intermittent mandatory ventilation breaths are required, the patient can usually be transferred to a spontaneous mode.

3 Decreasing the magnitude of set pressure in pressure-support mode.

Before extubation is considered, the patient's general condition should be stable or improving. The patient should be on 40% inspired oxygen or less with a minute volume at rest of less than 120 ml/kg/min producing a normal pH. The forced vital capacity should exceed 1000 ml and the patient should be able to generate a negative pressure within the circuit of 20 cmH$_2$O. Pulmonary secretions should be of small volume. Copious, thick secretions will delay extubation.

Acute lung injury/adult respiratory distress syndrome

The development of severe, life-threatening hypoxaemia, stiff lungs and bilateral infiltrates on chest X-ray in the absence of direct lung injury or infection was reported in 1967 and the term adult respiratory distress syndrome coined. The American-European Consensus Conference on adult respiratory distress syndrome (1994) has reported its recommendations on acute lung injury nomenclature. Acute lung injury is a syndrome of inflammation and increased permeability that is associated with a constellation of clinical, radiological and physiological abnormalities of acute onset that cannot be explained by, but may coexist with, left atrial or pulmonary capillary hypertension. It is associated most commonly with the sepsis syndrome, aspiration, primary pneumonia or multiple trauma. Less common associations are with multiple transfusions, fat embolism and pancreatitis. Adult respiratory distress syndrome, which should properly be acute (not adult) respiratory distress syndrome (Beale *et al.*, 1993) may be regarded as a severe form of acute lung injury.

The characteristic features of acute lung injury are:

Acute onset
Bilateral infiltrates on chest X-ray
Pulmonary capillary wedge pressure < 18 mmHg
No clinical evidence of left atrial enlargement
Arterial hypoxaemia to a P$_a$O$_2$/FIO$_2$ value < 300 mmHg (acute lung injury) or < 200 mmHg (adult respiratory distress syndrome)

Treatment of acute lung injury/adult respiratory distress syndrome is generally aimed at ensuring adequate arterial oxygen tensions by mechanical ventilatory support with positive end-expiratory pressure or continuous positive airway pressure and appropriate inspired oxygen, and protection of oxygen flux to the tissues by maintenance of an adequate cardiac output, guided by invasive monitoring. There is no specific treatment that aids resolution of the pulmonary disease process. Current concerns are avoidance of high inflation pressures and unnecessarily high inspired oxygen concentrations.

Several treatment regimens have been explored, or reintroduced, for the severe case in specialist centres. Nitric oxide, extra- or intracorporeal gas exchange may be beneficial in patients who have profound arterial hypoxaemia, acute lung injury or adult respiratory distress syndrome.

Nitric oxide

The oxides of nitrogen are currently under investigation for a wide range of pharmacological actions (Änggård, 1994; Gaston *et al.*, 1994; Vallance and Collier, 1994; Zapol *et al.*, 1994). Nitric oxide shows the greatest promise in ITU. Discovered to be the same as endothelial derived relaxing factor in 1987, nitric oxide (NO) is an ideal local transcellular messenger. Nitric oxide is synthesized in vascular endothelial cells from L-arginine and diffuses rapidly to nearby vascular smooth muscle. The physiological half-life is less than 5 seconds and it appears to be inactivated by haemoglobin. It is an extremely potent vasodilator, as well as being an important neurotransmitter and mediator of inflammatory cell cytotoxicity. Its vascular smooth muscle relaxation properties have been studied in ITU. When added in controlled concentrations to the inspired gas mixture, NO can be shown to lower pulmonary artery pressures (Rossaint *et al.*, 1993) and possibly promote radiological improvement in adult respiratory distress syndrome patients (Blomqvist *et al.*, 1993). It is not yet clear whether this pharmacological action is translated into worthwhile patient survival.

Extracorporeal gas exchange

These techniques (Van Meurs, Frankel and Pearl, 1992) are theoretically useful in pulmonary disease processes that are acutely severe, but known to resolve fully. Extracorporeal membrane oxygenation involves oxygenation of the blood outside the body. Initially used in 1972 it had a high mortality and fell into disuse. It has recently been reintroduced in paediatric patients with greater success (Delius, Bove and Meliones, 1992), but it is still a highly specialized technique. A slightly more useful technique is extracorporeal carbon-dioxide removal (Gattinoni *et al.*, 1986) with continued insufflation of oxygen to the lungs. This appears to have a lower morbidity because the extracoporeal circulation requires much less of a percentage of native cardiac output than with extracorporeal membrane oxygenation circuits and the lungs receive an adequate flow of oxygenated blood.

Intracorporeal gas exchange

Intracorporeal gas exchange with an intravenous oxygenator has also been described (Conrad *et al.*, 1993) with the oxygenator placed in a large vein.

Heart, circulation and fluid resuscitation

Assuming a haemoglobin concentration of 2.17 mmol/l (14 g/dl), arterial Po_2 of 13 kPa and saturation of 97%, the oxygen content of arterial blood is just under 20 ml oxygen/100 ml of arterial blood. With a normal resting cardiac output of 5 1/min, approximately 1000 ml O_2/minute is delivered to tissues, the oxygen flux. The balance of oxygen delivery and tissue demand in critically ill patients has been extensively researched and the use of this balance in determining the manner of resuscitation in ill patients has been proposed by Shoemaker *et al.* (1988). Briefly, this doctrine suggests that in seriously ill patients, oxygen delivery does not keep up with increased tissue demand, leading to the concept of supply dependent consumption. Tissue oxygen consumption is limited by supply, and augmentation of oxygen delivery by increasing cardiac output will lead to greater, beneficial tissue oxygen consumption. Ideally, oxygen delivery and consumption should be measured in all patients and the cardiac output artificially raised to the point at which tissue consumption levels out. An alternative and less cumbersome approach derived from survival studies is to plot oxygen delivery against consumption, indexed to body surface area square metres (m^2) and attempt to keep the value for delivery above 600 ml/m^2/minute and consumption above 170 ml/m^2/minute.

The attainment of a predetermined global supply/consumption oxygen balance in haemodynamic manipulations of all ill patients has declined in popularity (Russell and Phang, 1994) and has been replaced by a greater appreciation of regional perfusion. However, in ITU patients it is often necessary to answer the question, 'In this ill patient, what is the optimal cardiac output and if the body is incapable of producing or sustaining this cardiac output should it be raised artificially?' This form of cardiovascular measurement and manipulation has become common in the management of patients in ITU.

Monitoring cardiac function

Cardiac output may be measured invasively or non-invasively. Non-invasive techniques include Doppler flowmeters positioned in the sternal notch. A pulsed Doppler shift technique allows measurement of both flow velocity and the cross-sectional area of the aorta and thus calculation of cardiac output. Difficulties may arise in placement of the probe. Ideally, the angle between the ultrasonic beam and descending aorta should be zero. Impedance plethysmography measures the change in voltage across the chest in response to a high frequency current (usually 100 kHz). Electrodes placed around the neck and chest apply the current or record the ensuing voltage. Changes in transthoracic resistance are assumed to be mainly due to changes in blood volume.

Both the above techniques allow measurement of cardiac output non-invasively which, at best, correlates well with invasive measurements. Unfortunately, at times the correlation is poor and even if an accurate reading is obtained no information about cardiac chamber filling, pulmonary or systemic vascular resistance is gained. Assessment of cardiac function in ITU has been reviewed (Shephard, Brecker and Evans, 1994).

Invasive cardiac output measurements require the placement of a catheter in the pulmonary artery. Pulmonary artery catheters are used extensively in intensive therapy units and it is possible to monitor continuously the pulmonary artery pressure, mixed venous oxygen saturation and also make regular measurements of pulmonary artery wedge or occluded pressure, cardiac output and derived values such as pulmonary, systemic vascular resistance and cardiac function. In order to measure cardiac output, a known mass of indicator is injected intravenously and the concentration/time curve of indicator is used to calculate cardiac output. The first indicator was a dye, but a known mass of cold saline is used now. The indicator must be non-toxic, mix rapidly with blood, not alter the system under study and be suitable for repeated measurements. In the case of cold saline, rapid injection is made of a known volume (often 10 ml) of injectate at known temperature just proximal to the right ventricle. A thermistor attached to a catheter in the pulmonary artery measures the temperature/time curve.

The coefficient of variability with repeated measurements of a stable cardiac output can be minimized by attention to accuracy of the volume and temperature of injectate. The most accurate systems use an insulated syringe with measurement of injectate temperature. Each degree centigrade error produces an error of 3% at normal cardiac outputs. It is usual to perform three readings, with injection at the same point of the respiratory cycle and to average the readings. The readings should be within 10% of each other.

Information derived from a pulmonary artery catheter can be extremely useful (Mimoz *et al.*, 1994), but it is important to balance the risks of insertion of the catheter against the information obtained (Eidelman,

Pizov and Sprung, 1994). The catheter can be left *in situ* for some time, but after 4 days the incidence of infection increases sharply (Mermel and Maki, 1994). Monitoring the function of the right ventricle can be useful in some patients (Pinsky, 1993). The difficulty of knowing what global cardiac output is ideal in any particular patient has led to interest in regional perfusion.

Regional perfusion

The importance of splanchnic flow (see sepsis section later) initiated attempts to measure adequacy of gut blood flow/oxygenation. The gastric intramucosal pH (pHi) can be obtained by tonometry (Arnold *et al.*, 1994; Haglund, 1994). In this technique, a gastric tube with a distal, gas permeable, silicon balloon is inserted and the balloon filled with saline. After a 30 minute period of equilibration, the Pco_2 of the saline is measured in a blood gas analyser, together with an arterial blood sample for bicarbonate. These values are fed into a modified Henderson–Hasselbach equation and the intramucosal pH determined. Patients with an initially low pHi (<7.2) that does not increase with resuscitation have a higher mortality than those patients with a pHi initially normal (7.4) or becoming normal with resuscitation (Maynard, 1994). However, abnormally low pHi is a relatively non-specific predictor of poor outcome (Trinder *et al.*, 1995). Once the presence of splanchnic ischaemia has been identified, it may be possible to correct it. General measures to increase blood pressure/cardiac output and oxygen delivery may be adequate or specific manipulation of splanchnic blood flow may be required.

Fluid therapy

The choice of fluid for resuscitation of the shocked patient has been a source of dispute for at least a generation (Ross and Angaran, 1984). Despite a huge literature, the protagonists of crystalloid and colloid cannot agree. Fortunately, most clinicians are not so extreme in their views and use a mixture of crystalloid and colloid fluids. Some points seem beyond argument:

Colloids are more expensive than crystalloids
Colloids may cause anaphylactoid reactions (rarely)
The use of either solution in initial resuscitation allows blood to be used more effectively and safely later in the patient's care
Colloids are more efficient at restoring intravascular volume
Plasma oncotic pressure is better maintained with colloid, but this may or may not be clinically advantageous.

There is little to choose between the two groups of fluids in the resuscitation of hypovolaemic patients to standard end-points for heart rate, blood pressure and subjective assessments of perfusion. Obviously, if this is the case, there is no objective reason for preferring one colloid over another. However, we have no reason to be sure that the endpoints used to compare crystalloid and colloid resuscitation are appropriate.

Due to their longer intravascular half-life, colloids correct intravascular volume more quickly than crystalloids (Shoemaker *et al.*, 1981). Furthermore, it would be expected that crystalloid resuscitation would cause a greater increase in interstitial water than colloid (Hillman, 1986). Advocates of crystalloid resuscitation maintain that this peripheral oedema is of no consequence and that pulmonary oedema is no more likely after crystalloid than colloid. Interstitial oedema may decrease tissue oxygen tension. There are two reasons why this should happen. First, there is an increase in oxygen diffusion distance secondary to a waterlogged interstitium. Second, increased external pressure closes some capillary channels, thereby altering flow in others due to increased tissue pressure secondary to oedema. This fall in tissue oxygenation may slow wound healing, decrease tissue/organ function and reduce immunocompetence.

The most important point in resuscitation is to ensure that the patient has received adequate fluid. This will often mean transfusing three to four times the volume of blood lost when using crystalloid replacement or one and a half times to twice the volume using colloid. When appropriate, filling pressures and cardiac index should be measured using central venous and pulmonary artery pressure monitoring. Many studies have suggested that resuscitation to supranormal levels of cardiac index and tissue oxygen delivery may improve survival (Edwards *et al.*, 1989; Pinsky, 1993). Even if global perfusion appears satisfactory, regional hypoperfusion may exist, particularly in the splanchnic bed (Gottlieb *et al.*, 1983; Edouard *et al.*, 1994). The best clinical guide to good organ perfusion is a urinary output of at least 1 ml/kg/h without the influence of diuretics. Oliguria is an important clinical sign of hypovolaemia and should lead frequently to a fluid challenge and not administration of a loop diuretic. The sequelae of persistent hypovolaemia are tissue hypoxia, multiple organ dysfunction and death. The sequelae of fluid overload (congestive cardiac failure, pulmonary oedema and ventilator dependence) carry a much lower associated mortality.

Inotropes

Positive inotropes increase the force of myocardial contraction, improve cardiac function and increase cardiac output.

Dopamine

In low doses (2 μg/kg/min), dopamine has been used for many years for a renal protective effect, although there is doubt whether it can exert a protective effect on renal function (Baldwin, Henderson and Hickman, 1994; Lancet, 1994). Low doses of dopamine stimulate predominantly dopaminergic DA_1 and DA_2 receptors and the inotropic effect is associated with a marked increase in renal blood flow and sodium excretion. Higher infusion rates also stimulate adrenergic $beta_1$ and alpha receptors. At infusion rates greater than 10 μg/kg/min significant and deleterious peripheral vasoconstriction develops.

Dobutamine

Dobutamine appears to be a mild vasodilator at all doses and is the preferred inotrope in many instances, with the exception of sepsis where adrenaline can be useful. The importance of the splanchnic circulation has raised interest in dopexamine.

Dopexamine

Dopexamine, a dopamine analogue, stimulates predominantly DA_1 and adrenergic beta receptors and is therefore a (weak) inotrope which appears to increase splanchnic blood flow dramatically. Dopexamine certainly does improve oxygen flux in the postoperative period (Boyd, Grounds and Bennet, 1993) and may have a greater beneficial effect on the splanchnic bed than dopamine (Maynard *et al.*, 1992). Infusion of high doses of vasoactive compounds must be guided by information received from invasive monitoring.

Manipulation of the cardiovascular system should follow a logical sequence. In general this sequence is:

1 Is the cardiac output adequate? An inadequate cardiac output is suggested by hypotension, oliguria, cold peripheries and elevated serum lactate.
2 Is the low cardiac output due to hypovolaemia or poor myocardial function? A central venous pressure measurement will aid fluid administration. If it is high (> 12–14 mmHg) an inotrope such as dobutamine (5–20 μg/kg/min) is likely to be useful.
3 A pulmonary artery catheter will give much greater information and should be considered whenever intelligent manipulations based on central venous pressure measurements have failed to produce improvement.
4 Patients with sepsis have rapidly changing haemodynamic profiles and invasive monitoring with appropriate pharmacological support should be initiated early (see Sepsis section).

The brain, sedation and analgesia

The adult human brain receives a global blood flow of 50 ml/100 g/min. It accounts for approximately 20% of the total body oxygen consumption. Global cerebral blood flow is, through autoregulation, independent of perfusion pressure between mean arterial pressures of 60–120 mmHg, but is sensitive to changes in arterial carbon dioxide and oxygen tensions. The sympathetic system plays a minimal role in regulation of cerebral blood flow.

Since the brain is contained within a rigid cranium, the volumes of brain tissue, blood vessels and cerebrospinal fluid are interrelated. An increase in brain tissue volume due to oedema will either displace the other two components from the cranium or cause an increase in intracranial pressure. Elevation of intracranial pressure reduces cerebral blood flow. Cerebral perfusion pressure = mean arterial blood pressure − intracranial pressure.

In otolaryngological patients, common causes of severe brain dysfunction are:

1 Abscess formation or meningitis secondary to mastoid or sinus infection
2 Thrombosis of intracranial blood vessels
3 Interruption of arterial supply or venous drainage
4 Postoperative haematoma formation
5 Abnormal plasma biochemistry especially hyponataemia
6 Intracranial tumours.

It goes without saying that patients with brain dysfunction require treatment of the underlying condition. They also need regular assessment in a high dependency setting and specific treatment of raised intracranial pressure (if present).

Assessment of the patient

Patients with brain pathology or who have undergone operations within or near brain substance, require regular appraisal postoperatively to detect early deterioration. This appraisal can be made by observation of clinical signs (Smith, 1994) or measurement of intracranial pressure.

Clinical evaluation

This may be made objectively by measurement of pupil size and Glasgow coma scale scoring at regular intervals. The Glasgow coma scale score comprises the sum of numerical values for the functions of eye opening, best motor response and best verbal response. Hourly measurements should be performed during the most critical period and then reduced in frequency. Deterioration in Glasgow coma scale score is a worrying feature and patients must be moved to a high dependency area. CT scanning is invaluable to determine whether deterioration is due to a surgically remedial cause.

Intracranial pressure

Intracranial pressure can be measured directly by placement of a fluid-filled catheter within a lateral ventricle and connection to an external pressure transducer, or by placing the transducer itself in the subdural or extradural space. An intraventricular catheter and external pressure transducer allows CSF sampling for analysis and provides the most accurate, dependable pressure readings but at the cost of breaching the dura and subsequent risk of infection. Transducers placed via burr holes into the subarachnoid or subdural space usually provide clinically acceptable readings. The normal intracranial pressure is approximately 12 mmHg. Levels of 15–20 mmHg are reasonably elevated and levels of 40 mmHg and above carry a high mortality. The zero reference point for intracranial pressure measurements is not well established but the tragus provides a visible external reference point. It is important when calculating cerebral perfusion pressure that the transducers for arterial and intracranial pressures are zeroed to the same reference level. In a patient who is positioned head up, a substantial error will arise if the arterial blood pressure is measured at heart level and intracranial pressure at the head.

Treatment of the underlying condition may require antibiotics for infection, restoration of abnormal plasma biochemistry, control of diffuse cerebral oedema and, most importantly, surgical evacuation of intracranial space-occupying lesions such as haematoma and pus. In those patients in whom intracranial pressure is elevated, without a specific intracranial mass, the following methods may be used to optimize cerebral blood flow/control intracranial pressure:

1 Maintenance of normotension, slight head up posture
2 Avoidance of hypoxia and hypercarbia
3 Intermittent positive pressure ventilation to mild hypocarbia $P_a co_2$ 4 kPa
4 Intravenous mannitol 0.25–1 g/kg
5 Intravenous anaesthetic agents such as thiopentone
6 High dose dexamethasone (contentious).

Brain death criteria

In some patients the degree of brain damage is so great that recovery of vital brain-stem function is not possible. The tests for detection of this condition vary between countries and the criteria described are for an adult patient in the UK (Conference of Medical Royal Colleges and their Faculties, 1976). The criteria in babies or children have been described (Farrell and Levin, 1993).

Prerequisites for performing these tests are that a disease process is known to be present or have existed that could cause brain-stem death, the core temperature is greater than 35°C, no pharmacological sedation or muscle relaxation is present and plasma biochemistry is not unduly deranged. The patient, without exception, is comatose on full respiratory support.

The following tests and results indicate brain-stem death:

1 No pupillary response to bright light
2 No gag reflex
3 No carinal reflex
4 No corneal reflex
5 No motor response in the cranial nerve distribution to any somatic pain stimulus
6 No vestibular-ocular reflexes on rotation of the head
7 No eye movement in response to 20 ml of ice cold water injected into the ear after determining the patency of the external auditory canal
8 No respiratory movement in the presence of an arterial $P_a co_2$ in excess of 6.65 kPa and disconnection from the ventilator. A blood gas sample should confirm that the critical $P_a co_2$ was present during the period of observation. A constant flow of oxygen to the tracheal tube during the test will prevent hypoxaemia developing during disconnection.

These tests should be performed by two independent physicians, both experienced in this clinical area. One should be a consultant. A proforma helps to avoid errors in the strict method of testing. If the tests show no brain-stem activity, recovery is not possible. The relatives should be counselled and organ donation discussed.

The tests must be repeated, but there is no standard interval between the two sets of tests. A period of 24 hours is often used and assistance offered to the relatives during this time. Strict adherence to the prerequisites and protocols of testing will demonstrate the presence or absence of brain-stem activity. Absent brain-stem function, as judged by the above criteria, has never reversed and patient recovery is not possible. Ventilatory assistance is withdrawn or organ donation initiated. The time of death is the time that brain-stem death was established.

Sedation and analgesia

Patients in intensive care may require sedation, analgesia and muscle relaxation with opioids, benzodiazepines and non-depolarizing muscle relaxants respectively (Glynn, 1992; Shelley and Wang, 1992). For patients undergoing mechanical ventilation, current practice is to gain patient compliance by use of friendly modes of ventilation and low doses of opioids, benzodiazepines or anaesthetic agents. Muscle relaxation is used infrequently.

Opioids provide analgesia and some degree of sedation. The common side effects are respiratory depression, nausea and vomiting, constipation and miosis. Dependency is not a feature of their use perioperatively but may be a problem if used for several weeks. Respiratory depression may be convenient if patients are mechanically ventilated, or troublesome if breathing spontaneously. Particular care must be taken with the use of opioids in patients with brain dysfunction who are breathing spontaneously; the respiratory depression will exacerbate raised intracranial pressure. Useful drugs are morphine, papaveretum, fentanyl and alfentanil. The particular characteristics of these named drugs in addition to their analgesic activity are:

Morphine

Morphine is an opium alkaloid. It may be administered intravenously, intramuscularly or orally. Preparations of opium alkaloids such as *papaveretum* owe their major analgesic action to morphine. Mild histamine release may accompany the administration of high doses. The half life of elimination is 2–4 hours and the major source of elimination is hepatic metabolism, notably glucuronidation at carbons 3 and 6. Morphine-6-glucuronide is a pharmacologically active, potent opioid which is eliminated by renal excretion. Prolonged narcosis in patients with renal failure is due to this metabolite not the parent compound. Morphine is cheap, well known and dependable. Infusion rates of 2–6 mg/h are usual.

Fentanyl

Fentanyl is a synthetic phenylpiperidine. Cardiovascular stability is prominent and histamine release is minimal. Elimination is via hepatic metabolism and renal excretion of unchanged drug. The half life of elimination is similar to morphine at 2–4 hours.

Alfentanil

Alfentanil is related pharmacologically to fentanyl but has a shorter duration of action, the half life being 90 minutes. The peak onset of action is at 1 minute compared to 5 minutes for fentanyl. The usefulness of alfentanil lies in the intensity of analgesia that is provided by a bolus dose of 1–2 mg prior to turning, physiotherapy or tracheal tube suctioning in the mechanically ventilated patient, and the versatility of an infusion of an opioid with a short half-life and no active metabolites.

Benzodiazepines

Lorazepam, diazepam and midazolam are the drugs in this group that are most often used. The group as a whole provides sedation and amnesia, but no analgesia. Both diazepam and lorazepam have long durations of action, the former due to active metabolites. Midazolam offers considerable advantage over these two older drugs. The structure of midazolam is one which includes pH dependent ring opening. At a pH of 3, within the ampoule, the drug is water soluble, while at pH 7.4 the ring closes with restoration of lipid solubility. Sedation and amnesia are prominent actions of the drug. Hepatic clearance is high and the half-life is only 2 hours. The 1-hydroxy metabolite has some pharmacological activity but appears to be of importance only after prolonged infusions. Bolus administration of 1–5 mg produces rapid sedation but may be accompanied by hypotension caused by a reduction in systemic vascular resistance. In the mechanically ventilated patient, an infusion of 2–6 mg/h produces good quality sedation with minimal cardiovascular upset.

Anaesthetic agents

The only intravenous agent currently in use is di-isopropylphenol (Propofol). This drug has a high clearance and when given by infusion will provide rapidly adjustable levels of sedation. Cardiovascular depression is minimal during infusions, but may be prominent with bolus doses. Unfortunately, the drug is not water soluble and the lipid solubilizer has been implicated as the cause of irreversible metabolic acidosis and death in children receiving infusions over several days. It is recommended that the infusion rate should be kept within 4 mg/kg/h by concomitant use of opioids or benzodiazepines. It is an extremely useful drug in patients who are difficult to sedate in ITU.

Inhalational anaesthetic agents have been used (Spencer and Willatts, 1994). Nitrous oxide cannot be used because it interferes with vitamin B_{12} metabolism and causes bone marrow depression. The volatile agent, isoflurane, has been used with success, although it is relatively expensive. It is administered by calibrated vaporizer in the breathing circuit and produces sedation/anaesthesia. The drug appears to have little toxicity, probably because it is minimally metabolized. Enflurane is not useful because the inorganic fluoride metabolite is toxic to the kidney. A major disadvantage of using inhalational agents in ITU is the requirement to scavenge waste gases to minimize staff exposure to these agents.

Renal support

There are many factors associated with the development of acute renal failure in the ITU patient. In practice, most of these patients exhibit several of the factors listed and renal dysfunction can rarely be attributed to any single one. Common pharmacological causes of acute renal failure include high doses of some radiological contrast media, toxic plasma levels of some antibiotics, e.g. the aminoglycosides, the use of non-steroidal anti-inflammatory agents, cyclosporin A and antimitotics, e.g. cis-platinum and methotrexate (Parsons, 1980). As the understanding of renal pathophysiology has advanced, strategies have been developed which should reduce the incidence of acute renal failure. Adequate fluid replacement guided by central venous or pulmonary artery pressure, adequate blood transfusion, attention to oxygen transport and early nutritional support may all be important. The use of dopamine (2–3 μg/kg/min) or dopexamine (0.5–1.0 μg/kg/min) may increase renal blood flow and promote urine flow. Although such a strategy is often used in at risk patients there is no objective evidence that it prevents acute renal failure.

Indications for renal replacement therapy (dialysis) can be summarized as the presence of hyperkalaemia, fluid overload, metabolic acidosis or a high plasma level of urea and creatinine. The absolute values of the latter which trigger the decision to dialyse vary between centres. The techniques available are intermittent techniques such as peritoneal dialysis and haemodialysis and several continuous techniques such as continuous venovenous haemofiltration, continuous arteriovenous haemofiltration and continuous venovenous haemodialysis (Allen, 1990).

Peritoneal dialysis

Peritoneal dialysis was the original method for renal support and uses the peritoneal membrane as a dialysis membrane. Dialysis fluid is run into the peritoneal cavity, allowed to equilibrate with the blood in the peritoneal vasculature, then drained out. Peritoneal dialysis is simple, cheap and is usually associated with circulatory stability. It is contraindicated in abdominal sepsis and may also be contraindicated after previous abdominal surgery. The clearance of urea with this method is relatively inefficient and plasma urea may hardly decrease in severely catabolic patients. Major disadvantages with peritoneal dialysis are first, it can predispose to peritonitis and second, respiratory function is usually impaired due to abdominal distension and splinting of the diaphragm. The latter often necessitates the use of mechanical ventilation or prevents the withdrawal of mechanical ventilation.

Haemodialysis

This is by far the commonest method of renal replacement in ICU. It is usually performed for a 3 or 4 hour session on a daily or alternate day basis. It is a more efficient technique than peritoneal dialysis and may be particularly advantageous in the severely catabolic patient with acute renal failure in whom there is a very rapid rise of urea and creatinine. Haemodialysis was originally performed through surgical or plastic arteriovenous connections. For short term acute renal failure, haemodialysis is now usually achieved using a double lumen cannula inserted into a large vein, e.g. the femoral or subclavian veins.

The gastrointestinal tract
Stress ulcer prophylaxis

In critical illness, the reported incidence of macroscopic upper gastrointestinal tract bleeding is 5–15% (Shuman, Shuster and Zuckerman, 1987). There would appear to be many causes for this but the basis of the problem is an imbalance between the protective and destructive influences acting on the gastric/duodenal mucosa (Mackenzie, 1993). Hydrochloric acid and pepsin are the main destructive factors while gastric mucus, bicarbonate and endogenous prostaglandins are protective. Although stress ulceration is normally attributed to hyperacidity, most critically ill patients exhibit a reduction in acid secretion. It is more likely that background hypoperfusion and tissue hypoxia act to reduce the protective influences on the mucosa and thus compromise its integrity even in the face of a reduced threat (in terms of acidic attack). Historically, prevention of stress ulceration has concentrated on antagonism of gastric acidity, first with antacids (alkalis) administered intragastrically and later with histamine-2 receptor antagonists which are administered systemically. Recently the use of sucralfate, an agent which increases mucosal defences, has gained popularity.

Antacids

These are effective but need to be administered frequently (1–2 hourly). They are labour intensive and also add to the volume of material within the stomach. In addition they may cause diarrhoea, constipation or electrolyte disturbances depending on the salt(s) contained. In their favour, they are cheap and effective.

Histamine-2 receptor antagonists

These agents are usually administered intravenously in ITU and are not only as effective as antacids in reducing gastric acidity, but also reduce the volume of gastric secretions rather than adding to them. Many agents are available and differ mainly in their duration of action. *Ranitidine*, 50–100 mg 6 hourly, is a widely used regimen. Other agents in the group are cimetidine and famotidine. The *proton pump inhibitors* cause similar effects on gastric acid production but by a different mechanism.

Antacids, H$_2$ antagonists and proton pump inhibitors have their prophylactic effect by increasing gastric pH, ideally to > 3.5. This abolishes the bactericidal action of gastric secretions and predisposes to colonization of the stomach by Gram-negative bacilli originating further down the gastrointestinal tract. This may increase the incidence of Gram-negative pulmonary infection.

Sucralfate

This is a complex of sucrose octasulphate and aluminium hydroxide which has no direct effect on acid secretion but which seems to enhance protective factors by increasing endothelial mucus and bicarbonate production. It also adsorbs pepsin and bile salts. Sucralfate seems to increase the mucosal levels of protectant prostaglandins and stimulates endothelial cell proliferation and repair. It should be noted that the protectant effects of sucralfate are achieved while maintaining normal gastric acidity and this may safeguard against Gram-negative colonization. The use of sucralfate has been shown to reduce the incidence of nosocomial pneumonia by up to 50% in some patient groups (Driks et al., 1987).

A recently published study (Cook et al., 1994) in over 2200 patients found that only coagulopathy and respiratory failure predisposed to an increased risk of clinically significant gastrointestinal bleeding. Many intensivists now feel that, with improvements in mechanical ventilation, nutritional techniques, inotropic support of the circulation and prevention of infection, routine stress ulcer prophylaxis is no longer necessary. We need to confirm that the use of enteral nutrition in association with vasodilators (and potential oxygen radical scavengers) reduces the incidence of stress ulceration to such a low level that prophylactic measures become obsolete.

Nutritional support, the gut and multiorgan dysfunction syndrome

Simple starvation leads to the exhaustion of glycogen stores within 48 hours and an increase in glucose production from amino acids derived from breakdown of body proteins (gluconeogenesis). The glucose provided is used to fuel the brain and red blood cells which cannot normally utilize other substrates. This produces a rate of body protein breakdown which would be life-threatening if unchecked. Fortunately, in persistent uncomplicated starvation, the body switches to fat as the predominant energy source and the brain adapts to use ketones as a metabolic fuel, thereby allowing gluconeogenesis to slow down (Meguid, Collier and Howard, 1981). Unfortunately, in critical illness (particularly when complicated by sepsis) gluconeogenesis is not suppressed and this has to be fuelled by rapid protein breakdown – the so-called hypermetabolic or hypercatabolic state in which the body appears to be the victim of autocannibalism. Such protein breakdown has significant deleterious effects on organ function and outcome. By

providing exogenous glucose, amino acids and other nutrients it is hoped to modify this process.

Enteral and parenteral nutrition

Enteral nutrition is immunologically, nutritionally, and metabolically superior to feeding using the parenteral route. The present preference for enteral nutrition could be justified on the basis that it is less expensive, does not require central venous cannulation with its attendant complications and is less likely to produce fluid overload, hyperglycaemia or hypophosphataemia. While these points do represent advantages of enteral nutrition over the parenteral route, they are no longer viewed as the most significant. To appreciate fully the superiority of enteral nutrition we should consider the effects of critical illness and lack of luminal nutrients on the gastrointestinal tract.

Absorption and barrier function in critical illness

The mucosal cells of the gastrointestinal tract have one of the highest turnover rates of any body tissue. Endothelial renewal depends on the division and subsequent migration of stem cells within the mucosal crypts. An intact gut mucosa depends on a balance between cell renewal and exfoliation. It is recognized now that, even in critical illness, the gut remains physiologically and metabolically active to allow the controlled absorption of nutrients, while providing a barrier to the passage of toxins and bacteria from the lumen of the gut into the portal circulation. Barrier function is achieved by a series of elements: the intact mucosal layer with competent tight junctions between cells, lymphocytes, macrophages and neutrophils in the submucosa together with Peyers' patches and gut-generated IgA.

Contrary to clinical appearances, the gut is probably one of the first organs to suffer from the fall in perfusion and tissue oxygenation which takes place in many forms of critical illness (Wilmore et al., 1988). Hypoperfusion of the splanchnic circulatory bed may persist after apparently adequate fluid resuscitation (Gottlieb et al., 1983) and it would appear that even short periods of circulatory compromise may result in prolonged gut ischaemia/hypoxia (Edouard et al., 1994) with resultant cell necrosis and loss of mucosal integrity. This process may be exacerbated by starvation, change in gut flora due to the use of broad spectrum antibiotics and, possibly, reperfusion injury following periods of hypovolaemia and hypotension.

Bacterial translocation may happen following the loss of barrier function (often due to shock or sepsis), immunocompromise or alteration of gut flora. It is defined as the migration of bacteria across the intestinal mucosal barrier to the liver, spleen or mesenteric lymph nodes. Similarly endotoxin can cross the barrier when gut function is impaired. When such processes take place, the Kupffer cells in the liver prevent spill-over into the systemic circulation to a limited extent. However, when there is major dysfunction of the gut barrier, such spill-over happens because the liver is overwhelmed by the amount of bacteria and/or endotoxin presented and also because the underlying cause of gut barrier failure (e.g. hypoperfusion) will have simultaneously adversely affected the liver to prevent it from phagocytosing bacteria efficiently and removing endotoxin in the portal blood. Organisms which breech the mucosal element of the gut-barrier may be phagocytosed by macrophages and transported to the mesenteric lymph nodes. Yet again, if the microbial load is sufficient, these microorganisms may reach the circulation via lymph flow. Although translocation in man is not proven as a common phenomenon during critical illness, there are significant animal data and circumstantial evidence to support it. The presence of circulating endotoxin has itself been found to increase intestinal permeability in healthy humans (O'Dwyer *et al.*, 1988). According to the gut origin hypothesis for multiorgan dysfunction syndrome, the systemic circulation of bacteria/endotoxin causes macrophage activation, cytokine release, neutrophil protease release, free radical generation and complement activation – the systemic inflammatory response syndrome. This inflammatory response causes cellular injury, necrosis and ultimately multiple organ dysfunction.

Kudsk *et al.* (1983) showed that enterally fed rats had a higher survival rate than parenterally fed rats after *Escherichia coli*-induced peritonitis. Another study found that, although parenteral feeding was associated with greater weight gain and fat deposition, enteral nutrition was associated with greater intestinal mass and nitrogen content and, furthermore, that there was improved survival after haemorrhagic hypotension (Zaloga *et al.*, 1991). Moore *et al.* (1992) published a meta-analysis of eight studies which compared enteral and parenteral nutrition in surgical patients. Infective complications were significantly less frequent in the enteral nutrition groups and there was a lower incidence of pneumonia, intra-abdominal abscesses and, not unexpectedly, catheter sepsis.

It should be stressed that, even when catheter-related sepsis is excluded, parenteral nutrition is associated with a significantly higher incidence of infective complications than enteral nutrition. In animals, enteral nutrition is associated with less intestinal mucosal atrophy, liver dysfunction, bacterial translocation, greater immunocompetence and better survival after a variety of systemic insults.

Timing and method of delivering enteral nutrition

Which clinical findings should indicate the need for enteral feeding? The presence of bowel sounds, though comforting, is irrelevant. Many patients with no bowel sounds may tolerate and absorb nasogastric feeds. In contrast, gastric stasis, leading to high aspirates and vomiting, may be seen even when bowel sounds are present. Often a low nasogastric aspirate (< 250–300 ml in 24 hours) is the most appropriate prompt to initiate feeding.

After patients have suffered from a prolonged period of poor nutrition, initiation of feeding may produce severe hypophosphataemia and other electrolytic disturbances which can lead to acute respiratory failure, cardiac dysfunction, and neurological problems – the so-called *refeeding syndrome*. The early phases of enteral feeding require particular attention to metabolic and biochemical status.

Gastric stasis is a common problem which, increasingly, may be overcome by the use of feeding (surgical) jejunostomy tubes, nasoduodenal or nasojejunal tubes. Persuading feeding tubes to negotiate the pyloric canal and remain in position can be a problem. Within 24 hours of insertion only 15–20% of fine bore tubes spontaneously enter the duodenum from the stomach. Drugs which increase motility, such as metoclopramide or cisapride, have been advocated but have little objective evidence to support them. Endoscopic guidance or fluoroscopy are useful – the latter having a 95% success rate. With such strategies, it is possible to feed patients via the enteral route within 24 hours of major surgery. Grahm, Zadronzy and Harrington (1989) reported a controlled trial in head injured patients, which showed that aggressive early jejunal feeding was associated with fewer infective complications and shorter ITU and hospital stays than standard nasogastric feeding.

Most ITUs deliver enteral nutrition by continuous infusion into the gastrointestinal tract rather than bolus feeding. This reduces gastrointestinal side effects but may lead to increased Gram-negative colonization of the upper tract. The simple strategy of stopping enteral infusion for a period to permit a (bactericidal) decrease in intragastric pH has been shown to reduce the incidence of Gram-negative pulmonary infection (Lee, Chang and Jacobs, 1990). Current practice is to feed continuously for 18–20 hours and then have a 4–6 hour break, usually during the night.

The daily maintenance requirements vary between patients and in any given patient at different stages of their illness. Typical values for ITU patients for 24 hours are:

Water 35–40 ml/kg
Sodium 1–1.5 mmol/kg
Potassium 0.6–0.8 mmol/kg
Calories 20–30 kcal/kg
Nitrogen 0.2–0.3 g/kg (increased in severe illness)
Calorie: nitrogen ratio
  150:1 (moderate illness)
  100:1 (sepsis/multiorgan dysfunction syndrome/hypercatabolism).

Recent and future developments

Despite very aggressive nutritional support, it has proved impossible to prevent substantial body protein loss in severely catabolic patients for whom a different approach needs to be employed. If catabolism alters the body's requirements then, if those altered needs are addressed, the patient's anabolic response to severe illness may be enhanced.

Glutamine is the principal fuel for the enterocytes and also plays a significant role in immune function. Its concentration is approximately 30 times higher in skeletal muscle than in plasma. Muscle breakdown during acute illness releases vast quantities of endogenous glutamine. Despite this, tissue uptake is so great that circulating levels are low and remain so even into the recovery phase. Demand for glutamine during critical illness is such that it cannot be satisfied by endogenous supplies and therefore it should be viewed as a conditionally essential aminoacid. The use of oral glutamine in rats reduces bacterial translocation (Alverdy, Aoys and Moss, 1988) and when added to parenteral nutrition appears to enhance gut immune function. In addition, glutamine is a natural building block for the reducing agent glutathione and may have a role in reducing free radical activity.

In animals, improved immunocompetence has been associated with the use of specific nutrients such as arginine (Saito *et al.*, 1987), RNA and omega-3 fatty acids. Utilization of omega-6 fatty acids in the body results in the production of dienoic prostaglandins such as prostaglandin E2 which has an immunosuppressive effect due to its action on T cells. In contrast, omega-3 fatty acids alter prostaglandin synthesis from the dienoic to the trienoic pathway and reduce prostaglandin E2 levels. Guinea-pigs fed omega-3 fatty acids, had a reduced mortality after endotoxin administration (Mascioli *et al.*, 1988). It should be noted, however, that a recent study has suggested that rats receiving a diet enriched with omega-3 fatty acids had weaker operative wounds than 'control-fed' rats, 30 days after surgery (Albina, Gladen and Walsh, 1993). Daly *et al.* (1992) compared a supplemented feed containing all of these nutrients (Impact: Sandoz Nutrition Corp., Minneapolis) with a standard feed (Osmolite HN, Ross Laboratories, Columbus, Ohio) in 85 patients who had surgery for upper gastrointestinal malignancy. The supplemented feed, when compared with the standard feed, was associated with fewer infectious or wound complications, better lymphocyte mitogenesis at the seventh postoperative day and a significantly shorter hospital stay. It must be noted however that the supplemented group also had a higher calorie and nitrogen intake and better nitrogen balance.

In 1961, the administration of pituitary gland extract to a group of severely burned patients was found to reduce urinary nitrogen excretion and improve other nutritional parameters (Liljedahl *et al.*, 1961). By the 1980s recombinant human growth hormone was available and Manson and Wilmore (1986) showed, in a placebo-controlled study using normal subjects, that the beneficial effect on nitrogen balance could be achieved even with low calorie intakes. A similar improvement in nitrogen balance associated with the use of human growth hormone was demonstrated in a randomized placebo-controlled trial in patients receiving parenteral nutrition after major gastrointestinal surgery (Jiang *et al.*, 1989). When administered to children with burns, human growth hormone reduced the healing time of skin donor sites by up to 4 days when compared with injections of a saline placebo and, in the most severely burned, decreased the period in hospital from a mean of 46 to 32 days (Herndon *et al.*, 1990).

Sepsis

The usual clinical manifestations of septicaemia are hypotension, tachycardia, pyrexia and warm flushed peripheries. The early cardiovascular changes can be summarized by stating that there is peripheral vasodilatation with an elevated cardiac index, low arterial pressure and low filling pressures. Younger patients with more cardiac reserve, may well not become hypotensive due to their substantial ability to increase cardiac index. In resuscitation, the first priority is reversal of the effective hypovolaemia (see earlier).

Resuscitation

The aggressive infusion of colloid and/or crystalloid under the guidance of central venous or pulmonary artery wedge pressures will stabilize the condition in many patients. If further action is necessary then an inotrope is indicated. Both dopamine or dobutamine are used, although the former is often more effective in restoring blood pressure when used as the sole agent. Should it prove impossible to attain an adequate blood pressure then the problem is usually one of profound vasodilatation. In such cases a controlled infusion of a vasoconstrictor such as noradrenalin or phenylephrine may restore pressure and return coronary perfusion to normal. Dobutamine promotes greater improvements in perfusion than dopamine (Francis, Sharma and Hodges, 1982) and is the inotrope of choice when a vasoconstrictor has been added to maintain pressure. When using noradrenaline in this way, it is important to use a pulmonary artery flotation catheter to ensure that excessive vasoconstriction, assessed globally, does not take place. Even then there is no objective guide to the flow through regional capillary networks. The guiding principles of haemodynamic manipulations in sepsis are first, to restore normovolaemia, second, use an inotrope, e.g. dopamine and/or dobutamine, then third, use the smallest dose of noradrenalin which is compatible with acceptable blood pressure.

Even with the above measures, some patients remain grossly vasodilated, hypotensive and usually die of refractory cardiovascular failure. The role of nitric oxide (see earlier) in producing refractory vasodilatation is unclear. It is possible to envisage that patients who do not respond to vasoconstrictors might be under the influence of high NO production and may respond to an agent which blocked NO synthesis. No clinically suitable agent is yet available for this purpose.

Antimicrobials

Antibiotics should be administered as soon as possible. At this point the nature of the microorganisms concerned is usually not known. Therefore, it is standard practice to use double or even triple antibiotic therapy to cover all possible causative organisms. Fungi should not be forgotten as possible causative agents, especially in patients who have been on long-term broad spectrum antibacterial agents. The next step is to identify and remove potential sources of sepsis. Wounds should be examined and probed if necessary. All intravascular lines and the urinary catheter should be changed.

Investigating the source of infection

Often the source of sepsis is obvious. In other cases, however, full examination fails to reveal a problem. This group of patients needs persistent investigation. First, cultures should be taken from blood, sputum, urine, CSF and any surgical drains. A chest X-ray may reveal a pulmonary infection and/or the presence of fluid in the pleural cavity. If the latter is present, a diagnostic tap and/or paracentesis via a chest drain will be necessary. If cultures, X-ray and clinical examination are unrewarding, the location of an occult source of sepsis might be elsewhere, in the abdominal cavity (including the pelvis), the intracranial space or paranasal sinuses.

These possibilities can often be narrowed down further by otolaryngological evaluation and/or lumbar puncture. The abdominal cavity may be assessed non-invasively by either ultrasound, CT or a labelled white cell scan. After all three of these investigations have been performed and repeated there should be an 80% 'pick up' rate for septic foci within the abdomen/pelvis (Hinsdale and Jaffe, 1984). Once located, a septic focus may be obliterated either by radiologically-guided percutaneous drainage or by surgical laparotomy. There is still an indication for diagnostic laparotomy which will occasionally find a lesion previously missed by other forms of investigation. Laparotomy may need to be repeated after an interval before all sources of sepsis can be excluded.

Immunotherapy in sepsis

The translocation of gut organisms and endotoxin (see earlier) may well set the scene for later systemic sepsis and multiorgan dysfunction syndrome. Although the mechanisms by which Gram-negative bacteria and/or endotoxin gain entry to the systemic circulation are unclear, it does take place. Many researchers have addressed the effects of circulating endotoxin and cytokines, and mechanisms to reduce or abolish such effects. Endotoxin, a lipopolysaccharide, is a component of Gram-negative bacterial cell walls. It consists of a polysaccharide linked to a lipid segment (lipid A) which is identical in many Gram-negative organisms. This has allowed the development of antibodies against lipid A which are effective against endotoxin arising from a wide range of Gram-negative organisms. The use of such compounds straddles the border between prevention and treatment of infection. The most promising compound in this group was HA-1A, a human monoclonal antibody against endotoxin. In a large multicentre trial it appeared to reduce mortality in patients with Gram-negative bacteraemia, especially if this was associated with shock (Zeigler *et al.*, 1991). There has been much discussion regarding possible sources of error in this important study (Warren, Danner and Munford, 1992). Further work appears to refute the findings of Zeigler and her colleagues and suggests that there is a need to diagnose endotoxinaemia more readily at the bedside (McCloskey *et al.*, 1994).

Attention has moved to other mediators of sepsis – cytokines such as tumour necrosis factor (TNF), interleukins (IL) 1, 2 and 6. These cytokines are produced by macrophages after direct or indirect stimulation by endotoxin. They have damaging effects on cells both locally, at the point of production, and systemically. Experimentally, murine antibody to tumour necrosis factor has been shown to reduce the incidence of septic shock following a bacteraemic challenge (Tracy *et al.*, 1987; Exley, Cohen and Buurman, 1990). The concept of blocking the effects of tumour necrosis factor is, however, not as appealing as that of anti-endotoxins since tumour necrosis factor (unlike endotoxin), has a function in health within the circulation. Antagonism of tumour necrosis factor might be expected to have some surprising and unwelcome effects. It is significant that two anti-tumour necrosis factor agents have not yet progressed to full clinical trials.

Yet another approach is the use of interleukin receptor antagonist -IL1ra. Again, despite early promise, a recent trial has failed to produce convincing evidence of efficacy. Although monoclonal technology appears to show promise, we have yet to translate this into the clinical arena.

Scoring systems

In ITU, scoring systems have the potential to provide an objective way of measuring parameters such as severity of illness, physiological disturbance, organ failure, therapeutic intervention or multiple injury. Their main application is to facilitate comparison between different groups of patients (Palazzo and Patel, 1993). This may be important in the justification of resources or assessment of changes in management within a single ITU or for the comparison of outcomes in similar patients from different units. The most commonly applied scoring systems in intensive care today are the APACHE II scoring system and the therapeutic intervention scoring system.

Acute physiology and chronic health evaluation (APACHE) II system

The acute physiology and chronic health evaluation system was devised in 1981 and simplified in 1985 into the APACHE II scoring system (Knaus *et al.*, 1985). It attributes points to acute physiological disturbance, level of consciousness (based on Glasgow coma score), chronic health and age of the patient. The degree by which the physiological parameters diverge from the normal range dictates whether that parameter will score 1, 2, 3 or 4 points. There are 12 such acute parameters included in the system. In general the higher the APACHE II score the greater the severity of illness and the greater the likelihood of mortality. The APACHE II score can be included in a logistic regression equation along with the diagnostic category to derive a probability for hospital death. This aspect of its use has not been generally accepted and most authorities would concede that the APACHE II system may give guidance regarding the statistical chance of survival with a given severity of illness, but should not be used for prognostication in individual patients.

APACHE III has been developed in an attempt to improve the accuracy of prediction for hospital death. It requires considerably more data collection and is more complex than its predecessor. At present, its use is severely limited since the coefficients for each diagnostic category are not in the public domain.

Therapeutic intervention scoring system (TISS)

The therapeutic intervention scoring system (TISS) was introduced in 1974 as a method of measuring the utilization of intensive care resources and the nursing requirements of individual ITU patients. It was subsequently updated in 1983 and now comprises 76 therapeutic interventions for which points between 1 and 4 are allocated (Keene and Cullen, 1983). Changes in medical practice over time have created problems for the therapeutic intervention scoring system. Some therapeutic interventions have become less popular and fallen out of use, while new methods of treatment have been added. This has resulted in modification to the scoring system and many units have developed their own variation of it. Lack of uniformity is a major flaw within the therapeutic intervention scoring system. If consensus could be reached on a uniform scoring system, it would be extremely useful as it reflects nursing dependency and, to some degree, the cost of ITU treatment.

There are no perfect systems for the assessment of illness severity or its relationship with final outcome. The APACHE II system reflects the severity of illness and all the physiological abnormalities of the patient but takes no account of the amount of ITU support required to maintain that physiological status. The therapeutic intervention scoring system on the other hand reflects the amount of nursing and intensive therapy directed at the patient but takes no account of the severity of the patient's illness. Obviously if both these systems are used then a more complex assessment of the casemix in ITU is possible.

Many other scoring systems exist, e.g. the organ failure score, the simplified acute physiology score (SAPS) which has now been modified to SAPS 2. There are also scores for specific types of patients; PRISM for paediatric intensive care and injury severity score (ISS) and the TRISS methodology for trauma patients (Boyd, Tolson and Copes, 1987).

References

ALBINA, J. E., GLADDEN, P. and WALSH, W. R. (1993) Detrimental effects of omega-3 fatty acid-enriched diet on wound healing. *Parental and Enteral Nutrition*, **17**, 519–521

ALLEN, M. J. (1990) Renal replacement therapy in the intensive care unit. *Hospital Update*, **10**, 828–837

ALVERDY, J. C., AOYS, E. and MOSS, G. (1988) Total parenteral nutrition promotes bacterial translocation from the gut. *Surgery*, **104**, 185–190

ÄNGGÅORD, E. (1994) Nitric oxide: mediator, murderer, and medicine. *Lancet*, i, 1199–1206

ARNOLD, J., HENDRIKS, J., INCE, C. and BRUINING, H. (1994) Tonometry to assess the adequacy of splanchnic oxygenation in the critically ill patient. *Intensive Care Medicine*, **20**, 452–456

ASSOCIATION OF ANAESTHETISTS OF GREAT BRITAIN AND IRELAND (1991) The high dependency unit- acute care for the future.

BALDWIN, L., HENDERSON, A. and HICKMAN, P. (1994) Effect of postoperative low-dose dopamine on renal function after elective major vascular surgery. *Annals of Internal Medicine*, **120**, 744–747

BEALE, R. (1994) Weaning from mechanical ventilation, causes of difficulty and methods of assessing success. *British Journal of Intensive Care*, **4**, 168–175

BEALE, R., GROVER, E. R., SMITHIES. M. and BIHARI, D. (1993) Acute respiratory distress syndrome (ARDS): no more than a severe lung injury? *British Medical Journal*, **307**, 1335–1339

BLOMQVIST, H., WICKERTS, C. J., ANDREEN, M., ULLBERG, U., ÖRTQVIST, Å. and FROSTELL, C. (1993) Enhanced pneumonia resolution by inhalation of nitric oxide? *Acta Anaesthesiologica Scandinavica*, **37**, 110–114

BOYD, O., GROUNDS, R. M. and BENNETT, E. D. (1993) The use of dopexamine hydrochloride to increase oxygen delivery postoperatively. *Anesthesia and Analgesia*, **76**, 372–376

BOYD, C. R., TOLSON, M. A., and COPES, W. S. (1987) Evaluating trauma care: the TRISS method. *Journal of Trauma*, **27**, 370–378

CONFERENCE OF MEDICAL ROYAL COLLEGES AND THEIR FACULTIES (1976) Diagnosis of brain death. Statement issued by the honorary secretary of the Conference of Medical Royal Colleges and their Faculties in the United Kingdom. 1976. *British Medical Journal*, **2**, 1187–1188

CONRAD, S. A., EGGERSTEDT, J. M., MORRIS, V. F. and ROMERO, M. D. (1993) Prolonged intracorporeal support of gas exchange with an intravenacaval oxygenator. *Chest*, **103**, 158–161

COOK, D. J., FULLER, H. D., GUYATT, G. H., MARSHALL, J. C., LEASA, D., HALL, R. *et al.* (1994) Risk factors for gastrointestinal bleeding in critically ill patient. *New England Journal of Medicine*, **330**, 377–381

DALY, J. M., LIEBERMANN, M. D., GOLDFINE, J. SHOU, J., WEINTRAUB, F., ROSATO, E. F., *et al.* (1992) Enteral nutrition with supplemental arginine, RNA, and omega-3 fatty acids in patients after operation: immunologic, metabolic and clinical outcome. *Surgery*, **112**, 56–57

DELIUS, R. E., BOVE, E. L. and MELIONES, J. N. (1992) Use of extracorporeal life support in patients with congenital heart disease. *Critical Care Medicine*, **20**, 1216–1222

DRIKS, M. R., CRAVEN, D. E., CELLI, B. R., MANNING, M., GARVIN, G. M., KUNCHES, L. M., *et al.* (1987) Nosocomial pneumonia in intubated patients given sucralfate as compared with antacids or histamine type-2 blockers. *New England Journal of Medicine*, **317**, 1386–1392

EDOUARD, A. R., DEGREMONT, A-C., DURANTAEU, J., PUSSARD, E., BERDEAUX, A. and SAMII, K. (1994) Heterogeneous regional vascular responses to simulated transient hypovolaemia in man. *Intensive Care Medicine*, **20**, 414–420

EDWARDS, J. D., BROWN, G. C. S., NIGHTINGALE, P., SLATER, R. M. and FARRAGHER, E. B. *et al.* (1989) Use of survivor's cardiorespiratory values as therapeutic goals in septic shock. *Critical Care Medicine*, **17**, 1098–1103

EIDELMAN, L. A., PIZOV, R. and SPRUNG, C.L. (1994) Pulmonary artery catheterization – at the crossroads? *Critical Care Medicine*, **22**, 543–545

EUROPEAN SOCIETY OF INTENSIVE CARE MEDICINE TASK FORCE (1994) Guidelines for the utilisation of intensive care units. *Intensive Care Medicine*, **20**, 163–164

EXLEY, A. R., COHEN, J. and BUURMAN, W. (1990) Murine monoclonal antibody to recombinant human tumour necrosis factor in the treatment of severe septic shock. *Lancet*, i, 1275–1276

FARRELL, M. M. and LEVIN, D. L. (1993) Brain death in the pediatric patient: historical, sociological, medical, religious, cultural, legal and ethical considerations. *Critical Care Medicine*, **21**, 1951–1965

FRANCIS, G. S., SHARMA, B. and HODGES, M. (1982) Comparative hemodynamic effects of dopamine and dobutamine in patients with acute cardiogenic circulatory collapse. *American Heart Journal*, **103**, 995–1000

GASTON, B., DRAZEN, J. M., LOSCALZO, J. and STAMLER, J. S. (1994) The biology of nitrogen oxides in the airways. *American Journal of Respiratory and Critical Care Medicine*, **149**, 538–551

GATTINONI, L., PESENTI, A., MASCHERONI, D., MARCOLIN, R., FUMAGALLI, R., ROSSI, F. *et al.* (1986) Low-frequency positive-pressure ventilation with extracorporeal CO_2 removal in severe acute respiratory failure. *Journal of the American Medical Association*, **256**, 881–886

GLYNN, C. (1992) Pain control in intensive care units. *British Journal of Intensive Care*, **2**, 172–177

GOTTLIEB., M. E., SARFEH, I. J., STRATTON, H., GOLDMAN, M. L., NEWELL, J. C. and SHAH, D. M. (1983) Hepatic perfusion and splanchnic oxygen consumption in patients postinjury. *Journal of Trauma*, **23**, 836–843

GRAHM, T. W., ZADRONZY, D. B. and HARRINGTON, T. (1989) The benefits of early jejunal hyperalimentation in the head-injured patient. *Neurosurgery*, **25**, 729–735

GRENVIK, A., DOWNS, J., RÄSÄNEN, J. and SMITH, R. (eds) (1991) *Mechanical Ventilation and Assisted Respiration*. London: Churchill Livingstone

HAGLUND, U. (1994) Intramucosal pH. *Intensive Care Medicine*, **20**, 90–91

HAZARD, P. B. (1994) Further refinement of percutaneous tracheostomy technique. *Intensive Care Medicine*, **20**, 466–467

HERNDON, D. N., BARROW, R. E., KUNKEL, K. R., BROEMLING, L. and RUTAN, R. L. (1990) Effect of recombinant human growth hormone on donor site healing in severely burned children. *Annals of Surgery*, **212**, 424–431

HILLMAN, K. (1986) Colloid versus crystalloid fluid therapy in the critically ill. *Intensive and Critical Care Digest*, **5**, 7–9

HINSDALE, J. G. and JAFFE, B. M. (1984) Reoperation for intra-abdominal sepsis. *Annals of Surgery*, **199**, 31–36

JIANG, Z. M., HE, G. Z., ZHANG, S. Y., WANG, X. R. YANG, N. F. and ZHU, Y. *et al.* (1989) Low-dose growth hormone and hypocaloric nutrition attenuate the protein catabolic response after major operation. *Annals of Surgery*, **210**, 513–524

KEENE, A. R. and CULLEN, D. J. (1983) Therapeutic intervention scoring system; update. *Critical Care Medicine*, **11**, 1–3

KNAUS, W. A., DRAPER, E., WAGNER, D. P. and ZIMMERMAN, J. E. (1985) APACHE II: a severity of disease classification system. *Critical Care Medicine*, **13**, 818–829

KNAUS, W. A., DRAPER, E., WAGNER, D. P. and ZIMMERMAN, J. E. (1986) An evaluation of outcome from intensive care in major medical centres. *Annals of Internal Medicine*, **104**, 410–418

KUDSK, K. A., STONE, J. M., CARPENTER, G. and SHELDON, G. F. (1983) Enteral and parenteral feeding influences mortality after *E. coli* peritonitis in normal rats. *Journal of Trauma*, **23**, 605–609

LANCET (1994) Renal dose dopamine: a siren's song. *Lancet* ii, 7–8

LEE, B., CHANG, R. W. S. and JACOBS, S. (1990) Intermittent nasogastric feeding: a simple and effective method to reduce pneumonia among ventilated ICU patients. *Clinical Intensive Care*, **1**, 100–102

LILJEDAHL, S.-O., GEMZELL, C.-O., PLANTIN, L.-O. and BIRKE, G. (1961) Effect of growth hormone in patients with severe burns. *Acta Chirurgica Scandinavic*, **122**, 1–14

MCCLOSKEY, R. V., STRAUBE, R. C., SANDERS, C., SMITH, S. M., SMITH, C. R. and the CHESS TRIAL STUDY GROUP (1994) Treatment of septic shock with human monoclonal antibody HA–1A. *Annals of Internal Medicine*, **121**, 1–5

MACKENZIE, M. B. (1993) Stress ulcer prophylaxis: routine or targetted? *British Journal of Intensive Care*, **2**, 339–344

MANSON, J. M. and WILMORE, D. W. (1986) Positive nitrogen balance with human growth hormone and hypocaloric intravenous feeding. *Surgery*, **100**, 188–197

MASCIOLI, E., LEADER, L., FLORES, E., TRIMBO, S., BISTRIAN, B. and BLACKBURN, G. (1988) Enhanced survival to endotoxin in guinea pig fed IV fish oil emulsions. *Lipids*, **23**, 623–625

MAYNARD, N. D. (1994) Splanchnic ischaemia in the critically ill. *Critical Care International*, Sept/Oct., 12–18

MAYNARD, N. D., SMITHIES, M. N., MASON, R. and BIHARI, D. (1992) Dopexamine and gastric intramucosal pH in critically ill patients. *Intensive Care Medicine*, **18** (suppl 2), abstract 134

MEGUID, M. M., COLLIER, M. D. and HOWARD, U. (1981) Uncomplicated and stressed starvation. *Surgical Clinics of North America*, **61**, 529–543

MERMEL, L. A. and MAKI, D. G. (1994) Infectious complications of Swan–Ganz pulmonary artery catheters. *American Journal of Respiratory and Critical Care Medicine*, **149**, 1020–1036

MIMOZ, D., RAUSS, A., REKIK, N., BRUN-BUISSON, C., LEMAIRE, F. and BROCHARD, L. (1994) Pulmonary artery catheterization in critically ill patients: a prospective analysis of outcome changes associated with catheter-prompted changes in therapy. *Critical Care Medicine*, **22**, 573–579

MOORE, F. A., FELICIANO, D. V., ANDRASSY, R. J., MCARDLE, A. H. BOOTH, F. V. and MORGENSTEIN-WAGNER, T. B. *et al.* (1992) Early enteral feeding, compared with parenteral, reduces post-operative septic complications. *Annals of Surgery*, **216**, 172–183

O'DWYER, S. T., MICHIE, H. R., ZEIGLER, T. R., REVHAUG, A., SMITH, R. J. and WILMORE, D. W. (1988) A single dose of endotoxin increases intestinal permeability in healthy humans. *Archives of Surgery*, **123**, 1459–1464

PALAZZO, M. and PATEL, M. (1993) The use and interpretation of scoring systems in the ICU: parts 1 and 2. *British Journal of Intensive Care*, **2**, 255–260, 286–289

PARSONS, V. (1980) Recent advances in the management of acute renal failure. In: *Recent Advances in Critical Care Medicine*, Vol 3. edited by I. Ledingham. London: Churchill Livingstone

PINSKY, M. R. (1993) The role of the right ventricle in determining cardiac output in the critically ill. *Intensive Care Medicine*, **19**, 1–2

ROSS, A. D. and ANGARAN, D. M. (1984) Colloids vs crystalloids – a continuing controversy. *Drug Intelligence and Clinical Pharmacy*, **18**, 202–212

ROSSAINT, R., FALKE, K. J., LOPEZ, F., SLAMA, K., PISON, U. and ZAPOL, W. M. (1993) Inhaled nitric oxide for the adult respiratory distress syndrome. *New England Journal of Medicine*, **328**, 399–405

RUSSELL, J. A. and PHANG, P. T. (1994) The oxygen delivery/consumption controversy; approaches to management of the critically ill. *American Journal of Respiratory and Critical Care Medicine*, **149**, 533–537

SAITO, H., TROCKI, O., WANG, S. L., GONCE, S. J., JOFFE, S. N. and ALEXANDER, J. W. (1987) Metabolic and immune effects of dietary arginine supplementation after burn. *Archives of Surgery*, **12**, 784–789

SHANHOLTZ, C. and BROWER, R. (1994) Should inverse ratio ventilation be used in adult respiratory distress syndrome. *American Journal of Respiratory and Critical Care Medicine*, **149**, 1354–1358

SHELLEY, M. P. and WANG, D. Y. (1992) The assessment of sedation – a look at current methods and possible techniques for the future. *British Journal of Intensive Care*, **2**, 195–203

SHEPHARD, J. N., BRECKER, S. J. and EVANS, T. W. (1994) Bedside assessment of myocardial performance in the critically ill. *Intensive Care Medicine*, **20**, 513–521

SHOEMAKER, W. C., APPEL, P. L., KRAM, H. B., WAXMAN, K. and LEE, T.-S. (1988) Prospective trial of supranormal values of survivors as therapeutic goals in high-risk surgical patients. *Chest*, **94**, 1176–1186

SHOEMAKER, W. C., SCHLUCTER, M., HOPKINS, J. A., APPEL, P. A., SCHWARTZ, S. and CHANG, P. C. (1981) Comparison of the relative effectiveness of colloids and crystalloids in emergency resuscitation. *American Journal of Surgery*, **142**, 73–81

SHUMAN, R. B., SHUSTER, D. P. and ZUCKERMAN, G. R. (1987) Prophylactic therapy for stress ulcer bleeding. *Annals of Internal Medicine*, **106**, 562–567

SMITH, S. M. (1994) Examination of the central nervous system in the critically ill patient; important clinical signs and diagnoses. *British Journal of Intensive Care*, **4**, 116–121

SPENCER, E. M. and WILLATTS, S. M. (1994) Inhalational gases in the intensive care unit. *Clinical Intensive Care*, **5**, 21–28

THE AMERICAN-EUROPEAN CONSENSUS CONFERENCE ON ARDS (1994) Definitions, mechanisms, relevant outcomes and clinical trial coordintion. *American Journal of Respiratory and Critical Care Medicine*, **149**, 818–824

TOBIN, M. J. (1994) Current concepts. Mechanical ventilation. *New England Journal of Medicine*, **330**, 1056–1061

TRACY, K. J., FONG, Y., HEESE, D. G., MANOGUE, K. R., LEE, A. T., KUO, G. C. *et al.* (1987) Anti-cachetin/TNF monoclonal antibodies prevent septic shock during lethal bacteremia. *Nature*, **330**, 662–664

TRINDER, T. J., LAVERY, G. G., FEE, J. P. H. F. and LOWRY, K. G. (1995) Low gastric intramucosal pH: incidence and significance in intensive care patients. *Anaesthesia and Intensive Care*, **23**, 315–321

TUXEN, D. V. (1994) Permissive hypercapnic ventilation. *American Journal of Respiratory and Critical Care Medicine*, **150**, 870–874

VALLANCE, P. and COLLIER, J. (1994) Biology and clinical relevance of nitric oxide. *British Medical Journal*, **309**, 453–457

VAN MEURS, K. P., FRANKEL, L. R. and PEARL, R. G. (1992) Extracorporeal life support: issues of who, when, why, and how. *Critical Care Medicine*, **20**, 1200–1202

WARREN, H. S., DANNER, R. L. and MUNFORD, R. S. (1992) Anti-endotoxin monoclonal antibodies. *New England Journal of Medicine*, **326**, 1153–1157

WILMORE, D. W., SMITH, R. J., O'DWYER, S. T., JACOBS, D. O., ZEIGLER, T. R. and WANG, X. D. (1988) The gut: a central organ after surgical stress. *Surgery*, **104**, 917–923

WINKLER, W.-B., KARNIK, R., SEELMANN, O., HAVLICEK, J. and SLANY, J. (1994) Bedside percutaneous dilatational tracheostomy with endoscopic guidance: experience with 71 ICU patients. *Intensive Care Medicine*, **20**, 476–479

ZALOGA, G. P., KNOWLES, R., BLACK, K. W. and PRIELIPP, R. (1991) Total parenteral nutrition increases mortality after haemorrhage. *Critical Care Medicine*, **19**, 54–59

ZAPOL, W. M., RIMAR, S., GILLIS, N., MARLETTA, M. and BOSKEN, C. H. (1994) Nitric oxide and the lung. *American Journal of Respiratory and Critical Care Medicine*, **149**, 1375–1380

ZEIGLER, E. J., FISHER, C. J., SPRUNG, C. L., STRAUBE, R. C., SADOFF, J. C. and FOULKE, G. E. (1991) Treatment of gram-negative bacteremia and septic shock with HA-1A human monoclonal antibody against endotoxin. *New England Journal of Medicine*, **324**, 429–436

27

Anaesthesia

Henry J. L. Craig

Increasing range and complexity in otolaryngology in the past three decades have made greater demands on the skill and knowledge of the anaesthetist. There is no branch of surgery in which good communication and cooperation between surgeon and anaesthetist are more important for successful outcome. Problems in airway control are particularly likely in operations around the nose, pharynx, larynx and trachea as a consequence of the anaesthetist having to share the airway with the surgeon and, in addition, the airway may be compromised by disease. Following major head and neck surgery disruption of normal swallowing mechanisms, ablation of parathyroid and thyroid function, and compromised respiratory function frequently necessitate short or longer stays in the intensive care units postoperatively, with or without ventilatory control. Here the anaesthetist plays a vital part in patient recovery.

In this chapter both local and general anaesthetic techniques are discussed while anaesthesia for infants and young children is dealt with in Chapter 34 in Volume 6, Paediatric Otolaryngology. The aim of this chapter is not to try to teach surgeons general anaesthetic techniques but to help them to understand some of the anaesthetist's problems in this field.

Preoperative preparation

As in all surgery it is important to evaluate the physical condition of each patient and to achieve the healthiest possible state before surgery, this being an important determinant of peri- and postoperative morbidity and mortality. The modern trend is for shorter and shorter inpatient stays. Patients for minor or intermediate surgery, who are judged fit at an earlier outpatient general medical examination, can be admitted as day cases to specialized day surgery units

on the morning of operation, while those unsuited for day care can be kept in after operation in a conventional unit. In all major cases it is still usual to admit patients to hospital on the day before surgery, or earlier when associated medical problems cannot be investigated and treated on an outpatient basis.

History and physical examination

Assessment of general medical history with particular attention to cough, wheeze, sputum production, breathlessness, pain in the chest, drug therapy and tobacco and alcohol consumption is necessary. The use of a simple questionnaire to evaluate general medical health is useful; this can be completed by the patient at the outpatient department or, in the case of day surgery, at the time of admission to the unit. The physical examination should pay particular attention to the cardiovascular and respiratory systems.

Cardiovascular disease

Pre-existing cardiovascular disease is seldom a contraindication to general anaesthesia and surgery, provided optimum fitness is attained before operation. Avoidance of anxiety is important and good general anaesthesia, after adequate premedication, may be preferable to surgery under local anaesthesia. Adequate control of hypertension will ensure better stability of the blood pressure during anaesthesia (Prys-Roberts, Meloche and Foex, 1971), and therapy should be continued up to the time of operation. Cardiac failure must be fully treated before surgery; however even then the ultimate prognosis is poor.

Patients with stable angina are able to tolerate surgery and anaesthesia well, as myocardial work is decreased under general anaesthesia; however individuals with unstable poorly controlled angina, and those who experience pain at rest, are in a high risk category and surgery should, if possible, be postponed until their condition has been improved by drugs, coronary angioplasty or coronary artery bypass surgery. Patients with angina should have their usual coronary artery dilator drug included in the premedication. Elective surgery should, when possible, be postponed for 6 months after myocardial infarction.

A severe degree of heart block requires careful assessment by both anaesthetist and cardiologist, and the insertion of a pacemaker may be necessary before operation.

Respiratory disease

Upper respiratory tract infection is a contraindication to elective surgery, as it is a cause of excessive secretions together with hyperaemia and irritability of the respiratory tract, with a predisposition to laryngospasm and increased surgical bleeding. In the presence of an active chest infection anaesthesia should also be avoided and appropriate antibiotics administered. Patients with a chronic productive cough should have physiotherapy, and bronchodilators may improve respiratory function. However, some chronic infections, such as nasal discharge secondary to obstruction of the nasal passages, may never clear up without surgery, so it is essential that all factors are taken into consideration before the operation is postponed.

Asthmatic patients tolerate general anaesthesia well, as most inhalational agents are bronchodilators. The patient should use the usual bronchodilatory medication up to the time of operation, and premedication should avoid bronchoconstrictors such as morphine. Phenothiazines or benzodiazepines are suitable and an aminophylline suppository may be helpful. Postponement of surgery will be indicated in cases where the patient suffers an acute attack of bronchospasm immediately before the operation or during the induction of anaesthesia.

Diabetes

Diabetics should be properly controlled before surgery, and this is generally possible except in emergencies. Non-insulin-dependent diabetics, for minor or intermediate surgery, can usually be managed by omitting food and any oral hypoglycaemic agent on the day of operation, or the previous day in the case of long-acting agents (e.g. chlorpropamide). Before major operations it may be advisable to change to soluble insulin.

Insulin-dependent diabetics having minor surgery are best done first on the morning list, omitting both food and insulin preoperatively. Brief operations, with little postoperative upset (e.g. myringotomy), may allow early postoperative food intake and normal insulin administration, otherwise 5% dextrose can be infused with one-quarter to one-third of the usual insulin dose. A suitable regimen prior to intermediate and major surgery is to omit the insulin on the morning of the operation; measure the blood glucose level and administer a 5% dextrose solution with an amount of soluble insulin, determined by the blood sugar level, added to the dextrose, or administered subcutaneously, or as a separate infusion. The 5% dextrose solution is run at about 1.5 ml/kg/h with additional fluid, if required, being given as physiological saline. Many patients are able to return to oral feeding on the day of the operation, thus eliminating the need to add potassium to the infusion fluid. The blood glucose level should be checked immediately before and after operation, also intraoperatively during long procedures, and maintained at a relatively high level, around 10 mmol/l, reducing to 6–8 mmol/l postoperatively. Hypoglycaemia, which is difficult to detect in the unconscious patient, must always be avoided. For a comprehensive review of the perioperative management of diabetes the reader is referred to reviews by Walts *et al.* (1981) and Hirsch *et al.* (1991).

Pregnancy

Elective surgery is contraindicated in the first and last trimesters of pregnancy. Surgery causes a small increase in the risk of spontaneous abortion in the early stages, and if a miscarriage should happen the operation will certainly be blamed. In the final weeks of pregnancy increased intra-abdominal pressure may lead to respiratory embarrassment, and the risk of gastric regurgitation will be increased. In the middle trimester usually there is no contraindication to general anaesthesia.

Concurrent drug therapy

Concurrent drug therapy should be noted and given proper consideration, particularly for those on beta-adrenergic blocking drugs, calcium-channel blockers, monoamine oxidase inhibitors, corticosteroids, contraceptive drugs or tricyclic antidepressants.

Beta-adrenergic blocking drugs

The administration of beta-adrenergic blocking drugs, which are widely used in the treatment of hypertension and angina, should be continued up to the time of the operation. It may be advisable to substitute short-acting agents for long-acting members of the same group but, on the whole, problems are not usual when combined with modern anaesthetic agents. If necessary, adverse effects of beta-blockade can be controlled by drugs producing inotropic and chronotropic stimulation by way of alternative pathways.

Calcium-channel blocking drugs

Some calcium-channel blocking agents, such as nifedipine, are used in the treatment of angina and hypertension, while others, such as verapamil, are administered for the control of supraventricular arrhythmias. These drugs may have additive effects with the inhalational anaesthetics in depressing the myocardium and conductive pathways in the heart. Patients treated with calcium blocking drugs should continue this medication up to the time of surgery and be monitored for possible additive effects.

Monoamine oxidase inhibitors (MAOIs)

These drugs are quite frequently used to treat depression in patients resistant to the tricyclic antidepressants. Administration of pressor amines is contraindicated in the presence of monoamine oxidase inhibitors, as the combination will produce a dangerous hypertension. Use of nasal decongestants, such as ephedrine or phenylephrine, is contraindicated, as is adrenaline combined with local anaesthetic agents. Narcotics, particularly pethidine, can produce dangerous side effects such as excessive respiratory depression, hypo- or hypertension, sweating, nausea and collapse. In addition, any drug metabolized in the liver will be potentiated. If possible MAOI therapy should be stopped 3 weeks before administration of a general anaesthetic.

Tricyclic antidepressant drugs

These agents inhibit reuptake of noradrenalin into the presynaptic nerve terminals; most also have anticholinergic effects. Even in therapeutic doses, tricyclics may produce tachycardia and dysrhythmias, and the hypertensive response to directly acting sympathomimetic amines (e.g. adrenalin and noradrenalin) is increased. There is some increased risk of dysrhythmias and hypotension during anaesthesia, however therapy is usually not stopped before surgery. Centrally acting anticholinergic drugs (e.g. atropine, hyoscine) should be avoided in premedication as the additive effect may precipitate confusion, especially in the elderly. Adrenalin combined with local anaesthetic is not contraindicated, however, large doses should be avoided.

Corticosteroids

Patients on prolonged steroid therapy may suffer from adrenal suppression and require steroid cover during major surgery and in the immediate postoperative period. Minor surgery does not usually necessitate extra steroid cover; however, if thought necessary, a single dose of hydrocortisone at the time of premedication or during induction of anaesthesia will suffice.

Contraceptive pill

Patients on contraceptive therapy may be at greater risk of thromboembolic complications postoperatively than the general population. The hazard is probably minimal with modern low oestrogen preparations, however some authorities still advise cessation of therapy for one month prior to surgery. Where this is not possible prophylaxis with subcutaneous heparin or dextran infusion may be used.

Preoperative investigations

Routine laboratory tests in patients who are apparently healthy on history and clinical examination are invariably of little use, and a waste of resources. Investigations should only be ordered if the results are likely to yield information not revealed by the physical examination, and when the results are likely to alter the management of the patient.

Urine analysis should be performed on every patient, it is very inexpensive and will occasionally reveal urinary infection or an undiagnosed diabetic. Haemoglobin concentration should be measured when clinically indicated (by pallor, history of blood loss etc.), in all females, in males over 50 years and in all patients of African or Asian descent, in whom anaemia may indicate a haemoglobinopathy of the sickle cell type and will warrant further investigation. Haemoglobin concentration should also be measured in all patients before major surgery. Patients with a history of abnormal bleeding, anticoagulant therapy or liver disease should have appropriate blood coagulation tests and, if any abnormality is revealed, consultation with a haematologist may be necessary.

Urea and electrolyte concentrations should be measured in patients with a history of diarrhoea, vomiting or metabolic disease, in the presence of renal or hepatic disease, or an abnormal nutritional state, and in those receiving diuretics, digoxin, antihypertensive drugs, steroids or hypoglycaemic agents. Liver function tests are indicated in patients with hepatic disease, an abnormal nutritional state, metabolic disease, or with a history of high alcohol intake.

A chest X-ray is not required routinely in patients below 60 years of age, unless suggested by a history or physical signs of cardiac or pulmonary disease. Lung function tests, such as peak expiratory flow rate, forced vital capacity, forced expiratory volume over one second ($FEV_{1.0}$) and arterial blood gas analysis, may be helpful in monitoring response to treatment in patients with severe dyspnoea on mild or moderate exertion. Thoracic inlet X-rays are required in some cases of thyroid enlargement or other tumours in the base of the neck or upper mediastinum.

A 12-lead ECG should be obtained if there is a history or physical signs of cardiac disease, in the presence of hypertension and in all elderly patients.

Blood sugar estimations are required in all diabetics, in patients receiving corticosteroid drugs and those who suffer from vascular disease.

Preoperative medication

The objectives of premedication are to allay anxiety, decrease secretions, reduce postoperative nausea, dizziness and vomiting, and attenuate vagal and sympatho-adrenal responses. In certain circumstances a reduction in volume and an increase in pH of gastric contents may be desirable, e.g. pregnancy, hiatus hernia.

Sedative drugs

A good night's sleep before surgery is desirable and many patients require a short-acting hypnotic, such as temazepam 10–20 mg, to achieve this. Patients who are accustomed to taking night sedation should be given their usual drug in a slightly increased dose. A careful and reassuring explanation of the method of induction of anaesthesia, the operative procedure and the immediate postoperative period is more likely than any sedative drug to dispel apprehension. In some this reassurance may not be sufficient and anxiolytic medication may be required, the benzodiazepine drugs being very effective for this purpose.

Various drugs can be given 1–2 hours before surgery, depending on the patient's condition and the anaesthetist's individual preference, an oral anxiolytic drug such as lorazepam (2–4 mg) or temazepam (10–30 mg) being suitable. The elderly are not usually apprehensive and administration of sedative drugs may result in confusion.

Anticholinergic drugs

The use of anticholinergic drugs, such as atropine, which produce patient discomfort due to a dry mouth and loss of visual accommodation, are often omitted from routine premedication. However, if a dry mouth and throat are required during surgery, preoperative i.m. atropine is more effective than intraoperative i.v. injection. Bradycardia may develop during induction and maintenance of general anaesthesia, being particularly likely during laryngeal, aural and nasal stimulation and may, if severe, require i.v. atropine. Glycopyrrolate (5–10 μg/kg) is an alternative to atropine, providing both a better drying effect and more cardiostability (Mirakhur and Dundee, 1983). It is slower acting and so less suitable in an emergency situation of extreme bradycardia.

Prophylactic antibiotics

Bacteraemia is common during any oral or nasal operation, including endoscopy (Bayliss *et al.*, 1983),

and prevention of endocarditis is important in patients with heart valve lesions, prosthetic valves, septal defect or patent ductus arteriosus. Adult patients at risk, excluding those with prosthetic valves and those who have had endocarditis, are given amoxycillin 1 g i.m. 1 hour before operation, or i.v. during induction, followed by a single oral or i.m. dose of amoxycillin 500 mg 6 hours later. Patients with prosthetic valves or who have had endocarditis are at special risk, and should be given gentamicin 120 mg i.m. or i.v. immediately before induction in addition to amoxycillin. Patients who are already taking penicillin, or who are allergic to penicillin, can be given i.v. vancomycin 1 g over at least 100 minutes, then i.v. gentamicin 120 mg at induction, or 15 minutes before the procedure (Endocarditis Working Party, 1990).

Prophylactic anticoagulants

There is less risk of venous thrombosis after head and neck surgery than after major abdominal or thoracic procedures. Nevertheless, patients having prolonged operations with extensive dissection, or who are otherwise especially at risk, should be considered for prophylactic subcutaneous heparin; 5000 units being given before operation and 5000 units at 12-hourly intervals thereafter, until the patient is fully ambulant. This therapy will increase bleeding during operation and the risk of postoperative haemorrhage. Low molecular weight heparins are equally effective and their longer duration of action allows once daily administration (2000–4000 units), resulting in less painful and more convenient therapy.

Postoperative relief of pain

Pain is a complex sensation which is difficult to measure accurately and has a wide individual variation with important emotional and rational components. The emotional content will vary with the personality of the patient, the neurotic suffering more than the stoic. Anxiety is an important factor and preoperative explanation, reassurance and description of the pain relief techniques available will aid postoperative analgesia. While pain resulting from otolaryngological surgery is unlikely to be as severe as that following thoracic or upper abdominal operations, nevertheless, suffering can be considerable, and may be more severe following relatively limited procedures, such as uvulopalatopharyngoplasty, than after major head and neck dissection.

For the control of severe pain, i.m. opioids, on an as required basis, is not adequate, 60% of patients expressing dissatisfaction with the quality of postoperative analgesia derived from this technique. This is due to caution in dosage and frequency of administration for fear of undue respiratory depression, delay in administration due to nursing procedures, difficulty in matching the dose to the severity of the pain, variability in drug absorption and distribution, and the wide difference in inherent sensitivity of the opioid receptors in individual patients. The dose of morphine is limited by respiratory depression and, despite claims to the contrary, there is no evidence that any of the newer agonist/antagonist drugs produce analgesia equivalent to that of morphine with lesser degrees of respiratory depression. Some of these newer drugs produce a higher incidence of side effects, such as nausea, vomiting and sedation, than equi-analgesic doses of morphine. One of this group, buprenorphine, has some important differences from morphine. While being largely inactivated when taken by mouth, it is readily absorbed across mucous membranes and can be administered sublingually, 0.4 mg 6-hourly producing reasonable analgesia. A disadvantage is the degree of sedation produced, which is often unacceptable to ambulant patients. In low dosage buprenorphine antagonizes the action of morphine, so overlapping action must be avoided.

The quality of opioid analgesia can be improved by giving small doses i.v. as required, however, because of the risk of rapid induction of respiratory depression, this technique is largely limited to the postoperative recovery ward. Continuous infusion of adequate doses of opioids will provide good analgesia to patients on artificial ventilation in the intensive care unit, where respiratory depression is not a problem. However, in spontaneously breathing patients the dosage has to be determined on a trial and error basis, and a fixed rate of perfusion prescribed, carrying a great risk of respiratory depression, and so is not a suitable technique outside the intensive care or high dependency unit.

Severe postoperative pain in the spontaneously breathing subject is best managed by patient-controlled analgesia (PCA), using a specially designed syringe pump loaded with morphine (usually 2 mg/ml), or pethidine, combined with an antiemetic, controlled by the patient using a trigger device which results in a single set dose (usually 1 mg morphine) being administered intravenously. A minimal time interval between doses is set in the machine by the physician, usually 5–6 minutes, and the total maximum dose over a set period can also be programmed (Egan, 1990). Accidental triggering of the patient control can be prevented by requiring the patient to make two successive presses on the hand control within one second. A disadvantage of PCA is that the patient stops demanding opioid when asleep and the plasma concentration may fall below the analgesic threshold, the patient awakening in pain. To overcome this problem, some machines have the facility of a continuous low background infusion on which the patient superimposes boluses, however use of such a background infusion increases the incidence of episodes of undue respiratory depression. Success of PCA depends on proper instruction of the patient before operation, and on the patient's ability to cooperate and understand postoperatively.

Analgesic drugs, administered before operation, may convey some protection against afferent stimulation of the spinal cord and prostaglandin synthesis resulting from surgical insult, and give more effective pain relief than when given postoperatively (Wall, 1988; Campbell, 1990).

Non-steroidal anti-inflammatory drugs, NSAIDs (e.g. diclofenac sodium 75 mg i.m. or 100 mg as a rectal suppository; ketorolac 10 mg i.m. or i.v. followed by 10–30 mg 2–6 hourly, maximum 24 hour dose 90 mg, 60 mg in elderly, for a maximum period of 48 hours) while not adequate alone for the control of severe pain will, given perioperatively, control mild to moderate pain in the immediate postoperative period and reduce requirements of opioid analgesics for the control of severe pain (Ferreira, 1980). Contraindications to NSAIDs include hypovolaemia, coagulation disorders, peptic ulceration, asthma, renal impairment and heparin therapy (including low dose prophylactic heparin). NSAIDs inhibit platelet aggregation, prolong bleeding time and increase the risk of postoperative bleeding.

For control of mild to moderate pain in the later postoperative period oral preparations of paracetamol, either alone or combined with codeine phosphate or dihydrocodeine bitartrate, are usually adequate. Oral preparations are likely to be poorly absorbed in the immediate postoperative period due to delayed gastric emptying, especially so if opioids have been administered intraoperatively.

Regional blocks with local anaesthetic agents, while frequently used to provide pain relief after surgery on the trunk or limbs, are rarely used for this purpose in otolaryngology. However, some success in postoperative pain relief has been claimed following injection of bupivacaine into each anterior pillar of the fauces during tonsillectomy, and maxillary or cervical plexus block may be helpful after major head and neck surgery.

Local anaesthesia

Local anaesthesia and regional blocks play an important part in minor outpatient and day case surgery, and also in more major operations when specialist anaesthetic services are not available. Some of these procedures are used primarily to produce vasoconstriction, rather than analgesia, and are then frequently combined with general anaesthesia. Regional blocks are also used for postoperative analgesia using long-acting local anaesthetic agents, and for relief of intractable pain using either alcohol or phenol.

Pharmacology of local anaesthetic agents

Local effects

Drugs classified as local anaesthetics (aminoesters or aminoamides) produce reversible block of impulse transmission in a nerve by obstructing inflow of sodium ions through the nerve membrane, this flow being necessary for the conduction of an electrical impulse. The agents may be applied topically to mucosal surfaces, or injected around peripheral nerve endings, or in the vicinity of nerve trunks. An ideal agent should have adequate potency, short latency, good penetration, good diffusion, low toxicity and controllable duration of action with complete reversibility; it should also be water soluble and stable in solution to permit heat sterilization; in addition it should be non-irritant, non-antigenic and not interfere with wound healing. Excellent local anaesthetics are available, nevertheless the search for the ideal drug continues.

In myelinated nerve, the site of action of local anaesthetic drugs is at the nodes of Ranvier where the myelin sheath is thin or absent. Two or three adjacent nodes must be exposed to the agent (6–10 mm of nerve) as the electrical impulse is capable of jumping one or two nodes. A certain minimum concentration of local anaesthetic agent is needed to block impulse conduction within a reasonable time, the greater the diameter of the fibre the greater the concentration required. The duration of action depends on the firmness of the bond between the analgesic agent and the nerve membrane, and on the rate of drug removal, which is the result of dilution by tissue fluid, diffusion away from the nerve, bloodstream uptake and metabolic inactivation.

Local anaesthetic drugs in solution exist in two forms, the uncharged base and the charged cation, with the degree of ionization dependent on the pH of the solution and the buffering effect of the tissue fluid. The greater the acidity of the tissue fluid the higher is the ratio of ionized particles to free base, however only the lipid soluble free base can penetrate the fat barrier of the nerve sheath; thus a local anaesthetic drug injected into inflamed tissues, which have poor buffering properties and a low pH (pus is acid), tends to be ineffective.

All local anaesthetics, with the exception of lignocaine and cocaine, cause peripheral vasodilation by direct action on the arterioles; in contrast lignocaine has little effect, whereas cocaine causes vasoconstriction.

General systemic effects

Local anaesthetic agents have important actions on many systems in the body and these effects are sometimes used therapeutically, for example i.v. lignocaine used to control ventricular dysrhythmias. More often these actions are regarded as side or toxic effects depending on the severity of the patient's response, this in turn being determined both by the nature of the drug and the plasma concentration. Plasma concentration depends on dose and concentration of the local anaesthetic solution, the vascularity of the injection site (or mucosal surface) and the rate of removal from the plasma. The most important toxic manifestations develop in the central nervous and cardiovascular systems.

Central nervous system

Local anaesthetic agents pass readily from the bloodstream to the brain. At recommended clinical doses serum levels remain well below toxic concentrations, unless inadvertent intravascular injection occurs. Toxic plasma levels initially depress inhibitory cortical pathways and allow unopposed excitatory activity, with restlessness, visual and auditory disturbances (tinnitus), garrulousness, paraesthesia (especially perioral), slurred speech, shivering and muscular tremors leading to convulsions; a state of generalized central nervous system depression will follow. In the case of some drugs, such as lignocaine, the excitatory phase may not be manifest, with toxicity becoming apparent initially as depression with drowsiness and amnesia.

Cardiovascular system

The cardiovascular effects of local anaesthetics occur either indirectly by the inhibition of autonomic pathways, for example during epidural analgesia, or directly by depression of the myocardium and its conducting system, and relaxation of vascular smooth muscle. These direct actions result in slowing of the heart, a reduction in cardiac output and a fall in blood pressure.

Respiratory system

Central stimulation causes an increase in rate and depth of respiration, later, as the medulla becomes depressed, breathing becomes rapid and shallow. Respiration ceases during convulsions so, unless resuscitative measures are taken, severe hypoxia results.

Prevention and treatment of toxic effects

In otolaryngology the toxic effects of local anaesthetic agents are unlikely to be due to absolute overdosage, as large amounts are seldom injected. High plasma concentrations can result from direct intravascular injection, particularly intra-arterial, or from excessive amounts placed on vascular mucous membranes which facilitate rapid absorption. Intravascular injection can result in very rapid (10–20 seconds) appearance of toxic effects.

Clinical features are usually the result of central nervous system reactions to the agent, cardiovascular changes being due to resultant hypoxia. If signs of toxicity appear the infiltration of local anaesthetic must cease, 100% oxygen should be given via a face mask, and a good venous line secured (good practice dictates venous cannulation prior to any local anaesthetic procedure). Frequently such measures will be sufficient, however if muscle twitching continues 5–10 mg midazolam should be given i.v. An anaesthetist should be summoned so that if convulsions occur, in spite of this therapy, the patient can be paralysed with a myoneural blocking drug (muscle relaxant), the trachea intubated and respiration controlled. Cardiovascular depression, as indicated by hypotension and poor peripheral circulation, is treated by correction of hypoxia, moderate head-down tilt, infusion of crystalloid fluids and, if necessary, administration of inotropic agents.

Hypersensitivity reactions to local anaesthetic agents

Hypersensitivity reactions are rare, toxic reactions to small doses usually being the result of intravascular injection. True hypersensitivity reactions result in cardiovascular collapse, bronchospasm and cutaneous oedema. The treatment consists of i.v. adrenalin (1–5 ml 1:10 000) and rapid infusion of crystalloid or colloid solutions, plus artificial ventilation with 100% oxygen.

Local anaesthetic agents

A wide variety of local anaesthetic agents is available and it is usually possible to select a drug that will fulfil most of the requirements of any particular type of block. Properties of special concern are effectiveness, speed and duration of action, spreading power, toxicity and surface activity. Surgeons should limit their repertoire of local anaesthetic drugs in order to familiarize themselves thoroughly with the use of each one of them. In the following section only the most commonly used agents will be discussed.

Cocaine hydrochloride

Cocaine is an ester of benzoic acid which is metabolized in the body by plasma cholinesterase. It is heat labile and is broken down by autoclaving. Cocaine is used solely for topical application as it is too toxic for parenteral use. It provides excellent surface analgesia with a marked vasoconstrictor effect, due to its ability to block the reuptake of catecholamines released at adrenergic nerve endings; catecholamines thus accumulate at the active receptor sites. The effect of any additional sympathetic stimulation or exogenous catecholamines is potentiated and excessive sympathetic activity is responsible for many of the signs of cocaine toxicity. Stimulation of the central nervous system from above downwards causes euphoria and a reduction in the sense of fatigue; as this is an addictive effect the drug is in the controlled category. Medullary stimulation results in an increase in blood pressure and respiratory rate, followed by depression with coma or convulsions and respiratory failure. Cocaine sensitizes the myocardium to adrenaline, and toxic levels can cause ventricular fibrillation, the addition of adrenaline to cocaine increases the risk.

Cocaine is absorbed from mucosal surfaces, and while concentrated solutions, producing intense vasoconstriction, may be absorbed slowly, dilute preparations are considered to be safer. Cocaine is used as a 4–20% solution or as a 20% paste, the maximum dose being about 3 mg/kg with an absolute maximum of 200 mg in the fit adult. The duration of action is about 60 minutes. Because of toxicity its use is best confined to the nose, where only small quantities are required, topical analgesia of other surfaces, such as the larynx and trachea, can be more safely achieved using lignocaine.

Lignocaine hydrochloride

Lignocaine (Xylocaine, lidocaine USP) is an aminoacyl amide, a derivative of acetanalide, which is heat stable and can be autoclaved. It is metabolized in the liver, the metabolites being excreted in the urine. Lignocaine is a very effective local anaesthetic with a rapid onset of action and good diffusing properties. On injection it has a duration of action of about one hour, which can be prolonged to 2–3 hours by the addition of a vasoconstrictor.

Infiltration analgesia can be accomplished with 0.5% lignocaine, with or without the addition of adrenalin (1:200 000), while nerve blocks require 1–1.5%. The maximum dose depends on the concentration of solution used and on whether or not adrenalin is added; 3 mg/kg for 0.5% lignocaine (maximum dose 200 mg), 7 mg/kg when adrenalin is added (maximum dose 500 mg). These doses should be reduced when stronger solutions are used, when patients are elderly or not physically fit and when the injection is into very vascular regions.

Lignocaine is absorbed from mucous membranes and is a useful surface anaesthetic in concentrations of 2–4%. The 2% preparation is also available in viscous form for oral analgesia. The more effective 4% solution can be used in hand-operated sprays or in the form of nasal packs or applicators. There is also a pressurized 10% aerosol spray which gives 10 mg lignocaine per dose. Ointments and gels, in 2–5% concentrations, can be used for lubricating tubes and instruments. The maximum safe topical dose is about 3 mg/kg, with an upper limit of 200 mg in the fit adult. The onset of action is rapid but of short duration (approximately 20 minutes).

Prilocaine hydrochloride

Prilocaine (Citanest) while being less potent, less toxic and longer acting than lignocaine has similar actions, and is an effective mucosal surface anaesthetic. With large doses (over 500 mg) cyanosis may ensue as the result of the formation of methaemoglobin; this is harmless, unless accompanied by severe anaemia or circulatory impairment, and usually disappears within 24 hours. If necessary the condition can be treated with intravenous methylene blue (1 mg/kg). The maximum safe dose is 6 mg/kg (0.5% solution), with a vasoconstrictor 8 mg/kg, these doses being reduced in elderly and frail patients. Concentrations used are similar to those for lignocaine. The addition of adrenalin improves the duration and quality of the action of prilocaine but less impressively than with lignocaine.

Bupivacaine hydrochloride

Bupivacaine (Marcain) is a potent long-acting local anaesthetic, whose duration of action (about 4 hours) is only marginally increased by the addition of adrenalin (up to 6 hours). Residual analgesia may last up to 36 hours, a useful feature when postoperative pain relief is required. It is not an effective surface analgesic. Bupivacaine is about four times as potent as lignocaine, although this is offset by its greater toxicity. It is used in concentrations of 0.25–0.5% for peripheral nerve blocks, with or without adrenalin, the maximum safe dose being 2 mg/kg. In otolaryngology its principal use lies in regional nerve blocks when a prolonged action is required.

Other local anaesthetic agents

There are other local anaesthetic agents, some of which are just as effective as those described. Others, such as procaine which is less effective than lignocaine, and amethocaine which is more toxic, have been superseded by newer agents.

Vasoconstrictors

The addition of a vasoconstrictor to a local anaesthetic solution will reduce tissue bleeding, delay the rate of absorption, prolong the action and decrease the maximum plasma level attained, thereby reducing the risk of toxic effects.

Adrenalin

Adrenalin (epinephrine), the most commonly used vasoconstrictor, is present in many commercial preparations of lignocaine and bupivacaine. While these preparations are convenient the concentration of adrenalin is often too high, 1 in 80 000 being common, whereas 1 in 200 000 is all that is required. An antioxidant is usually added to prevent oxidation of adrenalin, resulting in a low solution pH, with a consequent decrease in free base and reduced penetration of nerve axons by the anaesthetic agent. A more satisfactory solution is to add adrenalin to the anaesthetic solution immediately before use.

The dose of adrenalin by injection should not exceed 0.01 mg/kg, with a total maximum of 0.5 mg (0.5 ml of 1 in 1000 solution) in the fit adult. High blood concentrations, usually the result of intravascular injection, may cause anxiety, vertigo, pallor and palpitations. Systolic blood pressure rises, diastolic pressure falls and cardiac output increases. Severe tachyarrhythmias may develop (which can terminate in ventricular fibrillation) reducing cardiac output and resulting in a fall in blood pressure with peripheral circulatory failure.

Infiltration of diluted adrenalin causes ischaemia of the skin and related tissues, however, vessels which supply muscle are dilated. The vasoconstrictor should not be infiltrated into tissues supplied by end arteries lest arterial insufficiency and tissue necrosis result.

Adrenalin is contraindicated in patients receiving agents which sensitize the myocardium to catecholamines (e.g. halothane and MAOIs), in advanced ischaemic heart disease, severe hypertension and thyrotoxicosis.

Felypressin

Felypressin (Octapressin), a synthetic vasoconstrictor, has low systemic toxicity and does not raise blood pressure or increase myocardial irritability. Onset of action is slow, taking up to 15 minutes for maximum vasoconstrictor effect. Felypressin is a possible alternative to adrenalin when that drug is contraindicated. It is more effective than adrenalin in prolonging the action of prilocaine, and is commercially available with 3% prilocaine in a 2 ml dental cartridge (felypressin 0.03 unit/ml).

Phenylephrine hydrochloride

Phenylephrine (Neosynephrine, Neophryn), a synthetic vasoconstrictor, is a weak agent compared with adrenalin; it is used in a concentration of 1 in 20 000. While it does not produce tachycardia it does sensitize the myocardium to catecholamines, and probably has the same contraindications to use as adrenalin.

Local anaesthetic techniques

The nose and paranasal sinuses

Topical anaesthesia, using 4–10% cocaine or 4% lignocaine with adrenalin, is widely used for minor surgery to the nose, such as the removal of polyps, local electrocautery and antral puncture. The nasal cavities are first sprayed with the anaesthetic solution, the patient having been warned not to swallow any excess for fear of gastric absorption, particularly important if cocaine is used. A few minutes later each side of the nose is carefully packed with half inch (1.27 cm) ribbon gauze soaked in the solution. The packs are removed after 10 minutes and a wool applicator, soaked in the anaesthetic solution, is inserted at an angle of 20° to the floor of the nose until bone is felt at a depth of 6–7 cm, the end now lying adjacent to the sphenopalatine foramen (Figure 27.1a). A second applicator is inserted along the anterior border of the nasal cavity until the anterior end of the cribriform plate is reached at a depth of about 5 cm (Figure 27.1b). A similar technique, with omission of the applicators, may be used to provide vasoconstriction before surgery under general anaesthesia.

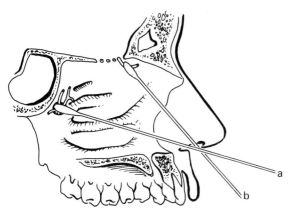

Figure 27.1 Applicators placed in nasal cavity in such a way that the tip of (a) is adjacent to the sphenopalatine foramen and (b) near the cribriform plate. (From Macintosh and Ostlere, 1955, by courtesy of the author and publisher)

For extensive surgery on the nose more thorough analgesia of the nasal mucosa may be required, using a modification of Moffet's technique (Curtiss, 1952). The nasal cavity is sprayed as before and the patient is then put into a supine position, with a pillow under the shoulders to extend the head until it is upside-down (Figure 27.2). The patient is told to breathe through the mouth and, using a special angulated cannula, 2 ml of 5% cocaine solution are injected into each side of the nasal cavity, as near to the roof of the nose as possible (Figure 27.3). The patient remains in this position for 10 minutes and then, after pinching the nose to prevent any solution being sniffed back and swallowed, is helped to roll into a prone position, with the head being kept down throughout. The remaining fluid drains out through the anterior nares and, if any runs down the back of the throat, the patient should be instructed to spit it out and not swallow it. The anaesthetic solution may extend

through the sphenopalatine foramen to the maxillary nerve, in which case analgesia will be sufficient for operations on the antrum, otherwise a separate maxillary nerve block is necessary for surgery in this region. The anterior ethmoidal nerve must also be blocked if the operation is likely to extend into the ethmoidal air cells. Infiltration of the columella of the nose with lignocaine through a fine needle will provide analgesia of the area not supplied by the anterior ethmoidal nerve and also help to separate mucous membrane from the septal cartilage, aiding septal surgery.

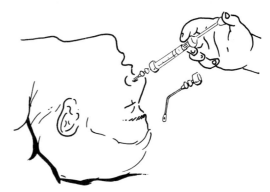

Figure 27.2 Position of the head before instillation of cocaine into the nasal cavity. (From Macintosh and Ostlere, 1955, by courtesy of the author and publisher)

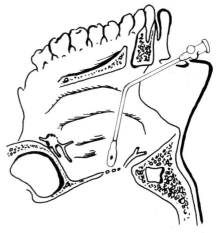

Figure 27.3 Angulated cannula in position for injection of cocaine into the nose. (From Macintosh and Ostlere, 1955, by courtesy of the author and publisher)

For external ethmoidectomy a block of the anterior ethmoidal and infratrochlear nerves, together with infiltration along the line of the incision, is required, while a maxillary nerve block is necessary if surgery is likely to extend into its territory.

A modified Moffet's technique can be used to produce vasoconstriction of the nasal mucosa under general anaesthesia. The procedure can be carried out after induction of anaesthesia, with the patient placed in the tonsillectomy position, any excess solution being removed by suction.

Maxillary nerve block

The maxillary division of the trigeminal nerve is blocked as it crosses the upper part of the pterygomaxillary fissure. An 8 cm needle, with a marker 5 cm from the tip, is inserted 1 cm below the inferior margin of the zygoma and overlying the anterior border of the masseter muscle, where a vertical line from the lateral orbital margin crosses a horizontal line through the middle of the upper lip (Figure 27.4). The needle is directed backwards at an angle of 30° from the horizontal and upwards and inwards, in such a direction that, when viewed from the front, the shaft of the needle lies in a plane which passes through the pupil (Figure 27.5). The marker indicates the maximum depth of insertion and the needle point will then lie in the pterygomaxillary fissure. The needle may be arrested at a depth of 4 cm by the upper part of the lateral pterygoid plate, however, even here an injection is effective. After an aspiration test, 4 ml of local anaesthetic solution are injected and a further 4 ml as the needle is slowly withdrawn over a distance of 1 cm.

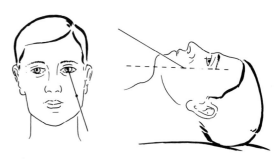

Figure 27.5 Maxillary nerve block. (From Macintosh and Ostlere, 1955, by courtesy of the author and publisher)

nerve in the upper half of the medial wall of the orbit, 2.5 cm from the orbital margin. A 5 cm needle, with a marker 2.5 cm from the tip, is inserted 1 cm above the inner canthus and directed horizontally backwards (Figure 27.6). The needle passes between the medial rectus and the inner wall of the orbit, well away from the eyeball. At a depth of 2.5 cm the tip lies close to the anterior ethmoidal nerve where it enters its foramen (Figure 27.7). One millilitre of local anaesthetic solution is injected and a further 1 ml as the needle is slowly withdrawn. If bone is encountered at a depth of less than 2.5 cm, the needle should be withdrawn almost to the skin before it is redirected.

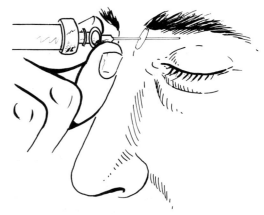

Figure 27.6 Anterior ethmoidal nerve block

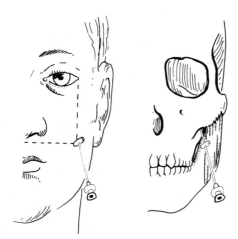

Figure 27.4 Maxillary nerve block (From Macintosh and Ostlere, 1955, by courtesy of the author and publisher)

Anterior ethmoidal nerve block

The anterior ethmoidal and infratrochlear nerves can be blocked together at their origin from the nasociliary

Pharynx, larynx and trachea

Topical anaesthesia can be used for direct laryngoscopy, and for tracheal intubation in the awake patient. A similar technique can be used for fibreoptic or rigid bronchoscopy, however, for the latter general anaesthesia is to be preferred. Topical anaesthesia of the oropharynx is obtained by oral administration of 5–10 ml of 2% Xylocaine viscous, instructing the patient to spread it around the mouth and retain it

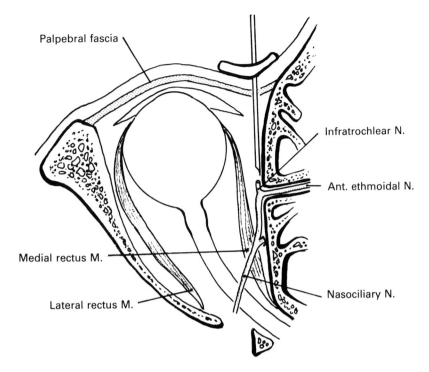

Palpebral fascia

Infratrochlear N.

Ant. ethmoidal N.

Medial rectus M.

Lateral rectus M.

Nasociliary N.

Figure 27.7 Course of needle for anterior ethmoidal nerve block

on the back of the tongue for a few minutes before spitting out any remaining fluid. With the patient sitting up, any remaining pharyngeal reflexes can be obtunded by spraying the soft palate and oropharynx with 4% lignocaine. With the tongue held forwards, a swab, soaked in 4% lignocaine and held by Krause's laryngeal forceps, is inserted in turn into each pyriform fossa by sliding it over the back of the tongue and keeping close to the lateral pharyngeal wall. Once in the fossa, the swab is held there for about 1 minute, to block the internal laryngeal nerve which at this point lies just deep to the mucosa. This will produce anaesthesia in the region extending as far as, and including, the upper surface of the vocal cords. Anaesthesia of the trachea can be obtained by spraying lignocaine through the cords under direct vision, or by injecting 1–2 ml 4% lignocaine through the cricothyroid membrane in the midline. With the latter technique, aspiration of air confirms the correct position of the needle, which must be withdrawn rapidly after the injection before the patient coughs. The total dose of lignocaine should not exceed 3 mg/ kg. Rigid bronchoscopy under topical anaesthesia is an unpleasant experience and as heavy a premedication as is consistent with the patient's ability to cooperate during the examination, and to cough on command at the end, should be administered. The

combination of an opioid and a sedative, such as diazepam or midazolam, is suitable.

With fibreoptic bronchoscopy a sedative premedication is normally not required. Usually the instrument is passed through the nose, requiring surface anaesthesia of the nose, pharynx, larynx and trachea. A 4% lignocaine aerosol spray from a hand nebulizer is used to anaesthetize the nose, and this usually penetrates to the pharynx and sometimes to the larynx. When the nose has become numb, the bronchoscope is introduced and advanced far enough into the pharynx to obtain a view of the vocal cords, which are then sprayed through the bronchoscope. After 1–2 minutes the instrument is passed through the cords into the trachea. If coughing occurs, small doses of 2% lignocaine are injected as the instrument is advanced.

Alternatively, excellent topical anaesthesia of the tracheobronchial tree can be obtained by using an aerosol in association with a ventilator. Most patients will accept positive pressure ventilation from a face mask for the few minutes that are required to nebulize 5 ml of 4% lignocaine (Newton and Edwards, 1979).

For tracheostomy simple infiltration of the skin and subcutaneous tissues in the region of the intended incision is usually adequate. If necessary, complete anaesthesia of the lower half of the neck can be obtained by blocking the clavicular branches of the superior cervical plexus by injecting about 5 ml of local anaesthetic solution just beneath the midpoint of the posterior border of the sternomastoid muscle. Deeper layers of the wound are managed by simple infiltration. Injection of 2–3 ml of 4% lignocaine transtracheally into the lumen will reduce coughing and straining when the trachea is opened.

Ear

Local anaesthesia has been used for almost all types of ear surgery and is effective for simple brief procedures. Long operations under local anaesthesia can be trying for both patient and surgeon. The delicate nature of the surgery and the use of the operating microscope necessitate the patient lying absolutely still, the slightest movement being greatly magnified. Advantages claimed are that an awake patient will be able to evaluate a hearing change and that a dry operating field can be maintained, however, for major ear surgery it has never been a popular technique in the UK. When the operation involves working near the labyrinth dizziness, nausea and even vomiting may make the procedure impossible.

Satisfactory anaesthesia of the tympanic membrane for myringotomy can be obtained by application of a eutectic mixture of 2.5% lignocaine and 2.5% prilocaine (EMLA cream). As animal experiments have shown ototoxic effects when the mixture is instilled into the middle ear, the manufacturers (Astra) do not recommend its use in situations where penetration or injection into the middle ear is possible. Minimal amounts of the cream should be instilled, and a technique using a 1 ml disposable tuberculin (or insulin) syringe and a 20 gauge cannula has been described (Bingham, Hawke and Halik, 1991). Using an aural speculum and microscope, 0.1–0.2 ml of cream is deposited on the site of the myringotomy and left for 15 minutes, before being removed with a small suction tip under direct vision. Using this technique, no evidence of ototoxicity has been found 1–12 months after the procedure.

For permeatal operations, analgesia can be obtained by permeatal injection of 0.5 ml of 1% lignocaine with adrenalin posteriorly, just lateral to the junction of the bony and cartilaginous parts of the meatus, while 0.25 ml of the anaesthetic are injected superiorly, inferiorly and anteriorly at the same depth. Analgesia is enhanced by two further injections of 0.2 ml superiorly and inferiorly, at points 5 mm lateral to the margin of the tympanic membrane. This technique will provide analgesia to the meatus adjacent to the drum, however more extensive blocks are required when other parts of the meatus, the auricle or skin over the mastoid are involved in the incision.

The auriculotemporal nerve can be blocked by injecting 1.5–2.0 ml lignocaine just anterior to the meatus. The operator's index finger is placed in the auditory canal and advanced until arrested by the bony part; the needle point is then advanced until it is adjacent to the tip of the finger (Figure 27.8). The great auricular and auricular nerves can be anaesthetized behind the pinna using a common skin puncture. A weal is raised in front of the lower anterior border of the mastoid process, a 7 cm needle is inserted and directed upwards, and 2–3 ml anaesthetic are placed between the mastoid process and the meatus. The needle is then withdrawn and redirected upwards and backwards to pass posteriorly to the ear canal until its tip is cranial to that structure; 2–4 ml of solution are injected as the needle is being withdrawn (Figure 27.9).

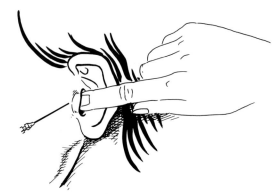

Figure 27.8 Nerve block of the auriculotemporal nerve. (From Morrison, Mirakhur and Craig, 1985, by courtesy of the publisher)

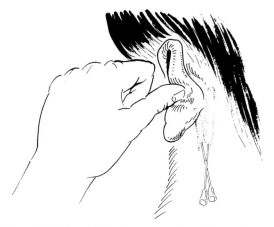

Figure 27.9 Nerve block of great auricular and auricular nerves. (From Morrison, Mirakhur and Craig, 1985, by courtesy of the publisher)

When anaesthesia is required within the tympanic cavity, 4–6 drops of sterile 4% lignocaine may be instilled; repeat of this process may be necessary as the irregular shape of the cavity may cause uneven distribution. Anaesthetic solutions in the middle ear may cause dizziness and nausea lasting up to 8 hours, and possible long-term ototoxic effects must caution against their use.

General anaesthesia

Drugs used in general anaesthesia

General anaesthetic agents can be divided into inhalational and intravenous groups, although some of the latter can be given by other routes. Inhalational agents can be subdivided into the gases and volatile liquids.

Nitrous oxide

Nitrous oxide is the only widely used anaesthetic gas. It is non-flammable, colourless, slightly heavier than air and has a sweetish odour. It is a weak anaesthetic agent and cannot alone produce surgical anaesthesia. Sub-anaesthetic concentrations (50%) with oxygen (50%) are used for analgesia (Entonox mixtures), while 60–70% nitrous oxide and oxygen, supplemented with other agents, is used for general anaesthesia. Nitrous oxide depresses the central nervous system, causes a slight depression of myocardial contractility which is counteracted by some alpha- and beta-adrenergic stimulation and, after prolonged use (24 hours), depression of bone marrow function.

Nitrous oxide is 34 times more soluble than nitrogen in the blood, and so will diffuse into any air-containing cavity more rapidly than nitrogen will exit. In the normal middle ear an increase in pressure (limited by the passive opening of the eustachian tube) and a slight increase in volume, due to the outward bulging of the tympanic membrane, will occur during inhalation of nitrous oxide. The rate of rise in pressure due to inhalation of 70% nitrous oxide is about 0.1–0.2 kPa/min (10–20 mm H_2O/min), reaching a maximum of 3.9 kPa (400 mm H_2O) in 30 minutes. The rate of pressure rise is increased if respiration is assisted, using a bag and mask, as gas can be forced into the ear cavity from the nasopharynx, and diffusion is even more rapid into ear clefts with an initial sub-atmospheric pressure (Drake-Lee, Casey and Ogg, 1983). However, nitrous oxide can have no effect on a middle ear cavity which is completely filled with fluid, as there is no air-containing space with which the gas can equilibrate; an unusual situation as some air remains, at least in the mastoid air cells, in most fluid-filled ear clefts (Gates and Cooper, 1980).

When nitrous oxide is discontinued, a negative pressure may develop as the gas diffuses out more rapidly than nitrogen can enter to replace it (O'Neill, 1980).

These pressure changes may be beneficial or harmful. An atelectatic membrane may be forced into a normal position and contour (Graham and Knight, 1981), and serous fluid may be displaced (Marshall and Cable, 1982). Tympanic membrane rupture has been reported after nitrous oxide inhalation, particularly in patients with ear pathology, also temporary conductive hearing losses, and displacement of ossicular reconstruction and tympanic membrane grafts (Man, Segal and Ezra, 1980). During middle ear surgery it may be advisable to discontinue nitrous oxide for a few minutes before the ear is closed with a tympanic graft, to avoid ballooning of the graft while it is being fixed in position and retraction of the graft postoperatively.

Halothane, enflurane and isoflurane

These volatile liquid, general anaesthetic agents, are all non-flammable. Halothane is twice as potent as enflurane, isoflurane occupying an intermediate position. All are administered from calibrated, temperature compensated vaporizers, each liquid having its own specific vaporizer. All three have a depressant effect on the respiratory and cardiovascular systems which is proportional to the depth of anaesthesia. The hypotension, which results from halothane administration, is due to myocardial depression and reduction in cardiac output, while with isoflurane it is due to vasodilatation and reduction in peripheral vascular resistance. Halothane sensitizes the myocardium to catecholamines and dysrhythmias are not infrequent, especially in the presence of hypercarbia. This agent is contraindicated if adrenalin infiltration is planned during surgery. Enflurane and isoflurane are more compatible with adrenalin, isoflurane being noted for the maintenance of a stable cardiac rhythm during anaesthesia.

Halothane may rarely cause gross disturbance of hepatic function with severe, often fatal, jaundice, the risk being greatest with repeated administrations. This hazard has resulted in a gradual decline in the use of halothane in adult anaesthesia.

Intravenous anaesthetic agents

Induction of anaesthesia is usually by the intravenous route, the two most commonly used agents being the barbiturate, sodium thiopentone and the phenol, propofol. Sodium thiopentone produces a smooth quiet induction in one arm–brain circulation time. Much emphasis has been placed on the respiratory and cardiovascular depressant effects of thiopentone, especially evident in poor risk patients, however the hypotensive effect can be minimized by slow administration and reduced dosage. As with all intravenous induction agents thiopentone should never be given by those unskilled in airway maintenance, tracheal intubation and artificial ventilation. Recovery from thiopentone results from redistribution of the drug in the body and not from rapid detoxication, 30% of the drug may be detected in the body after 24 hours making it unsuitable for repeated administration or prolonged infusion, and it is not ideal for day-case procedures.

Propofol, unlike thiopentone, is insoluble in water and is prepared as an emulsion in soya bean oil, egg phosphatide and glycerine. Pain on injection is not uncommon, especially if small veins are used, and can be minimized or prevented by admixture of 0.08 mg/kg lignocaine immediately prior to injection (Stafford, Hull and Wagstaff, 1991). Induction of anaesthesia is rapid, usually smooth and laryngospasm is uncommon. Hypotension and respiratory depression are more marked than with thiopentone. Redistribution and elimination of propofol is rapid and blood concentrations decline exponentially, most of the drug being metabolized in the liver, with little excreted unchanged. As propofol is non-cumulative patients awaken rapidly, even after days of administration. It can be given by infusion as the sole agent, or as a supplement to other agents, and is the best available induction agent for day-case surgery, having little or no hangover effect.

Many other drugs have been developed for intravenous anaesthesia but most have been discarded, either because they had no advantages over thiopentone, or produced sensitivity reactions in too high a percentage of patients, or had other toxic effects. Of these, three remain at present (1993), etomidate, which is rapidly metabolized and has the advantage of little depressant effect on the cardiovascular system, and the disadvantage of a high incidence of involuntary movement during induction; methohexitone, a barbiturate more rapidly eliminated than thiopentone but now largely superseded by propofol; and ketamine which produces a state of dissociative anaesthesia and is used mainly for paediatric anaesthesia.

Myoneural blocking drugs (muscle relaxants)

Myoneural blocking agents interrupt, at some stage, the normal sequence of acetylcholine release from motor nerve endings, with subsequent attachment to specific receptors in the motor end-plates of striated muscle fibres causing a brief (milliseconds) depolarization of the motor end-plate initiating muscle cell contraction. Since the introduction of tubocurarine into anaesthetic practice, a large number of myoneural blocking agents have been developed over the past five decades, all capable of producing profound

relaxation of striated muscle during light general anaesthesia.

Depolarizing muscle relaxants cause prolonged depolarization of the motor end-plate, preventing any subsequent depolarization and consequent contraction of the muscle fibre. Suxamethonium, the only depolarizing relaxant in common use, is administered when a short period of paralysis is required, for example to facilitate laryngoscopy and tracheal intubation.

Non-depolarizing, competitive blocking agents occupy the receptors on the motor end-plate, hindering access of acetylcholine and subsequent muscle contraction. This block may be partially or completely antagonized (depending on the degree of the block) by the anticholinesterase neostigmine, which delays the hydrolysis of acetylcholine, increasing the concentration at the motor end-plate. Of this group of competitive blockers, pancuronium is used to produce long periods of paralysis, its main disadvantage being the propensity to cause tachycardia. Atracurium, mivacurium and vecuronium are shorter-acting non-depolarizing blockers which do not have any significant effect on the cardiovascular system.

Analgesics

Longer-acting opioid analgesics (e.g. morphine, pethidine) are frequently given either intramuscularly before operation, or intravenously during surgery, to augment the effects of general anaesthetic agents and provide a carry-over analgesic effect into the postoperative period. Short-acting opioids, such as fentanyl (with a duration of action of 20 minutes with a single 1–2 μg/kg dose), or ultrashort-acting alfentanil (4–5 minutes action after 5–7 μg/kg), are also used intraoperatively to prevent reaction to painful stimuli. Opioids cause a dose-related respiratory depression, most marked after intravenous administration, which can be reversed (together with the analgesic effect) by naloxone (0.4 mg). While fentanyl is classed as a short-acting opioid, frequently repeated, or large, doses may cause delayed (6–8 hours) respiratory depression. Nausea and vomiting commonly occur after administration of opioids and require treatment with antiemetics.

Antiemetic drugs

About one-third of patients undergoing general anaesthesia suffer nausea, with or without vomiting, postoperatively. In certain types of surgery (e.g. operations on the middle ear) the proportion is very much higher. The cause may be peripheral or central, the latter arising either from the stimulation of the chemoreceptor trigger zone or by activation of the labyrinthine reflexes. Antiemetic drugs act either at the periphery, or on the vomiting centre, or both. The most useful drugs belong to the antihistamine (e.g. cyclizine), phenothiazine (e.g. perphenazine, prochlorperazine), butyrophenone (e.g. droperidol), anticholinergic (e.g. hyoscine, atropine) and gastrointestinal prokinetic (e.g. metoclopramide) groups. Side effects can occur with many of these agents and include acute dystonia-dyskinesia reactions, sedation and cardiovascular effects in a small proportion of cases; the incidence of extra-pyramidal effects with prochlorperazine being about 0.3%. Cyclizine, an effective antiemetic without extrapyramidal side effects, can be given parenterally as the lactate (50 mg every 6–8 hours) or orally as the hydrochloride. In severe cases of vomiting, such as that associated with labyrinthine disturbances, there is often an associated agitation, and the addition of a sedative drug, such as diazepam, can be helpful. In PCA metoclopramide can be mixed with morphine in a 1:2 ratio to reduce the incidence of nausea and vomiting. When opioids are used in premedication, the addition of an antiemetic will decrease the incidence of nausea and vomiting, particularly useful if atropine, which has an antiemetic action, has been omitted. More recently, drugs which act by highly selective and potent antagonism of 5-hydroxytryptamine$_3$ (5-HT$_3$) receptors in the brain have been found to be extremely effective antiemetic agents, particularly in the control of nausea and vomiting in patients receiving chemotherapeutic agents. One of this group, ondansetron, has also been used effectively in the control of postoperative nausea and vomiting (Leeser and Lip, 1991; Kenny *et al.*, 1992).

Techniques of general anaesthesia in otolaryngology

In otolaryngology, surgical access to the operative site usually precludes use of an anaesthetic face mask, so tracheal intubation via the mouth or nose, or placement of a laryngeal mask airway (LMA), is required. Tracheal intubation is facilitated by use of a muscle relaxant. Suxamethonium provides brief and profound relaxation, allowing rapid return of spontaneous respiration after the tube is in place, while longer-acting blockers, such as vecuronium or atracurium, may necessitate controlled ventilation for up to one hour, unless their action is terminated by neostigmine. Mivacurium has an intermediate duration of action of 15–20 minutes. Anaesthesia is maintained by administration of nitrous oxide, oxygen and an inhalational anaesthetic agent through the tracheal tube or LMA. In the adult a cuff is necessary on the tracheal tube to avoid leaks during controlled ventilation. Oral tracheal intubation is preferable to the nasal route, as the former avoids damage to delicate nasal mucosa and permits passage of a larger tube with reduced airway resistance. Intubation does not

guarantee a free airway as tubes can become kinked (less likely with modern preformed tubes), obstructed by secretions, or the tip partially or completely occluded by resting on the carina or against the wall of the trachea, the risk of the latter being reduced by side holes near the tip of the tube (Murphy's eyes). If the tube is too long it will pass into a bronchus, usually the right, resulting in one lung ventilation and oxygen desaturation, if too short it may be dislodged into the pharynx by flexion or rotation of the head during surgery. A tracheal tube does not ensure protection of the air passages from contamination by blood or secretions; a carefully placed throat pack and an inflated cuff on the tube, making an airtight seal with the tracheal wall, is necessary. Very rarely a traumatic intubation can cause damage to the pharyngeal mucosa and surgical emphysema may result, while dislocation of an arytenoid into the laryngeal inlet after traumatic intubation has resulted in obstruction and stridor after extubation (Tolley *et al.*, 1990).

The laryngeal mask airway, invented by Dr Brain, is made of silicone and consists of a plain tube with a distal cuff designed to obliterate the hypopharynx and the oesophageal isthmus, the flexible reinforced version differs only in having a narrower, more flexible and kink resistant tube, suitable for use with a split tongue plate gag (Figure 27.10). Correctly positioned the device is suitable for spontaneous respiration, ventilation of the lungs occurring through the tube and the larynx. Controlled ventilation is also possible if the inflation pressure does not increase to values which cause gases to bypass the inflated cuff, about 17–20 cm water pressure. While the device does not protect against regurgitation and aspiration of gastric contents (Brain *et al.*, 1985), a correctly placed LMA has been shown to protect the airway from contamination from above (John, Hill and Hughes, 1991). Advantages over conventional

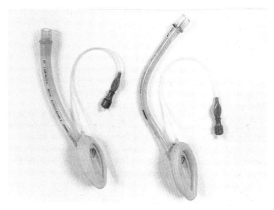

Figure 27.10 Laryngeal mask airways; standard type (left) and flexible kink resistant type (right)

tracheal intubation include avoidance of (a) the use of suxamethonium, (b) aspiration of blood into the trachea past uncuffed tubes, and (c) extubation at the end of surgery either under deep anaesthesia, leaving an unprotected insecure airway, or near awake extubation, risking excessive coughing, venous congestion and postoperative haemorrhage (Williams and Bailey, 1993).

Should anaesthetic hoses between the tracheal tube and the anaesthetic machine become disconnected during spontaneous respiration the patient will become too lightly anaesthetized, however, in a paralysed, ventilated patient, respiration will cease and life-threatening hypoxia result. Disconnections can occur easily and, while most anaesthetic machines are fitted with disconnection alarms these are not infallible, thus constant visual monitoring of apparatus and patient's respiration is necessary.

The aim is to establish and maintain a perfect airway otherwise, while minor degrees of obstruction may not be life threatening, the resultant venous congestion will increase bleeding. Light anaesthesia that results in coughing or straining will have the same effect.

Anaesthesia for adult tonsillectomy

As adenoidal tissue is normally absent in the adult a nasotracheal tube is suitable, however the use of a preformed oral tube, together with a gag with a split tongue plate, will avoid nasal trauma. A reinforced laryngeal mask airway is a possible alternative (Alexander, 1990). Spontaneous breathing is satisfactory and, when the standard tonsil position is used with the nasopharynx dependent to protect the airway from blood, a cuffed tube is not necessary. Stiff plastic nasal tubes should be softened in warm water before use to reduce trauma to the nasal mucosa.

Post-tonsillectomy bleeding

Re-operation to control secondary or reactionary haemorrhage after tonsillectomy presents a considerable hazard for the patient and poses formidable problems for the anaesthetist. Bleeding in the early postoperative period may be largely masked until blood loss is of significant proportions as the patient, drowsy or even asleep, may swallow blood as quickly as it is lost from the circulation, and the first external sign of bleeding may be vomiting of blood. When the problem is recognized a reliable wide bore intravenous line must be established, and blood should be taken for grouping and cross matching. It is ill advised to give sedative drugs in the hope that the bleeding will stop, as these tend to mask further haemorrhage and increase the risk of aspiration of blood into the respiratory tract. While blood transfusion is not often necessary, it is essential that blood volume is restored to near normal value with crystal-loid or plasma expanders (e.g. normal saline and starch solutions) before the patient is anaesthetized. Healthy patients will tolerate a haemoglobin of 8–9 g/100ml blood, provided the blood volume is satisfactory. While it must be assumed that the patient's stomach is full of blood, most subjects will be too distressed to tolerate the passage of a nasogastric tube and the attempt may further aggravate the bleeding.

Problems during induction of anaesthesia are the possibility of vomiting or regurgitation of blood, with danger of aspiration, active bleeding from the tonsil bed and blood clot in the pharynx obscuring the larynx, or even causing respiratory obstruction. Careful inspection of the oropharynx in the awake patient is necessary and, when no difficulty with intubation is anticipated, a rapid sequence intravenous technique is acceptable; that is, preoxygenation, an intravenous induction agent followed by suxamethonium, cricoid pressure being applied on loss of consciousness (to prevent passive regurgitation of stomach contents) and intubation, using a cuffed oral tube, avoiding positive pressure ventilation before the airway is secured. In the presence of active bleeding, or numerous large blood clots, it is advisable to maintain spontaneous respiration until there is no doubt that intubation can be achieved. Anaesthesia is induced with oxygen and halothane while the patient is in the head down left lateral position, cricoid pressure being applied by an assistant from the time of loss of consciousness. When the patient is deeply anaesthetized, direct laryngoscopy and intubation, again with a cuffed oral tube, is carried out. Adequate suction, a variety of working laryngoscopes and a range of tracheal tubes must be to hand. Most of the mishaps associated with pharyngeal bleeding occur as the result of loss of control of the airway.

Anaesthesia for the patient with an obstructed airway

Respiratory obstruction, of varying aetiology and severity, may occur in any part of the respiratory tract. With severe obstruction, in which obvious distress is evidenced by the use of the accessory muscles of respiration, the only safe method of inducing general anaesthesia is first to establish the airway in the conscious patient. If the obstruction lies in the region of the glottis, it may be possible to intubate the trachea under local anaesthesia using a fibreoptic bronchoscope. A nasotracheal tube of suitable size is threaded over the instrument and then, under local anaesthesia, the tube and endoscope are passed through the nose, the larynx visualized, and, once the tip of the instrument is through the glottis, the tube is pushed down into the trachea, thereafter rapidly inducing i.v. general anaesthesia. As the result of swelling and anatomical distortion, the procedure can be difficult and should only be attempted by those skilled in the use of this instrument. However, if the obstruction is higher, or trismus is present, then the only safe choice may be a tracheostomy performed under local anaesthesia. The cardinal rule is that general anaesthesia should not be induced until the airway is secured.

With lesser degrees of obstruction, induction of anaesthesia may be attempted with an inhalational technique, maintaining spontaneous respiration until direct laryngoscopy shows that intubation is possible. However facilities must be available for emergency cricothyroidectomy should this be necessary. Intravenous induction of anaesthesia in these circumstances is dangerous, as respiration can cease and it may not be possible to ventilate the patient or visualize the larynx.

Blind nasal intubation is of value in the unobstructed patient in whom laryngoscopy is impossible, e.g. a patient with a wired fractured mandible. However, this should not be attempted when the airway is compromised as it is unlikely to succeed because of the distorted anatomy, and may precipitate complete obstruction.

When a partially obstructed airway is present medication with opioids is dangerous as depression of the respiratory centre may lead to a complete cessation of respiration. In lesser degrees of respiratory embarrassment a benzodiazepine (e.g. temazepam) may be helpful.

Anaesthesia for nasal surgery

The principles of anaesthesia during surgery on the nose are those of faultless maintenance of anaesthesia and protection of the airway; with recognition of the probability of blood and debris draining into the pharynx during operation, of the possibility of systemic effects from the use of vasoconstrictor drugs, and the likelihood of preoperative and postoperative nasal obstruction. In addition the naso-cardiac reflex, mediated via the trigeminal and vagus nerves, can result in bradycardia, or even brief sinus arrest, following stimulation of the nasal mucosa (Baxandall and Thorn, 1988; Bailey, 1990).

A cuffed oral tracheal tube, together with a pharyngeal pack to prevent soiling of the respiratory tract, is standard practice. Alternatively a laryngeal mask airway can be used, together with a pack as an extra precaution against leakage of blood into the respiratory tract. Throat packs should be moistened with water, not with liquid paraffin or other insoluble lubricants which may cause lipid pneumonia if they enter the lungs. Spontaneous respiration is satisfactory for most nasal operations, however controlled ventilation, using muscle relaxants, is particularly suitable for long procedures and also in patients with an irritable respiratory tract, in whom deep anaesthesia would otherwise be necessary to prevent coughing or straining on the tracheal tube. When a laryngeal

mask airway is used, in conjunction with spontaneous respiration, it is important to avoid too light anaesthesia, which may result in coughing or laryngeal spasm and loss of control of the airway. Topical cocaine, or infiltration of adrenalin, contraindicates the use of halothane, enflurane or isoflurane being suitable alternatives as they are much less likely to cause dysrhythmias.

The patient should be placed in a slightly head-up position to reduce bleeding and improve surgical access. At the end of surgery care must be taken to remove the pharyngeal pack, clear the pharynx of blood by suction, turn the patient into the semi-prone position and insert a pharyngeal airway before removal of the tracheal tube. If a nasal pack is to be left in place its security must be checked to ensure that there is no likelihood of it becoming displaced and thus liable to be inhaled. A good airway, adequate anaesthesia, correct position of the patient and efficient use of topical vasoconstrictors are usually adequate to reduce bleeding to a minimum, however the occasional difficult rhinoplasty or extensive cancer surgery may suggest the use of a controlled hypotensive technique.

Anaesthesia for endoscopy

Laryngoscopy and microlaryngoscopy

During laryngoscopy, the surgeon requires a clear view, immobile cords and adequate space for inspection and instrumentation; while good anaesthetic practice demands overall safety, adequate respiratory exchange, protection of the lower airways and reliable and speedy recovery at the end of the procedure. Many different anaesthetic techniques have been described to try to meet these requirements. Light premedication, such as oral temazepam, is preferred to facilitate rapid postoperative recovery. Narcotics are best avoided if airway patency is suspect, and the precautions already described for induction in this situation must be taken. Most subjects for laryngoscopy have a clear airway and the main discussion about anaesthetic technique is whether or not a tracheal tube should be used and, if not, how adequate ventilation should be maintained.

Using a tracheal tube

Use of a small diameter oral or nasal cuffed tracheal tube secures the airway, provides protection from soiling and allows adequate ventilation. The 31-cm long, 4.5–6.5 mm internal diameter, tracheal tube, with a high volume (10 ml), low pressure cuff is suitable (Coplans, 1976). Airway resistance is high in small diameter tubes and controlled ventilation using muscle relaxants is necessary. Interference with surgical access is a disadvantage, particularly for lesions on the posterior aspect of the cords. Tubes can be occluded as the result of surgical manipulation and are a fire hazard when laser techniques are used.

Using a catheter

Instead of a tracheal tube, a small catheter (14 FG or smaller) can be positioned with the tip midway between the cords and the carina. After intravenous induction anaesthesia is deepened with an inhalational agent and the larynx and trachea thoroughly sprayed with 4% lignocaine before introduction of the catheter. Oxygen and anaesthetic agents are insufflated through the catheter, while the patient is allowed to breathe spontaneously (Hadaway, Page and Shortbridge, 1982). While the method may give better surgical access, disadvantages include lack of protection of the lower airway, some slight movement of the cords with respiration and the surgeon being subjected to exhaled anaesthetic gases.

Using jet ventilation techniques

To obtain an unobstructed view of the larynx during microlaryngoscopy Sanders' (1967) technique of low frequency jet ventilation can be used, anaesthesia being maintained with i.v. agents (e.g. propofol). The method uses the Venturi principle of entrainment of air by means of a tube within a tube, the larger tube being the trachea or laryngoscope. The gas (oxygen) in the inner tube is under pressure and thus expands at the point of exit, producing a suction effect which entrains the surrounding gas (air) in the larger tube, the result being a magnified gaseous thrust. Basic equipment consists of a bayonet fitting nipple plugged into the high pressure oxygen outlet, connected by high pressure tubing to a manual valve, which permits control of both the frequency and length of inspiration. From the valve plastic tubing connects the system to a jet ventilating needle or catheter. The size of the ventilating needle will vary according to the weight and age of the patient, a 14-gauge needle being suitable for most adults. Different points of delivery of the jet have been used and all have advantages and disadvantages.

If the tip of the jet is kept within the laryngoscope then, in order to maintain effective ventilation, the tip of the laryngoscope must be kept close to the cords and the lumen of the instrument kept in line with the axis of the trachea. Having the jet in this position avoids the need for a tube of any kind having to pass through the glottis. The cords must be fully relaxed and the lesion must not be so large as to cause mechanical obstruction to the air flow. Large tumours can have a ball valve effect, making ventilation ineffective. In these circumstances it is best to use a tracheal tube in the first instance, so that the bulk of the tumour can be surgically reduced before jet ventilation is started.

The tip of the jet can protrude beyond the laryngoscope, passing a short way through the glottis. There must be no obstruction to airflow back through the larynx, otherwise dangerously high intratracheal pressure can be generated with resultant barotrauma. A plastic nasal catheter can be used instead of a needle, the tip being placed 3–5 cm above the carina.

Jet ventilation techniques are not without risk and serious barotrauma has been reported (Craft *et al.*, 1990). The risk is increased if the jet exit is inside the trachea and any obstruction to expiration, small mucosal tears, or the use of too high gas pressures, further increases the hazards of surgical emphysema or pneumothorax. The risk is reduced if the tip of the jet is kept within the laryngoscope, precautions are taken to ensure that the airway is clear and ventilation is not started until the laryngoscope is in place and the relaxed unobstructed cords can be seen. In addition, gas can be forced down the oesophagus if the axis of the instrument is not kept in line with the trachea. Chest movements must be observed at all times and it is wise to commence with a low ventilating pressure (100–130 kPa). When using an intratracheal catheter, large volumes of gas can be jetted into the gastrointestinal tract if the catheter becomes displaced and, if a catheter with side holes is used, it is possible for gas to be forced down the oesophagus while the catheter tip still lies below the glottis and ventilation appears to be normal. If the catheter tip goes beyond the carina, one lung ventilation will result and dangerously high intrabronchial pressure may be generated. In addition to the dangers of gross abdominal distension, even small amounts of gas forced into the stomach will greatly increase the risk of regurgitation of gastric contents. If it is suspected that gas has entered the stomach, it is a wise precaution to pass a gastric tube and to keep it in place until the patient is awake. In patients with low lung compliance (e.g. obesity, chronic obstructive airways disease) low frequency jet ventilation systems may not be able to ensure adequate gas exchange and high frequency jet ventilation, or manual ventilation through a small cuffed tracheal tube, may be safer.

High frequency jet ventilators, cycling at about 60–80 breaths per minute with small tidal volumes (2–3 ml/kg body weight), can provide good gas exchange with low airway pressures (Smith, 1982). The gas can be delivered by a nasal or oral catheter with the tip well below the level of the cords (Babinski, Smith and Klain, 1980). A fairly stiff catheter, 3.5–4.0 mm in diameter is necessary, as fine flexible catheters may vibrate quite violently due to rapidly alternating pressures and can damage laryngeal or pharyngeal mucosa. Alternatively, a Teflon cannula can be inserted via a cricothyroid membrane or tracheal puncture, allowing unobstructed surgical access to the larynx (Klain, Kesyler and Stoll, 1983). The ventilator driving pressure can be varied (25–400 kPa), however while lower pressures decrease the vibratory cord movements they tend to produce less effective ventilation. The advantages over low frequency jet ventilation include a decreased risk of mucosal trauma, with reduced risk of surgical emphysema, and more effective ventilation in patients with respiratory disease. However, as with low frequency jet ventilation, gas delivered into the wrong location can cause serious problems (Sherry *et al.*, 1987). The risk can be reduced by using a high frequency ventilator with an airway-pressure-sensing device, which will immediately inhibit gas delivery following activation of the sensor when end-expiratory pressure fails to decrease below a user selected pre-set limit. Hence the machine will detect obstruction to expiration before large volumes of gas are pumped into the tissues (Smith, 1990).

Bronchoscopy

General anaesthetic techniques for bronchoscopy are as numerous and varied as those for laryngoscopy. The procedure may be therapeutic or diagnostic using a rigid or flexible instrument. As with laryngoscopy, the aim is to provide a quiet patient with fully obtunded gag and cough reflexes, who will quickly recover both consciousness and protective reflexes once the examination is completed. The choice of technique is dependent, to some degree, on the purpose of the examination, likely duration and the condition of the patient. Retention of spontaneous respiration is preferred in those cases where there is a foreign body, where there are copious secretions, or where a broncho-pleural fistula or cyst is present. With all techniques, sufficient general anaesthesia, topical anaesthesia and intravenous narcotics should be provided to prevent the occurrence of hypertension and dysrhythmias associated with stimulation of the tracheobronchial tree.

For rigid bronchoscopy anaesthesia can be induced in any suitable way and continued with the patient breathing a mixture of oxygen and inhalational agent. When sufficient depth of anaesthesia is obtained, the glottis and upper trachea are sprayed with a local anaesthetic solution and a ventilation pattern bronchoscope is inserted. Spontaneous respiration may continue with the anaesthetic mixture being delivered through the side port of the bronchoscope, with the eye-piece obturator in place as frequently as possible. Assisted or controlled ventilation is also possible under these circumstances. An alternative technique is the use of short-acting, (intermittent suxamethonium) or moderately long-acting (mivacurium), myoneural blocking agent with controlled ventilation throughout.

The low frequency jet injector technique can be used, the high pressure jet of oxygen being applied at the operator's end of an open bronchoscope and room air entrained during flow, so that the lungs are inflated with a mixture of oxygen and air. Ventilation

can be maintained in the absence of eye-pieces so the surgeon can work unimpeded, however blood and particulate matter may be blown down the tracheobronchial tree, and anaesthesia cannot easily be maintained with inhalational agents. The technique requires an anaesthetized and paralysed patient.

High frequency jet ventilation techniques have also been employed using rates of up to 300 breaths per minute (Smith, 1982; Vourc'h *et al.*, 1983). Movement in the bronchial tree is reduced to a minimum, a particular advantage during laser surgery, and there is little spread of blood and debris.

General anaesthesia is not commonly used for fibreoptic bronchoscopy, however the instrument can be passed through a tracheal tube, with ventilation continuing using the space between bronchoscope and tube wall, employing a 'chimney' or side arm connector for the breathing system. In patients with a tracheostomy it may be possible to pass the fibrescope through the nose or mouth and along the trachea behind the tracheostomy tube.

Bronchoscopy is well tolerated by patients who have no obvious reduction of cardiac or pulmonary reserves. However, in those with significant impairment, it is not a procedure to be undertaken lightly as complications can occur as a consequence of the inevitable increase in hypoxia. While trauma to the teeth and oropharyngeal tissue during the passage of the endoscope may result from inappropriate manipulation of the instrument, trauma to the tracheobronchial tree is more likely to be caused by coughing or movement of the patient. Bleeding, even of minor degree following biopsy, may pose a threat to life by obstructing the airway; therefore careful tracheobronchial suction through the bronchoscope must be continued until bleeding has stopped or become insignificant. Pneumothorax is rare, usually only occurring when excessive airway pressure has been allowed to develop as a result of ventilatory obstruction, or the use of injector ventilation with an inadequate expiratory airway.

Cardiovascular risks during laryngoscopy and bronchoscopy

Manipulation in and around the larynx and trachea, particularly when accompanied by supraglottic tissue tension, may cause a rise in blood pressure, tachycardia, dysrhythmias, myocardial ischaemia and even cardiac arrest. Increasing the duration of rigid laryngoscopy or bronchoscopy increases the pressor response, and while fibreoptic instrumentation causes less stimulation, hypertension still frequently occurs (Smith, Mackenzie and Scott-Knight, 1991). The risks are particularly great in the presence of coronary artery disease and uncontrolled hypertension. Hazards are reduced by preoperative treatment of hypertension, adequate anaesthesia, analgesia and ventilation, and careful monitoring. Adequate doses of short-acting opioids (fentanyl or alfentanil), given intravenously during induction, will attenuate the hypertensive response, as will the short-acting cardioselective beta-adrenergic blocking drug esmolol, given perioperatively as a single dose or by infusion (Ebert *et al.*, 1989; Vucevic, Purdy and Ellis, 1992). Tachycardia and the hypertensive response can also be moderated by careful application of topical anaesthesia to the mouth, pharynx, larynx and trachea after the patient loses consciousness. The procedure must be carried out slowly, one stage at a time, to avoid triggering the reflex; although tedious it may be of great value to the high risk patient. Too light levels of anaesthesia, hypercarbia or hypoxia increase the incidence of dysrhythmias. Tachycardia and hypertension are a dangerous combination, the former decreasing the time available for coronary artery perfusion of the deeper layers of the myocardium and the latter increasing the work load of the heart. Strong *et al.* (1974) reported an overall 1.5% incidence of myocardial infarction or ischaemia following microlaryngoscopy, with an incidence of 4% in patients with a history of cardiac disease. As many of these infarctions are symptomatically silent, a postoperative ECG is recommended for those patients thought to be at risk.

ECG, pulse oximetry and blood pressure monitoring are essential during laryngoscopy and bronchoscopy. If hypertension or dysrhythmias develop during laryngoscopy it may be necessary to release the suspension laryngoscope for a few minutes, deepen anaesthesia and sometimes give either beta-adrenergic or calcium-channel blocking drugs (Mikawa, Obara and Kusunoki, 1990).

Pharyngoscopy and oesophagoscopy

Tracheal intubation provides safety for the patient and good access for the surgeon. Adequate muscle relaxation is necessary for the passage of the oesophagoscope, and this will also prevent sudden movement which could result in laceration or perforation of the oesophagus while the endoscope is in place. Cardiac dysrhythmias sometimes occur as the instrument passes behind the heart, however they are rarely troublesome.

Anaesthesia for laser surgery

Laser surgery poses special problems for the anaesthetist. When rubber or plastic tubes are used they must be protected from the laser beam as, if hit directly or contacted by a beam reflected off a shiny metal surface, they are liable to be ignited. Flammable anaesthetic agents must not be used and it is wise to avoid high oxygen concentrations. Nitrous oxide, which supports combustion at high temperatures, is also contraindicated. Lubricants should be restricted to aqueous solutions as ointments and other greases are flammable. Combustible tracheal tubes can be protected against carbon dioxide (CO_2) lasers by wrapping in aluminium foil tape as far down as the cuff, or by covering in muslin soaked in saline. Cuffs, which should be inflated with saline rather than air, can be protected with saline-soaked cotton swabs, care being taken to ensure that all are removed at the end of the procedure. Plastic tracheostomy tubes can be protected in a similar manner. It is difficult to maintain effective protection of tracheal tubes at all times; gaps can appear between the layers of tape and, if the tape is broken, sharp edges can injure mucosa (Patil, Stenlurg and Zauder, 1979). Aluminium foil does not protect tubes from exposure to neodymium-yttrium aluminium garnet (Nd-YAG) laser beams, however clear polyvinyl chloride tubes with no markings are relatively resistant (Geffin *et al.*, 1986). Tubes made of silicone elastomer and coated with a layer of silicone containing reflective aluminium oxide, offer some resistance to CO_2 but not Nd-YAG lasers. Flexible all metal tubes with a double cuff are available, however, as the walls are relatively thick, surgical access is restricted, even with small internal diameter tubes. Fire hazards are removed by using jet ventilation through a metal cannula, or greatly reduced by jet ventilation via a Teflon cannula inserted through the cricothyroid membrane or trachea.

Anaesthesia for tracheostomy

The key to satisfactory tracheostomy is the prior securing of the airway by tracheal intubation or bronchoscopy, allowing the surgeon to perform an unhurried operation in an uncongested field. When the patient has significant airway obstruction before operation the technique for induction of anaesthesia alrady described for the patient with an obstructed airway must be used. While anaesthesia and a secure airway are always desirable for the optimum operating conditions, general anaesthesia may, in a very few cases, be too dangerous and the tracheostomy should then be performed under local anaesthesia. The anesthetist must never be persuaded to embark on a general anaesthetic against his better judgement, as he is the only person who can fully appreciate both the difficulties that may be encountered and the extent of his own experience and capability in overcoming them.

Anaesthesia for major head and neck surgery

Otolaryngology now includes major cancer and reconstructive operations on the nose, paranasal sinuses, mouth, pharynx, larynx, upper oesophagus and trachea, and intracranial procedures for removal of acoustic neuromas, vestibular nerve section and trans-sphenoidal hypophysectomy. The procedures are prolonged, often require extensive dissection, and many are associated with significant blood loss. As with all major surgery, perfect control of the airway, good reliable venous access for accurate fluid replacement and careful monitoring of vital functions during and after operation are essential.

Monitoring should include pulse oximetry to measure haemoglobin oxygen saturation, ECG display, end-tidal carbon dioxide concentration, inspired and expired oxygen and anaesthetic vapour concentration and blood pressure measurement, preferably using a direct method with radial artery cannulation. Central venous measurement can be useful both during and after operation to help estimate fluid replacement requirements. Central catheters are best placed via the infraclavicular approach to the subclavian vein, a neck approach being usually inside the surgical field. Catheter position must be checked preoperatively by radiography. A urinary catheter is necessary for accurate intraoperative urinary output measurement, while some intracranial procedures require spinal CSF drainage to reduce intracranial pressure. Long procedures may result in a fall in body temperature and this should be monitored by rectal or oesophageal temperature probes, and reduction in temperature minimized by using a heating blanket. The use of a peripheral nerve stimulator will provide a useful guide to the state of neuromuscular blockade and the timing of further doses of muscle relaxants.

Air embolism, although rare, is a potential complication. Air may be seen entering one of the neck veins, however the condition is best detected by observation of the end-tidal carbon dioxide concentration, which will fall rapidly should this mishap occur. A precordial Doppler flow transducer can also be used for the diagnosis, whereas hypotension, tachycardia and ECG changes (dysrhythmias and evidence of right heart strain) are late signs. Treatment consists of any measure that will increase venous pressure, such as continuous positive pressure ventilation and compression of the jugular veins. Nitrous oxide is discontinued and the patient ventilated with 100% oxygen and, as soon as practicable, is placed in the left lateral head-down position. It may be possible to aspirate air through the central venous catheter. In extreme cases external cardiac massage and transthoracic aspiration of air from the right ventricle, with needle and syringe, may be necessary. General supportive measures include the use of inotropic agents and correction of metabolic acidosis.

Patients should be transferred to an intensive care or high dependency unit after most major head and neck surgery.

Laryngectomy

Many patients for laryngectomy have chronic pulmonary pathology, require preoperative physiotherapy and, in some cases, bronchodilator drugs may be helpful. While obvious upper airway obstruction may not be present, a careful assessment of airway patency and possible difficulties in intubation of the trachea during induction of anaesthesia is necessary. Indirect or fibreoptic laryngoscopy can be helpful. Assessment at a prior laryngoscopy is useful, and should be recorded in the notes. Some patients develop oedema subsequent to laryngoscopy and biopsy, so a good airway at that time is not an absolute guarantee that all will be well a few days later. Very occasionally preliminary tracheostomy under local anaesthesia may be the safest course.

Care must be exercised during intubation to avoid trauma to the neoplastic area with consequent haemorrhage and possible tumour spread. A smaller tube than usual may be indicated. A north facing preformed tube is less likely to be occluded than a standard type. Once the airway is established problems are unlikely. If spontaneous respiration is used, then anaesthesia is based on an inhalational agent, however it is more usual to employ muscle relaxants and controlled ventilation throughout what is often a long operation in a poor risk patient. A few minutes before the trachea is divided the patient is ventilated with 100% oxygen and an inhalational agent. After tracheal division the oral tube is removed and a sterile cuffed tracheostomy tube, or a special preformed armoured tube (Figure 27.11), inserted into the trachea by the surgeon. The change-over should be performed as quickly and smoothly as possible. The surgeon who does not appreciate the need for speed in this manoeuvre may cause the anaesthetist considerable anxiety, as may the sudden discovery of a missing or inappropriate connection or piece of tubing. Care must be taken that blood does not enter the tracheostome. If spontaneous ventilation is allowed, anaesthesia must be deepened before the change-over period to avoid coughing, but as the patient is breathing throughout there is not the same urgency. Bleeding can be quite brisk at times and

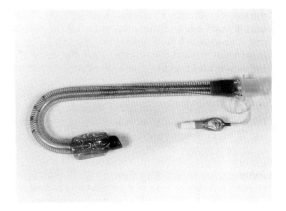

Figure 27.11 Preformed, cuffed, armoured tracheal tube for use during laryngectomy

blood loss can be significant, especially if a block dissection of neck glands is required. Good venous access with a wide bore cannula is mandatory, however blood lost can usually be adequately replaced with crystalloid or plasma expander fluids, blood transfusion being rarely necessary.

Pharyngolaryngectomy

Either a radical one-stage operation using a stomach 'pull-up' together with total oesophagectomy, or a more limited excision with a free jejunal graft and microvascular anastomosis, is the procedure used for the surgical treatment of some types of hypopharyngeal cancer. Anaemia, malnutrition and electrolyte imbalance may be present preoperatively, due to difficulty in swallowing food and even fluids. Nutrition can be improved, if necessary, by nasogastric feeding; parenteral nutrition is rarely required. As pre- and postoperative chest infection is not unusual, physiotherapy and attainment of maximum respiratory function is important preoperatively.

During operation access to the patient by the anaesthetist may be difficult because of the number of surgeons and their assistants. The anaesthetist may be very dependent on monitoring devices, however he must insist on having access to one arm on an armboard.

Controlled ventilation is used throughout, and while deliberate lowering of the arterial blood pressure may be helpful at certain stages this is not without risk in these debilitated patients; many feel it to be unnecessary and dangerous (Plant, 1982). Blood loss can be substantial, particularly during mobilization of the thoracic oesophagus, and may be largely concealed in the thorax. Dysrhythmias and dramatic falls in blood pressure, as the result of interference with venous return, are not infrequent at this stage. When the trachea becomes unsupported, after mobilization of the oesophagus, the fragile posterior wall may rupture at the site of the tracheostomy tube cuff, making inflation of the lungs difficult or impossible (Bains and Spiro, 1979). Manual ventilation of the lungs with 100% oxygen, until the stomach is drawn into the neck up to tamponade the leak, may cope with the situation, however a short cuffed tracheal or endobronchial tube may be necessary and should be available. The pleura on one or both sides may be torn during mobilization of the oesophagus requiring placement of chest drains.

Tracheal surgery

Elective operations involving excision of lesions with tracheal reconstruction, or emergency repair of the trachea following trauma, are a challenge to the anaesthetist. The problems of providing adequate oxygenation and facilitating carbon dioxide removal with an open trachea, combined with the need to provide good operating conditions, are formidable. Periods of hypoventilation may be unavoidable and monitoring is required to detect quickly the onset of hypoxaemia. Airway management may necessitate a multi-stage approach, each step being fully planned before surgery, with the nature, site and extent of the obstructed segment and proposed method of surgical repair all being taken into account.

The anaesthetic technique depends on the degree of narrowing of the trachea and the level of the lesion. Controlled ventilation, using a small bore uncuffed orotracheal tube inserted into the distal segment, is a suitable technique, provided that the narrowing is not too severe (Borgan and Privitera, 1976). If the trachea is deviated, the bevel of the tube should be cut in such a way that the opening does not lie against the tracheal wall. With a very tight stenosis it may be unwise to force through even a small diameter tube, for fear of subsequent bleeding and oedema. In such cases an ordinary tracheal tube is positioned just proximal to the stenosis.

When the presence of a tracheal tube interferes with the surgical access during the anastomosis, withdrawing the tube into the proximal segment and passing a catheter down the orotracheal tube into the distal segment of the trachea after its division, with ventilation being maintained by high frequency ventilation, may overcome the problem (Rogers *et al.*, 1985). When the stenosis is very low, two tubes may be passed, one down each bronchus. The catheters must be secured by a stitch to the tracheal or bronchial walls. As soon as the anastomosis is completed, the catheters should be withdrawn and ventilation continued through the tracheal tube. Alternatively, a cuffed tube may be inserted into the distal cut end of the trachea, or into a main bronchus (Kamvyssi-Dea *et al.*, 1975), which is then removed before completion of the anastomosis, at which time an orotracheal tube is passed down through the cut ends. A technique using spontaneous ventilation may occasionally be employed in high tracheal stenosis, however the danger of opening the pleurae during the operation must be borne in mind.

Anaesthesia during the period of the tracheal anastomosis is usually maintained with intravenous drugs (Vyas, Lyons and Dundee, 1983), except where a tracheal tube has been passed into the distal segment when inhalational agents can be used. When spontaneous ventilation is used, the wound is flooded with oxygen by way of a tracheal tube placed in the proximal segment during the anastomosis.

Maintenance of full power and control in the neck and pharyngeal musculature is important in the support of a traumatically disrupted trachea and the loss of this power, associated with induction of general anaesthesia, may result in airflow disruption. Preoperative visualization of the damaged area, using a fibreoptic bronchoscope under local anaesthesia, can be valuable in assessing the situation (Brierley, Oates and Bogod, 1991).

Controlled hypotension

Since the beginning of surgery bleeding has been a problem to the surgeon, when blood obscures the operative field and makes precise technique difficult, and to the anaesthetist, when the volume of blood lost is large. Surgical problems are greater when the operation involves very small structures, often in confined cavities such as the middle ear, when even very small amounts of blood make successful reconstructive surgery difficult or impossible. In this type of surgery a reduction in blood pressure is useful and may be essential, however indications for controlled hypotension in other head and neck procedures are less clear cut. The aim is to provide conditions that give the best operating field possible, without endangering in any way the life or well-being of the patient.

The exact relationship between the level of blood pressure and the degree of reduction of bleeding is not firmly established and there is no evidence that profound hypotension, with systolic pressures as low as 30 mmHg, is any more effective than more moderate and safer reduction (Donald, 1982). Venous oozing is an important component of operative bleeding and can be reduced by careful positioning of the patient, securing a free airway and ensuring a complete absence of coughing or straining. Local vasoconstriction, produced by infiltration of the operative site with adrenalin, can be as effective as hypotension in control of haemorrhage. Infection will result in vasodilatation and increased bleeding, which tends to be resistant to any of these measures of control.

Arterial pressure is directly proportional to cardiac output and peripheral resistance, being maintained, in normal circumstances, by the autonomic nervous system and hormonal control. These mechanisms tend to resist attempts to lower blood pressure; thus resistance to drugs and techniques aimed at producing hypotension is frequently encountered, especially in the young robust patient.

The ability of any given arterial pressure to maintain an adequate blood flow to vital organs, particularly the brain and heart, determines the safety of the technique. Both the brain and the heart are able to maintain their perfusion over a wide range of pressure change by local autoregulation, provided the vasculature is healthy and carbon dioxide tensions are kept in the normal range. Reduction in flow is unlikely, provided that arterial pressure is not reduced too rapidly (so that autoregulatory mechanisms have time to act), nor too low (less than 55–60 mmHg mean pressure). When a patient is tilted head up, to reduce venous pressure at the operation site, allowance should be made for the difference in arterial pressure between the point of measurement and the brain, allowing a 2 mmHg change in pressure for every 2.5 cm difference in vertical height.

When arterial pressure is reduced a fall in arterial oxygen tension occurs as a result of ventilation/perfusion inequalities in the lung. This is brought about by reduction in cardiac output, a fall in pulmonary blood pressure and depression of the normal hypoxic vasoconstrictor mechanism responsible for diverting pulmonary blood flow away from parts of the lung with a low alveolar oxygen tension. Thus, a high inspired oxygen concentration is advisable during hypotension, and evidence of significant impairment of lung function is a contraindication to the use of the technique.

Preoperative assessment is important to exclude cerebrovascular, cardiovascular or pulmonary disease. Hypertensive patients, even if well controlled, can be regarded as having a diseased cardiovascular system, and anaemia is also a contraindication. Diabetics are prone to atheroma and those with long-standing disease are not suitable for controlled hypotensive techniques, as are patients with a history of angina, coronary artery occlusion or cerebrovascular accident. Pregnancy, or the use of contraceptive medication, is also a contraindication. Competence of the circulation to the vital organs is erratically reduced by ageing and, as this is not clinically detectable, deliberate hypotension in the elderly is, if possible, to be avoided.

Blood pressure should not be reduced when this is thought to carry a significantly increased risk, as will be indicated by the general condition of the patient, the past history, or abnormal findings in ECG, chest X-ray, pulmonary function tests or routine blood analysis. When factors which increase wound bleeding are avoided, reasonably satisfactory results can often be obtained without recourse to reduction in arterial pressure.

Techniques of controlled hypotension

Blood pressure is reduced by lowering peripheral vascular resistance or cardiac output, or by a combination of both. Tilting the patient head up will hydrostatically decrease arterial and venous pressure at the operative site and pool blood in the lower parts of the body, decreasing venous return to the heart and cardiac output. Inhalational anaesthetic agents reduce blood pressure either by myocardial depression (halothane) or vasodilatation (isoflurane). Some muscle relaxants (pancuronium) increase heart rate, and hence cardiac output, and so are less suitable for hypotensive anaesthesia than others, with no effect on the heart rate or peripheral vascular resistance (vecuronium, atracurium).

Drugs used to lower blood pressure are many and varied, the four most commonly used being described below. With the exception of labetalol, all are administered by continuous infusion, blood pressure being controlled by the rate of delivery.

Trimetaphan camsylate

Trimetaphan camsylate has a direct dilatory effect on vascular smooth muscle and causes histamine release, however its hypotensive effect is mainly due to ganglionic blockade (Adams and Hewitt, 1982). Blood pressure falls within 4 minutes and the full effect is produced within 10 minutes of starting the infusion. Return to prehypotensive levels is usual within a few minutes of cessation of the infusion, however recovery can be delayed after prolonged administration and the use of large doses. The hypotensive effect is markedly potentiated by halothane and other inhalational agents. Tachycardia is frequently a problem, especially in young fit adults, resulting in increased cardiac output and difficulty in lowering arterial pressure. It can usually be controlled by beta-adrenergic blocking drugs.

Sodium nitroprusside

Sodium nitroprusside acts directly on vascular smooth muscle causing relaxation in both resistance and capacitance vessels. Action is rapid in onset and of short duration, the rapidity of response necessitating an accurate control of the rate of administration, preferably with an infusion pump. When administration ceases, arterial pressure rises spontaneously and rapidly, provided that significant blood loss has been replaced. While tachycardia can be troublesome, it can usually be controlled by adequate anaesthesia, analgesia, and administration of beta-adrenergic blocking drugs.

Rapid administration and large doses of nitroprusside (more than 1.5 mg/kg) can cause toxic effects as the result of cyanide release during metabolic breakdown. The rate of infusion should not exceed 10 μg/kg/min. In practice, only small doses are needed when use is made of the inhalational anaesthetic agents to potentiate the hypotensive effect. Nitroprusside is contraindicated in some patients with metabolic disorders, severe renal or hepatic disease, Leber's optic atrophy (a rare inherited disease), tobacco amblyopia and in the presence of neuropathies secondary to vitamin B_{12} deficiency, in all of whom cyanide metabolism is abnormal.

Nitroglycerin

Nitroglycerin (glyceryl trinitrate) produces dilatation of the peripheral veins, with a lesser dilatory effect on the resistance vessels. It has a slower onset of action than nitroprusside and a more prolonged effect; this can be an advantage in that it makes abrupt swings in pressure easier to avoid. The hypotensive action is potentiated by the inhalational agents and quite high concentrations are sometimes necessary to obtain adequate reduction in blood pressure in fit robust patients, who tend to be resistant.

Labetalol

Labetalol is an amide with both alpha- and beta-adrenergic blocking properties, decreasing blood pressure by a reduction in peripheral vascular resistance and by a decrease in cardiac output. The drug shows a remarkable synergism with the volatile anaesthetic agents in producing a hypotensive effect, and arterial pressure can be easily and quickly controlled by adjustment of the inspired concentration of the volatile agent. Blood pressure can be raised at the end of surgery by withdrawing the inhalational agent and, if necessary, giving atropine intravenously to increase the heart rate.

Monitoring during hypotensive anaesthesia

Careful monitoring is essential during controlled hypotension and, although particular attention must be paid to the level of arterial pressure, other vital observations must not be neglected.

Blood pressure

The method of pressure measurement depends on the hypotensive technique, the reduction of pressure desired and the nature of the surgery. When rapidly acting, powerful agents, such as nitroprusside, are used, direct blood pressure measurement via a radial artery cannula and pressure transducer, giving a beat by beat observation of the pressure, is required. While this is suitable for all techniques of controlled hypotension, when slower-acting, less powerful agents are used, to produce moderate falls in pressure, a non-invasive method of pressure measurement is adequate. Automatic blood pressure monitors, working on the oscillotonometry principle, are popular and becoming increasingly accurate, however these devices are unreliable at very low pressures.

Arterial oxygen saturation

Reliable pulse oximetry instruments, which measure the arterial oxygen saturation and pulse rate non-invasively and accurately to within $+/-$ 2%, are now available. The apparatus consists of a simple probe, attached to the finger or ear lobe, containing two light emitting diodes (red and infrared), with a single detector positioned on the opposite side of the digit. The proportion of light absorbed by haemoglobin depends on the light wave length and the ratio of oxyhaemoglobin to deoxyhaemoglobin. The instrument is so programmed that only the saturation of arterial blood is recorded. The device is simple to use and provides an overall assessment of the the integrity of all the systems involved in delivering oxygen to the tissues. Pulse oximetry should be regarded as mandatory for all patients having a general anaesthetic, being particularly valuable in those undergoing controlled hypotension.

ECG

A continuous display of the ECG is necessary during controlled hypotension to observe cardiac rhythm and detect myocardial ischaemia. A 12-lead preoperative ECG may be useful for comparison.

Carbon dioxide tension

A large decrease in arterial carbon dioxide tension, due to overventilation, may be hazardous in controlled hypotension as the resultant cerebral vasoconstriction will further decrease cerebral blood flow. End tidal carbon dioxide monitoring will act as an effective guide to the arterial gas tension.

Blood loss

Adequate replacement of blood lost is essential as the normal circulatory defence mechanisms, which compensate for a reduction in blood volume, are abolished by the hypotensive technique. During surgery where significant haemorrhage is likely, direct measurement of blood loss by weighing swabs and estimation of haemoglobin content of suction fluids is advisable. Central venous pressure measurement is helpful in monitoring fluid replacement, however central pressure can be reduced by some hypotensive agents.

Temperature

Body temperature should be monitored during long procedures; a mid-oesophageal or rectal probe is satisfactory.

References

ADAMS, A. P. and HEWITT, P. B. (1982) Clinical pharmacology of hypotensive agents. *International Anesthesiology Clinics*, **20**, 95–109

ALEXANDER, C. A. (1990) A modified intravent laryngeal mask for ENT and dental anaesthesia. *Anaesthesia*, **45**, 892–893

BABINSKI, M., SMITH, R. B. and KLAIN, M. (1980) High frequency jet ventilation for laryngoscopy. *Anesthesiology*, **52**, 178–180

BAILEY, P. L. (1990) Sinus arrest induced by trivial nasal stimulation during alfentanil-nitrous oxide anaesthesia. *British Journal of Anaesthesia*, **65**, 718–720.

BAINS, M. S. and SPIRO, R. H. (1979) Pharyngolaryngectomy, total extra thoracic esophagectomy and gastric transposition. *Surgery, Gynecology and Obstetrics*, **149**, 693–696

BAYLISS, R., CLARKE, C., OAKLEY, C. M, SOMERVILLE, W., WHITFIELD, A. G. W. and YOUNG, S. E. J. (1983) The microbiology and pathogenesis of infective endocarditis. *British Heart Journal*, **50**, 513–519

BAXANDALL, M. L. and THORN, J. L. (1988) The naso-cardiac reflex. *Anaesthesia*, **43**, 480–481

BINGHAM, B., HAWKE, M. and HALIK, J. (1991) The safety and efficacy of Emla Cream topical anesthesia for myringotomy and ventilation tube insertion. *Journal of Otolaryngology*, **20**, 193–195

BORGAN, C. P. and PRIVITERA, P. A. (1976) Resection of stenotic trachea; a case presentation. *Anesthesia and Analgesia*, **55**, 191–194

BRAIN, A. I. J., MCGHEE, T. D., MCATEER, E. J., THOMAS, A., ABU-SAAD, M. A. W. and BUSHMAN, J. A. (1985) The laryngeal mask airway. Development and preliminary trials of a new type of airway. *Anaesthesia*, **40**, 356–361

BRIERLEY, J. K., OATES, J. and BOGOD, D. G. (1991) Diagnostic and management dilemmas in a patient with tracheal trauma. *British Journal of Anaesthesia*, **66**, 724–727

CAMPBELL, W. I. (1990) Analgesic side effects and minor surgery: which analgesic for minor and day case surgery? *British Journal of Anaesthesia*, **64**, 617–620

COPLANS, M. P. (1976) A cuffed nasotracheal tube for microlaryngeal surgery. *Anaesthesia*, **31**, 430–431

CRAFT, T.M., CHAMBERS, P. H., WARD, M. E. and GOAT, V. A. (1990) Two cases of barotrauma associated with transtracheal jet ventilation. *British Journal of Anaesthesia*, **64**, 524–527

CURTISS, E. S. (1952) Postural nerve block for intra-nasal operations. *Lancet*, i, 989–991

DONALD, J. R. (1982) Induced hypotension and blood loss during surgery. *Journal of the Royal Society of Medicine*, **75**, 149–151

DRAKE-LEE, A. B., CASEY W. F. and OGG, T. W. (1983) Anaesthesia for myringotomy. *Anaesthesia*, **38**, 314–318

EBERT, J. P., PEARSON, J. D., GELMAN, S., HARRIS, C. and BRADLEY, E. L. (1989) Circulatory responses to laryngoscopy: the comparative effects of placebo, fentanyl and esmolol. *Canadian Journal of Anaesthesia*, **36**, 301–306

EGAN, K. J. (1990) What does it mean to be a patient 'in control'? In: *Patient Controlled Analgesia*, edited by F. M. FERRANTE, G. W. OSTHEIMER and B. G. COVINO. Oxford: Blackwell Scientific Publications. pp. 17–26

ENDOCARDITIS WORKING PARTY OF THE BRITISH SOCIETY FOR ANTIMICROBIAL CHEMOTHERAPY. (1990) Antibiotic prophylaxis of infective endocarditis. *Lancet*, i, 88–89

FERREIRA, S. H. (1980) Peripheral analgesia. Mechanism of the analgesic action of asprin like drugs and opiate-antagonists. *British Journal of Clinical Pharmacology*, **10**, 237s–245s

GATES, G. A. and COOPER, J. C. (1980) Effect of anesthetic gases on middle ear pressure in the presence of effusion. *Annals of Otology, Rhinology and Laryngology*, **89** (Suppl.), 62–64

GEFFIN, B., SHAPSHAY, S. M., BELLACK, G. S., HOBIN, K. and SETZER, S. E. (1986) Flammability of endotracheal tubes during Nd-YAG laser application in the airway. *Anesthesiology*, **65**, 511–515

GRAHAM, M. D. and KNIGHT, P. R. (1981) Atelectatic tympanic membrane reversal by nitrous oxide supplemented general anaesthesia and polyethylene ventilator tube insertion. *Laryngoscope*, **91**, 1469–1471

HADAWAY, E. G., PAGE, J. and SHORTBRIDGE, R. T. (1982) Anaesthesia for microsurgery of the larynx. *Annals of the Royal College of Surgeons of England*, **64**, 279–280

HIRSCH, I. B., MCGILL J. B., CRYER, P. E. and WHITE, P. F. (1991) Perioperative management of surgical patients with diabetes mellitus. *Anesthesiology*, **74**, 346–359

JOHN, R. E., HILL, S. and HUGHES, T. J. (1991) Airway protection by the laryngeal mask. *Anaesthesia*, **46**, 366–367

KAMVYSSI-DEA, S., KRITIKOU, P., EXARHOS, N. and SKALKEAS, G. (1975) Anaesthetic management of reconstruction of the lower portion of the trachea. *British Journal of Anaesthesia*, **47**, 82–84

KENNY, G. N. C., OATES, J. D. L., LEESER, J., ROWBOTHAM, D. J., LIP, H., RUST, M. *et al.* (1992) Efficacy of orally administered ondansetron in the prevention of postoperative nausea and vomiting: a dose ranging study. *British Journal of Anaesthesia*, **68**, 466–470

KLAIN, M., KESYLER, H. and STOLL, S. (1983) Transtracheal high frequency jet ventilation prevents aspiration. *Critical Care Medicine*, **11**, 170–172

LEESER, J. and LIP, H. (1991) Prevention of postoperative nausea and vomiting using ondansetron, a new selective 5 H-T$_3$ receptor antagonist. *Anesthesia and Analgesia*, **72**, 751–755

MACINTOSH, SIR R. and OSTLERE, M. (1955) *Local Analgesia: Head and Neck.* Edinburgh: E & S Livingstone

MAN, A., SEGAL, S. and EZRA, S. (1980) Ear injury caused by elevated intratympanic pressure during general anaesthesia. *Acta Anaesthesiologica Scandinavica*, **24**, 224–226

MARSHALL, F. P. F. and CABLE, H. R. (1982) The effect of nitrous oxide on middle ear effusions. *Journal of Laryngology and Otology*, **96**, 893–897

MIKAWA, K., OBARA, H. and KUSUNOKI, M. (1990) The effect of nicardipine on the cardiovascular response to tracheal intubation. *British Journal of Anaesthesia*, **64**, 240–242

MIRAKHUR, R. K. and DUNDEE, J. W. (1983) Glycopyrrolate: pharmacology and clinical use. *Anaesthesia*, **38**, 1195–1204

MORRISON, J. D., MIRAKHUR, R. K. and CRAIG, H. J. L. (1985) *Anaesthesia for Eye, Ear, Nose and Throat Surgery*, 2nd edn. Edinburgh: Churchill Livingstone

NEWTON, D. A. G. and EDWARDS, G. F. (1979) Route of induction and method of anaesthesia for fibreoptic bronchoscopy. *Chest*, **75**, 650

O'NEILL, G. (1980) Middle ear pressure measurements during nitrous oxide anaesthesia. *Clinical Otolaryngology*, **5**, 355

PATIL, V., STENLURG, L. C. and ZAUDER, H. L. (1979) A modified endotracheal tube for laser microsurgery. *Anesthesiology*, **51**, 571

PLANT, M. (1982) Anaesthesia for pharyngo-laryngectomy with extrathoracic oesophagectomy and gastric transposition. *Anaesthesia*, **37**, 1211–1213

PRYS-ROBERTS, C., MELOCHE, R. and FOEX, P. (1971) Studies of anaesthesia in relation to hypertension: 1. Cardiovascular responses of treated and untreated patients. *British Journal of Anaesthesia*, **43**, 122–137

ROGERS, R. C., GIBBONS, J., COSGROVE, J. and COPPEL, D. L. (1985) High frequency jet ventilation for surgery. *Anaesthesia*, **40**, 32–36

SANDERS, R. D. (1967) Two ventilating attachments for bronchoscopes. *Delaware State Medical Journal*, **39**, 170–176

SHERRY, K. M., KEELING, P. A., JONES, H. M. and AVELING, W. (1987) Insertion of intratracheal stents. Anaesthetic management using high frequency jet ventilation or cardiopulmonary bypass. *Anaesthesia*, **42**, 61–66

SMITH, B. E. (1990) Developments in the safe use of high frequency jet ventilation. *British Journal of Anaesthesia*, **65**, 735–736

SMITH, J. E., MACKENZIE, A. A. and SCOTT-KNIGHT, V. C. E. (1991) Comparison of two methods of fibrescope-guided tracheal intubation. *British Journal of Anaesthesia*, **66**, 546–550

SMITH, R. B. (1982) Ventilation at high respiratory frequencies. *Anaesthesia*, **37**, 1011–1018

STAFFORD, M. A., HULL, C. J. and WAGSTAFF, A. (1991) Effect of lignocaine on pain during injection of propofol. *British Journal of Anaesthesia*, **66**, 406P–407P

STRONG, M. S., VAUGHAN, C. W., MAHLER, D. L., JAFFE, D. R. and SULLIVAN, R. G. (1974) Cardiac complications of microsurgery of the larynx. *Laryngoscope*, **84**, 908–920

TOLLEY, N. S., CHEESMAN, T. D., MORGAN, D. and BROOKES, G. B. (1990) Dislocated arytenoid: an intubation induced injury. *Annals of the Royal College of Surgeons of England*, **72**, 353–356

VOURC'H, G., FISCHLER, M., MICHON, F., MELCHOIR, J. C. and SEIGNEUR, F. (1983) High frequency jet ventilation v. manual jet ventilation during bronchoscopy in patients with tracheo-bronchial stenosis. *British Journal of Anaesthesia*, **55**, 969–972

VUCEVIC, M., PURDY, G. M. and ELLIS, F. R. (1992) Esmolol hydrochloride for management of the cardiovascular stress responses to laryngoscopy and tracheal intubation. *British Journal of Anaesthesia*, **68**, 529–530

VYAS, A. B., LYONS, S. M. and DUNDEE, J. W. (1983) Continuous intravenous anaesthesia with Althesin for resection of tracheal stenosis. *Anaesthesia*, **38**, 132–135

WALL, P. D. (1988) The prevention of postoperative pain. *Pain*, **33**, 289–290

WALTS, L. F., MILLER, J., DAVIDSON, M. B. and BROWN, J. (1981) Perioperative management of diabetes mellitus. *Anesthesiology*, **55**, 104–109

WILLIAMS, P. J. and BAILEY, P. M. (1993) Comparison of the reinforced laryngeal mask airway and tracheal intubation for adenotonsillectomy. *British Journal of Anaesthesia*, **70**, 30–33

28

Biomaterials

J. J. Grote

Biomaterials are synthetic or treated materials employed to replace or augment tissues and organs. The potential usefulness of alloplastic materials in the fabrication of prostheses has been known for a long time; however, the adaptation of materials technology for the purposes of surgical implant manufacture did not take place until about 25 years ago (Calman, 1963).

Biomaterials science is the study of living and non-living materials. Biomaterials themselves have always been of interest to the otologist concerned with reconstructive middle ear surgery (Grote, 1984a). In the past, the results obtained from using alloplastic implant materials in the middle ear have been disappointing because of the problems associated with extrusion (Guildford, 1964; Portmann, 1967). Nevertheless, it is worth noting that the most successful middle ear reconstruction in otosclerosis patients has been that performed with alloplastic implants (Shea, 1969). The recent advances in biomaterials science and the concomitant increase in knowledge have effected a revival in the development of middle ear prostheses. Furthermore, in maxillofacial surgery, implants are being used for the reconstruction of bony defects. In cases of head and neck surgery and in rhinology, the use of biomaterials has so far been reported only in experimental studies.

Scientific methods and surgical criteria must be applied if good results with alloplastic materials are to be achieved; the interrelationship between these criteria, however, necessitates their combined application. The dissimilarity between the surgical aims and the demands made on implants used in orthopaedics and those used in otology will obviously be reflected in the different implant materials employed by surgeons in these respective fields. The same is true in the case of middle ear reconstruction, where the requirements for the reconstruction of the canal wall are different from those for an ossicular chain reconstruction.

The selection of alloplastics for reconstructive surgery is based on aspects derived from a variety of physical, chemical, biomechanical and surgical concepts (Homsy, 1970). With the ever increasing number of implants on the market, it is essential that the otolaryngologist has a fundamental knowledge of biomaterials science to complement his surgical aims.

Biocompatibility

The reaction of the body to the implant has to be studied in terms of both local and general reactions – the cytotoxicity of the implant material; however, the influence of the body on the prosthesis is also of importance. These reactions can eventually lead to degradation and loss of function. This phenomenon is called the biofunctionality of the implant.

Biocompatibility is the first prerequisite for a useful implant material and this must be tested extensively *in vitro*, in animal experiments, and in clinical studies with long postoperative follow-up periods. The final proof is the study of retrieved materials from patients.

Surface activity

An implant material can be regarded as bioinert if the body does not react at all to the implant material; as biotolerant if the body regards the implant material as a foreign body but, after incorporation, ceases to react to the implant; and as bioactive if the body has an active surface compatibility with the implant material, which leads to a firm integration between the body and the foreign material.

An implant material will always be placed in a wound and, therefore, normal wound reactions will inevitably take place (Silver, 1980). A foreign body will be encapsulated by a fibrous capsule with a varying number of reactive cells, particularly foreign body giant cells. In the case of a bioinert material, where no reaction to the surface of the body develops, the encapsulation will be in the form of only a small fibrous capsule, without further reaction taking place. A biotolerant material will have a good fibrous capsule around the implant material which is an indication of cellular activity. Giant cells, in particular, can be present even after long postoperative periods without compromising implant integration. A bioactive material will achieve a real bond with the surface of the surrounding tissue through active ion exchange which leads to a firm bond between the implant material and the body.

Structure

In the past, implant materials had a solid structure. However, during the last decade, several investigators have developed porous materials which enable the host tissue to grow into the pores of the implant, resulting in a good integration with the body (Friedenberg, 1963; Klawitter and Hulbert, 1971; Homsey and Anderson, 1976; Spector, Fleming and Kreutner, 1976). It was found that macropores of 100 μm were ideal for the ingrowth of fibrous tissue, especially of bone tissue, if adjacent to the implant material. Micropores of several micrometres seemed to be essential, particularly if the implant materials had to be resorbed and remodelled in living tissue. In contrast, the micropores can be a problem in those materials which are not meant for degradation.

It is important to understand that all materials will be affected by the body and will be resorbed to some degree, depending on the surface activity. If there is a large surface area, the response of the body tissue to the implant material will be greater, with the production of large numbers of macrophages and giant cells (Brown, Neel and Kern, 1979; Kerr, 1981). The corrosion of implants can lead to the release of potentially harmful substances into the body; e.g. metals such as nickel, cobalt, chromium and aluminium which can be released from metal implants, may cause allergic responses, for which nickel, in particular, is notorious (Barranco and Solomon, 1972; Benson, Goodwin and Brostoff, 1975). Polymers can undergo degradation as a result of water or lipid absorption by leaching low-molecular-weight molecules or by chain scission through oxidation or hydrolysis. It is probable that some additives, which are necessary for the stability of the polymer, will be released from the implant material and some of these can be very toxic (US Pharmacopeia XIX, 1975). Even ceramics, such as alumina, which are very inert, can release substances into the body which, in the case of alumina, can be stored in the brain. Small particles from the implant can stimulate a non-specific fibrocytic response, which leads to the destruction of surrounding tissue.

A most important criterion is the potential carcinogenic property of some substances which may be released, in particular from certain polymers. It has been demonstrated in animal experiments that large smooth surfaces may enhance the development of sarcomas, but the same is not reported from clinical studies (Oppenheimer *et al.*, 1964).

A foreign body placed in a wound can attract bacteria which colonize the surface of the implant in a protected environment that is ideal for the proliferation of such organisms, thereby rendering conventional antibiotic treatment ineffectual (Gristina *et al.*, 1976). Therefore, the behaviour of the implant material should also be studied in an infected environment.

Other aspects of the structure of the material which must be considered are the density and porosity (macropores and micropores). These influence integration, the wound reaction and remodelling capacity. In the case of ceramics, the crystallographic structure must also be indicated.

Generic names

Many implants are marketed with trade names, which give little or no information on the capacity of the material and, therefore, the generic name of the material used must be indicated. In addition to the generic names of the materials, the additives which might be part of the implant material must also be listed. The generic names can give the information on biocompatibility.

In reconstructive surgery, three classes of biomaterials are used: metals, polymers and ceramics. The different classes of biomaterials have both advantages and disadvantages with regard to biocompatibility, integration capacity and surgical application.

Metals

Metals are used less frequently in otolaryngology than in other disciplines. Over 100 years ago, it was noticed that metal, in the form of bullets, gave rise to inflammation, but occasionally the metal would be walled off in a pocket of scar tissue, thus creating few problems. However, metal implants were a considerable infection risk and caused a great deal of wound reaction; the exceptions were gold and silver devices, although their application had been restricted by the softness of these two metals. Metallurgic developments gave rise to a large variety of steel alloys (the patent for stainless steel was recorded in 1913), but none of the steels had sufficient resistance to corrosion. There are three classes of alloys: the cobalt-chromium group, the stainless steel group and the titanium group.

Cobalt-chromium alloys

These alloys were first invented by Haines. By the late 1930s, a cobalt-chromium alloy (Vitalium) began to be used in arthroplasty. After the Second World War, when knowledge about corrosion resistance had increased, metal implants achieved a wide application, especially in the field of orthopaedics. The cobalt-chromium alloy group is especially popular and is covered by several trade names, Vitalium being used most frequently. All cobalt-chromium alloys are corrosion resistant to tissues (Cohen, 1983). These types of prosthesis are generally not used in the middle ear but can be employed in maxillofacial surgery.

Stainless steels

According to the patent description of 1930, the definition of stainless steel is a steel that has a chromium content of between 11 and 30%, with the higher amount of chromium giving the steel a relative resistance to many corrosive fluids. The most corrosion resistant are those such as 316 low carbon steel and these are the most widely used.

Stainless steel prostheses, especially in the form of wire prostheses, are well known in middle ear surgery and have proven to be reliable, particularly when integrated into a mobile middle ear chain (Schuknecht, 1958). Stainless steel plates for the purpose of reconstruction are also used in maxillofacial surgery. However, these stainless steel prostheses never bond with the body.

Titanium

The development of a metal alloy based on titanium began during the Second World War when it was used in the aircraft industry. These metals are mostly used in orthopaedic devices. There is a reasonable level of corrosion resistance, but experience has shown that tissue surrounding the implant can become darkened which indicates an initial loss of titanium to the tissues. Titanium wires are used in middle ear surgery and bolts are used as a permanent transdermal device for the attachment of bone anchored hearing aids and cosmetic prostheses (Tjellström *et al.*, 1983).

Titanium inserted into human bone forms an intimate contact with it, a process called osseointegration. Calcium phosphate layers are formed on the passive oxide films of titanium and its alloys in a neutral electrolyte solution. Calcium phosphate is similar to apatite and it is this that gives it bioactivity and integration with bone (Hanawa and Ota, 1992).

In some metals, corrosion products can be observed in the cells around the implant. As with all implant materials, one important consideration is that concerning the possibility of the induction of malignancy. In orthopaedics, particularly, there are large numbers of patients who have had metal implants for long periods of time. There is no evidence to support an aetiological connection between the use of these metals and any type of neoplasm. A second very important aspect is that of hypersensitivity reactions to implants. Dermatologists are well aware of the sensitivity of some patients to certain metals, particularly nickel. However, whether that sensitivity also applies in the case of implants under the skin is not known. The conclusion must be that metal implants should not be widely used in otolaryngology, apart from their application in maxillofacial surgery and, in some cases, in middle ear surgery for reconstruction of the middle ear chain or bone anchorage. Integrated into a mobile middle ear chain remnant, these implants are reliable; placed against a mobile tympanic membrane, they are extruded (Plester, 1968).

Polymers

Large quantities of plastics were being manufactured as early as the 1930s and 1940s. The application of these industrial polymers to surgical procedures was dictated by both the availability of the product and the intuition of the clinician. The first use of a biomaterial in reconstructive middle ear surgery was by Wullstein in 1952. He implanted a columella of Palavit in the middle ear for the reconstruction of the middle ear chain. Initial hearing results were good but, in time, the implant was extruded. Commercial plastics such as polyethylene, Teflon and Silastic were also used, but only a few polymers were designed and tested specifically for surgical application. Later, many polymers were used for different types of columella reconstruction. By the end of the 1960s, the use of plastic implant materials was abandoned, particularly in reconstructive middle ear surgery, because of the high extrusion rate (Sheehy, 1965). Apart from the body's reaction to the different polymers, many materials used had been primarily intended for industrial use. These materials often contained low-molecular-weight impurities which were pharmacologically active.

Many classes of polymers are unsuitable for reconstructive surgery. In otolaryngology, the principal generic classes of interest are low density polyethylene (LDPE or LGP), high density polyethylene (HDPE or HDP), polytetrafluoroethylene (PTFE, also called Teflon) and polydimethyl-xylothene (Silastic). Some polymers may also consist of more than one chemical entity. To assess different polymers for their potential application in the field of reconstructive surgery it is necessary to subject them to a number of intradermal reaction tests and systemic toxicity tests. These tests are not very sensitive methods of assessing biocompatibility. More appropriate alternatives are procedures using tissue culture and cell growth inhibition (Autian, 1977). Long-term animal and clinical studies are essential. Following the implantation of polymer implants, chemical reactions as well as wound reaction take place which result in the formation of a fibrous capsule. The thickness of this capsule is an indication of the level of tolerance of the material. In the cellular infiltrate around the implant, the foreign body reaction with giant cells and macrophages is of primary importance. It has been shown that giant cell reaction around polymers continues for a long time. This foreign body reaction also takes place in the case of more tolerant materials, especially at sites where there is mechanical irritation (Kuijpers, 1984).

At the beginning of the 1970s, a new concept for implant materials was invented, namely the concept of the porous implant materials. Friedenberg (1963) was the first to report the possibility of adapting an open pore sponge material which, in his case, was made of polytetrafluoroethylene, for surgical reconstructive use. This initial work generated a great deal of further research into porous implant materials, especially where ingrowth was apparent when the material was in contact with the bony skeleton. Two porous alloplasts, Proplast and Plastipore, have been promoted in otolaryngology (Janeke and Shea, 1975; Shea, 1976). Proplast is a composite of polytetrafluoro-ethylene and carbon, while Plastipore is a trade name for a porous polyethylene polymer. These materials allowed ingrowth of fibrous tissue and capillaries during the first month of implantation and, if exposed to bone, bony ingrowth as well. During the implantation periods, the giant cells predominate in the transitional areas between implant and soft tissue (Figure 28.1). After longer survival periods, hyalinization of the fibrous tissue in the pores has been demonstrated in some studies (Kuijpers, 1984). The resorption of these materials by macrophages has also been demonstrated (Kerr, 1981). It has to be expected that a variety of other polymers will be developed in porous or solid form and that the same test results can be expected. Of the porous materials, total ossicular replacement prostheses (TORPS) and partial ossicular replacement prosthesis (PORPS), which are used as columellae between the footplate and the tympanic membrane, or between the stapes superstructure and the tympanic membrane, have been used in middle ear reconstructive surgery. An increase in extrusion rate has been reported unless cartilage is placed between the tympanic membrane and the prosthesis (Smyth *et al.*, 1978). Whether this can be blamed only on the materials or whether surgical procedures with regard to the columella technique are also culpable has not yet been established.

Silastic has been used for some time in otolaryngology, especially as plastic sheeting in the middle ear (Sheehy, 1973). Teflon is used in different situations in the middle ear as well as in head and neck surgery for augmentation of the vocal cords.

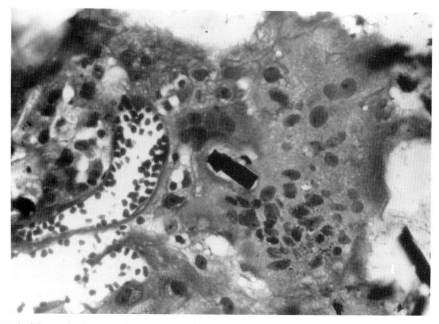

Figure 28.1 Marked foreign body giant cell reaction to Proplast implant. (Courtesy of A. G. Kerr)

It has to be admitted that precise knowledge of the surface chemistry and physics of different polymer implants does not yet exist. The chemical and physical reactions that take place in those areas where the implant is in contact with surrounding tissue, as well as with blood, deserve better understanding. Physical criteria have to be established in order to facilitate optimum selection of polymer materials for implantation. The search for bioactive polymers which bond directly with the body has started and will, no doubt, lead to new developments.

Ceramics

Biologically, most oxide ceramics are bioinert materials while glass and calcium phosphate ceramics are reactive materials. Some of these ceramics are used in otolaryngology.

Bioinert ceramics

The Al_2O_3 ceramic is a bioinert ceramic which is used in otolaryngology. It is a polycrystalline material which consists of corundum crystals. The advantage of this material is that it can be used under full load application. Although this is not of importance in the middle ear, it may be of significance in maxillofacial surgery. It has already been demonstrated in animal experiments that the implant is covered with a delicate membrane within 3 weeks; there is also a normal subepithelial cell layer with active fibroblast-collagen fibres and blood vessels. Because it is a bioinert ceramic, integration is less than with other implant materials, although a fibrous capsule develops. If used as an ossicular replacement, it has the advantage that it stays mobile. Prostheses of corundum crystals are very hard and not easy to shape; however, as has been proven in long-term clinical studies with columella prostheses, these bioinert materials behave well in the middle ear (Jahnke, Plester and Heimke, 1979). Other applications in maxillofacial surgery are being developed.

Bioactive ceramics

Glass ceramics

These ceramics were developed in order to achieve a direct chemical bond between the implant and the living tissues. They are available in different compositions of surface active glasses (Ceravital, Bioglass, and Macor). Each glass ceramic has its own distinct composition and the different reactivities can be explained in terms of individual composition. The basic reactivity depends on ion exchange at the surface of the implant material. The surface of glass ceramics is lysed after implantation and is coated with an amorphous gel layer, which probably contains SiO_2, CaO and P_2O_5 and is about 0.1 μm thick. Into this gel layer, the osteoblasts lay down and embed collagenous fibres. Calcium phosphate precipitates as apatite on the surface. This fixes the collagenous fibres on the surface of the implant, thereby preventing its further corrosion. All glass ceramics are degradable to a certain extent (Hench and Paschall, 1973).

Glass ceramics are used in otolaryngology mainly for reconstruction of the middle ear chain, in the form of columella prostheses (Reck, 1984). The long-term results show resorption and therefore loss of function.

Calcium phosphate ceramics

Because of their composition, calcium phosphate ceramics resemble bone tissue. These materials are used to fill defects in bone; Dreesman (1984) was the first to publish the clinical results. The problem is that the biomaterial usually disappears faster than new bone can fill the empty spaces. Different calcium phosphates have been studied and used in otolaryngology, e.g. B-whitlockite ($Ca_3[PO_4]_2$) and hydroxyapatite ($Ca_{10}[PO_4]_6[OH]_2$). Hydroxyapatite is present in bone tissue and B-whitlockite is present in the body in a soluble form and can, by means of sintering techniques, be reproduced in ceramic. A selection has to be made according to the reactivity of the body, but there is general agreement that calcium phosphate ceramics are very compatible with the body, especially with bony tissues (de Groot, 1981).

B-whitlockite

This is a tricalcium phosphate. It is a bioactive implant material and behaves in the same manner as all calcium phosphates in viable tissues. However, unlike hydroxyapatite, it seems to have a very variable degradation and remodelling. This is particularly noticeable when some impurities are present in the ceramic when remodelling cannot be controlled and trace elements of the implant are found in the macrophages around it. The degradation process takes place in two stages. Physicochemical dissolution of the necks between sintered powder particles results in individual particles being released, which are subsequently digested and presumably dissolved by cells. If degradation takes place rapidly, the cells cannot dissolve all particles intracellularly before they reach the lymph nodes. There is, therefore, a temporary presence of tricalcium phosphate crystals in the lymph nodes.

Tricalcium phosphates (B-whitlockite) have been used for the obliteration of mastoid cavities (Zöllner *et al.*, 1983; Wullstein, Schindler and Döll, 1984).

Hydroxyapatite

This has been studied extensively both *in vitro* and *in vivo*, and in long-term clinical studies (Grote, 1984b,

1986; van Blitterswijk *et al.*, 1986a, b). It has proven to be a bioactive material which achieves real integration with bone tissue without any encapsulation. There is controlled remodelling if a porous material is used and the mode of remodelling and resorption seem to be ideal for the composite for hydroxyapatite and tricalcium phosphate (HA/TCPA). These calcium phosphate ceramics can be made in porous as well as in dense forms, depending on the surgical requirements. The continuation of remodelling of the porous forms is also compatible in infected areas. The attachment of epithelium to dense apatite surfaces has been shown to take place by means of hemidesmosomes, while connective tissue fibres do not encapsulate the implant but run perpendicular to the ceramic surface.

Biologically, B-whitlockite or tricalcium phosphate ceramics behave in the same manner as hydroxyapatite, the one difference being that the B-whitlockite ceramic may be more biodegradable than hydroxyapatite. This means that an implant in bony tissue will be degraded in an uncertain way. Calcium phosphate materials are resorbed and remodelled in the same way as a living bone; in other words, they are resorbed and released by macrophages. Resorption and remodelling patterns are determined by both the macro- and micropores, which are dependent on the crystallography and stoichiometry of the calcium phosphate materials and on the sintering procedures. Another disadvantage of calcium phosphate ceramics is their brittleness. It has insufficient tensile strength and so is not useful as a replacement in large bony defects; only relatively small defects in bone, like those produced in maxillofacial surgery, can be repaired. The use of this ceramic in long-term clinical studies in middle ear surgery has validated its biocompatibility and usefulness. An extensive application in the fields of nasal and maxillofaical surgery has now begun.

Retrieved materials

The inspection of implants retrieved from reoperations on asymptomatic patients has demonstrated the biocompatibility of hydroxyapatite. Porous hydroxyapatite is changed into living bone tissue and late postoperative infections have no influence on this remodelled bone. However, there is less tendency to new bone formation in an infected operative site. Dense hydroxyapatite ossicles are integrated into the ossicular chain via fibrous connection or, if exposed to bare bone, by osseous connection. These new ossicles are covered with mucosa (van Blitterswijk *et al.*, 1986b).

Conclusions

Many criteria have to be met before an implant can be used effectively. The site where the implant is to be used largely determines the choice of material. The ideal implant should closely resemble the tissue it is designed to replace in such factors as size, shape and consistency. Its structure should not be affected by infection or the normal healing reaction. As the implant becomes established it should assume the characteristics of the tissue which it replaces or augments, thereby ensuring its permanent toleration by the body.

Autologous and homologous materials are often considered to be ideal for the reconstruction of defects in the body. However, after preservation techniques have been carried out, the remodelling of the body with these materials takes place in the same way as with alloplastic implant materials. Advances in biomaterials science will increase the fundamental knowledge of the surface activity of these alloplastic implant materials and of their interaction with the body. The more the material resembles the human body, the better will be its compatibility with the body. The surgical criteria employed in implantation techniques have to be developed and refined for different surgical areas. It is obvious that an increase in knowledge will lead to the development of innovative implant materials, devices and artificial organs in the near future. The prefabrication of these reliable materials will more than compete with all the problems associated with the transplantation of autologous materials and with the preservation and shaping of homologous materials.

References

AUTIAN, J. (1977) Toxocological testing of biomaterials. *Artificial Organs*, **1**, 59

BARRANCO, V. P. and SOLOMON, H. (1972) Eczematous dermatitis from nickel (letter). *Journal of the American Medical Association*, **220**, 1244

BENSON, M. K. D., GOODWIN, P. G. and BROSTOFF, J. (1975) Metal sensitivity in patients with joint replacement arthroplasties. *British Medical Journal*, **4**, 374–375

BROWN, B. L., NEEL, H. B. III and KERN, E. B. (1979) Implants of Supramid, Proplast and Plastipore and Silastic. *Archives of Otolaryngology*, **105**, 605–609

CALMAN, J. (1963) The use of inert plastic material in reconstructive surgery. *British Journal of Plastic Surgery*, **16**, 1

COHEN, J. (1983) Metal implants: historical background and biological response to implantation. In: *Biomaterials in Reconstructive Surgery*, edited by L. Rubin. St. Louis: C.V. Mosby Company. pp. 46–61

DE GROOT, K. (1981) Degradable ceramics. In: *Biocompatibility of Clinical Implants Materials*, vol. I, edited by D. F. Williams. Boca Raton, Fla: CRC Press. pp. 199–224

DREESMAN, H. (1984) Über Knochenplombierung. *Beitraege Klinik Chirurgica*, 9200

FRIEDENBERG, T. B. (1963) Bone growth into Teflon sponge. *Surgery, Gynecology and Obstetrics*, **116**, 588

GRISTINA, A. G., ROVERE, G. D., SJOHI, H. and NICASTRO, J. F. (1976) An *in vitro* study of bacterial response to inert and reactive metals and to methyl methacrylate. *Journal of Biomedical Materials Research*, **10**, 273–281

GROTE, J. J. (1984a) *Biomaterials in Otology*. Boston: Martinus Nijhoff Publishers

GROTE, J. J. (1984b) Tympanoplasty with calcium phosphate. *Archives of Otolaryngology*, **110**, 197

GROTE, J. J. (1986) Reconstruction of the middle ear with hydroxyapatite implants. *Annals of Otology, Rhinology and Laryngology*, **95** (suppl. 123), 1–12

GUILDFORD, F. R. (1964) Tympanoplasty: use of prosthesis in conduction mechanism. *Archives of Otolaryngology*, **80**, 80–86

HANAWA, I. and OTA, M. (1992). Characterization of surface-film formed on titanium in electrolyte using XPS. *Applied Surface Science*, **55**, 269–276

HENCH, L. L. and PASCHALL, H. A. (1973) Direct bond of bioactive glass ceramic materials to bone and muscle. *Journal of Biomedical Materials Research, Symp.*, **4**, 25–42

HOMSY, C. A. (1970) Biocompatibility in selection of materials for implantation. *Journal of Biomedical Materials Research*, **4**, 341–356

HOMSY, C. A. and ANDERSON, M. S. (1976) Functional stabilization of soft tissue and bone prostheses with a porous low modulus system. In: *Biocompatibility of Implant Materials*, edited by D. F. Williams. Tunbridge Wells: Sector Publications Ltd. p. 85

JAHNKE, K., PLESTER, D. and HEIMKE, G. (1979) Aluminium-oxide Keramik, ein bioinertes Material für die Mittelohrchirurgie. *Archives of Otorhinolaryngology*, **223**, 373–376

JANEKE, J. B. and SHEA, J. J. (1975) Self-stabilizing total ossicular replacement prostheses in tympanoplasty. *Laryngoscope*, **85**, 1550–1556

KERR, A. G. (1981) Proplast and Plastipore. *Clinical Otolaryngology*, **6**, 187–191

KLAWITTER, J. J. and HULBERT, S. F. (1971) Application of porous ceramics for the attachment of load bearing internal orthopedic application. *Journal of Biomedical Materials Research, Symp*, **2**, 161–229

KUIJPERS, W. (1984) Behaviour of bioimplants in the middle ear, an experimental study. In: *Biomaterials in Otology*, edited by J. J. Grote. Boston: Martinus Nijhoff Publishers. pp. 18–27

OPPENHEIMER, B. S., WILLWHITE, M., STOUT, A. P., DANISHEFSKY, I. and FISHMAN, M. M. (1964) A comparative study of the effects of imbedding cellophane and polystyrene films in rats. *Cancer Research*, **24**, 379

PLESTER, D. (1968) Die Anwendung prosthestischen Materialien im Mittelohr. *Laryngologie, Rhinologie und Otologie*, **102**, 105–109

PORTMANN, M. (1967) Management of ossicular chain defects. *Journal of Laryngology and Otology*, **81**, 1309–1323

RECK, R. (1984) Bioactive glass-ceramics in ear surgery. Animal studies and clinical results. *Laryngoscope*, **94**, (suppl. 33), 1–54

SCHUKNECHT, H. F. (1958) Stapedectomy and graft prostheses operation. *Acta Otolaryngologica*, **49**, 71–80

SHEA, J. J. (1969) A technique for stapes surgery in obliterative otosclerosis. *Otolaryngologic Clinics of North America*, **1**, 199–215

SHEA, J. J. (1976) Plastipore total ossicular replacement prosthesis. *Laryngoscope*, **86**, 239–240

SHEEHY, J. L. (1965) Ossicular problems in tympanoplasty. *Archives of Otolaryngology* **8**, 115–122

SHEEHY, J. L. (1973) Plastic sheeting in tympanoplasty. *Laryngoscope*, **83**, 1144

SILVER, I. A. (1980) The physiology of wound healing. In: *Wound Healing and Wound Infection*, edited by T. K. Hunt. New York: Appleton-Century Crofts. pp. 11–31

SMYTH, G. D., HASSARD, T. H., KERR, A. G. and HOULIHAN, F. (1978) Ossicular replacement prostheses. *Archives of Otolaryngology*, **104**, 345–351

SPECTOR, M., FLEMING, W. R. and KREUTNER, A. (1976) Bone ingrowth into porous high density polyethylene. *Journal of Biomedical Materials Research*, **7**, 595

TJELLSTRÖM, A., ROSENHALL, U., LINDSTRÖM, J., HALLEN, O., ALBREKTSSON, T. and BRÄNEMARK, P. I. (1983) Five years experience with skin penetrating bone anchored implants in the temporal bone. *Acta Otolaryngologica*, **95**, 568–575

US PHARMACOPEIA XIX (1975) *Biological Tests; Plastic Containers*. Easton, Pa: Mack Publishing Co

VAN BLITTERSWIJK, C. A., GROTE, J. J., KUIJPERS, W., DAEMS, W. TH. and DE GROOT, K. (1986a) Macropore tissue ingrowth: a quantitative and qualitative study on hydroxyapatite ceramic. *Biomaterials*, **7**, 137–144

VAN BLITTERSWIJK, C. A., KUIJPERS, W., DAEMS, W. TH. and GROTE, J. J. (1986b) Epithelial reactions to hydroxyapatite. *Acta Otolaryngologica*, **101**, 231–241

WULLSTEIN, H. L. (1952) Operationen am Mittelohr mit Hilfe des freien spaltlappen Transplantates. *Archives of Otolaryngology*, **161**, 422–435

WULLSTEIN, S. R., SCHINDLER, K. and DÖLL, W. (1984) Further observations on application of Plasticin in ear surgery. In: *Biomaterials in Otology*, edited by J. J. Grote. Boston: Martinus Nijhoff Publishers. pp. 250–261

ZÖLLNER, CH., STRUTZ, J., BECK, CHL., BÜSING, C. M., JAHNKE, K. and HEIMKE, G. (1983) Veródung des Wartenforsatzes mit poröser Trikalciumphosphat Keramik. *Laryngologie, Rhinologie und Otologie*, **62**, 106–111

29

Medical negligence in otolaryngology

Maurice Hawthorne and Ian Barker

The last decade has witnessed an upsurge in medical negligence litigation and otolaryngology, while not customarily thought of as a high risk specialty, has also become the subject of claims. This may not necessarily imply that there are more acts of negligence now than in the past, rather that there is an increase in the awareness of patients and an enhanced desire for accountability should things go wrong.

Not only may the doctor be called to account for his clinical decisions and acts, but he must be aware of the potential legal action that can arise with respect to racial and sexual discrimination, child abuse, the Misuse of Drugs Act and industrial compensatable disease.

Standard of skill and care

In determining whether a doctor has been negligent, the plaintiff must establish three things:

1 The doctor owed him a duty of care
2 There has been a breach of that duty
3 The plaintiff has suffered damage as a result of that breach of duty.

The second and third points are usually a matter for expert medical evidence. The first step of establishing a duty is more straight forward.

To establish a duty it is necessary for a doctor/ patient relationship to be in existence. There is no Good Samaritan law in the UK and doctors only have a legal responsibility to people they have agreed to treat. In general practice the agreement arises by virtue of accepting a patient onto one's list. In a hospital setting, the agreement either arises out of the doctor's Terms and Conditions of Employment or, with private patients, as a result of contract.

Patients tend to be seen by several different doctors and therefore, the question, *who owes the duty of care?*, may be a pertinent one. In the National Health Service, the employing authority will usually be named as first defendant as it would be liable to pay damages arising from any successful action by virtue of the principle of vicarious liability. Individual doctors may then be named as subsequent defendants.

An unresolved issue is who should be sued if a patient is placed on a waiting list, but suffers additional damage in the time it takes to receive a first appointment? Is the defendant the referring general practitioner, the Authority, or National Health Service Trust at whose clinic the patient is awaiting an appointment?

The standard of care required by law is that of the reasonably skilled and experienced doctor. The appropriate criterion is known as the Bolam test (Bolam v Friern Hospital Management Committee, 1957). This states: 'it is the standard of the ordinary skilled man exercising and professing to have that special skill. A man need not possess the highest expert skill; it is well-established law that it is sufficient if he exercises the ordinary skill of an ordinary competent man exercising that particular art'.

The standard of care relates to the specialty in which the doctor practises. A general practitioner will not be required to possess the skills of a specialist. An inexperienced doctor cannot rely on his lack of experience as a defence to alleged negligence (Wilsher v Essex Area Health Authority, 1988). However, a junior doctor may discharge his duty by seeking the help of a superior.

A doctor will not be negligent simply because he acted in a way that another doctor would not have done. The Bolam test establishes that a man is not negligent, if he is acting in accordance with a practice, merely because there is a body of medical opinion which would take a contrary view, provided there is a reasonable body of opinion which supports his practice.

While a doctor is under a duty to keep himself appraised of developments in his area, this is subject to the bounds of reasonableness. Failure to read one article, which might have prevented the negligent act could be excusable, while failure to be aware of new techniques that have become widespread may be inexcusable (Crawford v Board of Governors of the Charing Cross Hospital, 1953).

Consent

Much medical litigation results from the practitioner's failure to disclose adequate information about the risks inherent in a given procedure. Common law recognizes the principle that every person has the right to have his bodily integrity respected. There is a presumption that a person should not be exposed to risk unless he has voluntarily accepted that risk, based on adequate information and adequate comprehension.

In legal terms, every touching can be a potential battery, and to render any touching lawful, the doctor must obtain valid consent. Nevertheless, a doctor may still face an action in negligence for failure to give adequate information about the risks of the proposed therapy. The question of how much information must be given to the patient will vary from one situation to another, but is generally set by the professional standard according to the Bolam test, with doctors being arbiters of how much information should be given. Notably, in England and Wales, there is no notion of informed consent, as in North America, whereby the amount of information to be disclosed is dictated by what a patient would want to know.

This is modified to a degree by the case of Sidaway (Sidaway v Board of Governors of the Bethlem Royal Hospital, 1985) in which the House of Lords held that where the proposed treatment involved a substantial risk of grave or adverse consequences such that, notwithstanding any practice to the contrary, a patient's right to decide whether to consent to the treatment was so obvious that no prudent medical man could fail to warn of the risk, (save in emergency or some other sound clinical reason for non-disclosure), then it would be negligent not to warn.

Accordingly, the right of the doctor (acting in accordance with a reasonable body of medical opinion) to decide what the individual patient should be told remains enshrined in English case law. Such medical paternalism, which may be in the best interest of some of our patients is currently and repeatedly being questioned. The doctor should realize that in

Sidaway when the question, 'Is informed consent a part of English law?' was put to the five law lords, the answer was not unanimous. Scarman said 'Yes', Diplock said 'No' and Bridge, Keith and Templeman said 'Yes, with reservations'.

In assessing which material risks should be mentioned, doctors should consider the degree of probability of the risk materializing and seriousness of possible injury if it does. A risk, even if it is a mere possibility, should be disclosed if its occurrence would cause serious circumstances (Hopp v Lepp, 1979). Medical evidence will be necessary for the court to assess the degree of probability and the seriousness. A further medical factor upon which expert evidence will also be required is to assess the character of the risk, i.e. is this risk common to all surgery or is it specific to the particular operation? Special risks inherent in a recommended operation are more likely to be material.

The legal standard of disclosure required in response to direct questions is also set by the professional standard (Blyth v Bloomsbury Health Authority, 1993). Although the amount of information given must depend upon the circumstances, as a general proposition it is governed by the Bolam test (see above).

Children

Section 8(1) of the Family Law Reform Act (1969) provides that a person over 16 may give a valid consent to medical treatment as though he was an adult. As regards children under 16 years of age, the general principle is that laid down in the Gillick case (Gillick v West Norfolk and Wisbech Area Health Authority, 1986), that the parental right to determine whether or not a child under 16 should have medical treatment terminates when the child achieves a significant understanding and intelligence to enable him or her to understand fully what is proposed. Until such time, the *parents,* or others acting *in loco parentis,* may give their consent or refusal to medical treatment. Recent case law suggests that it may still be possible to treat a seemingly competent child who is refusing to give consent, providing someone else with the capacity to consent provides consent on the child's behalf (In re R, 1991 and in re W, 1992).

Mentally incompetent patients

Where a patient is unable to provide consent on his or her own behalf by reason of mental incapacity, no one else, including a court, may give consent on that person's behalf. The doctrine of necessity however, permits a doctor lawfully to operate on or give other treatment to adult incompetent patients, provided that the treatment is in their best interest, either to save their lives or to ensure improvement in their physical or mental health (In re F, 1990).

Jehovah's Witnesses

Certain groups of patients, including Jehovah's Witnesses, may refuse to receive blood transfusions or other life-saving therapies. The Court of Appeal has recently affirmed patients' rights to refuse medical treatment, even if this will result in their death. Nevertheless, for such a refusal to be effective, the court must be satisfied that at the time of refusal the patient's capacity is not diminished by illness or medication or given on the basis of false assumptions or misinformation. In the case of re T (1992), Lord Donaldson said: 'An adult patient who suffers from no mental incapacity has an absolute right to choose whether to consent to medical treatment, to refuse it or to choose one rather than another of the treatments being offered'.

A decision to refuse medical treatment does not have to be sensible, obviously rational or well considered, and in the case of a competent patient, a doctor cannot override the patient's wishes because he believes it to be in the patient's best interests.

Other special groups

Pregnant women, patients who are HIV positive or suffering from AIDS and the elderly do not represent special categories for the purposes of consent. Although the amount of information which has to be given to a patient varies from case to case, a decision to withhold information solely on paternalistic grounds that it may deter the patient from accepting the therapy may not be justified in law.

Proof of medical negligence

The onus lies upon the plaintiff to prove that the surgeon's treatment was negligent and that the negligence caused the injury. It is not sufficient simply to prove that the surgeon's actions were reprehensible or even reckless if the plaintiff cannot go on to show that his injury is directly attributable to the surgeon's poor performance. Hence, while it was clear that a casualty officer was negligent when he failed to examine a patient attending his department with the obvious signs of poisoning, there was a complete defence (Barnett v Chelsea & Kensington Hospital, 1968) when it was shown that there was no antidote to the poison taken by the patient.

The standard to which the plaintiff must prove his case is on the balance of probabilities. This means that the plaintiff must show that his version of events and expert analysis are more likely to be true than those put forward by the defence. If the case for each side is evenly balanced then the plaintiff will fail. Hence, where a patient suffers a nerve palsy that could equally have been due to negligence or could have been sustained as an inherent risk of the opera-

tion, even when performed with proper skill and care, the plaintiff's case should fail in the absence of some item of evidence to tip the scales in favour of negligence (Ashcroft v Mersey Regional Health Authority, 1985).

An apparent reversal of the burden of proof can happen where the likelihood of negligence is so obvious that it *'speaks for itself'* (*res ipsa loquitur*). In other words, a defendant may find that he is obliged to provide an explanation of the patient's injury that is consistent with reasonable care having been taken, even when the plaintiff has no positive evidence of negligence, where:

1 There is no evidence as to how or why the accident took place
2 The accident is such that it would not have happened without negligence
3 The defendant is proved to have been in control of the situation (Picard, 1984).

The doctrine first evolved in simple personal injury cases concerning falling objects (Byrne v Boadie, 1863; Scott v London & St Katherine's Docks, 1865; Pope v St Helen's Theatre, 1947), but has obvious attractions to a plaintiff in a medical case, where there may well be very real uncertainty as to how an injury came about, and where the often unconscious patient is entirely under the control of the medical team. Despite the fact that it is often pleaded, in England the doctrine has more often been conceded than litigated in medical cases, and so its ambit is unclear (Leigh, 1993). In practice, the Courts are reluctant to apply a doctrine derived from the relatively simple 'bumps and thumps' of stevedoring to the complex issues of causation found in medical litigation. It has been said: 'The human body is not a container filled with a material whose performance can be predictably charged . . . because of this, medical science has not yet reached the stage where the law ought to presume that a patient must come out of an operation as well or better than when he went into it' (Girard v Royal Columbian Hospital, 1976).

Thus as a matter of law, the onus of proving negligence will almost always fall on the plaintiff, though in cases where there is a strong and obvious inference of negligence from the very facts themselves, e.g. a retained swab (Mahon v Osborne, 1939),the defence may well find that onus discharged unless they are able to provide some alternative theory, not involving negligence, to answer the plaintiff's case.

The role of the expert

In simple terms this is to *give impartial advice and opinion.* When possible an expert should do his utmost to be retained on a regular basis by both plaintiff and defendant sides. This is not always easy when lawyers tend to concentrate on one side of the adversarial system or the other. Moves to establish an *approved list* of experts have been vehemently resisted by plaintiff solicitors, alleging that any list drawn up by the medical establishment is likely to be biased in favour of the doctor. However, the Association of Personal Injury Lawyers and Action for the Victims of Medical Accidents (AVMA) are able to provide advice on experts for plaintiff lawyers who are their members.

The expert is usually asked to elucidate the areas of medical contention within a case. Although the temptation is to be an arbitrator of medical colleagues, in court this is the province of the judge. Nevertheless, the expert will be asked to comment on whether the plaintiff's complaint has merit. When acting for the defence the expert will inevitably come across cases where defence is impossible. Here it is the expert's duty to advise that a speedy settlement is made to the aggrieved patient. This will have the secondary benefit of avoiding a colleague's professional shortcomings being exposed to public criticism in court. Rarely, some doctors expect their colleagues to defend them whatever the circumstances. Hence being an expert can lead to criticism or alienation by colleagues.

The credentials of the expert will be tested in court. It is extremely unwise for the expert to step outside his field. Should he be forced to comment outside his field of expertise he should add the rider that he is speaking only as an average medical practitioner. The expert will need to be conversant with up-to date research in his field. He needs to be aware of the various views on current practice even if these views are held by a minority of doctors.

Medical negligence cases can take an inordinate amount of time. Not only may the expert have to inspect all the records, examine the claimant, and prepare reports, he will have to do research, attend meetings with solicitors and counsel and attend court. A single case may, in unusual circumstances, take up to a 100 hours of time or more. The expert should never take on a case if he cannot afford the time.

In the case of the Ikarian Reefer (National Justice Compania Naviesa SA v Prudential Assurance Company Ltd, 1993), Cresswell stated that he considered that a misunderstanding on the part of some of the expert witnesses had taken place concerning their duties and responsibilities which had contributed to the length of the trial. Although this was a shipping case the seven duties and responsibilities laid down have equal validity for medical experts.

1 Expert evidence presented to the court should be, and should be seen to be, the independent product of the expert uninfluenced as to form or content by the exigencies of litigation.
2 Independent assistance should be provided to the court by way of objective unbiased opinion regarding matters within the expertise of the expert witness. (An expert witness should never assume the role of advocate.)
3 Facts or assumptions upon which the opinion was based should be stated together with material facts which could detract from the concluded opinion.
4 An expert witness should make it clear when a question or issue fell outside his expertise.
5 If the opinion was not properly researched because it was considered that insufficient data were available, then that had to be stated with an indication that the opinion was provisional. If the witness could not assert that the report contained the truth, the whole truth and nothing but the truth, then that quaiffication should be stated on the report.
6 If, after exchange of reports, an expert witness changed his mind on a material matter, then the change of view should be communicated to the other side through legal representatives without delay and, when appropriate, to the court.
7 Photographs, plans, survey reports and other documents referred to in the expert evidence had to be provided to the other side at the same time as exchange of reports.

The doctor as an expert witness

After preparation of the report, comment on specific claims and answering of interrogatories, the expert may wish to seek guidance on the case law pertaining to the circumstances. He should never shy away from discussing the case with the solicitor involved and if necessary request a meeting with counsel.

The purpose of expert opinion given in court is to persuade the judge that one side of a case has greater merit than the other. It is the judge who will decide between the two sides of the argument. The expert should not be tempted to usurp the role of the judge for this may do untold damage to his own side or at the very least earn a rebuke which may undermine his confidence.

In court the expert should wear conservative clothes. Evidence should be given in a straightforward, unequivocal manner. A personal view may be represented especially in response to a direct question but should always be tempered with information about acceptable alternative practice and opinion. He should always be prepared to concede points if it is appropriate to do so, and not to adhere rigidly to one view when that cannot be sustained. The expert often has difficult concepts to convey to the judge. The expert should not hesitate to use pictures, models or even video to illustrate a point but should avoid being seen as too flamboyant lest he discredits himself by not giving due respect to the court.

Counsel for the opposing side will attempt to undermine the evidence given by the expert or the standing of the expert in his profession. Above all, the expert must not see this as a personal insult lest he should lose his temper and hence his dignity.

Medicolegal reports

Before writing a report the expert should be aware of what the solicitor requires. Reports usually refer to one or more of the following six areas:

1 An initial statement on the possible merits of an allegation for a plaintiff before notes and other evidence are obtained
2 Liability
3 Causation
4 Current condition
5 Prognosis
6 Expert opinion on an area of medicine.

A quote should be given on the cost of the report in advance. Lawyers may have no concept of the cost in time and research to answer what to them may be the most simple of questions. The solicitor will not be pleased to receive a report of 100 pages with detailed bibliography costing £2000 when the damages sought are only £500 for a relatively minor event.

The report should be typed on A4 paper and double spaced. Each sheet should have the name of the plaintiff or defendant typed in the top right hand corner and be separately numbered. The names of the parties should be stated as should the requesting solicitor or insurance company. The standing of the expert should not be mentioned in the report but a short curriculum vitae should accompany the report. It is inadvisable to use the word *negligent* in the report. Negligence may be implied by using phrases such as *falling below an acceptable standard* or *followed a course of action that could not be supported by any body of medical opinion*. Phrases such as *reckless action* or *flagrant disregard* may have a special meaning and lead to criminal charges rather than a civil case.

Prior to disclosure of the expert's report it is permissible to discuss the report with counsel and amend it. However, it is not permissible for the lawyer to write the report (Whitehouse v Jordan, 1981). Inevitably the expert may need assistance with the actual wording from the barrister but it is not permissible for the barrister to alter or influence the opinion of the expert in the report. It is only proper that the barrister examines the expert's views and so test the conclusions. The lawyer may legitimately suggest alternative explanations to the expert. If the expert is convinced of such possibilities it is permissible to include them in the report. After this interchange the expert should feel confident to justify every word of his report.

The criminal law

Otolaryngologists rarely face criminal proceedings in connection with medical practice, but mention should be made to two types of criminal offence which may flow from medical treatment.

Involuntary manslaughter

In English Law there are, at present, two forms of involuntary manslaughter, as unlawful act manslaughter, and gross negligence manslaughter. The first, as the name suggests, has as a prerequisite an unlawful act on the part of the defendant, and is therefore highly unlikely to arise in the context of bona fide medical care. When clinicians are responsible for the death of a patient, it is the gross negligence form of manslaughter which might be considered by prosecuting authorities.

Until recently, the nature of the test in law to be applied for gross negligence manslaughter was most unclear. As a result of two decisions by the House of Lords in the early 1980s, significant confusion had arisen, so that in some cases, courts had applied a traditional gross negligence test to assess the culpability of a defendant and in other cases, what was known as a 'recklessness test' had been applied. Under the latter test, a defendant would be reckless if his actions created an obvious and serious risk (to the victim) and the defendant either appreciated the risk but went on to run it, or failed to appreciate the risk at all. In circumstances where a doctor had not appreciated the existence of a risk, perhaps through tiredness and overwork, conviction might still have resulted, and thus the test was considered a very harsh assessment of culpability.

In contrast, the traditional gross negligence test had no rigid formulation, and enabled excuses and mitigating circumstances which applied to a defendant to be put forward in assessing overall culpability.

The unsatisfactory state of affairs, whereby these two tests were seemingly available to trial judges, has now been resolved by judgments from the Court of Appeal and The House of Lords. Two cases of medical manslaughter were considered first by the Court of Appeal in 1993. The first case involved two junior doctors, Dr Prentice, a preregistration house officer, and Dr Sullman, a senior house officer. Dr Prentice, as part of chemotherapy treatment, injected vincristine intrathecally in error. He believed at the time he was acting under the supervision of Dr Sullman. For his part, Dr Sullman believed that he had only been asked to supervise the performance of the lumbar puncture, rather than administration of the drugs. As the Court of Appeal observed, the mitigating circumstances in relation to both doctors were many, but a version of the recklessness test had been put to the jury, resulting in their convictions. The second case involved an anaesthetist, Dr

Adamoko. In the course of an operation, an endotracheal tube became disconnected from the anaesthetic machine, and supply of oxygen to the patient was cut off. Dr Adamoko seemingly failed to appreciate the disconnection for a number of minutes, and the patient subsequently died. In that instance, the gross negligence test was put to the jury, and Dr Adamoko was convicted. The Court of Appeal determined that the appropriate test for involuntary manslaughter should be the gross negligence test, and accordingly the convictions of Dr Prentice and Dr Sullman were quashed. Dr Adamoko's conviction was upheld. Dr Adamoko therefore duly appealed to the House of Lords.

The House of Lords also upheld Dr Adamoko's conviction, confirming that the appropriate test for involuntary manslaughter should be that of gross negligence. When applying the gross negligence test a jury will now consider the following matters:

1 On the ordinary principles of the law of negligence, whether or not the defendant has been in breach of a duty of care to the deceased, and if so,
2 If the breach of duty, which involved a risk of serious injury or death, caused the death of the victim, and if so,
3 Whether the breach of duty should be categorized as gross negligence and therefore as a crime.

In assessing the third stage, the degree of culpability, the Court of Appeal had held as long ago as 1925 (R v Bateman) that mere civil negligence is not enough. It is necessary to establish that the negligence is clear, wicked, gross or similar epithet. That position was endorsed by the House of Lords in the Adamoko case. In attempting to assess culpability and describe culpable states of mind, the Court of Appeal (R v Prentice) had identified four states of mind which could be indicative of gross negligence:

1 Indifference to an obvious risk of injury to health
2 Actual foresight of the risk coupled with the determination nevertheless to run it
3 An appreciation of the risk coupled with an intention to avoid it, but also coupled with such a high degree of negligence in the attempted avoidance as the jury considers justifies conviction
4 Inattention or failure to advert to a serious risk which goes beyond mere inadvertence in respect of an obvious and important matter which the defendant's duty demanded he should address.

Proof of one of these states of mind is not of itself, however, indicative of guilt. The jury is still able to consider all the surrounding circumstances of the case, including mitigating factors and excuses put forward by a defendant in assessing culpability. As was indicated by Lord Mackay in delivering the leading judgment in the case of Dr Adamoko, the 'essence

of the matter which is supremely a jury question is whether having regard to the risk of death involved, the conduct of the defendant was so bad in all the circumstances as to amount in their judgment, to a criminal act or omission'.

Proposals for reform

At the conclusion of the judgment in the case of Drs Prentice and Sullman, the Court of Appeal indicated concern at the state of the law of involuntary manslaughter. The Court of Appeal asked that the Law Commission examine this area of law as a matter of urgency. To some extent, the concerns expressed by the Court of Appeal were remedied by the judgment of the House of Lords. Nevertheless the Law Commission has published a consultation paper and made preliminary proposals about reform in this area. In those preliminary proposals, the Commission suggests that unlawful act manslaughter should be abolished, and in place of gross negligence there should be two new offences. The first is described as subjective recklessness manslaughter, where the accused would be guilty of offence where he was aware of the risk that death or serious injury would occur, and unreasonably took that risk, with death then resulting. The Commission suggests that the maximum penalty which presently applies for manslaughter, life imprisonment, should also apply to this new offence.

The Law Commission then recommends a lesser offence which would be committed where:

1 The accused ought reasonably to have been aware of a significant risk that his conduct could result in death or serious injury
2 His conduct fell seriously and significantly below what could reasonably have been demanded of him in preventing that risk from occurring, or in preventing that risk, once in being, from resulting in the prohibited harm.

Insofar as the conduct of the defendant has to fall seriously and significantly below the standard to be expected, mere negligence again would be insufficient. The new formulation is an attempt to set out more clearly what is required to establish culpability, rather than having a loose formulation such as the gross negligence test. It is, however, not clear to what extent specific mitigating circumstances in any given case might be considered by a jury. The maximum sentence for this offence is 10 years.

In addition, the Law Commission made proposals concerning corporate manslaughter. To date, there have only been four prosecutions of corporations for manslaughter, and only one of those has been successful. There have been no prosecutions of health authorities, hospitals or trusts. Part of the difficulty relating to corporate responsibility in this area of law stems from the fact that it is necessary to point to a given individual as an appropriate controlling officer who would himself be guilty of gross negligence before prosecution of the company could be entertained. Aggregation of a series of minor errors or mistakes on the part of a number of individuals is not permitted to add up to criminal culpability on the part of the company.

In relation to the lesser offence, the Commission proposes that, in effect, aggregation would be permitted, and that identification of a principal officer would not be relevant. The Commission suggests that the corporation is only exposed to the question of whether it should have been aware of the significant risk because it chooses to engage in the operation in which that risk arises – including the running of the hospital. It is suggested that reference should be made to the company's organization, attitude and concern for safety in general and that it would be necessary, in considering culpability, to look at management systems to see if the necessary skills and systems are in place in relation to risks which might arise. Under this proposal, therefore, it would appear that trusts could be deemed guilty of corporate manslaughter through an aggregation of errors on the part of a number of employees, resulting in the death of a patient. The Law Commission's proposals are at a very preliminary stage, and may be modified as a result of a consultation process now under way. If in due course such proposals are recommended to Government, it is unlikely that they will be passed into law for at least a period of 2 years.

In Canada (The Annotated Tremear's Criminal Code, 1992), manslaughter may be committed where a doctor causes the death of a patient by, among other things, criminal negligence which may be committed where someone under a duty shows a wanton or reckless disregard for the lives or safety of others. The precise meaning of *wanton or reckless disregard* is in doubt. In a recent case (R v Tutton and Tutton, 1989) the Supreme Court of Canada was divided between those who considered that a defendant should have an intention to run a prohibited risk, or a wilful blindness to the risk, and those who considered that a marked and substantial departure from a standard of behaviour expected of a reasonably prudent individual would suffice.

In New Zealand (R v Yogasakaran, 1990), the test for manslaughter is that of mere negligence. A breach of the civil standard of care resulting in the death of a patient is all that is required. Similarly in Greece, the offence under the Greek Criminal Code (Greek Penal Code) is of causing death by negligence, mere civil negligence being sufficient. The charge is often seen as a precursor to civil proceedings, where a victim's family may make complaint to prosecuting authorities, effectively as part of the bargaining process for compensation.

Assault and battery

Charges of assault and battery are considered very infrequently by the prosecuting authorities in this jurisdiction in relation to medical practitioners. Courts are reluctant to consider actions in tort for battery arising out of a failure to obtain consent, let alone criminal charges. Very few doctors will intend to inflict harm on a patient, the overall aim being to provide some form of therapeutic benefit. However, where the clinician performs a procedure which goes substantially beyond that to which the patient has consented and that is known to the clinician, or the clinician foresees that might be the case, then such an offence may be made out even if of therapeutic benefit. In circumstances where surgical intervention takes place, an offence of greater seriousness than mere assault may result, e.g. assault causing grievous bodily harm.

Dealing with medical negligence claims

The first intimation of a claim against an otolaryngologist may well come in the form of a request for provision of medical records to a patient's solicitor. Thereafter, the clinician may hear nothing further until proceedings are to be served. At that time, solicitors will usually be instructed. The solicitor should obtain copies of all relevant records. He should meet the clinician to obtain instructions about the treatment of the patient and discuss the detailed allegations set out in the claim (Rules of the Supreme Court and the County Court Practice of Procedure).

Once a claim has been served, a defence must be submitted in response, indicating which allegations are accepted or denied and averring any further relevant information (Rules of the Supreme Court and the County Court Practice). In addition, the defendant's solicitors will be concerned to obtain guidance from experts swiftly, and once received, be able to form an initial view about whether or not the claim is defensible. The assessment of a claim at this stage will be facilitated by recent rule changes which have been made concerning the conduct of personal injury actions, including medical negligence litigation. These changes require that at the time of service of a writ, a plaintiff must also submit a medical report setting out the plaintiff's condition and prognosis, together with a Schedule of Special Damages said to result from any alleged negligence. Traditionally, such information was not available until much later in the litigation process. The change has resulted in defendant's solicitors being able to assess the potential value of a plaintiff's claim at an early stage. Accordingly, following that initial expert opinion, a settlement can be proposed early in the proceedings, if appropriate.

If settlement is desired but cannot be negotiated

between the solicitors, then the solicitors may try to settle the claim by what is known as a payment into Court. In making a payment into Court, the defendant can make an assessment of the damages which might be awarded in due course at trial, if negligence is established. If the trial judge awards a sum higher than the level of the payment-in, the plaintiff will receive his or her costs in the usual way. If, however, the sum awarded is the same or a lesser sum, then as a general rule, all costs of the action, including the defendant's costs, after the payment into Court, must be borne by the plaintiff. The plaintiff has 21 days to decide whether or not to accept the payment in. Thereafter the costs rules will apply. In cases where the plaintiff is legally aided, this device is of more limited assistance to a defendant. In other circumstances there may well be a strong incentive to a plaintiff to accept a payment into Court through fear of being prejudiced on costs in this way.

Following the service of a defence, in response to allegations contained in the Statement of Claim, both parties may raise requests for further information about their respective pleadings, and the plaintiff may choose to file a Reply to the Defence.

Directions concerning the conduct of a claim will be given by the Court, usually after the pleadings are completed. In the High Court, a formal hearing will take place to consider these directions, but in personal injury actions brought in the County Court, a series of so-called automatic directions is given by the Court. These are rarely, if ever, appropriate in medical negligence cases and it is therefore usual for the parties to apply to the Court for specific directions to be given. These directions will provide for, among other things, the disclosure of witness statements as to fact, and expert reports. Until relatively recently, in medical negligence actions, neither experts' reports nor witness statements were disclosed by one party to another. Only at trial, would the nature of the respective cases become clear. However, as a result of recent cases and changes in the procedural rules, expert reports and witness statements must now be disclosed, and this will be ordered by the Court at a directions hearing. It is usual for witness statements to be disclosed, followed shortly thereafter by expert reports, in order that experts can consider this information available from the other side in preparing the report. The exchange of both statements and reports gives a further opportunity for review of the case, both by plaintiff and medical defendant. At this stage the plaintiff may realize that the claim is weak and the case may be discontinued. Equally the defence may feel that the case is not defensible and settlement negotiations or a payment into Court may follow.

Trial and preparation for trial

If the exchange of witness statements and expert reports does not promote the settlement of a claim, then the case proceeds towards trial. In medical negligence actions, a fixed date for trial will usually be given by the Court because of the significant number of clinicians who may have to make themselves available, either as experts or as witnesses of fact.

By way of preparation for trial, both parties should arrange conferences with counsel in order to review the case in detail, and ensure all preparations are complete. If the defence considers that the case should be settled, or there are certain aspects of the case where a defendant may be vulnerable, a payment into Court may be made. The payment-in may be limited to those aspects of the claim where the defendant could be found liable. The plaintiff has 21 days within which to accept the payment-in before the penalty of costs starts to run. As a significant proportion of the costs of an action result from the trial itself, the defendants are usually anxious to make any payment into Court before 21 days in advance of the trial. Thereafter bundles of documents must be prepared for use in the Court by all parties, which will include the pleadings, medical records, witness statements and expert reports.

A proportion of cases are settled literally at the doors of the Court, the last opportunity for compromise before further significant costs of trial are incurred.

If no compromise can be reached, the trial will commence with an explanation of the case to the judge by counsel for the plaintiff, setting out the relevant events and the nature of the allegations. Plaintiff's counsel will then call witnesses of fact, usually followed then by expert witnesses. Each witness will be cross-examined in turn by the defence and then re-examined by plaintiff's counsel if necessary. When the plaintiff's evidence has been called, the defence case is then put in the same way and usually in the same order.

The trial judge may allow variation in this order of evidence, particularly in complex cases, so that witnesses for both sides are called first, to be followed then by experts. This will allow experts to hear all the evidence of fact before giving a final opinion. However, the present arrangements for disclosure of witness statements make such variation rare.

At the conclusion of the case, the judge will usually hear submissions from counsel on the law to be applied and the appropriate level of damages to be awarded if the plaintiff is successful. It is usual then for the judge to reserve judgment, to be delivered at a later day, as most negligence cases are complex and will require some consideration. Once judgment is given and if the plaintiff is successful, the judge will indicate the level of damages to be awarded. Only at that stage is the judge informed about any payment into Court which may have been made, and the costs to be awarded can then be considered.

them through the ear drum. A perforation does not automatically imply negligence as it may happen if the ear drum is inherently weak, if the patient moves, or by compression of deep meatal air when an occluding plug of wax is propelled towards the ear drum by the current of syringed water.

Facial nerve damage

There are risks of facial nerve damage inherent in a number of otological procedures, such as removal of acoustic neuroma or cholesteatoma. *This risk should be discussed with the patient.* There is still a significant body of medical opinion which would not discuss the relatively rare risk of facial paralysis in cholesteatoma surgery. Damage to the facial nerve may be an inevitable event when operating on malignancies, particularly in the parotid gland. This consequence should be discussed with the patient. Damage to the facial nerve as a result of surgery on the middle ear may be difficult to defend, however, damage to a dehiscent or an aberrant nerve should not of itself be considered negligent. Adequate irrigation with a correct drilling technique should prevent most palsies. Often it is not the way in which the paralysis was caused which was below an acceptable standard but the way in which the paralysis was managed. All too often no action is taken once the palsy has been sustained. In every case, neurophysiological investigation and reexploration of the damaged nerve must be considered and this action should be carefully annotated in the records. An urgent second opinion can be of great value and is rarely criticized.

Stapedectomy

This operation carries a risk of sensorineural hearing impairment with or without balance disruption. There is a risk of serious inner ear damage in 2–3% of cases. Patients must be warned of this risk and should always be offered the alternative of a hearing aid. Re-exploration should be carefully considered in the event of chronic postoperative vertigo or fluctuating hearing loss and this consideration should be recorded in the notes.

Risk of haemorrhage

There is an appreciable risk of haemorrhage in tonsillectomy, adenoidectomy and turbinate surgery. The public perception is that these operations are completely safe and so must be appraised of this risk and the possible need for blood transfusion. It is surprising how many parents change their minds about tonsillectomy when warned of a 0.5% risk of needing a blood transfusion. Most surgeons do not warn of this risk in these minor operations although death from haemorrhage has been recorded.

Ototoxicity

Deafness, tinnitus or vertigo are recognized side effects of certain drugs especially aminoglycoside antibiotics. Drugs may also be ototoxic to the developing fetus. The side effects of these drugs are well documented and their use should be monitored accordingly. Most cases arise from the use of these drugs in renal medicine, intensive care, orthopaedic and general surgical practice. Although blood levels are monitored, cases have arisen where results have been delayed or the patient's complaint of tinnitus or hearing loss has been ignored.

Laryngeal obstruction

Failure to detect, monitor and treat such obstructions may be fatal or lead to brain damage. In general practice or accident and emergency departments, negligence can arise when there is a failure to diagnose epiglottitis. There have been cases where patients have been sent home only to die from suffocation several hours later. Choosing to monitor a compromised airway, rather than securing the airway by tracheostomy or intubation, requires absolute confidence in the ability of those affording the nursing care and the resident medical staff to act promptly should the airway deteriorate. It can be difficult to defend death or brain damage arising as a result of inadequate monitoring.

Removal of swallowed or inhaled foreign bodies

Failure to detect a swallowed foreign body is a common cause for litigation. Non-removal can have serious if not fatal consequences. Endoscopy, especially rigid endoscopy, should be performed by adequately trained staff. Trainees should be closely supervised in this technique. Perforation of the oesophagus does not usually imply negligence as the foreign body can have caused the perforation itself. In addition, the presence of osteophytes or reduced spinal movement from arthritis may create additional hazards for the patient. The otolaryngologist must always bear the possibility of mediastinitis in mind because delay in diagnosis is often fatal. If the surgeon has the slightest suspicion, antibiotics must be commenced and the second opinion of a cardiothoracic surgeon considered and recorded. Failure to do this could be considered negligent.

The inhalation of foreign bodies, particularly by children, can cause asphyxiation. Extremely careful assessment, which should include X-rays, must be undertaken when a child presents with a history of a possible inhalation.

Vocal cord palsy

There is about a 1% chance of vocal cord palsy after thyroidectomy. This risk and the consequences of such damage should always be explained to the patient and recorded in their medical records.

Functional endoscopic sinus surgery

This relatively new technique has been employed by more and more surgeons over the last few years. There would seem to be a national learning curve and accidents have taken place which have resulted in damage to the orbital contents and anterior cranial fossa. This has led to a large number of negligence claims.

Submucosal diathermy to the inferior turbinates

This operation has a small but significant risk of damage from excessive use of diathermy. Negligent positioning of the needle has caused damage to orbital contents and, in some cases, blindness. Facial anaesthesia and burns to the nasal vestibule have been reported, cause disfiguring scars and result in litigation.

The future

With greater emphasis now being placed upon patient autonomy, we expect that otolaryngologists, along with other medical practitioners, will have to pay closer attention to the question of consent to the treatment of patients. This is likely to emerge in two particular areas: informed consent and unanticipated treatment during surgery.

The consent form

The present consent form recommended by the Department of Health (1992) specifies the nature of the procedure to be carried out and goes on to state that, 'any procedure in addition to the investigation or treatment prescribed on the form will only be carried out if it is necessary and in the patient's best interest'. This clearly gives a wide scope to the otolaryngologist. In future, we expect restrictions to the scope of the unspecified procedures, probably to circumstances where procedures which are immediately necessary to save life or prevent permanent damage to the patient's health, if not specifically set out on the consent form.

Informed consent

As indicated above the risks about which a patient should be advised respecting any given procedures are those which would be given by a responsible body of medical opinion. In Australia, the test relating to 'informed' consent has been modified recently (Rogers v Whitaker, 1993) so that medical practitioners are now under a duty to warn a patient of a

material risk inherent in the proposed treatment. Broadly speaking, a risk is material if in the circumstances of the particular case a reasonable person in the patient's position, if warned of the risk, would be likely to attach significance to it. The duty is still subject to therapeutic privilege. We anticipate that in due course developments may require more information to be given to the patient in this jurisdiction about risks inherent in treatment.

Negligence

Otolaryngologists may well have been concerned at the possibility that medical negligence actions in England and Wales will follow the pattern of the USA and that the perceived increase in the number of actions here may continue. However, with the reduction in the eligibility for legal aid (Legal Aid Handbook, 1993) many actions, which would have been funded by legal aid in the past, will now have to be funded privately. The introduction of contingency or conditional fees is unlikely to assist all those who are no longer eligible for legal aid. As an incentive for the plaintiff's solicitor, the conditional fee system (Courts and Legal Services Act, 1990) will allow the solicitor to claim twice the rate of fees the solicitor might have otherwise obtained in a successful action. There is a risk that the solicitor might receive no payment at all if the case is unsuccessful. Solicitors acting for patients are therefore likely to take on fewer claims (Preliminary Results of the Law Society Survey, 1993), concentrating on those where liability is obvious and can be quickly established. The result is likely to be that there will be no significant increase in the number of medical negligence actions in the short term. Indeed, it is possible that there will be a reduction at the expense of patients who might otherwise have had successful claims for compensation.

No-fault compensation

A number of proposals have been made for the introduction of a no-fault compensation system in recent years, including the introduction into Parliament of several Private Members Bills (Blair, 1993). The introduction of such a system in the future may well depend on the identity of the Government at any given time. At present, it does not appear to be part of government policy but we believe it is the subject of consideration at present. With the difficulties encountered with the New Zealand scheme, such a system in England and Wales would either prove very expensive or fail to deliver any real adequate compensation. An example of such restricted compensation on a no-fault basis comes in the payments made to those who have suffered vaccine damage, when standard payment for what can be massive brain damage is a mere £30 000 (Vaccine Damage Payments Act, 1979). The main criticism of a no-fault system is the lack of sanction against individual medical practitioners. However, systems proposed recently, including a joint proposal (1992) by AVMA (Action for the Victims of Medical Accidents) and ACHCEW (The Association of Community Health Councils of England and Wales) suggest the introduction of a Health Standards Inspectorate. It is proposed that such a body would have the ability not only to deal with compensation of medical accidents, but also to set and audit standards of health care, and further to discipline health care professionals. Calls for compensation would be made to a Compensation Commission, which would hold hearings on an inquisitorial rather than an adversarial basis.

If such a no-fault scheme were introduced, it would probably have to be in conjunction with a system of complaints investigation, disciplinary function and audit, in order to ensure the maintenance or improvement in standards. However, no-fault compensation should not be regarded as a panacea. Arguably, it merely moves the definition of what will result in compensation from negligence to a *mishap,* retaining a causation criterion. It will widen the scope of those to be compensated, but still provides a considerable hurdle. There would have to be increased funding with increased claims, or a reduction in the level of compensation. It appears that a move to a no-fault compensation scheme is unlikely to be made in the immediate future.

Complaints procedures

Complaints procedures in the National Health Service have recently been the subject of review by a committee chaired by Professor Alan Wilson. The committee has proposed that there should be a unified system to deal with complaints within the National Health Service, and sets out broad principles on which such a system might be based. It is suggested the key aspects of procedures should be set up by health departments, but individual institutions would then be able to establish their own procedures for dealing with complaints within those parameters.

Arbitration

There is very little arbitration in medical negligence at present of which we are aware. There may be some development on a voluntary basis in the medium term, but it is unlikely that this will be of any real challenge to the present civil litigation system. Arbitration is established as an alternative option to civil litigation in several jurisdictions in the USA and in a number of other countries such as Germany (Giesen, 1988). Legislation to introduce arbitration, certainly on a compulsory basis, in the National Health Service is unlikely. A consultation paper issued by the Department of Health (1991) invited comment on proposals for the introduction of a system of arbitration for the National Health Service. Arbitration under these proposals was to be based on submissions on paper, with no oral representation. Only limited legal aid was to be available in preparation of a case, which would have presented most complaints with a difficult task indeed in making any claim.

The proposals received widespread criticism (Hirst and Morrish, 1991; Peysner, 1991), with AVMA reportedly describing them as too lightweight, and it is believed that they have now been shelved. Arbitration could be put forward in the future as a possible solution for perceived difficulties in the existing civil system. However, if the changes introduced to legal aid financial eligibility produce no further increase in the numbers of actions, the pressure for changes including arbitration, is likely to be reduced significantly.

Acknowledgement

The authors of this chapter are most grateful to Julie Stone and Rex Forrester, their colleagues at Hempsons, without whose help and assistance this chapter could not have been produced.

References

A Health Standards Inspectorate: a proposal by ACHCEW and AVMA (1992) London: ACHCEW

Accident Compensation Acts (1972 & 1982) New Zealand

Accident Rehabilitation and Compensation Insurance Act (1992) New Zealand

Andrews v DPP (1937) Appeal Cases 576, PC

Ashcroft v Mersey Regional Health Authority [1985] 2 All England Reports 96

Barnett v Chelsea & Kensington Hospital [1968] 1 All England Reports 1068

Blair, L. (1993) *New Law Journal,* 1.l0.93, p. 1337

Blyth v Bloomsbury Health Authority [1993] 4 Medical Law Reports, Court of Appeal

Bolam v Friern Hospital Management Committee [1957] 1 Weekly Law Reports, 582

Byrne v Boadle (1863) 2 Hurlstone & Coltman's Exchequer Reports 722 (a barrel of flour)

Courts and Legal Services Act, S.58 (1990)

Crawford v Board of Governors of Charing Cross Hospital (1953) Times Law Reports, 8 December 1953, Court of Appeal

Department of Health (1991) Arbitration for Medical Negligence in the National Health Service. Discussion Paper, Department of Health.

Department of Health (1992) Health Circular (90)2 – revised 1992, Appendix A(1)

Glesen, D. (1988) In: *International Medical Malpractice Law,* paragraphs 1037–1052. Dordrecht, Boston and London: JCB Mohr, Tübingen & Martinus Nijhoff

Gillick v West Norfolk and Wisbech Area Health Authority [1986] Appeal Cases 112 House of Lords

Girard v Royal Columbian Hospital (1976) 66 Dominion Law Reports (3d) 676

Greek Penal Code, Article 302

Ham, C., Dingwall, R., Fenn, P. and Harris, D. (1988) In: *Medical Negligence: Compensation and Accountability.* London: Kings Fund Institute. pp 26–34

Hirst, S. and Morrish, A. (1991) Arbitrary justice. *New Law Journal,* 13.12.1991. pp. 1696, 1710

Hopp v Lepp (1979) 112 Dominion Law Reports 3d 67

In re F [1990] 2 Appeal Cases 1, House of Lords

In re R [1991] 4 All England Reports 177, Court of Appeal

In re T. Adult: Refusal of treatments [1992] 3 Weekly Law Reports 783

In re W [1992] 3 Weekly Law Reports 758

Kennedy, I. and Grubb, A. (1994) In: *Medical Law: Text & Material.* London: Butterworths. p. 512 f.f.

Kralj v McGrath [1986] All England Reports 54

Legal Aid Handbook (1993) Financial eligibility. London: Sweet and Maxwell. p. 455

Leigh, M.A.M.S. (1993) Res ipsa loquitur: what does it mean? *Medical Defence Union Journal,* 9, 66

Levitt v Hartlepool Area Health Authority (1993, unreported)

Lim v Camden Health Authority [1979] 2 All England Reports 910, House of Lords, per Lord Scarman

Livingston v Rawyards Coal Company (1880) 5 Appeal Cases 25 @ 39, House of Lords per Lord Blackburn

Lord Chancellor (1991) The Litigation Letter. Lecture to the Royal College of Physicians of Edinburgh, 4th June 1991. London: Legal Studies and Services Ltd

Lord Pearson (1978) Royal Commission on Civil Liability and Compensation for Personal Injury, Cmnd 7054. HMSO

Mahon v Osborne [1939] 2 Kings Bench 1450

National Justice Compania Naviesa SA v Prudential Assurance Company Ltd (Ikarian Reefer) (1993) *Times Law Reports,* 3rd March 1993

Patient Insurance Scheme 1975. Sweden

Peysner J. (1991) Medical negligence – A Trojan horse. *Solicitors Journal.* 6.12.1991, p. 1316

Picard (1984) Legal liability of doctors and hospitals in Canada, pp. 260–261, cited in Kennedy and Grubb, *Medical Law: Text & Material,* 1994, p. 465

Pope v St. Helen's Theatre (1947) Kings Bench 30 (the ceiling of a theatre)

Preliminary Results of the Law Society Survey of Personal Injury Specialists (1993) *Law Society Gazzette,* 29 September 1993, p. 3

R v Adamoko [1994] 3 Weekly Law Reports 288

R v Bateman (1925) 19 Criminal Appeal Reports 8, Court of Appeal

R v Prentice and Sullman [1994] QB 302

R v Tutton and Tutton (1989) 48 Canadian Criminal Cases (3d) 129, Canadian Supreme Court

R v Yogasakaran (1990) 1 New Zealand Law Reports 399, New Zealand Court of Appeal

Rogers v Whitaker (1993) 4 Medical Law Reports 79, High Court of Australia

Rules of the County Court (1994) Consulting editor, RCL Gregory. London: Butterworths

Rules of the Supreme Court (1995) General editor Sir Jack I. H. Jacobs. London: Sweet & Maxwell

Rules of the Supreme Court: Order 37 Rules 7–10. (1995) General editor Sir Jack I. H. Jacobs. London: Sweet & Maxwell

Sidaway v Board of Governors of the Bethlem Royal Hospital [1985] Appeal Cases 871, House of Lords

Scott v London & St. Katherine's Docks (1865) 3 Hurlstone & Coltman's Exchequer Reports 596 ExCh, (sugar bags)

The Annotated Tremear's Criminal Code (1992) Sections 219, 220, 222. Toronto, Calgary and Vancouver: Carswell

The Wilson review – Being Heard (1994) HMSO

Vaccine Damage Payments Act (1979) Statutory Sum Order 1991 No. 939

Ward v James [1965] 2 All England Reports 563, Court of Appeal

Whitehouse v Jordan [1981] 1 Weekly Law Reports 246, House of Lords

Wilsher v Essex Area Health Authority [1988] I All England Reports 871, House of Lords

Damages

A plaintiff having established negligence and having proved injury as a consequence, the question turns to the assessment of the compensation to be paid. The Court must award a sum of money that will, as nearly as possible, put the injured person in the same position as he would have been had he not been injured (Livingstone v Rawyards Coal Company, 1880). In some jurisdictions, notably the USA, an element of punitive damages may be awarded. Such an approach has been rejected in England and Wales (Kralj v McGrath, 1986).

Damages are broadly classified into two categories.

General damages

These include damages for pain, suffering and loss of amenity. This is the aspect of the plaintiff's loss which is not ascertainable by a mathematical calculation of economic loss and, in the past was determined by a jury (Ward v James, 1965). While the level of general damages will depend on the plaintiff's circumstances and the suffering which the particular injury has caused the individual, a general bracket for a particular injury will be determined with reference to awards (adjusted for inflation) from previously decided cases. Obviously, it is impossible to compensate someone for the loss of a limb or for a life of continual pain. The awards are essentially conventional figures. As a guide, the current conventional figure for injuries of the utmost severity is between £100 000 and £120 000, and so injuries of lesser significance will be a proportion of that maximum. In a recent case in Teesside, Levitt v Hartlepool Area Health Authority (1993), a minor born deaf was awarded £50 000 general damages which included her total hearing loss.

Special damages

These are the specific 'out-of-pocket' monetary expenses and losses which the plaintiff has incurred up until the date of the trial. These will include loss of earnings, medical expenses, travel costs and the cost of any special equipment consequent upon the injury. Often there will be a claim for losses expected in the future. *Future loss* is technically an item of general damages as its assessment is uncertain and it was formerly a matter for the jury to determine. As a matter of practice, the calculation of future loss is inseparable from that of past loss as many of the arguments are the same and one flows naturally to the other. The amount of money at issue will depend almost exclusively on the particular circumstances of the plaintiff (Lim v Camden Health Authority, 1979), guided by the principle that a plaintiff should only recover what he has lost as a result of the injury. He must prove that his expenditure was, or will be, reasonably necessary and that his needs cannot be met more cheaply by other reasonable means.

As a rule, English law seeks to compensate a plaintiff by way of a single lump sum award. This creates obvious problems where a plaintiff is likely to remain unemployed or requires continuing care for many years in the future. The only certain result is that the plaintiff will be either under or over compensated, depending on how circumstances unfold. This problem has not been solved, but ameliorated in certain cases. Where a plaintiff suffers a condition that may deteriorate significantly in the future, rather than receive a small sum to represent the risk, he can apply for an order for *provisional damages*, which leaves it open to the plaintiff to come back to court on a later date (Rules of the Supreme Court).

In very large claims where the plaintiff's life expectancy will determine the level of the award the risk can be borne by an insurance company by the purchase of an annuity. This is known as a *structured settlement.*

Comparison of different compensation systems

The English system of compensating those experiencing medical accidents has been the subject of criticism for some time. It is said that it is difficult to prove fault and that success may well be determined more by luck in obtaining helpful evidence. The litigation may be lengthy and expensive. Effectively, it is only available to the well off or to the poor who qualify for legal aid. A large section of the population who simply cannot afford to take on the significant risks and costs of medical litigation, even where their case is strong, is wholly excluded. The nature of the process is adversarial and can be distressing for all concerned.

The problem of delay is not as it was in the past, partly due to procedural changes, and partly due to greater degree of specialization and expertise of those advising plaintiffs. Nevertheless, while the 6–10 year delays between an action starting and its eventual hearing are now a thing of the past, the life of an action is still to be measured in years, rather than months.

The American contingency fee system has been proposed as a solution to the growing number of potential plaintiffs unable to obtain legal aid. However, the American experience shows that it has only limited practical application to medical negligence claims. While road traffic accident claims are relatively cheap to run, have a predictable outcome and are therefore attractive to lawyers on a contingency, medical negligence is seen as a particularly risky area. Accordingly lawyers may reject all but the clearest claims (Ham *et al*, 1988).

The inquisitorial system

The most obvious difference between the English and continental systems of justice is that in England and Wales, the parties are responsible for all the evidence that comes before the court, and the arguments that are advanced. The judge's role is to adjudicate between the parties on the basis of the cases they submit.

The procedure is inquisitorial on the Continent, more akin to an English Coroner's inquest. Judges are allowed and expected to take a much more active part in the proceedings. They may well be involved in the preparation of the case and will investigate the circumstances. The judge will identify and question witnesses himself. In continental legal systems it is normally the courts who appoint medical experts, though this does not necessarily debar the parties seeking their own expert opinions.

The English system is sometimes compared unfavourably to the European as a game of tactics presided over by an umpire rather than a search for the truth. In fact the difference is probably more of form rather than substance. In both systems there are different sides seeking to sway the judge this way or that and, so long as both sides have equal opportunity to investigate and present their case, the truth is just as likely to be found with one as with the other system. After all, the most acute analysis and criticism of each party's case is as likely, if not more, to come from their opponent as from a disinterested public servant.

No-fault compensation

The most radical solution to the problem of compensation is to abolish the concept of fault altogether. If there is to be an increase of the welfare state with emphasis on payments based on need rather than causation, a one to one payment based on negligence is increasingly difficult to justify in comparison to a national scheme of insurance. Every year several hundred babies are born with brain damage. In a very small number of cases this damage can be attributed to some negligence, in which case the parents of the child can expect to receive a sum in excess of £500 000 with which to care for the child. The rest receive nothing and must rely on state provision. Thus there is a windfall to one at the expense of the majority.

No-fault schemes have been introduced by both Sweden (Patient Insurance Scheme, 1975) and New Zealand (Accident Compensation Acts, 1972, 1983). The Swedish scheme is limited to injuries suffered as a result of medical treatment, but the amount of damages is assessed using the ordinary tort rules. Payments are relatively modest, as they merely supplement a comprehensive social welfare system. The patient retains the right to sue, but seldom exercises

it as a claim under the scheme is so much easier. The New Zealand scheme was much more radical and covered all *personal injuries by accident*; of which *medical misadventure* is but one aspect. Essentially, the only conditions excluded were those attributable solely to disease or old age. The price of comprehensiveness was the loss of the right to sue for any injury covered by the Act and significantly reduced awards available. The New Zealand system suffered from its own success and a recessionary economy unable to pay for it. In 1992 eligibility under the scheme was tightened considerably, including the definition of *medical error or mishap,* and while loss of earnings was properly compensated, the concept of general damages was abolished entirely (Accident Rehabilitation and Compensation Insurance Act, 1992).

The question of whether a no fault compensation scheme should be introduced in England was considered in the Pearson Report in 1978. The concept was rejected partly on the basis of the cost.

In 1994, Kennedy and Grubb calculated that the total cost of the present tort system could be estimated at £75M, of which £65M came from the NHS. This included both the actual damages paid and the costs incurred. They considered the cost of a Swedish style system would have been in the order of £117M. The Lord Chancellor, speaking in 1991, described a no-fault scheme as, 'tantamount to a policy of insurance of a kind which I do not see as a function of the State to provide'. It therefore appears unlikely that such a scheme will be implemented in the immediate future.

Specific kinds of medical negligence relating to otolaryngological surgery

Otolaryngology is a very wide-ranging specialty covering surgical and non-surgical medicine across a broad age spectrum, varying from major head and neck surgery to complex microsurgery. As well as the risks unique to this area, there will also be risks common to all specialties. These include failure to refer, failure to diagnose, failure to warn patients about inherent risks and the danger of accidents happening as a result of inadequate supervision. It is impossible to give an exhaustive list in a chapter such as this but given below are some of the areas in which litigation ensues on a regular basis.

Perforation of the tympanic membrane

This is particularly common in general practice as a result of syringing. In hospital practice perforations are sometimes inflicted when taking an impression for a hearing aid mould, but more commonly by accident and emergency staff attempting to remove foreign bodies from the ear and inadvertently pushing